Equine Reproductive Procedures

Equine Reproductive Procedures

Second Edition

Edited by

John Dascanio, VMD
Diplomate ACT and ABVP (Equine)
Senior Associate Dean for Academic and Student Affairs
Professor of Theriogenology
School of Veterinary Medicine
Texas Tech University
Amarillo, Texas, United States

Patrick McCue, DVM, PhD
Diplomate ACT
Iron Rose Ranch Professor of Equine Reproduction
Colorado State University
Equine Reproduction Laboratory
Fort Collins, Colorado, United States

WILEY Blackwell

This edition first published 2021

Edition History
John Wiley and Sons, Inc. (1e, 2014)

Registered Offices
John Wiley & Sons, Inc., 111 River Street, Hoboken, NJ 07030, USA
John Wiley & Sons Ltd, The Atrium, Southern Gate, Chichester, West Sussex, PO19 8SQ, UK

Editorial Office
111 River Street, Hoboken, NJ 07030, USA

For details of our global editorial offices, customer services, and more information about Wiley products visit us at www.wiley.com.

Wiley also publishes its books in a variety of electronic formats and by print-on-demand. Some content that appears in standard print versions of this book may not be available in other formats.

Library of Congress Cataloging-in-Publication Data

Names: Dascanio, John J. (John Joseph), 1961– editor. | McCue, Patrick M., editor. | Dascanio, John J. (John Joseph), 1961– Equine reproductive procedures.
Title: Equine reproductive procedures / edited by John Dascanio, Patrick McCue.
Description: 2nd edition. | Hoboken, NJ : Wiley-Blackwell, 2021. | Preceded by Equine reproductive procedures / John J. Dascanio, Patrick M. McCue. 2014 . | Includes bibliographical references and index.
Identifiers: LCCN 2020026465 (print) | LCCN 2020026466 (ebook) | ISBN 9781119555988 (cloth) | ISBN 9781119555971 (adobe pdf) | ISBN 9781119555933 (epub)
Subjects: MESH: Horses–physiology | Reproduction–physiology | Reproductive Techniques, Assisted–veterinary | Breeding
Classification: LCC SF768.2.H67 (print) | LCC SF768.2.H67 (ebook) | NLM SF768.2.H67 | DDC 636.1–dc23
LC record available at https://lccn.loc.gov/2020026465
LC ebook record available at https://lccn.loc.gov/2020026466

Cover Design: Wiley
Cover Images: (horses) Suzanne Sylvester / S. Sylvester Photography, LLC
(right) courtesy of Patrick McCue

Set in 9.5/12.5pt STIXTwoText by SPi Global, Pondicherry, India

MWEP410163031125

Contents

List of Contributors

Marco A. Alvarenga DVM, PhD
School of Veterinary Medicine
São Paulo State University
Botucatu, Brazil

Stacy Anderson DVM, MVSc, PhD, DACVS-LA
College of Veterinary Medicine
Lincoln Memorial University
Harrogate, TN, USA

Udeni B. R. Balasuriya BVSc, MS, PhD, FSLCVS
Department of Pathobiological Sciences
School of Veterinary Medicine
Louisiana State University
Baton Rouge, LA, USA

Jillian Bishop BS, Pharm D, BCPS
University of Kansas Health System
Lexexa, KS, USA

Anders Miki Bojesen DVM, PhD, DECVPS
Department of Veterinary and Animal Science
University of Copenhagen
Copenhagen, Denmark

Etta A. Bradecamp DVM, DACT, DABVP (Equine)
Rood and Riddle Equine Hospital
Lexington, KY, USA

Leonardo Brito DVM, PhD, DACT
Stgenetics
Middleton, WI, USA

Claire E. Card DVM, PhD, DACT
Department of Large Animal Clinical Sciences
Western College of Veterinary Medicine
University of Saskatchewan
Saskatchewan, Canada

Julie T. Cecere DVM, MS, DACT
Department of Small Animal Clinical Sciences
Virginia-Maryland College of Veterinary Medicine
Blacksburg, VA, USA

Undine Christmann Dr.Med.Vet., MS, MPH, PhD, DACVIM
College of Veterinary Medicine
Lincoln Memorial University
Harrogate, TN, USA

Peter F. Daels DVM, PhD, DACT, DECAR
Faculty of Veterinary Medicine
University of Gent
Merelbeke, Belgium

John J. Dascanio VMD, DACT, DABVP (Equine)
School of Veterinary Medicine
Texas Tech University
Amarillo, TX, USA

Pouya Dini DVM, PhD, DECAR, DACT
Department of Population Health and Reproduction
School of Veterinary Medicine
University of California-Davis
Davis, CA, USA

Ryan A. Ferris DVM, MS, DACT
Summit Equine
Gervais, OR, USA

Amanda I. Glazar PhD
Kynectiv, Inc.
Evergreen, CO, USA

Carlos M. Gradil DVM, MS, PhD, DACT
Cummings School of Veterinary Medicine
University of Massachusetts Veterinary and Animal Sciences
Amherst, MA, USA

Jennifer N. Hatzel DVM, MS, DACT
Equine Reproduction Laboratory
Colorado State University
Fort Collins, CO, USA

Dean A. Hendrickson DVM, MS, DACVS
Department of Clinical Sciences
College of Veterinary Medicine and Biomedical Sciences
Colorado State University
Fort Collins, CO, USA

Richard D. Holder DVM
Hagyard Equine Medical Institute
Lexington, KY, USA

G. Reed Holyoak DVM, PhD, DACT
Department of Veterinary Clinical Sciences
Oklahoma State University
Stillwater, OK, USA

Lauren Javernick DVM
Hagyard Equine Medical Institute
Lexington, KY, USA

Paul Loomis MS
Select Breeders Services
Chesapeake City, MD, USA

Charles Love DVM, PhD
Large Animal Clinical Sciences, College
of Veterinary Medicine and Biomedical Sciences,
Texas A&M University, College Station,
TX, USA

Kristina Lu VMD, DACT
Hagyard Equine Medical Institute
Lexington, KY, USA

Margo L. Macpherson DVM, MS, DACT
College of Veterinary Medicine
University of Florida
Gainesville, FL, USA

John Madigan DVM, MS, DACVIM, DACAW
School of Veterinary Medicine
University of California-Davis
Davis, CA, USA

Patrick M. McCue DVM, PhD, DACT
Equine Reproduction Laboratory
Colorado State University
Fort Collins, CO, USA

Sue M. McDonnell PhD, CAAB, Hon DACT
New Bolton Center
School of Veterinary Medicine
University of Pennsylvania
Kennett Square, PA, USA

Justin W. McNaughten BVMS, DACT
Rhinebeck Equine LLP
Rhinebeck, NY, USA

Lynda M. J. Miller DVM, PhD, DACT
College of Veterinary Medicine
Lincoln Memorial University
Harrowgate, TN, USA

Peter Morresey BVSC, MVM, MACVSc, DACT, DACVIM, CVA
Rood and Riddle Equine Hospital
Lexington, KY, USA

Morten Rønn Petersen DVM, PhD, DACT
The Fertility Clinic
University Hospital Copenhagen
Faculty of Health and Medical Sciences
University of Copenhagen
Copenhagen, Denmark

Rhonda A. Rathgeber DVM, PhD
Hagyard Equine Medical Institute
Lexington, KY, USA

Terje Raudsepp MS, PhD
Department of Veterinary Integrative Biosciences
College of Veterinary Medicine and Biomedical Sciences
Texas A&M University
College Station, TX, USA

Charles F. Scoggin DVM, MS, DACT
Rood and Riddle Equine Hospital
Lexington, KY, USA

Lorenzo G. T. M. Segabinazzi DVM, MS
School of Veterinary Medicine
São Paulo State University
Botucatu, Brazil

Sofie Sitters DVM
Amsterdam, The Netherlands

JoAnne Stokes BS
Equine Reproduction Laboratory
Colorado State University
Fort Collins, CO, USA

D. N. Rao Veeramachaneni BVSc, MScVet, PhD
Animal Reproduction and Biotechnology Laboratory
Colorado State University
Fort Collins, CO, USA

Karen Wolfsdorf DVM, DACT
Hagyard Equine Medical Institute
Lexington, KY, USA

Preface

This second edition of the *Equine Reproductive Procedures* book has been substantially updated with 39 new chapters, and a multitude of new diagnostic procedures and therapeutic protocols added to existing chapters. The overall goal has remained the same, which is to provide equine professionals with practical clinical information on basic and advanced techniques in the field of equine reproduction. It is our hope that veterinary students, graduate students, researchers in the field of equine reproduction and veterinarians in private practice will find the material in this book useful in their collective work.

The second edition is divided into sections on the Non-Pregnant Mare, Pregnant Mare, Postpartum Mare, Stallion and Newborn Foal. A total of 40 authors and co-authors contributed to the development of the book. In the first edition, we noted that approximately 90% of reproductive procedures used in the horse industry are nearly identical throughout the world. The other 10% varies according to the training and experience of the individual, geographic region, and availability of supplies and facilities. Hopefully we will all continue to learn throughout our careers from the knowledge and experience of others. Consequently, while the objective of this book is to provide examples of how reproductive procedures may be performed, it should not be construed that these are the only or the optimal methods to achieve diagnostic or therapeutic goals.

Again, we would like to thank the staff at Wiley Blackwell for their professional assistance in the development of this second edition. We would also like to acknowledge our many mentors and colleagues for providing academic and clinical guidance over the years. We owe our professional careers to their collective wisdom. Most importantly, we would also like to thank our families for their unwavering support. Thank you, Linda, Sarah, and Gabriel Dascanio! Thank you, Diane, Daniel, and Kelly McCue!

John Dascanio
Patrick McCue

Part I

Non-Pregnant Mare

1

Reproductive Evaluation

Patrick M. McCue

Equine Reproduction Laboratory, Colorado State University, USA

Introduction

The goals of a mare reproductive evaluation or breeding soundness examination (BSE) are to identify known or potential reproductive abnormalities and to evaluate the potential of a mare to become pregnant and carry a foal successfully to term. Mare reproductive examinations are performed in open (non-pregnant) mares prior to the onset of the breeding season, in problem mares during the breeding season, in barren mares at the end of the breeding season, as well as in mares with a history of embryonic loss, abortion, or other reproductive problems, or as part of a pre-purchase examination. The goal of this chapter is to provide an overview of the mare breeding soundness evaluation. Details on specific examinations will be covered in other chapters.

Equipment and Supplies

Obstetrical sleeve (non-sterile), obstetrical lubricant (non-sterile), tail wrap, metal bucket and plastic bag liner, non-irritant soap, roll cotton, vaginal speculum, obstetrical lubricant (sterile), obstetrical sleeve (sterile), uterine culture device, culture transport system (optional), uterine cytology device, glass slides, uterine biopsy forceps, formalin.

Examination Technique

Identification

All mares should be properly identified, and the breed, registration name, registration number, and date of birth recorded. Photographs should be taken or accurate drawings of markings and tattoos recorded.

Reproductive History

A complete breeding history should be obtained, including current reproductive status (maiden, open, barren, pregnant, or foaling), number of cycles bred during the last season, date of last breeding, breeding technique used (artificial insemination, natural cover, or pasture breeding), number of stallions, date of last foal, number of previous foals, and any previous history of abnormal estrous cycles, uterine infections, embryonic loss, or abortion.

Physical Examination

A general physical examination should be performed to assess whether the mare has the capacity to carry a foal to term. The evaluation should include, but is not limited to, examination of the oral cavity, eyes, and the respiratory, cardiac, and musculoskeletal systems. In addition, diet and body condition should be evaluated.

Perineal Conformation

See also Chapter 5. The external genitalia (vulva) should be evaluated for conformation and muscular tone. The optimal perineal conformation consists of a vulva in a nearly vertical position with two thirds of the vulva ventral to the brim of the pelvis. The muscular tone of the vulva should be sufficient to prevent or minimize aspiration of air into the vestibule or vagina. Horizontal sloping of the vulva secondary to recession of the anus or poor muscular tone to the labia of the vulva may predispose the mare to an ascending infection of the uterus.

Equine Reproductive Procedures, Second Edition. Edited by John Dascanio and Patrick McCue.

Estrous Detection

See also Chapter 2. The mare should be exposed to a stallion with good libido to evaluate estrous cycle stage. Adequate time should be taken to allow shy or nervous mares to express behavioral estrus. When teasing a mare with a foal, the foal must be restrained, and the mare may need to be restrained with a twitch before signs of estrus are exhibited.

Palpation Per Rectum

See also Chapter 7. The entire reproductive tract, including the cervix, uterus, and ovaries, should be thoroughly and systematically examined by palpation per rectum. The tone of the uterus and cervix, size and consistency of ovarian follicles, and the presence of a recent ovulation or a corpus hemorrhagicum should be recorded. The presence of abnormal ovarian, parovarian (i.e., fimbrial cysts), or uterine structures should be recorded.

Ultrasonography Per Rectum

See also Chapter 8. Manual palpation should be followed by a systematic ultrasound evaluation of the entire reproductive tract. Ultrasound is used in broodmares to visualize structures in the reproductive tract that cannot be palpated or differentiated on palpation per rectum, and in the early diagnosis of pregnancy, diagnosis of twins, and evaluation of potential ovarian or uterine pathology.

Vaginal Speculum Examination

See also Chapter 10. A vaginal speculum examination is performed to evaluate the anatomy of the vagina and the external os of the cervix. Speculum examination is useful in determination of the stage of the estrous cycle (via cervical morphology and vaginal mucous membrane changes), and detection of urine pooling and the presence of cervical/vaginal inflammation or discharge.

Digital Examination of the Cervix

See also Chapter 11. After the speculum examination is completed, the cervix should be examined manually for patency and the presence of abnormalities, such as adhesions, lacerations, or other cervical defects.

Uterine Culture

See also Chapter 12. Culture of the uterine lumen is usually performed in conjunction with cytology for the diagnosis of endometritis. Endometritis can be suspected in mares that exhibit an abnormally short estrous cycle, vaginal or cervical discharge, inflamed cervix on speculum examination, and free fluid in the uterus during diestrus detected on ultrasound.

Endometrial Cytology

See also Chapter 17. Cytologic evaluation of the uterus involves the collection and interpretation of cells lining the uterus (endometrium) and within the uterine lumen. Cytology is used in conjunction with culture and biopsy in the diagnosis of endometritis. Advantages of endometrial cytology for the diagnosis of endometritis include the ease of sample collection, low cost, and rapid availability of results.

Endometrial Biopsy

See also Chapter 19. Endometrial biopsy involves collection of a small sample of the uterine lining (endometrium) for histologic evaluation. It is primarily used as an aid in the diagnosis of uterine disease and as a prognostic indicator of the ability of a mare to carry a foal to term. An endometrial biopsy can also be used as the sample source for culture and cytologic evaluation.

Other Tests

The standard examination procedures in the mare BSE may not identify the cause of subfertility. Consequently, other examinations may be indicated (Table 1.1).

Additional Comments

Interpretation of the results of a mare BSE should take into account the mare's age, reproductive history, breed, stallion, breeding management, and other factors. Ultimately the goals are to determine the potential for fertility and detect abnormalities that may be associated with reduced fertility. Management and therapeutic options may be outlined to help optimize a successful outcome. It is important to emphasize that a mare BSE is only an evaluation of potential fertility and that the true assessment of fertility is the ability of the mare to conceive and carry a foal to term.

Table 1.1 Diagnostic tests that may be performed in addition to the standard tests in a mare breeding soundness evaluation.

Test	Indication
Chromosome analysis (karyotype)	Evaluate numeric or structural changes in chromosomes
Hormone analysis	Evaluate pituitary and/or ovarian endocrine function. Most commonly used to evaluate corpus luteum function and in the detection of an ovarian granulosa cell tumor
Hysteroscopy	Direct visualization of the interior of the uterus to detect intrauterine adhesions and other localized lesions, as well as inflammation and fibrosis
Laparoscopy	Direct visualization of the serosal surface of the ovary, oviduct, uterus, and abdominal cavity. Also used in ovarian biopsy, evaluation of oviductal patency, and the application of prostaglandin E_2 (PGE_2) to the oviductal surface
Low volume lavage	Collection of uterine samples for culture, cytology, and other evaluations (e.g., polymerase chain reaction). The effluent fluid may also be evaluated for clarity and pH
Oviductal flush	Performed by laparotomy, laparoscopy, or via videoendoscopy; used both diagnostically and therapeutically in suspected cases of oviductal blockage
Oviductal patency test	Deposition of fluorescent microbeads or starch granules onto the surface of the ovary or possibly within the infundibulum of the oviduct and subsequent examination of the uterine lumen for passage of the test material is used diagnostically to evaluate oviductal patency
Oviductal PGE_2 application	Direct application of PGE_2 can be used diagnostically and therapeutically in suspected cases of oviductal blockage
Ovarian biopsy	Laparoscopic collection of ovarian tissue for histologic evaluation may be used in the diagnosis of ovarian pathology
Test breed	Breeding to a highly fertile stallion can be used diagnostically to help determine if the mare is a cause of subfertility or infertility

Further Reading

LeBlanc MM, Lopate C, Knottenbelt D, Pascoe R. 2003. *The Mare. Equine Stud Farm Medicine and Surgery.* London: Elsevier, pp. 113–213.

McCue PM. 2008. The problem mare: management philosophy, diagnostic procedures, and therapeutic options. *J Eq Vet Sci* 28: 619–26.

2

Teasing

Patrick M. McCue

Equine Reproduction Laboratory, Colorado State University, USA

Introduction

The 21-day equine estrous cycle can be divided into two phases: estrus and diestrus, based on sexual receptivity to a stallion. Estrus is the period during which a mare is sexually receptive to the advances of a stallion. Behavioral estrus is stimulated by increasing levels of estradiol produced by the developing dominant follicle in the absence of progesterone. The average length of estrus has been reported to be 6.5 days, with a range of 4.5–8.9 days. Ovulation typically occurs 24–48 hours before the end of estrus. An increase in progesterone from the developing corpus luteum is responsible for the cessation of behavioral estrus. Behavioral diestrus largely overlaps the physiological luteal phase associated with high levels of progesterone produced by the corpus luteum.

Equipment and Supplies

Stallion, mare, lead shank, helmet, facilities (teasing rail, fence, chute, stall).

Technique

- A mare should be teased with a stallion that exhibits good libido in order to successfully evaluate estrous cycle stage.
- Adequate time should be taken to allow shy or nervous mares to express behavioral estrus.
- Knowledge of the mare's previous behavioral patterns may be helpful.
- In addition, observation of the mare's behavior with other horses in a pasture or paddock may indicate when a mare is in estrus.

Individual Teasing

An individual mare should be exposed to a stallion for an interval of time that is long enough for her to show estrus or diestrus types of behavior. It is preferable to have both the mare and stallion restrained for individual teasing; however, if only one handler is present, it is better to have the stallion restrained with the mare loose so that abnormal behaviors in the stallion may be corrected. Mares that remain indifferent may need to be teased longer, teased with a different stallion, or may just show more subtle signs. Mares may be reluctant initially and yet later show frank estrus behavior (i.e., "break down"). Sometimes full behavioral estrus is only expressed within a few hours of ovulation. It is also not unusual for a mare to fail to show signs of estrus while being directly teased to a stallion, and then break down as the stallion leaves. Mares may also display estrus at the mere sound or sight of a stallion. Mares with a foal by their side may be reluctant to display estrus behavior readily as they are concerned for their foal's safety.

Group Teasing

A stallion may be used to tease more than one mare concurrently if he is brought to the edge of a pen or turned out adjacent to a group of mares. Mares are allowed to approach the stallion at will in such a teasing program. However, some mares will not approach the stallion and will not express estrus when teased as part of a group. It may be necessary to tease such mares individually.

It is often not very efficient to tease mares as a group, since often the only mares that come to the fence or tease rail are assertive mares in heat or mares that want to attack the stallion. One may not be able to determine the heat status of mares that remain a distance from the stallion. It is generally more effective, but certainly more time

Equine Reproductive Procedures, Second Edition. Edited by John Dascanio and Patrick McCue.

consuming, to tease mares individually. Mares that are less dominant mares or further away from the fence or tease rail should still be observed for estrus behavior.

Behavioral Responses

Common behavioral responses of mares in estrus and diestrus are listed in Boxes 2.1 and 2.2 and shown in Figures 2.1 and 2.2.

Box 2.1 Common Behavioral Characteristics of Mares in Estrus

Tail raised and arched or deviated to one side
Rhythmic eversion of the labia and exposure of clitoris ("winking")
Passive urination
Ears relaxed and either held forward or in a neutral position
Rear limbs slightly abducted (i.e., wide-based stance)
Stifles and hocks flexed
Lowering of the pelvis (i.e., "squatting")
Leaning into fence or gate
Vocalization (squealing)
Calm behavior; does not try to bite or strike stallion

Box 2.2 Common Behavioral Characteristics of Mares in Diestrus

Tail held down or aggressively switched from side to side
Ears pinned back
Aggressive toward advances of the stallion
Biting at the stallion
Attempt to move away from the stallion
Squealing or vocalization
Calm behavior; does not try to bite or strike stallion

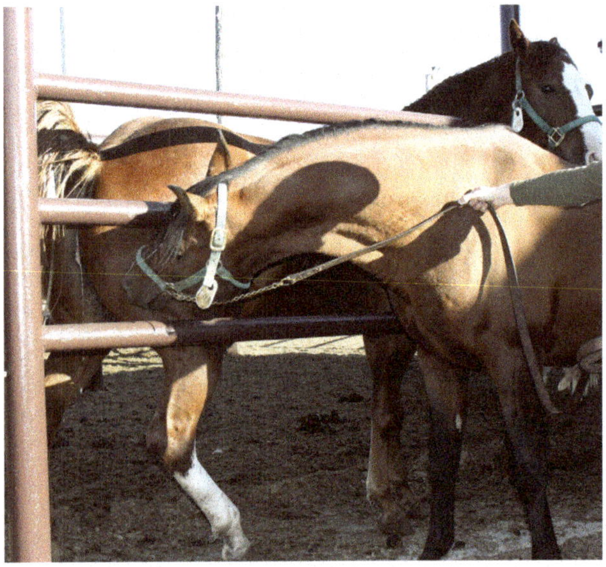

Figure 2.1 Mare in estrus (i.e., teasing in heat). Note the base-wide stance, raised tail, and urination.

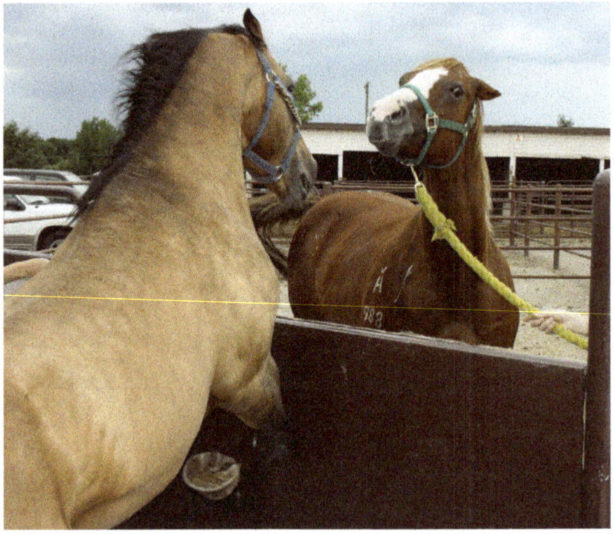

Figure 2.2 Mare in diestrus (i.e., out of heat) on far side of teasing wall. Note the ears and aggressive stance.

It should be noted that expression of estrus does not always indicate that a mare is in the follicular phase of the estrous cycle. Seasonally anovulatory mares, ovariectomized mares, and pregnant mares have all been reported to occasionally show signs of estrus when teased with a stallion. This may be due to submissive behavior or a lack of progesterone.

Records

Maintaining an accurate record of teasing behavior will be helpful when monitoring the estrous cycle of a mare. Notations can be made as to whether or not the mare exhibits overt, subtle, or no signs of estrus throughout a cycle (Table 2.1).

Table 2.1 Abbreviations for responses of a mare to a stallion (i.e., teasing behavior).

Abbreviation	Levels: Option 1	Levels: Option 2	Behavior
H	+	+++	In heat
O	–	–	Out of heat
H/O	+/–	++	Coming into or going out of heat
I		+	Indifferent

Silent Estrus

Maiden mares may not show heat well and foaling mares may not show heat at all unless the foal is restrained and/or safely away from the stallion. Subordinate mares may be inhibited from expressing estrus in the presence of a dominant mare. In addition, a mare may have a preference for, or an aversion toward, an individual stallion. Mares with "silent estrus" may have lower concentrations of estradiol 17 β than mares expressing normal estrus.

Additional Comments

There are many systems used for teasing mares, including chutes, rails, fences, pens, and paddocks. Keys to successful teasing are patience, persistence, and knowing the behavioral characteristics of each mare. Consequently, it is advantageous for the same individual(s) to tease mares each day, so that slight variations in individual responses can be recognized.

Further Reading

Ginther OJ. 1979. *Reproductive Biology of the Mare: Basic and Applied Aspects.* Ann Arbor, MI: McNaughton and Bunn, pp. 59–68.

McCue PM, Scoggin CF, Lindholm ARG. 2011. Estrus. In: McKinnon AO, Squires EL, Vaala WE, Varner DD (eds). *Equine Reproduction, 2nd edn. Ames, IA: Wiley Blackwell,* pp. 1716–27.

3

Tail Wrap and Preparation/Washing of the Perineum

John J. Dascanio

School of Veterinary Medicine, Texas Tech University, USA

Introduction

The mare's perineum should be washed prior to internal reproductive procedures and in preparation for foaling, to remove gross debris and to reduce bacterial numbers. In addition, the perineum is washed prior to perineal surgery such as the placement of a Caslick suture (vulvoplasty). The perineum is also washed as part of the minimum contamination breeding technique to reduce contamination of the uterus during natural cover or artificial insemination.

Equipment and Supplies

Tail wrap, tail rope, non-irritant soap, roll cotton, stainless steel bucket, plastic bag/bucket liner, paper towels, examination gloves.

Placement of a Tail Wrap

- A tail wrap should be placed prior to washing of the perineum. This may be a reusable neoprene wrap, Velcro® wrap, gauze wrap, flexible elastic wrap (Vetrap™), or an obstetrical sleeve.
- A reusable neoprene Velcro® wrap is cost effective and quick in application. It should be washed regularly with a disinfectant soap and dried before reuse. This is especially important if the wrap is used with different mare populations. The prevention of disease transmission is difficult with the reuse of this wrap without sanitation; thus, if there is a suspicion of such, a disposable tail wrap should be used.
- A gauze wrap is placed on the tail using one of two techniques. With both techniques the wrap goes from the base of the tail to a level just below the ventral commissure of the vulva. Technique one is to start at the top of the tail and with every circumferential wrap, flip some tail hairs upward so that they become trapped between successive layers (Figure 3.1). This prevents the tail wrap from slipping down the tail. This tail wrap

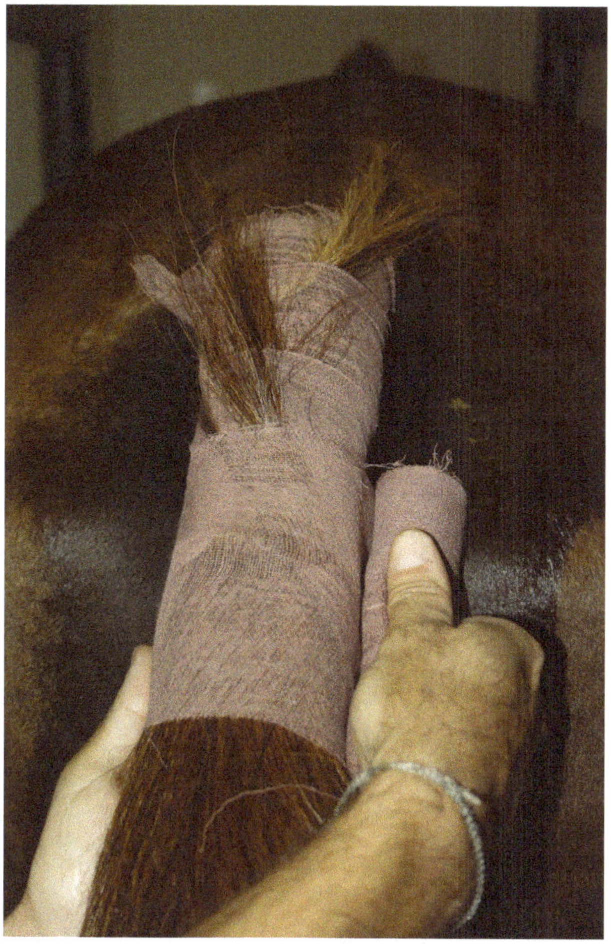

Figure 3.1 Gauze tail wrap with tail hairs flipped up to prevent sliding of the wrap down the tail.

Equine Reproductive Procedures, Second Edition. Edited by John Dascanio and Patrick McCue.

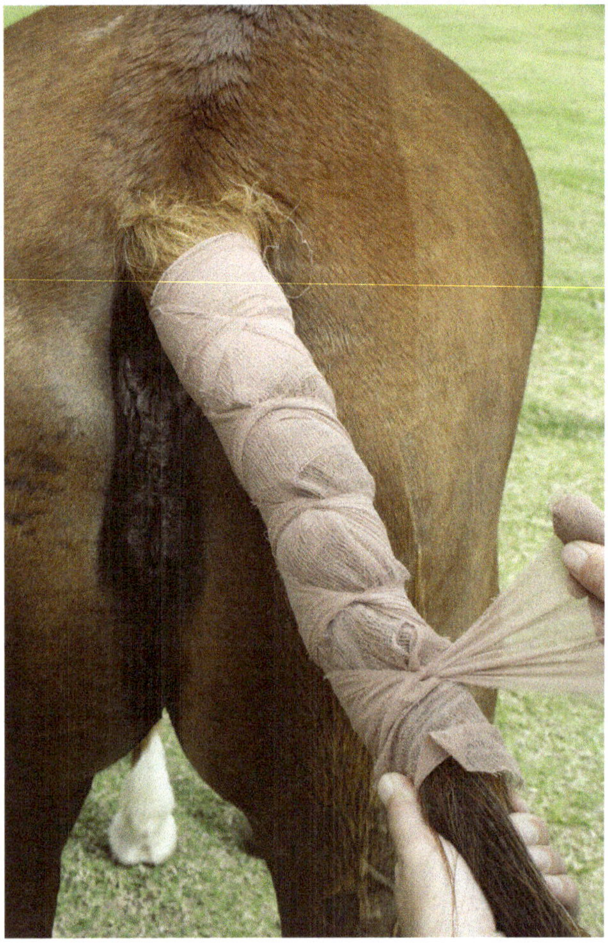

Figure 3.2 Gauze tail wrap twisted 360 degrees on the dorsum of the tail while the ventral aspect is wide.

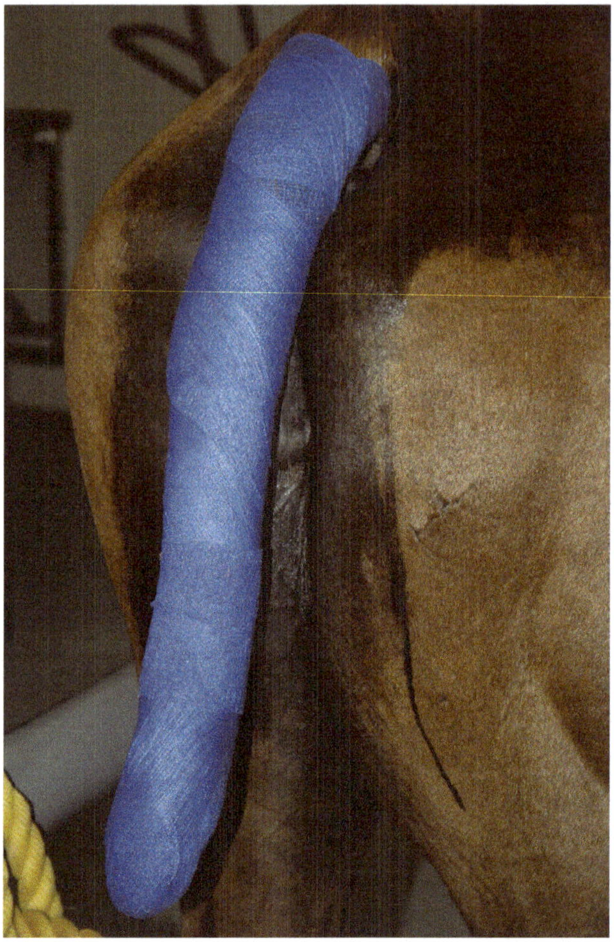

Figure 3.3 Elastic tail wrap encompassing the entire tail.

must be unwound to remove. The second type of gauze wrap starts at about the level of the ventral vulvar commissure (Figure 3.2). A small piece of gauze is left hanging and the wrap placed around the tail, moving upward to the tail base. Hair should not be included between layers, with each layer overlapping the previous slightly. Once at the tail base, the gauze is twisted 360 degrees so that the twisted part is on the dorsal tail, while the ventral aspect of the wrap remains flat and untwisted. This allows the twist to bite into the tail hair on the dorsum, preventing slippage of the wrap, while the flat underneath aspect prevents blood occlusion. The wrap is continued downward and is twisted upon every circumferential wrap ending at the point where the wrap began. The small hanging piece of gauze from the beginning is tied to the remaining wrap to prevent the wrap from coming loose. This wrap may be pulled from the top to slide down the tail and removed without having to unwind the wrap when the procedure is completed. This wrap acts like a Chinese finger trap.

- If an obstetrical sleeve is used for a tail wrap, the tail is placed entirely inside the sleeve. The sleeve may be split at the tail base and tied together to close the sleeve around the tail base, or elastic adhesive tape or an elastic band and clamp may be used to wrap around the sleeve at the tail base to secure it. This type of tail wrap is useful for mares with diarrhea to prevent soiling of the tail hairs.
- If a flexible elastic wrap is used such as Vetrap™, the wrap may either be used to wrap the entire tail or the upper portion (Figure 3.3). The entire tail is wrapped for a dystocia or a fetotomy to prevent tail hairs from interfering with the procedure. To place the entire tail in a wrap, fold the tail hairs so that the hairs do not extend beyond the tail stump. Wrap the elastic wrap around the tail/tail hairs so that no hair is visible along the entire tail length. This in effect creates a "club" with the tail wrapped completely.
- After wrapping, the tail is held to the side so that the perineum can be washed or the tail is tied to the mare (Figure 3.4).

- Alternative tail wrap techniques include use of a sock held in place by 5 cm (2 inch) medical tape (Figure 3.5) or a plastic bag (75 × 25 cm (30 × 10 inches)) held in place by 2.5 cm (1 inch) rubber tubing and a clamp (Figure 3.6). The wrapped tail can be held out of the way by using an elastic cord (Figure 3.7) or being tied to the mare as previously described.

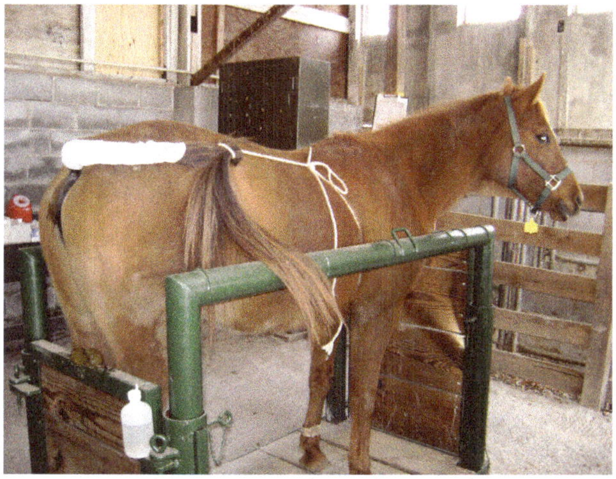

Figure 3.4 Tail wrap tied to the mare with quick release knots.

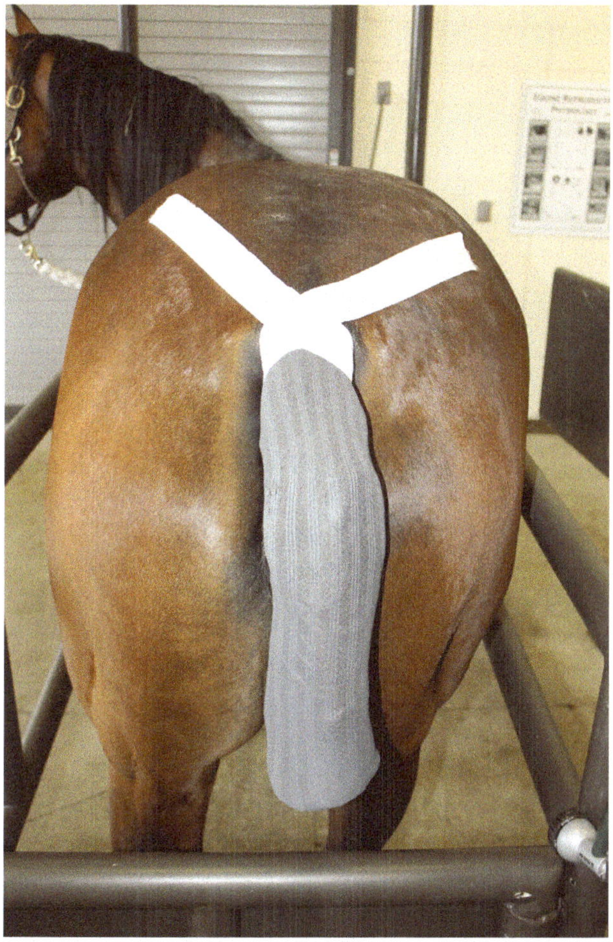

Figure 3.5 Tail wrap using a sock and secured with medical tape.

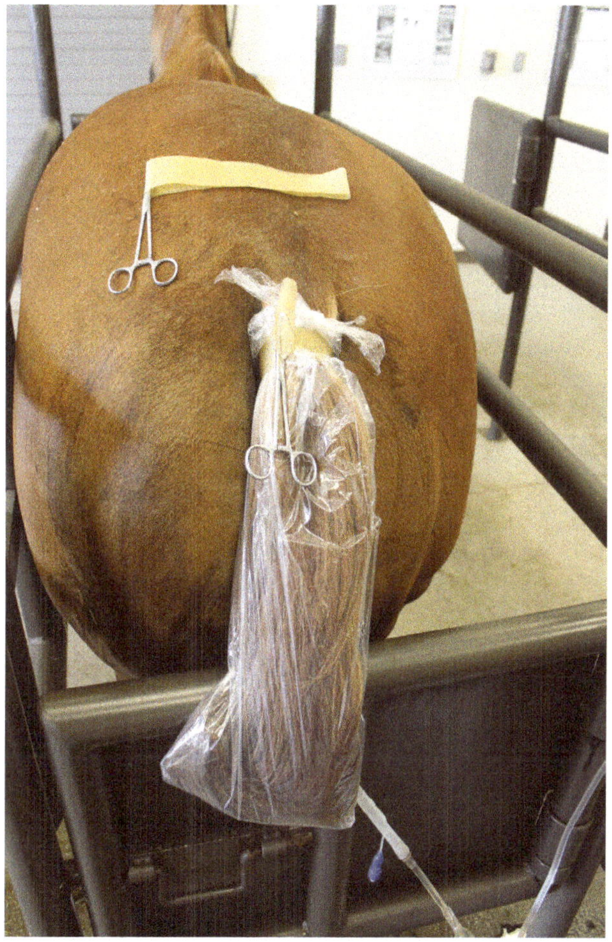

Figure 3.6 Tail wrap using a plastic bag and secured with rubber tubing and a clamp. An extra clamp is shown above the tail.

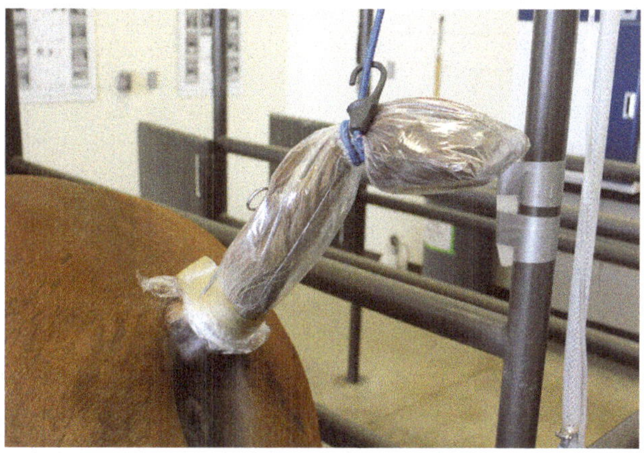

Figure 3.7 Wrapped tail held out of the way using an elastic cord.

Washing Perineum Technique

- Feces should be evacuated from the rectum prior to washing the perineum.
- The perineum is usually washed using one of two techniques: a bucket technique or a water hose technique.
- The bucket technique requires a clean bucket with a disposable liner. A small clean garbage bag works as a liner (Figure 3.8). The liner can be filled with warm water and the top tied to prevent spillage when carrying or to prevent dirt and dust from blowing into the water in a barn environment (Figure 3.9). When ready to use, simply open the plastic bag over the bucket. This also provides some biosecurity, with a new disposable liner used between horses or farms. The classic "clean hand, dirty hand" technique is used to wash the mare. Handfuls of loose cotton are placed into the bucket of water. The person washing the mare wears disposable examination gloves. The "clean" hand retrieves a piece of cotton and holds it away from the bucket over the "dirty" hand and allows the water to drip over the "dirty" hand. The "dirty" hand is massaged under the water flow to clean it of any dirt or debris. The cotton piece is then dropped from the "clean" hand into the "dirty" hand. The "dirty" hand is then used to wash the mare's perineum using concentric circles going outward from the vulva. A mild detergent may be used to help remove smegma and organic debris. The perineum is successively washed until the cotton washing the vulva appears clean after performing the wash. Typically three to four wash/rinse cycles are needed for the average mare. It is important to insure that all soap is rinsed from the perineum.
- The water hose technique is less labor intensive and involves fewer materials than the bucket technique and works well where there are stationary horse stocks. A

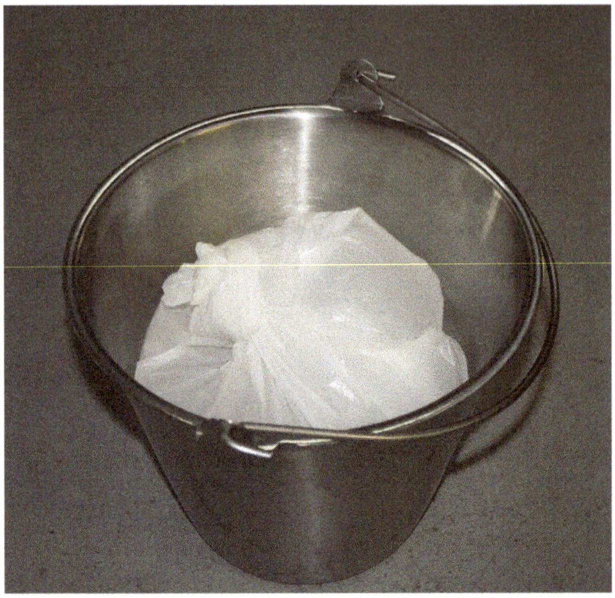

Figure 3.9 Bucket with liner closed to prevent dirt from contaminating water or to prevent water spillage when walking quickly with the bucket.

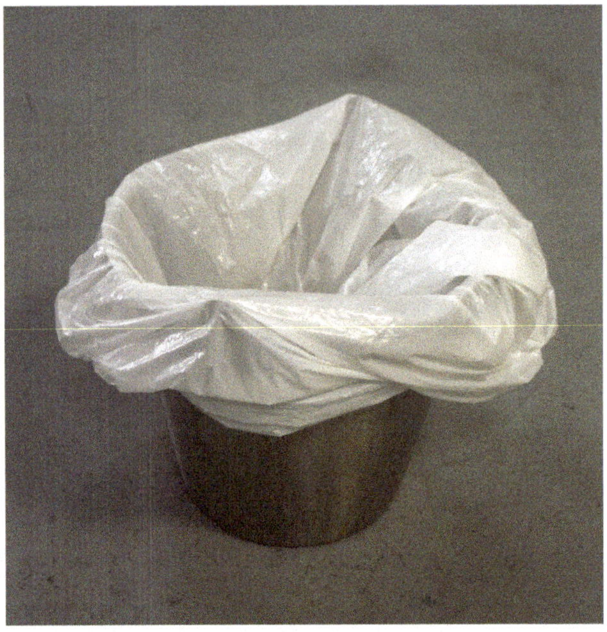

Figure 3.8 Bucket with liner to provide clean water for washing mares. All materials are disposed of between horses.

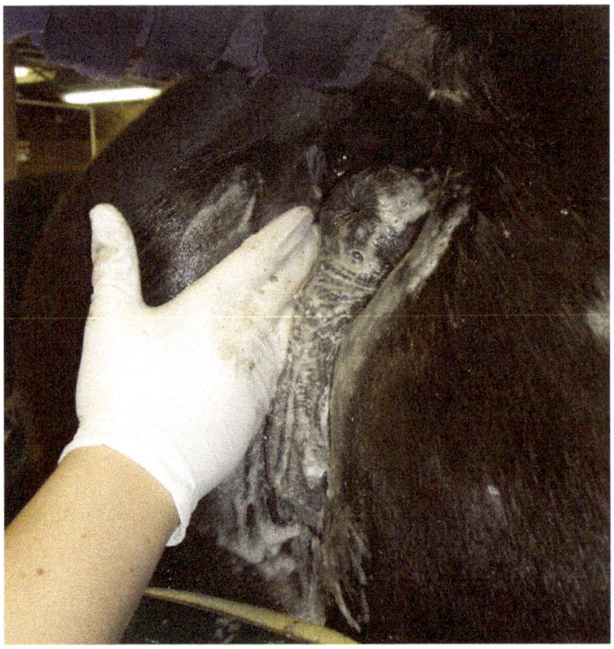

Figure 3.10 Washing the perineum with a gloved hand.

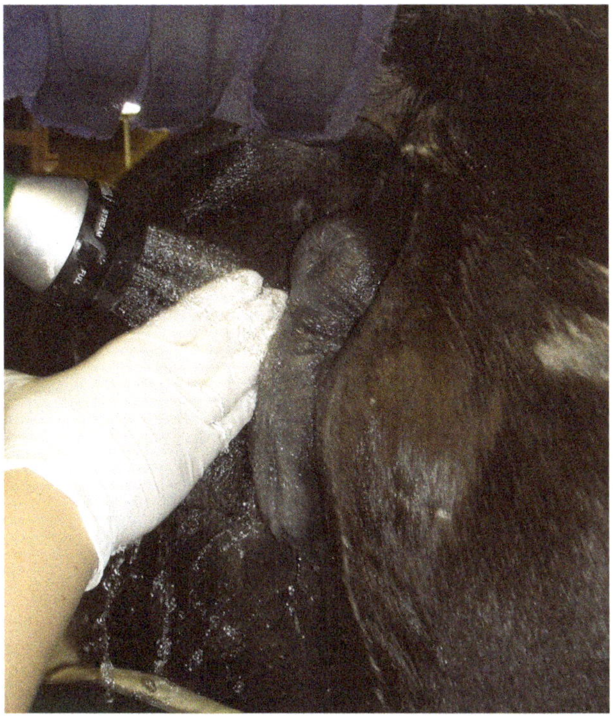

Figure 3.11 Rinsing the perineum with a gloved hand and a gentle shower spray. Note Velcro®/neoprene tail wrap.

gentle stream of water or a shower-type water nozzle should be used. Disposable examination gloves are placed on the hands and the perineum is rinsed with water to remove any gross debris. A mild detergent soap is placed directly on the labia or is placed on the back of the hand. The back of the hand and knuckles are used to vigorously scrub the perineum, using concentric circles going outward from the vulva (Figure 3.10). The gloved hand used to wash the mare is rinsed with the water hose. When rinsing the perineum with the water hose, the back of the hand/fingers may be used to help remove soap residue (Figure 3.11). The perineum is scrubbed until clean, usually involving three to four wash/rinse cycles.

- Once the mare has been cleaned adequately, a final wetted cotton piece is squeezed to remove most of the water and the lips of the vulva are separated. The cotton piece is then swiped from the dorsal to the ventral commissure just inside the mucosa to remove any debris that wicked in between the labia. This is done usually only once so as to avoid trauma to the mucosa. The perineum is dried with a clean paper towel in the same outward concentric pattern used to wash the mare.

Interpretation

- When washing the mare, care should be taken so that water running down the back legs does not cause the mare to kick outward.
- A disinfectant soap should not be routinely used in order to prevent killing normal skin flora and to prevent overgrowth of a pathogenic bacteria. A disinfectant soap may be used for surgical procedures.
- The perineum should be scrubbed from the labia to 15–30 cm outward from the labia so that if the mare moves when entering the vulva with a gloved arm, the gloved arm will remain clean.

4

Placement of a Tail Rope

John J. Dascanio

School of Veterinary Medicine, Texas Tech University, USA

Introduction

The mare's tail is often tied to the side to keep it from interfering with access to the rectum or reproductive tract. Horse tail hairs can be very abrasive to mucosal tissue or can lead to bacterial contamination from dirt/fecal contamination. In most cases the mare's tail should be tied to her body so that if she were to fall down or jump out of stocks, the tail would not be injured. If the tail is tied to a rigid structure, such as the stocks, it should be tied with an elastic cord that is attached to a lightweight piece of twine that would break when significant tension is placed on it.

Equipment and Supplies

Tail rope equal to 2× the length of the mare, bungee cord, tail wrap, twine.

Technique for Tying a Tail Rope

- Being careful to not stand behind the mare, the tail is grasped and the tail dock (or end) is located.
- The running end of the rope (short end) is laid across the tail hairs just caudal to the tail dock (Figure 4.1).
- The tail hairs are flipped upward and over the rope (Figure 4.2).
- The running end of the rope is passed under the tail and over the flipped tail hairs (Figure 4.3).
- A bight (loop) from the running end of the rope is tucked under the rope encompassing the tail and the standing part of the rope (longer end) is pulled to tighten the tail rope (Figures 4.4 and 4.5).
- The standing part of the rope is then passed over the mare's back so that if the tail is moved to the left side of the mare's body, the rope is passed over her back to her right shoulder. The rope is then passed between her front legs. It is then passed over her back and tied with a quick release knot at her back (Figure 4.6).
- This method works well when having to breed one mare, especially if there are no stocks around.
- Care should be exercised as some mares may find the rope around their chest constricting and may need time to acclimatize to it.

Technique for Using an Elastic Cord to Tie the Mare's Tail to the Stocks

- The mare's wrapped tail is encompassed by a stretchy cord such as a bungee cord with both ends of the bungee remaining free (Figure 4.7).

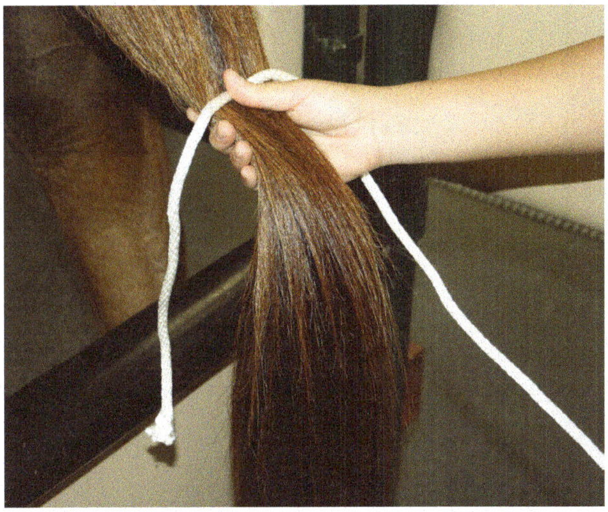

Figure 4.1 The running end of the rope (short end) is laid across the tail hairs just caudal to the tail dock.

Equine Reproductive Procedures, Second Edition. Edited by John Dascanio and Patrick McCue.

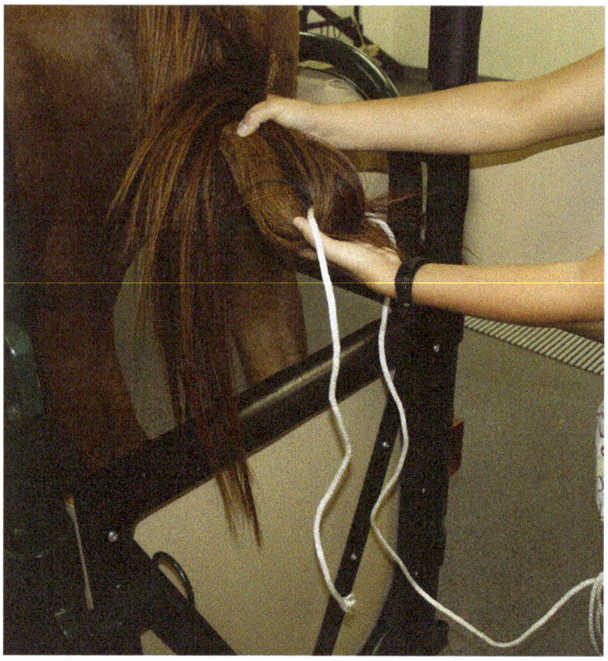

Figure 4.2 The tail hairs are flipped upward and over the rope.

- The bungee cord is hooked to a loop of twine attached to the stocks (Figure 4.8). The twine will break if too much tension is placed on it (due, for example, to the mare jumping out of the stocks). The bungee cord should never be directly attached to the stocks.

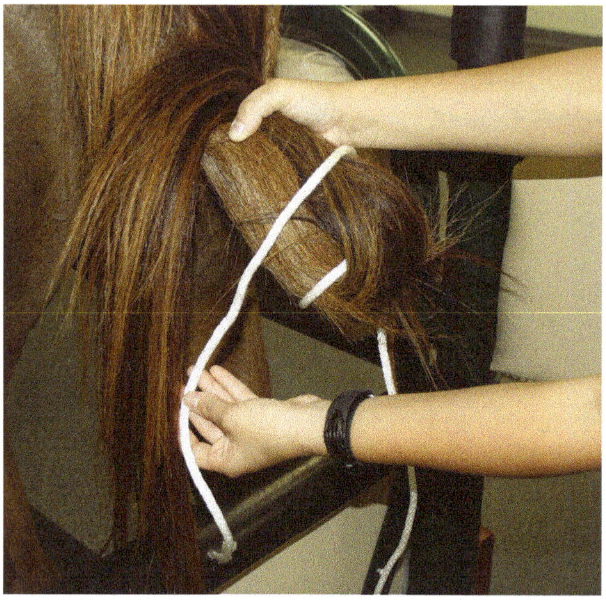

Figure 4.3 The running end of the rope is passed under the tail and over the flipped tail hairs.

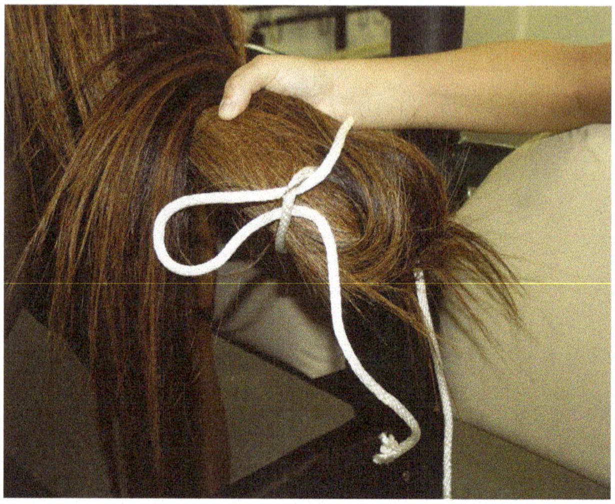

Figure 4.4 A bight (loop) from the running end of the rope is tucked under the rope encompassing the tail.

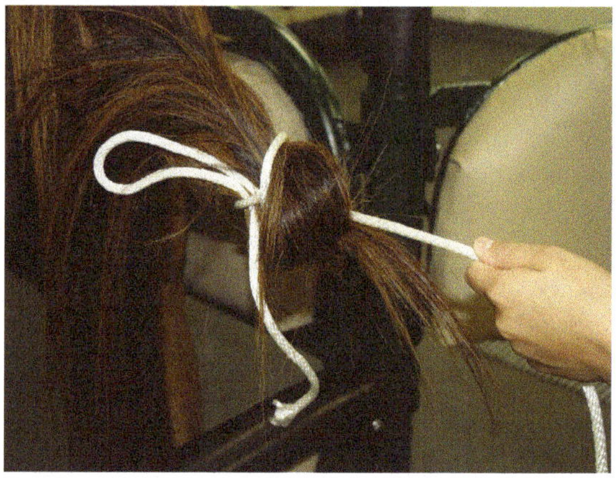

Figure 4.5 The standing part of the rope (longer end) is pulled to tighten the tail rope.

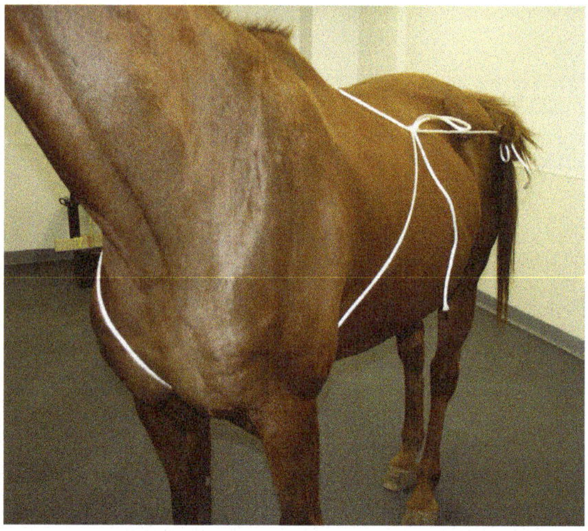

Figure 4.6 The standing part of the rope is passed over the mare' back to her right shoulder. The rope is then passed between her front legs. It is then passed over her back and tied with a quick release knot at her back.

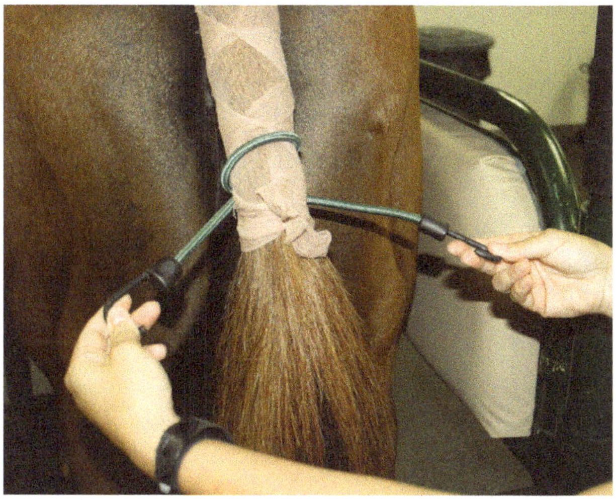

Figure 4.7 The mare's wrapped tail is encompassed by a stretchy cord such as a bungee cord with both ends of the bungee remaining free.

- The bungee cord is a much quicker method of holding the tail out of the way, especially if a Velcro® reusable tail wrap is used. This method works well when multiple mares are checked for cyclicity.

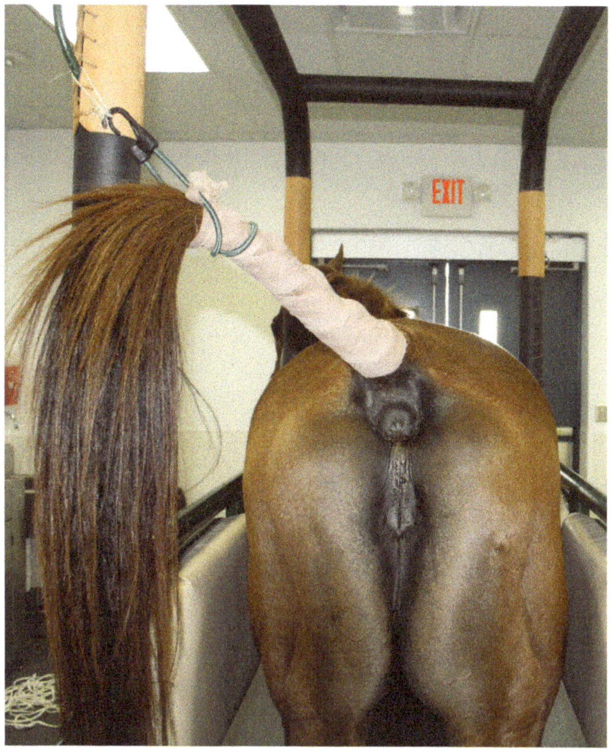

Figure 4.8 The bungee cord is hooked to a loop of twine attached to the stocks.

Further Reading

Leahy JR, Barrow P. 1953. *Restraint of Animals*, 2nd edn. Ithaca, NY: Cornell Campus Store.

5

Perineal Conformation Evaluation

John J. Dascanio

School of Veterinary Medicine, Texas Tech University, USA

Introduction

Perineal conformation evaluation is an integral part of the mare breeding soundness examination and should be performed in any mare presented for reproductive evaluation. While there could be defects present in the perineal area, such as from trauma, most commonly evaluation is directed to the vulva. The vulva serves as the first barrier to contamination of the reproductive tract. Defects in perineal conformation may predispose the reproductive tract to inflammation and infection.

Defects in perineal conformation are most often remedied by performing vulvoplasty (Caslick operation, Chapter 53). Alternative surgical perineal procedures include the Pouret operation, Slusher vestibuloplasty, or Gadd technique.

Equipment and Supplies

Tail wrap, exam gloves, flashlight.

Technique

- Wearing examination gloves, hold the tail to the side so as to visualize the anus, perineum, and vulva.
- Visualize the declination of the vulvar lips from vertical (Figure 5.1).
- Note any disruption to the labia such as from previous trauma or surgeries.
- Note any discharges from the vulva or on the skin ventral to the vulva. Purulent discharges may accumulate as a crusty discharge on the skin of the vulva and ventral perineum (Figure 5.2). Since the tail is usually relaxed and lying against the vulva, discharges often accumulate on the ventral aspect of the tail in the tail hairs. This area should be examined prior to placement of a tail wrap as a clue that there is a passive vaginal discharge.

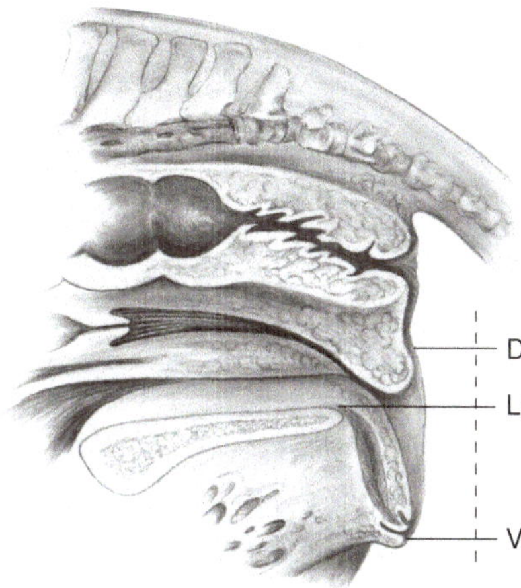

Figure 5.1 Normal conformation with two thirds of the vulvar opening lying below the level of the pelvic brim. Source: From Descanio JJ. 2011. External reproductive anatomy. In: McKinnon AO, Squires EL, Vaala WE, Varner DD (eds). *Equine Reproduction*, 2nd edn. Ames, IA: Wiley Blackwell, pp. 1577–81. Reproduced with the permission of John Wiley & Sons.

- Normal urine crystal/mucus accumulation on the ventral labia may appear as a chalky white discharge, especially evident when mares are in heat (Figure 5.3). There should be no discharge on the ventral skin or in the tail hairs since this is a normal finding.
- Wearing exam gloves, push the index fingers on either side of the labia to determine the relationship of the vulvar opening to the ventral pelvis.
- Place the thumbs on either side of the labia and pull the labia apart, exposing the vestibule to perform the Windsucker test (Figure 5.4) and thus test the integrity of the vestibulo-vaginal fold. The vestibulo-vaginal fold is a barrier to contamination of the anterior reproductive tract and should be intact in a normal mare. When the

Equine Reproductive Procedures, Second Edition. Edited by John Dascanio and Patrick McCue.

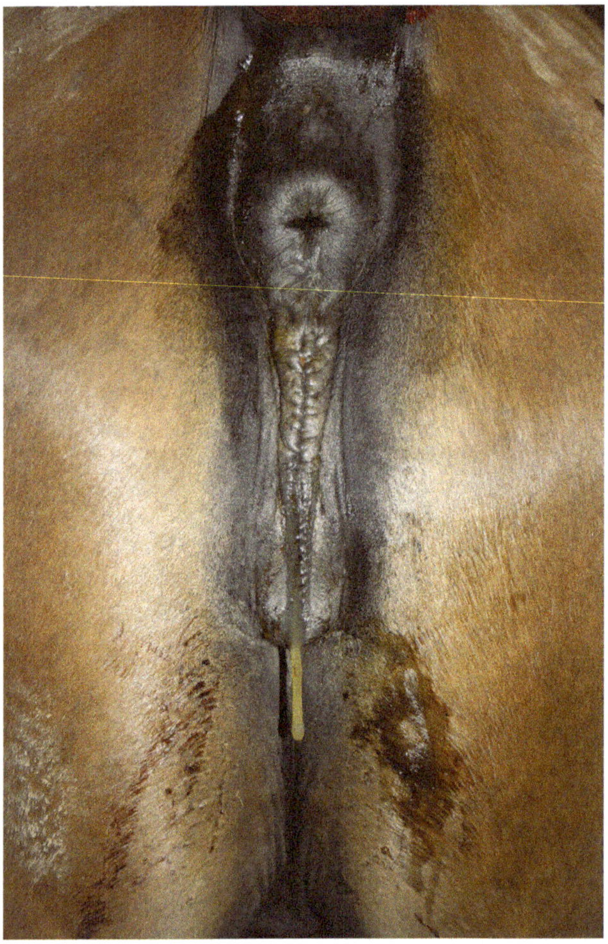

Figure 5.2 Mare with a purulent vaginal discharge and dried discharge on the inner aspect of the hind legs.

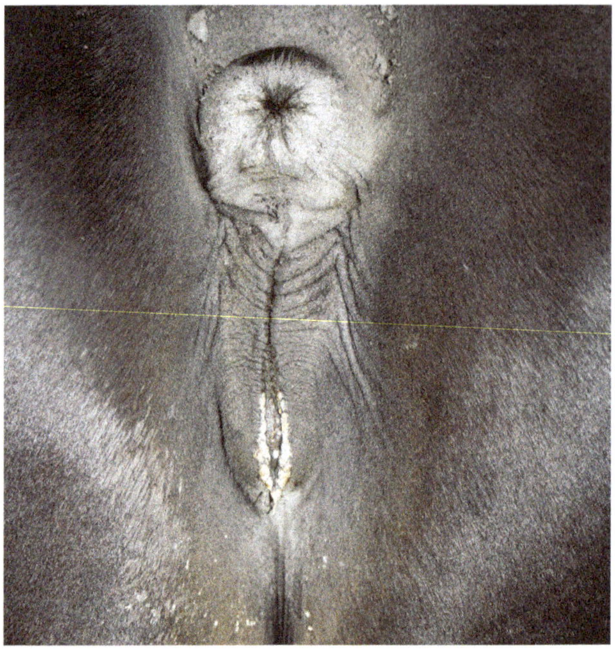

Figure 5.3 Normal chalky white discharge on the ventral labia from urination.

labia are separated, the vestibulo-vaginal fold will prevent air from entering the vagina. An in-rush of air or a "slurping" of air into the vagina occurs in mares with a non-functional vestibulo-vaginal fold.

Interpretation

- The vulva should be vertically orientated.
- The labia should meet without disruption of the mucosal seal.
- Two thirds or more of the vulvar opening should be below the pelvic brim.
- Upon separation of the vulvar lips and visualization of the vestibulo-vaginal fold, no air should enter the vagina.

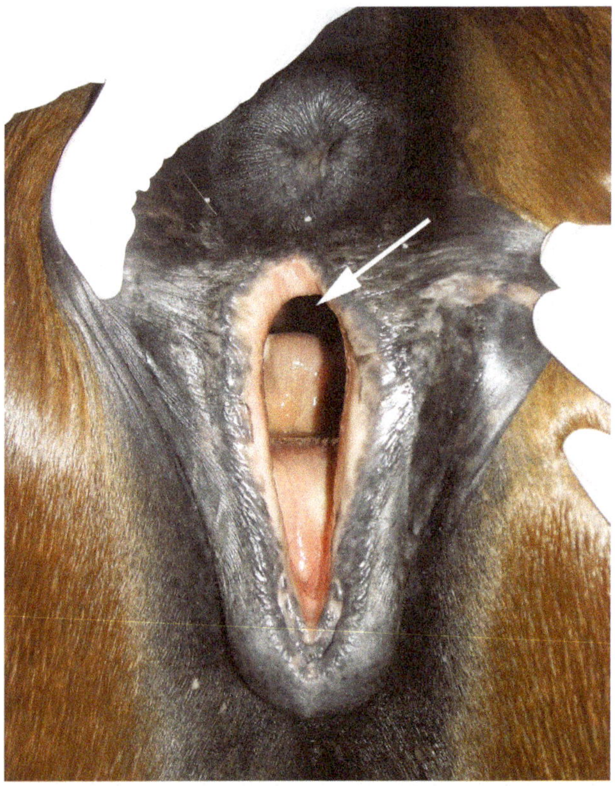

Figure 5.4 Mare with a positive Windsucker test. The arrow points at the opening into the cranial vagina. The vestibulo-vaginal fold is non-functional in this mare.

Reference

Dascanio JJ. 2011. External reproductive anatomy. In: McKinnon AO, Squires EL, Vaala WE, Varner DD (eds). Equine Reproduction, 2nd edn. Ames, IA: Wiley Blackwell, pp. 1577–81.

Further Reading

Gadd JD. 1975. The relationship of bacterial cultures, microscopic smear examination and medical treatment to surgical correction of barren mares. *Proc Annu Conv Am Assoc Eq Pract* 21: 362–8.

Pascoe RR. 1979. Observations on the length and angle of declination of the vulva and its relation to fertility in the mare. *J Reprod Fertil Suppl* 27: 299–305.

Pouret EJM. 1982. Surgical technique for the correction of pneumo- and urovagina. *Eq Vet J* 14: 249.

6

Removal of a Persistent Hymen

John J. Dascanio

School of Veterinary Medicine, Texas Tech University, USA

Introduction

The hymen may be a complete or partial tissue wall separating the vagina and vestibule. The hymen is usually ruptured at breeding or disrupted manually during artificial insemination. Once the hymen is opened, the remaining tissue is referred to as the vestibulo-vaginal fold. The purpose of the vestibulo-vaginal fold is to act as a one-way valve, helping to prevent air and contaminants from entering the vagina.

Occasionally, the hymen is very thick and accumulates a significant amount of secretions behind it. These secretions may be vaginal or uterine in origin. Typically, the secretions have a white liquid to mucoid consistency.

If the hymen does not rupture with digital pressure, a surgical procedure may be needed to open the thickened membrane. Care should be taken to ensure that there is a complete reproductive tract on the vaginal side of the hymen, as segmental aplasia of the reproductive tract could be present with thickened hymenal tissue. Transrectal ultrasound may be used to visualize accumulated fluid within the vagina/cervix/uterus to confirm the presence of the reproductive tract. Conversely, a small hole may be created in the hymen and an endoscope used to explore the tissue in front of the hymen to confirm that the vagina and cervix are present before expanding the incision in the hymen.

Equipment and Supplies

Tail wrap, tail rope, non-irritant soap, roll cotton, stainless steel bucket, disposable liner for bucket, paper towels, surgery gloves, basic surgical pack, sedation, local anesthetic, needles and syringes.

Technique

- Remove feces from the rectum.
- Place a tail wrap and a tail rope.
- Clean and dry the perineum (see Chapter 3).
- For a thin membrane hymen, a finger or blunt-tipped instrument such as the end of closed Metzenbaum scissors may be used to exert pressure on the central aspect of the hymen to disrupt it. The hand should be able to extend beyond the hymen to ensure that the hymen is opened adequately for breeding.
- For a thick membrane hymen, using Addison tissue forceps or towel forceps, grasp the hymen near its center and pull outward to evert it through the vulvar opening (Figure 6.1).

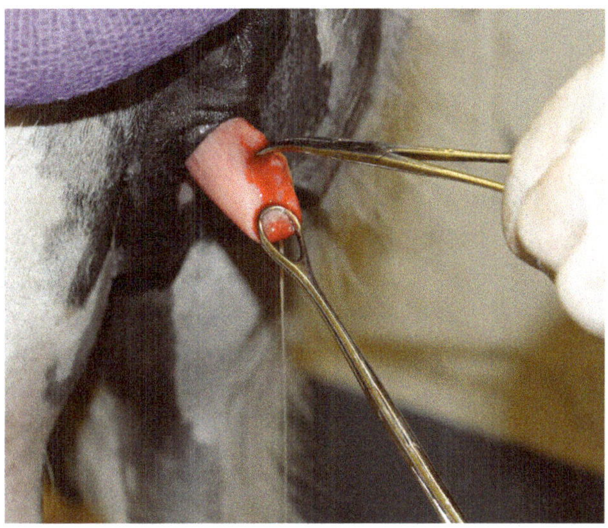

Figure 6.1 A thick hymen grasped with sponge forceps. A small hole was created with a scalpel blade and a creamy white discharge can be seen exiting the incision.

Equine Reproductive Procedures, Second Edition. Edited by John Dascanio and Patrick McCue.

- If the mare resents manipulation of the hymen, a local anesthetic may be infiltrated into the surrounding tissue or an epidural may be performed.
- For a thick hymen, a 1 cm hole is carefully created near the center of the hymen using a scapel or scissors.
- Any discharge from the cut hole should be noted at this time. Typically a white liquid will discharge, which is an accumulation of uterine/vaginal secretions.
- Using a finger, small speculum, or endoscope, examine the area just cranial to the hole in the hymen to confirm the presence of a normal reproductive tract. In some cases, agenesis of the reproductive tract may be present, and further surgical intervention should be discontinued. Confirmation of an intact reproductive tract may also be done with palpation and ultrasound examination per rectum.
- Once a normal reproductive tract is confirmed, the hole may be enlarged with Metzenbaum scissors so that a circular area of hymen is removed.
- Care should be taken to leave a rim of tissue around the hymen so as to not compromise the wall of the vestibule or vagina (Figure 6.2).
- Occasionally, it may be necessary to dilate the remaining tissue with the balloon from a Foley catheter to enlarge the vestibulo-vaginal area.

Interpretation

- A creamy white discharge with some hemorrhage may be present for a few days post-surgery.

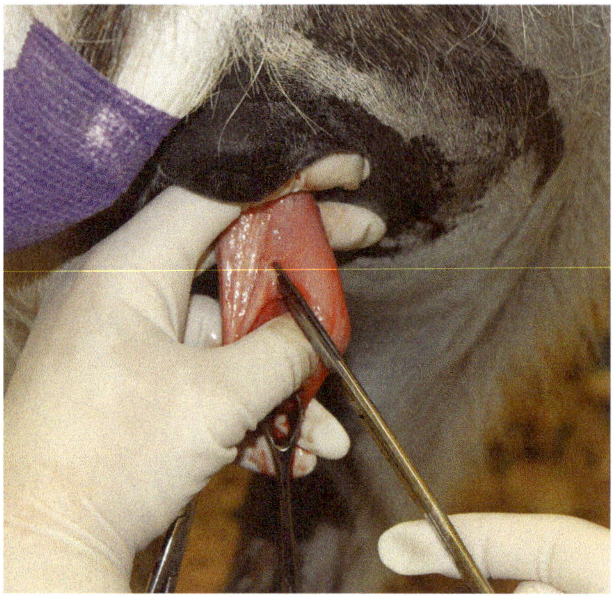

Figure 6.2 The incision is enlarged with Metzenbaum scissors and a circular piece of tissue removed from the central aspect of the hymen.

- The mare should not be bred immediately after surgery, but may be bred at the next estrus, to make sure that any pathology from the pressure from retained vaginal/uterine secretions can resolve first.
- Occasionally a stricture may form after removal of a significant hymen, which may require future dilation or possibly laser surgical removal.
- Generally, no aftercare is required.

7

Palpation of the Reproductive Tract

Patrick M. McCue

Equine Reproduction Laboratory, Colorado State University, USA

Introduction

Evaluation of the mare reproductive tract begins with a thorough and systematic manual palpation of the ovaries, uterus, and cervix per rectum. This may be followed by ultrasound evaluation of the reproductive tract and other procedures. Certain anatomic features such as softness of a pre-ovulatory follicle, sensitivity of the ovary in the peri-ovulatory period, tone in the uterus and cervix, and the presence of a parovarian cyst are easier to discern on palpation than on ultrasound.

Equipment and Supplies

Obstetrical sleeves (non-sterile), obstetrical lubricant, *N*-butylscopolammonium bromide (Buscopan®; Boehringer Ingelheim Vetmedica, Inc., St Joseph, MO, USA).

Palpation Technique

- It is important that the reproductive tract be examined in a systematic manner. The specific order of the exam is not as important as consistency and thoroughness of the examination.
- Administration of *N*-butylscopolammonium bromide (20–60 mg IV) may be indicated to induce relaxation of the smooth muscle of the rectum and facilitate a safe palpation of the reproductive tract.
- About 10–20 ml of obstetrical lubricant is applied to the palpation sleeve covering the hand and forearm. Fecal material in the rectum and distal small colon should be completely evacuated prior to manual palpation of the reproductive tract. Care should be exercised to not exert excessive focused pressure on the rectal wall to avoid rectal tears. In addition, the examiner should relax and make sure to not push forward when peristaltic contractions come over the hand and arm.
- The examination may begin by evaluating the size, tone, and consistency of the cervix. The uterus is then identified and one uterine horn is palpated from the uterine bifurcation to the horn tip, and the size, tone, and consistency noted. The ipsilateral ovary can then be grasped and thoroughly evaluated. The examination is subsequently repeated on the opposite side.
- In order to achieve an effective and meaningful ovarian palpation, the examiner must be able to feel all aspects of each ovary. It is significantly easier to palpate the contralateral ovary (i.e., the right ovary for a left-handed examiner) than the ipsilateral ovary.
- Any method used to hold the entire ovary that accomplishes the manual palpation examination is acceptable. One technique begins by sliding the cupped hand laterally along a uterine horn to the tip and then adjusting the open part of the hand in a cranial, lateral, and dorsal manner to contact and directly grasp the ovary (Figure 7.1).

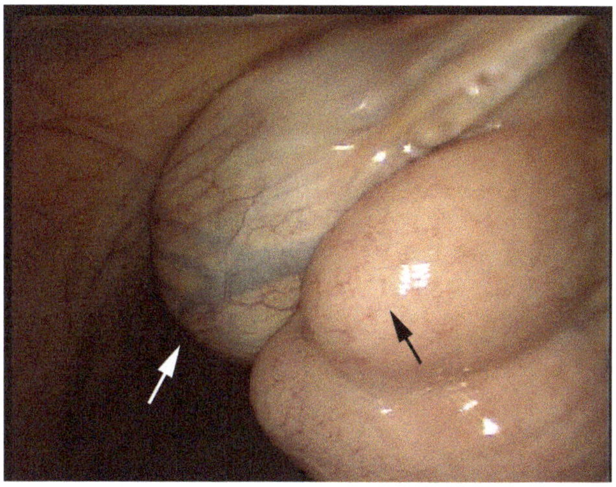

Figure 7.1 Palpation of the ovary (white arrow) as it is trapped against the pelvic wall with a hand within the rectum (black arrow) as viewed by laparoscopic camera.

Equine Reproductive Procedures, Second Edition. Edited by John Dascanio and Patrick McCue.

- If that is not successful, one can use the middle finger to "hook" the mesovarium above the ovary and use the flat part of the thumb on the caudal part of the ovary to push the ovary forward and dorsally from its location behind the mesometrium. One can then fully grasp the ovary for manual examination.
- If that technique does not work, one can subsequently place the middle finger of the palpating hand caudal to the ovary and then advance the finger cranially and medially to push the ovary forward. The examiner would then pronate their hand and rotate their shoulder to grasp the ovary from below.
- The goal of ovarian palpation should be to examine all aspects of the ovarian surface and ovulation fossa with gentle, firm, manual digital pressure (Figure 7.2). Follicles are recognized as smooth, dome-shaped, fluid-filled structures that protrude from the ovarian surface. Consistent and accurate determination of follicular diameter is important to monitor follicular growth and make sound breeding management decisions.
- A mare in estrus may have one or more developing follicles on either ovary. The dominant follicle will generally increase 3–5 mm in diameter each day.
- The diameter of the pre-ovulatory follicle is influenced significantly by breed. Quarter Horse and Arabian mares typically ovulate follicles 35–45 mm in diameter, while Thoroughbred mares ovulate follicles 45–55 mm in diameter, Warmblood mares ovulate follicles 45–60 mm in diameter, and draft breed mares usually ovulate follicles 50–60 mm in diameter.
- Individual mares are reasonably consistent with regard to ovulating follicles within a certain size range. However, some mares may occasionally ovulate small follicles, which can disrupt breeding plans. Initially the pre-ovulatory follicle will be firm on palpation, but the follicle will usually soften prior to ovulation.
- Occasionally an examiner will feel a large follicle collapse during manual palpation per rectum. More often, ovulation is diagnosed as an absence of a pre-existing large follicle, along with a depression in the ovary. The outer wall of the former follicle is often detectable around the boundary of the depression.
- The mare may also be sensitive to manipulation of the ovary for the first 24 hours after ovulation and occasionally just prior to ovulation. Gentle digital pressure on the ovulation site may elicit a noticeable response from the mare, such as lifting the ipsilateral hind leg or a slight muscular tremor.
- The lumen of the former follicle begins to fill with blood beginning 6–12 hours after ovulation, resulting in formation of the corpus hemorrhagicum (CH) (Figure 7.3). The CH may be discerned on manual palpation as a soft, spongy region in the ovary at the previous site of the large follicle.
- A CH can usually be detected for 2–3 days after ovulation. Clinically, detection of a CH indicates that ovulation occurred at least 6–12 hours previously and that it may be too late to breed if the mare has not been bred already.
- The mature corpus luteum of the mare is 2–3 cm in diameter and is contained within the substance of the ovary (i.e., there is no crown or papilla of luteal tissue palpable in the equine ovary) (Figure 7.4). Consequently, the mature corpus luteum cannot usually be palpated in the mare.
- A parovarian cyst can be differentiated from an ovarian follicle by manual palpation of a fluid-filled structure adjacent to, but separated from, the ovary (Figure 7.5).

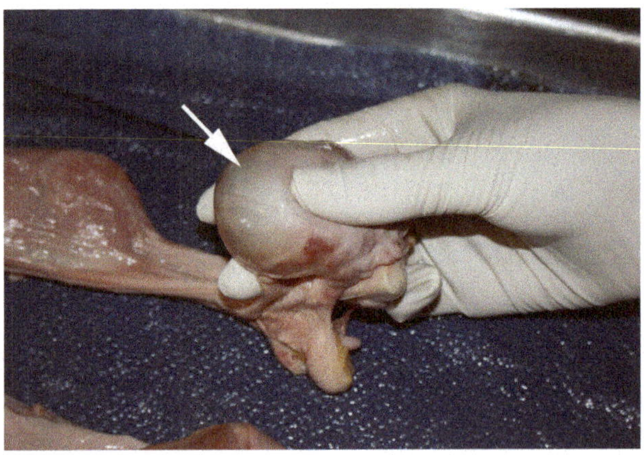

Figure 7.2 Manual palpation of a large follicle (arrow) within an ovary.

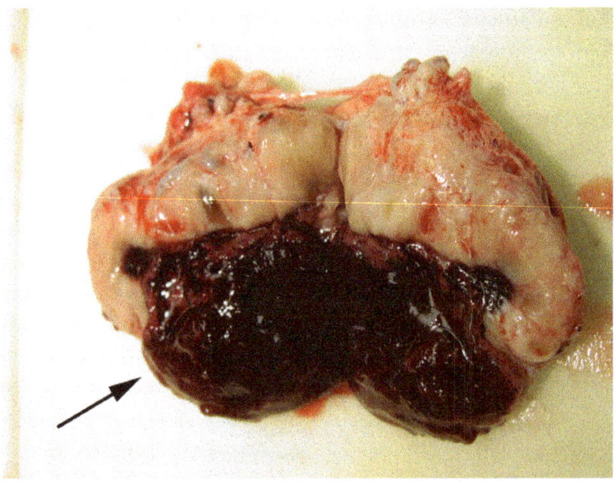

Figure 7.3 Corpus hemorrhagicum (arrow) within an ovary. Reproduced with permission from: Dr Anthony Claes.

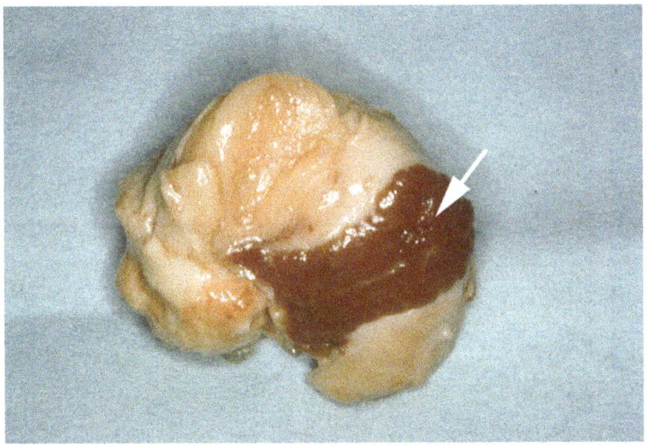

Figure 7.4 Corpus luteum (arrow) within an ovary.

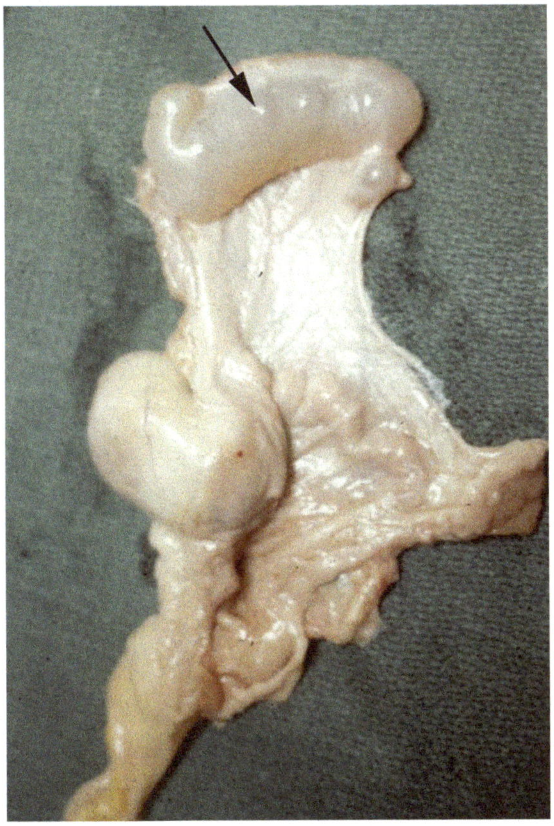

Figure 7.5 Parovarian cyst (arrow) adjacent to an ovary.

- The best way to manually examine the uterus is to advance the palpation arm cranially within the rectum beyond the uterus and then retract the arm while sweeping a cupped hand in a caudal–ventral direction. It is not necessary, nor advised, to retract the equine uterus into the pelvic canal as one would when palpating a cow uterus.
- Once the uterus is identified, move the cupped hand along one uterine horn in a lateral, cranial, and dorsal direction until the horn tip is reached. The uterine bifurcation is more dependent than the tips of the uterine horns. One should be able to discern uterine size, relative weight, and tone with the palm of the hand and fingertips. Repeat the evaluation on the other uterine horn.
- The uterus of a mare in estrus will develop a characteristic "heavy" or "doughy" feel as an increase in estradiol stimulates the development of endometrial edema (Figure 7.6). After ovulation, progesterone produced by the corpus luteum results in enhanced muscular tone of the uterus, which takes on a "tubular" feel. With careful palpation, edematous folds may be detected within the uterine horns of an estral mare.
- With the hand in the rectum to the level of the wrist, sweep the pelvic floor with a flat hand from a 3 o'clock to a 9 o'clock position, moving forward to about the mid forearm in the rectum until the tubular cervix is located. The cervix is best detected by flattening the hand and extending the fingers and pressing the cervix ventrally against the pelvic floor. The hand is moved back and forth laterally to evaluate cervical tone and length.
- The cervix of a mare in estrus is usually short and relaxed (i.e., without tone) and may be difficult to identify per rectum. After ovulation, an elevation in progesterone results in an increase in tone and length of the cervix. The cervix of a mare in diestrus is typically 8–10 cm in length and 2–4 cm in diameter, running cranial to caudal and "rolls" under manual digital pressure.
- The cervix of an older maiden mare may remain long and tight during estrus. Failure of cervical relaxation is one part of the "older maiden mare syndrome" that results in the retention of inflammatory fluid within the

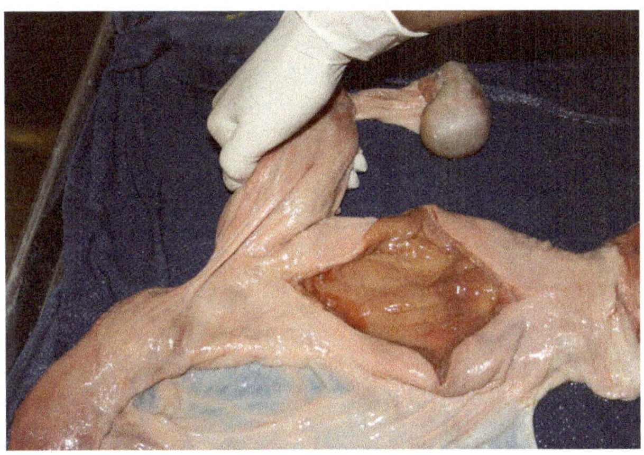

Figure 7.6 Palpation of the uterine horn using a cupped-hand technique. Note that the uterine body has been cut open in this specimen to view the endometrium.

uterus after breeding. Evaluation of cervical morphology and detection of cervical relaxation failure is important when formulating a reproduction management plan for an older maiden mare.

Additional Comments

It is important to learn manual palpation techniques and not just rely on imaging techniques, such as ultrasound, to evaluate the reproductive tract. Tactile differences in reproductive tissue may augment ultrasound findings.

Further Reading

Bowman TR. 2011. Directal rectal palpation. In: McKinnon AO, Squires EL, Vaala WE, Varner DD (eds). Equine Reproduction, 2nd edn. Ames, IA: Wiley Blackwell, pp. 1904–13.

8

Ultrasound Evaluation

Patrick M. McCue

Equine Reproduction Laboratory Colorado State University, USA

Introduction

Manual palpation should be followed by a systematic ultrasound evaluation of the entire reproductive tract. Ultrasound is used in broodmares to visualize structures in the reproductive tract that cannot be palpated or differentiated on palpation per rectum, such as detection of echogenic follicular fluid, endometrial cysts, and free fluid within the uterine lumen. In addition, ultrasonography is valuable in the early diagnosis of pregnancy, management of twins, and detection of potential ovarian or uterine pathology. Ultrasound also allows for critical evaluation of the events leading to ovulation, such as changes in follicular characteristics and grading of uterine edema.

Equipment and Supplies

Ultrasound machine, obstetrical sleeves (non-sterile), obstetrical lubricant (e.g. carboxymethylcellulose).

Technique

- Ultrasonography should be performed after manual palpation of the reproductive tract (see Chapter 7).
- The rectum should be free of fecal material prior to the ultrasound examination.
- Obstetrical lubricant is applied to the ultrasound probe and hand, and the probe is introduced into the rectum in the palm of the examiner's hand.
- A systematic examination of the reproductive tract should be performed. The uterus is identified in cross-section, and the probe is slowly moved from the base of one horn to the tip of that horn while observing the ultrasound image. The probe is often held at a 30–45 degree angle from horizontal so that the cranial tip of the probe is lower than the caudal part of the probe. The uterus is thus held between the probe and the body wall or pelvis for scanning.
- The probe is then manipulated to allow for complete visualization of the ovary ipsilateral to the uterine horn just examined.
- After the ovarian exam is completed, the ipsilateral horn tip is again identified and the probe is slowly passed distally along the uterine horn to the uterine bifurcation and then proximally up the opposite uterine horn (Figure 8.1).
- The position of the probe is again adjusted to evaluate the second ovary before descending back down the adjacent uterine horn.
- The final evaluation is of the uterine body, which is usually visualized in a longitudinal plane with a linear transducer.

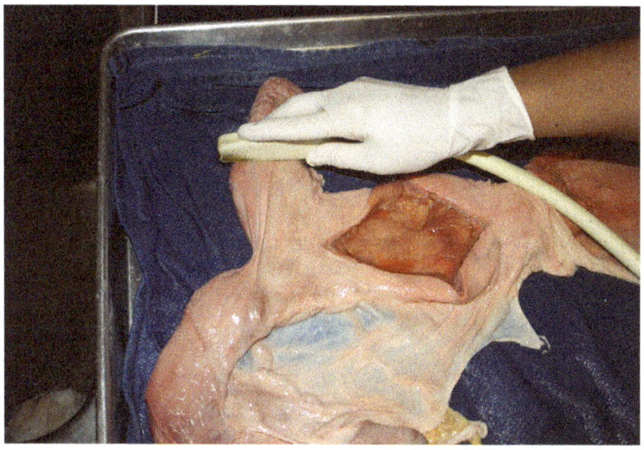

Figure 8.1 Technique for ultrasound examination of the mare reproductive tract. A linear array transducer is shown over the uterine horn. Note that the uterine body has been cut open in this specimen to view the endometrium.

Equine Reproductive Procedures, Second Edition. Edited by John Dascanio and Patrick McCue.

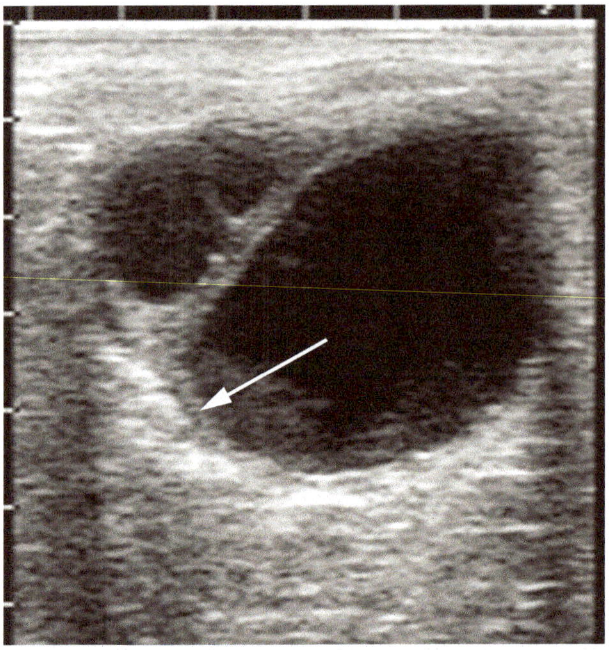

Figure 8.2 Ovarian follicles. The larger follicle is developing a thickened echogenic border (arrow).

- The entire reproductive tract should be examined in one continuous motion, avoiding disruption in visualization of any part of the tract. Small embryonic vesicles or small areas of pathology may be missed if a continuous scan of the reproductive tract is not performed.

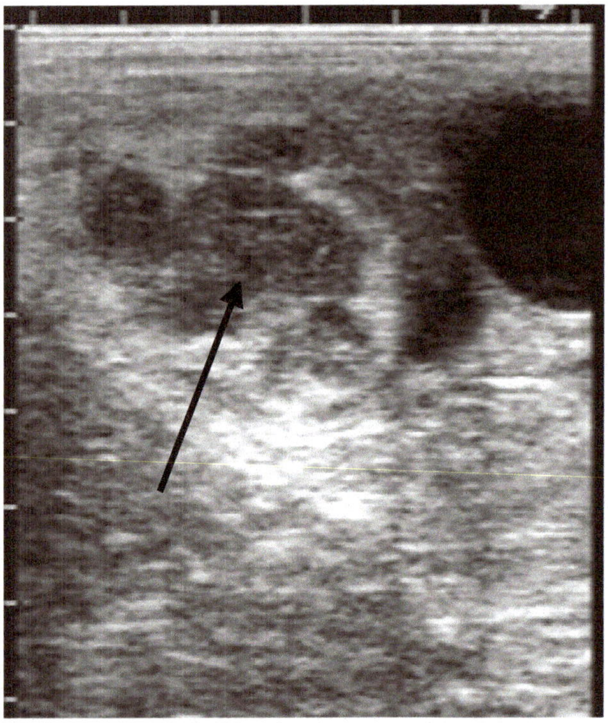

Figure 8.3 Corpus hemorrhagicum (arrow). The interior of the former follicular lumen is filled with echogenic material (i.e., clotted blood).

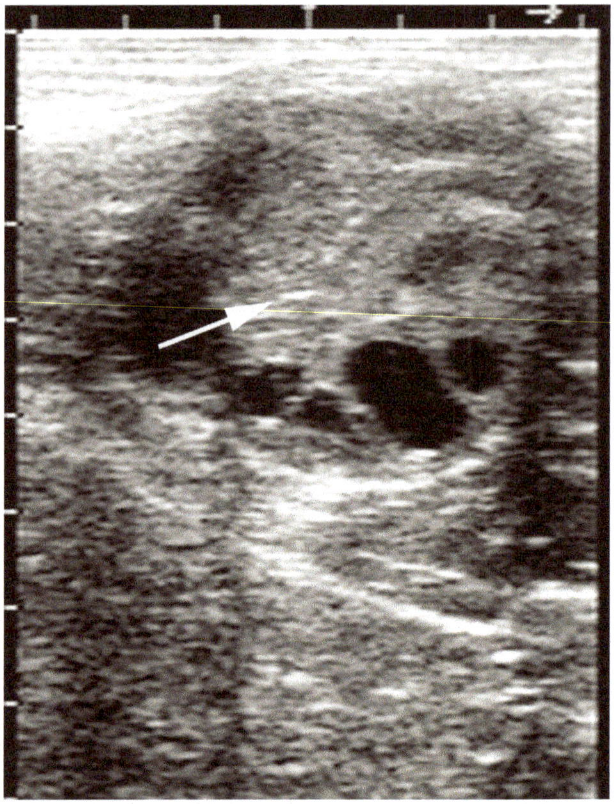

Figure 8.4 Mature corpus luteum (arrow) consisting of a solid structure of uniform echogenicity.

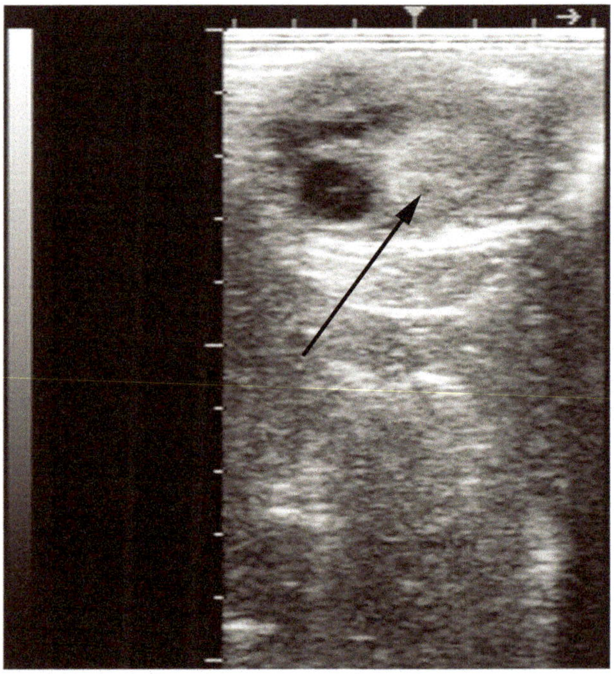

Figure 8.5 Regressing corpus luteum (arrow).

Interpretation

Ovarian Ultrasound Features

Normal ovarian structures routinely observed with ultrasound are various sizes of ovarian follicles, fresh ovulations, corpora hemorrhagica, corpora lutea, and regressing corpora albicans (Figures 8.2–8.5). Ovarian follicles contain clear follicular fluid, which results in a black image on ultrasound. Ovulation is initially detected as the absence of a previously noted large follicle in a mare in estrus. After ovulation, the follicle fills up with blood, forming the corpus hemorrhagicum. This structure is detected as a homogenous, diffusely gray image on ultrasound. The corpus hemorrhagicum matures into the corpus luteum within 2–5 days and takes on a more echogenic (whiter) ultrasonographic appearance.

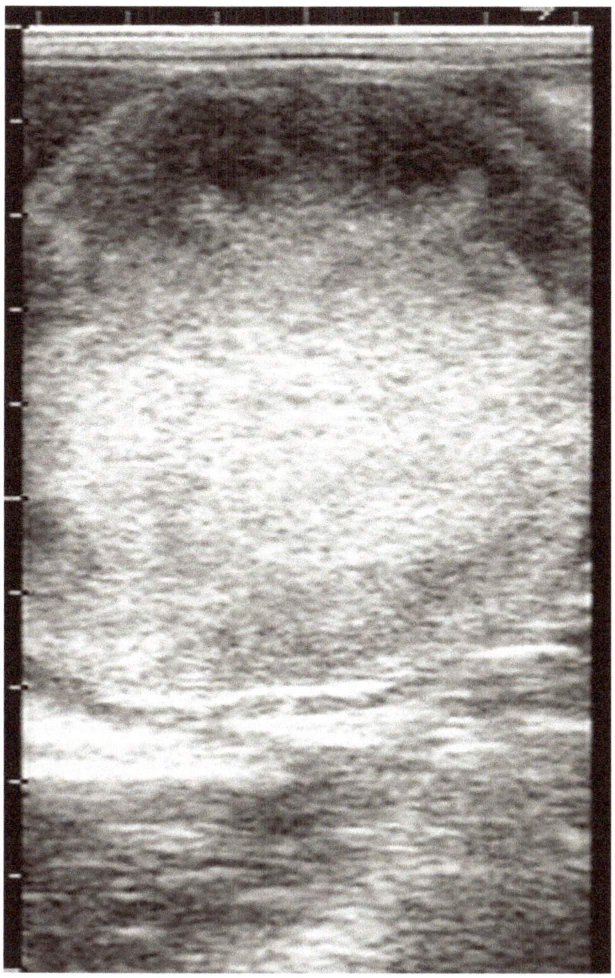

Figure 8.6 Hemorrhagic anovulatory follicle. The distinguishing feature was swirling, unclotted blood in the former follicular lumen.

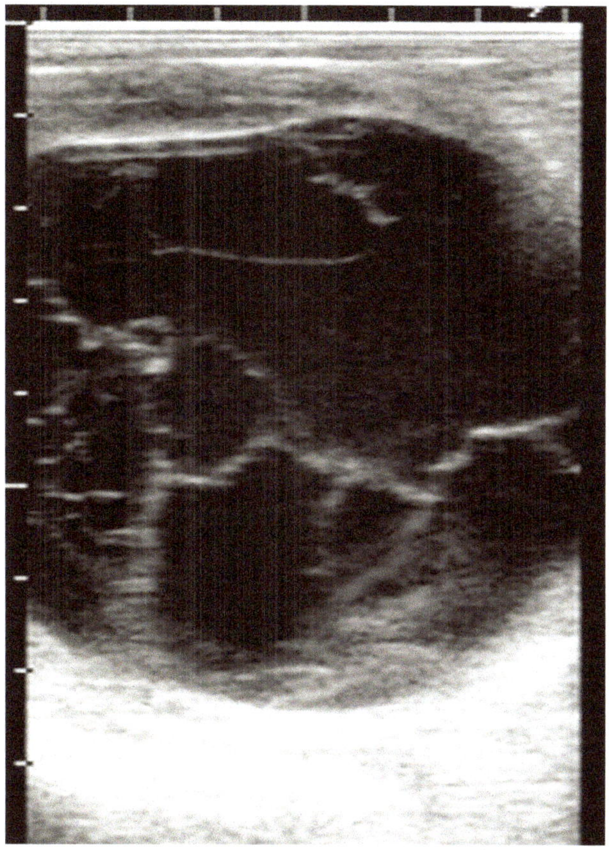

Figure 8.7 Echogenic strands within a follicular lumen early in the progression toward a luteinized anovulatory follicle.

Ultrasound can also help differentiate pathologic conditions of the ovary, such as persistent anovulatory follicles, ovarian tumors, and cystic structures (Figures 8.6–8.9). Persistent anovulatory follicles are initially recognized by the presence of multiple echogenic particles within the follicular fluid. Anovulatory follicles often subsequently develop numerous echogenic strands throughout the follicular lumen and usually completely fill in with echogenic material.

The most common ovarian tumor is the granulosa cell tumor, which is usually recognized as a large, multicystic structure with a small, inactive ovary present on the contralateral (opposite) side (Figures 8.10 and 8.11).

Uterine Ultrasound Features

Mares in estrus may have an edematous uterus and may have a small amount of free fluid present within the lumen of the uterus. Edema is best recognized on ultrasound of a cross-section of a uterine horn as a "sand dollar" or "spoke wheel" appearance. Edema indicates that elevated levels of estrogen and low levels of progesterone are present. Estrogen concentrations and degree of edema

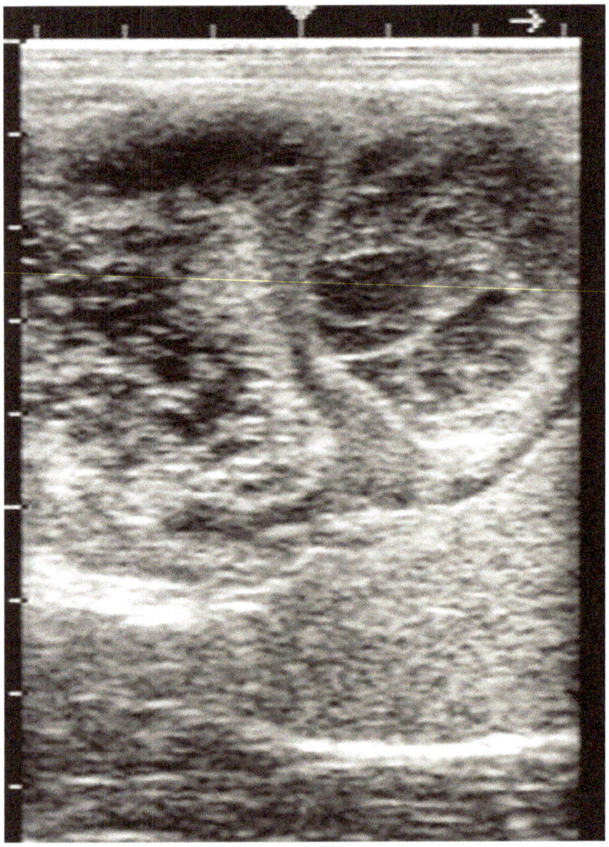

Figure 8.8 A pair of luteinized anovulatory follicles.

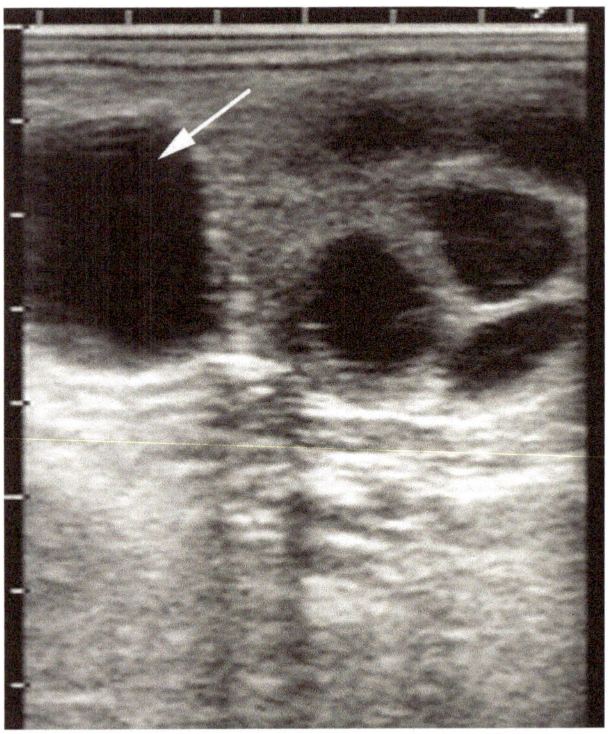

Figure 8.9 Parovarian cyst. The cystic structure (arrow) is adjacent to the ovary.

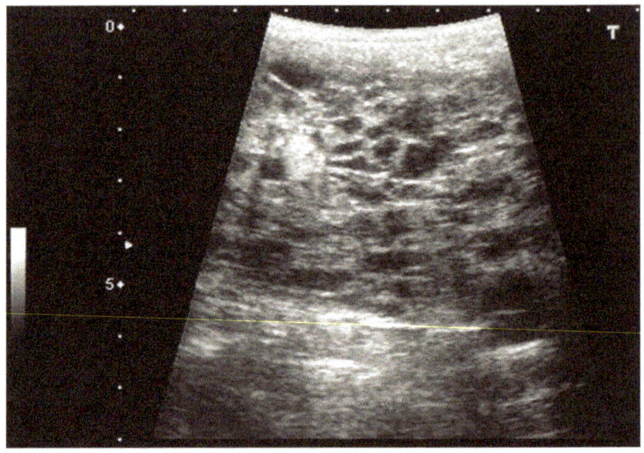

Figure 8.10 Granulosa cell tumor consisting of multiple cysts within an enlarged ovary.

increase during estrus and peak approximately 1 day prior to ovulation. Consequently, the degree of uterine edema may be used as an indicator of when to breed as well as a prognostic indicator of ovulation (Table 8.1). Uterine inflammation may be suspected if edema appears excessive or persists post-ovulation.

The uterus in diestrus is affected by elevated levels of progesterone and has a tubular, homogenous appearance without edema or free fluid within the uterine lumen. The presence of free fluid within the uterine lumen during diestrus is suggestive of inflammation and/or infection (Figure 8.12). Tables 8.2 and 8.3 show the classification of uterine fluid volume and its echogenic character.

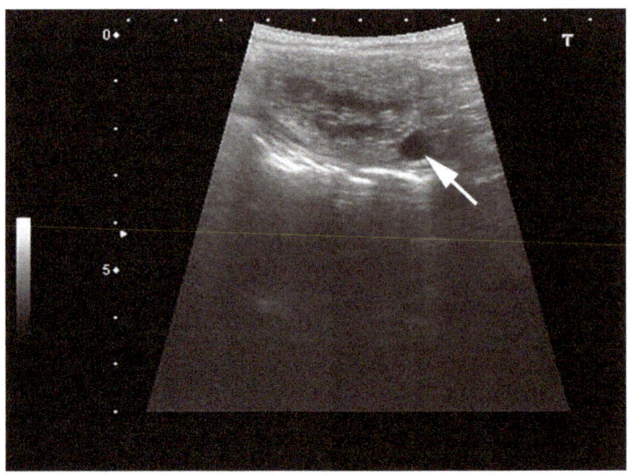

Figure 8.11 Normal ovary contralateral to the ovary with a granulosa cell tumor. This ovary is small and inactive (note only one small follicle is visible; arrow).

Table 8.1 A scoring system used to evaluate uterine edema in mares.

Edema Score	Edema Amount	Description	Ultrasonographic Image
0	None	No edema present; individual endometrial folds not discernable homogenous echotexture typical of diestrus or anestrus	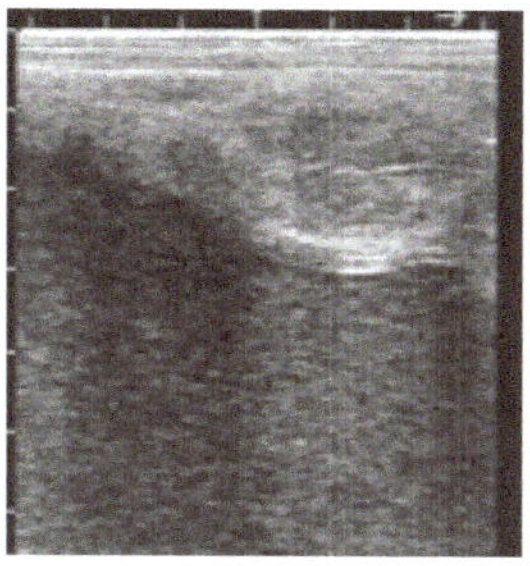
1	Slight	Endometrial folds easily observed in a light "spoke wheel" pattern; edema may be more evident in uterine horns than uterine body Typical of early estrus as the dominant follicle is developing or late estrus prior to or at the time of ovulation	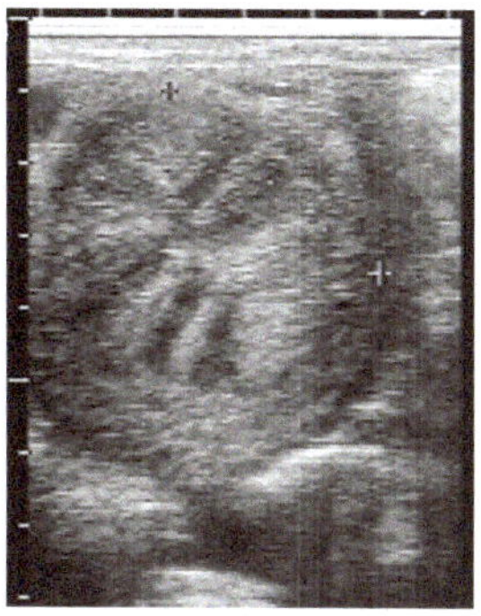
2	Moderate	Endometrial folds increased in thickness; edema pattern obvious throughout uterus Typical of mid-estrus and usually represents the peak estrogen effect noted 1–2 days prior to ovulation	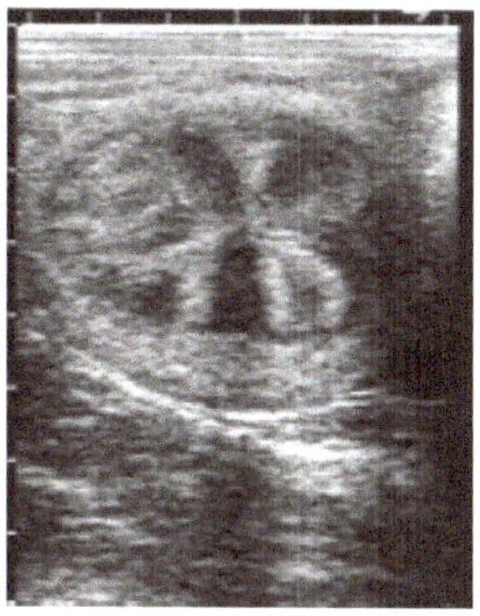
3	Heavy	Large distended endometrial folds; exaggerated degree of edema Not typical of a normal mare in estrus; may be associated with uterine inflammation; sometimes called hyperedema	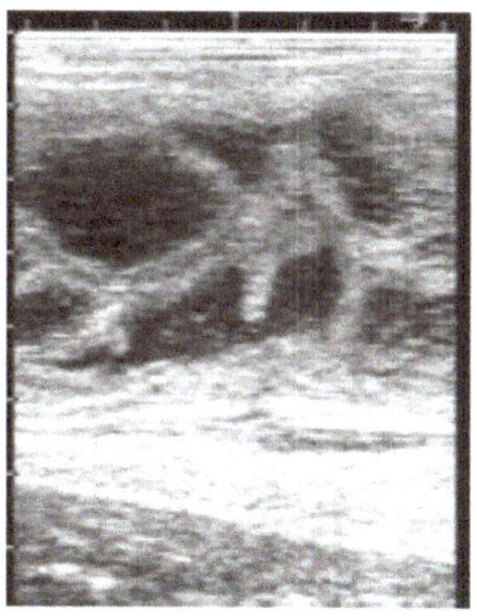

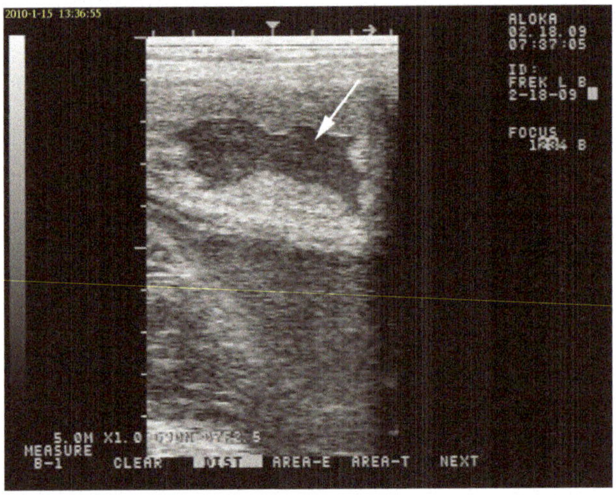

Figure 8.12 Echogenic fluid within the uterine lumen (arrow).

Table 8.2 Classification of uterine fluid volume.

Classification	Initials	Score
No fluid	0	0
Trace (<1.0 cm depth)	T	1
Small volume (1–2 cm depth)	S	2
Moderate volume (2.1–5 cm depth)	M	3
Large volume (>5.0 cm depth)	L	4

Table 8.3 Classification of the echogenic character of uterine fluid.

Classification	Score
No echogenic particles (i.e., clear)	4
Slightly echogenic (i.e., slightly cloudy)	3
Moderately echogenic	2
Highly echogenic	1

Further Reading

McCue PM, McKinnon AO. 2011. Ovarian abnormalities. In: McKinnon AO, Squires EL, Vaala WE, Varner DD (eds). *Equine Reproduction,* 2nd edn. Ames, IA: Wiley Blackwell, pp. 2123–36.

McKinnon AO, McCue PM. 2011. Uterine abnormalities. In: McKinnon AO, Squires EL, Vaala WE, Varner DD (eds). *Equine Reproduction,* 2nd edn. Ames, IA: Wiley Blackwell, pp. 2137–61.

9

Prediction of Ovulation

Patrick M. McCue

Equine Reproduction Laboratory, Colorado State University, USA

Introduction

A decision on when to breed a mare by live cover or artificial insemination is usually dependent on an accurate prediction of impending ovulation. Prediction of the time of ovulation may be accomplished by interpretation and integration of multiple factors for an individual mare. A majority of factors used to predict ovulation are based on normal physiological events in mares that have not been administered an ovulation induction agent.

Technique

- *Reproductive history.* An individual mare will often ovulate a follicle of approximately the same diameter each cycle. Consequently, data from previous cycles can often be used to predict follicle size at ovulation of subsequent cycles. Unfortunately, some mares will ovulate a dominant follicle during one estrous cycle that is of a very different size, either markedly smaller or larger, than follicles of other cycles. Prediction of ovulation is difficult in these mares and more than one breeding may be required so the cycle is not missed.
- *Season of year.* Follicular growth is often slower and the period of estrus longer during the first cycle of the year (short daylight length). Conversely, follicular growth is usually more rapid and the interval from onset of estrus to ovulation shorter during the middle of the physiological breeding season (long daylight length). Decisions on when to schedule mating or insemination need to be made earlier in the cycle during the middle of the breeding season.
- *Follicular growth pattern.* A dominant follicle will typically increase in diameter by 3–5 mm per day and occasionally up to 10 mm per day during early to mid-estrus. The follicle will reach its maximum diameter and subsequently remain approximately the same size for 2 or 3 days prior to ovulation in mares not administered an ovulation-inducing agent. This pattern is disrupted in mares receiving human chorionic gonadotropin (hCG) or gonadotropin-releasing hormone (GnRH) agonists, such as deslorelin or histrelin, as a developing dominant follicle may ovulate prior to attaining maximum diameter.
- *Diameter of follicle and breed.* The maximum diameter of the pre-ovulatory follicle can often be predicted based on mare size and breed. In general, mares of smaller light breeds will ovulate a follicle that is smaller in diameter than mares of larger breeds (Table 9.1). Friesian mares are notorious for developing very large follicles (i.e., 50 mm or greater) that remain present for several days prior to ovulation. A decision to administer an ovulation-inducing agent or when to cover or inseminate a mare should be based in part on breed and follicle diameter. For example, it would not be appropriate or effective to attempt to induce ovulation of a 35 mm follicle in a draft mare, but would be appropriate in an Arabian or Quarter Horse mare.
- *Softness of follicle.* A developing dominant follicle has a firm tone during the early and middle part of the normal growth phase. The dominant follicle usually becomes noticeably softer, as detected by manual palpation, within the 24-hour period prior to ovulation.

Table 9.1 Average diameter of pre-ovulatory follicles in various mare breeds.

Breed	Follicle Size at Ovulation (mm)
Arabian	35–45
Quarter Horse	35–45
Thoroughbred	45–55
Warmblood	45–60
Draft	50–60

Equine Reproductive Procedures, Second Edition. Edited by John Dascanio and Patrick McCue.

- *Number of days in estrus.* Mares are usually in estrus for 4–7 days and the interovulatory interval is approximately 21 days. Ovulation typically occurs 3–6 days after the onset of behavioral estrus. Mares are usually in heat for 1–2 days after ovulation, until the concentration of progesterone increases sufficiently to block behavioral estrus.
- *Interval from prostaglandin administration.* The average interval from prostaglandin $F_{2\alpha}$ (PGF) administration to the next spontaneous ovulation is approximately 5–11 days with an average interval of 8–9 days. It is important to understand that mares will return to estrus and ovulate in a reasonably predictable time period, based on the diameter of the largest follicle at the time of prostaglandin administration. As a consequence, ultrasound examination of the mare and recording follicle diameter at the time of PGF administration can be of great benefit in predicting when the mare should be bred and when ovulation may occur. In general, mares with small follicles at the time of PGF administration take longer to develop a dominant follicle and ovulate than mares with a larger follicle (Table 9.2).

It may be difficult to predict the interval to the next fertile ovulation in a mare with a large diestrous follicle (≥35 mm) at the time of PGF administration. Mares that ovulate a large diestrous follicle within 2 days after PGF will usually not express behavioral estrus, will not develop uterine edema, and the ovulation is generally not fertile. Mares that ovulate a large diestrous follicle more than 2 days after PGF will usually come into heat, develop uterine edema, and the ovulation is considered to be fertile. The third possibility is that the large diestrous follicle will regress and a different follicle will develop and eventually ovulate at a time interval related to the diameter of the next dominant follicle at the time of PGF administration.

Table 9.2 Interval from prostaglandin $F_{2\alpha}$ (PGF) administration to spontaneous ovulation based on follicle diameter at the time of treatment.

Follicle Diameter at PGF	Interval to Ovulation (days)
10 mm	10.4 ± 1.5 days
20 mm	9.2 ± 1.6 days
25 mm	8.2 ± 1.6 days
30 mm	7.1 ± 2.1 days
≥35 mm	*Possible outcomes* • 10% ovulate dominant follicle within 2 days • 80% ovulate dominant follicle 3 or more days after PGF; 68% of these ovulate within 3–6 days and 32% of these ovulate 7 or more days later • 10% regress the dominant follicle and develop another follicle that ovulates 10–12 days after PGF

- *Interval from hCG, deslorelin, or histrelin administration.* The duration from administration of hCG, deslorelin acetate, or histrelin to subsequent ovulation is reasonably consistent, provided that the guidelines for administration are followed. Administration of hCG will typically result in ovulation in 24–48 hours, with an average of 36 hours. Administration of deslorelin or histrelin will usually result in ovulation in 36–42 hours, with an average of 40 hours. Administration of an ovulation induction agent at an appropriate time during estrus will typically advance the ovulation by 1–2 days prior to the day of the expected spontaneous ovulation.
- *Uterine edema pattern during ultrasound examination.* Endometrial edema develops in response to the presence of estradiol and the absence of progesterone. In most mares, a predictable pattern of edema development and regression occurs during each heat period (Figure 9.1, see Chapter 8). Estradiol-17β concentrations and the amount of edema both peak 1–2 days prior to ovulation. Ovulation typically occurs when edema is in a stage of decline or is absent.
- *Thickness of the follicular wall.* Ultrasound examination of the developing dominant follicle will reveal a relatively thin follicular wall during early to mid-estrus. Final maturation of the follicle is associated with an increased thickness of the follicular wall due to an increase in vascularity around the follicle and pre-ovulatory luteinization of granulosa cells. In many cases a hypoechoic ring surrounds a more hyperechoic follicular wall. In contrast, the wall of a diestrus or early estrus follicle is not distinguishable from the surrounding ovarian tissue.
- *Shape of the follicle.* The pre-ovulatory follicle is typically round or slightly oval as viewed during a two-dimensional ultrasound evaluation. A "cone" or "point" may develop as the follicle tunnels toward the ovulation fossa in the hours preceding ovulation.
- *Vascularity with Doppler ultrasound.* Examination of the dominant follicle by Doppler ultrasound will reveal an increase in vascularity surrounding the follicle between 36 and 12 hours prior to ovulation followed by a decrease in color Doppler signals during the last 4 hours prior to ovulation (see Chapter 76).
- *Degree of cervical relaxation.* The physical characteristics of the cervix change throughout the estrous cycle due to the varied influence of estrogen and progesterone. These characteristics can be visualized on speculum examination and tone can be detected by manual palpation per rectum (see Chapter 10). A mare in heat, in the presence of estradiol 17β and an absence of progesterone will have a cervix that is relaxed and draped onto the floor of the

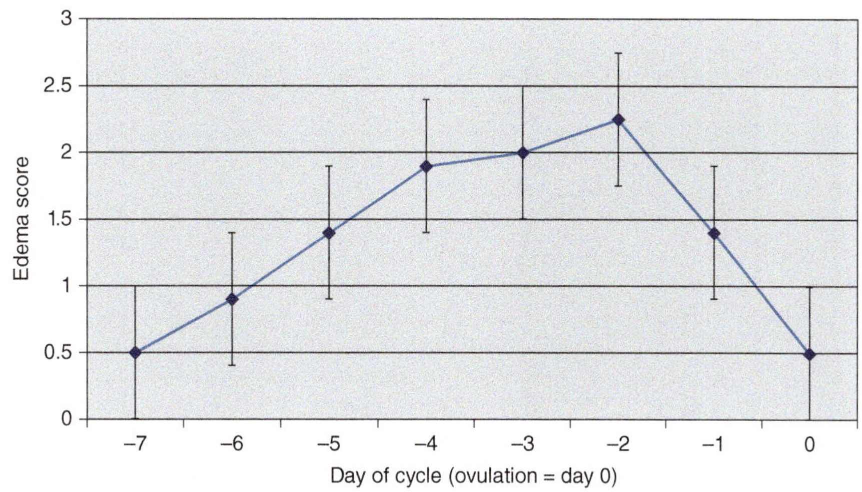

Figure 9.1 Pattern of endometrial edema relative to ovulation.

vagina, that is pink in color and moist. In contrast, a mare in diestrus will have a cervix that is high on the cranial vaginal wall and is closed tight, dry, and pale in color.

- *Peri-ovulatory ovarian pain on palpation*. Many mares will exhibit discomfort when the site of a fresh ovulation is palpated per rectum. Some mares will also be sensitive to palpation of the ovary as the time of ovulation approaches.

Further Reading

Ginther OJ. 1979. *Reproductive Biology of the Mare: Basic and Applied Aspects*. Cross Plains, WI: *Equiservices*.

McCue PM, Scoggin CF, Lindholm ARG. 2011. Estrus. In: McKinnon AO, Squires EL, Vaala WE, Varner DD (eds). *Equine Reproduction*, 2nd edn. Ames, IA: Wiley Blackwell, pp. 1716–27.

10

Speculum Examination of the Vagina

John J. Dascanio

School of Veterinary Medicine, Texas Tech University, USA

Introduction

A visual vaginal examination should be performed as part of a complete mare breeding soundness examination. A speculum examination may also be used to confirm the stage of the mare's estrous cycle and to observe the vagina for pathology such as urine pooling, varicosities, adhesions and cervical inflammation, or discharge. A disposable aluminum foil-covered tube speculum, a glass tube speculum (Figure 10.1), or a tri-valve Polansky (Caslick) speculum (Figure 10.2) may be used for the examination. The glass tube speculum tends to transmit more light into the vagina than the disposable aluminum tube speculum. The tri-valve Polansky (Caslick) speculum will provide a wider view of the cranial vagina and cervix, but may obscure the vagina in areas corresponding to the speculum arms.

The mare should have a relaxed external cervical os lying on the floor of the cranial vaginal vault and a pink, glistening vaginal mucosa during estrus. During diestrus, the external cervical os will be toned or closed and located high on the cranial wall of the vaginal vault, with a pale pink, dull, or dry vaginal mucosa. In anestrus, the cervix may be relaxed with a pale, dry mucous membrane. There should not be any discharge from the external cervical os and there should be no fluid accumulation on the floor of the vagina (e.g., urine pooling). The longer the speculum is in the vagina, the more air will irritate the mucosa, causing the mucous membranes to become redder and more congested. Infection may cause an increase in vascularity and redness to the vagina and yellow to white discharge may also be present from the cervical os. During pregnancy, the vagina will often have thick mucus present causing the vaginal walls to stick together. In addition, the cervix during pregnancy may have an accumulation of thick mucus visible (mucus plug).

Equipment and Supplies

Tail wrap, tail rope, non-irritant soap, roll cotton, stainless steel bucket, disposable liner bag for bucket, paper towels, exam gloves, sterilized glass speculum or disposable aluminum foil speculum, sterilized tri-valve Polansky (Caslick) speculum, sterile lubricant, light source, uterine culture swab, bacterial/fungal transport media.

Technique

- Remove feces from the rectum.
- Place a tail wrap and tie the tail out of the way (see Chapter 4).
- Clean and dry the perineum of the mare (see Chapter 3).
- Lubricate the end of the speculum with sterile lubricant. With the tube speculums, lubricant should not get into the lumen of the speculum so as to avoid obscuring visualization of the reproductive tract.

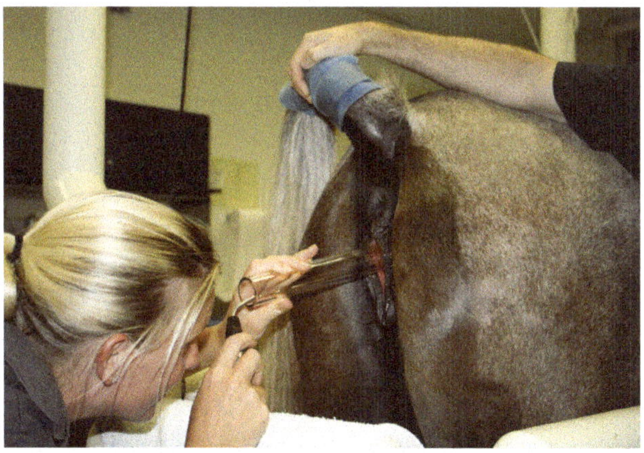

Figure 10.1 Use of a glass vaginal speculum.

Equine Reproductive Procedures, Second Edition. Edited by John Dascanio and Patrick McCue.

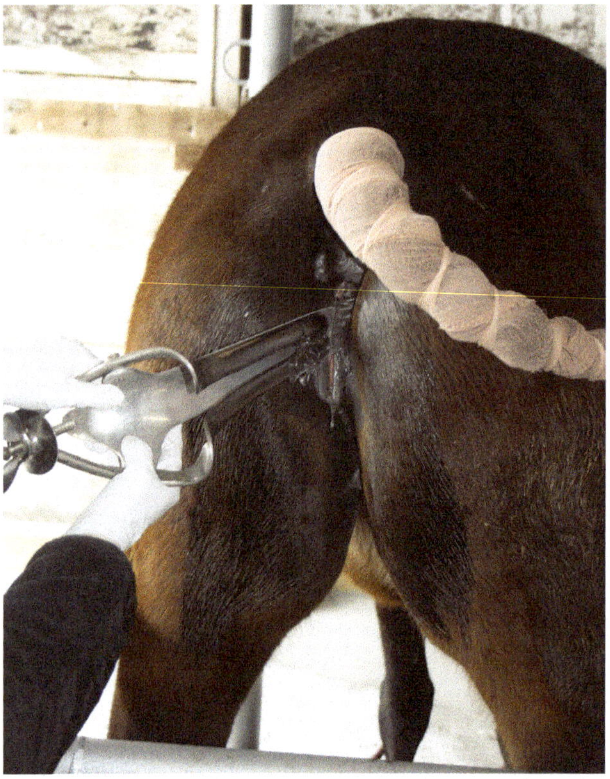

Figure 10.2 Inserting a tri-valve Polansky (Caslick) speculum.

- Wearing exam gloves, separate the lips of the vulva and insert the speculum in an upward manner to pass over the ventral pelvic brim.
- Once over the brim, bring the speculum to a horizontal orientation. Caution is advised when elevating the speculum to a horizontal plane as some mares will react when pressure is placed onto the perineal body.
- The tri-valve Polansky (Caslick) speculum is initially turned sideways to allow entry into the vulva (Figure 10.2) and then turned 90 degrees once over the then pelvic brim and past the vestibulo-vaginal fold. The tri-valve Polansky (Caslick) is advanced into the vagina and then opened by twisting the wing nut to extend the three arms outward (Figure 10.3).
- Some resistance will be encountered at the level of the vestibulo-vaginal fold. Slight forward pressure with some slight rotation will allow the speculum to enter the vagina.
- A light source is used to visualize the walls of the vagina and the cervix. The tube speculum may need to be moved in all directions and pushed inward or pulled outward to visualize all structures.
- Any purulent discharge should be sampled using a sterile uterine culture swab and submitted for bacterial/fungal identification in appropriate transport media.
- Visualization should continue while the tube speculum is removed from the vagina and vestibule.

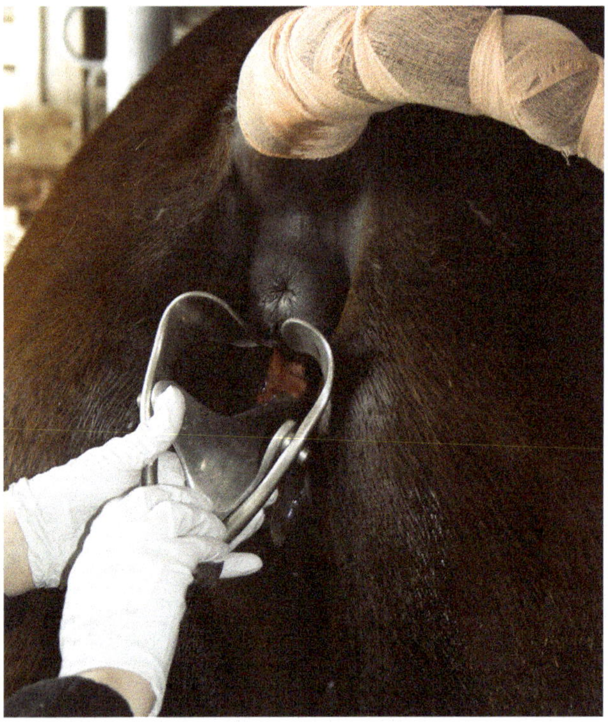

Figure 10.3 Turning the wing nut to open the tri-valve Polansky (Caslick) speculum.

Interpretation

- The vaginal membranes and cervix should appear as per the stage of the mare's estrous cycle.
- There should not be a purulent discharge from the cervix (Figure 10.4).

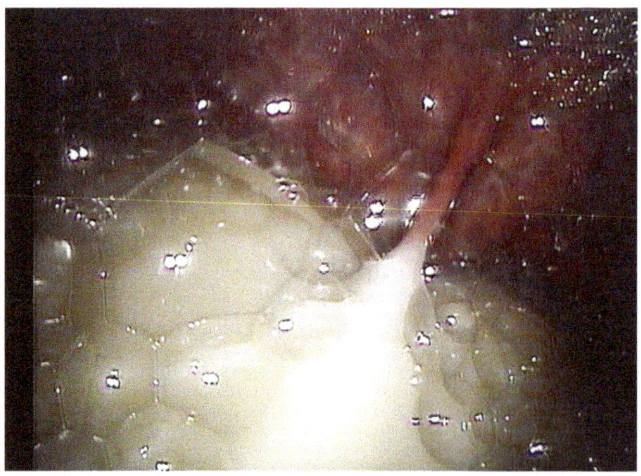

Figure 10.4 Discharge through the external os of the cervix in a mare with a pyometra.

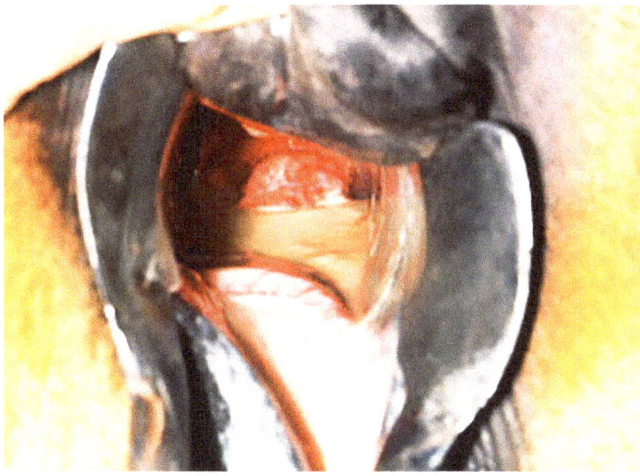

Figure 10.5 Urine in the cranial vaginal vault.

- There should not be any fluid accumulation on the floor of the vagina (Figure 10.5).
- No defects should be noted in the vagina or cervix such as adhesions, tissue disruption, or masses (Figure 10.6)

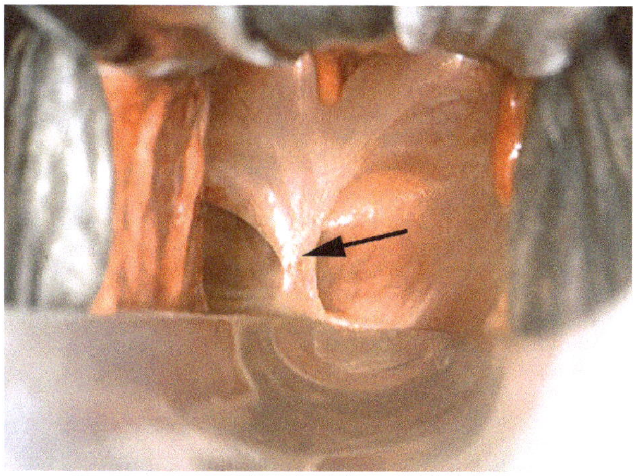

Figure 10.6 Adhesions covering the cervix of a mare secondary to a dystocia.

- The speculum should be examined upon removal for any abnormal discharges present on its surface.

Further Reading

Dascanio JJ. 2011. External reproductive anatomy. In: McKinnon AO, Squires EL, Vaala WE, Varner DD (eds). *Equine Reproduction,* 2nd edn. Ames, IA: Wiley Blackwell, pp. 1577–81.

Pascoe RR. 1979. Observations on the length and angle of declination of the vulva and its relation to fertility in the mare. *J Reprod Fertil Suppl* 27: 299–305.

11

Digital Examination of the Vagina/Cervix

Sofie Sitters

Amsterdam, The Netherlands

Introduction

Digital examination of the vagina and cervix is indicated when performing a breeding soundness examination on a mare and typically will be performed in conjunction with a speculum examination of the vagina and cervix. Unfortunately, digital examination of the cervix is often overlooked, rushed, or incompletely performed, although cervical abnormalities are a known cause of chronic infertility. A visualization of the cervix and external cervical os alone is insufficient to diagnose all cervical abnormalities. Digital palpation of the vagina and cervix will provide detailed information on subtle changes within the vaginal vault and will permit a more complete assessment of abnormalities of the external cervical os and the cervical lumen.

Thorough evaluation of the cervix is indicated in determining if a mare will make a suitable embryo transfer recipient. In these cases a digital examination of the cervix is important to establish if transcervical transfer of an embryo will be possible and if the cervix will functional normally to help maintain the ensuing pregnancy.

Digital examination of the vagina and cervix may also be indicated in postpartum mares in order to diagnose vaginal or cervical trauma. Cervical lacerations may occur during dystocia or during an apparently uneventful delivery. Pathology that may be detected with a manual examination includes lacerations, scar tissue formation, adhesions, fistula formation, cervical incompetence, tissue trauma, subcutaneous masses, and retained fetal membranes.

Palpation and ultrasonography of the reproductive tract per rectum is recommended prior to digital examination of the vagina and cervix to confirm that the mare is not pregnant. Performing vaginal examination in pregnant mares should be avoided as it may disrupt the natural mucosal seal and an iatrogenic ascending infection is a potential risk. In addition, manipulation of the cervix should be avoided in the late term pregnant mare due to the possibility of stimulating prostaglandin release and subsequent triggering of uterine contractions.

Equipment and Supplies

Tail wrap, tail rope, non-irritant soap, roll cotton, stainless steel bucket, disposable liner for bucket, paper towels, examination gloves, obstetrical sleeve, sterile water-soluble lubricant, surgery gloves.

Stage of Cycle

The goal of the exam dictates whether digital palpation of the vagina and cervix should be performed during estrus or diestrus. A digital examination of the vagina and cervix during estrus is indicated in the assessment of fertility in older maiden mares since failure of cervical relaxation is one factor attributed to reduced fertility. If reproductive failure due to a cervical laceration and/or adhesion is suspected, the examination is best conducted during diestrus when the cervix is normally closed under the influence of progesterone. A digital examination during diestrus allows assessment of the ability of the cervix to close and protect the uterus and a possible pregnancy from the external environment.

In the event of dystocia or other difficult birth, the examination is performed immediately after foaling to evaluate the cervix and vaginal vault for trauma.

Technique

- Remove feces from the mare's rectum.
- Place a tail wrap and tail rope on the mare (see Chapter 4).

Equine Reproductive Procedures, Second Edition. Edited by John Dascanio and Patrick McCue.

- Wearing examination gloves, clean and dry the perineum of the mare (see Chapter 3). Wear a clean obstetrical sleeve (turn inside-out) or a sterile obstetrical sleeve and apply sterile lubricant on the knuckles. A (sterile) surgeon's glove may be applied over the sleeve to aid in a more detailed palpation. The fingers of the obstetrical sleeve may be cut off with scissors before applying the surgeon's glove.
- Apply lubricant from the knuckles onto the vulva.
- Pass the fingers through the vulvar labia vertically and enter the vagina with a rotating movement, spreading lubricant on the inside of the vulva and preventing inward pulling of the vulvar lips and ventral aspect of the anal sphincter into the vagina. Avoid rubbing the hand or arm on the clitoris as this area harbors many bacteria.
- The vestibular vault will be entered first and has a ventro-dorsal slope. About wrist deep, the transverse vestibulo-vaginal fold will be passed and some resistance may be encountered in normal mares whilst doing so. This fold is a remnant of the hymen, which partitioned the vestibule from the vagina proper. It may extend for a variable distance up the lateral walls, and occasionally a persistent hymen is present.
- The external urethral orifice is located on the ventral midline under the transverse fold. Care should be taken not to dilate the opening with a finger or confuse it as being a continuation of the vagina or as being the external cervical os.
- The entire vaginal wall can be palpated using a flat hand in a systematic manner. Any abnormalities in the vaginal mucosa and vaginal musculature should be noted.
- Advance the hand cranially to the end of the vagina and locate the cervix and external cervical os. Insert the index finger into the cervical lumen and advance cranially evaluating tone, internal diameter, and direction of the cervical canal entering the uterus.
- Pull the index finger back to the level of the external cervical os and hold the opposing thumb on the outside of the cervical wall opposite the index finger. Exert slight compression between the two fingers on the cervical tissue in between them. Either rotate the two fingers together 360 degrees or rotate 180 degrees and then insert the thumb into the lumen, palpating the other half of the cervix between the thumb and opposing index finger on the outside of the cervix. Evaluate the complete vaginal/cervix area systematically to detect intravaginal and intracervical trans-luminal abnormalities.

Interpretation and Additional Comments

- In estrus, the vaginal and cervical surfaces will be moist and edematous. The cervix will be softened and dropped toward the vaginal floor. In diestrus, the cervical and vaginal surfaces will be dry and the external cervical os will project into the cranial vagina from high on the wall and is tightly contracted.
- The vestibulo-vaginal junction should be closed. However, if the examiner's hand slips easily into the anterior vagina, the mare may be predisposed to pneumovagina (see Chapter 5).
- The vaginal wall should be smooth and supple and lined by smooth vaginal mucosa. Vaginal trauma from a previous foaling or, less frequently, breeding accidents, might have caused vaginal scarring and adhesions, presenting as irregularities in the vaginal lining. Formation of scar tissue within the vaginal canal can be very extensive following dystocia and may nearly obliterate the vaginal canal, making vaginal penetration impossible in extreme cases. Scar tissue will feel firmer and non-confluent with the surrounding vaginal mucosa.
- Lacerations and tears of the vaginal wall may be present, caused by dystocia. In the case of small lesions, these may be felt more easily than seen. Fingers may slide into a blind pouch in the vagina where a fistula may be present from a foaling injury. These may occur with a direct communication to the rectum, into the retroperitoneal space or into the peritoneal cavity. Fistulas are more likely to enter the peritoneal cavity with a lesion of the cranial vagina or cervix and may result in peritonitis. Masses within the wall of the vagina may be hematomas related to trauma, abscessation, or tumor formation (e.g., leiomyoma).
- In maiden mares the hymen area should be palpated to ensure the absence of tissue bands formed by hymen remnants since these bands may contribute to a recto-vaginal perforation at parturition. However, these bands typically have no effect on fertility. Depending on the thickness and toughness of the hymen, it can be broken down easily with firm, steady pressure and digital dilation (see Chapter 6).
- Scars, adhesions, and lacerations may also involve the cervix. Cervical lacerations may involve the external os only or the entire length of the cervix. As long as the cervix has the ability to open and close normally, small tears

in the os are usually of minor importance. However, large lacerations involving the external os or the entire cervix are more significant and may require surgery to repair, restoring the cervical barrier to infection.

- Upon removal of the gloved hand from the vagina, the hand should be observed for abnormal discharges (purulent, bloody, etc.) or odors (infectious, necrotic, urine, etc.).

Further Reading

Carleton CL. 2006. Clinical examination of the nonpregnant equine female reproductive tract. In: Youngquist RS, Threlfall WR (eds). Current Therapy in Large Animal Theriogenology, 2nd edn. St Louis, MI: Saunders Elsevier, pp. 74–90.

Ginther OJ. 1992. Reproductive anatomy. In: Ginther OJ (ed.). Reproductive Biology of the Mare: Basic and Applied Aspects, 2nd edn. Cross Plains, WI: Equiservices, pp. 1–40.

Montilla HJ. 2012. Hymen, persistent. In: Wilson DA (ed.). Clinical Veterinary Advisor: the Horse. St Louis, MI: Saunders Elsevier, p. 278.

Pycock JF. 1993. Cervical function and uterine fluid accumulation in mares. *Eq Vet J* 25: 191.

Zent WW, Steiner JV. 2011. Vaginal examination. In: McKinnon AO, Squires EL, Vaala WE, Varner DD (eds). Equine Reproduction, 2nd edn. Ames, IA: Wiley Blackwell, pp. 1900–3.

12

Uterine Culture Collection: Swab/Brush

John J. Dascanio

School of Veterinary Medicine, Texas Tech University, USA

Introduction

Culture of the uterus is performed as part of the routine mare breeding soundness examination. It is also performed as part of an infertility workup, or upon request by a stallion owner prior to breeding, or as surveillance for disease. Culture may be performed via a standard uterine culture swab, from secretions obtained from a uterine brush, from a uterine biopsy, or from fluid obtained from a low volume uterine lavage.

The method for performing a uterine culture depends on a number of factors, such as cost, time to perform the procedure, and availability of equipment. Generally, a guarded or double-guarded swab or brush is routinely used to obtain a sample for culture, while a low volume uterine lavage would be indicated for an infertility workup in a problem mare or in a mare that is suspected of an infection, but has had a negative uterine swab/brush. With persistent or chronic infections, culture of a uterine biopsy may be warranted.

The best time to perform a uterine culture may be debatable, but is most often performed in early estrus. Cultures may be performed in diestrus, but prostaglandins should be administered after the collection procedure to lyse any luteal tissue and bring the mare into estrus, so that any contaminants introduced during the procedure may be eliminated.

Culture swabs should be immediately plated onto blood agar or other appropriate microbial culture media. If a culture swab is transported to a laboratory, it should be held at refrigerator temperature to prevent overgrowth of contaminants.

Equipment and Supplies

Tail wrap, tail rope, non-irritant soap, roll cotton, stainless steel bucket, disposable liner for bucket, paper towels, sterile lubricant, sterile obstetrical sleeve, guarded culture device (Kalayjian swab, single-guarded (Figure 12.1); McCullough swab, double-guarded (Figure 12.2); or uterine brush, guarded (Figure 12.3)), aerobic bacterial transport device.

Technique

- Remove feces from the rectum.
- Place a tail wrap and tie the tail out of the way (see Chapter 4).
- Clean and dry the perineum of the mare (see Chapter 3).
- Place a sterile obstetrical sleeve on the arm.
- Place the guarded culture device into the palm of the hand.
- Place sterile lubricant on the knuckles and down the length of the sleeve being careful not to get lubricant onto the palm. If the culture device becomes inundated with lubricant, it may be more difficult to obtain a diagnostic sample.
- Rub lubricant from the knuckles onto the vulva, straighten the fingers and insert through the vulva.
- Using a slight rotating motion, pass the hand into the vagina so that the mid-forearm is to about the level of the vulva. This should enable palpation of the external cervical os.

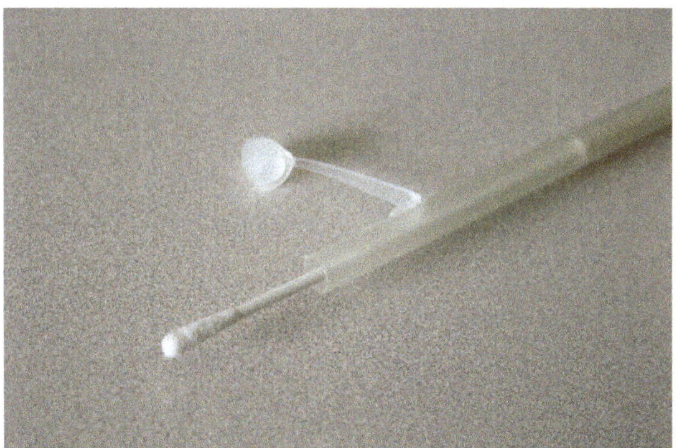

Figure 12.1 Kalayjian swab in the open position.

Equine Reproductive Procedures, Second Edition. Edited by John Dascanio and Patrick McCue.

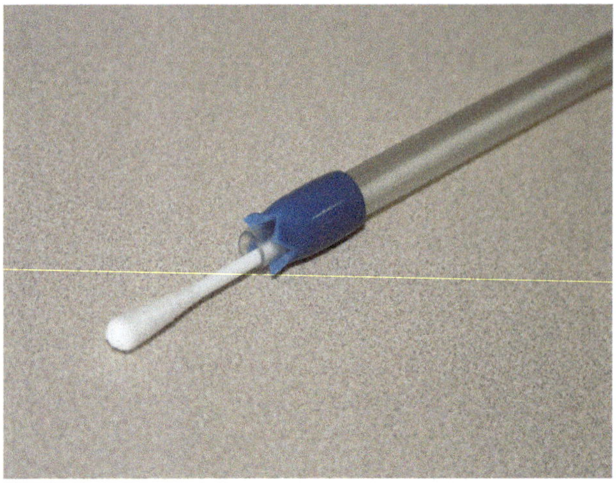

Figure 12.2 McCullough swab in the open position.

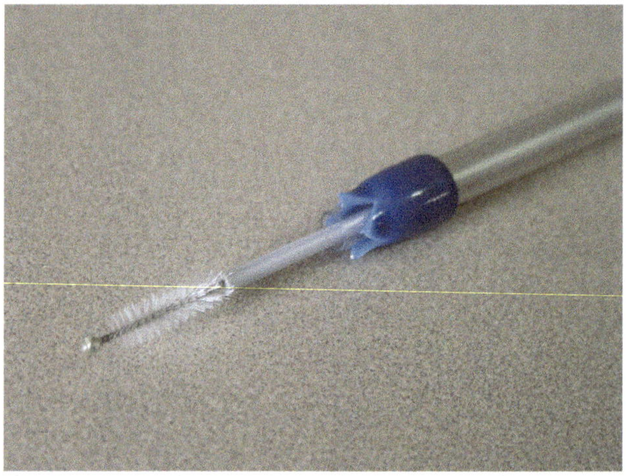

Figure 12.3 Uterine brush in the open position.

- Gently insert the index finger into the external cervical os. Sometimes the os may be off center, located slightly downward, or to the left or right of center.
- Pass the index finger through the cervix to the last knuckle (metacarpo-phalangeal joint). Usually one can detect when the fingertip enters the uterine body lumen. Pass the uterine culture instrument past the inserted index finger into the uterine body. Sometimes, if the cervical canal is under the influence of progesterone and is toned, the index finger may need to be removed prior to passing the culture device. The culture instrument may need to be pointed in a slightly downward direction when being passed through the cervix due to the dependent nature of the suspended uterus within the abdomen, especially in older broodmares.
- As most culture devices used today have a guard over the inserted end, the inner swab/brush is subsequently pushed forward through the cap/guard.
- Gently press the swab or brush in contact with the endometrium and gently rotate in one direction. It is recommended that the swab/brush be in contact with the endometrium for 10–15 seconds.
- The swab/brush is retracted back inside the outer guards and then the device is removed from the mare. Care should be taken when rotating the swab as excessive motion can result in breaking of the end of the swab (Figure 12.4).
- Once the culture instrument has been withdrawn from the external cervical os, a cupped hand should be placed over the device to limit vaginal contamination to the swab/brush.
- The swab should be immediately plated or transferred to a transport device with media such as a CultureSwab™ (Figure 12.5). Often the outer swab guard is removed from the inner guard before extending the swab/brush into a transport device to limit contamination from the outer guard.

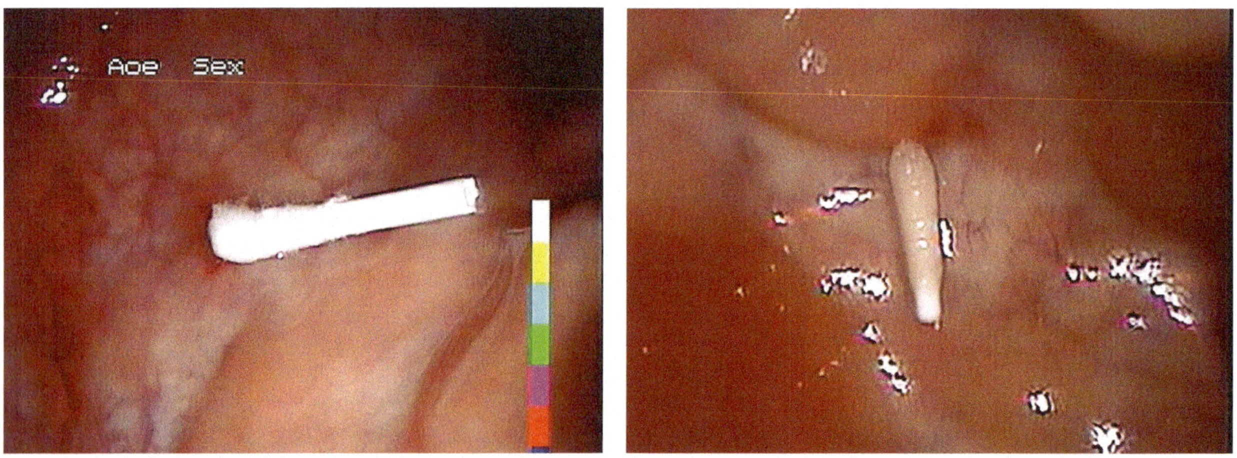

Figure 12.4 Tip of a uterine culture instrument broken off in the uterine lumen.

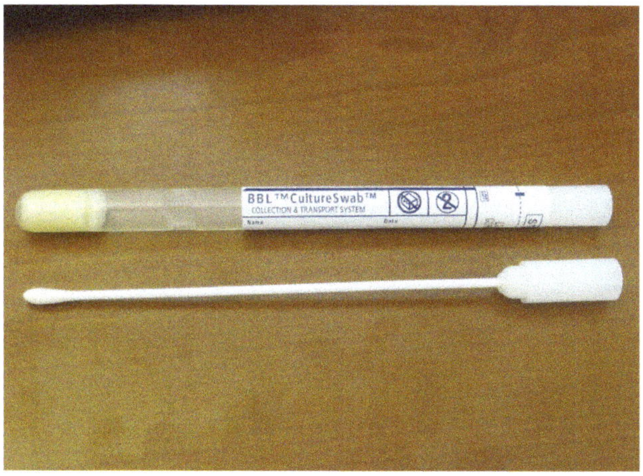

Figure 12.5 Transport device for uterine cultures.

Interpretation

- In mares with a dependent uterus, well over the brim of the pelvis, the swab may be subjected to the downward weight of the uterus, making breakage of the tip of the swab more likely. Breakage of the swab tip may occur particularly when the swab is rotated, thus caution should be used.
- Note any discharge present on the sterile sleeve when the gloved arm is pulled from the vagina. There should not be any purulent or hemorrhagic discharge, only the lubricant and clear mucous should be present.
- Ensure that the culture device is intact and that no part of the instrument was left within the mare's uterus/cervix/vagina.
- Note any discharge on the tip of the culture device. It is not uncommon to see some mild hemorrhage on the culture device as it rubbed against the endometrium.
- The most common pathogens of the equine uterus are *Streptococcus equi* subspecies *zooepidemicus, Escherichia coli, Klebsiella* species, *Pseudomonas aeruginosa,* and fungi, among others.
- Heavy growth of one organism may have more significance than light growth of multiple organisms.
- Uterine culture results should be correlated with uterine cytology and other reproductive findings to determine significance.

Further Reading

Hinrichs K, Cummings MR, Sertich, PL, Kenney RM. 1988. Clinical significance of aerobic bacterial flora of the uterus, vagina, vestibule, and clitoral fossa of clinically normal mares. *J Am Vet Med Assoc* 193(1): 72–5.

LeBlanc MM. 2010. Advances in the diagnosis and treatment of chronic infections and post-mating induced endometritis in the mare. *Reprod Dom Anim* 45(suppl. 2): 21–7.

Nielsen JM. 2005. Endometritis in the mare: a diagnostic study comparing cultures from swab and biopsy. *Theriogenology* 64(3): 510–18.

13

Antimicrobiotic Sensitivity Testing

Jillian Bishop[1] *and Patrick M. McCue*[2]

[1] *University of Kansas Health System, USA*
[2] *Equine Reproduction Laboratory, Colorado State University, USA*

Introduction

A Kirby–Bauer disk diffusion susceptibility test (agar disk diffusion test) is used to evaluate the effectiveness of specific antibiotics against aerobic bacterial organisms under *in vitro* culture conditions. A known quantity of bacteria are distributed evenly on the surface of the agar plate and a series of paper disks, each impregnated with one antibiotic, are placed on the surface of the agar plate. The zone of growth inhibition around each test disk is a measure of the sensitivity of the organism to the given antibiotic.

Equipment and Supplies

Mueller Hinton (MH) II agar plate: MH-II agar plates with 5% sheep blood for Gram-positive β-hemolytic organisms, MH-II agar plates without sheep blood for Gram-negative organisms; sterile swab; antibiotic disk dispenser; antibiotic sensitivity disks: ampicillin 10 μg, amikacin 10 μg, ceftiofur 30 μg, enrofloxacin 5 μg, gentamicin 10 μg, penicillin G 10 units, trimethoprim/sulfamethoxazole 23.75/1.25 μg, ticarcillin 75 μg with clavulanic acid; incubator; measuring device.

Technique

- Allow a Mueller Hinton (MH) II agar plate to equilibrate to room temperature. Label the plastic dish bottom (agar side) with the mare's name, source of sample, and date.
- If the bacterium of interest is Gram-positive and β-hemolytic, use a MH-II agar plate with 5% sheep's blood in order to visualize the colorless colonies and zones of inhibition (e.g., *Streptococcus equi* subspecies *zooepidemicus*).
- Option 1 for inoculating the MH-II agar plate:
  - Use a single cotton swab to pick up one to three isolated identical colonies from the original culture plate.
  - Streak the MH-II agar plate in a painting fashion until the entire plate has been swabbed with the bacteria (Figure 13.1). An example would be:
    - streak three parallel lines down the center of the plate
    - streak the entire plate going perpendicular to the primary three lines; try to cover the entire plate
    - rotate the plate 90 degrees and streak the entire plate again; try to cover the entire plate
    - rotate the plate 90 degrees and streak the entire plate one last time, ensuring a confluent coverage of the entire plate.
- Option 2 for inoculating the MH-II agar plate:
  - Prepare a bacterial suspension in saline, tryptic soy broth, or MH broth that contains between 1×10^8 and 2×10^8 CFU/ml of the bacteria in question.
    - Pick three to five isolated colonies from the primary plate.
    - Transfer the colonies into the media.
    - Adjust the turbidity to a 0.5 McFarland Standard.
    - Inoculate the plate with the bacterial suspension.
- For both options, use the following procedure. Place the antibiotic disk dispenser over the plate and depress the plunger to dispense the disks and gently tamp the antibiotic disks onto the agar surface.

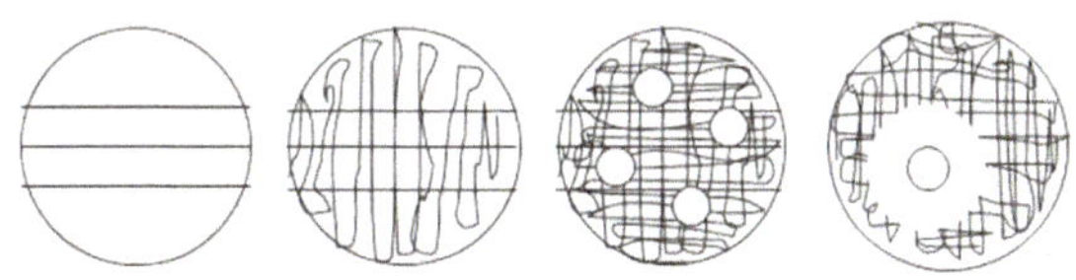

Figure 13.1 Pattern of bacterial streaking on a Mueller Hinton II agar plate and placement of antimicrobial disks.

Equine Reproductive Procedures, Second Edition. Edited by John Dascanio and Patrick McCue.

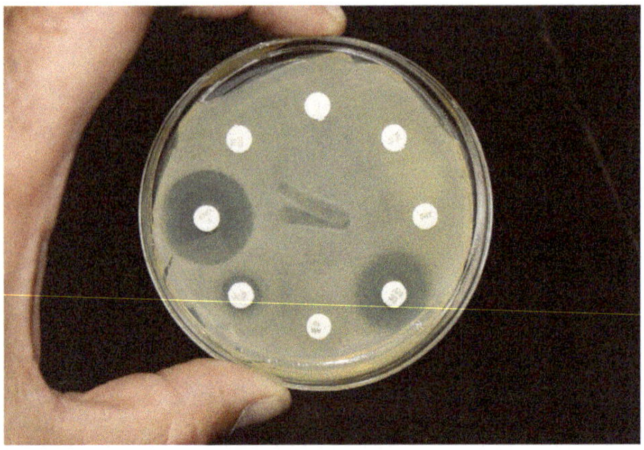

Figure 13.2 Antimicrobial susceptibility test. This bacterial organism was sensitive to two antibiotics, intermediate to one, and resistant to the other five antibiotics.

- Place the plate in an incubator, agar side up, for 24 hours at 37°C (99°F).
- After the incubation period, use a clear ruler to measure the diameter of the zone of inhibition around each disk (Figure 13.2). Measure on the bottom side of the plate viewing through the plate. If adjacent areas of inhibition overlap, measure the radius and multiple by 2.
- Record the results in millimeters. Always round up to the next millimeter.
- Compare the results with the standard zone of inhibition for each antibiotic provided by the manufacturer and report the result as resistant, intermediate, or susceptible. The zone of inhibition of bacterial growth is different for each antibiotic due to the differences in migration of the different-sized antibiotic molecules through the agar, the solubility of the antibiotic, and the diffusion properties.

Further Reading

Quinn PJ, Markey BK, Leonard FC, Hartigan P, Fanning S, FitzPatrick ES. 2011. Antibacterial agents. In: Veterinary Microbiology and Microbial Disease, 2nd edn. Chichester: Wiley Blackwell, pp. 143–8.

Ricketts SW. 2011. Uterine and clitoral cultures. In: McKinnon AO, Squires EL, Vaala WE, Varner DD (eds). Equine Reproduction, 2nd edn. Ames, IA: Wiley Blackwell, pp. 1963–78.

Songer J, Post K. 2005. Antimicrobial susceptibility testing and principles of antimicrobial therapy. In: Veterinary Microbiology Bacterial and Fungal Agents of Animal Disease. Amsterdam: Elsevier, pp. 21–31.

14

Microbiology: Microbial Culture

Patrick M. McCue[1] and Jillian Bishop[2]

[1]*Equine Reproduction Laboratory, Colorado State University, USA*
[2]*University of Kansas Health System, USA*

Introduction

A clinical microbiology laboratory can be set up at most veterinary practices to detect and identify common microbial pathogens encountered in equine reproduction. Microbial testing allows for early diagnosis of infectious endometritis and consequently the development and implementation of a therapeutic plan.

Equipment and Supplies

Incubator, refrigerator, biohazard waste container, biohazard bags, sterile cotton tip swabs/applicators, disposable inoculating loops, Vircon® disinfectant, quad plates (with tryptic soy agar (TSA) with 5% sheep blood, MacConkey II/TSA with 5% sheep blood, Gram-positive chromogenic agar, and Gram-negative chromogenic agar; Vetlab Supply, Inc., Palmetto Bay, FL, USA).

Technique

- The sample collected from the mare can be applied to either a single plate (i.e., tryptic soy agar (TSA) with 5% sheep blood), two individual plates (i.e., one with TSA with 5% sheep blood and the second with MacConkey II agar), or a "split plate" which has one half with TSA with 5% sheep blood and the other half with MacConkey II agar. MacConkey II agar is specific for Gram-negative bacteria (Table 14.1).
- In addition, the swab may be applied to a chromogenic agar. Bacterial or fungal colonies that grow on chromogenic agar will turn a specific color, dependent on the organism.
- Another option is to apply the sample onto an agar that is designed to promote growth of fungal organisms and inhibit development of bacterial organisms, such as Sabouraud agar. Incubation time varies widely for fungal organisms, and ranges from 2 days for some yeast organisms to 2–4 weeks for dimorphic fungi.

Table 14.1 Agar used in the culture of microbial organisms.

Agar type	Characteristics
Tryptic soy agar (TSA)	TSA is an all-purpose medium that supports the growth of bacteria that do not have a specific nutritional need. The addition of 5% sheep red blood cells to the agar allows for a visual differentiation of some bacterial organisms due to various types of hemolysis: • α-hemolysis: partial hemolysis, often appears as a zone of green, gray, or brown discoloration around the colony • β-hemolysis: clear, colorless zone caused by complete hemolysis of the red blood cells • γ-hemolysis: no detectable hemolysis
MacConkey II agar	MacConkey agar utilizes bile salts and crystal violet to inhibit the growth of most Gram-positive bacteria and most Gram-negative cocci, thus selecting for Gram-negative bacilli (i.e., rods). This agar can also be used as a visual differentiation medium based on the bacteria's ability or inability to ferment lactose. Organisms that ferment lactose produce acid that turns the acid indicator in the agar (phenol red) a reddish or pink color. Strong lactose fermenters will produce red colonies surrounded by a pink ring of precipitated bile salts. Non-lactose fermenters will produce colorless or transparent colonies. It is important for these plates to be checked by 24 hours as continued incubation will result in altered results as the bacteria use up the available lactose, resulting in misrepresented color characteristics

(Continued)

Equine Reproductive Procedures, Second Edition. Edited by John Dascanio and Patrick McCue.

Table 14.1 (Continued)

Agar type	Characteristics
Chromogenic agar	Chromogenic agar is an all-purpose medium. It is used for the presumptive identification of bacterial organisms based on the production of a color compound in the bacteria. Additional chromogenic media are available for use in fungal cultures. This type of media contains chromogens, or substrates, that release a particular colored compound when degraded by specific microbial enzymes. It is important to have a description of colors produced for a given company's chromogenic media as they may vary in the chromogens used in production of the media. Also, the color results should be interpreted within 24 hours as the colors may alter with continued incubation
Sabouraud agar	Sabouraud agar is a non-selective medium used for the cultivation of fungal organisms. The acidic pH and addition of chloramphenicol inhibits bacterial growth. The Emmons modification to the original formula has a higher pH and a reduced dextrose level to help in a greater recovery of fungi. It is advisable to utilize the added chloramphenicol if using the Sabouraud dextrose Emmons agar. Incubation time varies widely for fungal organisms, anywhere from 2 days for some yeast up to 2–4 weeks for dimorphic fungus. This difference is incubation time, along with colony morphology, can help in the presumptive identification of the organism
Mueller Hinton agar	Mueller Hinton agar is a non-selective medium used for antibiotic susceptibility testing using paper disks impregnated with a specific concentration of an antibiotic. This medium is low in sulfonamide, trimethoprim, and tetracycline inhibitors. It also provides satisfactory growth of most non-fastidious pathogens and demonstrates batch-to-batch reproducibility for standardized testing. The addition of 5% sheep red blood cells aids in the visualization of β-hemolytic bacterial growth

- Remove a quad plate of TSA with 5% sheep blood, MacConkey II agar, and Gram-positive and Gram-negative chromogenic agar from the refrigerator and allow it to equilibrate to room temperature. Label the bottom side of the agar plate with the mare's name, source of sample, and date.
- Streak all four quadrants with the sample swab on the inside of each corner of the plate (primary streak) (see Figure 14.1 as an example).
- With a new sterile swab, streak through the primary streak one or more times and continue to streak the second third of the plate (secondary streak).

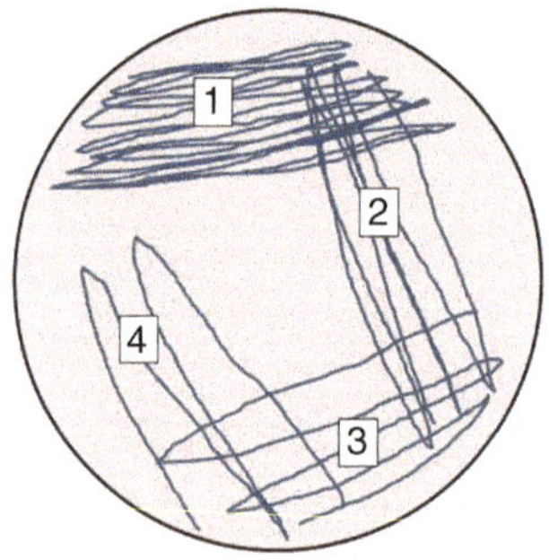

Inoculation of a streak plate

1. Initial inoculation - first streaks from culture swab typically yield heavy growth (if organisms are present)
2. A secondary streak through area 1 will yield lighter growth
3. A subsequent streak through area 2 will yield weaker microbial growth
4. The final streak through area 3 will yield growth of individual single colonies

Figure 14.1 Inoculation of a streak plate for cultivation of microbial organisms. This example shows how to streak one entire plate; a slight modification is required to streak each quadrant of a quad plate.

- With a new sterile swab, streak through the secondary streak one or more times and continue to streak the final third of the plate (tertiary streak). The concept is to separate the colonies so that individual colonies can be identified.
- Perform the same streaking pattern on the other quadrants.

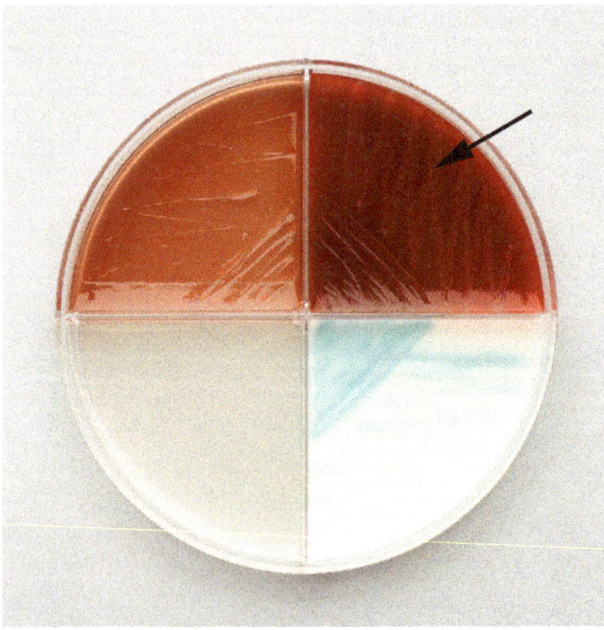

Figure 14.2 Culture of *Streptococcus equi* subspecies *zooepidemicus* on a quad plate with TSA with 5% sheep blood (upper right), MacConkey II agar (upper left), Gram-positive chromogenic agar (lower right), and Gram-negative chromogenic agar (lower left). Note the growth of small white colonies with β-hemolysis (black arrow) on blood agar, the lack of growth on MacConkey agar, and the small light blue colonies on the Gram-positive chromogenic agar.

- If additional agars are to be used, inoculate in the same manner as previously described.
- Incubate the plate(s), bottom side up in a 37°C (99°F) incubator for 20–24 hours.
- After incubation, observe the quad plate for the appearance of any colony growth and determine if more than one type of colony is present. Identify hemolytic activity of colonies developing on TSA agar. Determine if contaminants are present (e.g., where are the colonies located on the plate, are they actually touching a streak line, are there more than one type of colony?) (Figures 14.2–14.5; Table 14.2).
- Observe any additional inoculated agars for presumptive identification or growth of a fungal/yeast organism (i.e., Sabouraud agar).
- Characterize the amount of growth as either no growth, very light growth, light growth, moderate growth, or heavy growth.
- Plates with mixed growth should be subcultured and individual organisms subsequently identified.
- Plates should be cultured for a minimum of 72 hours before being discarded.

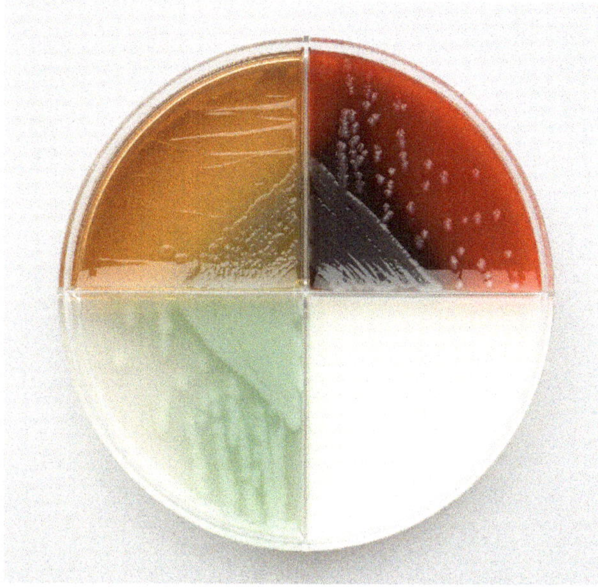

Figure 14.4 Culture of *Pseudomonas aeruginosa* on a quad plate with TSA with 5% sheep blood (upper right), MacConkey II agar (upper left), Gram-positive chromogenic agar (lower right), and Gram-negative chromogenic agar (lower left). Note the growth of flat metallic green-blue colonies on blood agar, the large pale greenish colonies on MacConkey agar, and the growth of transparent white to green colonies on Gram-negative chromogenic agar.

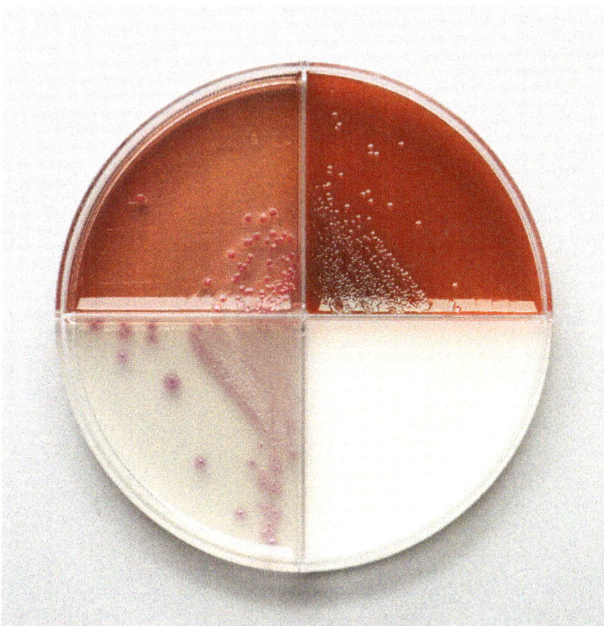

Figure 14.3 Culture of *Escherichia coli* on a quad plate with TSA with 5% sheep blood (upper right), MacConkey II agar (upper left), Gram-positive chromogenic agar (lower right), and Gram-negative chromogenic agar (lower left). Note the growth of cream-colored colonies without hemolysis on blood agar, the medium-sized pink colonies on MacConkey agar, and the pink to red colonies on Gram-negative chromogenic agar.

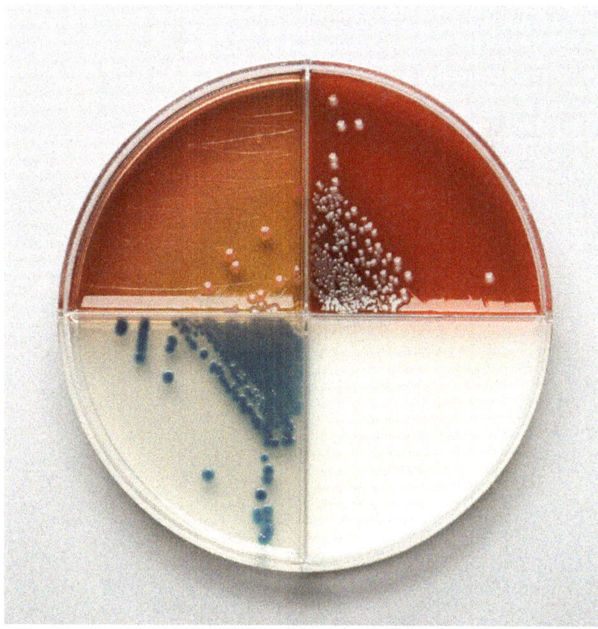

Figure 14.5 Culture of *Klebsiella pneumoniae* on a quad plate with TSA with 5% sheep blood (upper right), MacConkey II agar (upper left), Gram-positive chromogenic agar (lower right), and Gram-negative chromogenic agar (lower left). Note the growth of large gray mucoid colonies without hemolysis on blood agar, the large pink mucoid colonies on MacConkey agar, and the growth of large blue colonies with a slight pink halo on Gram-negative chromogenic agar.

Table 14.2 Culture characteristics for common microbial organisms associated with infectious equine endometritis.

Organism	Gram Stain	Morphology	TSA/5% Sheep Blood Agar	MacConkey Agar	Chromogenic Agar	Comments
Streptococcus equi subsp. *zooepidemicus*	Pos.	Cocci (ovoid, chains)	Small, white, round colonies (β-hemolysis) (0.5–1.0 mm)	No growth	Small, light blue colonies	
Escherichia coli	Neg.	Rods	Cream-colored colonies (α-hemolysis) (2–3 mm)	Medium sized, gray to pink colonies	Medium, pink to red colonies	
Klebsiella pneumoniae	Neg.	Rods	Large, gray, mucoid colonies (non-hemolytic) (2–4 mm)	Large, pink, mucoid colonies	Large, blue with slight pink halo colonies	
Pseudomonas aeruginosa	Neg.	Rods	Flat metallic blue colonies (β-hemolysis) (3–4 mm)	Large, pale greenish colonies	Transparent white to green colonies	Grape-like odor on blood agar; fluorescence with Wood's UV light
Staphylococcus aureus	Pos.	Cocci (round, clusters)	Medium, cream to gold colonies (± β-hemolysis) (2–3 mm)	No growth or limited growth of pink colonies	White to light yellow colonies	
Candida albicans			Soft, creamy, raised, glistening colonies			Beer-like odor; confirm with fungal agar (i.e., Sabouraud agar) for up to 7 days

Further Reading

Hartman DL, S Bliss. 2011. Laboratory methods for isolation and evaluation of bacteria, fungi and yeasts. In: McKinnon AO, Squires EL, Vaala WE, Varner DD (eds). Equine Reproduction, 2nd edn. Ames, IA: Wiley Blackwell, pp. 2674–81.

McKinnon AO, DP Beehan. 2011. Use of chromogenic agar to diagnose reproductive pathogens. In: McKinnon AO, Squires EL, Vaala WE, Varner DD (eds). Equine Reproduction, 2nd edn. Ames, IA: Wiley Blackwell, pp. 1979–87.

15

Microbiology: Gram Stain

Jillian Bishop[1] *and Patrick M. McCue*[2]

[1] *University of Kansas Health System, USA*
[2] *Equine Reproduction Laboratory, Colorado State University, USA*

Introduction

Gram staining is one of the initial steps used in the identification of bacterial organisms. The technique takes advantage of the chemical differences between bacterial cell walls, thereby making this a differential stain. Gram-positive bacteria stain a purple color due to the thick peptidoglycan layer and teichoic acids in the cell wall. This allows the bacteria to retain the primary stain once combined with the mordant, Gram iodine. The iodine reacts with the crystal violet that has already entered the cell, forming a large chemical complex that is not easily washed out of the cell.

Gram-negative bacteria stain a pink/red color since the cell wall contains a thinner peptidoglycan layer and an outer membrane of lipopolysaccharides. These characteristics of Gram-negative bacteria do not allow the cell to retain the crystal violet/Gram iodine complex after excess stain and mordant are rinsed off with water and the slide is decolorized using an isopropyl alcohol and acetone mixture. The alcohol dissolves parts of the lipid component of the outer membrane of the cell wall, creating "holes" in the cell membrane. Also, the much thinner and less complex peptidoglycan layer in the cell wall allows for the cell wall to be "leaky," thus allowing the stain complex to be rinsed out of the cell. A secondary stain, safranin, is added to the smear to allow for visualization of the otherwise colorless Gram-negative bacteria.

The most common Gram-positive bacteria cultured from the equine uterus are *Streptococcus equi* subspecies *zooepidemicus* and *Staphylococcus aureus*. The most common Gram-negative bacteria are *Escherichia coli*, *Pseudomonas aeruginosa*, and *Klebsiella pneumoniae*.

Equipment and Supplies

Glass slides (frosted), Gram stain kit with stabilized iodine, pencil, laboratory flame burner, deionized water in a squirt bottle, microscope, immersion oil.

Technique

- Label a glass slide with the mare's ID using a pencil.
- Use an inoculating loop to add 1 drop of deionized water to the slide.
- Use a sterile inoculating loop to pick up an isolated colony from the tryptic soy agar (TSA) side of the split plate and mix with the water on the slide. Use the loop to smear the mixture across the slide.
- Air-dry the slide completely.
- Heat-fix the slide by passing through a flame several times.
- Cover the dried and heat-fixed slide with crystal violet solution. Leave the stain on for 1 minute.
- Gently wash off the stain with a squirt bottle of deionized water. Be careful to spray the water around the smear, not directly on the smear, or the smear may rinse off.
- Cover the smear with Gram iodine solution. Leave the stain on for 1 minute.
- Gently wash off the iodine with the deionized water.
- Decolorize the slide using the Gram stain decolorizer. Hold the slide at an angle over the staining pan/bottle. Slowly dispense a few drops of decolorizer above the smear so that the decolorizer runs down over the smear. Blot the decolorizer that accumulates in the lower

Equine Reproductive Procedures, Second Edition. Edited by John Dascanio and Patrick McCue.

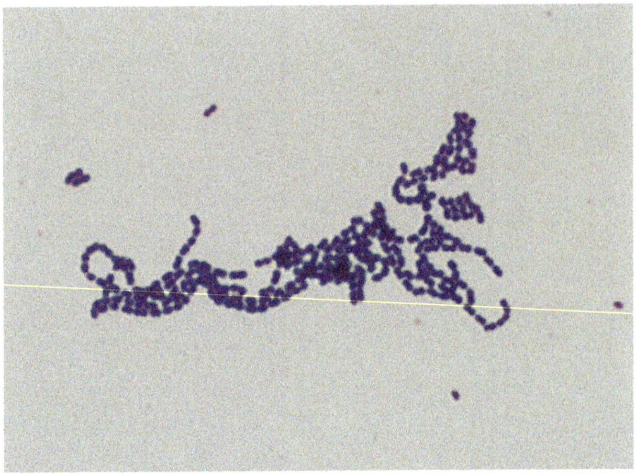

Figure 15.1 Gram-positive cocci in chains (*Streptococcus equi* subspecies *zooepidemicus*).

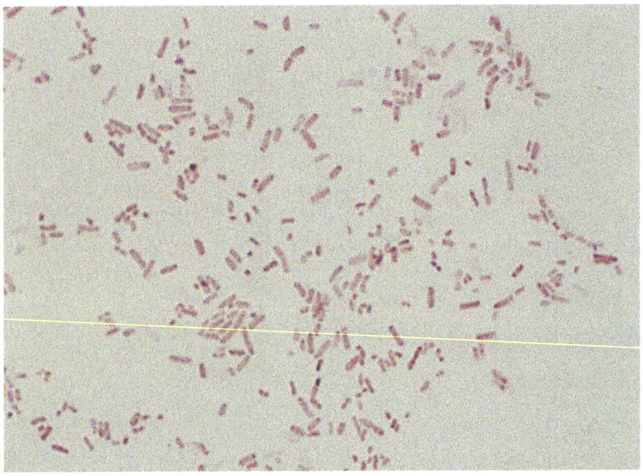

Figure 15.2 *Gram-negative rods* (Escherichia coli).

corner of the slide on a paper towel. The blotted decolorizer will be purple/blue in color at first. Apply more decolorizer, as above, just until the blotted decolorizer is colorless.

- Gently wash off the decolorizer with deionized water.
- Shake off any excess water, then cover the smear with the safranin solution. Leave the stain on for 1 minute.
- Gently wash off the safranin stain with deionized water.
- Gently blot the slides dry, using bibulous paper.
- Examine the stained smear with a compound microscope under oil immersion using the 100× objective.

Interpretation

Organisms staining dark blue or purple are Gram-positive (Figure 15.1). Organisms staining pink to red are Gram-negative (Figure 15.2).

Further Reading

Reddy CA, Beveridge TJ, Breznak JA. 2007. Methods for General and Molecular Microbiology, 3rd edn. Washington, DC: ASM Press.

Songer J, Post K. 2005. General principles of diagnosis. In: Veterinary Microbiology Bacterial and Fungal Agents of Animal Disease. Amsterdam: Elsevier, pp. 10–20.

16

qPCR Assay for the Diagnosis of Infectious Endometritis

Ryan A. Ferris[1] *and Patrick M. McCue*[2]

[1]*Summit, Equine, USA*
[2]*Equine Reproduction Laboratory, Colorado State University, USA*

Introduction

Infectious endometritis is a significant cause of reproductive inefficiency in mares. Bacterial endometritis is most commonly caused by *Streptococcus equi* subspecies *zooepidemicus*, *Escherichia coli*, *Pseudomonas aeruginosa*, and *Klebsiella pneumoniae*, whereas the most common pathogens of uterine fungal infections are *Candida* species, *Aspergillus* species, and *Mucor* species. Diagnosis of bacterial or fungal endometritis is traditionally based on a combination of reproductive history, clinical signs, physical examination, and results of ultrasound, uterine culture, cytology, and biopsy evaluations.

Unfortunately, standard uterine culture techniques do not always detect bacterial or fungal organisms that are present in a mare with infectious endometritis. Problems include presence of slow growing or fastidious bacterial organisms and the difficulty in culturing anaerobic bacterial organisms. In addition, some fungal organisms are notoriously difficult to grow in culture.

Polymerase chain reaction (PCR) can be used to detect minute quantities of the nucleotide sequence of deoxyribonucleic acid (DNA). DNA contains highly conserved regions that have been maintained throughout phylogenic development (i.e., common throughout the taxonomic kingdom level) and variant regions, which can be used for the identification of genus and species.

Real-time quantitative PCR (qPCR) assays work through primer probes specific for the conserved region of the 16S or 28S ribosomal DNA (rDNA) sequences for the detection of bacterial or fungal organisms, respectively. qPCR amplifies the target sequence of the rDNA, which is monitored in real time by measurement of increased fluorescence as the amplification process occurs. This allows for a semi-quantitative analysis as a high level of fluorescence early in the replication process indicates a greater number of original DNA targets. The final result of the qPCR reaction is millions of copies of an amplicon (i.e., the 16S or 28S rDNA regions that the primers targeted). This initial step allows for the determination of whether bacterial or fungal DNA is present or absent.

A second step involves DNA sequencing of the amplicon, which determines the order of nucleotides (G, A, T, and C) in a segment of DNA. Determination of the nucleotide sequence allows for the identification of the genus and species of bacterial or fungal organisms, as each organism has a genetically different DNA sequence.

Equipment and Supplies

Double-guarded culture swab or a low volume lavage to collect a uterine sample, sterile container (e.g. 15 ml conical tube or sterile glass tube), diagnostic laboratory.

Sample Collection Technique

- *Option 1.* Collect a swab sample of the endometrium and uterine lumen using traditional techniques (see Chapter 12). The swab tip is placed inside a sterile 15 ml centrifuge tube and submitted for qPCR analysis. The sample should be kept refrigerated or shipped on ice during transport to the laboratory to help maintain DNA integrity. Freezing or excessive heat should be avoided.
- *Option 2.* Collect a low volume uterine lavage sample using traditional techniques (see Chapter 18). Aliquot approximately equal volumes of the recovered effluent fluid into four separate 15 ml centrifuge tubes. The tubes are centrifuged at 600× g for 10 minutes. The supernatant

Equine Reproductive Procedures, Second Edition. Edited by John Dascanio and Patrick McCue.

is discarded and the residual pellets remaining at the bottom of the centrifuge tube are submitted for qPCR analysis, traditional microbial culture, and cytologic analysis. The pellet in the last centrifuge tube can be held for later analysis as needed.

qPCR and DNA Sequencing: The Basics

- This is a brief explanation of the qPCR process, each laboratory that performs qPCR will have slight modifications designed to optimize laboratory efficiency that are beyond the scope of this chapter.
- The ultimate goal of qPCR is to produce a large quantity of a specific genetic sequence that is approximately 100–150 nucleotide bases in length. The nucleotide sequence can then be "decoded" and evaluated against the nucleotide sequence of known microorganisms.
- The first step is to extract the DNA from the bacterial or fungal cells. The cells are first lysed to separate the DNA from other cellular material. The DNA is isolated by centrifugation or binding to magnetic beads. The quality and quantity of DNA recovered in the extraction process is imperative to the success of the qPCR assay. DNA extraction that has a low efficiency results in zero or very limited quantities of DNA available for detection by the qPCR assay, leading to the possibility of a false-negative diagnosis. Commercial kits are available that have been developed to maximize the DNA yield from a wide variety of samples.
- The DNA is placed into a special PCR tube.
- Primers consisting of short sequences of DNA, 15–30 nucleotides in length, designed to bind to the genetic sequence of interest, are added to the tube. Primers can be designed to detect all known organisms in a kingdom (i.e., the bacterial kingdom or the fungal kingdom). This may be advantageous as it allows detection of all known bacterial or fungal pathogens. However, it requires further diagnostic techniques to identify the specific organism.
- Alternatively, primers can be designed that are very specific and will detect a specific genus and species or even a specific gene. The advantage is that no further diagnostics are required. However, other potential pathogens could be missed if their DNA is not detected by a specific PCR assay.
- Forward and reverse primers are utilized to detect a small region of DNA. The DNA sequence between the two primers is subsequently replicated. In the case of equine endometritis, the goal is to detect either the 16S rDNA segment of bacteria or the 28S rDNA segment of fungal organisms.
  - Eubacterial primers previously used for the detection of bacterial DNA in equine uterine samples are:
- forward: 5′-TCCTACGGGAGGCAGCAGT-3′
- reverse: 5′-GGACTACCAGGGTATCTAATCCTGTT-3′.
  - Panfungal primers previously used for detection of fungal DNA in equine uterine samples are:
- forward: 5′-GCATAT-CAATAAGCGGAGGAAAAG-3
- reverse: 5′-TTAGCTTTAGATGRARTTTACCACC-3′.
- Nucleotides (A, C, G, T) are added to the PCR tube.
- DNA polymerase is added to the tube. The purpose of the DNA polymerase is to read the code of the extracted DNA and attach matching nucleotides. Commercial kits containing DNA polymerase and nucleotides are available to maximize the efficiency of the replication process.
- The PCR tube containing the DNA of interest, PCR primers, DNA polymerase, nucleotides, and SYBR green (fluorescent dye) are placed into a thermal cycler or transferred into a 96-well plate with other samples and loaded into a thermal cycler that will heat and cool the tube at specific times while monitoring the amplification of DNA within the tube.
- The initial step within the thermal cycler is to heat the tube to approximately 95°C, which will separate the DNA double helix into single-stranded DNA.
- The tube is then cooled down to approximately 50°C (122°F), which will allow the primers to lock or anneal onto their target sequence, if it is present in the PCR tube after extraction.
- Subsequently, the tube is heated to approximately 72°C (162°F) for one to several minutes, which will activate the DNA polymerase to synthesize a copy of the DNA strand template. DNA polymerase binds to the primers and only adds nucleotides in a 5′ to 3′ progression. The length of time for this step is directly dependent on the length of the gene of interest, for example it will take longer to replicate 450 base pairs of DNA than 100 base pairs. As the DNA polymerase is replicating the area of interest, a fluorescent signal is released that can be detected by the thermocycler. A stronger signal indicates that there are more copies of DNA being replicated at that specific qPCR replication cycle (Ct cycle). The fluorescent signaling provides a quantitative estimate of the amount of DNA in the sample.
- The process is then repeated over multiple cycles and an amplification curve is generated (Figure 16.1). It is estimated that 40 cycles will produce over 1 billion copies of the targeted DNA sequence from one original DNA sequence. As noted above, copies will only be produced

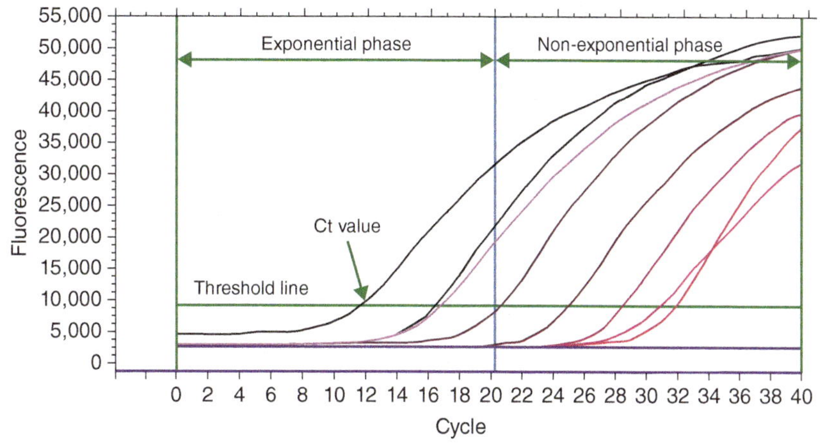

Figure 16.1 Example of an amplification curve detecting fungal DNA in a clinical sample. The *y* axis is the relative amount of fluorescence detected and the *x* axis is the number of replication cycles (Ct). There is one clinical sample (third line from the left) and seven control samples being evaluated in this particular amplification curve. The samples are going through an exponential phase of DNA replication and a corresponding amount of fluorescent signal is produced. The cycle in which the fluorescent signal surpasses the threshold is considered the Ct value in which the sample was positive. The exponential phase continues for 4–6 replication cycles before entering a plateau or non-exponential phase. The clinical sample had a Ct value of 17 which is near the control sample at Ct cycle 16 corresponding to approximately 1,000 CFU of *Candida albicans*. The amplicon was analyzed for genus and species identification and the organism was determined to be *Candida krusei*.

if the targeted DNA sequence was originally present in the initial tube after extraction. The entire time period for amplification is approximately 1–2 hours.

- The number of qPCR cycles or Ct cycles required to produce approximately 1 billion copies of the targeted DNA sequence can be used to estimate the relative concentration of microbial DNA in the original sample, providing for a semiquantitative evaluation.
- All qPCR assays should have controls with known colony-forming unit (CFU) standards to help control for day to day variation in extraction and replication of DNA. Additional controls of DNA-free water should be run in tandem with the unknown sample to determine if contamination has occurred during the extraction or amplification process. DNA-free water may exhibit evidence of contamination after approximately 35–37 Ct cycles. This key control is important to prevent a false-positive report to the clinician that submitted the sample.
- The end product of the qPCR replication process is called an amplicon.
- The amplicon consists of millions of copies of a DNA sequence. The DNA sequence of the amplicon can be submitted for DNA sequencing and compared against known published DNA sequences of microbial organisms using the web-based BLAST (Basic Local Alignment Search Tool) sequence-similarity tool.
- A genetic match of DNA sequences between the DNA replicated by qPCR and a published DNA sequence identifies the genus and species of the microbial organism recovered from the uterine sample.

Interpretation of qPCR Data

The number of threshold cycles (Ct cyles) required to replicate the original microbial DNA in the extracted sample (the template DNA) above the threshold level of detection (Figure 16.1) can be used to provide an approximation of the original DNA load. This can be used to provide an approximation of the number of microbial organisms in the original sample and the degree or severity of the infection (Table 16.1). Interpretation can be confounded by many factors including extraction efficiency, qPCR

Table 16.1 Interpretation of qPCR results relative to degree of infection in equine uterine samples based on studies performed at Colorado State University.

Number of Ct Cycles	Degree of Infection	Comments
≥35	None evident	Negative sample. If microbial DNA is detected, it is most likely due to contamination. Results need to be compared to negative controls
30–34	Mild	Low amount of bacterial DNA. Interpretation should include results of other diagnostic tests
20–30	Moderate	Presence of microbial DNA at a level consistent with infection
<20	Severe	A large amount of microbial DNA detected

sensitivity, contamination during sample collection, handling, storage, and processing, type of microbial organism, mare health status, and other factors.

The lower limit of detection of the bacterial organism *Streptococcus equi* subspecies *zooepidemicus* in equine uterine fluid has been reported to be 429×10^{-12} g, which is approximately 40 organisms worth of DNA. The lower limit of detection of DNA for the fungal organism *Candida albicans* has been reported to be 2×10^{-14} g. Since *C. albicans* contains approximately 37 fg of DNA, the qPCR assay theoretically has a detection limit of two yeast organisms.

Additional Comments

The advantages of qPCR assays to veterinary practitioners include rapid analysis of a sample (i.e., 2 hours) and the potential ability to detect the presence of microbial DNA in cases of infectious endometritis where traditional culture was unsuccessful. In our experience, the time interval from sample submission to identification of a positive or negative result for pathogen DNA is about 6 hours, with sequencing and final reporting of the causative agent approximately 24–48 hours later. Early detection of an infection will allow practitioners to make informed clinical decisions regarding antimicrobial therapy days before traditional culture results would be available. An added advantage of qPCR is that the assay offers the possibility of monitoring bacterial or fungal DNA levels during antimicrobial therapy. A reduction or absence of microbial DNA, as determined by qPCR, during therapy would indicate progress toward resolution.

A current limiting factor for qPCR analysis of equine samples is availability of the technology. Currently qPCR analysis is only available in selected diagnostic laboratories. However, it is anticipated that simple point-of-care (POC) molecular diagnostic qPCR systems that are currently available in human medicine will be incorporated into veterinary clinics in the near future.

Currently, qPCR assays typically cost around US $95 in most veterinary diagnostic laboratories, with results available in a few days. Microbial culture of fungal organisms and identification typically costs approximately $55, with results available in several days to weeks. One limitation of molecular assays is the inability to determine antimicrobial susceptibility patterns. Clinicians using qPCR to detect microbial organisms, such as fungal organisms, may use anecdotal experience to develop an appropriate treatment plan. As the mechanisms of resistance are better understood in fungal organisms, molecular techniques may be utilized to determine the potential for an organism to have inherent resistance to certain antifungal agents. We anticipate that in the future we should be able to detect, identify, and determine antifungal susceptibility patterns based on an organism's DNA signature.

Uterine samples collected for qPCR should be collected and handled with minimal contamination. Samples that are "sterile" may not have microbial growth, but the DNA of microbial pathogens may still be present. DNA contamination is one cause of a false-positive diagnosis when using a molecular-based assay. Steam autoclaving will reduce the amount of microbial DNA present on equipment. Glass blood tubes without anticoagulant and new 15 or 50 ml centrifugation tubes appear to have minimal microbial DNA.

The equine uterus has historically been noted to be a "privileged site" that should be free of all microbial organisms and therefore no microbial DNA should be present in uterine samples from "normal mares." However, recent studies have suggested that the equine uterus may contain a normal flora of non-pathogenic microorganisms.

Deep-seated infections and/or organisms in a biofilm may be present in an arrested state with a low replication rate, which may make detection difficult using traditional microbial culture. However, these quiescent organisms still contain DNA and may yield a positive qPCR result.

Detection of microbial DNA by qPCR and failure to detect organisms by traditional culture may be due to: (i) the ability of qPCR to amplify the DNA of non-viable organisms and free fungal DNA; (ii) the failure to provide the appropriate growth conditions for fungal organisms (agar, temperature, etc.); or (iii) the organism having an extremely low replication rate in which growth may take weeks to months.

Clinicians should use caution in interpreting the results of qPCR assays as they are often extremely sensitive and may detect DNA from dead organisms and may not match the clinical picture of a case. Negative controls may exhibit microbial DNA detection (i.e., contamination with dead bacterial DNA) by 35 or more Ct cycles. A "positive" signal from a clinical sample beginning at 35 Ct cycles or more should be considered to be the result of contamination. A sample is considered to contain organisms that are biologically relevant if microbial DNA is detected in the first 30 Ct cycles. Adequate controls of known organisms at set CFUs should be utilized to confirm that the qPCR assay is functioning normally and to estimate the organism load in a clinical sample.

Further Reading

Byrne BA. 2007. Laboratory diagnosis of bacterial infections. In: Sellon DC, Long MT (eds). Equine Infectious Diseases. St Louis, MI: Saunders Elsevier, pp. 236–44.

Ferris RA, Dern K, Veir JK, Hawley JR, Lappin MR, McCue PM. 2013. Development of a broad-range quantitative polymerase chain reaction assay to detect and identify fungal DNA in equine endometrial samples. *Am J Vet Res* 74: 161–5.

Ferris RA, Veir JK, Lappin MR, McCue PM. 2010. Development and clinical application of a broad range 16S quantitative PCR assay for detection of bacteria in the uterus of the mare. *Anim Reprod Sci* 121: S98–S100.

17

Uterine Cytology Collection: Swab/Brush

J. Dascanio[1] and Ryan A. Ferris[2]

[1] *School of Veterinary Medicine, Texas Tech University, USA*
[2] *Summit, Equine, USA*

Introduction

A cytologic examination of the uterus should always be performed in conjunction with a uterine culture. Cytologic evaluation of the uterus involves the collection and interpretation of cells lining the uterus (endometrium) and within the uterine lumen. Endometrial cytology is a rapid, inexpensive technique to detect the presence of endometritis in the mare.

There are circumstances whereby a uterine cytology may be normal (no inflammatory cells) and an infection is still present. These include isolated infections, deep-seated infections, or infections early in their course. It is also more common to have a negative cytology (i.e., no inflammatory cells) in the presence of an *Escherichia coli* infection than in the presence of a *Streptococcus equi* subspecies *zooepidemicus* infection.

Typically a guarded swab or a brush is used to obtain a uterine cytology sample; collection of a uterine sample with unguarded swabs may result in significant contamination from the vestibule, vagina, and cervix. A low volume uterine lavage may be more diagnostic than swab or brush samples in situations where isolated infections are present (see Chapter 18).

Equipment and Supplies

Tail wrap, tail rope, non-irritant soap, roll cotton, stainless steel bucket, disposable liner for bucket, paper towels, sterile lubricant, sterile sleeve, guarded culture device (Kalayjian swab, single-guarded; McCullough swab, double-guarded or uterine brush), microscope slides, modified Wright's stain (Diff-Quik® or equivalent), microscope.

Technique

- Remove feces from the rectum.
- Place a tail wrap and tie the tail out of the way (see Chapter 4).
- Clean and dry the perineum of the mare (see Chapter 3).
- Place a sterile sleeve on the arm.
- Place the guarded culture device into the palm of the hand.
- Place sterile lubricant on the knuckles and down the length of the sleeve being careful not to get lubricant onto the palm. If the culture device becomes inundated with lubricant, it may be more difficult to obtain a diagnostic sample.
- Rub lubricant from the knuckles onto the vulva, straighten the fingers and insert through the vulva, staying dorsal so as to not rub across the clitoris.
- Using a slight rotating motion, pass the hand into the vagina so that the mid-forearm is to about the level of the vulva. This should enable palpation of the external cervical os.
- Gently insert the index finger into the external cervical os. Sometimes the os may be off-center, located slightly downward, or to the left or right of center.
- Pass the index finger through the cervix to the last knuckle (metacarpo-phalangeal joint). Usually one can tell when the tip of the finger exits the internal cervical os and enters the uterine body lumen.
- Insert the uterine swab/brush instrument along the inserted index finger through the cervix and into the uterine lumen. Sometimes, if the cervical canal is under the influence of progesterone and is toned, the index finger may need to be removed prior to passing the culture device. Typically, the instrument would be pointed in a slightly downward direction when being passed through

Equine Reproductive Procedures, Second Edition. Edited by John Dascanio and Patrick McCue.

the cervix due to the dependent nature of the suspended uterus within the abdomen.

- The inner swab/brush is then advanced forward through the cap/guard.
- Allow the swab/brush to be in contact with the endometrium and uterine secretions for 10–15 seconds and then reverse the procedure to remove the device.
- Gentle rotation of the swab/brush may be indicated to pick up cells, but care should be taken to limit "heavy-handed" movements of the uterine culture swab as this may predispose to breaking of the end of the swab or may be associated with mild hemorrhage and contamination of the swab with blood.
- Once the culture instrument has been withdrawn from the external cervical os, a cupped hand should be placed over the device to limit vaginal cellular contamination to the swab/brush.
- If a single swab was used, the swab should be gently rolled over a sterile microscope slide (and can then still be used for uterine culture). If a sterile slide is not available, then a second swab may be used to obtain a uterine culture.
- If a single brush is used, a swab of the brush may be made for culture and then the brush rolled gently over a microscope slide. If the material discharged is thick, a second slide is placed over the first and gently pulled apart to create a smear.
- It is also common practice to collect two samples from a mare; first a swab for microbial culture and then a brush sample for endometrial cytology.
- Two slides are prepared from every sample in the event that one is broken prior to evaluation or if more than one stain is to be used.
- Microscope slides should be air-dried and may be fixed to preserve cellular architecture. The slides may then be stained with a modified Wright's stain such as Diff-Quik®.
- Additional stains that may be considered are a Gram stain or a fungus-specific stain such as Grocott methenamine silver (GMS) stain.

Interpretation

- A cytology brush may yield significantly more cells than a swab for interpretation.
- Distortion of cells may occur when a swab is rolled across a slide or during the collection of cells. This is more common if the swab is smeared instead of rolled across the slide.
- Note any discharge present on the sterile sleeve when the gloved arm is pulled from the vagina. There should not be any purulent or hemorrhagic discharge, only the lubricant and clear mucus should be present.
- Ensure that the culture device is intact and that no part of the instrument was left within the mare's reproductive tract. Breakage of the swab/brush is more likely when the device is placed into a dependent uterus (older broodmare) and rotated, causing undue stress on the device tip.
- Note any discharge on the tip of the culture device. It is not uncommon to see very mild hemorrhage on the culture device as it rubbed against the endometrium.
- Microscopic examination is performed at 400× (10× eye piece and 40× objective) magnification for uterine endometrial cells (individual cells and rafts of cells), white blood cells, debris, red blood cells, bacteria, yeast, fungal organisms, and spermatozoa. Evaluation at 1,000× (10× eye piece and 100× oil immersion objective) may be required to confirm the presence of bacterial and fungal pathogens initially detected at 400×.
- Evaluate slide quality (i.e., the presence of normal uterine epithelial cells as well as the presence and relative number of inflammatory cells (neutrophils, macrophages, lymphocytes, etc.) and any bacteria/fungi). If a low number of cells are present on the slide, the cytology should be repeated to obtain a diagnostic quality slide.
- The greater the ratio of neutrophils: uterine epithelial cells, the greater the degree of inflammation or endometritis.
- Neutrophils are primarily associated with acute inflammation, whereas macrophages, lymphocytes, and plasma cells are more common with chronic inflammation.
- The presence of inflammatory cells does not necessarily indicate infectious endometritis. Inflammatory cells may be present in cases of pneumo-uterus, reflux of urine into the uterus, or after normal procedures such as breeding, uterine lavage, or infusion. The case history and results of other diagnostic procedures should be considered in mares with a positive uterine cytology to differentiate infectious from non-infectious endometritis.
- The absence of inflammatory cells in a sample with an adequate number of normal endometrial cells generally indicates the absence of active inflammation. However, some bacteria, such as *Escherichia coli,* do not stimulate a large inflammatory response, whereas other bacteria, such as *Streptococcus equi* subspecies *zooepidemicus* are associated with a significant inflammatory response.

Uterine Epithelial Cells

Uterine epithelial cells (UECs) can range from cuboidal in anestrus to tall columnar during the estrous cycle. A majority of UECs are not ciliated, but ciliated cells are often observed in cytology preparations (Figure 17.1). A range of

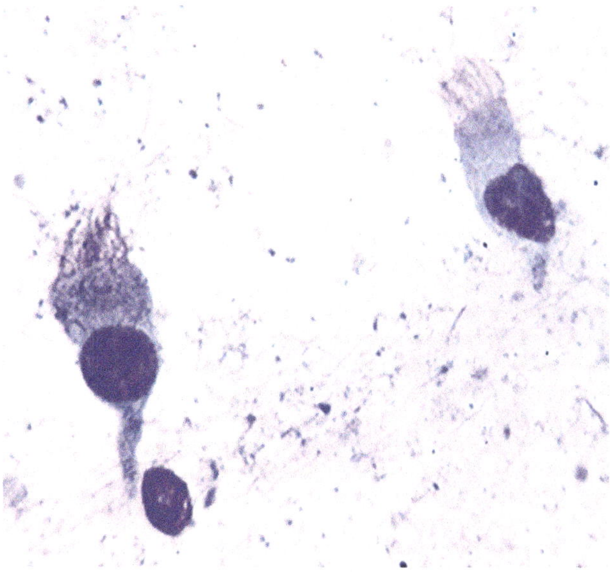

Figure 17.1 Ciliated tall columnar epithelial cells normally found in non-inflammatory uterine cytology.

UECs may be noted, including large rafts of cells, intact individual cells, or disrupted UECs (Figure 17.2). A large number of disrupted or degenerate UECs may indicate improper sample preparation, handling, or storage prior to staining or may be associated with a chronic uterine infection.

Debris

Debris may be classified as none/minimal (<25% of the slide), mild (25–50% of the slide), or moderate/severe (>75% of the slide). The presence of moderate to severe debris has been associated with bacterial endometritis.

White Blood Cells

- Neutrophils are the predominant white blood cells (WBCs) identified on uterine cytology preparations (Figure 17.3). Neutrophils are 10–12 μm in diameter (about twice as large as a red blood cell (RBC)), with a single nucleus that may be indented or divided into 3–5 lobes or segments.
- A cytology sample collected from a normal mare in estrus should have very few or no neutrophils; however, a rare neutrophil may be noted in association with blood contamination that occurred during the collection process. Neutrophils may be present in the uterine lumen following breeding, after uterine lavage or infusion, during the postpartum period, or in cases of endometritis.
- Other WBCs such as macrophages, lymphocytes, or eosinophils are not commonly found on equine uterine cytology preparations.
- Lymphocytes are approximately 7 μm in diameter (the same size as RBCs), are round to oval, and have only a small amount of cytoplasm (Figure 17.4).
- Macrophages are approximately 20 μm in diameter with abundant blue-staining cytoplasm filled with various-sized vacuoles (Figure 17.5). Lymphocytes and macrophages are found in in the postpartum mare and in chronic uterine infections.
- Eosinophils are 12–15 μm in diameter, with blue-staining cytoplasm that contains multiple pink or red granules (Figure 17.6). Eosinophils are found in cases of pneumovagina, fungal infections, or reflux of urine into the uterus.
- The average number of WBCs per high power field (hpf) is determined after evaluating at least 10 hpf in multiple areas of the slide, and is used to categorize the degree of inflammation (Table 17.1).
- Another method used to categorize the inflammatory response is the number of WBCs per UEC. A ratio of 1

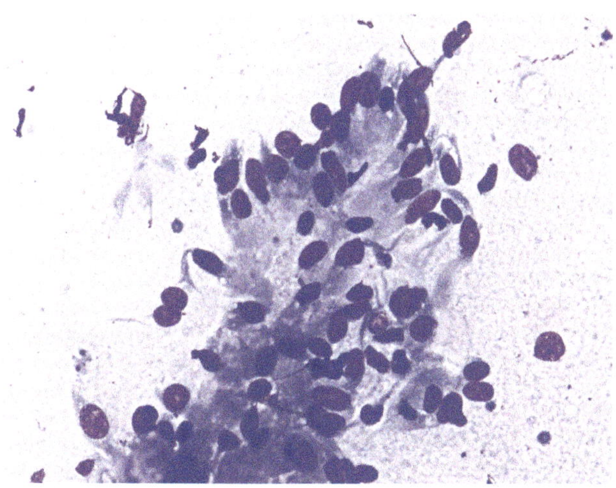

Figure 17.2 A raft of normal endometrial epithelial cells in an equine uterine cytology sample.

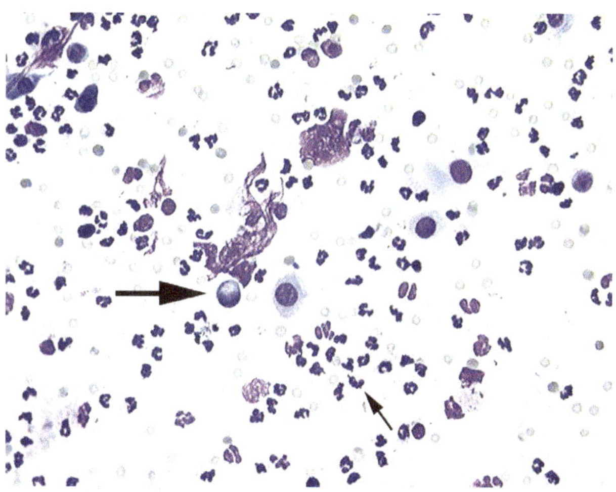

Figure 17.3 Inflammatory uterine cytology with quiescent macrophage (large arrow) and many neutrophils (small arrow).

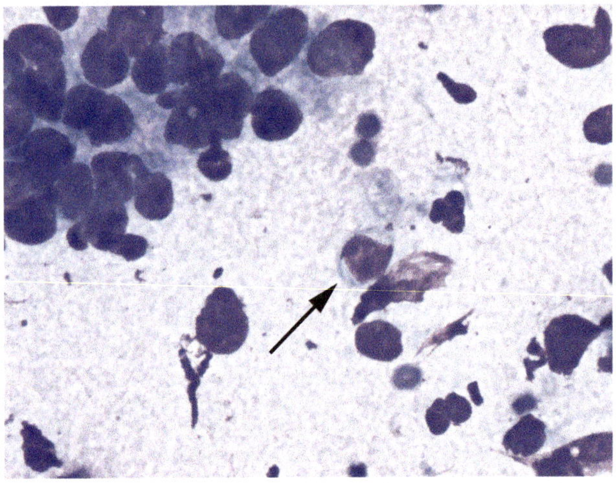

Figure 17.4 A lymphocyte (arrow) in a uterine cytology sample.

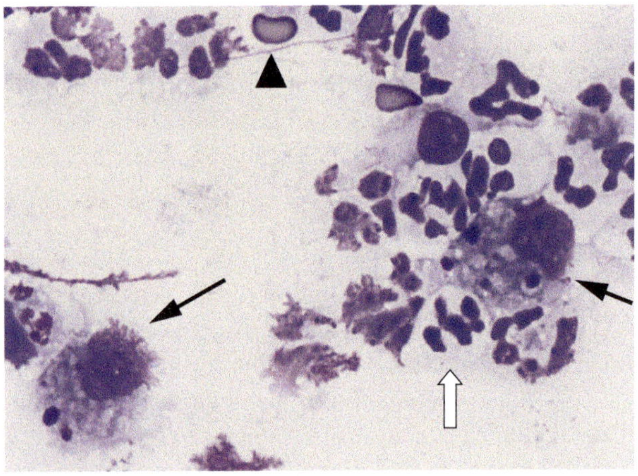

Figure 17.5 A pair of macrophages (solid arrows) in a uterine cytology sample along with neutrophils (open arrow) and red blood cells (arrow head).

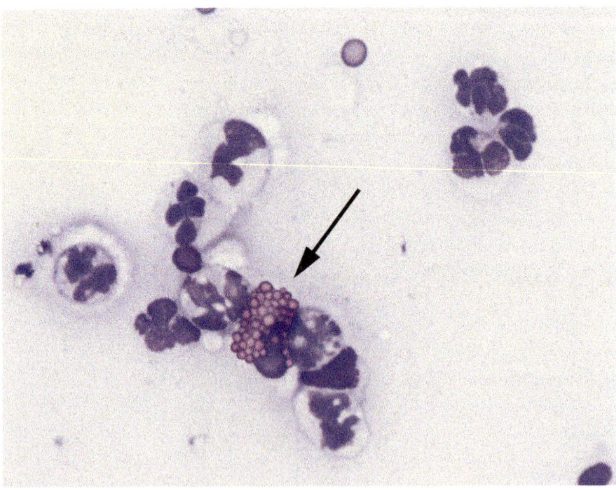

Figure 17.6 An eosinophil (arrow) in a uterine cytology sample along with neutrophils and a red blood cell.

Table 17.1 Description of the number of neutrophils per hpf with corresponding inflammation classification for samples collected from a brush/swab.

Number of Neutrophils per hpf	Classification
0 to rare	**Normal**
1–2	**Mild inflammation**
3–5	**Moderate inflammation**
>5	**Severe inflammation**

WBC to 20–40 epithelial cells has been used as a gauge of the degree of inflammation.

- Categorizing the degree of inflammation represented in a cytologic sample from a low volume lavage can be difficult. Centrifugation of the uterine effluent concentrates UECs, WBCs, microbial organisms, and debris into a pellet. The pellet is subsequently smeared onto a glass slide, stained and evaluated. A normal mare should have very few or no WBCs noted in the cytology from a low volume lavage. Mares with mild uterine inflammation often have >5–10 neutrophils per hpf, whereas mares with more severe inflammation usually have >10 neutrophils per hpf. The presence of microbial organisms should be interpreted with caution, as there is a higher risk potential for contamination during sample collection with a low volume lavage procedure versus the use of a double-guarded uterine swab or brush.

Red Blood Cells

- Red blood cells are 6 μm in diameter with a central pallor. These cells are commonly found in low numbers (i.e., <4/hpf) on routine cytologic evaluation.
- Excessive numbers of RBCs may indicate irritation to the endometrium from infection, infused compounds, or aggressive sampling technique.

Bacteria

- Bacteria can be visualized on a uterine cytology sample but often require 1,000× (10× eye piece and 100× oil immersion objective) magnification to differentiate them from debris. The presence of bacteria engulfed within WBCs can help determine if the bacteria are due to infectious endometritis or contamination.
- The four most common bacterial pathogens of the equine uterus are *Streptococcus equi* subspecies *zooepidemicus, Escherichia coli, Klebsiella pneumoniae,* and *Pseudomonas aeruginosa*.
- *Streptococcus equi* subspecies *zooepidemicus* are Gram-positive cocci approximately 1.0 μm in diameter that form chains of various length (Figure 17.7).

- *Escherichia coli, K. pneumoniae,* and *P. aeruginosa* are Gram-negative rods varying in size from 3 to 6 μm in length and cannot be differentiated accurately based on cytologic evaluation (Figure 17.8).

Fungal Organisms

- Yeast are typically 5–8 μm in size with a very distinct cell wall (100–200 nm) that forms a clear "halo" around the organism; this may be especially evident if the organism is surrounded by debris or other cells (Figure 17.9).
- Hyphate fungi are typically 3–5 μm in width and 8 μm in length. These individual cells are commonly linked together in long branching chains (Figures 17.10 and 17.11). In many instances, detection of a fungal organism on cytologic examination may be the only evidence of fungal endometritis, as organisms do not always grow on culture.

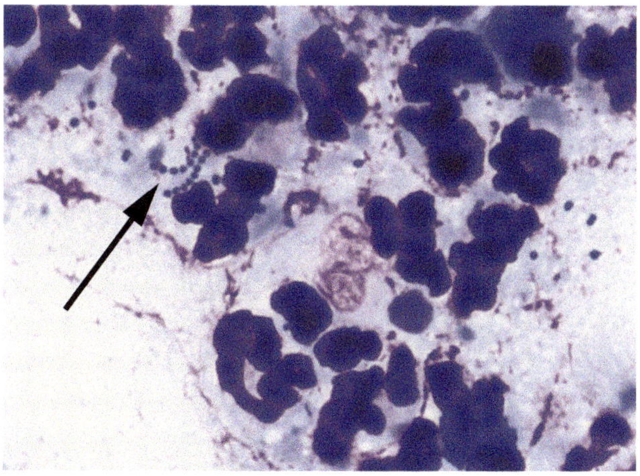

Figure 17.7 Chains of cocci (arrow) in a uterine cytology sample collected from a mare with a *Streptococcus equi* subspecies *zooepidemicus* infection.

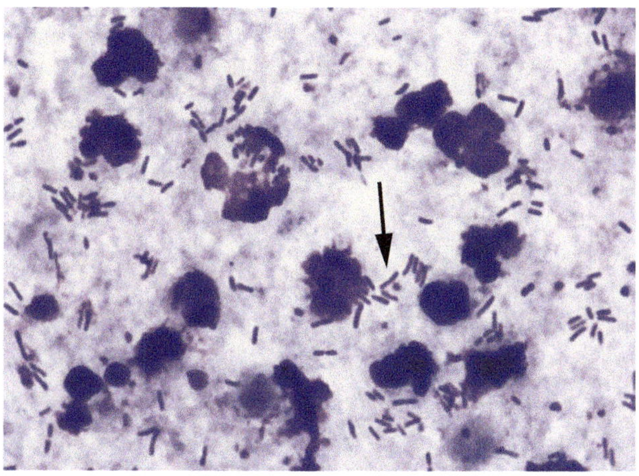

Figure 17.8 Gram-negative rods (arrow) in a uterine cytology sample collected from a mare with endometritis.

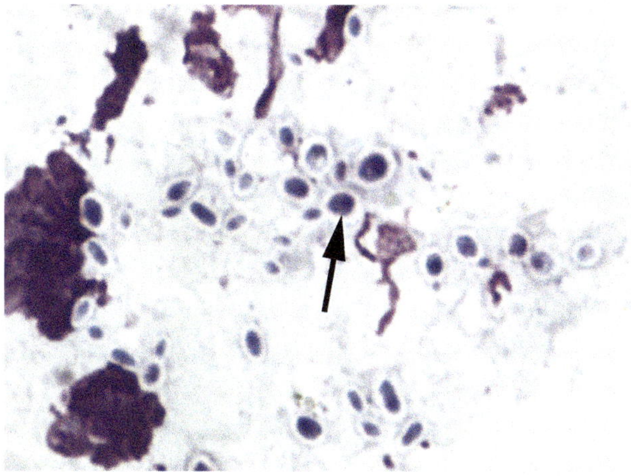

Figure 17.9 Yeast organisms *(Candida albicans)* (arrow) in a uterine cytology sample.

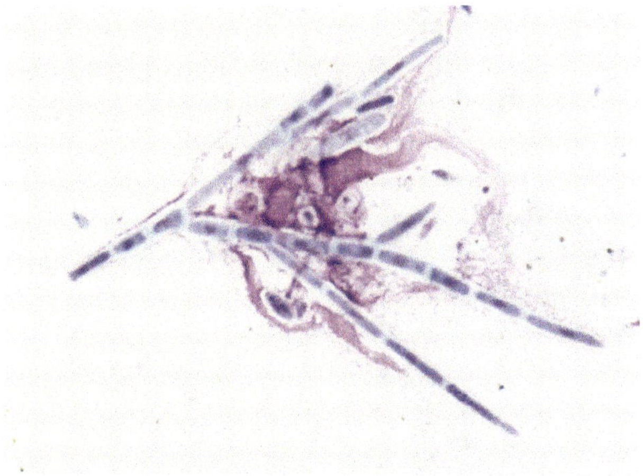

Figure 17.10 *Aspergillus fumigatus* organisms in a mare with fungal endometritis.

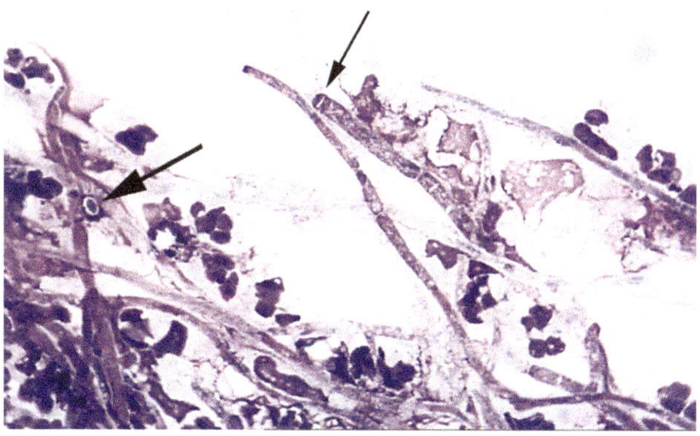

Figure 17.11 Yeast (large arrow) and hyphae (small arrow) with neutrophils in a mare with fungal endometritis.

Further Reading

Bourke M, Mills JN, Barnes AL. 2008. Collection of endometrial cells in the mare. *Aust Vet J* 75: 755–8.

Brook D. 1993. Uterine cytology. In: McKinnon AO, Voss JL (eds). Equine Reproduction. Philadelphia: Lea and Febiger, pp. 246–54.

Couto MS, Hughes JP. 1984. Technique and interpretation of cervical and endometrial cytology in the mare. *J Eq Vet Sci* 4: 265–73.

Dascanio J, Ley WB, Bowen JM. 1997. How to perform and interpret uterine cytology. *Proc Annu Conv Am Assoc Eq Pract* 43:182–6.

Riddle W, Leblanc M, Stromberg A. 2007. Relationships between uterine culture, cytology and pregnancy rates in a Thoroughbred practice. *Theriogenology* 68(3): 395–402.

18

Uterine Culture/Cytology: Low Volume Lavage

John J. Dascanio

School of Veterinary Medicine, Texas Tech University, USA

Introduction

Typically a double-guarded swab or a brush is used to obtain a sample for uterine culture or cytology. However, a low volume uterine lavage may be more diagnostic in situations where localized uterine infections are present or if an infection is suspected and no microbial growth was obtained after collection of a uterine sample with a guarded swab. The goal is to have the lavage fluid distribute throughout the uterine lumen and therefore "sample" the entire uterus instead of one specific region as would occur with a traditional swab. The negative aspects of performing a low volume uterine lavage are the extra time required to perform the procedure, the possibility of contamination since the tubing is not guarded, the need to have sterilized lavage tubing, and the centrifugation step used to concentrate the cellular material in the effluent.

Equipment and Supplies

Tail wrap, tail rope, non-irritant soap, roll cotton, stainless steel bucket, disposable liner for bucket, paper towels, obstetrical sleeve, obstetrical lubricant, examination gloves, sterile lubricant, sterile obstetrical sleeve, sterile 80 cm (30 inch) uterine lavage catheter, sterile single-line tubing, 50 ml centrifuge tubes, 150 or 250 ml sterile 0.9% sodium chloride or phosphate-buffered saline, catheter tipped 60 ml syringe, 60 ml syringe, microscope slides, Diff-Quik® stain, microscope, centrifuge, oxytocin, needles and syringes.

Technique

- Remove feces from the rectum.
- Place a tail wrap and tie the tail out of the way (see Chapter 4).
- Clean and dry the perineum of the mare (see Chapter 3).
- Don a sterile obstetrical sleeve.
- Place the end of an 80 cm uterine lavage catheter with a deflated 75 ml cuff into the palm of the hand.
- A 150–250 ml bag of 0.9% sodium chloride can be attached directly to the catheter and the catheter is filled prior to placement. This prevents air influx into the uterus and allows for better recovery of the lavage fluid. Alternatively, sterile, single-line tubing can be used to connect the bag of saline to the lavage catheter (Figure 18.1).
- Place sterile lubricant on the back of the gloved hand, being careful not to get lubricant onto the palm. If the end of the lavage tubing becomes inundated with lubricant, the lubricant may get into the sample thus interfering with interpretation of the cells.
- Rub lubricant from the knuckles on to the vulva, straighten the fingers and insert through the vulva, being careful to not rub the clitoris as this structure has a significant natural bacterial flora.

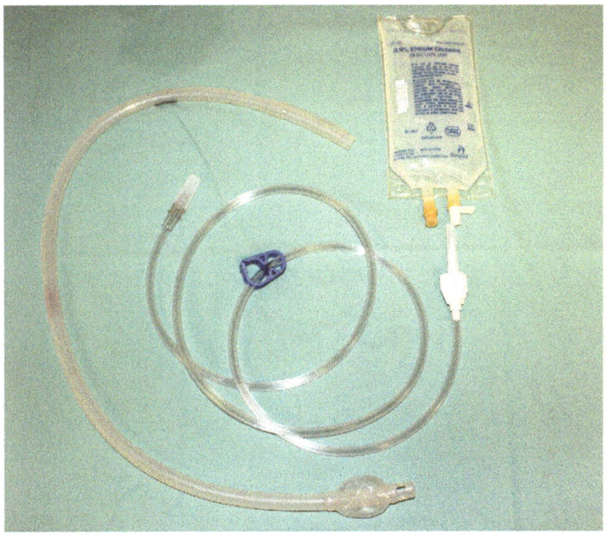

Figure 18.1 Low volume lavage supplies, including a uterine catheter, single-line tubing, and 150 ml bag of sterile saline.

Equine Reproductive Procedures, Second Edition. Edited by John Dascanio and Patrick McCue.

- Using a slight rotating motion, pass the hand into the vagina so that the mid-forearm is to about the level of the vulva. This should enable palpation of the external cervical os.
- Gently insert the index finger into the external cervical os. Sometimes the os may be off-center, located slightly downward, or to the left or right of center.
- Pass the index finger through the cervix to the last knuckle (metacarpo-phalangeal joint). Usually there is a feeling of entering the uterine body lumen when the tip of the finger exits the internal cervical os.
- Pass the uterine lavage catheter past the inserted index finger, past the internal cervical os, and into the caudal uterine body. Sometimes, if the cervical canal is under the influence of progesterone and is toned, the index finger may need to be removed prior to passing the lavage catheter. Typically, the catheter would be pointed in a slightly downward direction when being passed through the cervix due to the dependent nature of the suspended uterus within the abdomen. The cuff on the uterine catheter should be inflated with approximately 75 ml of air to prevent reflux of fluid into the vagina. The cuff should be gently snugged against the internal cervical os.
- The 150–250 ml bag of 0.9% sodium chloride or other sterile fluid is elevated to allow the fluid to flow by gravity into the uterus (Figure 18.2).
- The fluid is allowed to stay in the uterus for approximately 3 minutes to allow for distribution of fluid throughout the lumen.
- In addition, the uterus may be gently massaged per rectum to ensure distribution of the fluid. Care should be taken to not irritate the endometrium with the lavage catheter.
- The empty bag is subsequently lowered to allow a return of fluid via gravity flow (Figure 18.3). Gentle lifting of the uterus per rectum may increase return of fluid. If the fluid does not flow readily through the tubing, gentle aspiration with a catheter tipped 60 ml syringe may be used to initiate flow.
- A single 20 IU dose of oxytocin may be administered intravenously to stimulate uterine contractions and augment return of the uterine fluid.
- Once adequate fluid has been obtained, the clamp on the single-line tubing is closed or the catheter is disconnected to make sure that there is no contamination of the

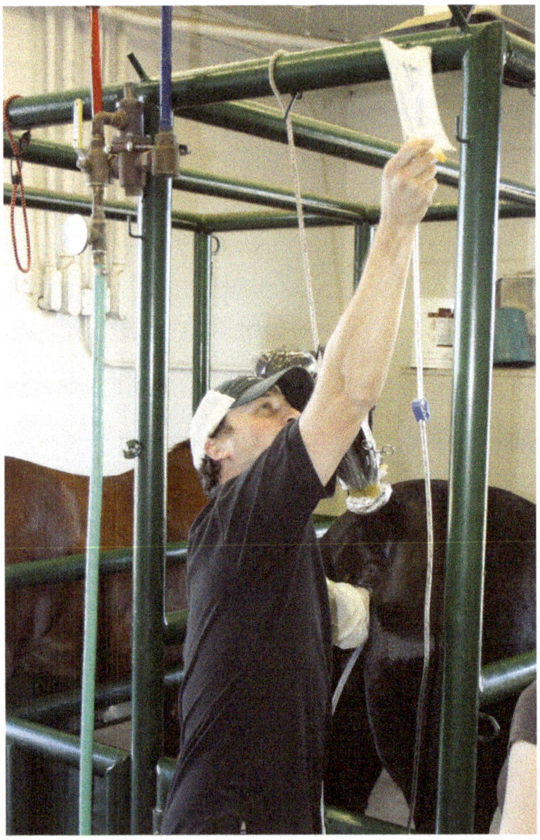

Figure 18.2 Infusion of sterile saline into the uterus by gravity flow for low volume lavage.

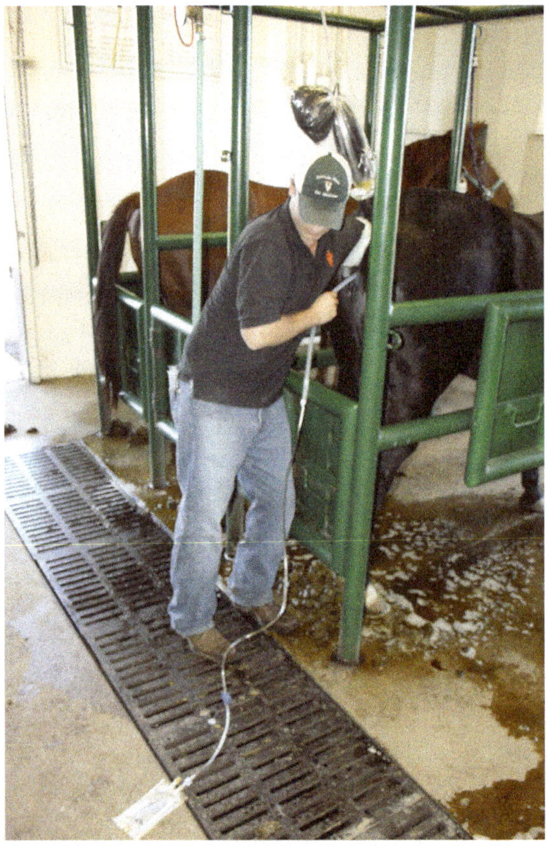

Figure 18.3 Recovery of fluid from the uterus during a low volume lavage procedure.

recovered fluid with bacteria from the vaginal vault or caudal reproductive tract.

- The cuff is subsequently deflated and the catheter removed from the reproductive tract.
- An alternative method involves passage of an insemination pipette into the uterus and the infusion of 60 ml of 0.9% sodium chloride via a syringe. The uterus is massaged to distribute the fluid and then the fluid is aspirated back into the syringe. Fluid recovery may be more difficult with this technique.
- Recovered fluid is placed into one or two 50 ml centrifuge tube(s) and centrifuged at 400× g for 10 minutes. Alternatively, the cellular material may be allowed to settle by gravity for a few hours.
- All but 5 ml of supernatant is removed and the pellet is re-suspended in the 5 ml of lavage fluid.
- Sterile culture swabs may be placed into the re-suspended lavage fluid to obtain samples for cytology and culture. The culture swab is transferred to a transport media and the cytology swab is gently rolled across a microscope slide. The slide is air-dried prior to staining with a modified Wright's stain such as Diff-Quik®.
- An additional sample may be obtained from the centrifuge tube for polymerase chain reaction (PCR) analysis for bacterial or fungal DNA.

Interpretation

- It is important that sufficient fluid is recovered from the uterus to be of diagnostic use.
- Enough fluid should pass through the lavage tubing so that assessment of the uterine environment is performed. Care should be taken to not just pass fluid into and out of the catheter without actually contacting the uterus.
- Note any discharge present on the sterile sleeve when the gloved arm is pulled from the vagina. There should not be any purulent or hemorrhagic discharge, only the lubricant and clear mucous should be present.
- The clarity and presence of debris and mucus should be noted in the effluent fluid recovered from the uterus. Typically, the recovered fluid is graded as clear, cloudy, or cloudy with mucus.
- Microscopic examination is performed at 400× (10× eye piece and 40× objective) magnification or under oil immersion at 1,000× (10× eye piece and 100× objective).
- Evaluate slide quality (e.g., the presence of normal uterine epithelial cells) as well as the presence and relative number of inflammatory cells (neutrophils, macrophages, lymphocytes, etc.) and any bacterial or fungal organisms.
- The amount of background debris and sediment appearing on stained slides from a low volume lavage is often greater than with swab or brush techniques. The amount of debris may be correlated with the degree of inflammation.
- The presence of >5–10 neutrophils per high power field is an indication of inflammation, providing that an adequate cellular sample was obtained.
- The greater the ratio of neutrophils : uterine epithelial cells, the greater the degree of inflammation or endometritis.
- Neutrophils are the primary white blood cells present with acute inflammation. Macrophages, lymphocytes, and plasma cells may be noted with chronic inflammation. Eosinophils may be noted in cases of fungal endometritis, urine pooling, or aspiration of air into the uterus.
- The absence of white blood cells (with normal endometrial cells present) often suggests that there is no inflammation present in the uterine lumen. However, some bacteria such as *Escherichia coli* and *Pseudomonas aeruginosa* may not stimulate a large inflammatory response and a "negative cytology" (i.e., the absence of white blood cells) may provide incorrect evidence of a "clean" or non-infected uterus. Consequently, it is recommended that both culture and cytology samples be collected and evaluated and not just one or the other.
- Please see Chapter 17 for further description of cell types found on cytology.

Further Reading

Ball BA, Shin SJ, Patten VH, Lein DH, Woods GL. 1988. Use of a low-volume uterine flush for microbiologic and cytologic examination of the mare's endometrium. *Theriogenology* 29: 1269–83.

Brook D. 1993. Uterine cytology. In: McKinnon AO, Voss JL (eds). Equine Reproduction. Philadelphia: Lea and Febiger, pp. 246–54.

Couto MS, Hughes JP. 1984. Technique and interpretation of cervical and endometrial cytology in the mare. *J Eq Vet Sci* 4: 265–73.

Leblanc MM, Magsig J, Stromberg AJ. 2007. Use of low-volume uterine flush for diagnosing endometritis in chronically infertile mares. *Theriogenology* 68: 403–12.

19

Endometrial Biopsy

Patrick M. McCue

Equine Reproduction Laboratory, Colorado State University, USA

Introduction

Biopsy of the uterine lining or endometrium is primarily used in the evaluation of uterine health, detection of uterine disease, and as a prognostic indicator of the ability of a mare to carry a foal to term. Endometrial biopsies are collected as part of a routine breeding soundness evaluation, as part of a pre-purchase evaluation of a potential broodmare, and in the examination of barren mares, problem breeding mares, and mares with a history of pregnancy loss. Samples may be collected prior to the onset of the breeding season, during the breeding season, or at the end of the breeding season. A biopsy may be collected during any stage of the estrous cycle, although individual veterinarians may prefer to collect samples when the mare is either in diestrus or in early estrus. It is important to record the stage of the mare's estrous cycle so that the pathologist evaluating the biopsy sample can interpret the architecture accordingly.

Endometrial biopsy samples may also be used for microbiological culture, cytologic evaluation, and detection of microbial DNA using reverse transcription polymerase chain reaction (RT-PCR) techniques.

Equipment and Supplies

Uterine biopsy instrument, sterile obstetrical sleeve, sterile obstetrical lubricant, formalin (10%) or Bouin's solution, alcohol (70%), 25 gauge needle to tease biopsy out of instrument.

Technique

- An ultrasound examination is recommended prior to biopsy collection to confirm that the mare is not pregnant and to help stage the mare's estrous cycle.
- The tail of the mare is wrapped and held out of the way (see Chapter 4).
- The perineal area is thoroughly cleansed using a nonresidual liquid soap, rinsed with clean water, and dried with paper towels (see Chapter 3).
- A sterile obstetrical sleeve with sterile lubricant is worn by the examiner.
- An endometrial biopsy instrument is held in a closed position within the hand, guided into the vagina, and then carefully passed through the cervix into the uterus.
- The examiner generally removes the arm guiding the biopsy instrument from the vagina and inserts the arm into the rectum to manually aid in placement of the instrument in the correct location. The biopsy location is usually at the base of one of the uterine horns or in an area of suspected pathology.
- The examiner then opens the cutting basket of the instrument and applies gentle ventral pressure on the rectum to push endometrial tissue inside the cutting basket. (Figure 19.1).

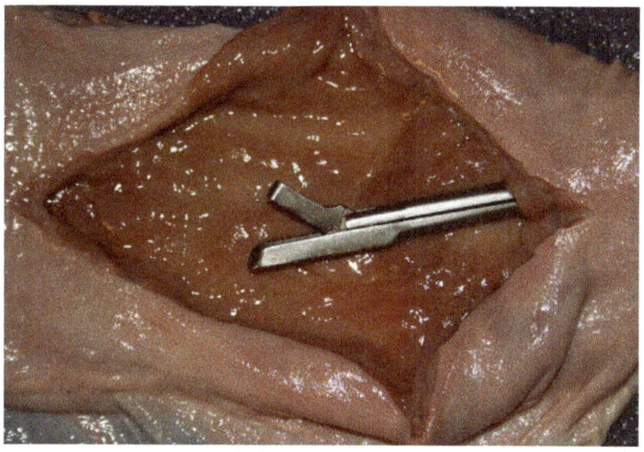

Figure 19.1 Endometrial biopsy instrument passed into the uterus of the mare. The basket is in the open position to take a sample.

Equine Reproductive Procedures, Second Edition. Edited by John Dascanio and Patrick McCue.

- The instrument is closed, collecting a small sample (0.25 × 1–2 cm) of endometrial tissue.
- The biopsy sample is placed into fixative solution (i.e., 10% formalin or Bouin's solution). A 25 gauge needle may be used to tease the sample out of the basket of the instrument. The container should be labeled with the name of the mare, collection date, and other pertinent information. If the biopsy sample is initially fixed in Bouin's solution, it should be transferred into 70% alcohol the following day.
- The fixed biopsy specimen is submitted to a pathology laboratory.
- A single biopsy sample collected from one site is generally representative of the entire endometrium. However, collection of multiple samples may be advantageous in mares where a long-standing infertility is present to better characterize the endometrium.
- The owner may be warned that the mare may have a slight vulvar hemorrhagic discharge post-biopsy for the first 24 hours.

Biopsy Interpretation

Histologic characteristics of the biopsy vary with the season and stage of the estrous cycle. Endometrial glands are inactive during seasonal anestrus and the luminal and glandular epithelial cells are either cuboidal or squamous. During estrus, the epithelial cells are usually columnar to tall columnar and considerable edema is present in the lamina propria. During diestrus, the epithelium varies from columnar to cuboidal, edema is absent, and the glandular branches are usually tortuous.

Endometrial biopsy samples are examined for the presence of inflammatory and degenerative changes. Inflammation is recognized by the accumulation of inflammatory cells in the endometrial tissue (Figure 19.2). Acute inflammation is recognized by the presence of polymorphonuclear leukocytes, whereas chronic inflammation is characterized by the presence of lymphocytes and other mononuclear cells in the endometrium. Inflammation may be infectious or non-infectious in origin, but is a potentially treatable pathologic condition which may respond to intrauterine or systemic therapy.

Endometrial glandular degeneration is most often recognized by a deposition of collagen in the form of fibrosis or scar tissue around the endometrial glands, often forming what are called glandular "nests." Other degenerative changes detected in biopsy evaluation include cystic dilation of glands, glandular necrosis, and accumulation of inspissated material within dilated glands (Figure 19.3). In contrast to inflammation, fibrosis represents a permanent, untreatable pathologic condition. In addition, a biofilm layer may be noted on the surface of endometrial biopsies collected from mares with endometritis that are fixed in Bouin's solution (Figure 19.4). Unfortunately, a biofilm is often washed away from endometrial biopsy samples fixed in formalin.

The endometrium is classified on a grading scale based on biopsy characteristics that ranges from I to III. Grade I endometrium is essentially normal, with minimal inflammation or fibrosis. Grade III endometrium includes severe inflammatory and/or fibrotic changes. Grade II is a broad category, often divided into subcategories IIA and IIB, encompassing all pathologic levels between grades I and III. It is possible for an improvement in endometrial grade

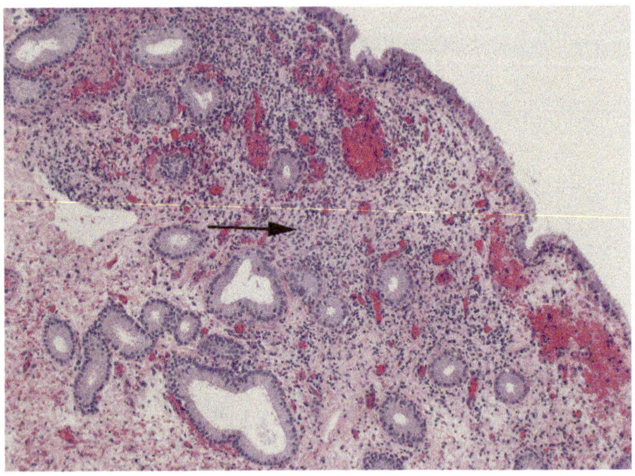

Figure 19.2 Endometrial biopsy from a mare with endometritis. Note the lymphocytic inflammatory cells infiltrating the endometrium (arrow).

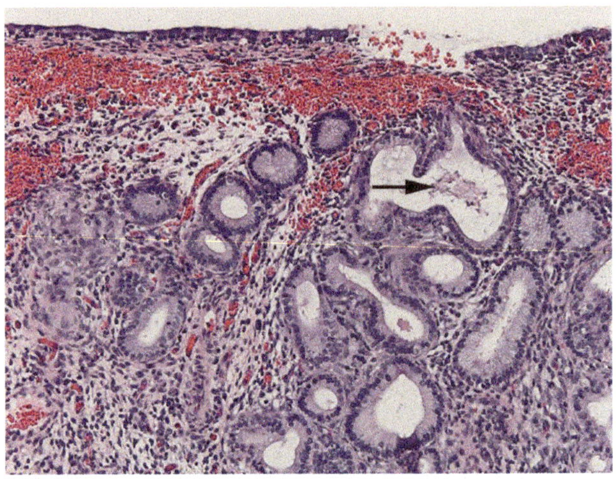

Figure 19.3 Endometrial biopsy (grade III) from a mare with severe fibrosis. Note the glandular nesting and inspissated material within the dilated glands (arrow).

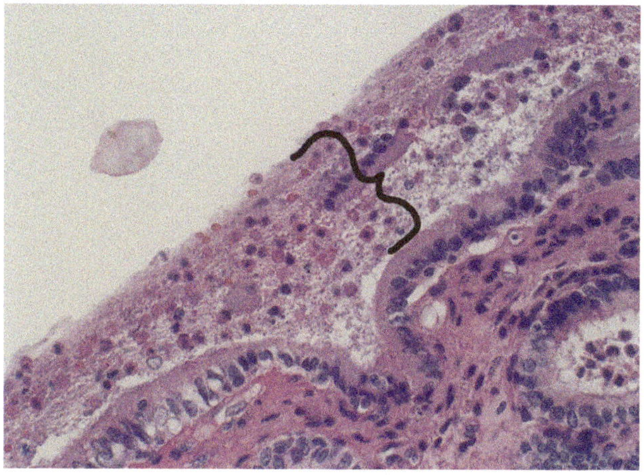

Figure 19.4 Biofilm (bracket) adhered to the endometrial surface of a mare with bacterial endometritis. Reproduced with permission from: Dr Ryan Ferris.

if the inflammation present is reduced or eliminated with proper treatment.

Additional information as to the potential cause of endometrial pathology is often available from diagnostic tests performed in conjunction with the biopsy, such as ultrasonography, speculum examination, uterine culture, and uterine cytology. As noted previously, fibrosis or scar tissue

Table 19.1 Expected foaling rates of mares according to endometrial biopsy grade.

Category	Degree of Endometrial Change	Expected Foaling Rate (%)
I	Absent	80–90
IIa	Mild	50–80
IIb	Moderate	10–50
III	Severe	<10

Adapted from Kenney and Doig (1986).

is considered a permanent condition. However, if the biopsy score is adversely affected by inflammation, successful treatment could result in improvement of the endometrial grade on a subsequent evaluation.

The endometrial biopsy is often used to determine the prognosis for a mare to carry a foal to term. Expected foaling rates for each endometrial biopsy category are given in Table 19.1. Initial pregnancy rates decrease and pregnancy loss rates increase with each advanced grade of pathologic condition. Many additional factors, such as stallion and broodmare management, also play critical roles in conception and maintenance of pregnancy.

Reference

Kenney RM, Doig PA. 1986. Equine endometrial biopsy. In: Morrow DA (ed.). Current Therapy in Theriogenology. Philadelphia: WB Saunders, pp. 723–9.

Further Reading

Kenney RM. 1978. Cyclic and pathologic changes of the mare endometrium as detected by biopsy, with a note on early embryonic death. *J Am Vet Med Assoc* 172: 241–62.

Love CC. 2011. Endometrial biopsy. In: McKinnon AO, Squires EL, Vaala WE, Varner DD (eds). Equine Reproduction, 2nd edn. Ames, IA: Wiley Blackwell, pp. 1929–39.

20

Hysteroscopic Examination of the Uterus

Patrick M. McCue

Equine Reproduction Laboratory, Colorado State University, USA

Introduction

Hysteroscopy is the term used for direct visualization of the interior of the uterus using a videoendoscope or fiberoptic endoscope. The true value of an endoscopic examination is detection of pathologic abnormalities within the uterine lumen that cannot be diagnosed by traditional diagnostic techniques. Such abnormalities include intrauterine adhesions (Figure 20.1), retained endometrial cups (Figure 20.2), localized lesions, and focal sites of infection. Endometrial cysts, free fluid within the uterine lumen, and foreign bodies are usually detectable by ultrasound. Similarly, a majority of infectious, inflammatory, and degenerative conditions of the uterus can be detected by culture, cytology, or biopsy.

The major obstacle preventing widespread use of this technique is cost of the equipment.

Equipment and Supplies

Tail wrap, non-irritant soap, roll cotton, stainless steel bucket, disposable liner for bucket, paper towels, exam gloves, gluteraldehyde disinfectant, sterile saline, obstetrical sleeve, obstetrical lubricant, endoscope (videoendoscope or fiberoptic endoscope), obstetrical sleeves (sterile), sterile obstetrical lubricant, sedation (e.g. detomidine hydrochloride and butorphanol tartrate).

Technique

- The endoscope should be cold sterilized before use. This may be accomplished by cold sterilization in an activated solution of 2.4% glutaraldehyde (Cidex®); the endoscope is then thoroughly rinsed with 0.9% sterile saline.
- The mare should be restrained in examination stocks and sedated (i.e., 5 mg of detomidine hydrochloride plus 5 mg of butorphanol tartrate IV for a 450 kg mare).
- Remove feces from the rectum to prevent contamination of equipment during untimely defecation.
- Wrap the tail and then thoroughly wash the perineal area using a non-residual liquid soap, rinse with warm water, and dry with paper towels (see Chapters 3 & 4).
- Apply a small amount of obstetrical lubricant to the gloved hand holding the endoscope.
- Manually guide the endoscope into the vagina and gently pass through the cervix into the uterus. The vagina and cervical lumen should be visualized for any discharges (Figure 20.3).
- Distend the uterine lumen with air to allow for visualization of the uterine lumen. It will be necessary to hold the

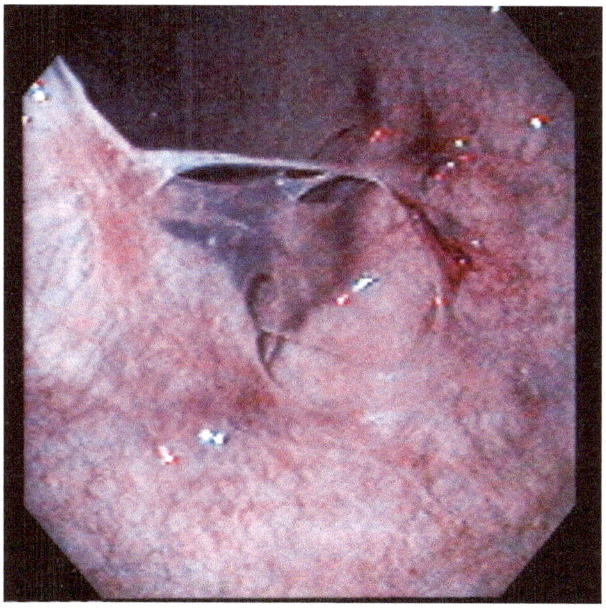

Figure 20.1 Intrauterine adhesions in a mare viewed through an endoscope.

Equine Reproductive Procedures, Second Edition. Edited by John Dascanio and Patrick McCue.

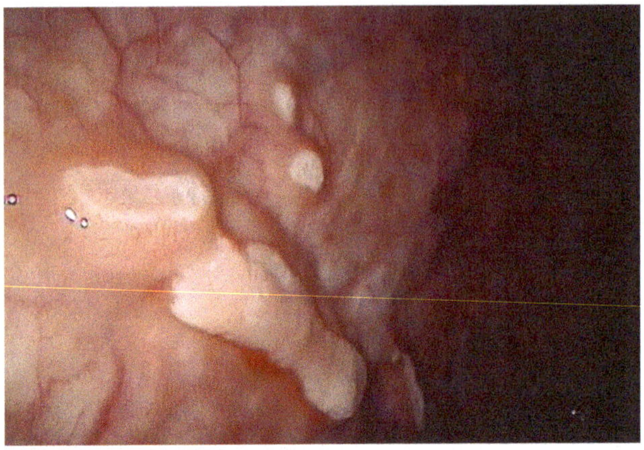

Figure 20.2 Endometrial cups viewed through an endoscope in a mare that lost her pregnancy.

cervix closed around the endoscope to maintain insufflation of the uterus. This may be difficult if the mare is in estrus with a relaxed cervix.

- Examine the body of the uterus and bifurcation first (Figure 20.4).
- Subsequently pass the endoscope up each uterine horn to the tip (Figure 20.5). It should be possible to view the utero-tubular junction (UTJ) at the tip of each horn (Figure 20.6).
- Samples for culture and histology can be obtained through the biopsy port of the endoscope using a double lumen sterile brush such as those used for tracheal diagnostic sampling.

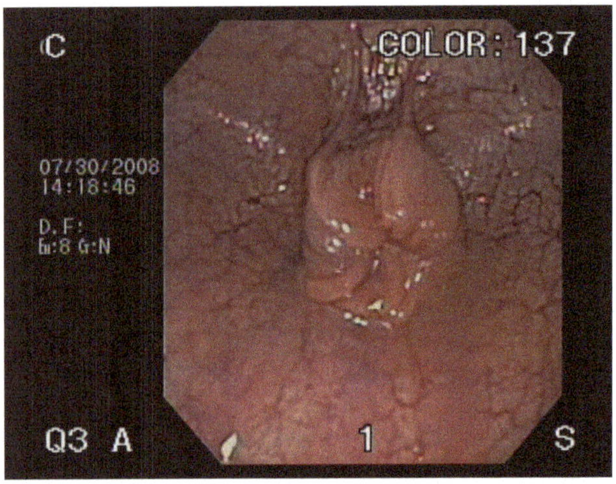

Figure 20.3 Normal mare's cervix viewed by endoscopy.

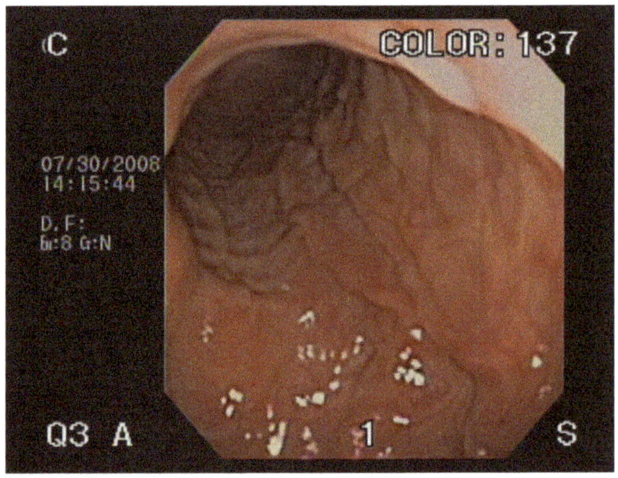

Figure 20.5 Hysteroscopic view of a normal mare's uterine horn.

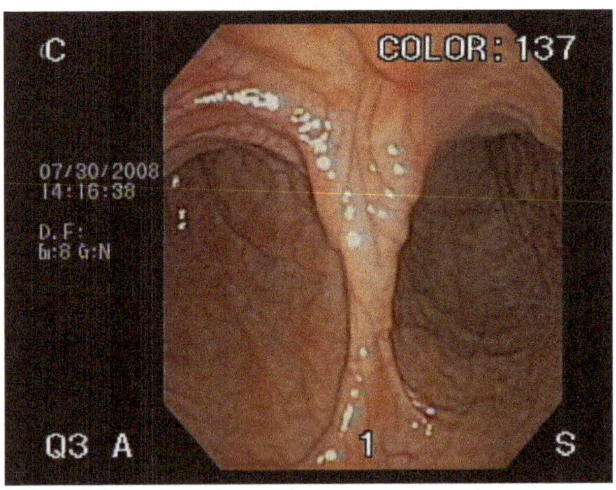

Figure 20.4 Hysteroscopic view of a normal mare's uterine bifurcation.

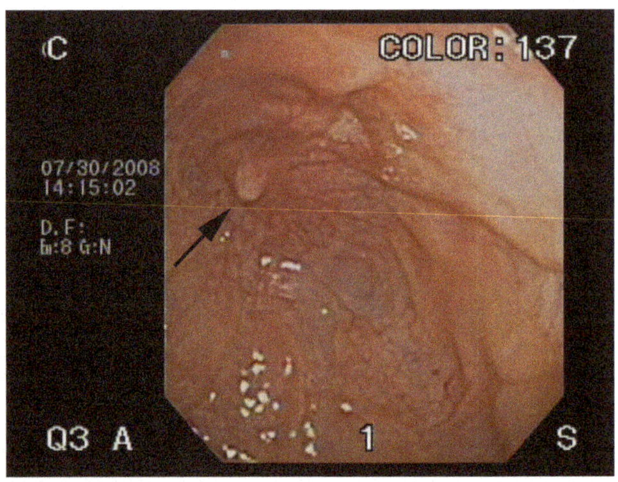

Figure 20.6 Hysteroscopic view of a normal mare's utero-tubal papilla (arrow) visible at the end of one uterine horn.

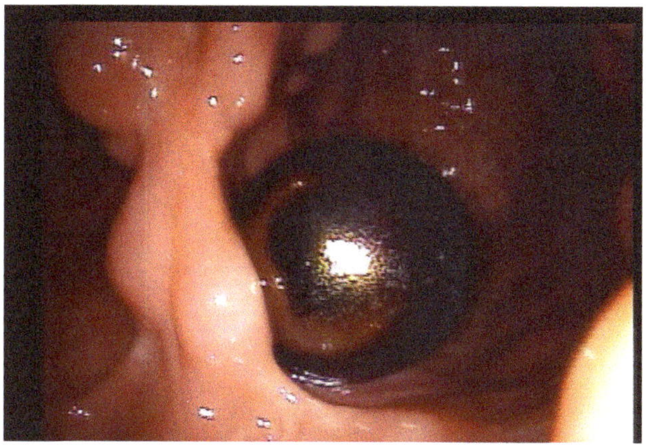

Figure 20.7 Marble within the uterine lumen viewed by an endoscope.

- It is recommended that broad-spectrum antibiotics be infused into the uterus after the endoscopic procedure. If the mare was examined during diestrus, it is important to administer a dose of prostaglandins to return the mare to estrus, thus clearing any contaminants and placing the mare into a phase of her cycle better suited to clear bacteria.

Additional Comments

Foreign bodies, such as a marble or the tip of a culture instrument, are easily visualized with an endoscope (Figures 20.7 and 20.8). Videoendoscopy can also be used to deposit a small volume of concentrated spermatozoa at the UTJ as part of a low dose, deep horn insemination protocol. Laser ablation and other types of management of endometrial cysts are also performed using an endoscope. Finally, videoendoscopy can be used to facilitate cannulation of the UTJ to flush the oviducts of mares suspected of oviductal blockage (see Chapter 32).

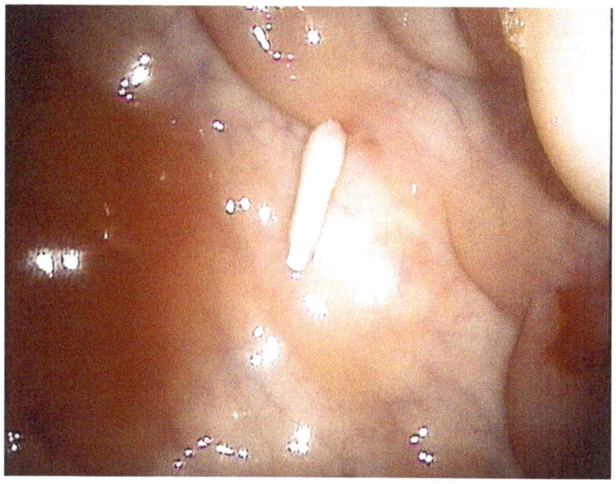

Figure 20.8 Tip of a uterine culture instrument in the uterine lumen viewed by an endoscope.

Further Reading

Bracher V, Allen WR. 1992. Videoendoscopic evaluation of the mare's uterus: I. Findings in normal fertile mares. *Eq Vet J* 24: 274–8.

Bracher V, Mathias S, Allen WR. 1992. Videoendoscopic evaluation of the mare's uterus: II. Findings in normal fertile mares. *Eq Vet J* 24: 279–84.

Card CE. 2011. Endoscopic examination. In: McKinnon AO, Squires EL, Vaala WE, Varner DD (eds). Equine Reproduction, 2nd edn. Ames, IA: Wiley Blackwell, pp. 1940–50.

Inoue Y, Sekiguchi M. 2018. Clinical application of hysteroscopic hydrotubation for unexplained infertility in the mare. *Eq Vet J* 50: 470–3.

Lindsey AC, Morris LHA, Allen WR, Shenk JL, Squires EL, Bruemmer JE. 2002. Hysteroscopic insemination of mares with low numbers of nonsorted or flow sorted spermatozoa. *Eq Vet J* 34: 128–32.

Rambags BPB, Stout TAE. 2005. Transcervical endoscope-guided emptying of a transmural uterine cyst in a mare. *Vet Record* 156: 679–82.

21

Endometrial Cyst Removal

John J. Dascanio

School of Veterinary Medicine, Texas Tech University, USA

Introduction

Endometrial or uterine cysts may be glandular or lymphatic in origin and may range from a few millimeters to as large as 20 cm. The presence of cysts usually indicates a degree of uterine pathology, with affected mares having an increase in uterine biopsy score due in part to increased fibrosis. Cysts may have a negative effect on fertility due to prevention of embryo migration, thus interfering with maternal recognition of pregnancy, interference with early embryonic histotroph absorption, and interference with placentation. Removal of cysts that are large in size or multiple in number may have a positive effect on fertility. Removal of cysts has been described using a snare, laser hysteroscopy, loop cautery, or uterine biopsy instrument. Uterine lavage and infusion of intrauterine antibiotics may be performed after cysts are removed.

Equipment and Supplies

Tail wrap, non-irritant soap, roll cotton, stainless steel bucket, disposable liner for bucket, paper towels, exam gloves, flunixin meglumine, sedatives, artificial insemination pipettes, No. 3 polyamide suture material, tape, sterile uterine biopsy instrument, obstetrical sleeve, sterile obstetrical lubricant, endoscope, gluteraldehyde disinfectant, chlorhexadine solution, sterile saline, laser fibers, electrocautery unit, loop cautery fiber.

Techniques

General Preparation

- Remove feces from the rectum and document the size and location of each endometrial cyst using transrectal ultrasound (Figure 21.1).
- Place a tail wrap and tail rope onto the mare (see Chapter 4).
- Wearing examination gloves, clean and dry the perineum of the mare (see Chapter 3).
- The mare is usually sedated using a combination of xylazine (0.33–0.44 mg/kg IV) or detomidine (0.0088–0.011 mg/kg IV) plus butorphanol tartrate (0.011–0.022 mg/kg IV).

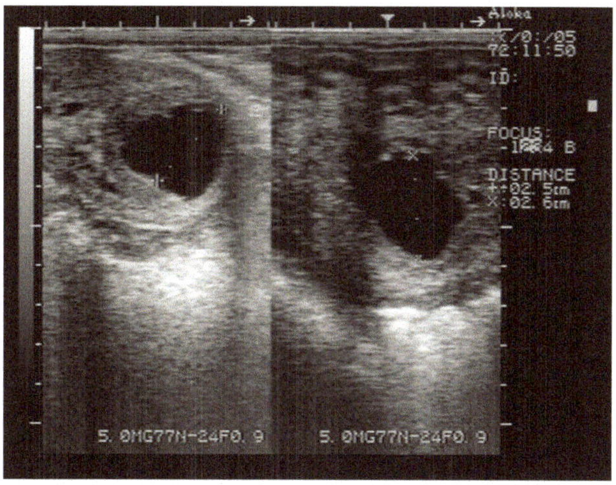

Figure 21.1 Two ultrasound images of endometrial cysts of 2.5 and 2.6 cm diameter in a mare.

Equine Reproductive Procedures, Second Edition. Edited by John Dascanio and Patrick McCue.

- Flunixin meglumine may be administered (1.1 mg/kg IV) to minimize the inflammation caused by removal of the cyst(s).

Snare Removal

- The mare should be in estrus so that the cervix is dilated to allow passage of a small hand into the uterus.
- Large endometrial cysts that are pedunculated (lymphatic cysts) may be removed using a snare technique.
- A snare is fashioned using two artificial insemination pipettes attached together side by side using tape. No. 3 polyamide suture material is threaded through the end of one pipette and back into the other pipette so that there is a loop going between the two pipettes (Figure 21.2). The length of the suture material should be 3× the length of the pipettes.
- Cold sterilize the snare apparatus in dilute chlorhexidine solution (approximately 12 ml chlorhexidine in 500 ml sterile saline) for 15 minutes and rinse with sterile saline.
- Place a sterile obstetrical sleeve on one arm and place sterile lubricant on the back of the gloved hand and down the sleeve.
- With the gloved hand, the end of the snare apparatus is passed through the cervix into the uterus and the loop is fitted around the base of the pedunculated cyst. Cervical dilation may be achieved with slow constant pressure with the hand in a mare in estrus.
- The loop is tightened by pushing the pipettes inward against the pedicle of the cyst while pulling outward on the suture material.
- The suture material is subsequently moved back and forth to cut through the cyst stalk and the cyst is then removed by hand (Figure 21.2).

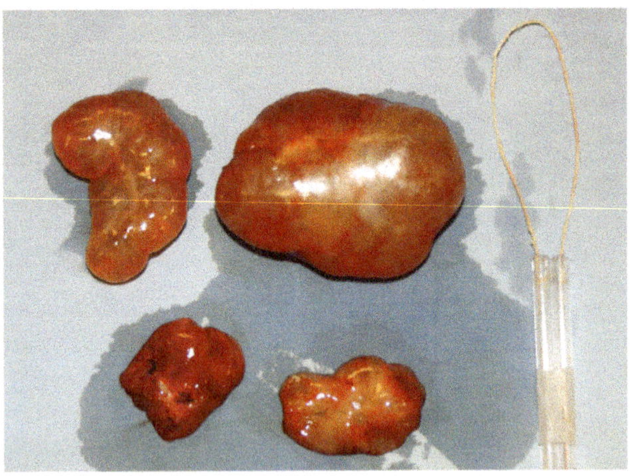

Figure 21.2 Lymphatic cysts removed using a snare. The snare is to the right of the cysts.

Endoscope Preparation

- The mare should be in diestrus, with a closed cervix, to allow insufflation of the uterus for visualization.
- Cold sterilize a 1 m long, 11 mm diameter endoscope in an activated solution of 2.4% glutaraldehyde (Cidex®) and rinse thoroughly with sterile saline making sure to properly clean and rinse the accessory channel.
- Place a sterile obstetrical sleeve on one arm and hold the end of the endoscope in this gloved hand. A second operator will be necessary to work the endoscope controls.
- Place sterile lubricant on the back of the gloved hand and down the sleeve, being careful to not get lubricant on the camera end of the endoscope.
- Separate the vulvar labia and introduce the gloved hand/endoscope into the vestibule, through the vestibulo-vaginal fold, and into the vagina and through the cervix.
- Examine the entire uterine lumen for pathology including cysts, discharge, and adhesions (Figure 21.3).
- Prostaglandins should be administered intramuscularly after the procedure to bring the mare into estrus to help clear any uterine contaminants from the procedure.

Laser Removal

- The uterus is insufflated with either carbon dioxide (Nd:YAG laser) or warm, sterile, lactated Ringer's solution (diode laser) for the procedure.
- For the Nd:YAG laser, a 2.1 mm diameter coaxial transmitting tube (600 μm diameter non-contact glass laser fiber) is passed through the accessory channel of the endoscope. Carbon dioxide is then passed through the tubing surrounding the laser fiber to insufflate the uterus. The laser is positioned about 1 cm from the cyst

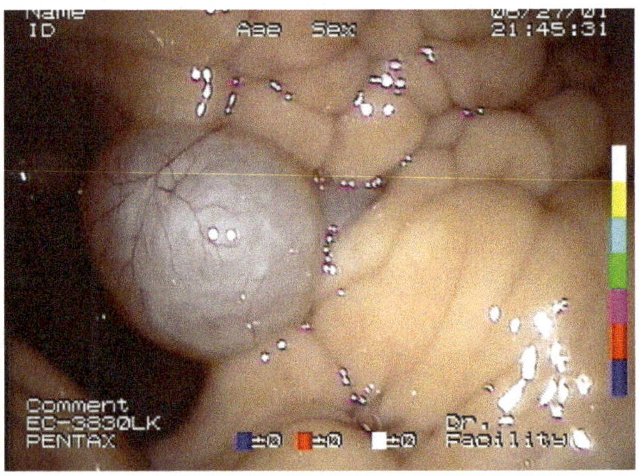

Figure 21.3 Uterine cyst viewed through a videoendoscope.

to be treated. The power is set to continuous mode at 50 W to blanch the surface of the cyst. The power is then elevated to 100 W and the cyst is punctured. The fluid is allowed to drain from the cyst and the remaining cyst membrane is photo-ablated. Exposure times are from 1 to 5 seconds. The procedure may need to be repeated later that day or the next day if visualization becomes obscured due to smoke within the lumen when multiple cysts are present. An attempt to eliminate smoke may be performed with a suction device attached to the accessory channel with the laser fiber removed.
- For a diode laser, the laser is set to 12–14 W for smaller cysts and 14–18 W for larger cysts.

Electrocautery Cyst Removal

- The uterus is insufflated with warm, sterile, lactated Ringer's solution.
- A monopolar electrocautery 5 cm loop is passed through the accessory channel of the endoscope.
- The loop is attached to an electrosurgical unit and the grounding plate is attached to the gluteal area on the mare. The grounding plate should have conductive gel placed underneath, with the hair shaved over the area to create minimal resistance.
- The loop is passed over the cyst and slightly tightened around the base of the cyst.
- A coagulation current is passed through the loop, while the loop is pulled through the base of the cyst.
- The detached cyst is removed using the cautery loop with the current turned off; a small biopsy instrument or a tissue retrieval basket is passed through the accessory channel of the endoscope. Once the tissue is grasped, the entire end of the endoscope is removed from the reproductive tract, being careful to not drop the piece of tissue.

Cyst Removal Using a Uterine Biopsy Instrument

- Don a sterile obstetrical sleeve and place some sterile lubricant on the back of the hand and down the arm of the sleeve.
- Place the end of a sterile uterine biopsy instrument in the palm of the hand and introduce the biopsy instrument per vagina through the cervix and into the uterus.
- While keeping the biopsy instrument in the uterus, remove the hand and place it per rectum so as to palpate the end of the biopsy instrument in the uterus.
- If the cyst is palpable, the biopsy instrument may be guided to the area of the cyst and the jaws of the instrument opened and closed over the cyst to disrupt it. A slight pull or tug on the biopsy instrument may be necessary to disrupt the cyst, being careful not to pull the biopsy instrument out of the cervix until the procedure is complete.
- If there are numerous cysts or it is difficult to palpate the cyst per rectum, then an ultrasound probe may be used to visualize the cyst and to coordinate placement of the biopsy instrument to disrupt the various cysts.

Needle Removal

Alternatively, a needle with an extension set and syringe attached may be manually placed into a cyst to remove fluid in a mare in estrus, but this may not result in permanent resolution.

Interpretation

- Biopsy or needle disruption of cysts results in temporary deflation of cysts; cysts often reoccur as the secretory lining of the cyst may not be removed adequately.
- Excess cautery or laser contact should be avoided so as to not create a full thickness transmural necrosis of the uterine wall, potentially leading to adhesion formation or peritonitis.
- Mares with uterine cysts typically have an increased biopsy score and may have a degree of endometrosis (chronic degenerative changes).
- Mares should be re-examined with transrectal ultrasound at 7–10 days after treatment to document any remaining cysts that may need to be treated.

Further Reading

Bilkslager AT, Tate LP, Weinstock D. 1993. Effects of neodymium:yttrium aluminum garnet laser irradiation on endometrium and on endometrial cysts in six mares. *Vet Surg* 22: 351–6.

Brook D, Frankel K. 1987. Electrocoagulative removal of endometrial cysts in the mare. *J Eq Vet Sci* 7: 77–81.

Deluca CA, Gee EK, McCue PM. 2009. How to remove large endometrial cysts with an improvised snare: a simple technique for practitioners. *Proc Annu Conv Am Assoc Eq Pract* 55: 328–30.

Eilts BE, Scholl DT, Paccamonti DL, *et al*. 1995. Prevalence of endometrial cysts and their effect on fertility. *Biol Reprod Mono* 1: 527–32.

Scherrer N. 2015. Treatment of uterine cysts with diode laser photoablation in a Thoroughbred broodmare population. *Proc Annu Conv Am Assoc Eq Pract* 61: 469.

Stanton MB, Steiner JV, Pugh DG. 2004. Endometrial cysts in the mare. *J Eq Vet Sci* 24: 14–19.

Wilson DL. 1985. Diagnostic and therapeutic hysteroscopy for endometrial cysts in mares. *Vet Med* 80: 59–63.

22

Chromosomal Analysis

Terje Raudsepp

College of Veterinary Medicine and Biomedical Sciences, Texas A&M University, USA

Introduction

In every cell, the genetic material, DNA, is packaged with the help of diverse proteins into distinct structures – the chromosomes. Chromosomes are located in the cell nucleus and show species-specific features in number, size, and appearance. The chromosome complement of a cell of a species is called the karyotype and the field of science studying the chromosomes is cytogenetics.

The diploid (2n) chromosome number for the normal horse is 64 and includes 31 pairs of autosomes and a pair of sex chromosomes. Female horses have two X chromosomes and male horses have one X and one Y chromosome. Thus, normal female and male horse karyotypes are denoted as 64,XX and 64,XY, respectively. Half of chromosomes are inherited from the sire, the other half from the dam.

Changes in chromosome number and morphology directly affect the viability of zygotes and embryos, normal development, and the formation of gametes. Changes in the number of autosomes such as trisomies are typically lethal, but if present in live-born foals are accompanied by multiple and severe congenital malformations and primary infertility. Structural rearrangements of chromosomes, known as translocations, may have only a mild effect on the carrier, but can significantly affect both male and female fertility. Abnormal number or structure of sex chromosomes can cause infertility and/or disorders of sexual development (Raudsepp & Chowdhary 2016).

The aim of clinical chromosome analysis is to determine whether or not a horse has a normal set of chromosomes. The analysis is usually carried out on animals with various reproductive and/or developmental disorders to ascertain possible causes of abnormalities. Additionally, cytogenetic tests are ordered by insurance companies, horse breeders, and owners to evaluate potential breeding stallions, broodmares, or the horses to be purchased. A more recent addition to equine clinical cytogenetics is the evaluation of chromosomal stability in stem cell lines that are produced for stem cell therapy.

Chromosomal analysis includes counting the diploid (2n) chromosome number, arranging chromosomes into a karyotype, and evaluating chromosome morphology according to their banding patterns following the international system of chromosomal nomenclature for the horse (ISCNH) (Bowling *et al.* 1997). The analysis also determines whether or not the chromosomal (genetic) sex agrees with the gonadal and phenotypic sex.

This chapter describes the methods that are used for clinical cytogenetic analysis in horses. This includes a list of the basic required equipment and supplies for an equine cytogenetics laboratory, a detailed step-wise methodology for the preparation of metaphase chromosome spreads from different tissues, and a description of the main principles and methods of chromosome analysis. Finally, advanced chromosome analysis approaches and future perspectives of equine clinical cytogenetics are briefly discussed.

Chromosomal Analysis Techniques

Sample collection and shipping

Note: the underlying principle of chromosome analysis is cell division during which metaphase chromosome spreads can be obtained. Therefore, the material (blood, tissue, biopsy, etc.) for chromosome analysis must contain live cells and be free of bacterial and fungal contamination. This is why chromosome analysis cannot be done from hair or frozen tissues.

- Peripheral blood (~20 ml) is collected in green top (for cell cultures) and purple top (for DNA isolation) Vacutainer®

Equine Reproductive Procedures, Second Edition. Edited by John Dascanio and Patrick McCue.

Equipment and Supplies

Laboratory equipment

Laminar flow hood for sterile cell culture work, CO_2 incubator regulated at 37°C (99°F), clinical centrifuge with a swing-out rotor for 15 ml conical centrifuge tubes, water pump for liquid aspiration, water bath, a set of adjustable volume laboratory micropipettes, autoclave, refrigerator-freezer, heating plate or hot oven, inverted light microscope with 20× and 40× phase-contrast objectives, light microscope with a 20× phase-contrast objective and a 100× objective, equipped with a CCD (charge-coupled device) camera and image analysis software to capture metaphase spreads and arrange karyotypes.

Supplies for cell cultures

7–10 ml sodium or lithium heparin (green top) and EDTA (purple top) Vacutainer® tubes and 20 gauge needles for Vacutainer® tubes for blood collection, sterile forceps and small scissors, sterile Petri dishes, sterile T25 and T75 cell culture flasks, sterile conical 15 ml centrifuge tubes, sterile serologic pipettes(1, 2, 5, and 10 ml), culture medium for blood lymphocytes: RPMI medium 1640 with Glutamax™ and 25 mM HEPES buffer (Gibco™; Life Technologies Ltd, Grand Island, NY, USA) supplemented with 30% fetal bovine serum (FBS; various suppliers), 1× antibiotic–antimycotic solution (100× stock; Gibco), 1% pokeweed mitogen (lectin from *Phytolacca americana*; Sigma Aldrich, Burlington, MA, USA). (Larger quantities (500 ml) of ready-to-use media can be prepared and stored in 9 ml aliquots in sterile 15 ml screw-cap centrifuge tubes at −20°C. The tubes should be defrosted only once.) Culture medium for fibroblasts: minimum essential medium (MEM) α with Glutamax™ (Gibco) and nucleosides supplemented with 10–20% FBS and 1× antibiotic–antimycotic solution, sterile Hanks' balanced salt solution (HBSS; Gibco), sterile 0.25% trypsin-EDTA (Gibco).

Supplies for cell harvest and chromosome preparations

Ethidium bromide 1 mg/ml solution in double distilled water (ddH_2O) (optional; prevents chromosome condensation), demecolcine solution to stop the movement of cell spindle and capture chromosomes at metaphase (10 mg/ml in HBSS (Sigma-Aldrich, St Louis, MO, USA)), hypotonic solution to burst cytoplasm and release the chromosomes (optimal hypotonic solution (Genial Helix, Chester, UK) or 0.067 M KCl solution in ddH_2O), fixative: methanol/glacial acetic acid in a ratio of 3:1, pre-cleaned double-frosted microscope slides, fine-tip plastic transfer pipettes, Coplin jars.

Supplies for chromosome staining and banding

Giemsa stain (KaryoMAX® Giemsa Satin Solution; Gibco), Gurr buffer tablets (Gibco), 0.125% trypsin (stock 2.5%; Gibco), 0.1N HCl, 5% $Ba(OH)_2$ in water, 2× saline sodium citrate (SSC) (stock 20× SSC).

tubes, wrapped individually in paper towels to prevent breakage, and shipped with refrigerator packs (do not freeze!). Shipping should be overnight or as fast as possible. Blood older than 7–10 days may not be suitable for cell cultures.

- A skin biopsy is collected for transport into sterile tubes containing collection medium: 10 ml HBSS supplemented with 2× antibiotic–antimycotic solution.
- Cell lines: pre-established cell lines can be shipped frozen in cryovials on dry ice or in culture flasks at room temperature. Culture flasks must be completely filled with medium to prevent detachment and damage of cells during transport.

Peripheral blood lymphocyte cultures

- Upon arrival, blood samples should stand at room temperature for 30 minutes to sediment the red blood cells. The buffy coat, with lymphocytes, is seen as a thin white layer between the red blood cells and plasma.
- Under sterile conditions, add 1 ml of plasma with the buffy coat to pre-warmed (37°C) 9 ml cell culture media in a 15 ml centrifuge tube. Mix the tube and incubate for 72 hours at 37°C. Gently invert the cultures twice a day. Note: only blood collected in Na- or Li-heparin Vacutainer® tubes is suitable for cell cultures.
- Start cell harvest at 68 hours of culture following the procedures described under "Cell harvest."

Primary fibroblast cultures

- Place a tissue biopsy, with a small amount of collection medium, into a sterile Petri dish and mince with sterile forceps and scissors to the size of 2–4 mm^2. Wash the pieces 10 times in sterile collection medium (use a succession of Petri dishes).
- Transfer the pieces of tissue into T25 flasks, approximately 4–6 pieces per flask. Add 0.5 ml culture medium and incubate at 37°C with 5% CO_2 overnight. The pieces should get attached on the next day.

- Check the pieces under an inverted microscope every day for the outgrowth of fibroblast cells, as well as for possible contamination. In the latter case, the cultures should be discarded.
- Wash the pieces with HBSS/2× antibiotics–antimycotics and change medium (0.5 ml) every day. Do not let the pieces dry out. The first cells typically appear in a week.
- When outgrowth is sufficient (~100 fibroblast cells around most of the pieces), remove the tissue pieces, aspirate the culture medium and wash the flasks twice with 5 ml of HBSS. Add 1 ml 0.25% trypsin-EDTA and incubate for 5–10 minutes at 37°C to detach the cells. Without removing trypsin, add 2 ml culture medium, transfer the cells into a new T25 flask, add 5 ml fresh medium, and incubate at 37°C in 5% CO_2. Check the cultures every day and change media every 2–3 days.
- The cells can be grown in T25 flasks or, if more cells are needed, in T75 flasks. The transfer of cells from T25 to T75 is done with 0.25% trypsin-EDTA as described in the previous step.
- Cultures are ready for harvest when they are semiconfluent (~60–70%) and contain many mitotic cells visible as round, enlarged, partially detached bodies. Non-diving fibroblasts appear as elongated bodies attached to the surface (Figure 22.1).

Note: Even though procurement and handling of biopsies and setting up primary fibroblast cultures is more laborious and time consuming compared with lymphocyte cultures, the advantage is that live fibroblasts can be cryopreserved in liquid nitrogen and used years later for additional cytogenetic studies and various advanced molecular analyses.

Stem cell lines

- Stem cell lines are developed elsewhere and usually sent for chromosome analysis as attached semiconfluent cultures in T75 flasks.
- Upon arrival, all transport medium is removed and replaced with 10 ml regular cell culture medium (specified by the stem cell laboratory).
- The cells are grown at 37°C in 5% CO_2, inspected every day, and harvested when many mitotic cells are visible (Figure 22.1).

Cell harvest

- Add ethidium bromide solution (100 µl per 10 ml culture; final concentration 10 µg/ml) and demecolcine solution (100 µl per 10 ml culture; final concentration 0.1 µg/ml) directly into cell culture tubes or flasks and incubate for 2 hours at 37°C.

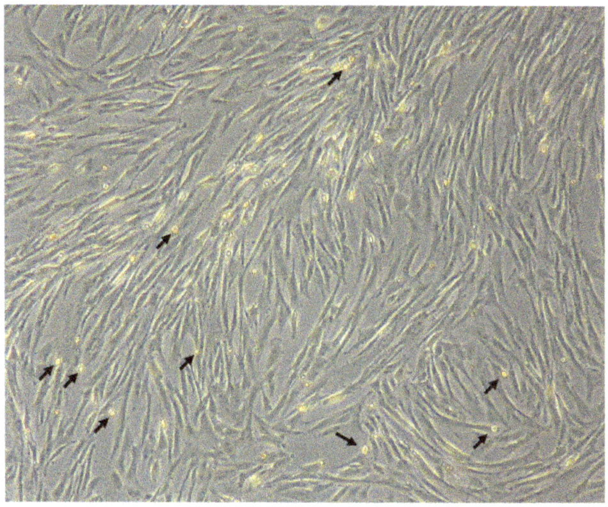

Figure 22.1 A semiconfluent horse fibroblast cell culture showing many dividing cells (round and bright; arrows); magnification 20×.

- Blood cultures are grown in centrifuge tubes and can proceed directly to the next step. Cells in T25 or T75 cultures flasks need to be transferred into centrifuge tubes as follows: tap the flasks vigorously to detach loosely attached cells and transfer medium with loose cells into a centrifuge tube. Next, detach the remaining cells with trypsin as described above (see "Primary fibroblast cultures") and transfer the cells into another centrifuge tube. Use more tubes if necessary.
- Spin the cells at 100× *g* for 10 minutes and aspirate the supernatant leaving ~1 ml medium at the bottom. Re-suspend the cell pellet gently with a plastic fine-tip pipette.
- Add 2–3 ml pre-warmed (37°C) hypotonic solution, gently mix the cells with a pipette, and take the volume to 10 ml. Incubate for 20–30 minutes at 37°C.
- Add 500 µl of cold fixative directly into the hypotonic solution and spin the cells down at 100× g for 10 minutes.
- Aspirate the supernatant and gently re-suspend the cells so that no clumps remain; add ~1 ml fresh fixative and mix the cells again; take the fixative volume to 5 ml, spin the cells at 100× g for 10 minutes, aspirate the supernatant, and repeat the fixation step three more times.
- Aspirate most of the supernatant, leaving cells in ~200 µl fixative. Re-suspend the cells by gentle pipetting and transfer the fixed cell suspension from 15 ml centrifuge tubes into 1.5–2.0 ml microcentrifuge tubes. Store the cell suspensions at −20°C (−4°F) until needed.

Chromosome preparations

- Glass slides for chromosome preparations must be precleaned by soaking overnight in glass cleaning solution (chromic-sulphuric acid) followed by overnight rinsing under running tap water. Clean slides are stored in distilled H_2O at 4°C (39°F) until needed. A slide is clean when a water film spreads evenly over the glass surface.

- To make chromosome preparations, drop approximately 10 μl of fixed cell suspension on one end of a wet slide and allow it to spread on the slide. Let the slide air-dry and check it under a light microscope using 20× phase contrast objective for the number and quality of metaphase spreads. If the number of spreads is low, the cell suspension should be concentrated by centrifugation. If the metaphases are surrounded by cytoplasm and chromosomes are not spread, wash the cells with fixative for 2–3 more times. Slides can be stored in air-tight boxes containing desiccant at –20°C for several years.

Giemsa staining

The method is used for basic chromosome analysis and is usually sufficient for counting the chromosome number and arranging horse chromosomes roughly into a karyotype.

- Stain the slides in 4% Giemsa solution in Gurr buffer for 5 minutes.
- Rinse the stain gently off with distilled water and air-dry.

G-banding

The method produces distinct banding patterns characteristic to individual horse chromosomes (Figures 22.2 and 22.3) and is used for refined chromosome analysis. It

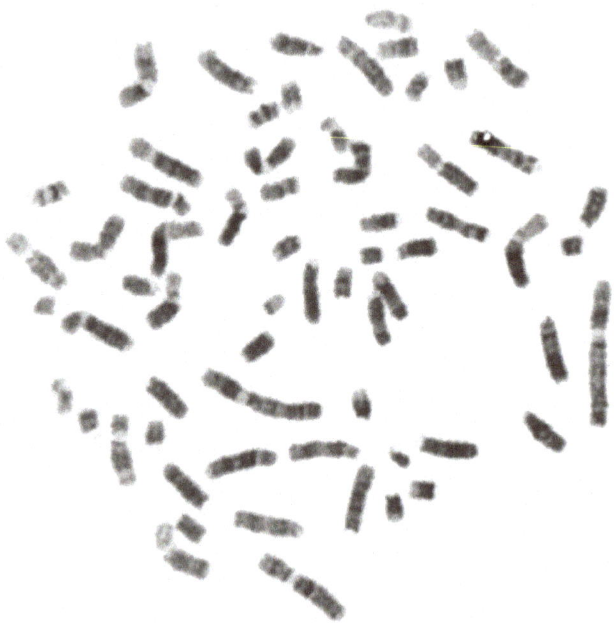

Figure 22.2 A G-banded metaphase spread of a normal male horse; magnification 1,000×.

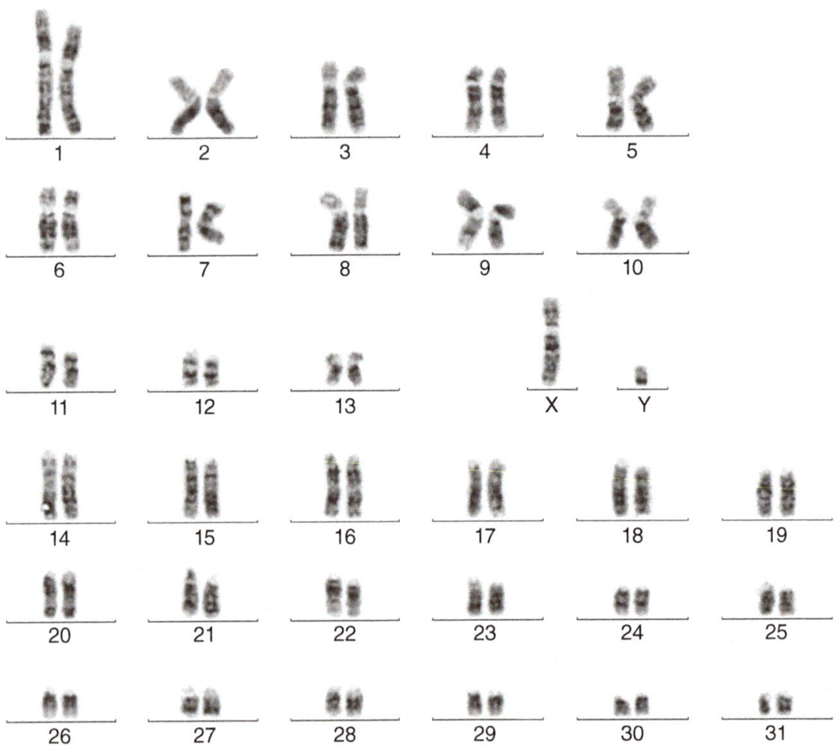

Figure 22.3 G-banded chromosomes of a normal male horse arranged into a karyotype.

allows chromosome identification, arranging them into a karyotype following the international nomenclature (Bowling *et al.* 1997), and detecting numeric and structural abnormalities. There are many modifications to the original G-banding method (Seabright 1971). The following procedure is used for G-banding at the Molecular Cytogenetics Laboratory at Texas A&M University.

- Bake slides on a hot plate at 70°C (158°F) for 10–20 minutes and allow to cool.
- Dip the slides in HBSS for 1 minute.
- Treat the slides with 0.125% trypsin working solution in HBSS for 1–5 seconds.
- Dip the slides in HBSS containing 2% FBS for 1 minute.
- Dip the slides in Gurr buffer for 1 minute.
- Stain the slides in 4% Giemsa in Gurr buffer for 5 minutes and air-dry.
- Check the quality of chromosomes and G-banding under a microscope and adjust the time of trypsin treatment and Giemsa staining if necessary.

C-banding

This method specifically highlights centromeric regions of all chromosomes and produces distinct staining pattern on horse sex chromosomes (Figure 22.4). C-banding is used to further verify the number and morphology of sex chromosomes. The method was originally developed by Arrighi and Hsu (1971) and includes the following steps:

- Treat the slides with 0.1 N HCl at room temperature for 3 minutes and rinse in distilled water.
- Treat the slides in 5% $Ba(OH)_2$ at 60°C (140°F) for 3 minutes and rinse in distilled water.

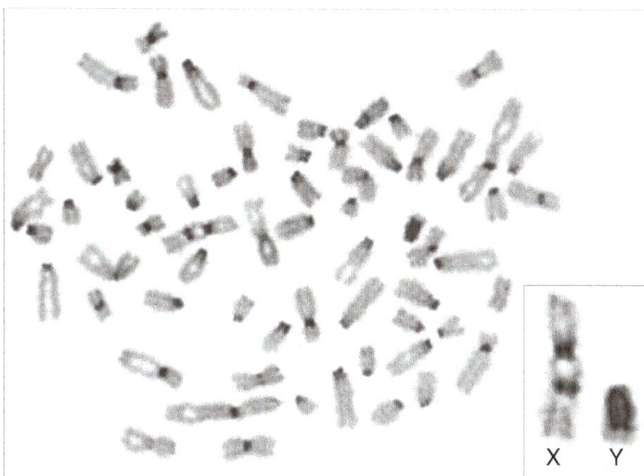

Figure 22.4 A C-banded metaphase spread of a male horse; distinct C-bands of the X and the Y chromosomes are highlighted at the lower right.

- Treat the slides for 5 minutes in 2× SSC at 60°C and rinse in distilled water.
- Stain the slides in 4% Giemsa in Gurr buffer for 1 hour, rinse gently in distilled water, and air-dry.

Note: timings of treatment steps for C-banding can vary between slides and individuals and may need adjustment.

Microscopy and image analysis

Normally, images of at least 30 metaphase spreads are captured and analyzed for each case and five representative cells are karyotyped.

Other Procedures

Polymerase Chain Reaction Test for the *SRY* Gene

In addition to chromosome analysis and karyotyping, it is a common practice in horse cytogenetics laboratories to test each case for the presence or absence of the *SRY* gene in the Y chromosome. The procedure involves polymerase chain reaction (PCR) with *SRY* primers and the genomic DNA of the horse in question. The test is useful for cases of sex reversal where a sterile female horse has XY sex chromosomes, with or without the *SRY* gene. The PCR test can also discover female horses that are mosaic or chimeric for a cell line carrying the Y chromosome.

Chromosome Analysis Time Line

Chromosome analysis from blood lymphocytes typically takes 10 working days; analysis from cell lines may take longer depending on the progression of cell cultures. The procedures and the turnaround time for the basic chromosome analysis, however, varies between service laboratories and depends on the complexity of each individual case.

Advanced Chromosome Analysis

In cases of aneuploidies (trisomies) or structural rearrangements (large deletions, translocations), fluorescence *in situ* hybridization (FISH) may be applied to confirm and refine the findings. The method uses fluorescently tagged DNA probes that are specific to individual horse chromosomes. These probes are hybridized to metaphase chromosome spreads and the results are observed under a fluorescence microscope. For example, FISH is particularly useful to identify small chromosomes involved in trisomies (Figure 22.5) or to determine the break and fusion points underlying structural rearrangements. However, the use of molecular cytogenetic methods is costly, laborious, and sets high demands on the microscopy and imaging systems,

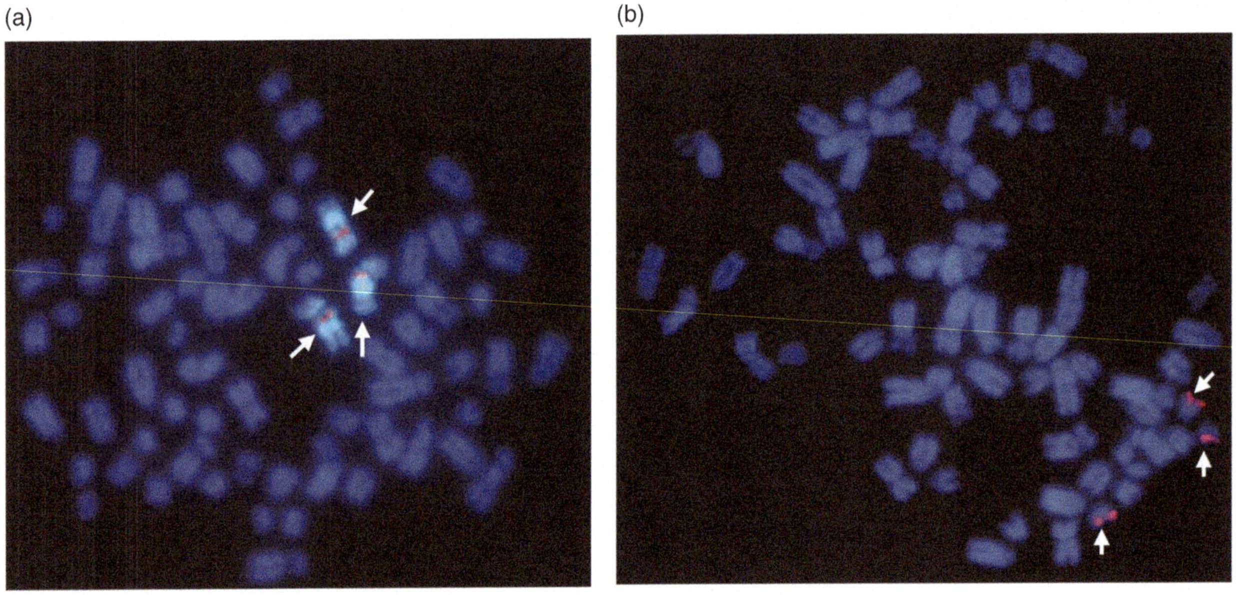

Figure 22.5 Fluorescence *in situ* hybridization (FISH) (a) with horse X chromosome probes (green and red; arrows) in an infertile mare with X-trisomy (65,XXX) and (b) with horse chromosome 30 probes (red; arrows) in a developmentally abnormal colt carrying three copies of chromosome 30 (65,XY+30).

as well as on the skills of the personnel. Therefore, molecular methods are mainly used for research and less frequently for basic chromosome analysis service.

International Horse Clinical Cytogenetic Laboratories

Only a handful of laboratories worldwide offer chromosome analysis services for horses (Table 22.1). The type of analyses offered are quite similar, although specific requirements for samples, methods used, turnaround time, and cost may vary between laboratories.

Additional Comments and Future Perspectives

With the availability of the horse genome reference sequence for the past 10 years, several new cutting edge technologies have emerged for horse genome and chromosome analysis. Single nucleotide polymorphism (SNP) arrays can detect aneuploidies and small sub-chromosomal deletions and duplications at a resolution not achieved by conventional karyotyping or FISH. An even more powerful approach is next generation sequencing (NGS), which allows the analysis of the whole genome sequence of an individual horse. Although SNP arrays and NGS are widely used in horse disease genetics, their application in clinical cytogenetics has been limited, likely because of the relatively high cost and demanding bioinformatics. Also, neither platform is able to ascertain cell to cell variations or accurately resolve mosaic/chimeric cytogenetic patterns.

Perhaps the most promising technology for next generation cytogenetics is the BioNano Genomics Irys® System, which utilizes nanochannel technology and high resolution imaging of high molecular weight DNA. The platform

Table 22.1 Horse clinical cytogenetics service laboratories in different countries.

Country, City	Laboratory	Director/Principal Investigator	Contact
Poland, Krakow	Department of Animal Reproduction, Anatomy and Genomics, University of Agriculture	Monika Bugno Poniewierska	monika.bugno.poniewierska@gmail.com
Spain, Cordoba	Department of Genetics, University of Cordoba	Miguel Moreno-Millán	Ge1momim@uco.es
Canada, Guelph	KARYOTEKK, University of Guelph	Allan W. King	info@karyotekk.com; http://www.karyotekk.com/home
USA, Texas, College Station	Molecular Cytogenetics, Texas A&M University	Terje Raudsepp	http://vetmed.tamu.edu/labs/cytogenics-genomics

can detect almost any structural or numeric changes in the genome, including balanced translocations and inversions. It is anticipated that the BioNano Irys® System will fill a role between cytogenetics and NGS, given that the estimated price per sample will get close to that of conventional clinical cytogenetic analysis.

Despite the promises of novel technology, it is unlikely that it will entirely replace conventional and FISH-based chromosome analysis in horses. Traditional cytogenetics is still the most straightforward and cost-effective approach and will remain the gold standard for the initial evaluation of breeding animals and individuals with reproductive or developmental disorders.

References

Arrighi FE, Hsu TC. 1971. Localization of heterochromatin in human chromosomes. *Cytogenetics* 10: 81–6.

Bowling AT, Breen M, Chowdhary BP, *et al.* 1997. International system for cytogenetic nomenclature of the domestic horse. Report of the Third International Committee for the Standardization of the domestic horse karyotype, Davis, CA, USA, 1996. *Chromosome Res* 5: 433–43.

Raudsepp T, Chowdhary BP. 2016. Chromosome aberrations and fertility disorders in domestic animals. *Annu Rev Anim Biosci* 4: 15–43.

Seabright M. 1971. A rapid banding technique for human chromosomes. *Lancet* 2: 971–2.

Further Reading

Durkin K, Raudsepp T, Chowdhary B. 2011. Cytogenetic evaluation of the stallion. In: McKinnon AO, Squires EL, Vaala WE, Varner DD (eds). Equine Reproduction, 2nd edn. Ames, IA: Wiley Blackwell, pp. 1462–8.

Lear TL. 2014. Chromosomal analysis. In: Dascanio J, McCue P (eds). Equine Reproductive Procedures, 1st edn. Oxford: John Wiley & Sons, Inc., pp. 77–82.

Lear TL, McGee RB. 2012. Disorders of sexual development in the domestic horse, *Equus caballus. Sex Dev* 6: 61–71.

Lear TL, Villagomez DAF. 2011. Cytogenetic evaluation of mares and foals. In: McKinnon AO, Squires EL, Vaala WE, Varner DD (eds). Equine Reproduction, 2nd edn. Ames, IA: Wiley Blackwell, pp. 1951–62.

Szczerbal I, Switonski M. 2016. Chromosome abnormalities in domestic animals as causes of disorders of sex development or impaired fertility. *IntechOpen*, doi: 10.5772/62053.

23

Endocrinological Examination

Patrick M. McCue

Equine Reproduction Laboratory, Colorado State University, USA

Introduction

Analysis of reproductive hormones in the non-pregnant mare is most commonly performed to stage the estrous cycle, evaluate corpus luteum function, and to diagnose ovarian abnormalities. Endocrine tests available for the analysis of clinical samples that may be valuable in equine practice include progesterone, inhibin, testosterone, anti-Mullerian hormone, total estrogens, conjugated estrogens, adrenocorticotrophic hormone (ACTH), and cortisol. Additional tests that may be available in specialized laboratories include equine chorionic gonadotropin, follicle-stimulating hormone, luteinizing hormone, prolactin, and relaxin.

Traditionally, blood samples and either serum or plasma samples are collected and submitted to a diagnostic laboratory for analysis. In some instances, such as wild or feral equids, endocrine analysis of urine or feces may be necessary to provide a diagnosis.

Equipment and Supplies

Vacutainer® tubes (10 ml): serum (red top tube without anticoagulant), plasma (green top tube with heparin); Vacutainer® needles, Vacutainer® needle guide, centrifuge, disposable pipettes.

Technique

- Collection of one blood sample is generally sufficient. However, because of potential variability in hormone levels in individual animals, the submission of paired samples collected at different times of the day or on subsequent days may be beneficial.
- Blood collected in a Vacutainer® tube without anticoagulant should be allowed to clot for 30 minutes. The tube should be centrifuged at 1500–1800× g and the serum aspirated with a disposable pipette and placed into a separate sterile tube for storage or shipment to an endocrine laboratory.
- Blood collected in a Vacutainer® tube containing an anticoagulant may be centrifuged immediately and the plasma subsequently transferred into a separate sterile tube using a disposable pipette.

Interpretation

- Progesterone concentrations of <0.25 ng/ml indicate an absence of luteal tissue, while concentrations >1 ng/ml indicate the presence of an active corpus luteum.
- A progesterone level between 0.25 and 1.0 ng/ml indicates the presence of a limited amount of active luteal tissue. This may be sufficient to keep a mare out of heat or keep edema from forming within endometrial tissue.
- Testosterone levels range between 20 and 45 pg/ml in the non-pregnant mare. Levels are higher in estrus and parallel levels of estradiol-17β. Approximately 50–60% of mares with ovarian granulosa/theca cell tumors have elevated concentrations of testosterone and affected mares usually exhibit aggressive or stallion-like behavior. The specific tumor type in these mares is a granulosa/theca cell tumor and the testosterone is produced by the theca cells. Mares with a granulosa cell tumor without a theca cell component will have low testosterone levels.
- Inhibin levels range from 2 to 60 pg/ml in the non-pregnant mare. Concentrations are highest in estrus and decline rapidly after ovulation. Inhibin is elevated in approximately 90% of mares with granulosa cell tumors.
- A diagnostic panel consisting of inhibin, testosterone, and progesterone is commonly used to detect the presence, or suggest the absence, of an ovarian granulosa cell

Equine Reproductive Procedures, Second Edition. Edited by John Dascanio and Patrick McCue.

tumor (Table 23.1). Elevation in progesterone indicates the presence of luteal tissue and suggests that a tumor is not likely to be present.

- Equine chorionic gonadotropin levels may be evaluated to determine pregnancy status or determine the presence or absence of retained endometrial cups in non-pregnant mares. Mares may exhibit abnormal estrous cycles and repeated cycles with hemorrhagic or luteinized anovulatory follicles.
- Anti-Müllerian hormone (AMH) testing is performed primarily to detect the presence of granulosa cell tumors of the ovary. The concentration of AMH in a mare with a granulosa cell tumor is higher than that in normal mares. The sensitivity of an elevated AMH level for the presence of a granulosa cell tumor has been reported to be 98%.
- Another potential use for an AMH test could be to determine the presence or absence of ovaries in a mare. AMH levels should be at baseline concentrations in an ovariectomized mare, but would be detectable in an intact mare.
- ACTH and cortisol levels may be useful in evaluating mares suspected of pituitary pars intermedia dysfunction (PPID) or equine Cushing's disease. Concentrations of ACTH and cortisol are commonly elevated in mares with PPID. A dexamethasone suppression test is considered the gold standard for PPID diagnosis. Affected mares may exhibit failure of follicular development, ovulation failure, or reduced fertility.

Table 23.1 Granulosa cell tumor (GCT) diagnostic panel of hormone reference ranges. Note that reference ranges from individual laboratories may vary slightly.

Hormone	Normal Range	% Elevated in Mares with GCTs
Anti-Müllerian hormone	0.1–6.9 ng/ml	98%
Inhibin	2–60 pg/ml	90%
Testosterone	20–45 pg/ml	50–60%
Progesterone	<1.0 ng/ml in estrus or anestrus >1.0 ng/ml in diestrus or pregnancy	<1%

Further Reading

Almeida J, Ball BA, Conley AJ, *et al.* 2011. Biological and clinical significance of anti-Mullerian hormone determination in blood serum of the mare. *Theriogenology* 76: 1393–403.

Anderson RA, Nelson SM, Wallace WHB. 2012. Measuring anti-Müllerian hormone for the assessment of ovarian reserve: when and for whom is it indicated? *Maturitas* 71: 28–33.

McCue PM, Roser JF, Munro CJ, *et al.* 2006. Granulosa cell tumors of the equine ovary. *Vet Clin North Am Eq Pract* 22: 799–817.

24

Laparoscopic Examination of the Female Reproductive Track with Ovarian Biopsy

Dean A. Hendrickson

College of Veterinary Medicine and Biomedical Sciences, Colorado State University, USA

Introduction

Laparoscopy is a minimally invasive procedure used in the evaluation and treatment of a large variety of medical conditions in the horse. Laparoscopy allows the objective visual assessment of the ovaries, uterine body and horns, and broad ligament. Examples of how laparoscopy can be used in the area of equine reproduction include ovary evaluation and removal, ovarian biopsy, evaluation of the oviduct, delivery of microspheres into the infundibulum of the oviduct, and application of prostaglandin E_2 (PGE_2) to the surface of the oviducts. The primary disadvantages of laparoscopy are the initial cost of the equipment and the specialized surgical training required.

Technique

- The mare should be held off-feed for at least 12 hours, or placed in a low residue diet for 18–24 hours, prior to surgery.
- The mare is restrained in the stocks and a 14 gauge IV catheter placed in either jugular vein. The mare is then sedated with a combination of detomidine hydrochloride (0.01 mg/kg IV) and butorphanol tartrate (0.01 mg/kg IV) or similar sedatives. Timing of the initial sedation will depend upon the mare's degree of cooperation.
- A transrectal exam should be performed prior to surgery in order to determine the amount of ingesta in the colon and the location and size of the spleen and cecum relative to the anticipated sites of the portals as well as the size of the ovaries.
- The paralumbar fossa(s) are clipped and prepared for surgery. The landmarks for the surgical area in the paralumbar fossa are:
  - Cranially – last four ribs.
  - Dorsally – above the transverse processes of the lumbar vertebrae.
  - Caudally – caudal to the tuber coxae.
  - Ventrally – skin fold of the flank.
- The chosen paralumbar fossa(s) is (are) completely clipped and cleaned using an antiseptic scrub or non-

Equipment and Supplies

Hair clippers, antiseptic scrub, sterile towels and drapes, 0.9% saline (1 liter bag), xylazine hydrochloride, butorphanol tartrate, detomidine hydrochloride, 14 gauge IV catheter and extension set, 2% lidocaine, 60 ml syringe, 20 gauge 4 cm (1.5 inch) needles, no. 10 scalpel blade, basic surgical instruments.

Laparoscopy equipment

0 or 30 degrees, 10 mm OD, 57 cm (22 inch) (preferred) or 33 cm (13 inch) long scope, 5 mm ID reducing cannulas, 10 mm ID cannulas with matching obturators (blunt tips reduce the possibility of bowel puncture) with one-way valve systems, atraumatic grasping forceps, 10 mm OD scissors, 10 mm OD electrosurgical forceps, 10 mm OD laparoscopic grasping forceps, 10 mm OD laparoscopic biopsy forceps, 10 mm OD laparoscopic retractors. Endoscopy tower: monitor, camera, 300 W xenon light source with long large diameter light cable, CO_2 insufflator, digital or analog recorder (optional but recommended), printer (optional but recommended).

Equine Reproductive Procedures, Second Edition. Edited by John Dascanio and Patrick McCue.

residual liquid soap, rinsed with water, and dried with sterile towels.

- This is followed by a sterile preparation of the surgical site with povidone-iodine and alcohol or chlorhexidine and sterile saline.
- The fossa is then desensitized using regional anesthesia with lidocaine or by direct infiltration of the proposed laparoscope and instrument portal sites.
- A 1 liter bag of isotonic saline with 20 mg of detomidine is prepared and a continuous intravenous infusion of this solution is started and titrated to effect.
- If both flanks are prepared for surgery, the surgery is generally started on the left side in order to take advantage of the location of the spleen to reduce the possibility of visceral perforation.
- The first 1.5 cm long incision is actually the middle portal and should be located at the level of the proximal border of the internal abdominal oblique muscle, midway between the last rib and the coxal tuberosity, aiming slightly caudally. At this position, it is possible to use the endoscope to observe the creation of the other portals, making it safer for the mare (Figure 24.1).
- To avoid inadvertently insufflating the retroperitoneal space, a cannula with a blunt obturator is inserted through the paralumbar fossa prior to insufflation of the abdominal cavity. The laparoscope is inserted to confirm the location of the cannula within the peritoneal cavity. The endoTIP (endoscopic threaded imaging port) cannula also provides optical control of the cannula's insertion.
- Insufflation can be initiated or maintained once the cannula is in the peritoneal space. Normally, the peritoneal space is insufflated with CO_2 to about 10–12 mmHg of pressure. Regardless of the chosen technique, if performed correctly, studies have identified that this momentary iatrogenic intra-abdominal hypertension is not harmful for the sedated horse.
- If insufflation is performed through the 10 mm trocar and the abdominal cavity can be immediately visualized and explored, the additional portals can be created while monitoring the insertion of the other cannulas by direct visualization with the laparoscope. It is difficult to see the cannulas from the ipsilateral flank.
- The telescope is positioned in the dorsal portal and initial evaluation of the abdominal cavity and the female reproductive tract should be performed in a systematic manner.
- Ovarian and uterine size, shape, and overall appearance should be evaluated, and obvious space-occupying masses, tears, adhesions, and any other external abnormalities should be documented by means of photography and/or video recording. If a visual diagnosis alone is not enough for a therapeutic plan, a biopsy of the affected area, ovaries, uterus, or supportive tissues should be considered.

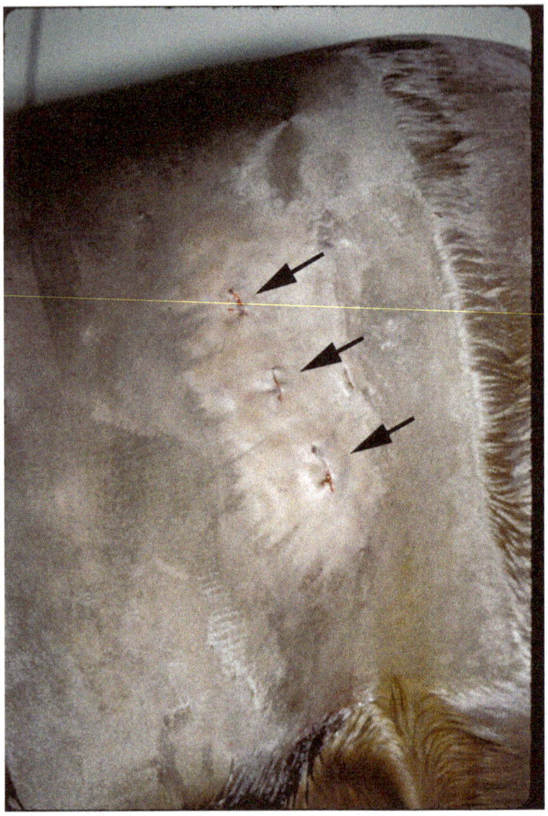

Figure 24.1 Sites for insertion of trocars (arrows) in the paralumbar fossa for general abdominal laparoscopy.

Ovarian Biopsy Technique

- The area to be biopsied is selected and a laparoscopy aspiration needle is inserted through one of the instrument portals. A syringe with 2% lidocaine or mepivicaine is then connected to the Luer lock end of the needle and is pushed into the selected area. A moderate amount of anesthetic is then injected (2–5 ml) as the needle is retracted; 2–3 minutes should lapse before attempting to collect the sample.
- Once sufficient time after local anesthesia has lapsed, the ovary or uterus should be secured by applying an atraumatic grasping forceps to the organ itself or to its suspensory ligament.
- The biopsy instrument is then introduced through a second portal and with the organ secured the instrument is then opened and pushed into the organ. Once in position, the jaw of the biopsy forceps is closed firmly to

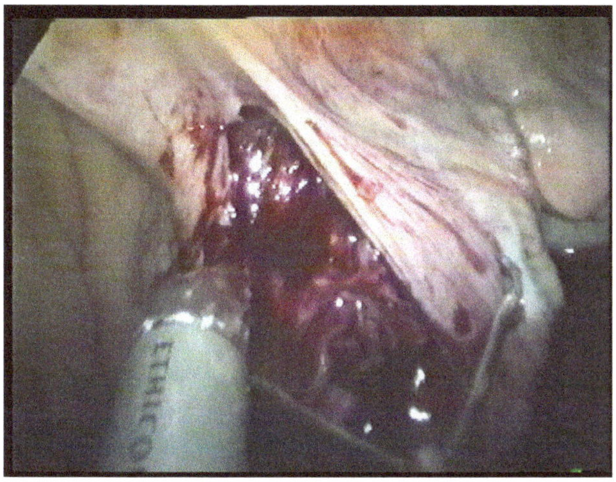

Figure 24.2 Collection of an ovarian biopsy.

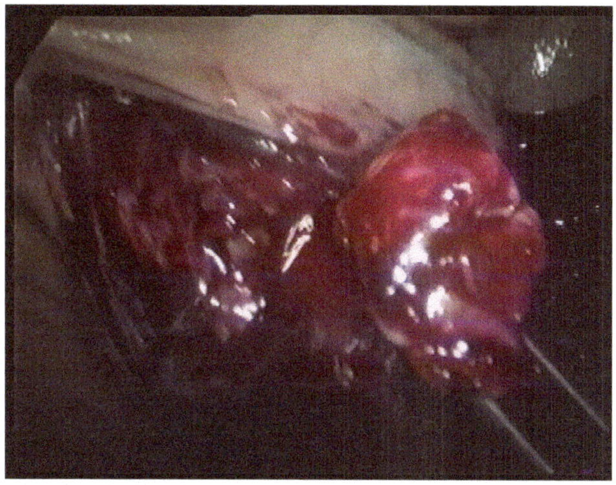

Figure 24.3 Removal of an ovarian biopsy sample.

collect a small sample (1–2 cm) of tissue (Figures 24.2 and 24.3).

- Bleeding can be controlled with an electrosurgical forceps. The ovary and/or uterus should be observed for at least 3–4 minutes to ensure that all bleeding has stopped prior to removing the instruments from the abdomen. Another option is to use a hernia stapling device to staple the capsule of the ovary back together.
- The biopsy sample is then placed into fixative solution (i.e., 10% formalin). The container should be labeled with the name of the mare, collection date, and other pertinent information.
- The fixed biopsy specimen can then be submitted to a pathology laboratory.
- The instruments are withdrawn and the skin incision site is sutured closed.
- Postoperative care may include administration of a non-steroidal anti-inflammatory drug, such as flunixin meglumine (1.0 mg/kg IV), and, as needed based on the individual clinical case, administration of antimicrobial agents. The horse should be examined periodically after the conclusion of the procedure to monitor comfort level as well as localized swelling, pain, heat, or discharge at the incision sites.

Further Reading

Caron JP. 2009. Equine laparoscopic surgery: here to stay? *Eq Vet Educ* 21(6): 301–2.

Caron JP. 2012. Equine laparoscopy: equipment and basic principles. *Compend Contin Educ Vet* 34(3): E1–E7.

Fisher AT, Jr. 2001. Equine Diagnostic and Surgical Laparoscopy. Philadelphia: WB Saunders.

Hendrickson DA. 2012a. A review of equine laparoscopy. ISRN Vet Sci 2012: article ID 492650.

Hendrickson DA. 2012b. Diagnostic techniques. In: Ragle CA (ed.). Advances in Equine Laparoscopy. Ames, IA: Wiley Blackwell, pp. 83–91.

25

Evaluation of the Mammary Gland

Patrick M. McCue

Equine Reproduction Laboratory, Colorado State University, USA

Introduction

The mammary gland plays a key role in allowing the fetus to survive outside the uterus. It is responsible for providing the neonate with colostral antibodies critical to survival and supplies nutrition to the foal during the first few months of life. The equine mammary gland is located high in the inguinal region of the mare. The equine mammary gland is divided into left and right halves by a connective tissue septum, each with a glandular body and teat. The glandular portion of each half is further divided by fibroelastic capsules into cranial and caudal lobes. Each of the two teats serves a cranial and caudal lobe of mammary tissue and has two teat orifices (Figure 25.1).

Abnormalities of the equine mammary gland include agalactia, premature lactation, inappropriate lactation, and mastitis. Less common issues include abscessation, neoplasia, and trauma.

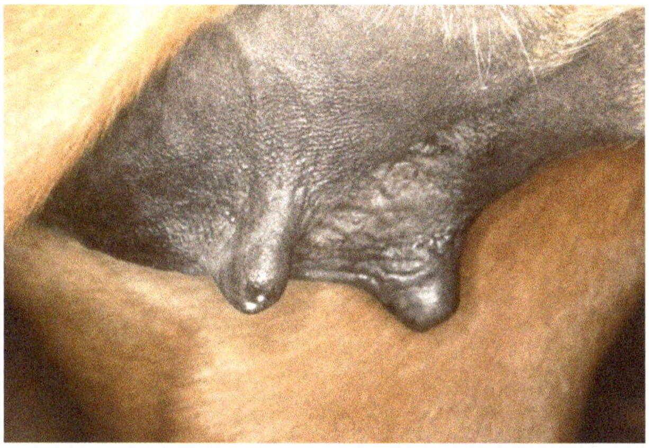

Figure 25.1 Mammary gland of a mare. Note the two teat orifices visible on the end of the right teat.

Equipment and Supplies

Exam glove, alcohol swabs, sterile container (red top tube, urine cup, etc.), culture transport system, glass microscope slides, cytology stain, microscope, ultrasound.

Techinque

- A visual assessment of the mammary gland should be performed initially. Udder size, shape, and symmetry should be assessed and related to the reproductive status of the mare (non-pregnant, late-term pregnant, postpartum, post-weaning, etc.).
- The pregnant mare's udder will increase in size over the last 4–6 weeks of gestation. Nulliparous mares may not have much udder development until 1–2 weeks prior to parturition or even not until parturition. Fescue toxicosis should be ruled out in cases of poor udder development.
- Foals born to mares with abnormally large teats may have difficulty nursing due to an inability to form a proper suction. These foals should be watched closely for adequate ingestion of milk and weighed daily to ensure intake.
- A manual examination of the udder should be performed next. A hot, swollen, painful quarter is consistent with acute mastitis (Figure 25.2). In addition, edema may be present cranial to the udder in affected mares (Figure 25.3). Edema may also be present in normal mares near foaling as the blood vessels to the udder develop, due to the position of the *in utero* foal decreasing venous return and due to mare inactivity in late pregnancy.
- Mares with inappropriate lactation or galactorrhea, such as may occur secondary to pituitary pars intermedia dysfunction, often have a small to moderate amount of mammary secretion produced in all four quarters and the overall gland is not hot or painful (Figure 25.4).

Equine Reproductive Procedures, Second Edition. Edited by John Dascanio and Patrick McCue.

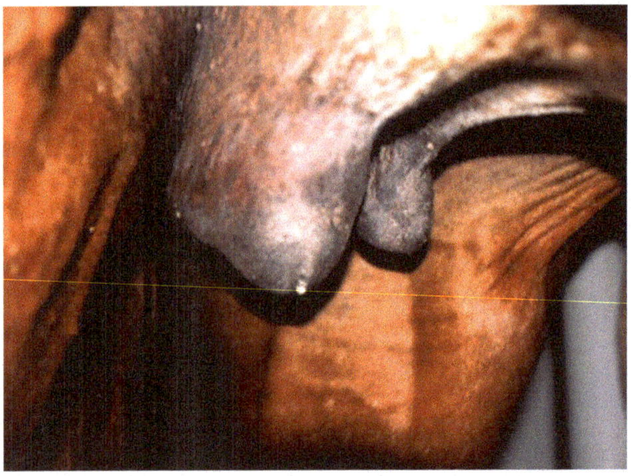

Figure 25.2 Enlargement of the right rear quarter of a mare secondary to mastitis.

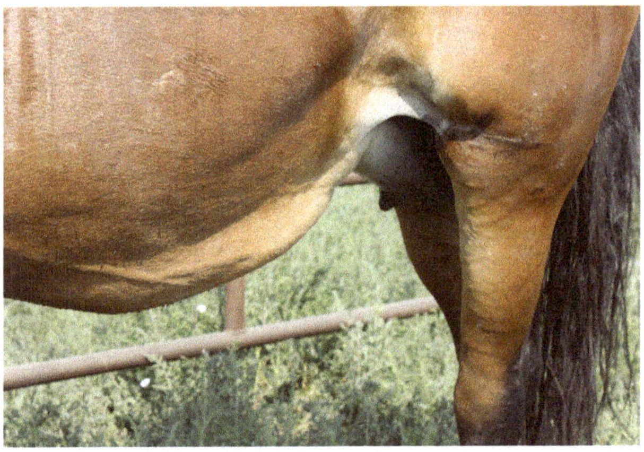

Figure 25.3 Edema cranial to the udder in a mare with mastitis.

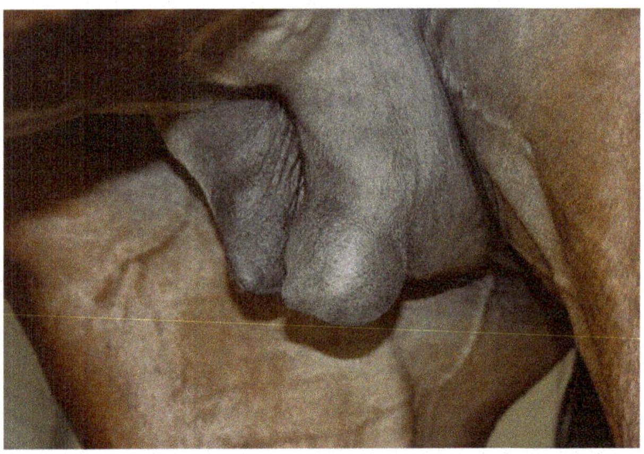

Figure 25.4 Enlargement of the entire udder in a mare with galactorrhea secondary to pituitary pars intermedia dysfunction.

Sometimes, normal, older multiparous mares may have large teat or gland cisterns that fill with secretions without active lactation or pregnancy.

- Mammary fluid should be expressed and the character of the fluid assessed. Mastitic fluid is typically thick, white to slightly yellow in color (Figure 25.5), and may be blood tinged.
- A cytologic evaluation of the mammary fluid may be indicated if mastitis or neoplasia is suspected. Mare milk produced during normal lactation and mammary secretion from a non-pregnant, non-foaling mare with inappropriate lactation should not have a large number of white blood cells on cytology. In contrast, white blood cells are abundant in mares with mastitis (Figure 25.6).
- The teat should be cleaned of dirt/debris and the end disinfected with an alcohol swab prior to expression of milk for bacteriological culture (see Chapter 106).
- Secretions should be collected from the teat into a sterile container.

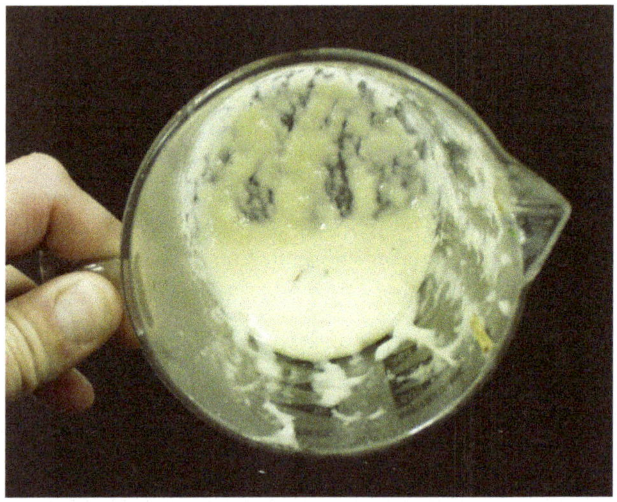

Figure 25.5 Thick inflammatory fluid expressed from the udder of a mare with mastitis.

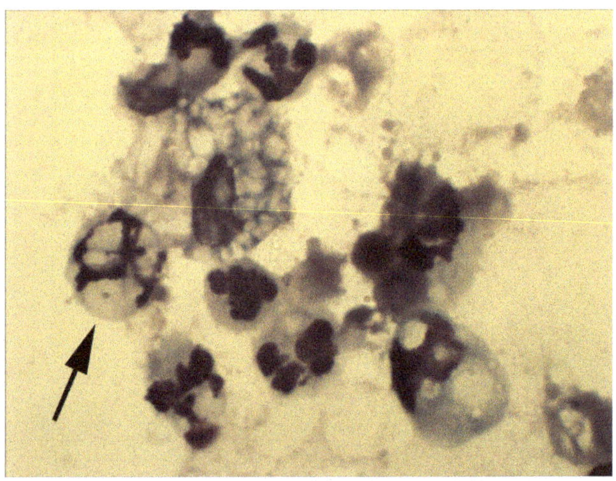

Figure 25.6 Cytologic evaluation of mammary fluid from a mare with mastitis. Note the large number of degenerated white blood cells (arrow).

- A culture of mammary secretion should be performed if mastitis is suspected. Equine mastitis is usually bacterial in origin and the most common organisms are *Streptococcus equi* subspecies *zooepidemicus* and *Staphylococcus* species. Gram-negative organisms such as *Escherichia coli* and *Klebsiella* species are less commonly isolated.
- An ultrasound examination may be performed following manual assessment of the mammary gland to evaluate a region for a potential mammary tumor or abscess. Application of isopropyl alcohol to the skin may be needed to provide adequate probe contact.
- Biopsy of the mammary gland may be indicated for histologic verification of neoplasia. However, tumors of the equine mammary gland are rare and consequently biopsies of the udder are rarely performed.
- At weaning the foal should be removed from the mare and the mare should not be milked. The active pressure within the aveoli will cause milk production to cease. Some mares may experience slight pain for 1–2 days upon removal of the foal.

Further Reading

Gee EK, McCue PM. 2011. Mastitis. In: McKinnon AO, Squires EL, Vaala WE, Varner DD (eds). Equine Reproduction, 2nd edn. Ames, IA: Wiley Blackwell, pp. 2738–41.

McCue PM, Sitters S. 2011. Lactation. In: McKinnon AO, Squires EL, Vaala WE, Varner DD (eds). Equine Reproduction, 2nd edn. Ames, IA: Wiley Blackwell, pp. 2277–90.

Waldridge BM, Ward TA. 1999. Ultrasound examination of the equine mammary gland. *Eq Pract* 21: 10–13.

26

Antisperm Antibody Testing

Patrick M. McCue

Equine Reproduction Laboratory, Colorado State University, USA

Introduction

Antisperm antibodies (ASAs) have been suggested to be a cause of infertility in both males and females of a number of species, including mice, rabbits, cattle, horses, humans, and other species. IgG, IgA, and IgM antibodies directed against sperm antigens have been detected in various fluids and tissues.

Published studies have reported that 13–77% of women with unexplained infertility have ASAs detected in their serum. Mechanical or chemical disruption of the mucosal layer of the female genital tract has been proposed as the mechanism by which exposure to the "foreign" sperm antigen occurs. An immune response subsequently develops following exposure to sperm antigens.

Potential mechanisms by which ASAs may adversely affect fertility in the female of various species include:

- Prevention of sperm from undergoing capacitation.
- Prevention of sperm binding to the oocyte.
- Prevention of sperm from undergoing the acrosome reaction.
- Prevention of sperm from penetration of the zona pellucida.
- Interference with early embryonic development.
- Interference with maintenance of the pregnancy.

Technique

Assays for ASAs in various species include immunobead assays, mixed antiglobulin reaction tests, enzyme-linked immunosorbant assays, immunofluorescence tests, tube-slide agglutination tests, tray agglutination tests, flow cytometry, and radiolabeled agglutination tests. Pitfalls and false-positive results have apparently been associated with all of the diagnostic tests for ASAs.

There are currently no diagnostic laboratories offering tests to determine the presence or absence of ASAs in equine serum or seminal plasma.

Additional Comments

In the horse, two case reports have associated the presence of ASAs in subfertile stallions that experienced testicular trauma. One study evaluated the prevalence of ASAs in a population of mares and reported that 10.2% of horses had ASAs in their serum. A pair of studies evaluated the immune response of mares actively immunized against stallion sperm cells. The authors concluded that IgG antibodies, and to a lesser extent IgA antibodies, against sperm cells increased following immunization, but there was no apparent decrease in fertility. A recent study reported that the percentage of IgG antibody bound spermatozoa were higher in non-satisfactory breeder stallions than in satisfactory breeder stallions.

Clearly, additional studies are needed to determine the incidence of ASAs in mares with a history of subfertility or infertility. Furthermore, the relationship (if any) between the presence of ASAs and failure to conceive or failure to remain pregnant needs further investigation.

Equine Reproductive Procedures, Second Edition. Edited by John Dascanio and Patrick McCue.

Further Reading

Day MJ. 1996. Detection of equine antisperm antibodies by indirect immunofluorescence and the tube-slide agglutination test. *Eq Vet J* 28: 494–6.

Ferrer MS, George A, Miller LMJ, *et al.* 2014. Diagnosis of sperm-bound anti-sperm antibodies by flow cytometry and their association with semen quality. *J Eq Vet Sci* 34: 57.

Lee C, Nie GJ, Joo HS, Momont H. 1993. An enzyme-linked immunosorbent assay (ELISA) for the detection of antisperm antibodies in horse serum. *Theriogenology* 40: 1117–26.

Mazumdar S, Levine AS. 1998. Antisperm antibodies: etiology, pathogenesis, diagnosis, and treatment. *Fertil Steril* 70: 799–810.

Nie GJ, Lee C, Momont HW, Joo HS. 1993. Equine antisperm antibodies (EASA): preliminary study of the clinical response following breeding in immunized mares. *Theriogenology* 40: 1107–16.

Papa FO, Alvarenga MA, Lopes MD, Campos Filho EP. 1990. Infertility of autoimmune origin in a stallion. *Eq Vet J* 22: 145–6.

Risvanli A, Cetin H, Apaydin AM, Kkorkmaz O, Atli MO, Timurkan H. 2005. Prevalence of anti-sperm antibodies in mares in the south-eastern Anatolian of Turkey. *Bull Vet Inst Pulawy* 49: 45–8.

Zhang J, Ricketts SW, Tanner SJ. 1990. Antisperm antibodies in the semen of a stallion following testicular trauma. *Eq Vet J* 22: 138-41.

27

Starch Granule Test for the Evaluation of Oviductal Patency

Sofie Sitters[1] and John J. Dascanio[2]

[1]*Amsterdam, The Netherlands*
[2]*School of Veterinary Medicine, Texas Tech University, USA*

Introduction

The oviduct plays a critical role during fertilization and early embryonic development. Consequently, pathologic conditions of the oviduct such as salpingitis, hydrosalpinx, and occlusion can adversely affect fertility of mares.

Blockage of the oviducts by masses of collagen, fibroblast cells, and other cellular and non-cellular debris has been described. These oviductal masses can become a physical obstruction to both the upward passage of sperm and the downward passage of an embryo after fertilization. Diagnosis, however, of a blocked oviduct may be difficult and is sometimes suspected after exclusion of other possibilities for infertility in a mare.

This chapter describes the starch granule test for the diagnosis of oviductal patency. The starch granule test involves the deposition of a starch suspension onto the ovarian surface (through a transabdominal approach with a long needle) and the subsequent recovery of starch from the uterus or cervix. One oviduct can be tested at a time.

Equipment and Supplies

Surgical scrub, clippers, sterile soluble starch powder (1 g), sterile water (10 ml), sterile saline, 2% lidocaine, 2% Lugol's iodine, microscope slides, coverslips, microscope, 14 gauge 5 cm (2 inch) needle, 18 gauge 12.5 cm (5 inch) spinal needle, syringes, obstetrical sleeve, obstetrical lubricant, sterile lavage tubing (optional).

Technique

- The mare should be in diestrus for the procedure. Estrual mares may have a delay in oviductal transport.
- A suspension of starch granules is made by mixing 1 g of sterile soluble starch powder in 10 ml of sterile water.
- The flank of the mare is clipped and a sterile prep performed.
- 5 ml of 2% lidocaine is infiltrated subcutaneously and into deeper muscle layers in the flank area corresponding to the needle puncture for starch deposition.
- As an optional procedure, one can create a puncture hole through the skin with either a small scalpel blade or a 14 gauge needle.
- The ovary is held per rectum against the ipsilateral flank and a percutaneous needle puncture is made through the skin, or the previous puncture hole, with an 18 gauge 12.5 cm (5 inch) spinal needle to deposit 5 ml of starch solution on the ovarian surface.
- The external cervical os and vagina are flushed with 10 ml of sterile saline beginning 24 hours after application of the starch solution (original description of the test). The fluid is recovered by aspiration back into the syringe.
- Alternatively, the uterus of the mare could be lavaged with sterile saline through a catheter and inflatable cuff. The recovered fluid is allowed to sediment or is centrifuged.
- An aliquot of the recovered fluid is placed onto a microscope slide and stained using a few drops of 2% Lugol's iodine. A coverslip is then placed over the admixture.
- The solution is examined with conventional light microscopy with the 10× objective for the presence of stained starch granules (dark blue granules).
- The presence of starch granules in the uterine fluid suggests that the oviduct is patent.
- Another option for deposition of the starch granules onto the surface of the ovary would be via laparoscopy or a transvaginal needle.

Equine Reproductive Procedures, Second Edition. Edited by John Dascanio and Patrick McCue.

Additional Comments

The starch granule procedure is relatively easy to perform and does not require specialized equipment, technology, or training. However, the starch granule test requires individual testing of each oviduct on separate estrous cycles. The rate of transport through the oviduct is decreased significantly if the starch granules are applied at the time of ovulation. In the original report, granules were evident in the vagina of all mares by 24 hours, except when applied onto an ovulating ovary, in which case granules were not identified until at least 4 days later. The starch mixture contains granules of varying size (4–120 μm diameter), but only small granules (6–56 μm) are usually recovered from the uterus or cervix. These granules are significantly smaller than an early equine embryo (150–250 μm). There is considerable variability in the transport and recovery of all markers. As with other tests evaluating natural oviductal transport of markers, the starch granule test is not considered to be highly reliable or accurate in the detection of oviductal blockage.

Further Reading

Allen WE, Kessy BM, Noakes DE. 1979. Evaluation of uterine tube function in pony mares. *Vet Rec* 105: 364–6.

Kenney RM. 1993. A review of the pathology of the equine oviduct. *Eq Vet J Suppl* 15: 42–6.

Liu IKM, Lantz KC, Schalafke S, *et al.* 1990. Clinical observations of oviductal masses in the mare. *Proc Annu Conv Am Assoc Eq Pract* 36: 41–5.

Tsutsumi Y, Suzuki H, Takeda T, Terami Y. 1979. Evidence of the origin of the gelatinous masses in the oviducts of mares. *J Reprod Fertil* 57: 287–90.

28

Fluorescent Microspheres Test for Evaluation of Oviductal Patency

Sofie Sitters[1] *and John J. Dascanio*[2]

[1] *Amsterday, The Netherlands*
[2] *School of Veterinary Medicine, Texas Tech University, USA*

Introduction

Blockage of one or both oviducts with intraluminal gelatinous masses can result in reduction of fertility in the mare. The starch granule test has limitations for evaluation of oviductal patency in the mare. One limitation is the inability to evaluate both oviducts simultaneously. A second concern is the size variation of the starch granules that typically seem to pass through the tested oviducts and that these granules are significantly smaller than the diameter of an early equine embryo.

Consequently, fluorescent microspheres have been used as an alternative to evaluate oviductal patency. The clear advantage of using fluorescent microspheres over the starch granule test is that use of two colors of beads can discriminate between patency of the left and right oviduct, making it possible to demonstrate patency of both the mare's oviducts in a single procedure. A solution containing fluorescent microspheres is deposited onto the surface of the ovary using a transvaginal ultrasound probe and needle or applied into the proximal oviductal lumen via a laparoscope. This technique requires access to either a fluorescent microscope or a flow cytometer.

Equipment and Supplies

Examination gloves, tail wrap, tail rope, non-irritant soap, bucket, disposable bucket liner, roll cotton, obstetrical sleeves, obstetrical lubricant, twitch, sedation, fluorescent microspheres (15 µm in diameter) in two colors (i.e., red and green). Option 1: ultrasound with transvaginal probe and 60 cm (24 inch) 18 gauge single channel needle. Option 2: laparoscope and 8 Fr catheter. Uterine lavage catheter, 0.9% sterile saline or lactated Ringer's solution, flow cytometer or fluorescent microscope.

Transvaginal Ultrasound Technique

- The mare should be in diestrus for the procedure. Estrual mares may have a delay in oviductal transport.
- A tail wrap and tail rope are placed and the perineum washed in standard fashion (see Chapter 3 & Chapter 4).
- The vaginal vault is rinsed with 500 ml solution of sterile saline containing 0.05% povidone-iodine followed by a rinse with 450 ml sterile saline containing 50 ml of 2% lidocaine.
- A sterilized transvaginal probe is passed into the anterior vagina.
- One ovary is grasped per rectum and stabilized near the probe head.
- The 18 gauge 60 cm (24 inch) single channel needle is passed along the channel of the probe and the vaginal wall is punctured. A twitch may be applied prior to this or sedation provided to the mare, since puncture of the vaginal wall may cause a response by the mare.
- 5 ml of sterile saline containing 2 million fluorescent microspheres (Triton Technology, Inc., San Diego, CA, USA) is deposited over the surface of the ovary. One color of fluorescent microspheres may be applied to the left ovary and a different color microsphere is applied to the right ovary.
- The uterus is lavaged 24 and/or 48 hours later with 1 liter of sterile saline.
- The recovered fluid is centrifuged at 1,500 rpm for 10 minutes.
- The pellet is resuspended in 5 ml sterile saline.
- The sample is evaluated by flow cytometry for the presence and fluorescence pattern of microspheres. Alternatively, the presence of beads may be detected by fluorescent microscopy.

Equine Reproductive Procedures, Second Edition. Edited by John Dascanio and Patrick McCue.

Laparoscope Technique

- Mares are evaluated during diestrus.
- The standard preparation for standing flank laparoscopy is performed (see Chapter 24).
- The ostium of the oviduct is grasped with forceps.
- An 8 Fr polypropylene catheter passed through the biopsy channel is used to cannulate the proximal oviduct.
- Approximately 1 ml of solution containing 2 million fluorescent microspheres in 0.5% carboxymethylcellulose is infused into the oviduct (when possible) or spread onto the mucosal surface of the infundibulum.
- A second procedure is performed on the opposite ovary using a new catheter and different colored microspheres.
- The uterus is lavaged 48 hours after surgery with three 1-liter flushes of lactated Ringer's solution. The fluid is recovered into a 5-liter graduated cylinder.
- The beads are allowed to settle for 1 hour and the supernatant decanted.
- 100 ml of fluid is aspirated from the bottom and transferred into two 50 ml centrifuge tubes.
  The tubes are centrifuged for 10 minutes at 500× g.
- The supernatant is removed, and the pellets are combined and examined for the presence of beads by fluorescent microscopy.

Additional Comments

In a study using laparoscopy, fluorescent beads were recovered from the uterus of 86% of mares with oviducts without plugs (determined by flushing excised oviducts at necropsy) as compared with only 29% of mares with oviducts containing plugs. Interestingly, 92.8% of oviducts contained beads of both colors, suggesting intraperitoneal bead movement. Ultimately, the study noted a 71.4% ability of the test to correctly detect a mare with plugs (test sensitivity) and an 85.7% ability of the procedure to correctly detect a mare without plugs (test specificity). The absence of fluorescent beads in the uterine lumen is suggestive of, but not conclusive evidence for, a blocked oviduct.

As with the starch granule test, the diameter of the microspheres used in the published studies are considerably smaller, at 15 μm, than an oocyte or early developing oviductal stage embryo (150–250 μm) and may not be the ideal size for the detection of a mass that would impede embryo transport distally through the isthmus and into the uterus.

Transvaginal deposition may result in a variable amount of beads entering the infundibulum; whereas, laparoscopic cannulation results in more accurate placement of beads. Laparoscopic deposition does, however, require a certain technical skill and specialized equipment. Laparoscopic deposition of beads also allows for direct observation of the oviduct. Mares with oviductal pathology may exhibit oviductal swelling, and an increase in vascularity or adhesions.

Further Reading

Arnold CE, Love CC. 2013. Laparoscopic evaluation of oviductal patency in the standing mare. *Theriogenology* 79: 905–10.

Kollmann M, Rotting A, Heberling A, Sieme H. 2011. Laparoscopic techniques for investigating the equine oviduct. *Eq Vet J* 43: 106–11.

Ley WB, Bowen JM, Purswell BJ, *et al.* 1998. Modified technique to evaluate uterine tubal patency in the mare. *Proc Annu Conv Am Assoc Eq Pract* 44: 73–104.

29

Oviductal Flush Procedure for the Evaluation of Oviductal Patency

Sofie Sitters[1] *and Patrick M. McCue*[2]

[1] *Amsterdam, The Netherlands*
[2] *Equine Reproduction Laboratory, Colorado State University, USA*

Introduction

Blockage of one or both oviducts with intraluminal gelatinous mases consisting of a mixture of collagen, fibroblast cells, and other debris, can result in reduction of fertility in the mare. Access to the oviduct for both diagnostic and therapeutic purposes is limited. As discussed in Chapters 27 and 28, both the diagnostic starch granule test and the fluorescent microspheres test have their limitations for the evaluation of oviductal patency in the mare and neither method treats a potentially blocked oviduct.

Flushing of the oviduct has been performed as both a diagnostic and a therapeutic procedure. Techniques have included retrograde flushing from the utero-tubular junction (UTJ) proximally toward the infundibulum and normograde flushing from the infundibulum distally toward the uterus using either a standing flank laparoscopic or ventral midline laparotomy approach. In addition, retrograde flushing of the oviduct via the UTJ is possible using a standing hysteroscopic approach (see Chapter 32).

Oviductal flush techniques are reserved for mares that have a prolonged history of infertility, with good breeding management, bred to fertile stallion(s), and that have no other significant reproductive abnormalities noted during a breeding soundness evaluation.

Retrograde Oviductal Flush (Laparotomy Approach) Technique

Performed under general anesthesia.

- The mare is fasted for 24 hours prior to surgery.
- Antibiotics and flunixin meglumine (1.1 mg/kg, IV, s.i.d.) are administered prior to surgery and after surgery as needed.
- The mare is placed under general anesthesia and in dorsal recumbency.
- The ventral abdomen is clipped free of hair.
- A standard surgical prep is made over the ventral abdomen.
- Two paramedian incisions are made in the caudal ventral abdomen through the skin and blunt dissection is used to pass through the external and internal abdominal oblique muscles.
- A hand is passed into the abdomen and the adjacent ovary and uterine horn tip are exteriorized.
- A small incision is made near the uterine horn tip and the uterus is everted to expose the papilla of the UTJ.
- The papilla is cannulated with the blunt-ended catheter.
- The oviduct is flushed retrograde with sterile saline containing fluorescein dye.
- The infundibulum end of the oviduct is observed for the presence of colored saline which may contain masses.
- The procedures are repeated on the contralateral oviduct.
- The uterus and abdomen are closed in a routine manner.

Comments

Cannulation of the papilla of the UTJ is technically difficult to perform. The original paper (Zent *et al.* 1993) indicated that the flush procedure was successful in five of eight mares, with oviductal masses observed in the flush fluid from both oviducts in all five mares. Three of the mares eventually had live foals. Note that the retrograde oviductal flush is also possible via a hysteroscopic approach in the standing mare.

Equine Reproductive Procedures, Second Edition. Edited by John Dascanio and Patrick McCue.

Equipment and Supplies

Antibiotics, non-steroidal anti-inflammatory drugs, sedation, local anesthetic, and general anesthesia use vary with each procedure.

Retrograde oviductal flush, laparotomy approach

Surgical scrub, examination gloves, clippers, standard surgical supplies for abdominal surgery, sterile saline, 1.3 cm (0.5 inch) 24 gauge blunt-ended catheter, fluorescein dye (add one fluorescein ophthalmic strip to 10 ml of sterile saline), 12 ml syringe.

Normograde oviductal flush, laparotomy approach

Surgical scrub, examination gloves, clippers, standard surgical supplies for abdominal surgery, Doyen intestinal forceps, 8.0 Fr Foley catheter 30 cm (12 inch) with 5.0 ml balloon cuff (no. V-PFC8-30; Cook Veterinary Products, Inc., Bloomington, IN, USA), sterile saline, new methylene blue dye, 20 ml syringe.

Normograde oviductal flush, laparoscopic approach

Standard equipment and supplies for a standing laparoscopic surgery: detomidine hydrochloride, butorphanol tartrate, laparoscopic Babcock forceps or oviductal forceps (×2), 7 Fr balloon catheter (Willy Rŭsch GmbH, Kernen i.R., Germany), sterile saline, methylene blue dye, 20 ml syringe, videoendoscope to evaluate the uterine lumen after the flush procedure.

Retrograde oviductal flush, hysteroscopic approach

Examination gloves, tail wrap, tail rope, non-irritant soap, bucket, disposable bucket liner, roll cotton, sterile surgical gloves, long sterile sleeves, indigo carmine solution (5 ml, 4 mg/ml indigo carmoine injection), oviduct catheter: 200 cm (79 inch) polyethylene tube (1.7 mm OD) with a 22 gauge 4.45 cm (1.75 inch) injection catheter attached at one end and a 20 gauge 3.8 cm (1.5 inch) needle connected to a 5 ml syringe (filled with dye) at the opposite end, guidewire for human angiography (0.46 mm diameter, 220 cm (87 inches) long, RF-GA18263; Terumo, Surrey, UK), standard supplies for abdominocentesis, spectrophotometer, sterile flexible videoendoscope, videoprocessor, light source.

Optional (vaginotomy)

Scalpel, second sterile flexible endoscope.

Normograde Oviductal Flush (Laparotomy Approach) Technique

Performed under general anesthesia.

- The mare is fasted for 24 hours prior to surgery.
- Antibiotics and flunixin meglumine (1.1 mg/kg IV, s.i.d.) are administered prior to surgery and for 3 days after surgery.
- The mare is placed under general anesthesia and in dorsal recumbency and a pelvic tilt apparatus applied to gain better access to the reproductive tract.
- The ventral abdomen is clipped free of hair.
- A standard surgical prep is made over the ventral abdomen.
- A 10 cm incision is made along the ventral midline just cranial to the udder.
- One ovary and uterine horn are exteriorized and examined for gross pathology.
- Doyen intestinal forceps are placed on the uterine horn 5 cm from the cranial tip to occlude the uterine horn.
- An 8.0 Fr balloon-tipped catheter is passed into the infundibulum of the oviduct and down to the ampulla region and the cuff inflated with approximately 1.0–1.5 ml of air.
- 20 ml of sterile saline with new methylene blue dye is slowly injected through the catheter as the catheter is held in the oviduct by the application of manual pressure proximal to the balloon.
- Patency of the oviduct may be confirmed by the techniques below:
  - Injection and aspiration of 10–20 ml of sterile saline into the occluded cranial uterine horn to detect the presence of dye.
  - Injection of 20 ml of air through the catheterized oviduct and listening for the sound of air "gurgling" through the UTJ into the uterine lumen.
  - The advantage of performing these confirmation procedures is that additional flushing could be performed if the oviduct is not yet patent.
  - Alternatively, an endoscopic examination of the uterine lumen could be used to visualize the dye. This could be accomplished by a second set of personnel during surgery while the horse is under general anesthesia.
- The procedures are repeated on the contralateral oviduct.
- The abdomen is closed in a routine manner.

Comments

Oviductal lavage may cause dislodgment of oviductal blockages and may therefore be therapeutic. Caution should be used to not overly dilate the oviduct or exert excessive pressure. Severely occluded oviducts may rupture during the flush procedure. A unilateral ovariectomy may be performed in the event of irreversible occlusion or oviductal rupture. An initial report (Bennett *et al.* 2002) using this technique noted that eight of 12 mares diagnosed with bilateral occlusions and five of six mares with unilateral oviductal occlusion became pregnant on the first cycle after the flush procedure.

Normograde Oviductal Flush (Laparoscopic Approach) Technique

Standing procedure.

- The mare is fasted for 24 hours prior to surgery.
- Antibiotics and flunixin meglumine (1.1 mg/kg, IV, s.i.d.) are administered prior to surgery and after surgery as needed.
- The mare is appropriately sedated; additional sedation may be required and administered as needed. In the original paper a combination of detomidine hydrochloride (0.01 mg/kg, IV) and butorphanol tartrate (0.01 mg/kg, IV) were administered.
- The paralumbar fossa is prepared for laparoscopic surgery.
- A local anesthetic is placed into the locations for the portal sites.
- Three instrument portals are created and one portal for the laparoscope (Figure 29.1). The abdomen is insufflated with CO_2 to allow for visualization of the internal abdominal structures.
- A pair of laparoscopic Babcock forceps or oviductal forceps are used to grasp and open the edges of the infundibulum to view the ostium of the oviduct.
- The balloon catheter is inserted into a guide sleeve and passed into the ostium and advanced distally toward the ampulla.
- The cuff is inflated with 1.0–1.5 ml of air.
- One Babcock forceps is removed from the infundibulum and repositioned behind the balloon cuff to secure the catheter in place during the flush procedure
- The oviduct is flushed with 20 ml of sterile methylene blue solution.
- The procedure is subsequently performed on the contralateral oviduct.
- Hysteroscopy to visualize the oviductal papilla is performed during the flush to determine if the dye solution passed through each oviduct into the uterus.
- The portal incisions are closed in a routine manner.

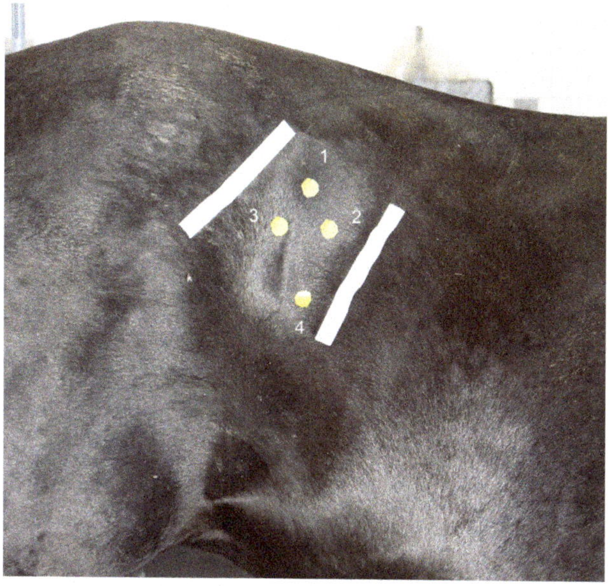

Figure 29.1 Landmarks for instrument portals: 1 is the laparoscopic portal; 2 and 3 are locations for the portals for the forceps; and 4 is the portal for the guide sleeve and catheter.

Comments

The original paper (Köllmann *et al.* 2011) compared flank laparoscopy with a transvaginal laparoscopic approach. The transvaginal approach was not successful and consequently is not discussed in this chapter. The major advantages of the laparoscopic procedure as compared with laparotomy are elimination of the need for general anesthesia and a minimally invasive approach. Disadvantages include costs of laparoscopic equipment and the clinical expertise needed to perform the procedure.

Additional Comments

Overall, flushing the oviducts provides diagnostic information on oviductal patency and at the same time often provides therapeutic intervention in affected mares. In regard to the latter, it has been suggested that removing oviductal masses via the normograde approach may be more difficult compared with the retrograde approach, as the luminal diameter of the isthmus is significantly smaller than the ampulla.

A concern for all the approaches discussed is the need to provide significant pressure during the flush to successfully relieve blockage(s) without rupturing the oviduct. It may be possible to reduce the risk by systemic administration of *N*-butylscopolammonium bromide and/or local application of prostaglandin E_2 gel onto the surface of the oviduct or the UTJ prior to the flush.

To avoid this risk of rupture of the oviduct altogether, the purely therapeutic option of applicating PGE_2 to either the oviductal surface or the UTJ (without first checking oviductal patency) can also be considered in mares suspected of having oviductal issues (see Chapters 30 and 31).

References

Bennett SD, Griffin RL, Rhoads WS. 2002. Surgical evaluation of oviduct disease and patency in the mare. *Proc Annu Conv Am Assoc Eq Pract* 48: 347–9.

Kollmann M, Rötting A, Heberling A, Sieme H. 2011. Laparoscopic techniques for investigating the equine oviduct. *Eq Vet J* 43: 106–11.

Zent WW, Liu IKM, Spirito MA. 1993. Oviduct flushing as a treatment for infertility in the mare. *Eq Vet J Suppl* 15: 47–8.

Further Reading

Arnold CE, Love CC. 2013. Laparoscopic evaluation of oviductal patency in the standing mare. *Theriogenology* 79: 905–10.

Bennett SD. 2007. Diagnosis of oviductal disorders and diagnostic techniques. In: Samper JC, Pycock JF, McKinnon AO (eds). Current Therapy in Equine Reproduction. St Louis, MI: Saunders Elsevier, pp. 78–82.

Inoue Y. 2013. Hysteroscopic hydrotubation of the equine oviduct. *Eq Vet J* 45:761–65.

Inoue Y, Sekiguchi M. 2018. Clinical application of hysteroscopic hydrotubation for unexplained fertility in the mare. *Eq Vet J* 50: 470–3.

30

Prostaglandin E_2 Treatment for Blocked Oviducts

Patrick M. McCue,[1] Sofie Sitters[2] and Charles F. Scoggin[3]

[1] *Equine Reproduction Laboratory, Colorado State University, USA*
[2] *Amsterdam, The Netherlands*
[3] *Rood and Riddle Equine Hospital, USA*

Introduction

Studies have reported that oviducts (uterine tubes) of middle aged and older mares may contain gelatinous masses of collagen, fibroblasts, and debris which can occlude the lumen of the oviduct. This may lead to a reduction in fertility by either preventing sperm from reaching the site of fertilization or preventing embryos from reaching the uterus. The frequency with which clinical obstructions occur is unknown. However, clinical studies have reported that topical administration of prostaglandin E_2 (PGE_2) onto the surface of the oviduct in mares with unexplained fertility has resulted in a resumption in fertility in a high proportion of treated mares.

The technique is performed via laparoscopy and involves direct visualization of the serosal surface of the oviduct, ovary, and their mesenteric attachments. It is performed with standing sedation and local anesthesia.

Equine embryos secrete PGE_2 which promotes passage of the embryo through the oviductal isthmus into the uterus. Unfertilized oocytes and non-viable embryos do not produce PGE_2 and are consequently retained at the junction of the ampulla and isthmus. This chapter describes the technique of laparoscopic application of PGE_2 onto the oviductal surface.

Equipment and Supplies

Surgical pack including sterile drapes, suture material, and/or stapler; scalpel blade; sterile surgery gloves; sterile plastic embryo transfer pipette and 0.5 ml straw; laparoscopic instrumentation – laparoscope: 57 cm or 30 cm × 10 mm, 30 degrees; light source: 300 W xenon with large diameter light cord; video camera and monitor; insufflator: at least 6 l/min (20 l/min preferred); trocars/cannulas: 7.5 and 11.5 mm diameter × 20 cm long. Endolaparoscopic Babcock atraumatic grasping forceps (45 cm (7.5 inch) long); dinoprostone cervical gel (Prepidil® Gel; Pharmacia and Upjohn/Pfizer, New York, USA); disposable 0.5 ml Cassou gun; 0.5 ml semen straws; 2% lidocaine; antibiotics; non-steroidal anti-inflammatory drugs; needles; syringes; surgical scrub; examination gloves.

Technique

- The mare is fasted for 24 hours prior to treatment.
- The mare is placed in stocks designed to allow access to the flank area.
- The paralumbar areas are surgically prepared.
- Antibiotics and a non-steroidal anti-inflammatory agent are administered prior to surgery; treatment may continue after surgery as needed.
- Detomidine hydrochloride (0.01 mg/kg IV) is administered for sedation.
- A local anesthetic such as 2% lidocaine hydrochloride is injected under the skin and infiltrated into the abdominal muscles and surface of the peritoneum in the two instrumental portal sites in the paralumbar region. Local anesthesia may also be accomplished with an inverted "L" in the paralumbar fossa.
- A 1–2.5 cm (0.5–1 inch) skin incision is made 10–15 cm (4–6 inches) below the dorsal aspect of the tuber coxae.
- A trochar and cannula are passed through the skin incision and inserted into the abdominal cavity.
- A 10 mm OD rigid laparoscope with a 30-degree viewing angle is inserted into the peritoneal cavity.
- The abdomen is distended by insufflation with CO_2 gas to allow for visualization of the ipsilateral ovary, oviduct, and uterine horn.
- A second (7.5 mm OD) trochar and cannula are passed into the abdominal cavity 5–10 cm (2–4 inches) dorsal to the laparoscope.

Equine Reproductive Procedures, Second Edition. Edited by John Dascanio and Patrick McCue.

- Atraumatic forceps are used to grasp and manipulate the ovary and expose the full length of the oviduct.
- The forceps are removed and replaced with a sterile disposable embryo transfer gun containing a 0.5 ml straw loaded with PGE_2 gel.
- The gel is slowly extruded onto the surface of the oviduct from the infundibulum to the utero-tubular junction, but especially along the isthmus region (Figure 30.1).
- The application is repeated using a second disposable embryo transfer gun yielding a total dosage of 1.0 ml (0.2 mg) of PGE_2 gel on one oviduct.
- The procedure is subsequently performed on the contralateral oviduct.
- The CO_2 gas is released from the abdomen and all cannulas are removed and the skin incisions are closed with sutures or staples.

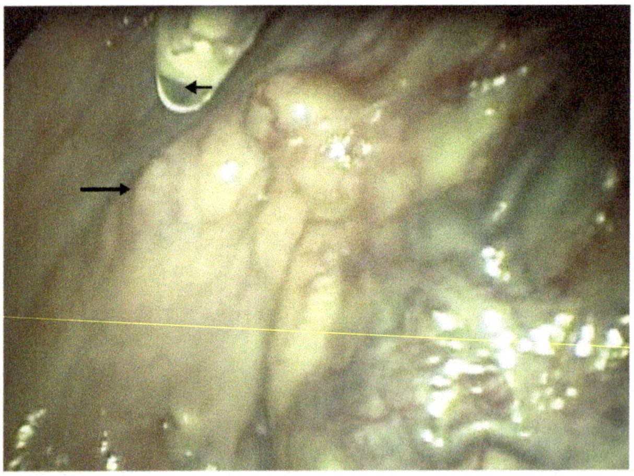

Figure 30.1 Application of PGE_2 gel (small arrow) onto surface of the oviduct (large arrow).

Additional Comments

The procedure has been successfully performed in mares in behavioral estrus and in mares in diestrus. In the original study by Allen *et al.* (2006), 14 of 15 mares (93%) treated with PGE_2 conceived to matings in either the same or subsequent breeding season after having previously been barren for multiple seasons for unknown reasons. In a report by Ortis *et al.* (2013), embryos were recovered or pregnancies were obtained from 24 of 28 barren mares treated with topical PGE_2.

Proper selection of candidate mares is one of the most important considerations for potential PGE_2 treatment. Blockage of the oviduct(s) should be considered as a cause for infertility in a mare that has historically produced live foals if all other common causes of infertility are evaluated first and addressed.

References

Allen WR, Wilsher S, Morris L, *et al.* 2006a. Laparoscopic application of PGE_2 to re-establish oviductal patency and fertility in infertile mares: a preliminary study. *Eq Vet J* 38: 454–9.

Ortis HA, Foss RR, McCue PM, Bradecamp EA, Ferris RA, Hendrickson DA. 2013. Laparoscopic application of PGE_2 to the uterine tube surface enhances fertility in selected subfertile mares. *J Eq Vet Sci* 33(11): 896–900.

Further Reading

Allen WR, Wilsher S, Morris L, *et al.* 2006b. Re-establishment of oviductal patency and fertility in infertile mares. *Anim Reprod Sci* 94: 242–3.

Robinson SJ, Neal H, Allen WR. 2000. Modulation of oviductal transport in mares by local application of prostaglandin E2. *J Reprod Fertil* 56:587–92.

Weber JA, Freeman DA, Vanderwall DK, Woods GL. 1991. Prostaglandin E_2 secretion by oviductal transport-stage equine embryos. *Biol Reprod* 45: 540–3.

31

Prostaglandin E_1 Treatment for Blocked Oviducts

Patrick M. McCue[1] and Charles F. Scoggin[2]

[1]*Equine Reproduction Laboratory, Colorado State University, USA*
[2]*Rood and Riddle Equine Hospital, USA*

Introduction

Pathology of the equine oviducts is considered to be relatively uncommon. Confirmative diagnosis is tedious and expensive, and, in many instances, is made via exclusion of more common causes of infertility. Despite the rarity of oviductal disease, studies using dissected specimens have demonsrated a relatively high incidence of collagenous masses within the lumen of the oviducts. Furthermore, clinical reports have demonstrated that treatment for suspected cases of oviductal obstructions can improve pregnancy or embryo recovery rates in mares.

Methods to relieve oviductal obstructions or treat idiopathic infertility include flushing of the oviductal lumen or topical application of prostaglandin E_2 (PGE_2) to the serosal surface of the oviducts (see Chapters 30 and 32). A newer and separate technique involves deposition of misprostol (PGE_1) onto the oviductal papillae or utero-tubular junction (UTJ) by deep horn uterine infusion, using a similar technique as a deep horn insemination (see Chapter 48). The procedure can be performed either during diestrus or estrus, and involves passing a long flexible insemination pipette to the tip of a uterine horn, followed by infusion of PGE_1 in the region of the oviductal papilla. Ultrasound guidance can be utilized to confirm pipette placement, and the procedure is subsequently repeated in the opposite horn. Immediately following deposition of PGE_1, the horn can be held off or the base of the horn lifted dorsad to promote diffusion of PGE_1 onto each papilla.

The use of this technique has not been compared with other methods of treating oviductal obstructions or unexplained infertility. A recent clinical study reported 68.2% success rate in obtaining pregnancies or recovering embryos within two cycles following PGE_1 treatment in a small subset of infertile mares. This result appears similar to other methods, with a primary advantage being much lower costs relative to laparoscopy or hydrotubation. Additional studies are needed to confirm the efficacy of PGE_1 therapy for blocked oviducts or idiopathic infertility.

Equipment and Supplies

Misoprostol tablets (200 µg/tab; Cytotec®, Pfizer, Inc., New York, USA), sterile water, 12 ml syringe, deep horn insemination pipette, sterile obstetrical sleeves, examination gloves, obstetrical lube. Optional: ultrasound with 5 MHz rectal probe.

Technique

- The mare is restrained appropriately and her tail wrapped (see Chapter 4).
- The rectum is evacuated and the perineum prepared routinely for a clean vaginal procedure (see Chapter 3).
- A 200 µg tablet of misoprostol is dissolved in 3 ml of sterile water and the solution drawn up into a sterile, long, flexible insemination pipette attached to a sterile 12 ml syringe.
- Using a sterile obstetrical sleeve and sterile lubricant, the insemination pipette is passed through the cervix and directed up a uterine horn.
- The arm is withdrawn from the vagina and is then placed in the rectum to direct the pipette up the tip of the horn. Note: transrectal ultrasound can be used to confirm location of pipette tip.
- Once the tip of the pipette is in the proper location, the misoprostol solution is infused. During and immediately following infusion, the tip of the horn can be held off or the base of the horn can be elevated dorsad to assist the solution in coming into contact with the uterine tube papillae.

Equine Reproductive Procedures, Second Edition. Edited by John Dascanio and Patrick McCue.

- Once complete, the tip of the pipette is withdrawn from the horn and redirected up to the tip of the other horn, and additional PGE_1 is deposited as previously described.
- Evaluation of the mare the following day is highly recommended. Some mares may experience an inflammatory response to this treatment, necessitating the use of ecbolics and/or uterine lavage.

Additional Comments

- The procedure can be performed in estrus or diestrus.
- Mares can be bred or inseminated as early as the day after PGE_1 infusion.

Further Reading

Allen WR, Wilsher S, Morris L, *et al.* 2006. Re-establishment of oviductal patency and fertility in infertile mares. *Anim Reprod Sci* 94: 242–3.

Allen WR, Wilsher S, Morris L, *et al.* 2006. Laparoscopic application of PGE_2 to re-establish oviductal patency and fertility in infertile mares: a preliminary study. *Eq Vet J* 38: 454–9.

Alvarenga MA, Segabinazzi LG. 2018. Application of misprostol as a treatment of unexplained infertility in mares. *J Eq Vet Sci* 71: 46–50.

Bradecamp EA, Schnobrich MR. 2016. Hysteroscopic hydrotubation of the oviducts as a treatment for idiopathic infertility in the mare – a retrospective study. *Proc Annu Conv Soc Theriogenol* 8(3): 337.

Inoue Y. 2013. Hysteroscopic hydrotubation of the equine oviduct. *Eq Vet J* 45: 761–5.

Inoue Y, Sekiguchi M. 2017. Clinical application of hysteroscopic hydrotubation for unexplained infertility in the mare. *Eq Vet J* 50: 470–3.

Ortis HA, Foss RR, McCue PM, Bradecamp EA, Ferris RA, Hendrickson DA. 2013. Laparoscopic application of PGE_2 to the uterine tube surface enhances fertility in selected subfertile mares. *J Eq Vet Sci* 33(11): 896–900.

Tsunami Y, Suzuki H, Takeda T, *et al.* 1979. Evidence of the origin of the gelatinous masses in the oviducts of mares. *J Reprod Fertil* 57: 287–90.

32

Hysteroscopic Hydrotubation of the Oviducts

Charles F. Scoggin

Rood and Riddle Equine Hospital, USA

Introduction

Hysteroscopic hydrotubation of the oviducts (uterine tubes) involves catheterizing the oviductal papillae (utero-tubular junction) and flushing the oviducts in a retrograde fashion via endoscopic guidance. This technique is performed in confirmed or suspected cases of oviductal obstructions or in mares with unexplained infertility. Clinical studies in mares carrying their own pregnancy and embryo donors mares reported an ~80% success rate, in terms of either pregnancy or embryo recovery rates, within two cycles following the hydrotubation procedure.

In the author's practice, this procedure is performed during diestrus or under the influence of progesterone when the cervix is tight to prevent air from escaping the uterine lumen during insufflation. It also requires a minimum of three experienced individuals: one person to pass the endoscope, another to drive the endoscope, and a third to operate the catheter and perform the flushing. The procedure is usually performed on each oviduct, after which the uterus is typically lavaged with lactated Ringer's solution (LRS) and the mare administered a luteolytic dose of prostaglandin $F_{2\alpha}$. Treatment with antibiotics and anti-inflammatory drugs may also be performed at the discretion of the clinician. Follow-up therapy with daily lavages for 1–3 days post-hydrotubation is recommended to reduce the risk of iatrogenic endometritis.

Equipment and Supplies

Sedation, previously sterilized 1 or 1.5 m flexible videoendoscope, 200 cm (79 inch) polyethylene tube with 1.7 mm OD (Hibiki high class grade size 5) with a 22 gauge 2.45 cm (1 inch) injection catheter attached to one end, 0.46 diameter and 220 cm (87 inch) long angiocatheter guidewire (Nit-Vu® Angiodynamics®, Latham, New York, USA), 12 ml plastic syringes, 20 g × 4 cm (1.5 inch) needles, sterile obstetrical sleeves, examination gloves and sterile obstetrical lubricant, lactated Ringer's solution, uterine lavage tubing, prostaglandin $F_{2\alpha}$.

Technique

- The mare is placed in stocks and sedated appropriately.
- The mare's rectum is evacuated and her perineum prepared routinely for a clean vaginal procedure (see Chapter 3).
- Using a sterile obstetrical sleeve and sterile lube, a 1 m flexible endoscope is advanced through the cervix and the uterus insufflated with air.
- The scope is passed up to the tip of one horn and the papilla at the utero-tubular junction is identified (Figure 32.1).
- The catheter is fed through the injection port of the endoscope and, with the assistance of the guidewire, the orifice of the papilla is cannulated and the catheter is advanced over the wire and seated in place a few millimeters into the oviductal papilla (Figure 32.2).
- The guidewire is withdrawn, and a 20 gauge 4 cm (1.5 inch) needle attached to a syringe with 10 ml of LRS is secured onto the opposite end of the catheter. Fluid is then pulsed through the tube and into the oviduct. Note: it is not uncommon to experience significant resistance when pulsing fluid through the oviduct. This can be counteracted by gentle rotation and slight withdrawal and advancement of the catheter system until fluid flows more freely. Movements should be relatively fine to avoid unseating the catheter.
- The procedure is repeated on the contralateral oviductal papilla.
- The uterus is lavaged with LRS (see Chapter 34) at the conclusion of the procedure and once daily for 2–3 subsequent days.

Equine Reproductive Procedures, Second Edition. Edited by John Dascanio and Patrick McCue.

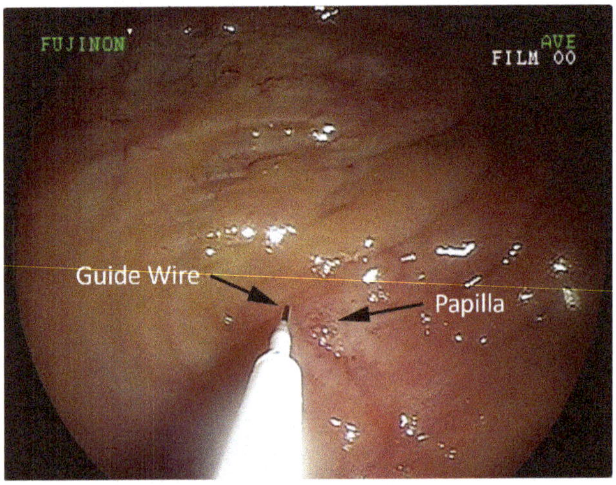

Figure 32.1 Hysteroscopic view of hydrotubation of the uterine tubes. The guidewire has been advanced a few millimeters from the distal tip of the catheter to facilitate cannulation of the orifice of the uterine tube papilla.

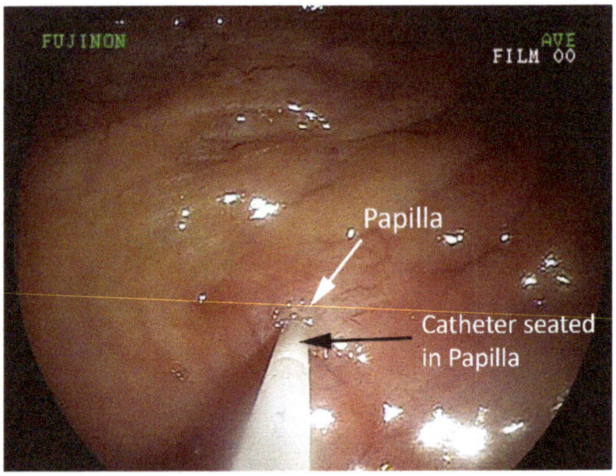

Figure 32.2 Hysteroscopic view of the hydrotubation procedure with the catheter seated in the uterine tube papilla.

- Prostaglandin $F_{2\alpha}$ is administered intramuscularly to bring the mare back into estrus and allow her to clean out any contamination.

The oviduct is an important link between the ovary and uterus, and is the site of fertilization *in vivo*. Past research has shown that oviductal masses are not uncommon in mares, but the extent to which these masses can block or interfere with fertilization is unknown and likely only affects a small subset of mares. An accurate diagnosis of oviductal obstruction is difficult, and a presumptive diagnosis is often made by excluding other causes of subfertility. Consequently, diagnosis is often foregone and treatment is instead pursued to resolve potentially blocked oviducts.

Further Reading

Bradecamp EA, Schnobrich MR. 2016. Hysteroscopic hydrotubation of the oviducts as a treatment for idiopathic infertility in the mare – a retrospective study. *Proc Annu Conv Soc Theriogenol* 8(3): 337.

Inoue Y. 2013. Hysteroscopic hydrotubation of the equine oviduct. *Eq Vet J* 45: 761–5.

Inoue Y, Sekiguchi M. 2017. Clinical application of hysteroscopic hydrotubation for unexplained infertility in the mare. *Eq Vet J* 50: 470–3.

33

Transvaginal Ovarian Biopsy

Claire E. Card

Western College of Veterinary Medicine, University of Saskatchewan, Canada

Introduction

Transvaginal ovarian biopsy (TVOB) is one method to determine the nature of an ovarian abnormality. The TVOB technique requires specialized equipment including a transvaginal ultrasound unit, a modified spring-loaded biopsy instrument (Figure 33.1), and personnel trained to perform the procedure. The procedure is indicated when there are ovarian abnormalities of an unknown nature identified by palpation or transrectal ultrasound examination of the ovary. It is also indicated when an ovarian tumor cannot be identified and when ovarian tumor serum biomarker analyses are discordant with the ultrasonographic appearance of the ovary or clinical signs.

The success rate in obtaining samples using this procedure is high. However, the diagnostic value of the ovarian samples is dependent on obtaining samples from the target location and is somewhat limited by the small size of the biopsies obtained (Figure 33.2). Complications associated with the biopsy procedure are uncommon.

Alternative procedures to TVOB to ascertain the nature of an ovarian abnormality include laparoscopic ovarian biopsy and ovariectomy. Ovariectomy is irreversible and may limit fertility.

Equipment and Supplies

Tail wrap, tail rope, non-irritant soap, roll cotton, stainless steel bucket, paper towels, exam gloves, sterile surgery gloves, sterile rectal sleeves, sterile lubricant, sedation, sterile towel, 14 g × 65 cm (25.5 inch) biopsy instrument, convex or linear array transvaginal ultrasound probe (7.5 or 10 mHz) self-contained or with a housing, 70% isopropyl alcohol, sterile saline, formalin, sample vials, sterile glass slides, pencil, sedation, *N*-butylscopolammonium bromide.

Technique

- The self-contained probe should be wiped with 70% isopropyl alcohol. The biopsy channel should be similarly cold sterilized and then rinsed with sterile saline or a sterile pipette should be inserted into the biopsy channel so the biopsy instrument does not contact an unclean surface.
- If ultrasound probe housing is used it should be cold sterilized for a minimum of 10 minutes and the solution vigorously rinsed off with sterile water. The probe to be inserted in the housing should be wiped with 70% isopropyl alcohol and the unit assembled using sterile gloves.
- The distal 10 cm (4 inch) of the biopsy instrument should be cold sterilized with the sample notch exposed. The immersed end of the biopsy instrument should be rinsed with sterile saline and the remaining needle length and handle wiped with 70% isopropyl alcohol or disinfectant wipes and placed on a sterile towel.
- Place the mare in stocks to provide adequate restraint from lateral movement.
- Wrap the tail and remove feces from the rectum (see Chapter 4). Administer *N*-butylscopolammonium bromide at 0.15 mg/kg slowly IV to relax the rectum.
- Tie the mare's tail to the side, and remove the feces. Perform an ultrasound examination to determine the ovary or ovaries to be biopsied and the target location to be sampled.
- Prepare the mare's perineum by washing and then drying the perineum (see Chapter 3).
- Administer sedation consisting of xylazine (0.3–0.4 mg/kg IV) combined with butorphanol (0.01–0.02 mg/kg IV), or detomidine (0.01–0.02 mg/kg IV) combined with butorphanol (0.01–0.02 mg/kg IV). Position the mare's head to prevent airway obstruction when the head drops due to the sedation.

Equine Reproductive Procedures, Second Edition. Edited by John Dascanio and Patrick McCue.

(a)

(b)

(c) (d)

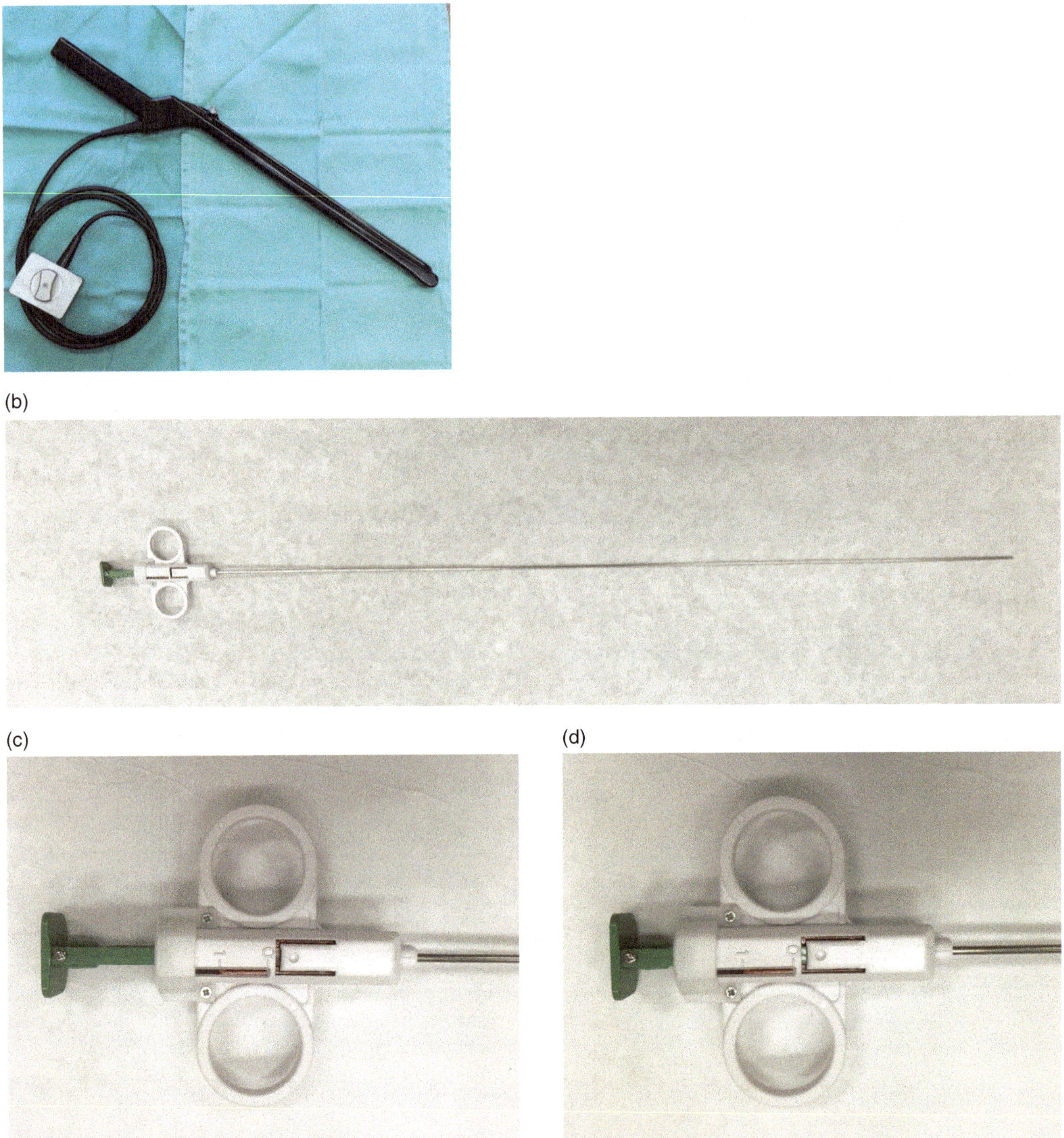

Figure 33.1 Self-contained transvaginal ultrasound probe (a), custom modified spring-loaded 65 cm biopsy instrument (b), and handle of biopsy device when cocked (c) and when advanced to the first stop (d).

- Sterile lubricant should be applied to the surface of the probe. The self-contained vaginal probe or the assembled probe, may be placed into a sterile sleeve, and inserted into the vagina. Alternatively, the examiner may wear a sterile rectal sleeve and shield the end of the probe while placing it lateral to the cervix, ipsilateral to the ovary to be biopsied. The opening to the biopsy port is covered with a sterile towel to prevent fecal contamination.
- The examiner's hand is then placed in the rectum, the feces evacuated, and the ovary to be biopsied is positioned adjacent to the vaginal probe. This may be accomplished by moving the ovary deeper into the abdomen

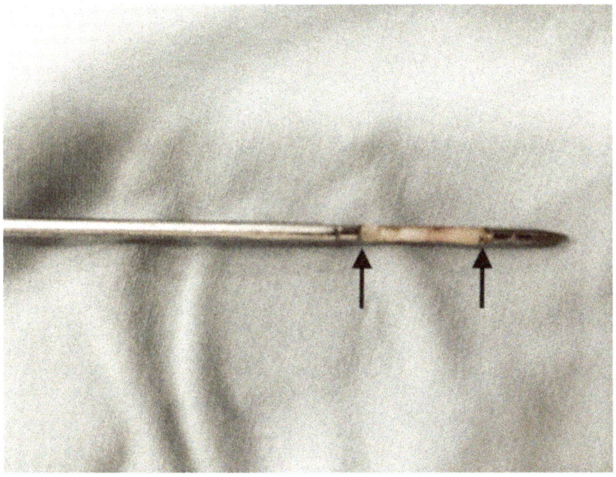

Figure 33.2 Biopsy device tip with sample notch exposed (arrows) revealing a core ovarian biopsy.

and then moving the ovary dorsally over the broad ligament.

- The ovary is examined using ultrasound and the target area to be biopsied is identified. The biopsy guide may be used to assist in obtaining the biopsy, by positioning the ovary so the biopsy guide lines bisect the area to be sampled.
- The assistant, wearing surgical gloves, cocks the biopsy instrument and lubricates the tip with a small amount of sterile lubricant. The tip of the biopsy instrument is inserted into the biopsy channel of the self-contained probe, or ultrasound housing, and advanced until resistance is felt. Slight intermittent pressure against the vaginal wall will help identify the position of the tip of the biopsy instrument in relationship to the target area on the ovary as viewed on the ultrasound.
- The examiner, with their hand in the rectum, steadies the ovary firmly against the ultrasound probe. The assistant estimates the distance to the target area to be biopsied.
- The needle is advanced into the ovary a smooth quick motion to the approximate depth needed to reach the target area.
- The tip of the biopsy instrument may be positioned 2 cm (0.75 inch) behind the ovarian target area and fired (the one step method) or the tip of the biopsy instrument may be advanced to the first stop, which exposes the notch on the biopsy device's needle, and then fired (two step method).
- The biopsy instrument is removed from the ovary and placed on the sterile field. The biopsy instrument is cocked and advanced to the first stop to expose the sample notch. The sample is removed from the notch using small (22 or 25 gauge) needles. Any of the following may be performed with the sample: imprints may be made on a sterile slide for cytology, it may be placed in formalin for histopathology, or the sample may be snap frozen in liquid nitrogen for mRNA analysis. The biopsy instrument is returned to the shielded position, re-lubricated, and the process repeated to obtain 3–5 good biopsy cores from the target area per ovary.
- It is recommended that a physical examination (temperature, pulse, respiration rate) is performed on the mare daily for 3 days post-procedure to monitor for any complications.

Interpretation

- There is a slight risk of significant vaginal bleeding from the biopsy needle penetration. There is small risk of peritonitis arising due to the biopsy instrument penetrating the vaginal wall, which contains bacterial flora.
- There is a slight risk of rectal puncture arising from overzealous penetration of the ovary, failure to position the biopsy instrument accurately, accidentally firing the biopsy instrument, or mare movement.
- Antibiotics and anti-inflammatory drugs are typically not administered following this procedure. If a rectal puncture has occurred then non-steroidal anti-inflammatory therapy for 3 days and trimethoprim sulfa (30 mg/kg by mouth) twice daily for 7–10 days, or other broad-spectrum antibiotic therapy may be indicated.

Further Reading

Aerts JMJ, Oste M, Bols PEJ. 2005. Development and practical applications of a method for repeated transvaginal, ultrasound-guided biopsy collection of the bovine ovary. *Theriogenology* 64: 947–57.

Diel de Amorim M, Nairn LD, Manning S, Dedden I, Ripley E, Card C. 2016. Evaluation of diagnostic utility, safety considerations, and effect on fertility of transvaginal ultrasound-guided ovarian biopsy in mares. *Theriogenology* 5(6): 1030–6.

Gastal, GA, Alves BG, Alves, KA, *et al.* 2017. Ovarian fragment sizes affect viability and morphology of preantral follicles during storage at 4°C. *Reproduction* 153(5): 577–87.

Murase H, Ball B, Tangyuenyong S, *et al.* 2018. Serum anti-müllerian hormone concentrations in mares with granulosa cell tumors versus other ovarian abnormalities. *J Eq Vet Sci* 60: 6–10.

Slough TL, Rispoli LA, Carnevale EM, Niswender GD, Bruemmer J. 2011. Temporal gene expression in equine corpora lutea based on serial biopsies in vivo. *J Anim Sci* 89: 389–96.

Velez IC, Arnold C, Jacobson CC, *et al.* 2012. Effects of repeated transvaginal aspiration of immature follicles on mare health and ovarian status. *Eq Vet J Suppl* 44: 78–83.

34

Uterine Lavage

John J. Dascanio

School of Veterinary Medicine, Texas Tech University, USA

Introduction

Lavage of the equine uterus is used primarily to remove debris, infectious organisms, and fluid from the uterine lumen. The adage "dilution is the solution to the pollution" is applicable to the uterus for decreasing bacterial numbers, inflammatory cells, and removal of debris with lavage.

Mares in estrus may be lavaged one or more days prior to breeding to remove accumulated fluid or as part of a therapeutic plan for mares with infectious endometritis. It is common to lavage a mare with 1–3 liters or more of sterile 0.9% saline or lactated Ringer's solution (LRS). In general, the uterus is lavaged until the effluent is clear. The lavage procedure may have to be repeated on sequential days.

If a uterine lavage is required immediately prior to breeding or insemination, it is recommended that LRS be used instead of 0.9% saline. Research has shown that pregnancy rates are higher if LRS is used immediately prior to breeding than if saline is used. Lavage fluids may be warmed (to 42–45°C, 108–113°F) to help with removal of viscous fluids and to prevent discomfort or cramping by the mare. The tubing should be a "closed" system with no requirement to pull the tubing apart to attach bags for lavage once the procedure begins.

A uterine lavage may be required after breeding or insemination in mares with persistent mating-induced endometritis (PMIE). The lavage is generally performed 4–6 hours after mating in mares with a known history of PMIE or the next day in other affected mares. The goal is to remove dead sperm, inflammatory cells, debris, and other material and prevent or limit the sperm-induced inflammatory response. Uterine lavage may be performed without significant detrimental effects on pregnancy up to 2 days after ovulation. In some selected cases a lavage may have to be performed 3 or even 4 days after ovulation, but routine lavage on those dates should be discouraged so as to limit uterine inflammation prior to entrance of the embryo into the uterus from the oviduct.

In the postpartum mare, a uterine lavage may be performed in the event of a retained placenta, prolonged discharge of lochia, or metritis.

Equipment and Supplies

Tail wrap, non-irritant soap, roll cotton, stainless steel bucket, disposable liner for bucket, paper towels, examination gloves, 1–5 liters of lavage solution, uterine lavage catheter with inflatable cuff, "Y" extension tubing with spike, double-ended "Christmas tree" adapter (if needed), collection bottle or graduated cylinder, sterile obstetrical sleeve, sterile obstetrical lubricant.

Technique

- Remove feces from the rectum.
- Place a tail wrap and tail rope on the mare (see Chapter 4).
- Wearing examination gloves, clean and dry the perineum of the mare (see Chapter 3).
- Hang the lavage fluids so that they are above the level of the mare's uterus to augment gravity flow.
- Attach the "Y" tubing to the fluid bag using either the spike (if present) or a sterile double-ended adaptor (Figures 34.1 and 34.2).
- Attach the "Y" tubing to the lavage catheter and fill the line and catheter with fluid. The cuff on the lavage tubing may be inflated to ensure it will hold air and then be deflated for placement (Figure 34.3).
- Place the end of the sterile lavage tubing into the palm of the gloved hand.

Equine Reproductive Procedures, Second Edition. Edited by John Dascanio and Patrick McCue.

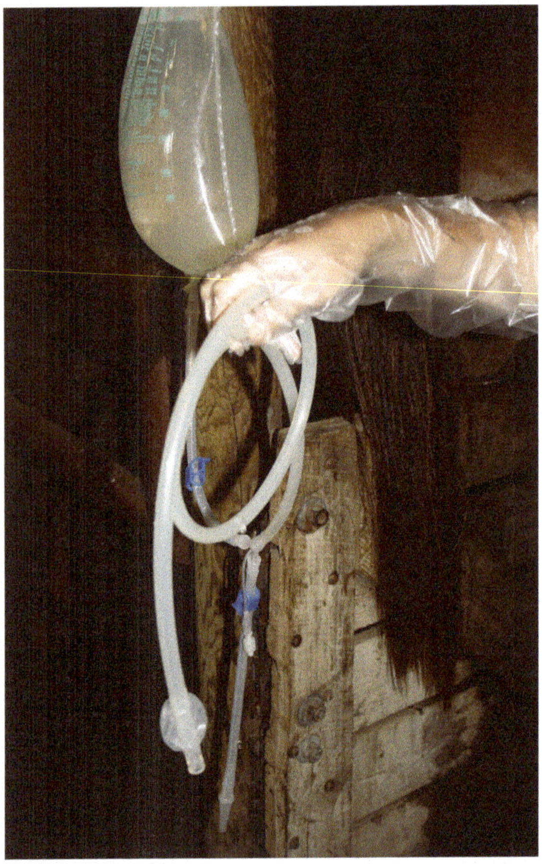

Figure 34.1 Lavage solution hung next to a mare with the uterine lavage tubing attached. The clamps are present on the ingress and egress tubing to control fluid flow.

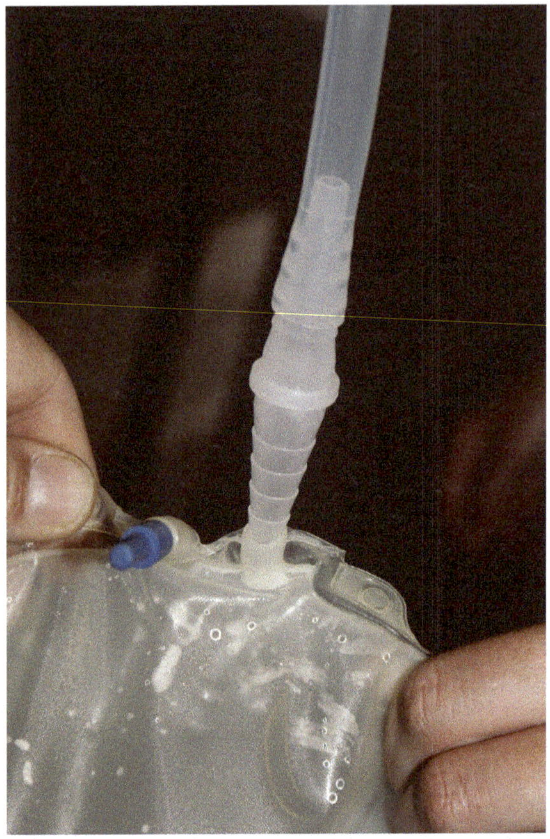

Figure 34.2 Double-ended "Christmas tree" adapter attached to the uterine lavage tubing and the cutoff end of the injection port of a fluid bag.

- Open the clamp on the ingress lavage tubing to fill the tubing with fluid. This will prevent placing air within the mare's uterus once fluid lavage commences.
- Place a sterile obstetrical sleeve on the arm.
- Place sterile lubricant on the knuckles and down the length of the sleeve.
- Rub lubricant from the knuckles onto the vulva, straighten the fingers, and insert the hand and tubing through the vulva, being careful to not rub the clitoris.
- Using a slight rotating motion, pass the hand into the vagina so that the mid-forearm is to about the level of the vulva. This should enable palpation of the external cervical os.
- Gently insert the index finger into the external cervical os. Sometimes the os may be off-center, located slightly downward, or to the left or right of center.
- Using the hand outside the reproductive tract, feed the tubing forward while using the hand inside the mare to guide the tubing into the cervical lumen.
- Once the tubing is past the internal cervical os, the cuff in the tubing may be inflated with air. Usually 30–75 ml of air is sufficient for most uterine lavage catheters. The cuff may be gently pulled back snugly against the internal cervical os to prevent fluid loss. It may be necessary to hold the external cervical os closed over the catheter in mares in estrus and postpartum mares to prevent reflux of lavage fluid into the vagina.

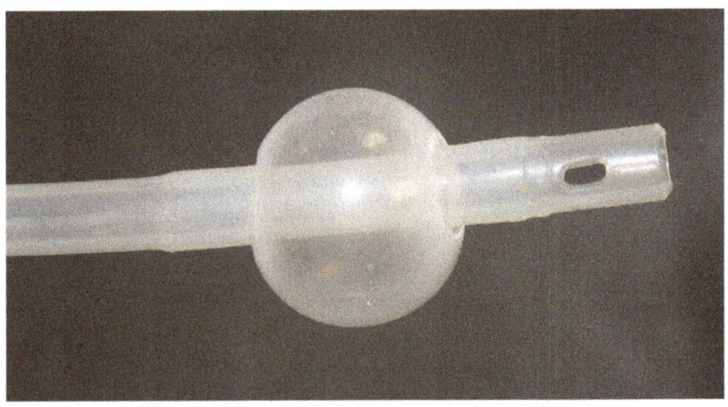

Figure 34.3 Inflated air cuff on the end of the uterine lavage tubing.

- The clamp on the ingress tubing is opened and the uterus is filled with fluid until either the flow stops, the mare becomes uncomfortable, or a specific volume has been instilled. Typically the uterus of most non-pregnant

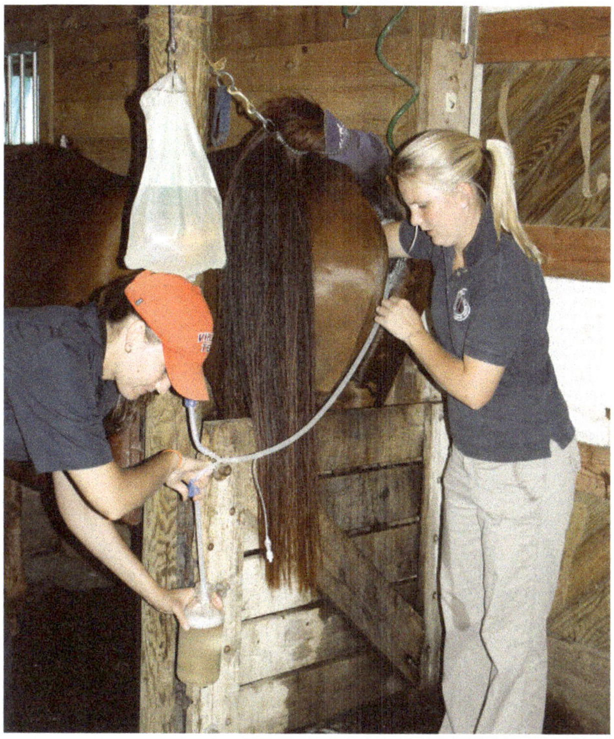

Figure 34.4 Uterine lavage of a mare post-breeding with "Y" tubing. The lavage solution may be raised higher to augment gravity flow into the mare's uterus.

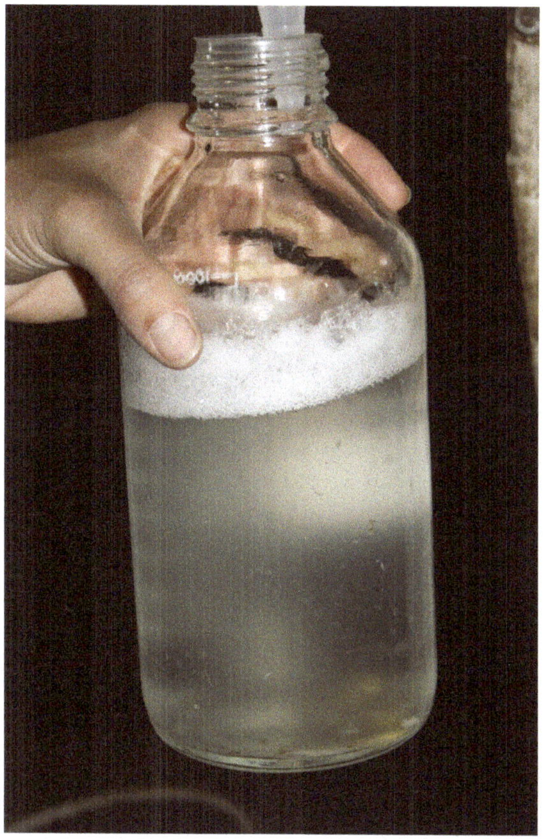

Figure 34.5 Cloudy uterine lavage return solution.

mares will hold 1–2 liters of fluid without major discomfort. This volume increases with parity. Postpartum mares will accommodate 3–5 liters per lavage or more. A sterile or disinfected equine stomach tube may be used in postpartum mares to reach dependent areas of the uterus and to provide a large bore tube for debris removal.

- Once the uterus is filled, the ingress clamp is shut and the egress clamp is opened. The end of the egress tubing should be lower than the mare's reproductive tract to allow for gravity flow of fluid out of the uterus.
- In most instances fluid egress occurs uneventfully. It may be necessary to adjust or manipulate the uterine catheter slightly per vagina by rotating the catheter 180 degrees, by advancing the catheter slightly, by directing the catheter tip ventrally, or by retracting the catheter slightly to keep the catheter within the fluid pocket and to free the catheter from the endometrium.
- In some instances, fluid recovery is difficult. A technique that works well in these mares is to deflate the cuff, advance the catheter deeply into the uterus as additional fluid is being infused, and recover fluid from the most dependent part of the uterus (i.e., below the pelvic brim) instead of adjacent to the internal cervical os.
- Administration of oxytocin (20 IU IV) may aid in fluid recovery by stimulation of uterine contractions.
- It is also common to massage the uterus or to lift a uterine horn per rectum to move fluid toward the catheter. Ultrasound imaging can be used to monitor fluid recovery and locate pockets of fluid still within the uterine lumen.
- The fluid should be recovered into a clear container so that the degree of cloudiness and amount of debris can be subjectively evaluated (Figures 34.4 and 34.5). In addition, quantification of the amount of fluid returned will allow determination of how much fluid remains within the uterus.
- It is common to repeat the uterine lavage until the effluent fluid is clear.
- A transrectal ultrasound examination may be performed at the end of the lavage, while the uterine catheter is still in place, to confirm whether or not the uterus is free of fluid.
- Once lavage is complete, the cuff is deflated and the catheter is gently removed from the reproductive tract.

Additives to the Lavage Solution

- In most cases the uterus is lavaged without additions to the lavage fluid.

- Potential additions include:
  - Povidone-iodine (1–5 ml of 10% povidone-iodine per liter of lavage fluid) as a general disinfectant.
  - White vinegar (2%) (20 ml per liter of sterile saline) to acidify the lavage fluid in mares with fungal endometritis.

Interpretation

- If the fluid returned at the end of all the lavages is still not clear, lavage should be performed at the next examination of the mare, typically the next day.
- If the first lavage returns clear fluid, no subsequent lavages are necessary. Occasionally, the material within the uterus is very viscous and does not readily mix with the lavage solution. Thus, it may seem as though clear fluid is returned when in reality the lavage solution did not mix adequately with the uterine fluid. This should be taken into consideration from pre-lavage ultrasound examinations demonstrating hyperechoic fluid within the uterine lumen. Massage of the uterus per rectum during lavage or the use of warm lavage solution may aid in the removal of viscous fluids.
- Ultrasound may be used to determine how much lavage solution is present within the uterine lumen in order to guide the lavage tubing into that area to remove the fluid. Occasionally, the cuff may need to be deflated to allow movement of the tubing into dependent areas of the uterine body and horns.
- Ultrasound after the lavage procedure may demonstrate air in the uterus as a consequence of the procedure.

Further Reading

Brinkso SP, Varner DD, Blanchard TL. 1991. The effect of uterine lavage performed four hours post insemination on pregnancy rate in mares. *Theriogenology* 35: 1111–19.

Vanderwall DK, Woods GL. 2003. Effect on fertility of uterine lavage performed immediately prior to insemination in mares. *J Am Vet Med Assoc* 222: 1108–10.

35

Uterine Infusion

John J. Dascanio

School of Veterinary Medicine, Texas Tech University, USA

Introduction

Infusion of the uterus is most commonly performed to deposit semen into the uterus of the mare as part of an artificial insemination program. In addition, it may be used for the instillation of antibiotics, *n*-acetylcysteine, Tris-EDTA, dimethyl sulfoxide (DMSO), or other drugs or compounds. Infusion is unlike lavage in that the liquid instilled is not removed, but allowed to remain for either a set period of time, after which a uterine lavage is performed to remove the substance, or it is left to be absorbed or removed by natural mechanisms. These natural mechanisms include uterine contraction, lymphatic removal, engulfment by inflammatory cells, mucociliary clearance, and gravity flow. Infusion may be performed with a pipette and syringe or may utilize extension tubing between a pipette and a small bag of fluids.

Equipment and Supplies

Tail wrap, non-irritant soap, roll cotton, stainless steel bucket, disposable liner for bucket, paper towels, exam gloves, solution for infusion, uterine infusion pipette, syringes, sterile obstetrical sleeve, sterile obstetrical lubricant.

Technique

- Remove the feces from the rectum.
- Place a tail wrap and tail rope on the mare (see Chapter 4).
- Wearing examination gloves, clean and dry the perineum of the mare (see Chapter 3).
- Place a sterile obstetrical sleeve on the arm.
- Place the end of the sterile pipette into the palm of the gloved hand and cover the pipette end with the thumb. There are different models and lengths of pipettes depending on the procedure performed and the distance to the mare's uterus (Figure 35.1). Some pipettes have a large rounded end or provide a flexible attachment for a syringe (Figure 35.2).
- Place sterile lubricant on the knuckles and down the length of the sleeve.
- Rub lubricant from the knuckles onto the vulva, straighten the fingers, and insert the hand and pipette through the vulva, being careful to not rub the clitoris.
- Using a slight rotational motion, pass the hand into the vagina so that the mid-forearm is to about the level of the vulva. This should enable palpation of the external cervical os.
- Using the index finger, gently insert the index finger into the external cervical os. Sometimes the os may be off-center, located slightly downward, or to the left or right of center. The index finger may be inserted to the metacarpo-phalangeal joint.
- Using the contralateral hand, the pipette is manipulated so that it passes next to the inserted finger and into the uterine lumen.
- The hand within the vagina may help to direct the pipette downwards or sideways to augment passage through the cervix. The cervical lumen often is directed downward due to the pull of the uterus, especially in multiparous mares.
- The hand within the vagina may grasp the pipette to hold it steady while a syringe or extension tubing is attached.
- The substance to be administered is infused through the pipette and into the uterine lumen.
- Sometimes the pipette has a flexible end to which the syringe is attached, allowing the syringe to be orientated vertically during infusion. If a small amount of air is included in the syringe prior to infusion, then the vertical syringe orientation will allow for the air to pass after

Equine Reproductive Procedures, Second Edition. Edited by John Dascanio and Patrick McCue.

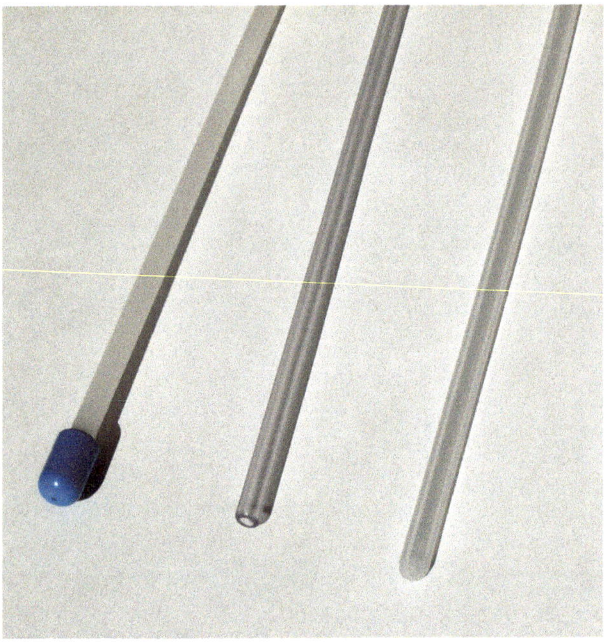

Figure 35.1 Intrauterine ends of various types of pipettes. From left to right: universal pipette (Minitube USA, Inc., Verona, WI, USA), In-Fu-Zee™ pipette (Patterson Veterinary Supply, Inc., Greeley, CO, USA), and IMV Flexible Equine Catheter (IMV Technologies USA, Maple Grove, MN, USA).

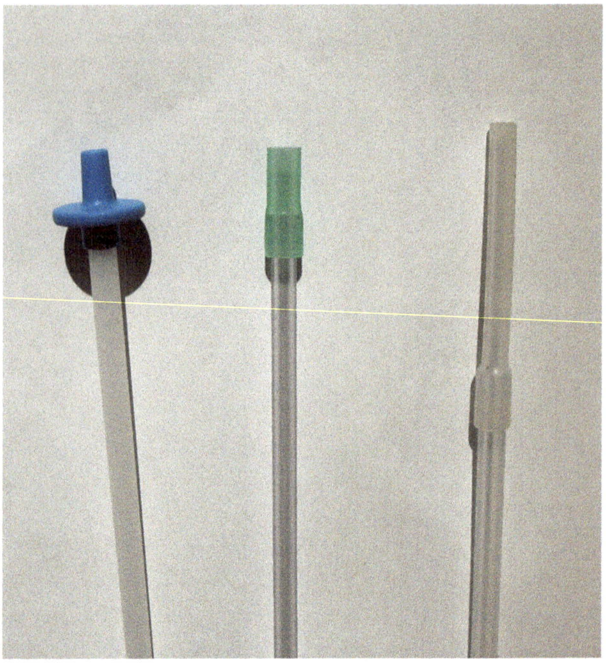

Figure 35.2 Ends of pipettes to which a syringe is attached. From left to right: universal pipette, In-Fu-Zee™ pipette, and IMV Flexible Equine Catheter. The IMV pipette has a flexible piece of plastic to allow vertical orientation of the syringe during infusion.

the liquid, flushing the liquid out of the pipette. If the flexible attachment is not present, then the syringe may be unattached, some air added, and then reattached to flush the pipette. Extra air should not be pushed into the uterus as this may cause uterine inflammation. Most pipettes hold between 4 and 6 ml of liquid.

- The pipette is withdrawn after infusion and the external cervical os may be held closed circumferentially with slight digital pressure or elevated slightly for about 10–15 seconds to prevent backflow of material out of the dilated cervix.

Interpretation

- A reflux of fluid may be felt with the hand in the vagina or the finger in the cervix during uterine infusion. If this occurs, the pipette should immediately be repositioned further inward and in a downward direction and the cervix raised dorsally with the fingers to prevent further loss of fluid.
- The gloved hand should be examined upon retraction from the vagina for any abnormal discharges or odor.
- Smaller pipettes are about 57 cm (22.5 inches) in length. Longer infusion pipettes (65 and 75 cm (25.5 and 29.5 inches) in length) are available for Warmblood and draft horses.
- The volume of the infusion should be held to no more than 150–200 ml total volume to avoid reflux of fluid back through the cervix. The propensity for reflux is also correlated with the size of the uterus, parity of the mare, and physical location of the uterus in relation to the pelvic canal.

Further Reading

Bennett DG, Poland HJ, Kaneps AJ, Snyder SP. 1980. Reaction of the equine endometrium to intrauterine infusion. *Proc Annu Conv Am Assoc Eq Pract* 26: 135–9.

36

Therapeutics for Infectious Endometritis

Ryan A. Ferris

Summit, Equine, USA

Introduction

Clinical cases of bacterial endometritis can be divided into acute and chronic infections. Acute endometritis will be defined as cases in which mares are exposed to bacterial pathogens and an initial infection develops. The term chronic endometritis will be defined as cases where acute bacterial endometritis was detected, appropriate therapy initiated, yet the infection continues to persist despite treatment.

Acute Bacterial Endometritis

Mares with acute bacterial endometritis appear systemically healthy, may have intrauterine fluid present on transrectal ultrasound examination, fluid in the vaginal vault on speculum examination, or a vulvar discharge. Speculum examination may reveal a reddened cervix and a cervical discharge. Normally, the mare's uterus can rapidly clear contamination by bacterial or fungal organisms without development of a persistent infection. However, any breakdown in the defense mechanisms of the reproductive tract predisposes a mare to a uterine infection. Increased numbers of bacteria reaching the endometrium due to abnormalities of the perineum, vestibulo-vaginal seal, or cervix may result in development of an infection. A decrease in the ability of the myometrium to produce effective contractions will also result in retention or reduced clearance of inflammatory fluid and contaminants from the uterus. Other mechanisms that may predispose to uterine infections include failure of cervical dilation, decrease lymph drainage, and a dependent uterine position. Finally, a breakdown in the innate immune system reduces the immune response toward pathogens in the uterus. All of these factors individually or in combination contribute to development of bacterial endometritis.

Intrauterine Antibiotic Therapy

The therapeutic plan for a mare with bacterial endometritis is to aid the uterus in clearing the infectious agent(s) and inflammatory debris. If a large volume of uterine fluid is present, a uterine lavage should be performed prior to antibiotic treatment (see Chapter 34). The goal of the lavage is to reduce the number of infectious organisms, remove inflammatory debris from the uterus, and potentially enhance luminal defense mechanisms by inducing local irritation and influx of polymorphonuclear neutrophils into the uterine lumen. Uterine lavage may be performed using sterile saline (0.9%) or lactated Ringer's solution (or similar sterile fluid).

Uterine lavage is often followed by intrauterine infusion of antibiotics. A common protocol consists of three intrauterine treatments 24 hours apart (i.e., 3 days of therapy). Ideally, the choice of intrauterine agent(s) should be based on antimicrobial susceptibility patterns following culture of a pathogenic organism. Empirical therapy may be initiated before the acquisition of antibiotic sensitivity results, in clinical situations in which a culture was not collected, or if the culture was negative and a bacterial infection is still suspected.

Choices for empirical therapy include a combination of a β-lactam antibiotic (i.e., a penicillin derivative) plus an aminoglycoside or a single broad-spectrum antibiotic with efficacy against Gram-positive and Gram-negative organisms (Table 36.1). Antimicrobial therapy should be adjusted once results of uterine culture and antimicrobial susceptibility tests are available.

Equine Reproductive Procedures, Second Edition. Edited by John Dascanio and Patrick McCue.

Table 36.1 Antibiotics for intrauterine therapy.

Medication	Dosage, Route, Frequency	Indications
Amikacin sulfate (250 mg/ml)	1–2 g; buffer with 10–20 ml 8.4% sodium bicarbonate then qs to 60 ml with sterile saline	Antibiotic (Gram-negative spectrum)
Ampicillin (1 g vial)	1–2 g, reconstitute in 60 ml sterile saline	Antibiotic (Gram-positive spectrum primarily)
Ceftiofur sodium	1 g, reconstitute with 20–60 ml sterile water	Antibiotic (broad-spectrum)
Gentamicin (100 mg/ml)	1–2 g; buffer with 10–20 ml 8.4 % sodium bicarbonate	Antibiotic (Gram-negative spectrum)
Penicillin (potassium) (5 million units/vial)	5 million units, reconstitute in 60 ml sterile saline	Antibiotic (Gram-positive spectrum)
Penicillin (procaine) (300,000 units/ml)	15 ml, dilute to 60 ml in sterile saline	Antibiotic (Gram-positive spectrum)
Ticarcillin/clavulanic acid (3.1 g/vial)	3.1 g, reconstitute to 60 ml with sterile saline	Antibiotic combination; clavulanate blocks penicillinase; used for Gram-positive organisms and *Pseudomonas aeruginosa*

Ecbolics such as oxytocin or cloprostenol sodium should not be given concurrently with antibiotic infusion, as this may cause a majority of the antibiotics to be immediately evacuated from the uterus.

Systemic Antibiotic Therapy

Systemic therapy may be considered in cases where the bacteria are deep seated within the endometrium, if antimicrobial susceptibility tests indicate that the only effective antimicrobial agent is one that has to be administered systemically, or in cases in which the veterinarian or mare owner prefers systemic therapy over repeated intrauterine therapy. Options for systemic antibiotic therapy are presented in Table 36.2. Systemic therapy is usually administered for 5–7 days or longer.

Follow-Up Examination

It is important to perform a follow-up reproductive evaluation during the next estrous cycle after the mare has been treated. The exam should include transrectal ultrasonography, speculum examination, uterine culture, and uterine cytology. It is not uncommon for antimicrobial therapy to fail to eliminate the original microbial organism or for detection of a different pathogenic organism.

Additional Therapy

Any treatment plan for infectious endometritis needs to address issues with perineal conformation (see Chapter 5). Procedures to correct anatomic issues include a Caslick, perineal body reconstruction, or cervical laceration repair.

Table 36.2 Systemic antibiotics.

Medication	Dosage, Route, Frequency	Indications
Ceftiofur sodium (50 mg/ml)	1.1–2.2 mg/kg IV or IM, q 12 hours	Antibiotic (broad-spectrum)
Ceftiofur crystalline free acid (200 mg/ml)	3.0 mg ceftiofur equivalents/kg IM; retreat in 4 days if needed	Antibiotic (broad-spectrum)
Enrofloxacin (50 or 100 mg/ml)	5 mg/kg IV, q 24 hours or 7.5 mg/kg PO, q 24 hours	Antibiotic (broad-spectrum); used in the treatment of endometritis caused by resistant *Pseudomonas* species. Note: intrauterine therapy of the commercial bovine product is associated with severe necrosis and is not recommended

Mares with less than two thirds of the vulva below the pelvic brim or >10 degrees of angulation of the vulva warrant placement of a Caslick (see Chapter 53). Severe cases with minimal to no vulva below the pelvic brim or >60 degrees of angulation to the vulva warrant perineal body reconstruction.

References

Dascanio JJ. 2011. How and when to treat endometritis with systemic or local antibiotics. *AAEP Proc* 57: 24–31.

Gores-Lindholm AR, LeBlanc MM, Causey R, *et al.* 2013. Relationships between intrauterine infusion of N-acetylcysteine, equine endometrial pathology, neutrophil function, post-breeding therapy, and reproductive performance. *Theriogenology* 80: 218–27.

LeBlanc MM. 2010. Advances in the diagnosis and treatment of chronic infectious and post-mating-induced endometritis in the mare. *Reprod Domest Anim* 45(suppl 2): 21–7.

LeBlanc MM, Causey RC. 2009. Clinical and subclinical endometritis in the mare: both threats to fertility. *Reprod Domest Anim* 44(suppl 3): 10–22.

37

Bacterial Biofilm and Endometritis

Ryan A. Ferris

Summit, Equine, USA

Introduction

Bacteria are capable of living in two different lifestyles: planktonic or biofilm states. Planktonic bacteria are single bacterial cells free floating in a suspension. Bacteria in this lifestyle utilize available nutrients for procreation. These individual bacteria are relatively susceptible to recognition and degradation by the host immune system, susceptible to changes in environment (desiccation, lack of nutrients, etc.), and are sensitive to antibiotics. However, the planktonic cell paradigm does not accurately reflect the growth of bacteria associated with a biofilm.

A biofilm is an aggregate of microbial cells adherent to a surface, embedded within a complex matrix of extracellular polymeric substances (EPS) which may include nucleic acids, proteins, polysaccharides (exopolysaccarides), and lipids of microbial origin as well as host components. Biofilms are essentially three-dimensional structures with microorganisms living within a coordinated functional community. Bacteria within a biofilm are protected from the host immune system as white blood cells have reduced ability for movement and function, and the thick layer of exopolysaccaride prevents antibodies from reaching bacteria deep within the biofilm. Biofilms protect bacteria from antibiotics by providing a diffusion barrier or gradient that decreases the amount of antibiotics that reach the protected bacterial colonies.

Antimicrobial agents must traverse through a layer of thick EPS, DNA, RNA, lipids, and proteins in order to reach bacteria living deep within this protective barrier. Bacteria in the outer region may be killed, but a decrease in the level of antibiotics reaching the inner layer bacteria contributes to the formation of a bacterial nidus for chronic infection. In addition, the biofilm creates a microenvironment that slows down the metabolism, and therefore the replication rate of bacteria, which also makes them more resistant to antimicrobial agents. Biofilm development is likely to contribute to chronic or recurrent equine uterine infections.

Equine Biofilms

Evaluation of bacteria isolated from the equine uterus suggests that the majority of isolates of *Streptococcus equi* subspecies *zooepidemicus*, *Escherichia coli*, *Pseudomonas aeruginosa*, and *Klebsiella pneumoniae* are capable of producing a biofilm *in vitro*. Biofilm infections are often multifocal, with the greatest amount of adherent material located between the endometrial tissue folds and in the uterine horns. The bacteria in biofilms are at greater numbers deep within the endometrial glands as compared with the luminal surface. Treatments should be designed to penetrate deep into the glands and tissues to effectively clear the pathogenic organisms.

Diagnostic Tests

Currently there is not a specific commercial clinical assay to detect the presence or absence of a bacterial biofilm. The difficult part in detecting an *in vivo* biofilm is that a majority of the biofilm matrix is made up of host cells. Additionally, the biofilm communities are not a ubiquitous coating, but small pin-point plaques. Endometrial culture, cytology, and biopsy are collected blindly and a biofilm-associated infection will only be detected if the instrument collects a sample where one of these biofilm plaques is present. This results in a high rate of false-negative samples from mares with a biofilm infection.

Culture and cytology alone are unable to differentiate a biofilm and planktonic-associated bacterial infection. A uterine biopsy can be evaluated for the presence of

Equine Reproductive Procedures, Second Edition. Edited by John Dascanio and Patrick McCue.

adherent material, which is strongly suggestive of a biofilm-associated infection. The biopsy sample should be placed in to Bouin's solution in order to maintain the integrity of the adherent material. Unfortunately, biofilm material is not retained on uterine biopsy samples preserved in 10% formalin.

Clinically, a biofilm may be suspected if a uterine infection is treated appropriately, including antibiotic therapy based on antimicrobial susceptibility tests, and yet the infection persists or reoccurs.

Treatment Options for Biofilms

A series of *in vitro* studies have been conducted to assess biofilm dispersal and/or bacterial killing for antibiotics and non-antibiotic agents alone or in combination against Gram-negative bacteria. *In vitro* studies indicated that a combination of antibiotics and non-antibiotic agents, such as Tris-EDTA or dimethyl sulfoxide (DMSO), were more effective against a bacterial biofilm than treatment with either an antibiotic or a non-antibiotic agent alone. Preparation of antibiotic/non-antibiotic combinations are presented in Table 37.1. Intrauterine treatments should be infused once per day for 3 consecutive days.

It is important to note that some non-antibiotic agents and antibiotics should *not* be combined in the same syringe. For example, *in vitro* data indicated that mixing acetylcysteine with antibiotics in the same syringe resulted in reduced activity of the antibiotics.

Antibiotic sensitivity testing is recommended for all Gram-negative organisms. Bacteria inherently resistant to an antibiotic will still be resistant when that antibiotic is used in combination with a non-antibiotic agent.

Table 37.1 Antibiotic and non-antibiotic combinations for the treatment of biofilm-associated bacterial endometritis in mares.

Tris-EDTA

- Tris-EDTA: final concentration in the syringe should be 50 mM Tris and 3.5 mM EDTA
- Note: Tris-EDTA and Tricide® are similar; however Tricide® is not equivalent to Tris-EDTA in regard to bacterial killing
- To make Tris-EDTA: 480 ml (16 oz) bottle of Dechra Triz-EDTA crystals; add 240 ml (8 oz) of sterile water (this is different to the bottle instructions). The 2× concentration of Tris-EDTA solution will be further diluted by the antibiotics below to the proper final concentration

Antibiotic	Drug Amount	Tris EDTA	QS	Final Volume	Notes
Amikacin (250 mg/ml)	4 ml (1 g)	30 ml	16 ml sterile fluid (saline, LRS, sterile H_2O)	60 ml	10 ml of 8.4% sodium bicarbonate should be added to the amikacin
Ceftiofur (1 g reconstituted in 20 ml)	20 ml (1 g)	30 ml	10 ml sterile fluid (sterile H_2O)	60 ml	

Hydrogen peroxide (H_2O_2)

- H_2O_2: 1% final concentration in the syringe
- A 3% stock solution is available at many drug stores and veterinary distributors

Antibiotic	Drug Amount	H_2O_2	QS	Final Volume	Notes
Amikacin (250 mg/ml)	4 ml (1 g)	20 ml	26 ml sterile fluid (saline, LRS, sterile H_2O)	60 ml	10 ml of 8.4% sodium bicarbonate should be added to the amikacin
Ciprofloxacin (10 mg/ml)	40 ml (400 mg)	20 ml	0	60 ml	

Dimethyl sulfoxide (DMSO)

- DMSO: 30% final concentration in the syringe
- 99% stock solution is used for calculations below

Antibiotic	Drug Amount	DMSO	QS	Final Volume	Notes
Ceftiofur (1 g reconstituted in 20 ml)	20 ml (1 g)	20 ml	20 ml sterile fluid (sterile H_2O)	60 ml	
Ciprofloxacin (10 mg/ml)	40 ml (400 mg)	20 ml	0	60 ml	

LRS, lactated Ringer's solution.

Further Reading

Costerton JW, Stewart PS, Greenberg EP. 1999. Bacterial biofilms: a common cause of persistent infections. *Science* 284: 1318–22.

Ferris RA, McCue PM, Borlee GI, Loncar KD, Hennet ML, Borlee BR. 2016. In vitro efficacy of nonantibiotic treatments on biofilm disruption of Gram-negative pathogens and an in vivo model of infectious endometritis utilizing isolates from the equine uterus. *J Clin Microbiol* 54: 631–9.

LeBlanc MM. 2010. Advances in the diagnosis and treatment of chronic infectious and post-mating-induced endometritis in the mare. *Reprod Domest Anim* 45: 21–7.

Lindsay D, Holy von A. 2006. Bacterial biofilms within the clinical setting: what healthcare professionals should know. *J Hosp Infect* 64: 313–25.

Loncar KD, Ferris RA, McCue PM, Borlee GI, Hennet ML, Borlee BR. 2017. In vitro biofilm disruption and bacterial killing using non-antibiotic compounds against Gram-negative equine uterine pathogens. *J Eq Vet Sci* 53: 94–9.

Petersen MR, Nielsen JM, Lehn-Jensen H, Bojesen AM. 2009. Streptococcus equi subspecies zooepidemicus resides deep in the chronically infected endometrium of mares. *Clin Theriogenol* 1: 161–5.

Petersen MR, Skive B, Christoffersen M, *et al.* 2015. Activation of persistent Streptococcus equi subspecies zooepidemicus in mares with subclinical endometritis. *Vet Microbiol* 179: 119–25.

38

Latent Uterine Bacterial Infections

Morten Rønn Petersen[1] *and Anders Miki Bojesen*[2]

[1] *University Hospital Copenhagen, University of Copenhagen, Denmark*
[2] *University of Copenhagen, Denmark*

Introduction

During the reproductive career of the mare, the uterus is repeatedly challenged by microorganisms, particularly in relation to breeding and foaling. In situations with suboptimal closure of the vulvar, vestibular, and/or cervical seal, the microbial exposure is intensified.

When diagnosing equine endometritis, the diagnostic method will affect sensitivity and specificity results (see Chapters 12 and 16–19). While *Escherichia coli* is the most prevalent species isolated using low volume uterine lavage (LeBlanc *et al.* 2007), an endometrial biopsy has been reported to be superior in regard to detection of β-hemolytic *Streptococcus equi* subspecies *zooepidemicus* (Nielsen 2005). This likely reflects the preferred bacterial localization, with *E. coli* localized on the luminal epithelium and *Streptococcus* species within or below the luminal epithelia in a multifocal distribution (Petersen *et al.* 2009).

The multifocal endometrial distribution that *Streptococcus* species has in some chronically infected mares has been demonstrated to reach millimeters into the endometrium making diagnostics using commonly employed techniques (e.g., swabs) inadequate. This is of particular importance in mares with a low level of infection, decreasing the chance of "collecting" bacteria when recovering a diagnostic sample. Suspicion of infection despite repeated negative diagnostic tests may yet prompt antimicrobial treatment in this group of problem mares. However antibiotic treatment, systemic and/or uterine has little or no effect, as the *Streptococcus* species are metabolic inactive and dormant, which makes them tolerant to even very high levels of antibiotics (Petersen *et al.* 2015). The presence of dormant *Streptococcus* species in the uterine lining indicates that such mares are latently infected. Latent infections have been defined as an "asymptomatic infection capable of showing symptoms under some circumstances or if activated" (*Farlex Partner Medical Dictionary* 2012).

The specialized growth medium, bActivate (Bojesen and Petersen Biotech, Copenhagen, Denmark), is capable of resuscitating dormant bacteria, particularly *Streptococcus* species, and thus allows subsequent diagnostics of latent endometritis. Following intrauterine instillation of bActivate, active growth of dormant in-active *Streptococcus* species within the endometrium is stimulated (Petersen *et al.* 2015). Induction of the bacterial metabolism and growth allows detection of the bacteria at the uterine luminal surface using regular diagnostic techniques in mares that previously have been found to be culture negative (Figure 38.1). The metabolically active bacteria also regain susceptibility to regular antibiotic treatment, thus allowing for the efficient clearance of the infection (Skriver & Larsen 2019).

By spending one estrus undergoing activation and treatment, the mare is ready for breeding in the following cycle. Inclusion of bActivate to aid diagnostics and treatment of latent infections in problem mares on a large well-managed Thoroughbred breeding farm demonstrated an increase in fertility and reduction of pregnancy loss compared with historic data (Petersen *et al.* 2018).

Equipment and Supplies

Tail wrap, tail rope, non-irritant soap, roll cotton, stainless steel bucket, disposable liner for bucket, paper towels, sterile lubricant, sterile obstetrical sleeve, equipment for low volume uterine lavage (see Chapter 18), bActivate. Infusion pipette, syringes, needles, intrauterine or systemic antibiotics as needed.

Equine Reproductive Procedures, Second Edition. Edited by John Dascanio and Patrick McCue.

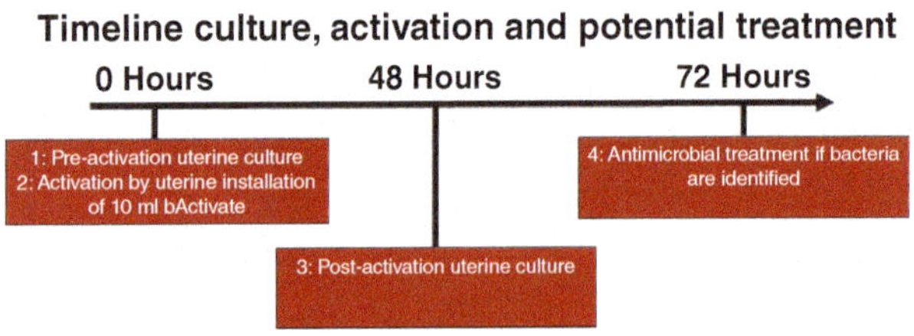

Figure 38.1 Diagnostic and treatment protocol for the use of bActivate.

Technique

- Remove feces from the rectum.
- Place a tail wrap and tie the tail out of the way (see Chapter 4).
- Clean and dry the perineum of the mare (see Chapter 3).
- Place a sterile obstetrical sleeve on the arm
- Uterine culture and activation is initiated during early estrus to allow treatment to be completed no later than 3 days following ovulation (Figure 38.1).
- *0 hours*. The mare's perineum is prepared and a low volume uterine lavage is performed (see Chapter 18). Infuse 10 ml of bActivate into the uterus.
- *48 hours*. The mare's perineum is prepared and a low volume uterine lavage is performed (see Chapter 18).
- *72 hours*. The mare's perineum is prepared and antimicrobial treatment initiated if bacteria are identified (see next section).

Interpretation of Findings and Selection of Antibiotics

The mare is defined as having latent infected if more bacteria are isolated 48 hours after activation compared with immediately before activation (0 hours). In some mares, no bacteria are identified prior to activation whereas heavy growth is seen at 48 hours after activation. In other mares, a low number of colonies are detected at 0 hours, which increases to medium growth (i.e., 20–50 colonies) at 48 hours. An increasing number of colonies isolated 48 hours after activation indicates initial presence of a latent infection with dormant bacteria. Systemic antibiotics are recommended in latent infected mares following activation and diagnosis. Systemic antibiotics allow clearance of active bacteria located deep within the endometrium. Procaine penicillin G is the antibiotic of choice if *Streptococcus* species are isolated, and should be administered twice daily for 3 days (22,000 IU/kg IM, b.i.d.).

Beta-hemolytic *Streptococcus* species are the most commonly isolated pathogens in latent infected mares. It is, however, not uncommon to observe growth of *E. coli* on the pre-activation uterine sample, but only *Streptococcus* species following activation. In such cases, uterine choice of antibiotics should consider bacteria isolated both before and after activation. For optimal treatment effect, it is crucial to select both uterine and systemic antibiotics. Intrauterine antibiotics are necessary to help clear the luminal part of the infection. Uterine lavage can be helpful, especially in the initial days of treatment, to help physically clean the uterine lumen, as some mares will generate a substantial amount of fluid and purulent debris following activation. Uterine ecbolics, such as 10 IU of oxytocin administered intramuscularly, can also be advantageous in treatment.

Disclosure

Anders Miki Bojesen and Morten Petersen invented, produce, and sell bActivate, www.bactivate.eu (last accessed June 2020).

References

Farlex Partner Medical Dictionary, 2012.

LeBlanc MM, Magsig J, Stromberg AJ. 2007. Use of a low-volume uterine flush for diagnosing endometritis in chronically infertile mares. *Theriogenology* 68(3): 403–12.

Nielsen JM. 2005. Endometritis in the mare: a diagnostic study comparing cultures from swab and biopsy. *Theriogenology* 64(3): 510–18.

Petersen MR, Nielsen JM, Lehn-Jensen H, Bojesen AM. 2009. *Streptococcus equi* subsp. *zooepidemicus* resides deep in the chronically infected endometrium of mares. *Clin Theriogenol* 1: 393–409.

Petersen MR, Skive B, Christoffersen M, *et al.* 2015. Activation of persistent *Streptococcus equi* subspecies *zooepidemicus* in mares with subclinical endometritis. *Vet Microbiol* 179(1/2): 119–25.

Petersen, MR, Rosenbrock, A, Osborne, M, Bojesen AM. 2018. High prevalence of subclinical endometritis in problem mares – effect of activation and treatment on fertility. *ISER Proc* 66: 117.

Skriver A, Larsen RB. 2019. *The effect of activation and treatment of uterine persistent Streptococcus equi subspecies zooepidemicus in barren mares.* DVM thesis. Frederiksberg, Denmark: University of Copenhagen.

39

Acupuncture in Mare Reproduction

Kristina Lu and Lauren Javernick

Hagyard Equine Medical Institute, USA

Introduction

The use of acupuncture and traditional Chinese veterinary medicine (TCVM) are considered complimentary, not as an alternative, to a complete medical evaluation and treatment. It is possible to place needles in acupuncture points without studying the theory, but the results will not be as profound. When combining accurate needle placement with a correct TCVM diagnosis (bian zheng), the response can be amazing and sometimes appear miraculous. The bian zheng is the animal's pattern and is based on their tongue, pulse character, constitution, symptoms, temperature, and response to their environment.

TCVM requires harmony within the animal's body and between the animal and its environment. Harmony exists in TCVM within several different medical theories. To start, the yin and yang need to be in harmony. Yin is the dark area within the yin/yang symbol and a few examples of what it represents include substantial objects/organs, a quiet resting type energy, women, the moon, dark, and cold. Yang is the white area and symbolizes activity/organs' activities, men, the sun, light, and heat. The opposite colored dots represent the opposing energy within the yin or yang. All yin has yang and all yang has yin. For example, the heart muscle and organ would be considered yin, but the activity of pumping blood would be yang. In TCVM, disease exists when the animal is not balanced between yin and yang, and achieving balance is the practitioner's goal.

The five element theory of TCVM is based on the Chinese elements: wood, fire, earth, metal, and water. An animal's constitution often falls within one of these five elements and can often lead to certain disharmonies. Wood animals are competitive, dominant, often athletic, and prone to anger when stressed. Fire animals are overly friendly, hyperactive, center of attention, and prone to drama. Earth animals are laid back, friendly, unbothered, and prone to laziness. Metal animals like everything in their place, controlling, routine orientated, and prone to being aloof. Water animals are timid, scared, fearful, and prone to being fear-biters/kickers. The 12 zang-fu organs/meridians of Chinese medicine fall within these elements and are listed below in Table 39.1 with their abbreviations. These abbreviations will serve as the meridian abbreviations when describing acupuncture points. Two additional, extraordinary, meridian channels utilized for mare reproduction acupuncture are also listed in Table 39.1. The five element theory relies on balance between the elements and the meridians/

Table 39.1 The 12 organs/meridians of Chinese medicine.

	Number of Points	TCVM Element
Zang (yin) organs/meridians		
Lung (LU)	11	Metal
Spleen (SP)	21	Earth
Heart (HT)	9	Fire
Kidney (KID)	27	Water
Pericardium (PC)	9	Fire
Liver (LIV)	14	Wood
Fu (yang) organs/meridians		
Large intestine (LI)	20	Metal
Stomach (ST)	45	Earth
Small intestine (SI)	19	Fire
Bladder (BL)	67	Water
Triple heather (TH)	23	Fire
Gallbladder (GB)	44	Wood
Extraordinary channels		
Governing vessel (GV)	28	–
Conception vessel (CV)	24	–

Equine Reproductive Procedures, Second Edition. Edited by John Dascanio and Patrick McCue.

organs within these elements. Each element can affect another element and a disharmony leads to imbalance, which leads to disease. An example would be that chronic stress and anger causes a disharmony in the wood element, which often can lead to gastrointestinal upset or disharmony in the earth element.

The last theory discussed in this very brief summary of TCVM is that of the eight principles that incorporate (i) yin and yang; (ii) interior or exterior; (iii) hot or cold; and (iv) excess or deficiency. This theory identifies disharmonies in the four substances of Chinese medicine: qi, yin, blood, and yang. When dealing with the eight principles it is important to identify with the bian zheng – whether the animal is excess or deficient or cold or hot. Failure to properly identify the bian zheng can lessen the response to acupuncture or in some cases, especially with the use of Chinese herbal therapies, can make animals much worse. For example, an excess condition should never be tonified and a deficient condition should never be drained. Several opportunities exist for training in acupuncture and TCVM. For the best results with problem mares, consultation with a trained practitioner is highly recommended.

Three commonly used acupuncture regimes are discussed here and include mares with fluid pre- and post-breeding, urine poolers, and pregnancy maintenance. The measurement "cun" in horses is roughly two finger widths or the size of the last rib. The anatomic references are a guide and get the practitioner within the area. Training and practice allow the practitioner to accurately find the acupuncture points. A few acupuncture points will be discussed that are commonly utilized, but for best results the practitioner should use an accurate TCVM bian zheng and individualized treatment.

Equipment and Supplies

Electroacupuncture unit with a minimum of three cords with frequencies ranging from 20 to 120 Hz; needles: 28 gauge 75 mm solid core stainless steel acupuncture needles, 28 gauge 50 mm solid core stainless steel acupuncture needles, 28 gauge 4 cm (1.5 inch) hypodermic needles; syringes: 3, 5, and 10 ml; oxytocin 20 units/ml; vitamin B_{12} solution 1,000 μg/ml; lip chain or twitch if needed; tranquilizer if needed.

Restraint and Tranquilization

A lip chain is preferred because the procedure takes 20–30 minutes. Occasionally a mare does not tolerate the needle placement, but seems to enjoy the electrostimulation. These are the animals that would benefit from a twitch restraint because the needle placement is relatively short in duration.

Tranquilizer (3 mg detomidine hydrochloride and 3 mg butorphanol tartrate intravenously) is used occasionally if the animal is too fractious for placement of the needles or for the electrical stimulation. Tranquilizer has been shown to diminish the response to acupuncture and should be utilized only when necessary.

Pre- and Post-Breeding Uterine Fluid Technique

Acupuncture Points

- GB-21: calming point. Halfway along the cranial edge of the scapula; 50–75 mm acupuncture needle.
- Bai hui: lumbosacral space; 50 mm acupuncture needle.
- Shen shu: located 2 cun lateral from the lumbosacral space. Bilateral; 75 mm acupuncture needles.
- Shen peng: located 2 cun lateral to the spine and 2 cun cranial to shen shu. Bilateral; 75 mm acupuncture needles.
- Shen jiao: located 2 cun lateral to the spine and 2 cun caudal to shen shu. Bilateral; 75 mm acupuncture needles.
- GV-2: located at the epidural space cranial to the tail.
- Tail points: two points located along both sides of the tail. Needle placement is along the tail base, parallel to the spine; 50 mm acupuncture needles.

Procedure

Electroacupuncture for 15 minutes with a minimum frequency of 20 Hz up to 80 Hz. Intensity is animal dependent, but some degree of muscle fasciculation should be observed. The following points are most commonly utilized.

- GB-21: dry needle.
- Electroacupuncture connecting:
  - Shen shu: ipsilateral tail point. Bilateral.
  - Bai hui: GV-2.
  - For additional stimulus, shen peng: ipsilateral shen jiao. Bilateral.
- Oxytocin: 10 units placed at bai hui using a 25 gauge 4 cm (1.5 inch) hypodermic needle.
- Additional acupoints utilized:
  - SP-6: caudal to the tibial border 3 cun proximal to medial malleolus. Master point for urogenital tract; 50 mm acupuncture dry needle or 3 ml 1,000 μg vitamin B_{12} with 25 g 4 cm (1.5 inch) hypodermic needle.

- SP-9: level of patellar ligaments, 0.5 cun in front of saphenous vein. For incontinence. 50 mm acupuncture dry needle. Note: SP-6 and SP-9 are both good points for a pattern with damp heat.
- KID-3: in large depression between the medial malleolus and calcaneal tuber opposite BL-60. 50 mm dry acupuncture needle. Two points (KID-3 and BL-60) may be used together if the mare has any lameness issues on top of infertility. Great point for yin deficiency too.
- BL-23: level of L2–L3, 3 cun from midline. 50 mm acupuncture dry needle. Association point for KID.
- Yan chi: halfway between the tuber coxae and shen peng (see above for location). For male and female infertility, and hindquarter pain. 75 mm dry acupuncture needle.
- CV-1: between the anus and vulva. Indicated for infertility and incontinence. 5 ml of 1,000 μg vitamin B_{12} with a 25 gauge 4 cm (1.5 inch) hypodermic needle.
- "Tings:" if an excess condition exists, the bleeding of tings (jing well points) is also recommended and should be based on the pattern diagnosis.

Treatment Regime

Electroacupuncture with oxytocin should be performed the day before breeding and the day after breeding. If the mare is going to be bred late in the day, then treatment on the day of breeding would be beneficial. Electroacupuncture is utilized every other day; if treating consecutive days choose different acupuncture points to maximize the effect. If the mare is known to have problems clearing fluid, then treatment can begin when the cervix starts to open. For post-breeding fluid acupuncture, utilize the day following breeding and up to day 5 post-ovulation on an every other day schedule.

Urine Poolers

The points and treatment regime are similar for urine poolers as for mares with fluid. Acute urine poolers from trauma/foaling trauma seem to respond better than chronic urine poolers. If the mare is an acute urine pooler, treat her weekly during diestrus and then do a more focused treatment (see previous section) during estrus.

Acupuncture Points

- BL-28: S2–S3 3 cun from midline. 75 mm solid acupuncture needles. Incontinence, bladder association point.
- BL-40: in the popliteal fossa. He-sea point descending the bladder qi for incontinence. The master point for caudal back and hip pain.
- BL-54: halfway between the lumbosacral space and the greater trochanter in a large depression. 75 mm acupuncture needle. Good for urinary disorders and any hind limb lameness.

Procedure

Perform 15 minutes of electroacupuncture 80 Hz at the following points:

- Shen shu: tail point, bilateral.
- Bai hui: GV-2.
- BL-54: ipsilateral BL 40, bilateral.
- BL-28: bilateral.
- CV-1: 5 ml of 1,000 μg vitamin B_{12} with a 25 gauge 4 cm (1.5 inch) hypodermic needle.
- Oxytocin: 10 units placed at bai hui using a 25 gauge 4 cm (1.5 inch) hypodermic needle.

Pregnancy Maintenance

TCVM patterns commonly seen with abortion include kidney deficiency, blood stasis, and spleen qi deficiency. Pregnancy loss in the first trimester is often associated with blood or jing (essence, prenatal qi) deficiency and kidney deficiency, while pregnancy loss beyond the first trimester is often associated with liver blood stasis or sinking/collapsing Spleen qi (Macioca 1989, p. 161). Kidney jing deficiency may be associated with a red tongue and pulse that is floating and empty or best felt superficially and is soft. The degree of kidney yin deficiency and kidney yang deficiency are also important to assess. Liver blood stasis is associated with a tongue that is purple, especially on the sides, and a wiry pulse. Sinking spleen qi can manifest with a pale tongue that may be swollen on the sides and a weak pulse. Also look for clues, such as decreased appetite or loose manure. These patterns, as well as constitutional points, are ideally addressed prior to pregnancy with additional treatment during pregnancy as needed. Signalment and history are also important factors, such as mare age, history and gestational stage of previous abortions, and history of endometritis or other reproductive pathology during breeding. Mares typically present with a combination of patterns and variable underlying causes, thus points are chosen that best suit the individual.

Potential Points for Treating Liver Blood Stasis

- GB43 (regulates liver qi): located on the lateral aspect of the hind limb distal to the fetlock joint.
- LIV-3 (regulates liver qi and blood): located on the hind cranio-medial cannon bone, one third of the distance from the tarsus to the fetlock.
- LIV-8 (tonifies liver qi and blood): located in a depression 2 cun cranio-medial and proximal to the popliteal fossa.
- BL-18 (regulates liver blood): two points at the 13th and 14th intercostal spaces 3 cun lateral to the dorsal midline.
- BL-17 (gathering point for blood, regulates blood with dry needle): at the 12th intercostal space 3 cun lateral to dorsal midline.
- SP-10 (regulates blood): 2 cun proximal to the proximo-medial border of the patella.
- Ren/CV-6 (regulates qi and moves blood in the abdomen, used in women with abdominal pain): on ventral midline 1.5 cun caudal to the umbilicus.
  (Macioca 1989, p. 219.)

Potential Acupuncture Points for Treating Spleen Qi Deficiency

- Bai hui (raises qi, moxa): on dorsal midline at the lumbosacral space.
- ST-36 (tonifies spleen qi): 0.5 cun lateral to the tibial crest.
- SP-3 (tonifies spleen qi, source point of spleen): distal to the distal end of the hind limb medial splint bone.
- SP-6 (tonifies spleen qi): 3 cun proximal to the medial malleolus, caudal to the tibia, 0.5 cun posterior of the saphenous vein.
- BL-20 and BL-21 (tonify spleen qi, important for chronic conditions): at the 17th intercostal space and caudal to the last rib 3 cun lateral to the dorsal midline.
- Ren/CV-12 (tonifies spleen qi): 4 cun cranial to the umbilicus.
  (Macioca 1989, pp. 242–4.)

Potential Acupuncture Points for Treating Kidney Jing Deficiency

- KI-3 (tonifies kidney yin and jing): between the medial malleolus and calcaneal tuberosity.
- KI-6 (tonifies kidney yin): in a depression between the calcaneal tuberosity and talus.
- LU-7 right (regulates the conception vessel): cranio-medial radius cranial to the cephalic vein at the level of the distal edge of the chestnut.
- Ren/CV-4 (tonifies jing): 3 cun caudal to the umbilicus.
- BL-23 (tonifies kidneys): at the 2nd lumbar intervertebral space 3 cun lateral to the dorsal midline.
- Du/GV-4 (tonifies yang aspect of jing): on the dorsal midline at the L2–L3 intervertebral space.
  (Maciocia 1989, pp. 252–7.)

Potential Acupuncture Points for Use During Mare Pregnancy

- Baihui (calms the mind).
- BL-18 and BL-19 (harmonizes the liver, association points of liver and gallbladder): BL-19 is at the 15th intercostal space 3 cun lateral to the dorsal midline.
- BL-20 and BL-21 (tonifies spleen qi, association points of spleen and stomach).
- Qi-hai-shu (tonifies spleen qi): at the 16th intercostal space between the longissimus dorsi and iliocostalis muscles.
- Da-feng-men, tian-men, an-shen (calms the mind, used for fetal restlessness): da-feng men is a triangle of points with the apex at the rostral forelock and legs of 0.5 cun; tian-men is at the atlanto-occipital joint; an-shen is in a depression behind the ears.
  (Xie & Preast 2007, pp. 324–5.)

Several points are listed in the veterinary literature as being contraindicated in pregnant animals, including points around the abdomen and lumbosacral region:

- Du/CV-1 through 6, yan-chi, BL-23 through 28, BL-52, LI-4, SP-6, BL-60, BL-40, ST-36, and BL-67.
  (Xie & Preast 2007, p. 325)

Additional Comments

There are many acupuncture points available that would be beneficial in treating problem mares. This summary represents the points most commonly utilized. There are mares that tolerate acupuncture well during the peak of estrus, but can be fractious during other times. Always proceed with caution and utilize an experienced handler when acupuncturing a mare. Not discussed is the use of Chinese herbal medications for use with the problem mare. These are incredibly effective when combined with acupuncture to treat a diagnosed bian zheng (pattern). The herbal remedy most commonly used for pregnancy maintenance is based on the classical formula bai zhu san (Xie 2008, p. 71).

References

Maciocia G. 1989. The Foundations of Chinese Medicine. London: Churchill Livingstone.

Xie H. 2008. Chinese Veterinary Herbal Handbook, 2nd edn. Reddick, FL: Chi Institute.

Xie H, Preast V. 2007. Xie's Veterinary Acupuncture. Oxford: Blackwell Publishing.

Further Reading

Maciocia G. 2011. Obstetrics and Gynecology in Chinese Medicine, 2nd edn. London: Churchill Livingstone.

Xie H, Preast V. Traditional Chinese Veterinary Medicine. Reddick, FL, Chi Institute.

40

Restraint for Breeding

John J. Dascanio

School of Veterinary Medicine, Texas Tech University, USA

Introduction

Mares may be pasture bred, bred by live cover in hand, or bred by artificial insemination. Live cover breeding in hand entails some type of restraint of the mare. This may range from tying the mare to a post or breeding rail and handling only the stallion, to handling both the mare and stallion by different individuals. Ultimately the goal is to facilitate a safe and successful mating.

If the mare is in good heat and is experienced (i.e., not a maiden mare), it may only be necessary to restrain the mare by holding the lead rope during a live cover. If the mare is nervous, frightened, or inexperienced, it may be beneficial to administer a mild tranquilizer 5–10 minutes prior to the live cover attempt. If this is not sufficient, a lip twitch may be applied to the mare to facilitate mating.

In some breeding operations, breeding hobbles are routinely placed on the mare to prevent the mare from injuring the stallion. Removal of hind shoes (if present), padding the hind feet, or placement of felt pads on the hind feet may be required in some breeding operations.

Mares to be used as a jump mare for semen collection should be in good heat, show receptivity to the stallion, and be easy/safe to handle. An ovariectomized mare can provide a consistent, reliable behavior pattern for semen collection, which may be enhanced with the occasional administration of estradiol (3–10 mg IM administered anywhere from once per week to once per month or longer as needed).

Equipment and Supplies

Twitch, leg rope, xylazine, detomidine, butorphanol, acepromazine, hobbles, needles, syringes.

Technique

- A large, flat area with good footing should be used for breeding activities.
- Two handlers may sometimes be necessary on either side of the mare's head to prevent the mare from moving sideways, away from the mounting stallion.
- A common level of restraint for a mare would be the application of a chain shank over her nose and the use of a lip twitch. A long-handled twitch allows placement of the distal end of the twitch into the mare's shoulder to provide a pivot point if necessary to turn the mare.
- A front leg leather strap or rope may also be used to help prevent movement and potential kicking by the mare. It should be noted that with this method the mare can still kick with her hind legs, but may be delayed in action. The strap is placed on the pastern of the left front leg with a quick release knot. The leg is elevated and the strap is wrapped around the upper leg and then lower leg to keep the leg flexed at the carpus (Figures 40.1 and 40.2). The wrapped leg is usually released when the stallion mounts the mare so that she can stand on all four feet.
- Tranquilization may also be administered for restraint. Typically a xylazine (0.33–0.44 mg/kg IV) and butorphanol (0.011–0.022 mg/kg IV) combination is used to provide sedation and a degree of immobility for the mare. Alternatively, acepromazine (0.044–0.066 mg/kg IV) or detomidine (0.0088–0.011 mg/kg IV) may be used.
- Hobbles may be used to restrain the mare from kicking (Figure 40.3). Hobbles are attached to the rear legs of the mare at the level of the fetlock or hock, depending on the type of hobbles available. The two rear leg buckles are secured and the neck collar is subsequently placed on

Equine Reproductive Procedures, Second Edition. Edited by John Dascanio and Patrick McCue.

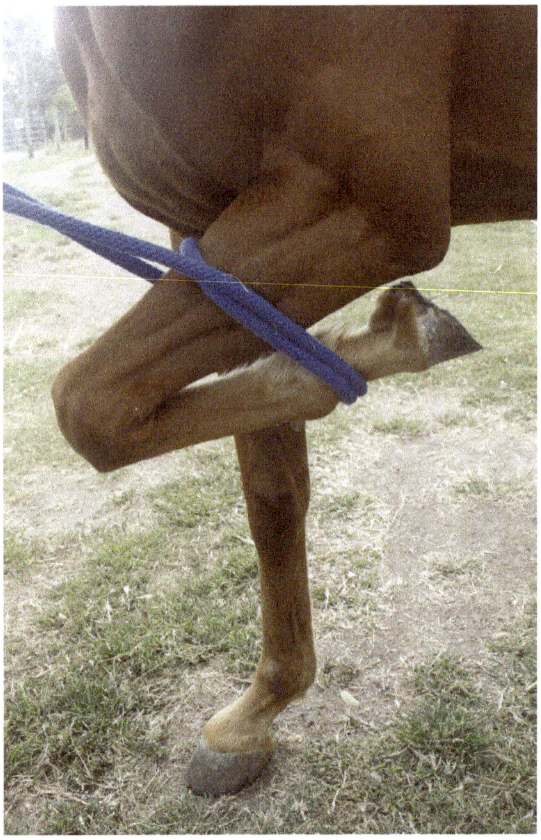

Figure 40.1 Rope wrapped around the pastern and forearm. The free ends of the rope are held by the mare handler.

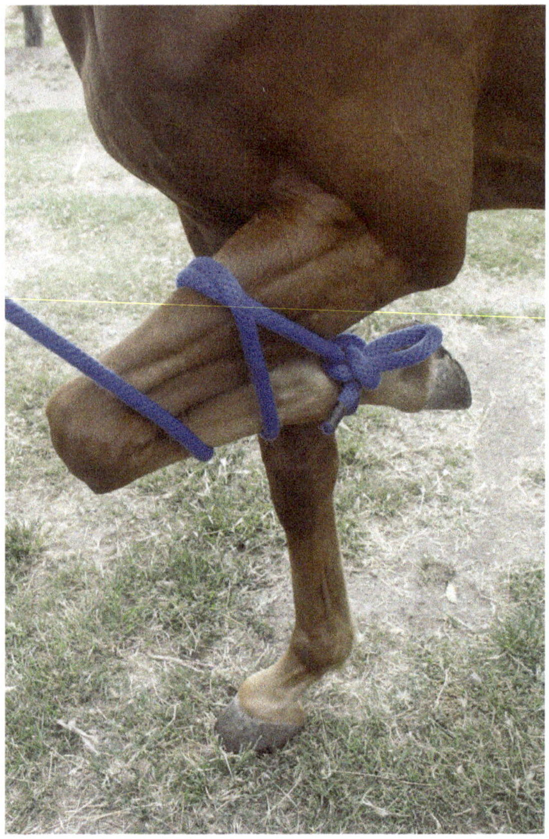

Figure 40.2 Rope wrapped around the pastern and forearm. One end is tied to the pastern with a quick release knot and other end is held by the mare handler.

the mare and a rope with a quick release cleat is attached to the buckle. When hobbles are first placed on the mare, the ropes should be very loose so that the mare may be walked to get used to the presence of the apparatus. The ropes are slowly tightened and the mare walked each time so that she gets used to progressively less ability to move. Since there is some ability to move even with hobbles placed on a mare, kicking may still be possible, but in a limited fashion.

Interpretation

- Mare teasing activity may provide an idea of the degree of restraint required before a stallion mounts.
- Prior knowledge of previous breeding activity and normal behavior should dictate the required restraint techniques.
- It is important for the mare handler to keep the mare's hind end centered when the stallion mounts so that the stallion will be properly aligned with the mare.

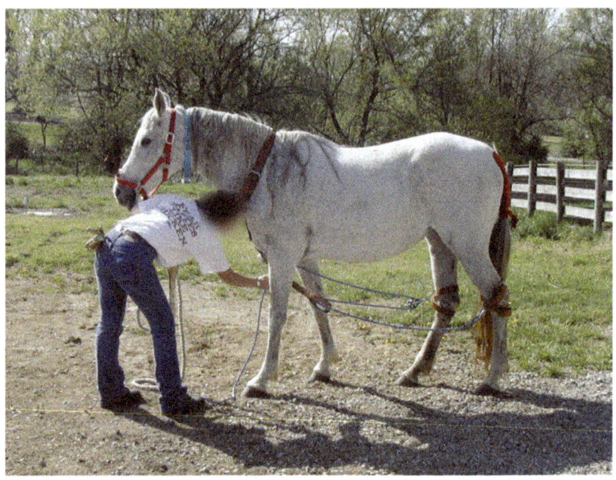

Figure 40.3 Mare with hobbles and tail wrap in preparation for breeding.

- When using hobbles, a sharp pocket knife should be available to cut ropes in case the horses get entangled during breeding.

41

Natural Service: Pasture Breeding

Patrick M. McCue

Equine Reproduction Laboratory, Colorado State University, USA

Introduction

Mares may be bred by natural service (also referred to as live cover or natural cover) during pasture breeding or hand mating. Natural cover is the only breeding technique allowed by the Jockey Club in Thoroughbred mares if the foal is to be registered (Section V, Rule 1D).

The advantages of pasture breeding (the stallion turned out onto pasture with the mares) are decreased horse handling, decreased expenses for personnel, and decreased breeding expenses. With pasture breeding, the stallion is responsible for estrus detection and experienced pasture stallions will rarely attempt to breed a mare that is not in heat. An inexperienced stallion will quickly learn equine social skills in a pasture of seasoned broodmares as he will be aggressively turned away from mares not in estrus. In general, most pasture-breeding stallions are very tolerant of foals and have good parental instincts.

Disadvantages of pasture breeding include potential for injury to the stallion or the mares, inability to detect reproductive problems with either the stallion or the mares while they are turned out together, spread of disease through the herd, and lack of an accurate conception date for calculation of a potential foaling date.

Pasture Breeding Programs

- A stallion is typically turned out with a band of up to 15–20 mares for approximately 90 days or more beginning in May or June in North America. Mares housed outside in North America under ambient light conditions may not begin regular estrous cycles until April or early May depending on geographic latitude.
- Typically, a group or band of mares is put together in the spring and allowed to establish their social hierarchy. A week or so later a stallion is introduced to the group (Figure 41.1).
- Stallions may mate a mare in estrus multiple times per day in a pasture-breeding situation (Figure 41.2).
- If a stallion is young or inexperienced, it may be beneficial to first turn him out with a single, older, experienced mare in good heat so that he may gain breeding experience.
- Ideally, pasture-bred mares should be examined for pregnancy by transrectal ultrasonograpy a minimum of 14 days after the stallion was removed from his harem.
- However, in many instances no pregnancy exams are performed at all on pasture-bred mares. An owner may simply wait until the following spring or summer to observe which mares produce foals.

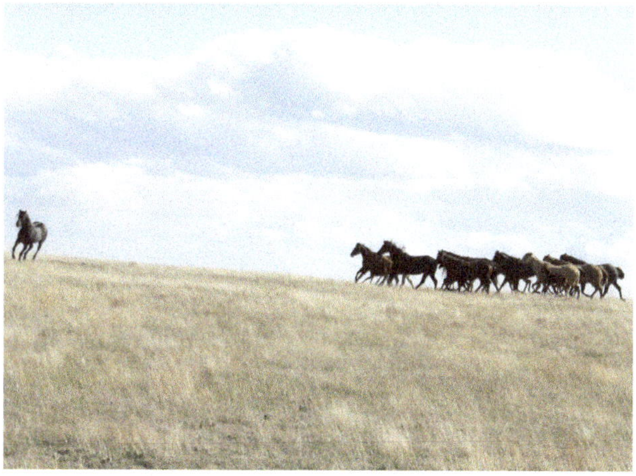

Figure 41.1 Stallion (left) gathering his harem of mares.

Equine Reproductive Procedures, Second Edition. Edited by John Dascanio and Patrick McCue.

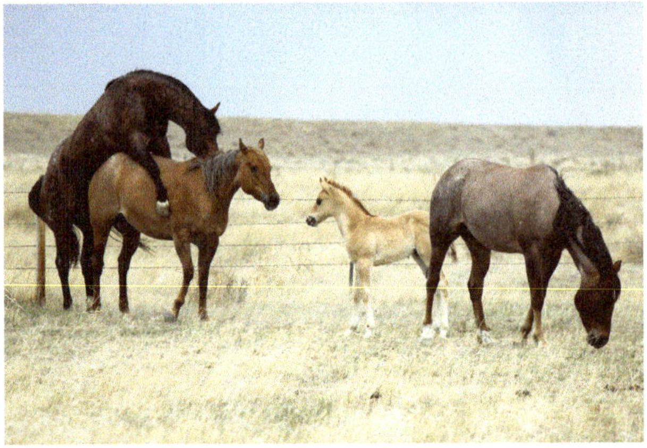

Figure 41.2 Stallion mating a mare with a foal at her side. The mare was part of a band of 20 mares turned out onto a large pasture.

- A potential pitfall with a minimalistic approach to pasture breeding (i.e., no examination of the stallion prior to turnout, no examination of open mares prior to turnout, and no pregnancy exams during turnout or after the stallion is removed) is that fertility issues of the stallion or individual mares can result in a decreased foal crop. In addition, if a mare is not pregnant after being bred over two to three cycles with one stallion, she may become pregnant if given an opportunity to be mated to another stallion. In addition, if the mare is pastured on endophyte-infected fescue grass, it does not allow removal of her from the pasture or an alternative feed source to be fed in the last 30–45 days of gestation.

Further Reading

Umphenour NW, P McCarthy, TL Blanchard. 2011. Management of stallions in natural-service programs. In: McKinnon AO, Squires EL, Vaala WE, Varner DD (eds). Equine Reproduction, 2nd edn. Ames, IA: Wiley Blackwell, pp. 1208–27.

42

Natural Service: In-hand Breeding

Charles F. Scoggin

Rood and Riddle Equine Hospital, USA

Introduction

A natural service or live-cover mating is mandated in Thoroughbred mares by the Jockey Club (Section V, Rule 1D). In other horse breeds, mares may be bred by live cover or artificial insemination.

Hand mating (also known as "in-hand breeding" or "breeding in-hand") implies that both the stallion and mare are handled and restrained in a controlled breeding environment. Advantages of hand breeding over pasture breeding are that a mating can be scheduled and confirmed, the mare can be examined before and after breeding, a dismount sample could be collected from the stallion to examine for live spermatozoa, and, at least theoretically, hand breeding offers less risk to the stallion than pasture breeding.

Disadvantages of hand breeding are the time required for satisfactory examination and teasing of mares, number of personnel involved in the breeding process, and potential risk of injury to personnel and horses in the breeding shed.

Equipment and Supplies

Items for the mare
Leather halter with identification, chain shank with a leather lead, twitch, leather leg strap or breeding hobbles (optional), non-spermicidal lubricant, kick boots (optional), leather neck apron (optional), breeding rolls of various sizes.
Items for the stallion
Leather halter with identification, breeding bridle or chain shank with a leather lead.
Items for breeding shed personnel
Helmet, equestrian safety vest, heavy duty work boots.
Items for semen analysis
Microscope equipped with a phase-contrast lens and warming stage, pre-warmed microscope slides and coverslips, disposable plastic pipettes.

Technique

- The mare owner/agent presents the proper paperwork (breeding shed form, statement of a clean uterine culture (if required), CEM (contagious equine metritis) status (if required), etc.) to the breeding shed attendant.
- The mare is introduced to a teaser stallion via a padded partition to evaluate her for signs of estrus. She is subsequently placed in examination stocks, her tail is wrapped, and her perineum cleansed with a non-residual soap, rinsed with warm water, and dried with a clean paper towel. The wash should extend to the area between the mare's hind legs in case the penis becomes ventrally deviated during the breeding. The tail wrap is intended to keep tail hairs out of the way and to prevent the hairs from injuring the penis of the stallion during intromission.
- If a maiden mare is being bred for the first time (i.e., a first-trip maiden mare), a teaser stallion will be brought in to test-jump her to determine if she will tolerate mounting by a commercial stallion (Figure 42.1). The purpose is to protect the breeding stallion from injury if the mare is not in heat or will not stand to be mounted.
- The mare is led into the breeding shed and her identification is checked to ensure that she is being bred to the proper stallion. The chain portion of the lead shank is placed in the mare's mouth or over her nose, and a twitch is applied to the mare's nose.
- Non-spermicidal lubricant is placed on the vulvar lips to assist with intromission of the stallion's penis. A leather leg strap is looped around the mare's left front limb so as to encircle the mid-radius and pastern, and the free end is held tight by one of the breeding shed attendants (Figure 42.2). Alternatively, breeding hobbles may be placed on the mare.

Equine Reproductive Procedures, Second Edition. Edited by John Dascanio and Patrick McCue.

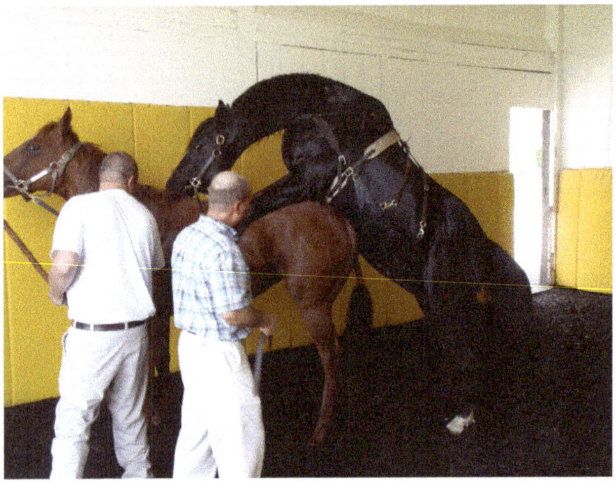

Figure 42.1 Evaluation of a mare for live-cover breeding using a teaser stallion.

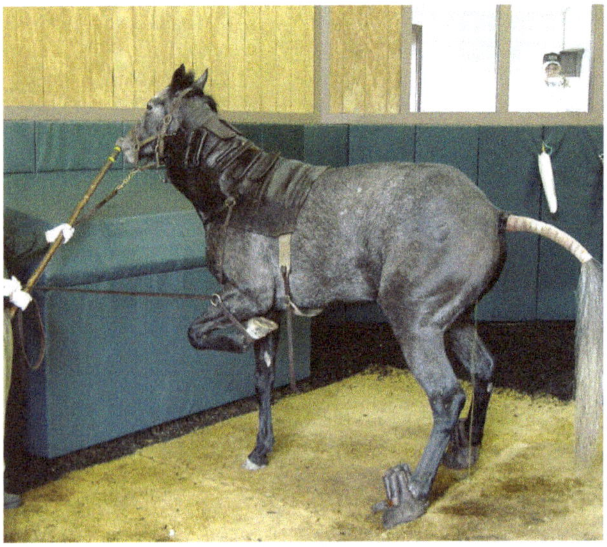

Figure 42.2 Mare wearing a neck apron and kick boots while restrained with a twitch and leg strap prior to mating.

- The stallion is led (either with a breeding bridle or a chain shank placed in the mouth or over the nose) into the breeding shed and his penis is rinsed with warm water (without soap) and either dried with a towel or allowed to air-dry. Washing of the stallion is part of the minimum contamination breeding technique that should be practiced with hand mating. Repeatedly washing the penis of a stallion with soap, especially disinfectant soaps, may eliminate normal skin bacteria and promote overgrowth of potentially pathogenic bacteria on the penis (see Chapter 123).
- The stallion is then introduced to the left flank of the mare. The stallion is allowed to interact with the mare as needed from the left flank to the perineum.
- Once the stallion is deemed ready for breeding (e.g., firm erection and obvious interest in the mare) he is allowed to mount the mare. Just prior to mounting, an attendant on the right or "off" side of the mare grasps the mare's tail and pulls it laterally to prevent it from interfering with penetration of the stallion's penis.
- If necessary, a breeding roll is placed by this same attendant above the penis against the mare's perineum just before the stallion enters her. This will prevent undue or excessive intromission by the stallion and potential trauma to the cranial vagina. Following intromission, tension is released from the leg strap holding the mare's left limb up, thereby allowing the mare to place her leg back on the ground. Occasionally the breeding attendant may have to guide the penis into the vulva with a gloved hand.
- The stallion will perform a series of thrusts, and ejaculation is usually characterized by "flagging" of the stallion's tail (Figure 42.3).
- Once flagging is observed, one of the attendants will step to the left flank of the mare and collect a sample of semen in a clean, pre-warmed collection container (e.g., disposable specimen cup) from the stallion as he dismounts the mare. The attendant takes this sample to a nearby room with a microscope where it is evaluated for the presence of spermatozoa to confirm ejaculation. Once the presence of live, motile sperm is detected, the breeding is considered to be complete. Examination of the dismount sample can provide information on sperm motility, concentration, and morphology. The dismount sample may be filtered, a semen extender added, and the mare bred in accordance with reinforcement breeding guidelines (see Chapter 44).

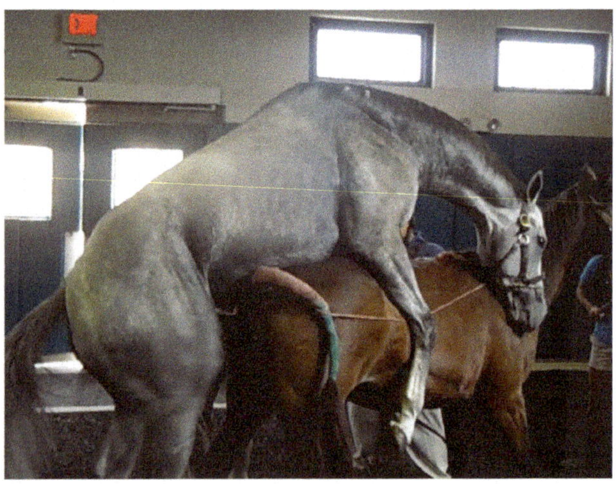

Figure 42.3 Live cover of a mare by a stallion.

- When the stallion dismounts, he is immediately moved away from the mare to prevent the occasional unwanted physical or aggressive behavior that may be initiated by either of the two horses.

Additional Comments

In commercial Thoroughbred breeding programs, most mares will only receive one cover per cycle due to the busy schedules of the stallions. This requires fairly intensive mare management, requiring them to be checked regularly by palpation and/or ultrasonography to determine the optimal day of breeding. Ovulation induction agents are also commonly used and timed so that the mare ovulates within 12–24 hours after mating. In lower volume programs, mares can be bred on their 2nd or 3rd day of estrus and mated every other day until the mare is no longer receptive to the stallion.

Natural service requires a minimum of three qualified individuals. One person is responsible for handling the stallion, another person restrains the mare, while the third person is responsible for directing the stallion into the mare (i.e., ensuring intromission occurs).

Further Reading

Umphenour NW, McCarthy P, Blanchard TL. 2011. Management of stallions in natural service programs. In: McKinnon AO, Squires EL, Vaala WE, Varner DD (eds). Equine Reproduction, 2nd edn. Ames, IA: Wiley Blackwell, pp. 1208–27.

43

Breeding Stitches

Charles F. Scoggin

Rood and Riddle Equine Hospital, USA

Introduction

A breeding stitch is sometimes placed in the vulva of a mare following a Caslick operation. The purpose of this stitch is to alleviate potential stress or tension on the primary Caslick suture line. This stitch is utilized most commonly in live-cover operations to avoid repeated replacement of a Caslick stitch for breeding. It can also be used in mares with a Caslick that require additional vaginal procedures, such as artificial insemination, uterine lavage, or intrauterine infusion, avoiding continual removal of the primary suture line. Indications for use include perineal lacerations, poor perineal conformation, pnemovagina, and urovagina.

The choice of suture is somewhat clinician dependent. The author prefers No. 3 nylon with a swaged-on needle. Alternatively, No. 0, 1, or 2 can be double-threaded using an eyed needle.

Equipment and Supplies

No. 3 nylon non-absorbable sterile suture with half-circle reverse cutting swaged-on needle; alternatively, No. 0, 1, or 2 nylone suture with half-circle reverse cutting eyed needle; needle holders or drivers, scissors.

Techniques

Technique 1

- Following placement of the Caslick suture (see Chapter 53), an area 2 cm (0.75 inch) above the ventral aspect of the suture line is located.
- The stitch is started 2 cm (0.75 inch) lateral to this location on one side of the vulvar labia. The needle containing No. 3 nylon suture is passed into the skin, directed

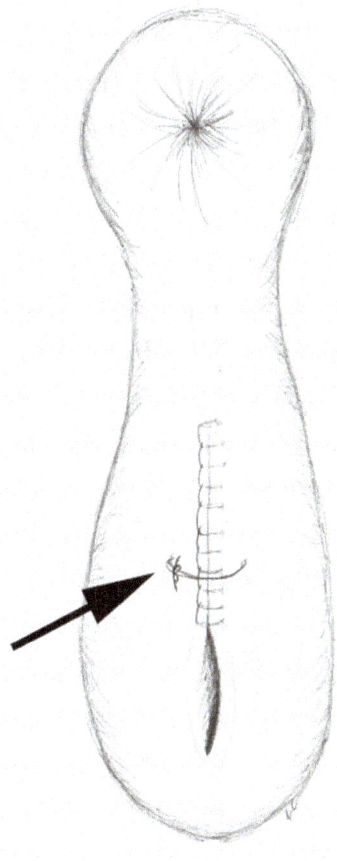

Figure 43.1 Schematic of a breeding stitch (arrow) encircling a region just below the distal third of a traditional Caslick suture.

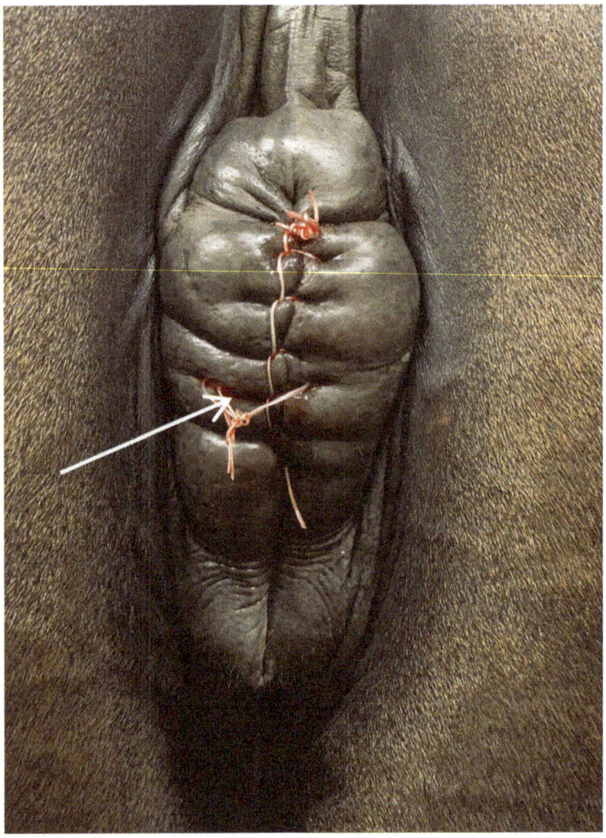

Figure 43.2 Breeding stitch (arrow) just placed in a Thoroughbred mare after a traditional Caslick procedure.

through the submucosa underneath the Caslick suture, and exited on the contralateral vulvar labia directly horizontal to the site of entrance.

- A square knot is tied, but care is taken not to pull it too tight (the clinician should be able to place 1–2 fingers within the loop). The free ends of the suture are then cut to free the needle and trim excess suture material (Figure 43.1).
- The site for placement should have already been scrubbed and desensitized from the prior Caslick procedure, but can be repeated if deemed necessary.

Technique 2

- A strand of No. 0, 1, or 2 suture approximately 25–30 cm (10–12 inches) in length is threaded through the needle so that both ends are of equal length to create a double-stranded stitch.
- Following placement of the Caslick suture, an area 2 cm above the ventral aspect of the suture line is located.
- The stitch is then started 2 cm lateral to this location on one side of the vulvar labia. The needle is passed into the skin, directed through the submucosa underneath the Caslick suture, and exited on the contralateral vulvar labia directly horizontal to the site of entrance.
- A square knot is then hand-tied, but care is taken to not pull it too tight (the clinician should be able to place 1–2 fingers within the loop). The free ends of the suture are then cut to free the needle and trim excess suture material (Figure 43.2).
- The site for placement should have already been scrubbed and desensitized from the prior Caslick procedure, but can be repeated if deemed necessary.

Additional Comments

Location of the stitch is important, especially if the mare is going to be bred in the near future. If located too far distal, it could potentially injure the stallion's penis during intromission. The stitch is usually removed after breeding or after satisfactory healing of the primary incision.

Further Reading

Bradecamp EA. 2011. Pneumovagina. In: McKinnon AO, Squires EL, Vaala WE, Varner DD (eds). Equine Reproduction, 2nd edn. Ames, IA: Wiley Blackwell, pp. 2537–44.

44

Reinforcement Breeding

Charles F. Scoggin

Rood and Riddle Equine Hospital, USA

Introduction

The use of assisted reproductive techniques, such as artificial insemination and embryo transfer, are forbidden under the current rules of the Jockey Club, which is the sole certifying breed registry for Thoroughbred horses in North America (Box 44.1). Foals can only be registered with the Jockey Club following conception via live-cover or natural service matings.

However, there is a permissible technique whereby semen from a stallion can be obtained as he is dismounting the mare and the semen subsequently deposited back into the reproductive tract of the mare that was just bred by that stallion. Semen extender is often added to this dismount sample prior to deposition into the mare's uterus. This technique is commonly termed "reinforcement breeding" and is described here.

Indications for a reinforcement breeding include both mare and stallion factors. For instance, a reinforcement breeding may increase the effective "dosage" of spermatozoa per breeding, thereby populating the mare's reproductive tract with an increased number of sperm cells. The addition of extender may increase spermatozoal longevity, while the presence of antibiotics may reduce the incidence of post-mating-induced endometritis. Mares with a fibrotic or dysfunctional cervix may also benefit from a reinforcement breeding to ensure that semen is deposited into the uterus and not the vagina.

The choice of semen extender is not a trivial matter. Testing in different extenders is recommended prior to the season to determine which extender(s) each stallion performs best in with respect to longevity and viability (see Chapter 147). While rare, some stallions may experience a drop in pregnancy rates when reinforcement breedings are used, in which case the practice should be discontinued.

Equipment and Supplies

Clean styrofoam cups (240 ml, 8 oz), Timentin® (3.1 g ticarcillin and clavulanate potassium), semen extender, sterile sample collection cups (120 ml, 4 oz), 63.5 cm (25 inch) sterile insemination pipettes, 20 ml sterile plastic syringes, sterile obstetrical sleeves, sterile non-spermicidal lubricant, disposable nylon mesh gel filters.

Box 44.1 The Jockey Club, Registry, Section V, Rule 1D

To be eligible for registration, a foal must be the result of a stallion's breeding with a broodmare (which is the physical mounting of a broodmare by a stallion with intromission of the penis and ejaculation of semen into the reproductive tract). As an aid to the breeding, a portion of the ejaculate produced by the stallion during such mating may immediately be placed in the uterus of the broodmare being bred. A natural gestation must take place in, and delivery must be from, the body of the same broodmare in which the foal was conceived. Without limiting the above, any foal resulting from or produced by the processes of artificial insemination, embryo transfer or transplant, cloning or any other form of genetic manipulation not herein specified, shall not be eligible for registration.

Source: Jockey Club. 2008. *The American Stud Book: Principal Rules and Requirements*. Section V, Rule 1D. The Jockey Club (Registry).

Equine Reproductive Procedures, Second Edition. Edited by John Dascanio and Patrick McCue.

Technique

- Semen extender is prepared by adding 13 ml of sterile physiological saline to a 3.1 g vial of Timentin® resulting in a concentration of approximately 200 mg/ml ticarcillin and 6.7 mg/ml clavulanic acid. A total of 1.0 ml of this solution is added to a 200 ml bottle of INRA-96® semen extender (IMV Technologies USA, Maple Grove, MN, USA) to yield a final concentration of 1 mg/ml ticarcillin and 0.0335 mg/ml clavulanic acid within the semen extender; 15 ml of the prepared semen extender is then aliquoted into a 120 ml sterile specimen cup.
- A dismount sample is collected at the conclusion of a natural cover mating by first holding a clean disposable cup just below the ventral aspect of the vulva to collect semen expelled upon withdrawl of the penis and subsequently by directing the tip of the stallion's penis into the cup to collect the remaining ejaculate.
- The dismount sample is evaluated and processed while the mare is placed into a set of stocks where her perineum is washed and dried (see Chapter 3).
- A very small (approximately 20 μl) aliquot of the dismount sample is placed on a pre-warmed microscope slide, and a coverslip is applied over the top of the sample. The sample is evaluated with a phase-contrast microscope to determine the presence of live spermatozoa, as well as a subjective estimation of the total and progressive motility of the spermatozoa (see Chapter 130).
- The remaining dismount sample is then filtered through a nylon mesh filter into a sterile specimen cup containing approximately 15 ml of warmed semen extender.
- The resulting mixture is drawn into a sterile plastic syringe and a sterile insemination pipette is attached to the syringe.
- The extended dismount sample is then deposited directly into the body of the uterus of the mare that had just been covered (see Chapter 45). As the pipette is withdrawn, negative pressure is applied to the syringe to retrieve any ejaculate remaining within the vaginal vault. The resulting aspirate is grossly evaluated as it is being drawn through the pipette and into the syringe. If it appears to be of normal character and color, it is then also deposited into the body of the uterus. If it appears to be grossly abnormal, such as appearing hemorrhagic or tainted with urine, then it is retrieved from the vaginal vault and discarded.

Additional Comments

It has been reported that reinforcement breeding may enhance pregnancy rates in Thoroughbred mares. Higher pregnancy rates were observed in mares in which reinforcement breeding was performed compared with those in which it was not performed. A report also indicted that improved pregnancy rates were dependent upon the estimated total number of spermatozoa within the reinforcement breeding dose.

Further Reading

Blanchard TL, Love CC, Thompson JA, *et al.* 2006. Role of reinforcement breeding in a natural service mating program. *Proc Annu Conv Am Assoc Eq Pract* 52: 384–6.

Jockey Club. 2008. *The American Stud Book: Principal Rules and Requirements.* Section V, Subsection 1D. The Jockey Club (Registry).

LeBlanc MM. 2008. The chronically infertile mare. *Proc Annu Conv Am Assoc Eq Pract* 54: 391–407.

45

Breeding with Fresh or Cooled Semen

John J. Dascanio[1] and Patrick M. McCue[2]

[1]*School of Veterinary Medicine, Texas Tech University, USA*
[2]*Equine Reproduction Laboratory, Colorado State University, USA*

Introduction

Artificial insemination allows for an opportunity to evaluate the stallion's semen prior to breeding, ensures that live motile spermatozoa are placed in the uterus of the mare, and utilizes minimal contamination techniques during the breeding process. Mares may be inseminated with fresh semen, cooled-stored semen, or frozen-thawed semen. This chapter will focus on insemination of mares with fresh and cooled-stored semen.

Equipment and Supplies

Tail wrap, tail rope, obstetrical sleeve, obstetrical lubricant, non-irritant soap, roll cotton, stainless steel bucket, disposable liner for bucket, paper towels, exam gloves, sterile obstetrical sleeve, sterile obstetrical lubricant, semen, microscope, microscope slides, coverslips, disposable pipettes, insemination pipette, all-plastic syringes.

Pre-Insemination Technique

- Collect a semen sample.
- Filter the semen with a semen filter to remove gel and debris.
- Evaluate the semen for volume, concentration, and motility (total and progressive).
- Calculate a breeding dose. A minimum of 500 million progressively motile sperm (PMS) are recommended for a fresh insemination dose.
- For fresh semen, an appropriate semen extender should be added to the raw semen. A minimum ratio of 1:1 (semen : extender) is recommended. It is common to extend semen to a concentration of 25–50 million PMS/ml.
- If cooled semen is to be used, it is recommended that a total of 1 billion PMS be packaged per dose at a concentration of 25–50 million PMS/ml. This should result in a total volume of 40–60 ml per dose. One to two doses of cooled semen are typically sent in one shipment for a given mare. Cooled semen is generally shipped by overnight courier or by counter to counter (same day) airline delivery.
- Light breed mares, such as Quarter Horses and Arabians, are typically inseminated when they are in heat with a follicle 35 mm or greater and edema is present in the uterus visible on ultrasound. The pre-ovulatory follicle of Warmblood mares and draft horse mares generally attains a significantly larger diameter and breeding decisions are adjusted accordingly.
- It is common to administer an ovulation-inducing medication at the time of breeding or possibly the day before breeding to provide a timed insemination. See Chapter 57 for ovulation induction protocols.

Insemination Technique

- Remove feces from the mare's rectum.
- Place a tail wrap and tail rope on the mare (see Chapter 4).
- Wearing examination gloves, clean and dry the perineum of the mare (see Chapter 3).
- The semen sample should be thoroughly mixed prior to aspiration into an insemination all-plastic syringe and pipette.
- A notation should be made of any sediment within the semen container such as excessive smegma, urine crystals, or other organic debris that does not appear to be an opaque white-to-cream-colored semen pellet. With cooled semen, a small aliquot of semen (<0.25 ml)

Equine Reproductive Procedures, Second Edition. Edited by John Dascanio and Patrick McCue.

should be warmed for 10 minutes and examined under a microscope to evaluate sperm motility.

- A small amount of air equal to the volume of the pipette (3–5 ml depending on pipette length) may be aspirated into the syringe already containing the semen to be deposited. This will be used after insemination to clear the pipette of semen.
- Attach an insemination pipette to the syringe. Although not necessary, the pipette may be prefilled with semen prior to placement into the mare to avoid air from entering the uterus. Avoid losing the air previously aspirated into the syringe with the semen.
- Don a sterile obstetrical sleeve and place a sterile, water-soluble lubricant on the outside of the hand and down the arm.
- The tip of the insemination pipette is placed into the palm of the hand with the obstetrical sleeve (Figure 45.1).
- The sleeved hand is inserted through the vulvar labia and advanced to the external cervical os. Typically this is to the depth of approximately mid-forearm. A slight rotational motion may be used to help spread lubricant within the reproductive tract and aid in forward movement of the arm.
- The lumen of the external cervical os is located with the index finger (Figure 45.2). The os of the cervix may be directed slightly downward or off to one side. Careful exploration will provide eventual access to the lumen.

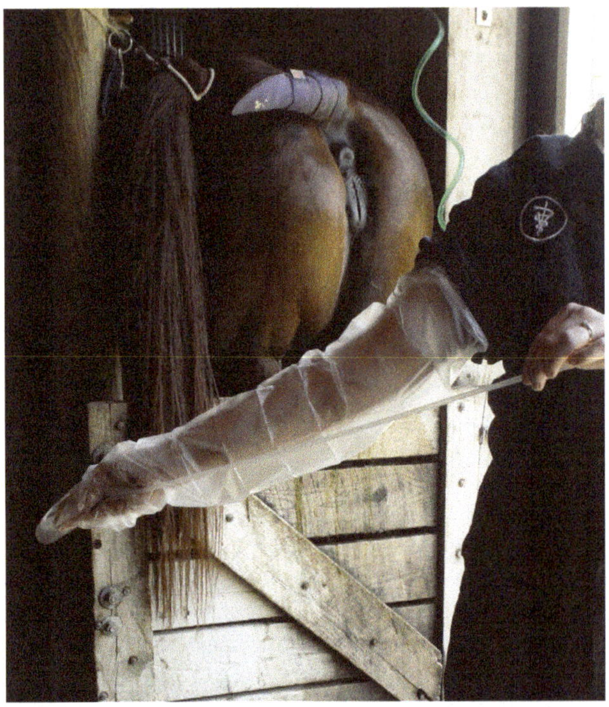

Figure 45.1 Placement of an insemination pipette into the hand for placement into the mare's reproductive tract.

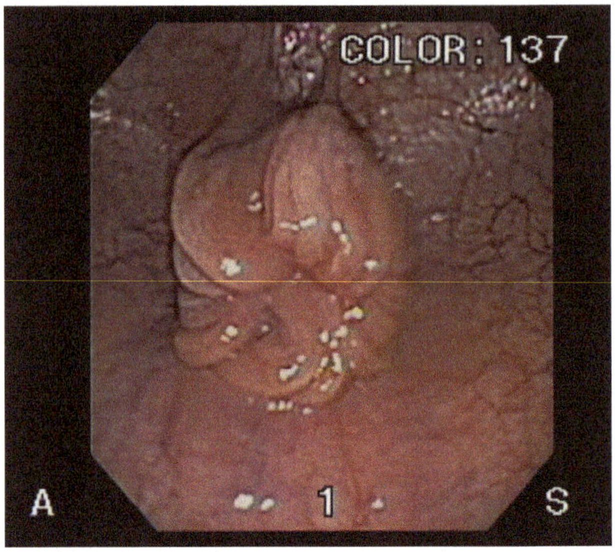

Figure 45.2 External cervical os. The cervical canal is located in the center of the cervix.

- Place the index finger into the cervical canal, using a probing maneuver to locate the direction of the canal. The cervical canal is not always directly straight and may slightly curve, especially downward in a multiparous mare.
- Using the hand outside the mare, holding the body of the pipette, direct the tip of the pipette into the cervical lumen past the inserted index finger (Figure 45.3). The pipette may be advanced a few centimeters past the index finger to ensure placement in the uterine lumen. Sometimes downward pressure on the pipette within the cervix with the inserted index finger may help direct the pipette tip into a downward sloping cervical canal.
- Start slow pressure on the syringe plunger, pushing semen through the pipette and into the uterus. If there is

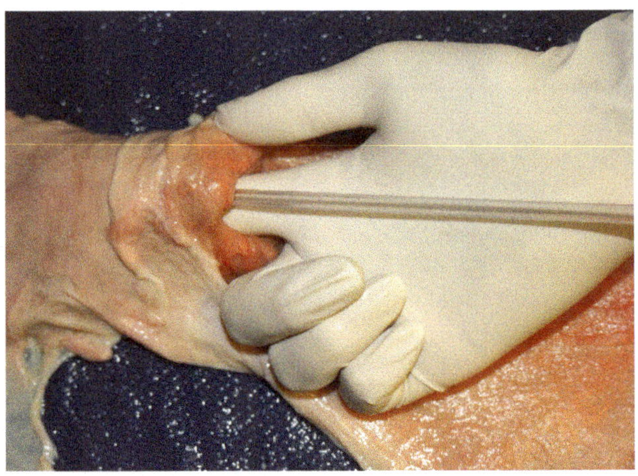

Figure 45.3 Introduction of an artificial insemination pipette along the index finger and through the cervical canal into the uterus.

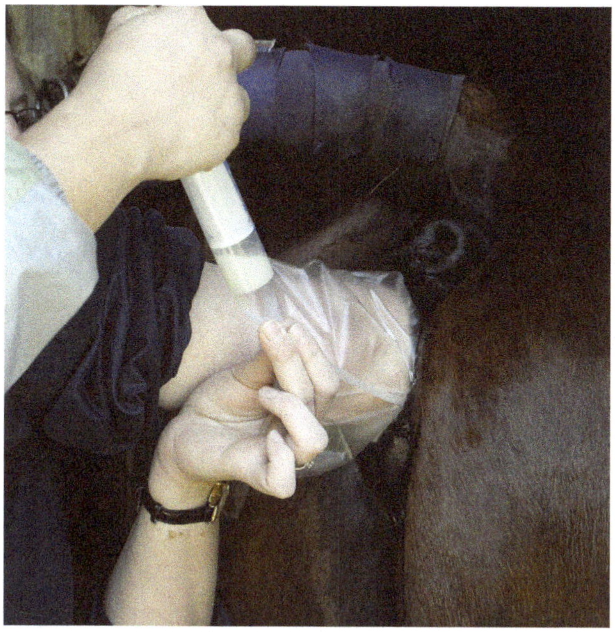

Figure 45.4 Vertical orientation of the syringe during insemination to allow passage of air after the inseminant.

a feeling that semen is back-flowing out the cervix into the vagina, reposition the tip of the pipette further into the cervix and into the uterus.

- When getting close to depositing the entire contents of the syringe, hold the syringe more vertically so that the air in the syringe is the last to enter the pipette, thus flushing the contained semen into the uterus (Figure 45.4). If no air was in the syringe, then once the insemination is complete, pull the syringe off the pipette, aspirate 3–5 ml of air, reattach, and push the remaining semen from the pipette into the uterus.
- The insemination pipette is withdrawn from the cervix along with the index finger.
- Optionally, prior to removal of the hand and pipette from the vagina, the external cervical os may be held closed for 10–15 seconds to prevent immediate back-flow of the inseminate.
- Lubricant is wiped off the mare's perineum and the tail wrap and tail tie removed.
- The mare should have a repeat ultrasound examination in 24 hours to determine if ovulation occurred and to note any accumulation of fluid in the uterus that may need to be treated.

Interpretation

- The goal with fresh semen is to inseminate the mare within 48 hours prior to ovulation.
- The goal with cooled-stored semen is to inseminate the mare within 24–48 hours prior to ovulation.
- Compare the motility of the semen at the time of processing to the motility at the time of breeding. If there is a significant drop in motility (>30–50%) with 24 hours of storage, alternative methods for semen processing should be considered such as centrifugation, gradient centrifugation, or use of an alternative extender.
- Examine the sterile obstetrical sleeve after removal from the vagina for any discharges (purulent, bloody, etc.) or foul odor (urine, necrotic tissue) that may indicate reproductive tract pathology.
- Avoid pushing excessive amounts of air into the uterus in order to clear the pipette of semen. This may lead to uterine inflammation. Air will be hyperechoic with a ventral shadow on ultrasound; detection of air in the uterus is commonly found if the mare is examined by ultrasound within a few hours of breeding.
- Back-flow of semen out of the cervix may be more common with the use of a large volume (>60 ml) of inseminant.
- Occasionally, the mare may urinate after breeding as a consequence of having the procedure performed. This is not desirable, especially in mares with very dependent uterus as urine may enter the dilated cervix. If this occurs regularly in a particular mare with breeding, the mare may be walked for a few minutes post-insemination to prevent immediate urination.
- Significant discoloration of the semen pellet in the shipping container may indicate inadequate washing of the stallion prior to collection, with a potential increase in deposition of organic material and bacteria into the mare's reproductive tract.

Further Reading

Brinsko SP. 2011. Semen collection techniques and insemination procedures. In: McKinnon AO, Squires EL, Vaala WE, Varner DD (eds). Equine Reproduction, 2nd edn. Ames, IA: Wiley Blackwell, pp. 1268–77.

Hughes JP, Loy RG. 1970. Artificial insemination in the equine. A comparison of natural breeding and artificial insemination of mares using semen from six stallions. *Cornell Vet* 60: 463–75.

Pickett BW, Shiner KA. 1994. Recent developments in artificial insemination in horses. *Livestock Prod Sci* 40: 31–6.

Sieme H, Bonk A, Hamann H, Klug E, Katila T. 2004. The effects of different insemination regimes on fertility in mares. *Theriogenology* 62: 915–28.

46

Insemination Through a Vaginal Speculum

Patrick M. McCue

Equine Reproduction Laboratory, Colorado State University, USA

Introduction

Mares can be inseminated through a vaginal speculum if the mare has had an episioplasty or Caslick procedure (i.e., "sutured"), or if for some reason it is not possible to insert the hand into the vagina. Consequently, the Caslick would not have to be opened for insemination and subsequently re-sutured. Some mares may have to be lightly sedated or restrained for this procedure.

Equipment and Supplies

Tail wrap, tail rope, non-irritant soap, roll cotton, stainless steel bucket, plastic bag/bucket liner, paper towels, examination gloves, sterile vaginal speculum, sterile obstetrical lubricant, light source, insemination pipette, syringe.

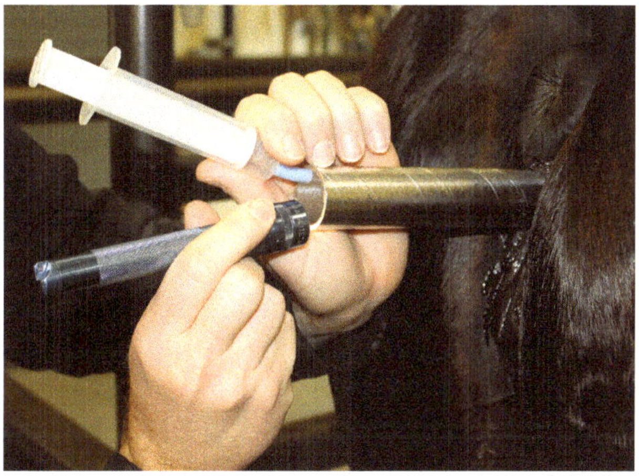

Figure 46.1 Viewing the cervix through a disposable speculum during insemination.

Technique

- The tail should be wrapped and the perineum cleansed and dried (see Chapter 3).
- A sterile vaginal speculum is lubricated and slowly inserted into the vulva initially at an upward angle. Once the speculum has passed the floor of the pelvis, the speculum is then moved to a horizontal position and inserted slowly through the vestibulo-vaginal fold into the vaginal vault.
- A penlight or other light source is used to illuminate the vaginal vault (Figure 46.1).
- The cervix is visually located and the insemination pipette, with the syringe containing the semen attached, is introduced through the speculum and into the external cervical os (Figure 46.2).
- The pipette is slowly advanced through the cervical canal into the uterine body.

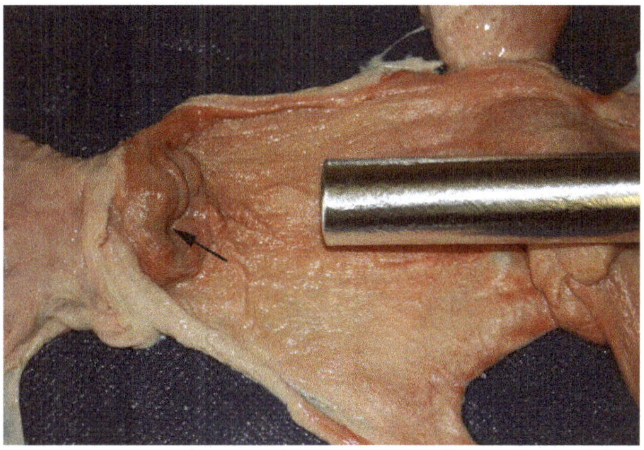

Figure 46.2 Position of the speculum prior to passage of the insemination pipette. Note the location of the external cervical os (arrow).

Equine Reproductive Procedures, Second Edition. Edited by John Dascanio and Patrick McCue.

- Once the insemination pipette is positioned appropriately, the semen is expelled by depressing the plunger of the syringe. The cervix should be visualized during semen deposition to make sure there is not efflux of semen from the external cervical os. If this occurs, then the pipette should be repositioned into the uterus prior to further insemination.

Additional Comments

- Mares will usually allow the passage of a vaginal speculum without issue.
- A mare with a Caslick may exhibit discomfort when the speculum is raised into a horizontal position as pressure is placed on the co-joined aspect of the dorsal commissure of the vulva.
- It may be difficult in some mares to pass the pipette into the external os of the cervix. The distal end of the speculum may be used to "guide" the pipette tip to the appropriate position. Once the tip is correctly placed, the pipette can usually be easily advanced into the uterus. A pipette tip with a bulbous end may be easier to pass forward than a narrow-tipped pipette which may get caught in tissue folds. Extending the cervix caudally may help with passage of the pipette. This would require use of long-handled forceps to gently grasp and extend the external os caudally.

Further Reading

Wilsher S, Allen WR. 2004. An improved method for nonsurgical embryo transfer in the mare. *Eq Vet Educ* 16: 39–44.

Zent WW, Steiner JV. 2011. Vaginal examination. In: McKinnon AO, Squires EL, Vaala WE, Varner DD (eds). Equine Reproduction, 2nd edn. Ames, IA: Wiley Blackwell, pp. 1900–3.

47

Breeding with Frozen Semen

John J. Dascanio

School of Veterinary Medicine, Texas Tech University, USA

Introduction

Frozen semen use has increased in the equine industry due to the availability of commercial freezing extenders, standardized protocols for freezing semen, and the development of practical mare management strategies for the use of frozen semen. There is often a large variation in the fertility rates between stallions with frozen-thawed semen. This can be controlled to a degree with diligent selection of stallion candidates and freezing procedures to maximize post-thaw spermatozoal viability. In addition, the selection of mares may influence the success rate of frozen semen. Pregnancy rates may be lower in mares with a history of subfertility, mares predisposed to delayed uterine clearance, and in aged mares. Proper timing of insemination is required as frozen-thawed semen has a limited longevity, so that semen should be inseminated within 12 hours prior to ovulation and within 6–8 hours after ovulation.

Equipment and Supplies

Tail wrap, tail rope, non-irritant soap, roll cotton, stainless steel bucket, disposable liner for bucket, paper towels, exam gloves, obstetrical sleeve, obstetrical lubricant, semen, microscope, microscope slides, coverslips, disposable pipettes, insemination pipette, all-plastic syringes, sterile water-soluble lubricant, sterile obstetrical sleeve, syringes, needles, ovulatory drugs, water bath, thermometer, straw cutter.

Administration of an Ovulation Induction Agent

- Light breed mares such as Quarter Horses and Arabians are typically administered an ovulation-inducing agent when they are in heat with a follicle 35 mm or greater and uterine edema is visible on ultrasound. The pre-ovulatory follicle of Warmblood mares and draft horse mares generally attain a significantly larger diameter and breeding decisions are adjusted accordingly.
- Administration of an ovulatory induction agent is recommended to promote a timed ovulation in order to facilitate mare management (see Chapter 57 for ovulation induction protocols).

Management Strategy with One Dose of Semen Available per Cycle

- If only one dose of frozen-thawed equine semen is available, the insemination is typically performed immediately after ovulation is detected. If the mare is inseminated prior to an anticipated ovulation and the mare does not ovulate for 12–24 hours or more after insemination, pregnancy rates will be lower. The possibility of pregnancy will be non-existent if the mare is inseminated but does not ovulate at all.
- A practical mare management strategy when one dose of semen is available is to administer deslorelin acetate at 8:00 pm, with the anticipation that ovulation will occur at 12:00 pm (noon) approximately 40 hours later. The mare should be examined periodically the day after deslorelin administration and then early in the morning the day she is supposed to ovulate. If the management protocol works as anticipated, the dominant follicle will still be present in the morning and the mare will have a fresh ovulation detected when examined at approximately 12:00 pm. The dose of semen is subsequently thawed and the mare inseminated.
- Another option is to thaw one half of the dose, if using multiple straws per dose, and inseminate prior to the anticipated ovulation. The other half of the dose is used after ovulation has been confirmed. A potential

Equine Reproductive Procedures, Second Edition. Edited by John Dascanio and Patrick McCue.

disadvantage of this strategy is if the mare fails to ovulate on schedule or fails to ovulate at all and a portion of the semen is wasted. This technique also relies on adequate spermatozoal numbers in the dose.

Management Strategy with Two Doses of Semen Available per Cycle

- If two doses of frozen semen are available for a given estrous cycle, one dose may be inseminated immediately prior to the anticipated ovulation and the second dose inseminated after ovulation has been confirmed.
- A practical mare management strategy when two doses of frozen semen are available is to administer deslorelin acetate at 8:00 am, with the anticipation that ovulation will occur at 12:00 am (midnight) approximately 40 hours later. The mare should be examined periodically the day after deslorelin administration and the mare inseminated in the evening (approximately 32–36 hours later). The mare is examined early in the morning the next day and she is re-inseminated if a fresh ovulation is detected (approximately 46–48 hours).
- A similar management strategy using human chorionic gonadotropin (hCG) would be to administer hCG at 12:00 pm with the anticipation that ovulation will occur at 12:00 am, approximately 36 hours later.
- An alternative technique would be timed inseminations at 24 and 40 hours post-ovulatory agent administration. If the mare did not ovulate between the 24- and 40-hour examinations, the second dose would be withheld until ovulation occurs. If the mare did ovulate, then the second dose is given at 40 hours. If the ovulatory agent is given at 4:00 pm, the mare would be bred at 4:00 pm the next day (24 hours) and 8:00 am the following day (40 hours).
- With these management strategies or modifications thereof, the mare is immediately inseminated if ovulation is detected earlier than anticipated.
- If the mare has not ovulated by the predicted time, she should be examined at regular intervals, such as every 4–6 hours, and the second dose inseminated after ovulation is detected.

Breeding Technique

- Prepare the mare for insemination using standard hygiene techniques. The feces of the mare should be removed from the rectum if deep horn insemination is to be performed (see Chapter 48).
- Thaw the semen according to directions from the facility that froze the semen (see Chapter 155).
- The method used to deliver the semen into the uterus depends on the number of straws, type of straw, type of pipette, and experience of the inseminator.
- If one 0.5 ml straw is to be inseminated, the best method is direct deposition with a pipette that allows the user to place the straw within the pipette and the use of a metal stylet to advance the cotton plug within the end of the straw and expel the semen (Figures 47.1 and 47.2). This same method can be used if multiple straws are to be inseminated. The pipette can remain in the uterus of the mare and thawed straws sequentially reloaded into the pipette for deposition into the uterus. This method is

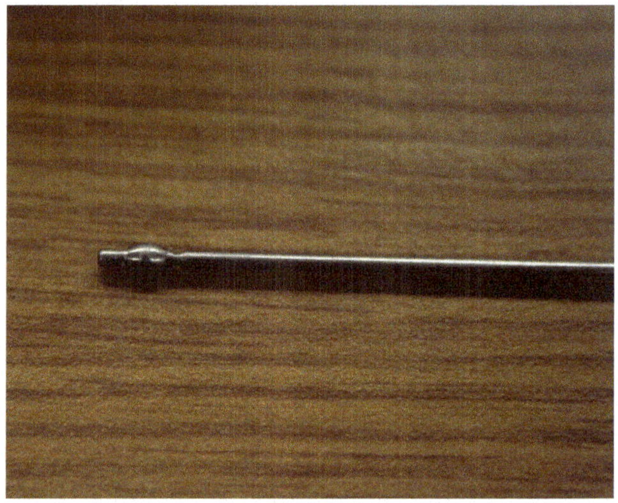

Figure 47.1 End of the stylet that will be inserted into the straw inside the breeding pipette (Minitube®). The enlarged metal ball on the end of the pipette will push the cotton pledget through the straw to push semen out the pipette.

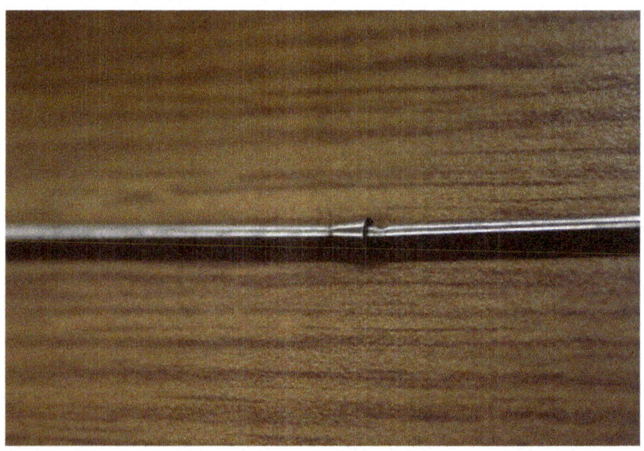

Figure 47.2 The cone on the stylet shaft that will catch the semen straw. Upon insertion of the stylet into the semen straw, the cone will hold the straw for removal of the straw from the pipette so an additional straw may be inserted for multiple straw breedings (Minitube®).

considered by many to be superior over other methods as it optimizes delivery of the entire semen dose into the uterus. If there is semen remaining in the straw, a drop should be placed on a warmed microscope slide and examined for motility.

- An alternative technique is to dispense the thawed semen into a warmed vessel such as a test tube or centrifuge tube. This may be used when multiple 0.5 ml straws are to be thawed or with the use of 2.5–5 ml macrostraws, goblets, or packets. A pre-warmed pipette is then inserted into the tube and the semen aspirated into the pipette.
- Prior to insemination a small drop of semen may be placed on a warmed microscope slide and examined for motility.
- Frozen-thawed semen may be deposited in the uterine body using standard insemination procedures (see Chapter 45).
- Deep horn insemination, with deposition of semen close to the utero-tubular junction, may be the best technique for the frozen-thawed semen of some stallions to optimize pregnancy rates (see Chapter 48). This may include stallions with poor post-thaw motility, stallions with a history of low fertility, or when a limited number of straws are utilized.

Interpretation

- With direct insemination of straws within a pipette using a metal stylet, 92–96% of semen is deposited within the reproductive tract. With aspiration of semen into a pipette and subsequent deposition, 76–87% of semen is deposited depending on the type of insemination pipette and number of straws per dose. With the placement of semen into a syringe with deposition through a pipette, 29–79% of the dose is delivered. Loss is from wetting of surfaces that cannot be recovered when working with low volumes (0.5–2 ml) (Figure 47.3).
- Frozen semen may also be stored in goblets, packets, or large straws. Instructions for proper thawing of the semen should accompany delivery of the semen and should be followed to optimize post-thaw viability of the spermatozoa.

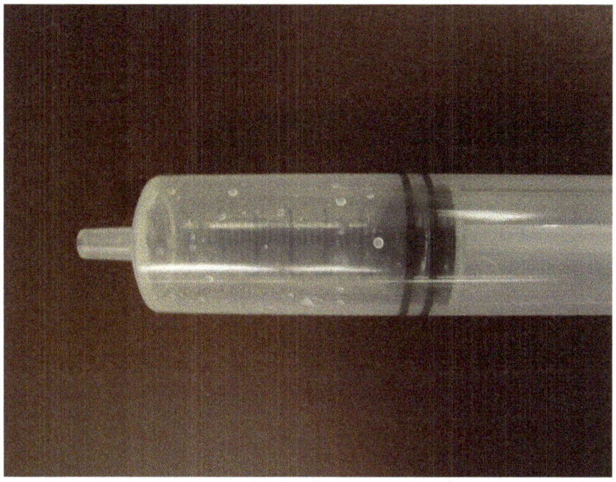

Figure 47.3 Semen remaining in the syringe if semen is drawn into the syringe for insemination. This technique should be avoided as it results in less than optimum semen volume delivery.

- Examine the sterile obstetrical sleeve after removal from the vagina for any discharges (purulent, bloody, etc.) or foul odor (urine, necrotic tissue) that may indicate reproductive tract pathology.
- Avoid pushing excessive amounts of air into the uterus in order to clear the pipette of semen. This may lead to uterine inflammation. Air will be hyperechoic with an acoustic shadow on ultrasound, particularly if the mare is examined within a few hours of breeding.
- Examine the mare the day after insemination to determine if there is any fluid accumulation and inflammation from breeding with frozen semen. The post-mating inflammatory reaction may be greater in mares bred with frozen semen than in mares bred with fresh or cooled semen due to the absence of seminal plasma. Treatment may include uterine lavage and/or administration of an ecbolic agent such as oxytocin or cloprostenol.
- Occasionally, the mare may urinate after breeding as a consequence of having the procedure performed. This is not desirable, especially in mares with a very dependent uterus as urine may enter the dilated cervix. If this occurs regularly in a particular mare with breeding, the mare may be walked for a few minutes post-insemination to prevent immediate urination.

Further Reading

Dascanio JJ, Kasimanickam R. 2008. Breeding the mare with frozen semen. *Eq Vet Educ* 20: 667–72.

Dascanio JJ, Kasimanickam R, Milburn S, Canerossi A, Splan R. 2006. Retention of liquid within insemination equipment using various equine frozen semen insemination methods and two semen freezing extenders. *J Eq Vet Sci* 26: 305–9.

Loomis PR. 2007. Techniques and applications of artificial insemination with frozen equine semen. *J Eq Vet Sci* 6: 139–42.

Miller CD. 2008. Optimizing the use of frozen-thawed equine semen. *Theriogenology* 70: 463–8.

48

Deep Horn Insemination

John J. Dascanio

School of Veterinary Medicine, Texas Tech University, USA

Introduction

Deep horn insemination is a technique that may be used to deliver spermatozoa to the tip of the uterine horn in close proximity to the utero-tubal junction. The procedure is most often used when the volume of semen is low or when frozen-thawed semen is inseminated. The insemination pipette is passed through the uterine body and up the ipsilateral horn of the ovary with the ovulatory follicle.

The pipette used should have a blunt tip, be long enough to reach the tip of the uterine horn, and be flexible. The dose to be inseminated should be aspirated into the end of the pipette if not already pre-packaged into 0.5 ml straws. There appears to be no advantage of using hysteroscopic insemination over manual deep horn insemination unless the number of spermatozoa is less than 5 million.

Deep horn insemination requires skill and practice in the correct placement of the pipette and transrectal manipulation of the pipette after insertion into the uterus, but the procedure can be accomplished on a farm with a little practice.

Equipment and Supplies

Tail wrap, tail rope, non-irritant soap, roll cotton, stainless steel bucket, disposable liner for bucket, paper towels, examination gloves, sterile obstetrical sleeve, obstetrical sleeve, sterile water-soluble lubricant, insemination pipette, syringes, semen.

Technique

- Remove feces from the mare's rectum.
- Place a tail wrap and tail rope on the mare (see Chapter 4).
- Wearing examination gloves, clean and dry the perineum of the mare (see Chapter 3).
- Place an insemination pipette in a warm incubator at 37°C (99°F). This will warm the plastic pipette, allowing it to be curled easily, if that is desired. If this is not possible, placement in the sun on a vehicle dashboard or on a vehicle dashboard with the defroster set to warm will suffice.
- Remove the pipette from the incubator (or warm area) and curl it either in a large arc or into a circle (Figure 48.1). Relax the pipette and it should retain the curvature (Figure 48.2). The curve in the pipette will help in placement into the chosen uterine horn.
- The pipette is advanced through the cervix into the uterine body using traditional techniques.
- The gloved hand is removed from the vagina and placed into the rectum of the mare.

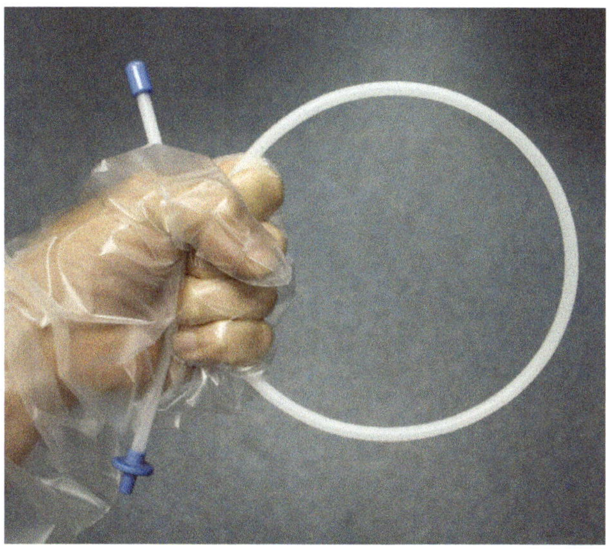

Figure 48.1 Bending of an artificial insemination pipette after removing from the incubator.

Equine Reproductive Procedures, Second Edition. Edited by John Dascanio and Patrick McCue.

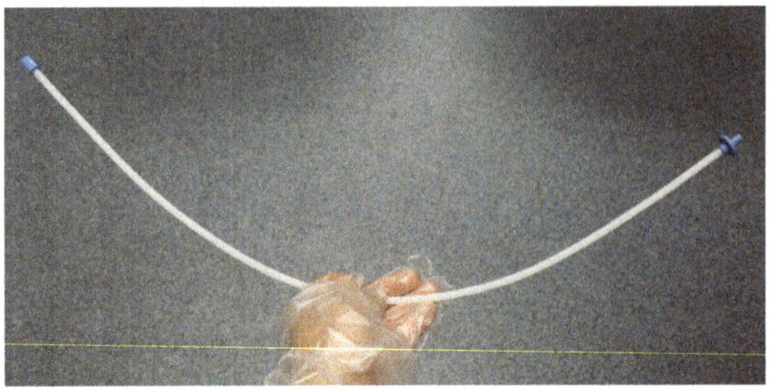

Figure 48.2 Bend that remains in the pipette after curling. This bend aids in the placement of the pipette into the correct uterine horn.

- The tip of the pipette is located per rectum and advanced into the correct uterine horn. The curve of the pipette and manual manipulation are used to guide the pipette.
- Lifting or straightening the uterine horn per rectum may help with passage of the pipette into and proximally up the uterine horn.
- The pipette should be advanced until it reaches the tip of the uterine horn as confirmed by palpation.
- Inseminate the mare and withdraw the pipette.

Interpretation

- When using the metal stylet within the Minitube® insemination pipette for frozen-thawed semen, the curvature of the pipette may slightly inhibit the passage of the metal stylet. Once the pipette is properly placed at the tip of the horn, some straightening of the pipette with the hand per rectum may be attempted to aid in passing the metal stylet to advance a semen straw into place.
- Use of a specifically designed deep horn insemination catheter, with a tip palpable per rectum, may aid in accurate placement (sterile AI deep horn catheter, IMV Technologies USA, Maple Grove, MN, USA).
- Excessive air should be avoided from entering the uterus during the procedure as this may result in uterine inflammation. Holding a clean gloved finger over the open end of the pipette or placement of an empty 3 ml syringe onto the pipette will prevent excessive air entry.
- When larger volumes of semen are used (>5 ml) there does not seem to be an advantage to using a deep horn insemination technique as the semen tends to gravitate toward the uterine bifurcation after insemination.

Further Reading

Brinsko SP, Rigby SL, Lindsey AC, Blanchard TL, Love CC. 2003. Pregnancy rates in mares following hysteroscopic or transrectally-guided insemination with low sperm numbers at the utero-tubal papilla. *Theriogenology* 59: 1001–9.

Schmidt AR. 2011. How to breed mares with frozen semen by deep horn insemination. *Proc Annu Conv Am Assoc Eq Pract* 57: 48–51.

49

Hysteroscopic (Low Dose) Insemination

Patrick M. McCue

Equine Reproduction Laboratory, Colorado State University, USA

Introduction

A normal fertile stallion will deposit 2–10 billion or more spermatozoa into the reproductive tract of a mare after a natural service ejaculation. In contrast, the standard minimum artificial insemination dose using fresh semen is 500 million progressively motile sperm (PMS).

In some instances it may be necessary to inseminate a mare with a dramatically lower than usual number of sperm. This may be the case when a very limited number of frozen semen straws are available, if a stallion has a low sperm count in his ejaculate, or if the book of mares for a given day is higher than the number of insemination doses collected from a stallion.

Acceptable pregnancy rates can be achieved using "low dose insemination techniques" in which 5–50 million or more spermatozoa, in volumes ranging from less than 0.1 ml up to 1–2 ml, are deposited into the uterus of a mare. The primary advantage of the hysteroscopic low dose insemination technique is direct visualization and precise deposition of a small volume of concentrated semen directly onto the utero-tubal junction. Disadvantages include the initial cost of the videoendoscope, the time required to set up, perform, and clean up after the procedure, and the requirement for multiple trained personnel.

Equipment and Supplies

Videoendoscope, catheter (210 cm, 83 inch), syringe (3 ml), centrifuge, semen extender, glass vial, obstetrical sleeve (sterile), obstetrical lubricant (sterile), sterile saline, glutaraldehyde solution.

Technique

- Timing of a low dose insemination is an important part of the success of the process. The goal is to deposit semen immediately before ovulation is predicted to occur or immediately after ovulation has been confirmed. Induce a timed ovulation with human chorionic gonadotropin (hCG), deslorelin, or histrelin.
- The mare is placed in examination stocks and sedated. A combination of detomidine hydrochloride (5 mg) plus butorphanol tartrate (5 mg) administered intravenously is usually effective for a light breed horse.
- The tail of the mare is wrapped and held out of the way (see Chapter 4).
- The mare's perineal area is thoroughly scrubbed using a non-residual soap and rinsed with clean water and dried with disposable paper towels (see Chapter 3).
- Semen should be processed and readily available. This may entail centrifugation of semen and re-suspension in a very small volume of extender (i.e., 50–100 million PMS re-suspended in a total volume of 0.2–0.5 ml) or thawing a single straw of frozen semen.
- The endoscope should be cold sterilized before use. This may be accomplished by cold sterilization in an activated solution of 2.4% glutaraldehyde (Cidex®); the endoscope is then thoroughly rinsed with 0.9% sterile saline.
- A special catheter (210 cm, 83 inches) (Figure 49.1) is passed down the working channel of the endoscope until the tip of the catheter exits the endoscope.
- The low volume semen sample is aspirated into the distal end of the catheter.
- The catheter is withdrawn into the endoscope.
- A sterile obstetrical sleeve is worn by the person passing the endoscope.

Equine Reproductive Procedures, Second Edition. Edited by John Dascanio and Patrick McCue.

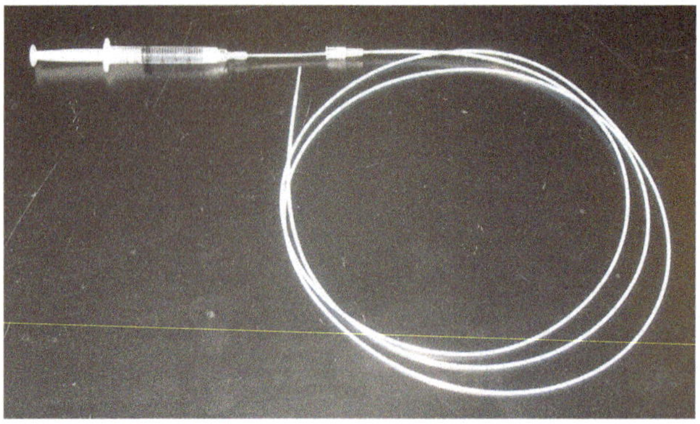

Figure 49.1 Catheter used to deposit semen on the utero-tubular junction. The catheter is passed through the biopsy channel of a videoendoscope.

- A small volume of sterile obstetrical lubricant is applied to the back of the gloved hand.
- The endoscope is protected in the palm of the hand while being passed through the vulva and into the vaginal vault.
- The working end of the endoscope is passed through the cervix into the uterine body.
- The cervix is held in a closed position while the uterine lumen is inflated using the endoscope with sufficient room air to distend the lumen and allow visualization and passage of the scope up the uterine horn ipsilateral to the antral follicle.
- Once the uterus is inflated, the uterine bifurcation should be visible (Figure 49.2).
- The endoscope is subsequently passed up the lumen of the horn adjacent to the ovary containing the pre-ovulatory follicle (Figure 49.3).
- The utero-tubal junction is visualized at the distal end of the uterine horn (Figure 49.4).

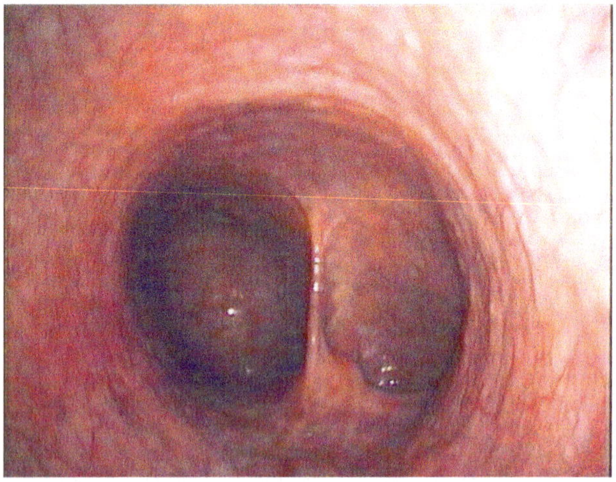

Figure 49.2 Uterine bifurcation as viewed through a videoendoscope.

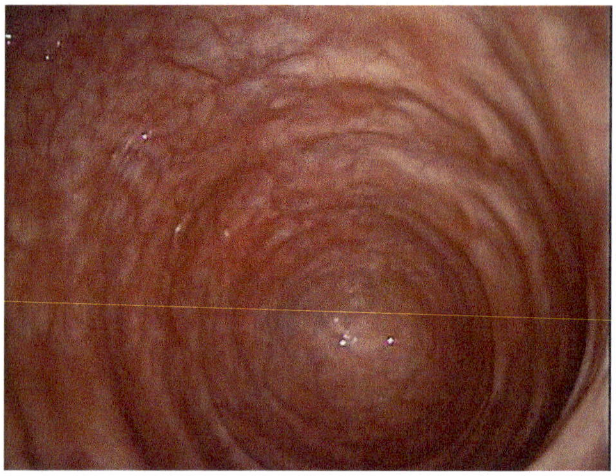

Figure 49.3 A dilated uterine horn as viewed through a videoendoscope.

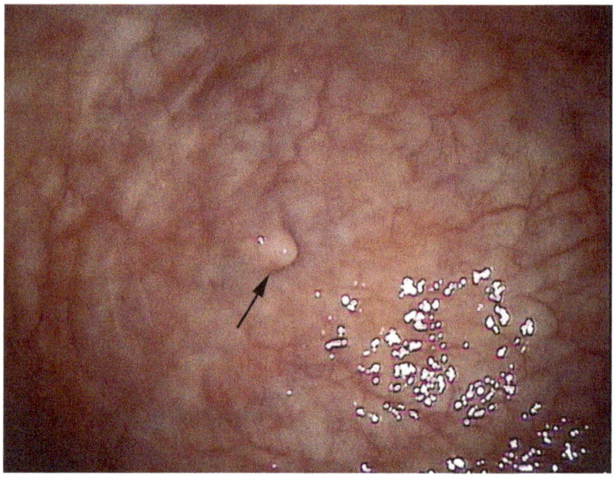

Figure 49.4 Utero-tubal junction (arrow) viewed through a videoendoscope.

- The catheter tip is advanced out of the endoscope until the tip gently touches the papilla.
- The small volume of extended semen is then slowly deposited directly onto the papilla.
- The endoscope is withdrawn to the caudal uterine body and the air in the uterus is evacuated.

Additional Comments

Insemination of less than 100 million motile spermatozoa using a traditional technique is likely to result in a low pregnancy rate per cycle. However, pregnancy rates of 50–75% have been obtained with insemination doses of

5–25 million PMS using a hysteroscopic insemination technique.

There is no significant difference in pregnancy rate between the manual deep horn low dose technique and the hysteroscopic low dose insemination technique. Both methods can yield acceptable pregnancy rates using low numbers of spermatozoa if the stallion has good inherent fertility. However, low dose insemination techniques may have reduced effectiveness when used with subfertile stallions or with less than 5 million total spermatozoa.

Further Reading

Brinsko SP, Rigby SL, Lindsey AC, Blanchard TL, Love CC, Varner DD. 2003. Pregnancy rates in mares following hysteroscopic or transrectally-guided insemination with low sperm numbers at the utero-tubal papilla. *Theriogenology* 59: 1001–9.

Lindsey AC, Morris LH, Allen WR, Schenk JL, Squires EL. 2002. Hysteroscopic insemination of mares with low numbers of nonsorted or flow cytometrically sorted spermatozoa. *Eq Vet J* 34: 128–32.

Morris LHA, SK Lyle. 2011. Low dose insemination. In: McKinnon AO, Squires EL, Vaala WE, Varner DD (eds). Equine Reproduction, 2nd edn. Ames, IA: Wiley Blackwell, pp. 3036–41.

50

Transvaginal Oocyte Pickup

Jennifer N. Hatzel

Equine Reproduction Laboratory, Colorado State University, USA

Introduction

Transvaginal oocyte pickup (OPU) of the mare has become an increasingly common clinical procedure applicable to both academic and private breeding facilities around the world. Reasons for submitting a mare or stallion into an OPU program include: infertility, production and "storing" of valuable embryos during the "non-breeding season," working around scheduling conflicts during competition season, and to optimize the use of limited amounts of frozen semen. Oocytes that are collected with this procedure can be utilized for oocyte transfer or, more commonly, intracytoplasmic sperm injection (ICSI) for *in vitro* production of embryos. Once at an appropriate stage of development (early blastocyst or blastocyst), ICSI-derived embryos are transferred transcervically into a recipient mare, which ideally ovulated 4 or 5 days previously.

Although collection of oocytes has become more common, established facilities that can perform ICSI are less common. Consequently, oocytes collected at one location are routinely transported to a center for sperm injection and initial embryo culture. In general terms, there are two different types of oocytes that are collected: (i) mature oocytes collected from the pre-ovulatory dominant ovarian follicle; and (ii) immature oocytes collected from smaller ovarian follicles.

Collecting a maturing oocyte from the pre-ovulatory dominant follicle of a mare has advantages and disadvantages. The primary advantage is that the mare provides her own hormonal milieu in preparation for that oocyte to ovulate and, therefore, may result in a better oocyte. These oocytes also tend to be easier to harvest as the granulosa cells surrounding the oocyte have begun to naturally loosen in preparation for impending ovulation. However, as the oocyte has been initiated to mature, they become more sensitive to temperature fluctuations and must be maintained at body temperature (38°C, 100°F) even during transportation, requiring a portable incubator if shipping to another facility for ICSI. In order to identify a pre-ovulatory follicle for OPU, the mare's cycle must be monitored via transrectal ultrasonography and ovulation induction medications administered when she has a large (>33 mm) follicle and uterine edema present. Most mares will only present with one and occasionally two dominant follicles. These oocytes are also ready for ICSI at 40 hours following ovulation induction drug administration, making a shipment window tight for certain facilities. Some practices find this to be a less efficient method.

Due to more relaxed logistical organization and oocyte handling, practices often opt to collect immature oocytes from multiple small follicles. This technique has advantages and disadvantages. Small follicle collections are conducted at various time points within a mare's cycle regardless of her estrous cycle stage. OPU sessions typically are performed at approximately 14-day intervals. The immature status of the oocytes collected results in less sensitivity to temperature alterations and the oocytes can be transported at room temperature (22°C, 71.5°F) in commercially available devices. The main disadvantage for this collection technique involves the collection process itself. As these follicles were not stimulated by either endogenous or exogenous hormones, the oocytes are tightly adhered to the follicular wall and require physical exfoliation to collect, which decreases the collection rate per follicle and can potentially cause trauma to the ovarian tissue. Finally, immature oocytes require *in vitro* maturation and only a percentage successfully mature into metaphase II and are eligible for the ICSI procedure.

Equine Reproductive Procedures, Second Edition. Edited by John Dascanio and Patrick McCue.

Equipment and Supplies

Halter and lead rope, twitch, non-steroidal anti-inflammatory drugs (flunixin meglumine), *N*-butylscopolammonium, sedation (acepromazine, xylazine, detomidine, butorphanol), antibiotics, ovulation induction drugs (human chorionic gonadotropin and deslorelin), set of sturdy palpation stocks, tail wrap, exam gloves, povidone-iodine scrub, 10 × 10 cm (4 × 4 inch) gauze squares, palpation sleeves, non-sterile obstetrical lube, ultrasound unit with appropriate transvaginal aspiration handle encasing a micro-convex or linear probe with corresponding needle guide, 12 gauge double-lumen equine follicle aspiration needle, foot-peddle-operated suction system, pre-warmed sterile collection bottle (250 ml), warming container to hold collection bottle, sterile lube, pre-warmed complete embryo flush media with heparin, controlled flushing set, sterile palpation sleeve, all-plastic syringe for flushing, heating plates (37°C, 99°F), stage warmer for dissecting microscope, dissecting microscope with 10–20× magnification, pre-warmed polystyrene Petri dishes (150 × 25 mm), 0.25 ml pre-warmed γ-irradiated semen straw, 0.25 ml straw adapter to connect to a 1 ml tuberculin syringe, pre-warmed washing media (commercial embryo-holding medium or lab made), pre-warmed polystyrene Petri dish (35 × 10 mm), sterile urinary catheter (immature collections), pre-warmed sterile 75 μm embryo filter dish (immature collections).

Technique

- Mares selected for collection of maturing oocytes from dominant follicles will be monitored through transrectal ultrasonography and prepared upon identification of a follicle at least 33 mm in diameter, the presence of uterine edema, and cervical palpation associated with the estrus phase of her cycle.
- Human chorionic gonadotropin (2000 IU IV) and deslorelin acetate (0.9 mg IM) are both administered; it is important that the OPU session be scheduled 20–24 hours later.
- For pre-ovulatory follicle aspiration procedures, the mare is placed into a set of stocks and the tail wrapped and held to the side while the perineum is washed with a gloved hand and povidone-iodine scrub (see Chapter 3).
- The perineum is dried with paper towels and a small amount of clean 10 × 10 cm (4 × 4 inch) gauze squares deposited into the caudal vestibule to capture fecal material and lube during manure extraction.
- A new palpation sleeve is utilized to manually remove as much manure from the mare's rectum as possible and a transrectal ultrasound examination is performed to identify that the pre-ovulatory follicle is still present. Air within the rectum can be removed at this time with a dose syringe (or similar device) to facilitate transrectal manipulations.
- Sedation medication is typically administered with either xylazine hydrochloride (150–400 mg IV) or detomidine hydrochloride (5–7 mg IV) along with butorphanol (5–10 mg IV).
- The perineum is thoroughly washed again with a gloved hand and povidone-iodine scrub, dried, and the gauze removed from the vestibule; if there is evidence of fecal contamination, the vestibule is swept again with cotton and water.
- Prior to initiation of the OPU procedure, all lab equipment must be equilibrated, organized, and pre-warmed to body temperature (37°C).
- Once the mare is ready, the aspiration needle setup is prepped by carefully positioning the rubber stopper into the warmed collection bottle pre-rinsed with complete embryo flush media and attaching a new all-plastic 12 ml syringe to the outflow line; all connections are checked for tightness and the entire apparatus removed from sterile packaging. The needle is carefully positioned into the needle guide of the transvaginal aspiration (TVA) handle at this time.
- The inflow line is connected to a controlled flushing set attached to a pre-warmed bag of complete embryo flush media with the addition of heparin (5–20 IU/ml) and a 30 ml all-plastic syringe is attached for the purpose of pushing fluid into the follicle during the procedure (Figure 50.1).
- Suction is connected to the inflow needle of the rubber stopper attached to the collection bottle, now placed within a warmed container.
- The TVA handle is picked up by the OPU operator donning a sterile palpation sleeve and the needle advanced

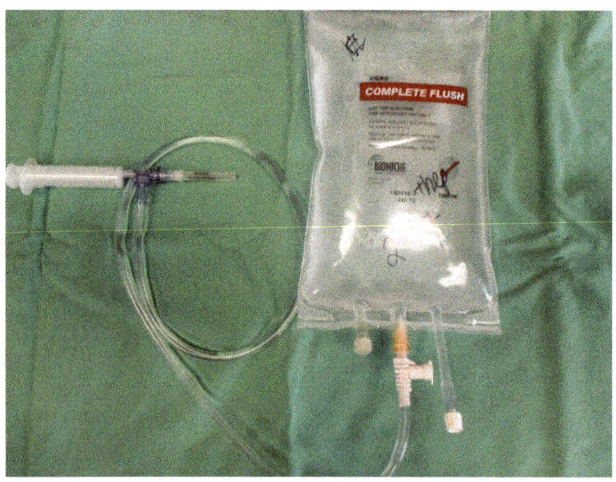

Figure 50.1 A sterile controlled flushing set is spiked into a pre-warmed bag of complete embryo flush media with 5–20 IU/ml heparin; this is prepared just prior to initiation of the OPU procedure.

out of the front of the needle guide; the assistant pushes fluid through the inflow line to prime the line and ensure that no air is present.

- The needle is repositioned within the guide and the *N*-butylscopolammonium (100–150 mg IV) is administered immediately prior to placement of the TVA probe/handle into the vagina with sterile lube, positioning it lateral to the cervix and ipsilateral to the ovary being aspirated.
- The operator removes their hand from the vagina, applies non-sterile obstetrical lube, and replaces their arm within the rectum to manipulate the ovary, such that it is flipped over to rest upon the dorsal aspect of the broad ligament and pulled caudally toward the ultrasound transducer head against the peritoneal surface of the vaginal wall (Figure 50.2).
- Ensuring there are no other structures in line with the path of the needle (bowel, oviduct, ovulation fossa), the operator will palpate the surface of the ovary to identify the large pre-ovulatory follicle and position it against the dorsal aspect of the ultrasound probe directly against the needle guide, which can be visualized with ultrasound.
- Upon satisfactory positioning, the horse handler applies a nose twitch and the OPU operator advances the needle well into the follicle antrum; suction is initiated by the assistant immediately at 120–175 mmHg.
- Amber-colored follicular fluid will begin collecting within the warmed bottle and as the follicle wall collapses, the assistant will begin pushing media into the follicle to continue a steady flow of fluid into and out of the follicle.

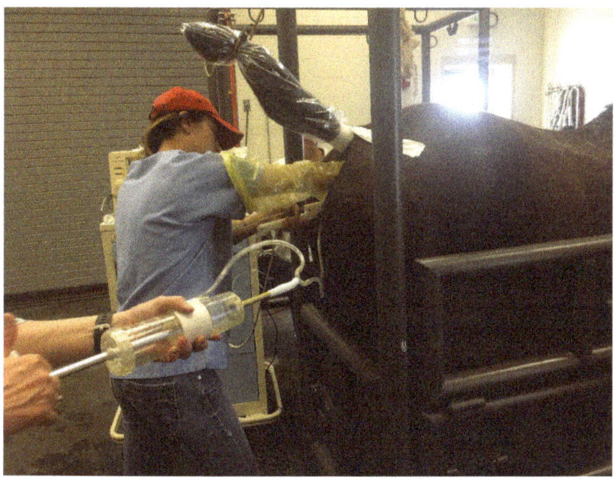

Figure 50.2 Positioning the TVA handle encasing the ultrasound probe per vagina, lateral to the cervix. Note the assistant with dosing syringe setup to assist with rectal air removal as needed.

- The OPU operator will begin massaging the follicle per rectum in an attempt to dislodge the cumulus–oocyte complex (COC) from the follicle wall and capture it within the suction line.
- Upon completion of the full amount of the 30 ml all-plastic syringe, the suction is paused and fluid alone is pushed into the follicle in an effort to observe it filling back up almost to its original size before suction is initiated again. This cycle will be continued three or four times, depending upon positioning and the behavior of the mare; meanwhile the collection fluid will eventually become hemorrhagic in color.
- Once the follicle has been satisfactorily rinsed and ample amounts of mature granulosa cells are observed within the collection bottle, the suction is discontinued and the needle is withdrawn.
- If immature follicles are also to be collected, the rubber stopper is relocated to a different clean, sterile, pre-rinsed, warmed collection bottle and the full bottle is capped and placed within a warming incubator to be searched later for the oocyte(s).
- Immature follicles are identified on ultrasound and aligned as previously described, but massaging the follicle is more aggressive, with the addition of rapid manual needle twisting within the antrum and/or full ovarian movement to exfoliate the interior follicular wall, as immature oocytes are tightly adhered.
- The assistant will additionally facilitate by applying pulses of fluid at 3-4 ml volumes, with intermittent suction applied, which will cause more turbulence in the follicle, and assist with dislodgment of the COC. This procedure is repeated 6–10 times per follicle.
- Once all available follicles have been aspirated, the needle is retracted back into the needle guide, the nose twitch relieved, and the TVA probe/handle removed from the vagina.
- The tail wrap is removed and flunixin meglumine administered (300–500 mg IV). The mare is allowed to recover in the stocks until awake enough to return to a stall for further recovery from sedation.
- Ensure removal of all hay and feed from the stall to allow recovery from sedation without potential esophageal choke and initiate a short re-feeding protocol throughout the afternoon/evening.
- The collection bottle containing the mature oocyte can be distributed amongst 4+ pre-warmed, large, polystyrene Petri dishes (150 × 25 mm) and searched for the oftentimes clear COC that disperses the more hemorrhagic surrounding fluid. The COC structures can often be observed with the naked eye (Figure 50.3).
- Other clear regions within the dish are collections of granulosa cells, which should be evaluated thoroughly under

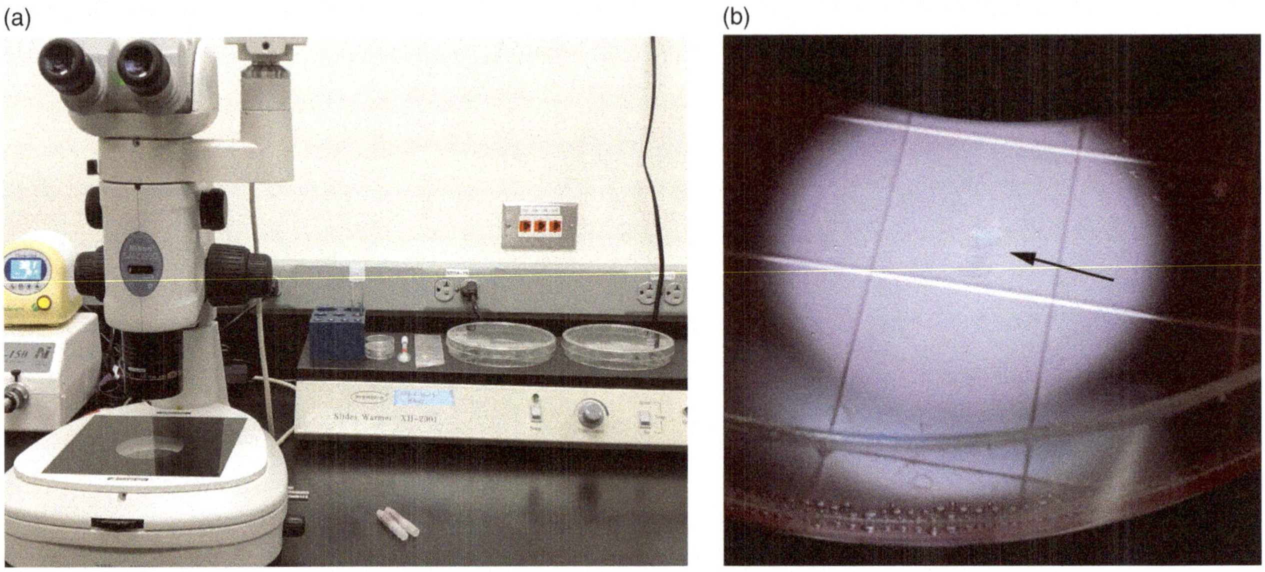

Figure 50.3 (a) Lab equipment (dissecting microscope with heated stage, 150 × 25 mm polystyrene Petri dishes, 35 × 10 mm polystyrene Petri dishes, 0.25 ml semen straws, urethral adapter attached to 1 ml tuberculin syringe and warming plate) prepared for oocyte searching. (b) Pre-ovulatory oocyte identified by the clear COC (arrow).

10–20× magnification upon a heated stage by exploration with a 22 gauge needle. Upon identification, mature oocytes are recognized due to the expansion of surrounding cumulus cells and a central gray-colored oocyte.

- The collection bottle containing the immature oocytes should be poured through a pre-warmed 75 μm embryo collection cup and thoroughly rinsed to remove as much blood as possible, which will greatly facilitate identification of the more compacted immature COC (Figure 50.4). Immature oocytes are recognized by the compacted nature of surrounding cumulus cells and a darker oocyte (Figure 50.5).

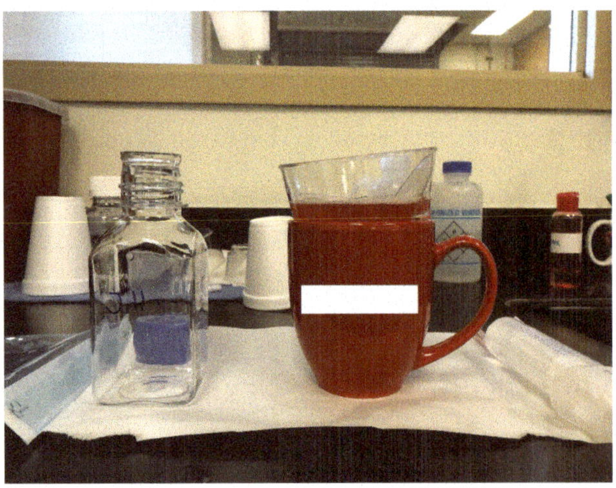

Figure 50.4 Pre-warmed 75 μm embryo filtration cup with contents of immature oocyte collection cup poured through for easier identification of this type of oocyte population.

- All identified oocytes can be manipulated and picked up with a pre-warmed 0.25 ml, γ-irradiated semen straw attached to a urethral catheter connector and a 1 ml tuberculin syringe or a P20 micropipette.
- Oocytes should each be placed within warmed wash media in a smaller polystyrene Petri dish (35 × 10 mm) (either in commercially available embryo-holding medium or lab-prepared medium) and deposited in several clean locations of the Petri dish to facilitate removal of blood or debris.
- At this time, oocytes should be placed within either lab-prepared supportive media (typically M199 with Hanks' salts buffered for room atmosphere) at 38°C (maturing oocytes from a hormone-stimulated pre-ovulatory follicle) or a commercial embryo-holding media at room temperature (immature oocytes) to facilitate shipping to an ICSI facility (see Chapter 51).

Interpretation and Additional Comments

- Despite the recent popularity of these procedures, it is imperative to remember that OPU is invasive and should not be taken lightly.
- If a bacterial endometritis is diagnosed, a vaginal lavage with 1 liter of saline is recommended prior to and after the OPU session; in addition antibiotics (such as a long-acting ceftiofur) should be administered.

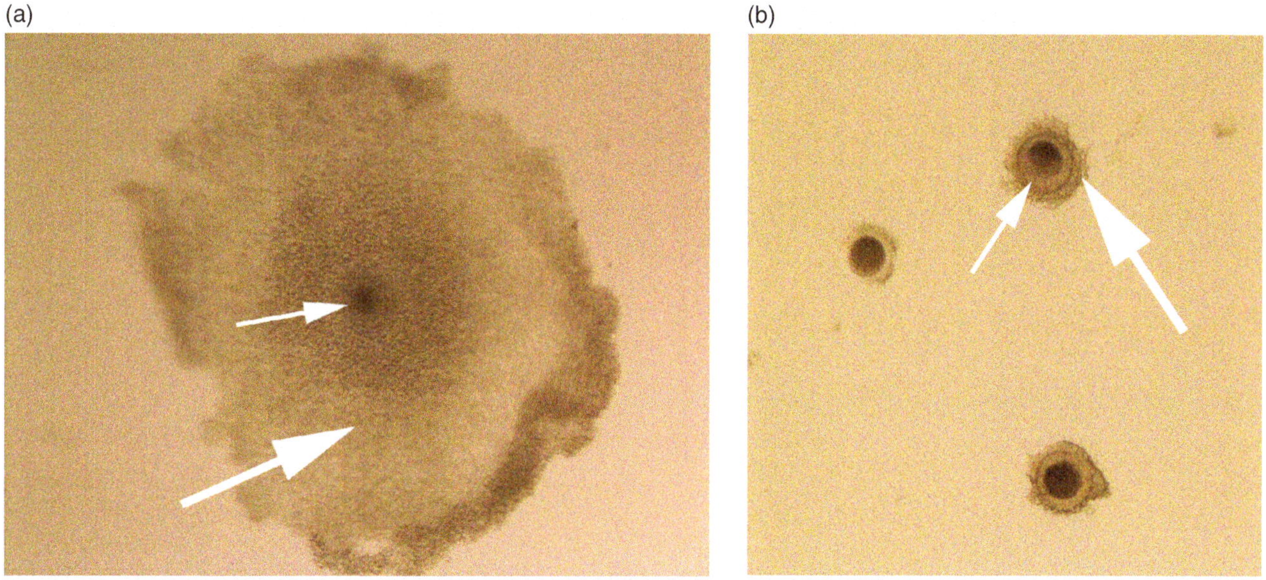

Figure 50.5 (a) Image of maturing oocyte recovered from a hormone-stimulated pre-ovulatory follicle; note the expanding cumulus cells (large white arrow) surrounding the oocyte (small white arrow). (b) Image of immature oocytes identified following filtration; note the tight layer of cumulus cells (large white arrow) surrounding the oocyte (small white arrow).

- Ideally, ovarian positioning for immature follicle collection should maximize the accessibility of several follicles with one ovarian puncture if possible.
- Placement of a urinary catheter maybe helpful to facilitate bladder emptying prior to and during aspiration of immature oocytes.
- All ovarian movements should be achieved without rectal irritation and the operator should diligently check their sleeve at the conclusion of each procedure for any evidence of hemorrhage.

Further Reading

Carnevale EM. 2016. Advances in collection, transport and maturation of equine oocytes for assisted reproductive techniques. *Vet Clin North Am Eq Pract* 32: 379–99.

Hinrichs, K. 2013. Assisted reproduction techniques in the horse. *Reprod Fertil Dev* 25: 80–93.

Foss R, Ortis H, Hinrichs K. 2013. Effect of potential oocyte transport protocols on blastocyst rates after intracytoplasmic sperm injection in the horse. *Eq Vet J* 45: 39–43.

51

Packaging and transport of oocytes

Jennifer N. Hatzel

Equine Reproduction Laboratory, Colorado State University, USA

Introduction

With the expansion of transvaginal oocyte pickup (OPU), clinicians around the world are becoming more comfortable with the collection and identification of equine oocytes. However, the expense of equipment and technical support required for intracytoplasmic sperm injection (ICSI) is often cost prohibitive for many laboratories and clinics, requiring the shipment of collected oocytes to a nearby facility offering ICSI services. Once collected and identified, both maturing oocytes from pre-ovulatory follicles and immature oocytes from smaller follicles can be packaged within appropriate media and shipped in a variety of isothermic containers.

Although the collection and identification of maturing oocytes from large dominant follicles can be easier, shipping conditions tend to be a bit more complicated. The oocyte continues maturing after collection and is temperature sensitive and therefore requires special media and a portable incubator. The ICSI procedure is typically performed 40–44 hours following the administration of ovulation induction medications such as human chorionic gonadotropin (hCG) and deslorelin acetate. Therefore, it is recommended that these medications are administered the evening before the OPU is performed. The oocyte(s) is/are collected the following afternoon, packaged, and shipped out as soon as possible to arrive at the ICSI facility early the following day. Due to the difficulties in providing a gassed environment during transportation, most facilities receive maturing oocytes in a medium buffered for room atmosphere. As these oocytes are sensitive to temperature changes, they are shipped within a portable incubator maintained at 38°C (100°F).

Most clinicians performing transvaginal OPU now prefer to collect and ship immature oocytes due to the ease of logistics involved with shipping. This population is typically comprised of a greater total number of oocytes, is less sensitive to temperature fluctuations, and is less constrained to timing requirements. Collection and shipment of immature oocytes evolved through the need to maintain oocytes in an arrested state of development, holding them without meiotic progression. A commercial embryo-holding medium is typically used for maintaining and transporting these oocytes. The collection of oocytes from an individual mare can be packaged together in a container and secured within a variety of commercially available shipping containers. Currently, immature oocytes are shipped in containers maintaining room temperature (22–25°C, 71.5–77°F) during transit. Ideally, these oocytes will arrive at an ICSI facility early the following morning and immediately placed within maturational medium upon arrival, with the intention for sperm injection the following day. Both ground shipping options and direct flights (counter to

Equipment and Supplies

Medium buffered for room atmosphere for maturing oocytes (M199 with Hanks' salts, 20% newborn calf serum, 25 μg/ml gentamicin, and 0.3 mmol/l sodium pyruvate), commercially available embryo-holding medium for immature oocytes (Syngro®, Vetoquinol USA, Inc., Fort Worth, TX, USA; or EmCare™, ICPbio Reproduction, Spring Valley, WI, USA), 0.25 ml gamma irradiated semen straws, urethral adapter for 1 ml tuberculin syringe, P20 micropipette with appropriate sterile tips, non-toxic container for holding oocytes (5 ml polystyrene tube with snap cap for mature oocytes or 1 ml sterile borosilicate glass vial for immature oocytes), parafilm, labelling tape, marker, 15 ml conical tube, isothermic shipping container that can maintain room temperature during transport (e.g., Equitainer® or EquOcyte®; Hamilton Biovet LLC, Ipswich, MA, USA), and/or portable incubator (e.g., MicroQ; MicroQ Technologies LLC, Scottsdale, AZ, USA).

Equine Reproductive Procedures, Second Edition. Edited by John Dascanio and Patrick McCue.

counter) are appropriate methods for shipping either oocyte type, but containers will be subjected to various environmental factors such as extreme temperatures and other acclimate weather conditions.

Technique

- Identify either immature or mature oocytes (see Chapter 50) following the transvaginal oocyte collection procedure and thoroughly wash to remove blood within the rinse media.
- For mature oocytes with expanded granulosa/cumulus cells surrounding the oocyte: rinse the tip of a 0.25 ml straw attached to a urethral adapter with 1 ml tuberculin syringe with warmed medium (38°C, 100°F) chosen for transportation of maturing oocytes and maintain a small amount in the very tip in order to manipulate the oocyte.
- For immature oocytes with compacted cumulus and very few granulosa cells: rinse the tip of a P20 micropipette with room temperature media chosen for transportation of immature oocytes and maintain a very small amount in the tip in order to manipulate these oocytes.
- Isolate the mature oocyte and gently pick it up with a 0.25 ml straw, maintaining the small amount of fluid prior to picking it up, to be expelled following the oocyte.
- Isolate immature oocytes and pick up multiple oocytes using the P20 micropipette.
- Gently dispense the mature oocyte into the bottom of a 5 ml polystyrene tube prefilled with warm medium to ensure enough nutrients are available for this oocyte as it continues the maturation process during transit.
- Gently dispense immature oocytes towards the bottom of a glass 1 ml vial prefilled with room temperature medium utilized for transport, taking care not to pull fluid back and forth in and out of the pipette as oocytes can stick to the plastic tip of the pipette.
- Fill the remaining portion of the vial with appropriate media for both scenarios taking care to leave a small amount of air once the lid is replaced to accommodate pressure changes during airline transportation.
- Tightly snap or screw on the cap of the vial in place and secure with parafilm.
- Place the glass vial or plastic tube within the 15 ml conical tube and fill completely with either room temperature (immature) or warmed (mature) complete flush media to provide secondary protection in the event the container holding the oocyte(s) leaks, and as an insulation against mechanical trauma during transport.
- Secure the lid to this tube and wrap with parafilm.

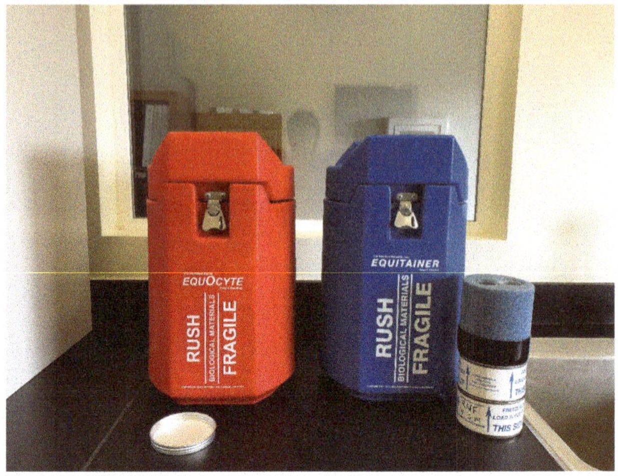

Figure 51.1 Two examples of isothermic containers utilized for shipment of oocytes: the EquOcyte® (left) and Equitainer® (right).

- Wrap this tube with a piece of tape containing: the donor mare's registered name, the date, and the number of oocytes contained within the container (if applicable).
- Place the entire tube securely into an appropriate tube holder within either a portable incubator pre-equilibrated and set to 37°C (99°F) (for mature oocytes) or travel incubator intended to maintain room temperature (for immature oocytes) (Figure 51.1).
- Ensure the tube(s) are surrounded with appropriate padding for the particular incubator to minimize movement during transportation. Place with it the appropriate documentation for the oocytes, containing: the donor mare's registered name, the stallion chosen for ICSI, the date oocytes were collected, the owner's name/contact information, and number of oocytes expected within the packaging.
- Close and latch the incubator and secure with additional locks, latches, or tape as needed for individual shipping containers.

Additional Comments

- Do not ship immature oocytes at body temperature unless they are kept within appropriate maturation medium and the receiving ICSI facility is prepared to perform the sperm injection at the appropriate time.
- Collection of equine oocytes and shipment to a facility providing ICSI services can establish a successful assisted reproductive technique program for a private practice.

Further Reading

Carnevale EM. 2016. Advances in collection, transport and maturation of equine oocytes for assisted reproductive techniques. *Vet Clin North Am Eq Pract* 32: 379–99.

Foss R, Ortis H, Hinrichs K. 2013. Effect of potential oocyte transport protocols on blastocyst rates after intracytoplasmic sperm injection in the horse. *Eq Vet J* 45: 39–43.

Hinrichs K. 2010. Application of assisted reproductive technologies (ART) to clinical practice. *Proc Annu Conv Am Assoc Eq Pract* 56: 195–206.

52

Intracytoplasmic Sperm Injection

Jennifer N. Hatzel and JoAnne Stokes

Equine Reproduction Laboratory, Colorado State University, USA

Introduction

Intracytoplasmic sperm injection (ICSI) has been an effective method for producing foals and has been commercially available since the early 2000s. Traditional *in vitro* fertilization (IVF), placing equine oocytes into a Petri dish with equine sperm, has not proven to be a consistent and successful method for creating equine embryos. These ineffective IVF procedures in the horse have promoted the use of ICSI for a certain population of mares and stallions. Reasons for entering a mare into an ICSI program include: infertility issues associated with cervical damage, chronic endometritis, oviductal issues, continual hemorrhagic anovulatory follicle production, damage incurred during a dystocia, conflict with a busy competition schedule, banking valuable genetics during the traditional "off season," and, to an extent, age-related subfertility. Frozen supply of semen from stallions presented to an ICSI program is typically low in quantity, due to death or old age of that stallion.

One of the advantages of utilizing ICSI for stallions with a limited amount of frozen semen is the potential to cut a single straw of frozen semen and utilize 6–10 pieces of a "cut straw" to be thawed individually. Another option is to thaw an entire straw of frozen semen, dilute the contents to approximately 1 million sperm/ml and refreeze multiple dilute straws from the original to create "ICSI only" doses (see Chapter 154). The additional refreezing process incurs damage to a population of sperm cells, but successful pregnancies and live foals have resulted from this process and success is highly variable between stallions and ejaculates.

The overall success rate of oocyte pickup (OPU), oocyte maturation, and ICSI procedures can vary greatly between individual stallion and mare combinations. Although multiple oocytes can often be collected from a single OPU procedure, the entire cohort represents a diverse population with varying stages of development and not all oocytes will mature or form blastocysts from an individual ICSI procedure. Additionally, the costs for procedures and overall logistics can be overwhelming for clients. It is imperative for the clinician collecting oocytes to manage the owner's expectations appropriately in addition to communicating with the ICSI facility throughout the process. These assisted reproduction procedures are especially valuable for mares and stallions where traditional and additional assisted reproductive techniques have failed to produce a live foal.

Equipment and Supplies

Trained ICSI technician with experience in equine oocyte micromanipulation and *in vitro* oocyte and embryo culture, lab-prepared maturation media (M199 with Earle's salts, 25 µg/ml gentamicin, 10% fetal bovine serum, 15 ng/ml follicle-stimulating hormone, 1 µg/ml luteinizing hormone, 50 ng/ml equine growth factor, 100 ng/ml insulin growth factor, 1 µg/ml estrogen, and 500 ng/ml progesterone), polystyrene cell culture dishes of various sizes, four-well polystyrene cell culture plates, warming incubator with CO_2, cell stripping pipetter, stripping pipette tips in a variety of sizes, hyaluronidase for denuding oocytes, G-IVF™ (Vitrolife, Inc., Englewood, CO, USA) sperm prep media, G-MOPS™ (Vitrolife, Inc., Englewood, CO, USA) benchtop media with bovine serum albumin (BSA) for sperm prep, adjustable micropipettes with corresponding sterile tips (P1000, P200, P100, P20), sterile oil utilized for covering of media during and following ICSI, 5–10% polyvinylpyrrolidone (PVP) medium for sperm holding, holding pipette (120–140 µm) for micromanipulation of oocytes, injection pipette (5–6 µm) for microinjection with Piezo drill capabilities, commercial embryo culture medium, incubator with mixed medical grade gas (5% O_2, 7% CO_2, and the remainder N_2) at 38.2°C (100.8°F) for embryo culture.

Technique

- Oocytes from dominant maturing follicles will undergo the ICSI process approximately 40 hours following

Equine Reproductive Procedures, Second Edition. Edited by John Dascanio and Patrick McCue.

gonadotropin stimulation of the donor mare; typically, the morning after oocyte collection.

- Oocytes collected from immature follicles will undergo the ICSI process after approximately 30 hours of culture in maturational media. This includes in-house immature oocytes placed immediately into maturation medium with hormones following OPU or oocytes sent to an ICSI facility from outside practitioners in holding medium, typically the afternoon following placement into the maturation medium.
- From both populations, once the appropriate time is reached, the dish containing the oocyte(s) is removed from the incubator and identification of oocytes is confirmed.
- The oocyte is evaluated under a dissecting microscope and transferred to a drop of hyaluronidase (200 IU) in G-MOPS™ with BSA.
- The expanded cumulus cells surrounding the oocyte are removed (denuded) by hand pipetting with a stripper pipetter tip. A larger tip size is chosen initially to encompass the cumulus–oocyte complex and slowly scaled down to eventually only encompass the oocyte as cumulus cells are shed.
- Oocytes that have achieved maturation to metaphase II, identified by the extrusion of the first polar body, are placed back into their maturation media and into the incubator to await ICSI within the hour.
- Semen preparation takes place next, usually with frozen semen as it is often more convenient to utilize for ICSI than obtaining fresh or cooled semen.
- A swim-up procedure is the method of choice for sperm selection when an adequate population of viable sperm cells are available.
- A cut portion of an original frozen straw of semen is thawed by placing under 1 ml of pre-equilibrated G-IVF™ medium at 38.2°C (100.8°F) within a 5 ml snap-top tube maintained within a 7% CO_2 incubator.
- The tube is incubated at 38.2°C (100.8°F) for approximately 15 minutes to allow live motile spermatozoa ample opportunity to "swim up" after thawing.
- The top supernatant is pulled out and placed into a 15 ml conical tube with an additional 2 ml of pre-equilibrated G-IVF™ and centrifuged at 327× g for 5 minutes.
- The resulting supernatant is removed following centrifugation and the sperm pellet re-suspended in the remaining medium to be used for ICSI.
- A direct dilution procedure is utilized if sperm numbers are low and individual sperm cells are difficult to identify.
- Either a full frozen straw of "ICSI dose" semen or a cut portion of an original straw is thawed and placed within a drop of warmed G-MOPS™ media.
- From this droplet, several progressively motile sperm cells are identified and selected for ICSI.
- An ICSI dish is prepared and labeled prior to preparing the gametes, through utilization of the lid of a 35 × 10 mm polystyrene Petri dish, whereupon droplets prepared for holding oocytes and sperm are maintained under oil.
- The paperwork and identification of both the mare and stallion is confirmed again prior to performing the ICSI procedure.
- Upon confirmation, the ICSI dish is positioned upon the heated stage (38.2°C (100.8°F)) of an inverted microscope with micromanipulation capabilities.
- 1 µl of sperm preparation is placed in 3 µl of PVP medium to act as the sperm holding droplet.
- The dish containing the mature oocyte(s) is removed from the incubator and identification of the donor mare is once again confirmed before any oocytes are removed and placed within the holding medium droplet on the ICSI dish.
- The oocyte is positioned at the tip of a holding pipette and is held by a small amount of suction.
- A single sperm with subjectively normal morphology and motility is selected out of the 5% PVP droplet and pulled into the injection pipette tail-first. Once the midpiece has entered the pipette, the Piezo drill is pulsed several times to effectively immobilize the sperm.
- The injection pipette containing the immobilized sperm is returned to the droplet containing the oocyte.
- The oocyte is maneuvered using the injection pipette into a position such that the polar body is located directly in the 12 or 6 o'clock position and the clearest portion of ooplasm is nearest the holding pipette (Figure 52.1).
- Once in position, the operator utilizes the Piezo drill to bore through a portion of the zona pellucida directly

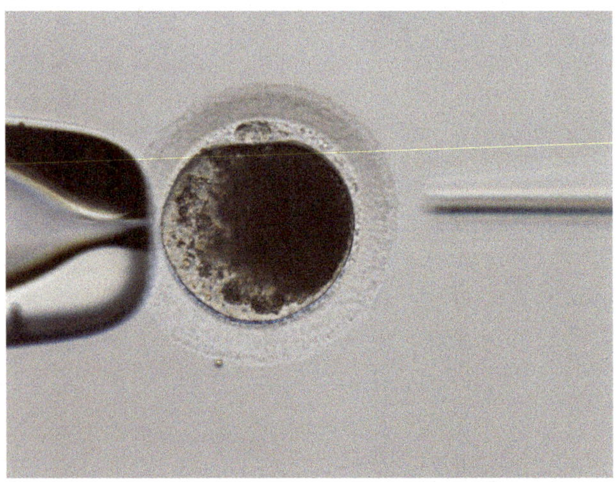

Figure 52.1 Equine oocyte held in place with suction from a holding pipette (left) positioning the oocyte with the polar body at 12 o'clock and an injection pipette (right) poised for ICSI.

across from where the holding pipette is holding the oocyte, and casts the zona fragment aside, creating a tunnel towards the oocyte plasma membrane.

- The selected sperm cell is then pushed down to be positioned at the tip of the injection pipette, which is then inserted back through the tunnel of zona pellucida and into the oocyte. A single Piezo pulse is applied and a small amount of ooplasm is aspirated up the injection pipette to confirm the ooplasmic membrane is broken.
- The tip of the injection pipette is advanced to the far side of the oocyte closest to the holding pipette and the sperm is deposited.
- The oocyte(s) that undergo the ICSI procedure is/are placed into a 30 μl droplet of post-ICSI embryo culture medium. This is pre-equilibrated and appropriately labeled within a 60 × 15 mm polystyrene Petri dish.
- Presumptive zygotes are placed within these droplets of media (up to two per drop) and are cultured within a mixed gas incubator at 38.2°C (100.8°F).
- Evidence of cleavage is evaluated 24 hours following ICSI in order to appropriately prepare recipient mares. If available, one recipient mare with a pre-ovulatory follicle and strong uterine edema will be administered an ovulation induction agent to stimulate ovulation approximately 2 days after the cleavage evaluation.
- Cleaved embryos are evaluated again 5 days following ICSI for continued growth and development and are transferred into a clean droplet of culture media.
- Most *in vitro* produced embryos reach blastocyst stage appropriate for transcervical transfer into a recipient mare on days 7–9 post-injection.

Interpretation and Additional Comments

- Both the owner of the mare and the facility performing the ICSI procedure should be under contractual agreement highlighting: the donor mare's registered name, the stallion(s) of choice, the potential risks of the procedure, the destination of any embryos derived, and the costs estimated for each component of the procedure.
- Labeling all lab equipment containing both oocytes and sperm with appropriate mare and stallion identification, respectively, is one of the most important practices within an ICSI lab.
- It is important to remember that oocytes collected from smaller immature follicles are at a variety of stages and will not all mature successfully for the ICSI procedure to be performed.
- Cooled/shipped semen from an actively breeding stallion may also be used, but will need to be coordinated to arrive the day before ICSI or early the morning of the ICSI procedure, which can be problematic if logistics become complicated.
- Although production of ICSI-derived embryos is not as efficient as other techniques, such as artificial insemination or embryo transfer, it provides an alternative method for mares and stallions where these traditional methods to obtain a live foal have failed.

Further Reading

Hinrichs K. 2010. Application of assisted reproductive technologies (ART) to clinical practice. *ProcAm Assoc Eq Pract* 56: 195–206.

Hinrichs K. 2013. Assisted reproduction techniques in the horse. *Reprod Fertil Dev* 25: 80–93.

Rader K, Choi YH, Hinrichs K. 2016. Intracytoplasmic sperm injection, embryo culture, and transfer of in vitro-produced blastocysts. *Vet ClinNorth Am Eq Pract* 32: 401–13.

53

Caslick Operation or Vulvoplasty

John J. Dascanio

School of Veterinary Medicine, Texas Tech University, USA

Introduction

Defects in perineal conformation involving abnormal declination of the labia or defects in mucosal apposition of the labia are most often remedied by performing a vulvoplasty (Caslick operation). Other conditions, such as a positive Windsucker test (incompetent vestibulo-vaginal fold) may also warrant vulvoplasty. Occasionally, mares may have no obvious perineal abnormalities, but may have a vulvoplasty performed as a preventative measure. This is especially true in young racehorses that have little intrapelvic fat and thus have an acquired angulation of the vulva.

Equipment and Supplies

Tail wrap, tail rope, non-irritant soap, roll cotton, stainless steel bucket, disposable liner for bucket, paper towels, exam gloves, twitch, skin stapler, staple removal device, local anesthetic, sterile surgery gloves, surgical pack, suture material with a cutting needle, topical disinfectant spray.

Initial Stage of Technique

- Remove feces from the rectum.
- Place a tail wrap and tail rope (see Chapter 4).
- Clean and dry the perineum of the mare (see Chapter 3).
- Place a twitch on the mare if needed. Sedation is not normally needed, but may be administered.

Temporary Staple Technique

- Wearing examination gloves, grasp the dorsal vulvar commissure and pull it upward to align both the vulvar labia in close apposition (Figure 53.1).
- Using a surgical skin staple gun, place individual staples 1 cm (0.4 inches) apart, starting at the dorsal commissure and proceeding downward (Figure 53.2). There is no incision of the mucosa with this technique.
- The line of staples should extend to below the level of the pelvic floor while still allowing approximately 6 cm (2.4 inch) of open vulva to allow for urination (Figure 53.3).
- The mare may become more resistant to stapling as the procedure progresses, so proceed with caution.

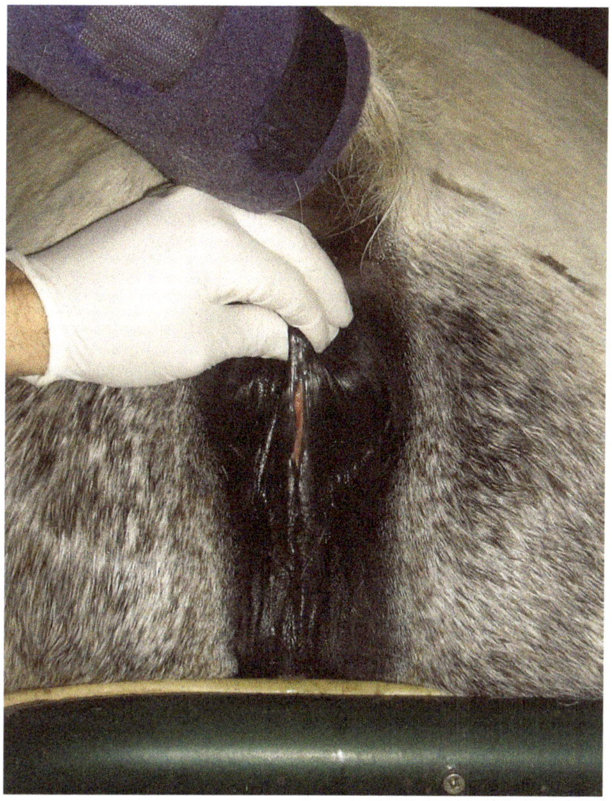

Figure 53.1 Grasping the dorsal commissure of the vulva in preparation for staple vulvoplasty.

Equine Reproductive Procedures, Second Edition. Edited by John Dascanio and Patrick McCue.

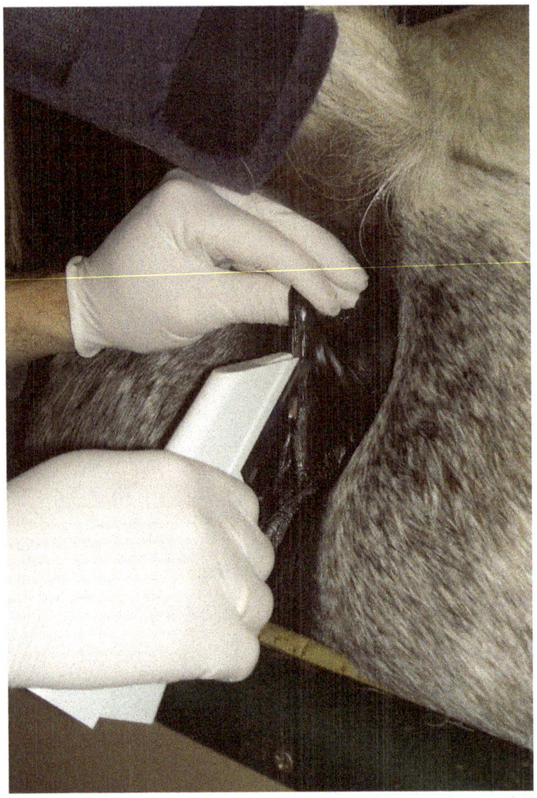

Figure 53.2 Placement of skin staples in the vulvar labia for staple vulvoplasty.

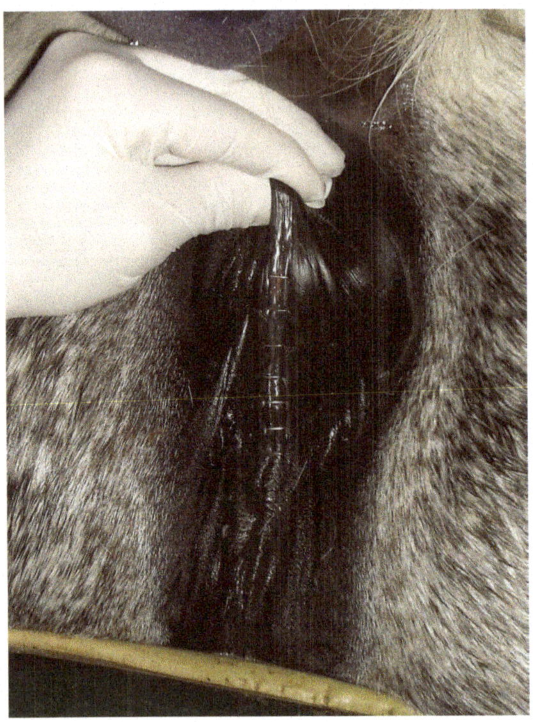

Figure 53.3 Finished temporary vulvoplasty.

- The staples provide a temporary vulvoplasty that may be removed and replaced to allow for breeding or treatment of the uterus. Once the mare has been confirmed pregnant, a permanent vulvoplasty may be placed.

Comments

- The staples will remain present for days to months depending on the mare's behavior and how well the staples are placed.
- Occasionally, single staples may fall out and need to be replaced to maintain the integrity of the vulvoplasty.
- Removal and replacement of staples for uterine therapy or for breeding may be accomplished with restraint using a twitch.
- A permanent vulvoplasty (Caslick operation) may be performed at any time.

Permanent Suture Technique

- The goal of the traditional Caslick procedure is to provide permanent apposition and healing of the dorsal aspect of the left and right vulva to minimize bacterial contamination and aspiration of air.
- Wearing examination gloves, grasp the vulvar lips and instill a local anesthetic (lidocaine or carbocaine) at the mucocutaneous junction on both sides, starting at the most ventral aspect of the vulvoplasty and proceeding upward to the dorsal commissure, using a 20 gauge 4 cm (1.5 inch) needle with a total of approximately 20 ml of local anesthetic.
- The most ventral extent of the vulvoplasty should extend below the level of the pelvic floor while still allowing approximately 4–5 cm (1.5–2 inches) of open vulva to allow for urination.
- A final wash of the perineum may be performed.
- There are two methods to incise the vulvar mucosa. In the first, a 0.5 cm (0.2 inch) strip of mucosa at the mucocutaneous junction is removed from the left and right labia, making sure to remain on the mucosa and to not involve the skin (Figure 53.4). The two strips are joined at the dorsal commissure. In the second method, a scalpel blade is used to make an upside down "U"-shaped incision in the same fashion as the removal of a strip of mucosa, but without removal of any tissue.
- The two labia are sutured together with suture material fixed to a cutting needle using a Ford interlocking or similar suture pattern (Figure 53.5). The type and size of the suture material depends on clinician preference and can range from 2-0 to No. 2. The use of non-absorbable

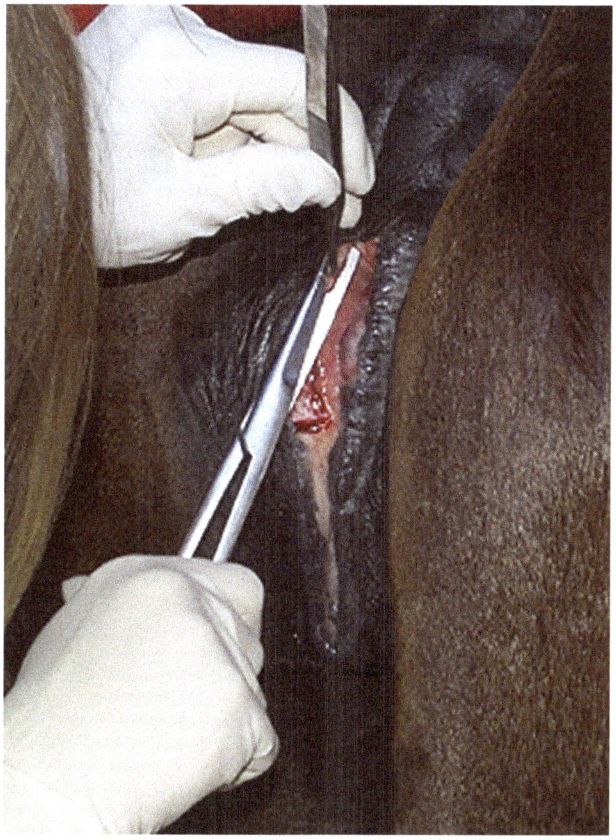

Figure 53.4 Trimming mucosa from the inner labia.

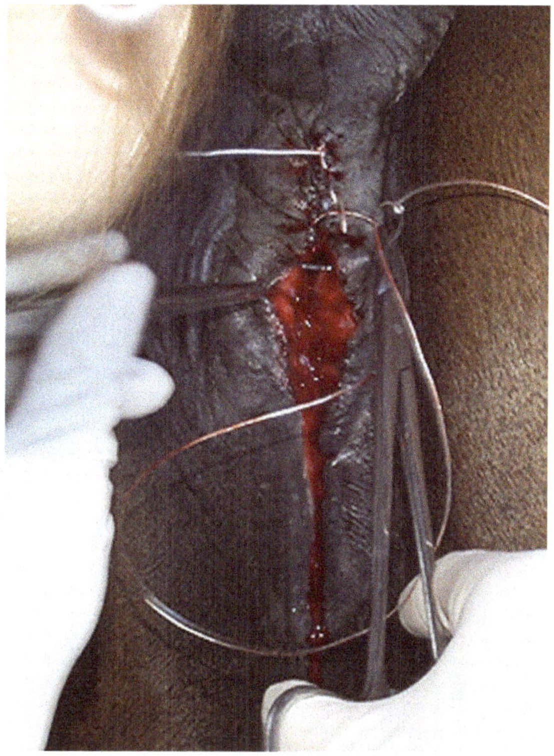

Figure 53.5 Suturing the labia together.

sutures requires that suture material be removed in about 2 weeks. Alternatively, the use of absorbable suture material alleviates the need for suture removal. Sutures should be placed approximately 0.5–1 cm (0.2–0.4 inches) apart and about 0.5–1 cm from the cut edge of the mucosa.

- A topical water-resistant aerosol bandage (such as an aluminum powder spray) may be applied over the completed surgical site if desired.
- Sutures (non-absorbable suture material) should be removed in approximately 14 days.
- The healed vulvoplasty will remain intact until opened. If the mare is pregnant, the Caslick must be opened 10–14 days prior to the due date or earlier if the mare shows clinical signs of parturition.
- Removal or opening of the vulvoplasty can be performed with the mare in stocks or restrained while standing in a stall. If the membrane is thick, a local anesthetic may be infused in a line along the area to be incised. If the membrane is thin, it may be incised with sharp Metzenbaum scissors without prior infusion of local anesthesia (Figures 53.6 and 53.7). In most instances, and certainly in the peripartum mare, the vulva is opened completely to the level of the original dorsal

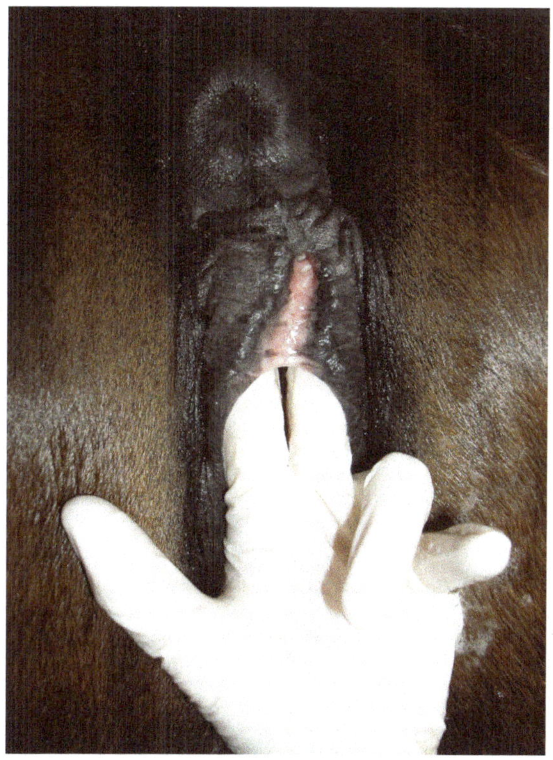

Figure 53.6 Placement of fingers for the removal of the vulvoplasty.

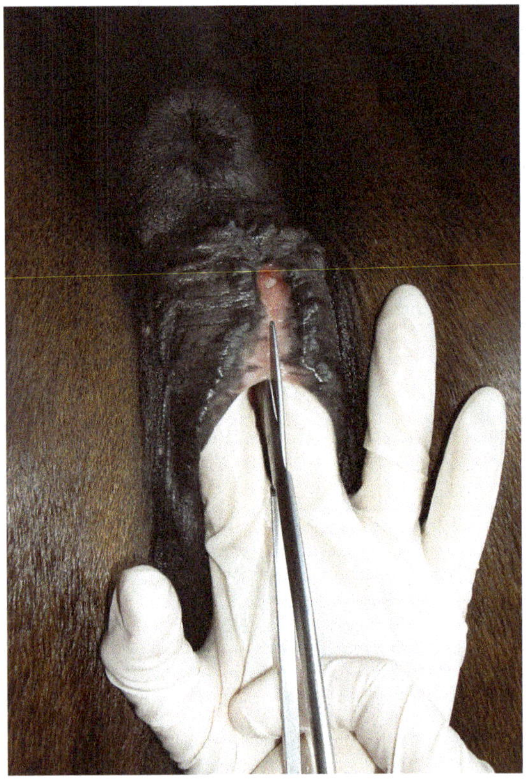

Figure 53.7 Cutting the co-joined mucosa to remove the vulvoplasty.

commissure. In contrast, the vulva may be partially opened if the goal is to facilitate breeding or uterine therapy in a non-pregnant mare. Additional options to be considered when opening a Caslick include sedation of the mare, applying a twitch, placing a tail wrap, evacuating the rectum of feces, and washing the perineum.

- One should be advised to stand to the side of the mare when opening the Caslick to avoid injury. No aftercare is required after cutting the mucosa.

Comments

- At the time of suture removal, the seal may be evaluated by placing two gloved fingers underneath the joined vulvar lips to examine for area(s) that are not co-joined. If the areas are greater than 2 cm (0.75 inches), a second surgery may be required.
- Mares with urovagina may have more urine retention with a vulvoplasty due to the decrease in effective vulvar opening.
- Scar tissue may form if the initial incision involves the vulvar skin, making subsequent vulvoplasties more difficult to perform.
- Mares may be bred through a speculum, bypassing the need to remove a Caslick (see Chapter 46).

Further Reading

Pascoe RR. 1979. Observations on the length and angle of declination of the vulva and its relation to fertility in the mare. *J Reprod Fertil Suppl* 27: 299–305.

Purswell BJ, Moll HD. 1999. Surgery of the vulva and perineum. In: Wolfe DF, Moll HD (eds). Large Animal Urogenital Surgery. Baltimore: Williams and Wilkins, pp. 91–5.

54

Contagious Equine Metritis Testing

John J. Dascanio

School of Veterinary Medicine, Texas Tech University, USA

Introduction

Contagious equine metritis (CEM) is a sexually transmitted infectious disease caused by the organism *Taylorella equigenitalis,* a Gram-negative bacterium. *T. equigenitalis* has been detected in many countries around the world and causes infertility and abortions in mares. Infected mares may exhibit a thick, mucopurulent vulvar discharge, while stallions do not generally exhibit clinical signs of the disease. The organism may be transmitted between stallion and mare during live cover, from stallion to mare during artificial insemination, or between stallions via contaminated breeding equipment during semen collection.

Mares may be tested as part of a surveillance program for CEM or during a disease outbreak. CEM may be treated and eradicated through the use of antiseptics and antibiotics. Horses imported from countries positive for CEM are required to go through a quarantine and treatment protocol. Diagnostic tests must be negative for *T. equigenitalis* prior to release from quarantine for CEM-positive mares or those from CEM-positive countries. *T. equigenitalis* may be detected by bacterial culture or serology, and a certified laboratory must be used for CEM testing.

A disinfectant scrub should not be used prior to collecting test samples as this may kill the *Taylorella* bacteria in the sample, leading to a false-negative test. In addition, systemic antibiotics should not be given to a horse that is undergoing CEM testing as this may result in an inaccurate diagnosis. A minimum of 7 days must elapse between the last antibiotic administration and CEM testing. All samples should be placed into Amies transport media with charcoal and transported to the testing laboratory for evaluation within 48 hours of collection. Treatment may not begin until after culture results are returned in case a culture has to be repeated due to inconclusive culture results. If treated, a 21-day period must elapse prior to re-culture.

Note that all testing and treatments must be performed in accordance with approved Animal and Plant Health Inspection Service/United States Department of Agriculture (APHIS/USDA) protocols or the country of residence. In addition, procedures for qualifying and testing CEM-negative test mares for stallions to breed should conform to AHIS/USDA guidelines or the country of residence. See the AHPIS/USDA website for current information (https://www.aphis.usda.gov/aphis/ourfocus/animalhealth/animal-disease-information/equine/cem/contagious-equine-metritis; last accessed October 2020.).

Equipment and Supplies

Tail wrap, non-irritant soap, roll cotton, stainless steel bucket, disposable liner for bucket, paper towels, examination gloves, 2.5% squalene cleansing solution, curved tip 12 ml syringe, 2% chlorhexidine scrub, ultrafine sterile swabs 14 cm (5.5 inch) long by 0.6 mm (0.025 inch) diameter, Amies charcoal transport media with culture swab, uterine culture swab, 2% chlorhexidine ointment.

Mare Diagnosis

- Collect serum for the complement fixation test.
- Collect swabs from the clitoral sinus and clitoral fossa for bacterial culture in accordance with the schedule from AHPIS/USDA (Figures 54.1 and 54.2). Each sample should be performed with a separate sterile swab. Only remove organic debris with a clean disposable paper towel or by using minimal sterile water, if needed, prior to culture. A 14 cm long by 0.6 mm diameter sterile ultrafine swab must be used for the clitoral sinuses as a regular culture swab is too large to fit into the sinuses.
- After performing the last series of clitoral cultures, place a tail wrap and wash the perineum with a mild

Equine Reproductive Procedures, Second Edition. Edited by John Dascanio and Patrick McCue.

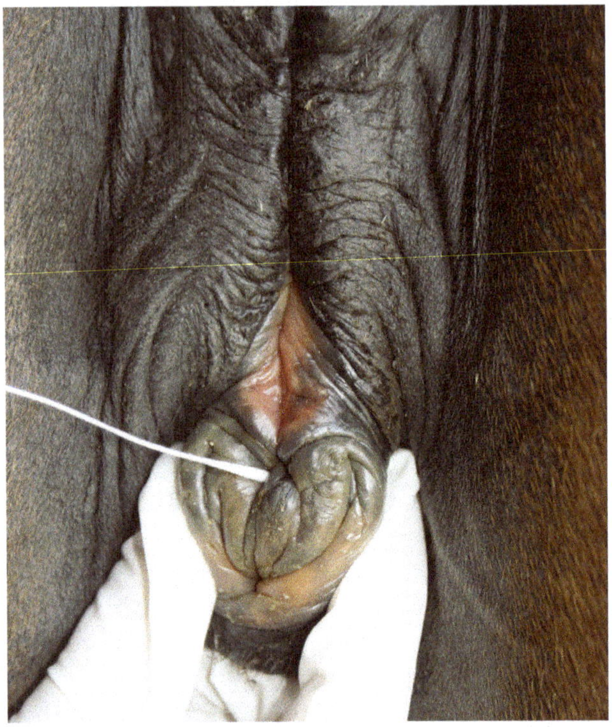

Figure 54.1 Culture of the central clitoral sinus using an ultrafine culture swab.

disinfectant and rinse liberally. A disposable bucket liner and examination gloves should be used during the washing procedure to prevent transfer of pathogens to other horses. Using a guarded uterine culture swab, collect a bacterial culture swab of the cervix or endometrium.

- If the mare is pregnant at the time of testing, the clitoral cultures may be performed, but the cervical or endometrial culture should be performed post-foaling.
- Foals born to positive mares must remain under quarantine until tested negative for CEM.

Mare Treatment

- Pregnant mares may be treated pre-foaling or after foaling. Pre-foaling treatment, especially for culture-positive mares, may decrease the likelihood that the foal will become infected, but does not exclude the foal from testing.
- Manually express any smegma from the central clitoral sinuses by squeezing the clitoris between the thumb and index finger while gently pulling down and out.
- Infuse the two lateral and the central clitoral sinuses with 0.5 ml of a 2.5% squalene cleansing solution (ceruminolytic agent) to remove any retained smegma.
- Lavage the clitoral sinuses with approximately 5ml of warm sterile saline to remove any debris and the cleansing solution using a curved tip 12 ml sterile syringe (Figure 54.3).

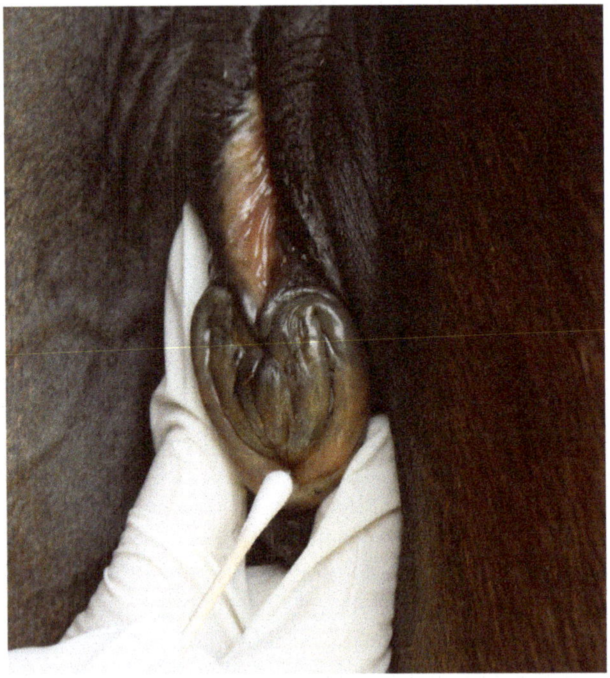

Figure 54.2 Culture of the clitoral fossa.

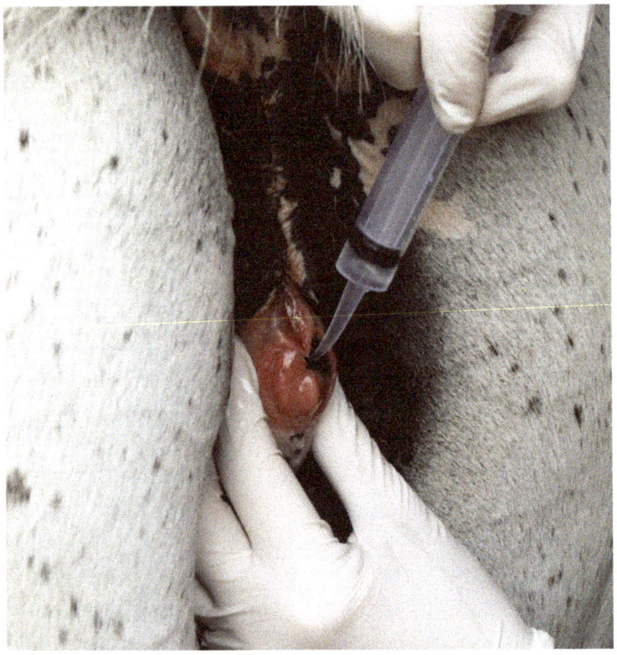

Figure 54.3 Flushing the central clitoral fossa using a curved tip syringe.

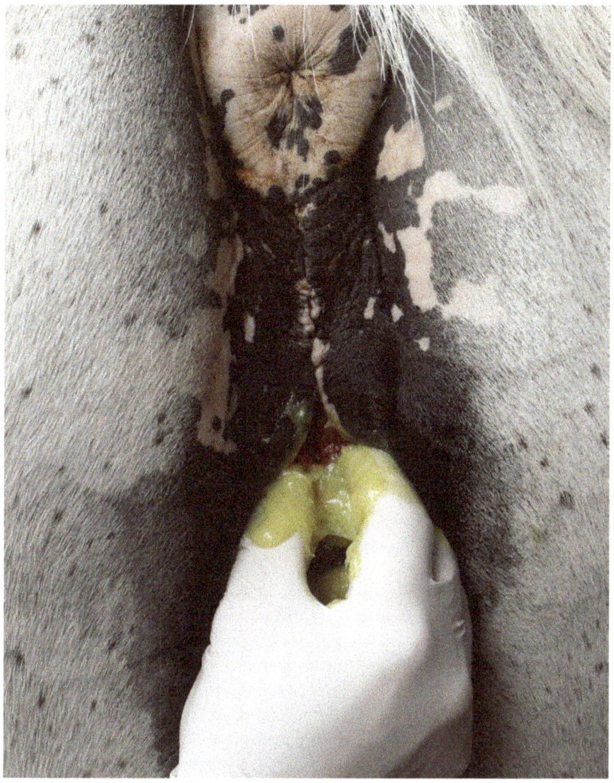

Figure 54.4 Packing the clitoris with 0.2% nitrofurazone antibiotic ointment.

- Clean and scrub the clitoral sinuses and clitoral fossa with a 2% chlorhexidine solution using a 5-minute scrub. Rinse the washed areas with warm sterile saline.
- Pack the clitoral fossa and sinuses with a 0.2% nitrofurazone ointment or a silver sulfadiazine ointment (Figure 54.4). Manually work the ointment into the clitoral sinuses with gloved fingers.
- Repeat the chlorhexidine scrub and packing according to the AHPIS/USDA timetable and instructions. Infusion of the clitoral sinuses with the cleansing solution only needs to be done on the first day of treatment.
- Mares that were positive for *T. equigenitalis* will require a complete culture series for the clitoris and cervix or endometrium after treatment is concluded to demonstrate treatment efficacy.

Stallion Diagnosis

- The serum complement fixation test is not used for stallions since they do not develop an immune response.
- Stallions may be shipped to an approved facility with mares that can be bred as part of the testing process.

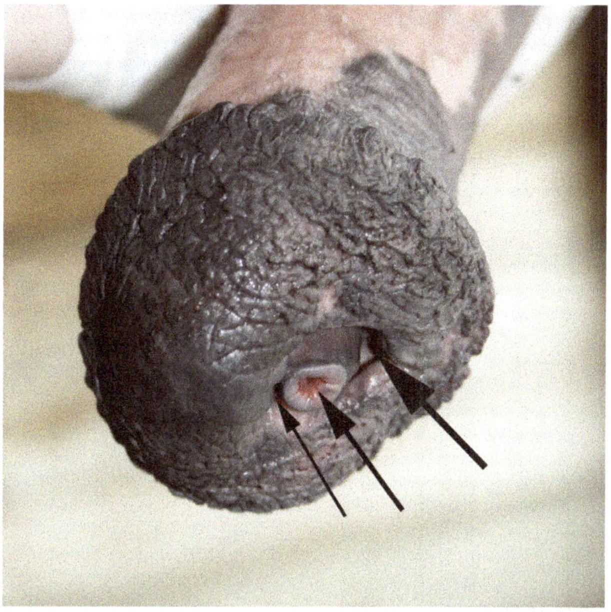

Figure 54.5 Culture locations on the distal penis: urethral sinus (thin arrow) located dorsal to urethra, urethra (central arrow), and fossa glandis (large arrow).

- The prepuce near the base of the penis, urethral sinus, fossa glandis (also called the urethral fossa), and the distal urethra should each be cultured separately using a sterile swab (Figure 54.5). Only remove organic debris with a clean disposable paper towel or by using minimal sterile water, if needed, prior to culture. One to three cultures may be required by animal health officials. Disposable examination gloves should be used when handling the stallion's genitalia.
- If the stallion is positive on any culture, treatment may be initiated immediately before any test breeding.
- If the stallion is negative on all cultures, the next step is to test breed two CEM-negative mares by live cover. The mares will subsequently undergo clitoral cultures according to the AHPIS/USDA timetable and instructions. The two test mares will have a blood sample collected for complement fixation testing and cultures of the clitoral area and cervix/uterus as described earlier.

Stallion Treatment

- Clean the prepuce, penis, fossa glandis, and urethral sinus with 2% chlorhexidine, with the penis erect, once a day according to the AHPIS/USDA timetable and instructions.
- Each day after cleaning, coat (pack) the prepuce, penis, fossa glandis, and urethral sinus with 0.2% nitrofurazone ointment or a silver sulfadiazine ointment.

Further Reading

APHIS (Animal and Plant Health Inspection Service). 2015. APHIS Veterinary Services Fact Sheet. *Contagious Equine Metritis*. September.

Erdman MM, Creekmore LH, Fox PE, *et al.* 2011. Diagnostic and epidemiologic analysis of the 2008–2010 investigation of a multi-year outbreak of contagious equine metritis in the United States. *Prev Vet Med* 101: 219–28.

Luddy S, Kutzler MA. 2010. Contagious equine metritis within the United States: a review of the 2008 outbreak. *J Eq Vet Sci* 30: 393–400.

Timoney PJ. 1996. Contagious equine metritis. *Comp Immun Microbiol Infect Dis* 19: 199–204.

55

Management of Seasonal Anestrus: Artificial Photoperiod

Patrick M. McCue

Equine Reproduction Laboratory, Colorado State University, USA

Introduction

The natural or physiological breeding season of mares extends from April to October in the northern hemisphere. A majority of mares enter a state of ovarian inactivity, or seasonal anestrus, during the winter months. The mean calendar date of the first spontaneous ovulation of the year in anestrous mares maintained under ambient light conditions in North America ranges from the middle of March to early May.

Mares housed under a stimulatory artificial photoperiod will ovulate earlier in the year and potentially cycle and ovulate more often during the breeding season than mares maintained under ambient light conditions. The physiological mechanism by which artificial photoperiod works is through interruption of the normal pattern of melatonin secretion from the pineal gland. Melatonin is secreted during the hours of darkness. Extending the duration of light exposure will reduce the duration of melatonin secretion, which will subsequently stimulate hypothalamic production of gonadotropin-releasing hormone (GnRH).

Equipment and Supplies

Lights (incandescent or fluorescent), automatic timer (optional).

Technique

- Mares in the northern hemisphere (especially above 23 degrees latitude) should be stabled under lights beginning on December 1 (June 1 in the southern hemisphere) to advance the first ovulation of the year to early February. The duration from onset of artificial light exposure to ovulation is approximately 60–70 days.
- Provide a minimum light intensity of 10 foot-candles (approximately 100 lux). A 100–200 W incandescent bulb in a 3.6 × 3.6 m (~12 × 12 feet) box stall should be sufficient. Alternatively, fluorescent lights are also effective (Figure 55.1).

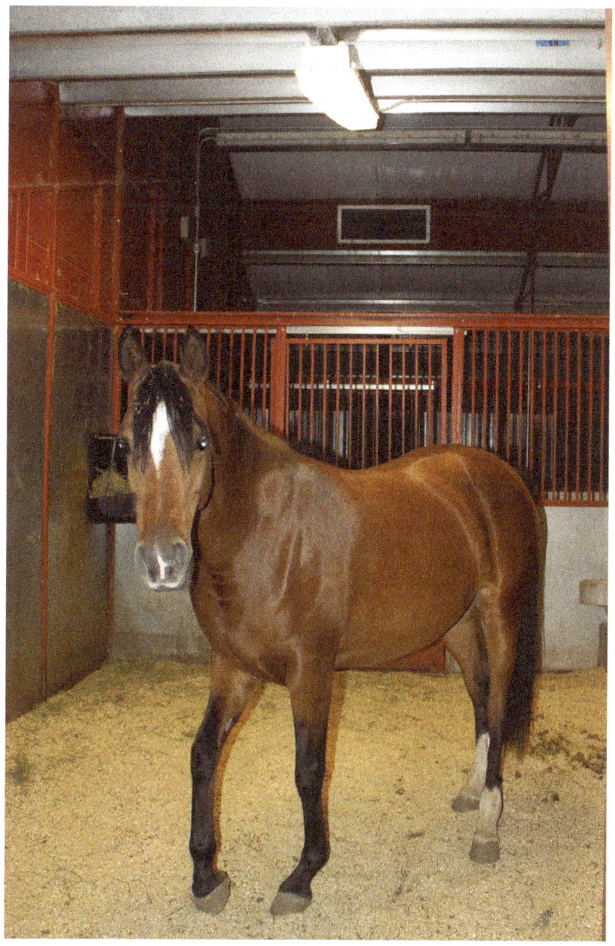

Figure 55.1 Mare in box stall with a fluorescent light overhead.

Equine Reproductive Procedures, Second Edition. Edited by John Dascanio and Patrick McCue.

- It may be most convenient to set timer(s) to turn the lights on just prior to dusk and shut the lights off at 11:00 pm. The goal is to provide 16 hours of light and allow 8 hours of darkness.
- Alternatively, one can provide 2.5–6 hours of additional light exposure after dusk.

Additional Comments

Exposure of deep anestrous mares to just 35 days of a stimulatory artificial photoperiod (14.5 hours light and 9.5 hours dark, 100 lux) beginning December 20 was reported to be equally effective in advancing the first ovulation of the season in pony mares as compared to "permanent" long day (14.5 hours light, 9.5 hours dark) exposure.

Anestrous mares housed indoors, exposed to a stimulatory artificial light program and induced to ovulate may revert to anestrus if moved outdoors under ambient light conditions after the first photoperiod-induced ovulation of the year.

Exposure of mares to lights for 1–2 hours during a "photosensitive" phase beginning either 8 or 9.5 hours after the onset of darkness has been noted to stimulate follicular development in anestrus mares. The term "skeletal lighting" has been used to describe this type of artificial photoperiod regimen.

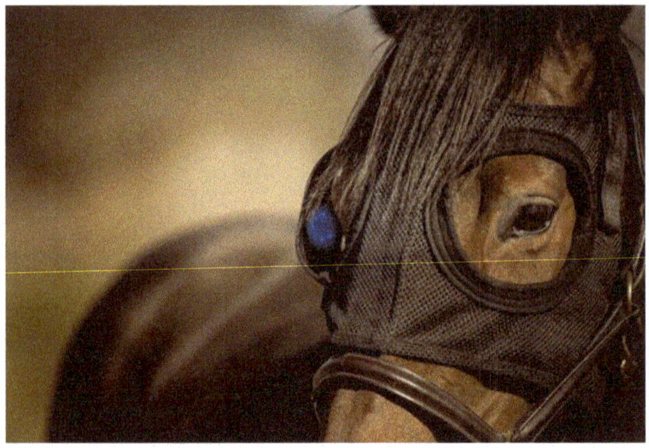

Figure 55.2 Mare wearing a mask emitting a blue light into one eye.

Recently the use of a light mask (Figure 55.2) equipped with a LED emitting a blue light at a peak wavelength of 468 nm directed at one eye was shown to alter the pattern of melatonin secretion and advance the onset of the breeding season (Equilume Ltd, Kildare, Ireland).

Further Reading

Burkhardt J. 1947. Transition from anoestrus in the mare and the effect of artificial lighting. *J Agric Sci Camb* 37: 64–8.

McCue PM, Logan NL, Magee C. 2007. Management of the transition period: physiology and artificial photoperiod. *Eq Vet Educ* 19: 146–50.

Palmer E, Driancourt MA, Ortavant R. 1982. Photoperiodic stimulation of the mare during winter anoestrus. *J Reprod Fertil Suppl* 32: 275–82.

Walsh CM, Prendergast RL, Sheridan JT, Murphy BA. 2013. Blue light from light-emitting diodes directed at a single eye elicits a dose-dependent suppression of melatonin in horses. *Vet J* 196: 231–5.

56

Management of Seasonal Anestrus: Hormone Therapy

Patrick M. McCue

Equine Reproduction Laboratory, Colorado State University, USA

Introduction

An artificial photoperiod is the most common technique used to advance the first ovulation of the year in seasonally anestrous mares. However, light therapy is not universally effective as improper phototherapy may limit efficacy and not all mares respond to light therapy. In addition, many mares are not maintained under lights in the winter months and yet owners still want them bred early in the season.

Equipment and Supplies

Syringes (variety), needles, hormones (see text).

Technique

A variety of hormone therapies have been reported to stimulate follicular development in anestrous mares and advance the date of the first ovulation of the year (Table 56.1).

Table 56.1 Medications and dosage regimens that have been used in the management of transitional mares.

Altrenogest	0.044 mg/kg PO, s.i.d.
Buserelin (GnRH agonist)	10–100 μg IM or SC, b.i.d.
Deslorelin (GnRH agonist)	25–125 μg IM, b.i.d.
Domperidone	1.1 mg/kg PO, s.i.d.
Equine FSH	6.25–12.5 mg IM, b.i.d.
Recombinant equine FSH	0.65 mg IM, b.i.d.
GnRH (native)	50–500 μg IM, b.i.d. to t.i.d.
Goserelin (GnRH agonist)	One third to one half of a 3.6 mg implant, SC, once
hCG	2,500 units IV, once
Histrelin	25–125 μg IM, b.i.d.
Progesterone	150 mg IM, s.i.d.
Progesterone plus estradiol	150 mg progesterone plus 5 mg estrogen, IM
Sulpiride	sulpiride 0.5 to 1.0 mg/kg IM, s.i.d or b.i.d.

FSH, follicle-stimulating hormone; GnRH, gonadotropin-releasing hormone; hCG, human chorionic gonadotrophin.

Gonadotropin-Releasing Hormone (GnRH)

- Administration of GnRH or GnRH analogs can be effective if administered two to three times daily by intramuscular injection.
- Response to GnRH administration in anestrous mares is related to follicle size at the onset of treatment or the depth of anestrus (deep anestrus versus transition). Typically, mares in transition are more likely to respond than mares in deep anestrus. Increasing GnRH dose and/or treatment frequency tends to increase follicular development, percentage of mares that ovulate, and/or number of ovulations.
- Deep anestrous mares induced to ovulate with GnRH may return to anestrus after the conclusion of therapy. In contrast, transitional mares are more likely to continue to cycle after a GnRH-induced ovulation.

Equine Reproductive Procedures, Second Edition. Edited by John Dascanio and Patrick McCue.

- The corpus luteum that forms after a GnRH-induced ovulation in an anestrous mare is similar to the one that forms following spontaneous ovulation in a cycling mare. Ovulations induced with GnRH in anestrous mares are generally considered to be fertile.

Follicle-Stimulating Hormone (FSH)

- An extract prepared from equine pituitaries (equine pituitary extract) was reported to stimulate follicular development in anestrous mares and induce ovulation of multiple follicles. The interval to ovulation was lower and the ovulation rate higher in transitional mares as compared with deep anestrous mares.
- Purified equine FSH was subsequently shown to stimulate follicular development and advance the first ovulation of the year in transitional mares. Twice daily therapy was more effective than once daily therapy.
- A recombinant equine FSH (reFSH) was also shown to stimulate follicular development in deep anestrous mares. Ovulations were induced in approximately 75% of treated mares by administration of human chorionic gonadotropin (hCG). A high percentage of mares ovulated multiple follicles.

Ovulation-Inducing Agents

- hCG has been reported to be effective in inducing ovulation in late transitional mares with large follicles (i.e., >35 mm).
- Deslorelin acetate, a potent agonist of GnRH, has also been used to induce ovulation of late transitional follicles with large follicles (i.e., >35 mm).
- If an ovulation-inducing agent is not administered when a large dominant follicle is present in a transitional mare, the follicle may regress without ovulation, a new follicular wave would eventually develop, and the ultimate result may be a longer transition period.

Progesterone and Progestin

- Conflicting reports exist as to the efficacy of progesterone in advancing the first ovulation of the year. A majority of studies indicate that progesterone therapy will not stimulate follicular development in deep anestrous mares, but may synchronize the return to estrus when administered to late transitional mares.
- A combination of progesterone and estradiol may be used to "program" transitional mares to ovulate in a predictable time window.
- Insertion of a progesterone-infused device, termed a controlled internal drug release (CIDR®) or a progesterone releasing intrauterine device (PRID®) into the vaginal vault of transitional mares has been reported to stimulate development of ovarian follicles Initial studies were conducted using CIDRs designed for cattle. One commercial vaginal device designed for mares (Cue-Mare®) containing 1.72 g of progesterone is available in New Zealand. Controlled clinical research trials reported that mares treated with the intravaginal progesterone insert were bred earlier in the breeding season than untreated mares and overall a higher seasonal pregnancy rate was obtained in treated mares. There was no difference in first service conception rate between treated and control mares.

Prolactin

- Administration of ovine prolactin or recombinant porcine prolactin (rpPRL) has been reported to advance follicular development in anestrous mares.

Dopamine Antagonists

- The administration of a dopamine antagonist, such as domperidone or sulpiride, stimulates an increase in plasma prolactin concentrations. This effect is potentiated by the administration of estradiol prior to treatment. Prolactin acts directly on the ovary to stimulate expression of gonadotropin receptors. Pituitary gonadotropin (FSH and luteinizing hormone) secretion is not altered by dopamine antagonist therapy, but treated mares are more sensitive to endogenous gonadotropins due to increased numbers of gonadotropin receptors which may stimulate follicular development.
- Dopamine antagonist treatment is not universally successful in stimulating follicular development in anestrous mares. The success rate is likely to be higher in transitional mares and mares maintained indoors under a stimulatory artificial photoperiod and/or in warmer climates.

Additional Comments

The use of a stimulatory artificial photoperiod in conjunction with GnRH agonists, progestins, dopamine antagonists, and/or hCG is common in equine practice. Administration of GnRH agonists and reFSH appear to hold the most potential for inducing follicle development and ovulation in a relatively short time period (i.e., <2 weeks). Dopamine antagonists may not be effective under all management conditions and the duration of treatment may be prolonged (i.e., >4 weeks). Progesterone therapy is effective at suppressing estrus and synchronizing ovulation when administered to mares late in transition.

Further Reading

Grimmett JB, Hanlon DW, Duris GF, Jochle W. 2002. A new intravaginal progesterone-releasing device (Cue-Mare™) for controlling the estrous cycle in mares. *Theriogenology* 58: 585–7.

McCue PM, Logan NL, Magee C. 2007. Management of the transition period: hormone therapy. *Eq Vet Educ* 19: 215–21.

Newcombe JR. 2002. Field observations on the use of a progesterone-releasing intravaginal device to induce estrus and ovulation in seasonally anestrous mares. *J Eq Vet Sci* 22(9): 378–82.

Sharp DC. 2011. Vernal transition into the breeding season. In: McKinnon AO, Squires EL, Vaala WE, Varner DD (eds). Equine Reproduction, 2nd edn. Ames, IA: Wiley Blackwell, pp. 1704–15.

57

Hormone Therapy in Cycling Mares

Patrick M. McCue

Equine Reproduction Laboratory, Colorado State University, USA

Introduction

A wide variety of therapeutic agents are used in mares to induce ovulation, cause regression of a corpus luteum, stimulate uterine contractions to evacuate fluid, bring mares into estrus, block expression of estrus, and in other aspects of broodmare management. The objective of this chapter is to discuss the clinical application of hormone therapy in the mare. Drug dosages, frequency, and routes of administration are presented in Appendix 3.

Gonadotropin-Releasing Hormone and GnRH Agonists

Native or natural gonadotropin-releasing hormone (GnRH) is a small (10 amino acid) peptide produced in the hypothalamus. In the horse, there is limited clinical use for exogenous natural GnRH. Low doses of native GnRH (i.e., 10–25 μg) may be used as a physiological challenge to evaluate pituitary function by measuring the output of luteinizing hormone (LH) and follicle-stimulating hormone (FSH).

Potent agonists of GnRH, such as deslorelin, buserelin, and histrelin, are used in broodmare practice to induce a timed ovulation in cycling mares in estrus. The mechanism of action of any GnRH agonist is the stimulation of LH secretion from the anterior pituitary, which subsequently causes follicle maturation and ovulation. Administration of a GnRH agonist will also cause secretion of FSH, which is not needed to induce ovulation.

Deslorelin is a small molecule (nine amino acids) and consequently mares do not develop antibodies against the peptide. Therefore, deslorelin may be administered to mares over multiple estrous cycles within a single breeding season without a decrease in efficacy. Deslorelin is available in a sustained release suspension and a sustained release implant.

- SucroMate™ (Thorn BioScience LLC, Louisville, KY, USA) is a commercial product containing deslorelin acetate in a sustained release suspension. Administration of the manufacturer's recommended dose of 1.8 mg (1.0 ml) as an intramuscular injection is effective in inducing ovulation in light horse mares in estrus that have a follicle ≥35 mm in diameter. Approximately 85–95% of mares will ovulate within 48 hours after treatment. The average interval from treatment to ovulation is approximately 40–42 hours. Ovulation has been successfully induced by administration of deslorelin in doses ranging from 0.5 to 1.8 mg.
- Ovuplant™ is a commercial product containing deslorelin acetate as a sustained release subcutaneous implant. Each implant pellet contains 2.1 mg of deslorelin. Approximately 85–95% of mares in estrus with a follicle >35 mm in diameter will ovulate within 48 hours after implant insertion (Figure 57.1). Delayed return to estrus has been reported in some mares that received prostaglandins in diestrus following an ovulation induced by Ovuplant™. This effect is apparently due to temporary downregulation of pituitary function secondary to prolonged secretion of deslorelin from the implant. Insertion of the implant in the vulva and removal of the implant 48 hours later after ovulation is confirmed will prevent the downregulation and delayed return to estrus.

Histrelin is another potent GnRH agonist used to induce ovulation in estrual mares. Doses of histrelin range from 0.5 to 1.0 mg, and the average interval from administration to ovulation is 40 hours. Histrelin is available from various compounding pharmacies.

The administration of low dose buserelin therapy (i.e., 10 μg in an aqueous solution) to mares in the middle of

Equine Reproductive Procedures, Second Edition. Edited by John Dascanio and Patrick McCue.

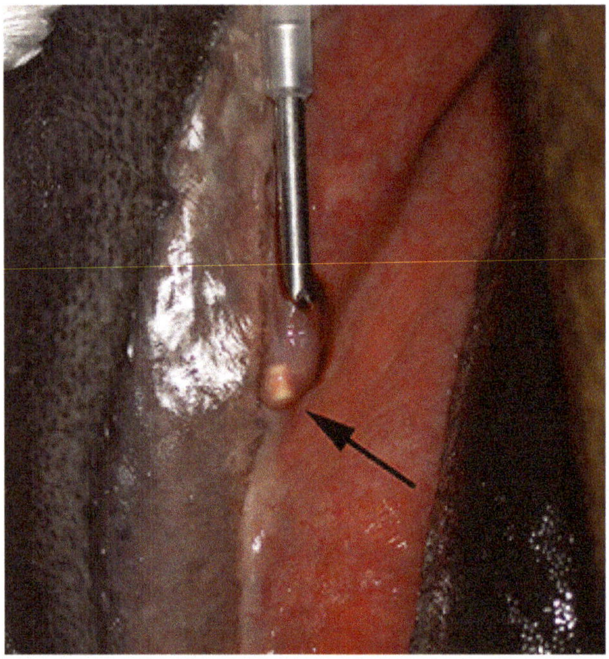

Figure 57.1 Insertion of an Ovuplant™ implant (arrow) in the vulvar mucosa.

diestrus (i.e., a single dose on days 8 to 12 or daily doses from day 8 to 12) has been associated with an increase in per cycle pregnancy rates of approximately 10%.

In addition, twice daily administration of low dose deslorelin or histrelin (i.e., 10–50 μg in an aqueous solution) has been shown to stimulate follicular development in seasonally anestrous and transitional mares. The interval from onset of treatment to development of a dominant follicle ≥35 mm in diameter is approximately 5–7 days. It is recommended that human chorionic gonadotropin (hCG) be subsequently administered to induce ovulation of the dominant follicle. Administration of 100 μg of deslorelin acetate twice daily to cycling mares beginning in mid-diestrus when the largest follicles are 20–25 mm in diameter has been associated with an increase in the percentage of mares with double ovulations.

Human Chorionic Gonadotropin

Human chorionic gonadotropin is a large glycoprotein hormone used primarily to induce ovulation in mares. The biological action of this human-origin hormone is due to its inherent LH-like biological activity. Administration of hCG to an estral mare with a follicle ≥35 mm in diameter and uterine edema will usually induce ovulation an average of 36 hours (24–48 hours) after treatment. A wide dose range of hCG has been used successfully for induction of ovulation (1,000–3,300 units) and the drug may be given intravenously or as an intramuscular injection. A common dosage is 2,500 units administered intravenously.

The hormone will induce a timed ovulation in 80–90% of mares. hCG is most effective in young mares that have not received the hormone previously and in middle-aged to older mares receiving the hormone for the first two or three times within a single breeding season. However, the efficacy may be somewhat reduced if hCG is given to a mare repeatedly during the same breeding season (i.e., the mare may not ovulate in the predicted time period). A comparison of efficacy of deslorelin and hCG for induction of ovulation is presented in Table 57.1.

Table 57.1 Comparison of hCG and deslorelin for the induction of ovulation in mares.

Group	n	Follicle (mm)	Interval to Ovulation (days)	% Ovulation Within 48 hours
Saline	19	38.9 ± 2.2	3.1 ± 1.6[a]	36.8%[a]
hCG	128	40.3 ± 2.9	2.0 ± 0.7[b]	88.3%[b]
Deslorelin	101	40.4 ± 2.8	1.9 ± 0.7[b]	90.1%[b]

[a,b] Data within a column with different superscripts are significantly different (P <0.05).

Follicle-Stimulating Hormone

Superovulation, or stimulation of multiple ovulations, has been an elusive goal in the mare. Purified equine FSH (eFSH; equine pituitary derived) and recombinant equine FSH (reFSH) have both been effective in inducing multiple ovulations in horses. The recommended protocol is to administer FSH twice daily beginning approximately 5–7 days after ovulation, beginning when the diameter of the largest follicle is approximately 20 mm. Prostaglandins are administered on the second day of FSH therapy. Treatment with FSH should be discontinued once follicles reach 32–35 mm in diameter and mares are allowed to "coast" without hormone therapy for 24–36 hours. hCG or deslorelin is subsequently administered to induce synchronous ovulations.

Equine FSH and reFSH have also been used to stimulate follicular development in anestrous and transitional mares, mares exhibiting postpartum anestrus, and acyclic mares during the physiological breeding season.

Unfortunately, the availability of commercial eFSH products has been intermittent. Porcine, ovine, and other FSH products are not effective in the mare.

Progesterone and Progestins

Progesterone (P_4) and progestins are naturally produced by the ovarian corpus luteum and the equine placenta. Progesterone-type hormones are primarily used in horses to suppress behavioral estrus, to synchronize estrus in a group of mares, and to help maintain pregnancy in problem mares. Progesterone has a potent negative feedback effect on pituitary LH secretion and estradiol has a similar negative feedback suppression of pituitary FSH secretion. The combination of progesterone and estradiol (P&E) suppresses both LH and FSH and results in a marked decrease in ovarian follicular development and the suppression of estrus. The combination works especially well for synchronizing the reproductive cycles of mares.

Short-acting progesterone products are administered intramuscularly once daily. A dose of 100–150 mg (i.e., 2–3 ml) is required to maintain blood progesterone levels high enough to suppress estrus (i.e., >1.0 ng/ml).

A long-acting product containing natural progesterone that may be administered once every 7 days to maintain pregnancy in mares is available from some compounding pharmacies. Administration of 1,500 mg of long-acting progesterone (150 or 300 mg/ml) is effective at maintaining progesterone levels ≥4.0 ng/ml for about 7 days and above 1.0 ng/ml for about 10 days in the absence of endogenous progesterone. Anecdotal reports indicate that some mares may have a mild to significant inflammatory response at the injection site. In addition, some mares receiving long-acting progesterone have experienced a delay in the inter-ovulatory interval, possibly associated with a prolonged suppression of LH. It should be noted that long-acting progesterone products from most compounding pharmacies have not been evaluated adequately and may not all provide the same blood levels or therapeutic results.

Subcutaneous implants (e.g., Synovex® S or C; Zoetis, Florham Park, NJ, USA) containing natural progesterone and an estrogen, designed to promote weight gain and increased feed efficiency in cattle, are not effective in the suppression of estrus in mares. There is not enough progesterone released by the implants to provide blood levels of progesterone high enough to be effective at estrous suppression.

Altrenogest is a synthetic progestin approved for use in the horse for the suppression of estrus. It is also commonly used in the management of the transition period, estrous synchronization, treatment of luteal insufficiency, management of high risk pregnancies, and management of twins. Altrenogest will not be detected by most standard progesterone assays. Consequently, it is possible to determine the level of endogenous progesterone in a mare being treated with altrenogest. Some compounding pharmacies advertise an injectable form of altrenogest for the suppression of estrus or maintenance of pregnancy. In many cases no controlled pharmacokinetic or clinical efficacy studies have been performed or published.

Inadequate production of progesterone by the corpus luteum has been proposed to be a contributing factor to early embryonic loss in mares. "Progesterone insufficiency" is a controversial topic. Progesterone levels ≥4.0 ng/ml are generally considered adequate to maintain pregnancy. Mares with concentrations below 4.0 ng/ml may be at increased risk of pregnancy loss. Therapy consists of progesterone supplementation and is usually initiated either 1 or 2 days after ovulation is detected or after ultrasonographic pregnancy diagnosis (i.e., day 14). Therapy is generally continued until day 100 to 120 of pregnancy, at which time production of progestogens by the placenta is adequate to maintain pregnancy. Alternatively, exogenous progestin therapy can be discontinued if levels of endogenous progesterone are ≥4.0 ng/ml.

Other synthetic progestins, such as medroxyprogesterone acetate, hydroxyprogesterone caproate, norgestomet, and megesterol acetate have been administered to mares in an attempt to block estrus or maintain pregnancy. Unfortunately, there is no clinical evidence that synthetic progestins other than altrenogest are effective in either the suppression of estrus or the maintenance of pregnancy in mares.

Progesterone-releasing devices originally designed to be inserted into the vaginal vault of cattle (i.e., PRID®, CIDR®) and devices specifically designed for use in mares (i.e., Cue-Mare®) have been used in cycling mares to suppress estrus, synchronize estrus, and assist with maintenance of pregnancy. Insertion leads to a rapid rise of serum progesterone and a concomitant decrease in pituitary LH secretion, followed by a slow decline in progesterone levels until the device is removed 7–10 days later. Use of vaginal inserts in mares is commonly associated with a mild vaginitis, but rarely with an ascending endometritis.

Estrogens

Estrogens are produced by granulosa cells of the developing follicles of cycling mares. Estrogens are also secreted by the corpus luteum of pregnant mares under the influence of equine chorionic gonadotropin (eCG) and the fetal–placental unit.

The primary clinical indication for estrogen therapy in the non-cycling, non-pregnant mare is stimulation of behavioral estrus. Approximately 5–10 mg of estradiol-17β or estradiol cypionate may be administered periodically to an ovariectomized or seasonally anestrous mare to stimulate behavioral estrus and allow the mare to be used as a tease mare or jump mare for semen collection. Estradiol administration will also result in a profound increase in uterine edema and will promote cervical relaxation.

Estradiol will not stimulate behavioral estrus when administered to a cycling mare in diestrus when progesterone levels are elevated.

Estradiol has a negative feedback effect on pituitary FSH secretion and will consequently suppress follicular development if administered to an intact mare. Estradiol is used in conjunction with progesterone (P&E therapy) to synchronize estrus in cycling mares and to "program" transitional mares housed under lights.

Conjugated estrogens (i.e., estradiol cypionate or estradiol valerate) will have a longer half-life and similar biological effects as the natural hormone estradiol 17β.

Prostaglandins

Prostaglandin $F_{2\alpha}$ ($PGF_{2\alpha}$)

Pulsatile secretion of endogenous $PGF_{2\alpha}$ from the endometrium approximately 14 days after ovulation results in the regression of the corpus luteum in a non-pregnant mare. The administration of exogenous $PGF_{2\alpha}$ is used clinically to either cause destruction of the corpus luteum (luteolysis) or to stimulate uterine contractions. The most common $PGF_{2\alpha}$ medications currently available are cloprostenol sodium and dinoprost tromethamine. Potential side effects of $PGF_{2\alpha}$ administration are transient sweating, abdominal cramping, and diarrhea.

Clinical uses of $PGF_{2\alpha}$ that are based on the luteolytic effect are short cycling, estrous synchronization, treatment of persistent corpora lutea, and termination of pregnancy. Complete luteolyis is achieved if $PGF_{2\alpha}$ is administered when the ovarian corpus luteum is mature, or from approximately 5 days post-ovulation onward.

Administration of $PGF_{2\alpha}$ will cause luteolysis and allow a mare the opportunity to come into heat.

The actual biological mechanism of return to estrus is dependent on pituitary FSH secretion, follicular development, and estradiol synthesis and secretion. $PGF_{2\alpha}$ administration will not cause a mare without an active corpus luteum (i.e., an anestrus or acyclic mare) to come into heat.

The interval from administration of $PGF_{2\alpha}$ to subsequent ovulation is largely dependent on the diameter of the largest follicle at the time of hormone administration. Mares with small follicles at the time of $PGF_{2\alpha}$ treatment will generally take longer to develop a dominant follicle and to ovulate than a mare with a moderate-sized follicle (Table 57.2). The follicle destined to be the ovulatory follicle typically increases by 3–5 mm per day.

Table 57.2 Interval from prostaglandin $F_{2\alpha}$ ($PGF_{2\alpha}$) administration to ovulation in mares with various sized follicles.

Follicle Diameter at $PGF_{2\alpha}$ Administration	Interval from $PGF_{2\alpha}$ to Subsequent Ovulation
<15 mm	10–1 2 days
20–25 mm	7–10 days
≥35 mm	a. Follicle ovulates within 48 hours b. Follicle ovulates after 48 hours c. Follicle regresses and is replaced by another follicle

Three clinical scenarios are possible in mares with large (i.e., ≥35 mm) diestrous follicles at the time of $PGF_{2\alpha}$ administration. The dominant follicle may ovulate within 48 hours and the mare will not have a chance to come into behavioral estrus or develop significant uterine edema. This is generally not considered to be a fertile ovulation. A second scenario is that the dominant follicle can continue to develop, the mare will show behavioral estrus, and a fertile ovulation will occur 3–6 days after $PGF_{2\alpha}$ administration. The third scenario is that the large diestrous follicle regresses after $PGF_{2\alpha}$ administration and another follicular wave develops, leading to eventual replacement with another dominant follicle. The duration from $PGF_{2\alpha}$ to ovulation in the last scenario is 7–10 days or more.

The primary clinical indication for the uterine contraction effect of $PGF_{2\alpha}$ is the treatment of uterine fluid accumulation or persistent mating-induced endometritis. A single intramuscular dose of $PGF_{2\alpha}$ will cause uterine contractions for 2–4 hours. The efficacy of $PGF_{2\alpha}$ therapy in evacuating uterine fluid may be better than oxytocin in some individual mares.

$PGF_{2\alpha}$ should not be routinely administered after ovulation is detected as the hormone will interfere with development of the corpus luteum and will decrease pregnancy rates. In individual clinical cases, $PGF_{2\alpha}$ has been administered in the post-ovulation period to facilitate uterine clearance and the mare administered altrenogest to help maintain the pregnancy.

Prostaglandin E_1 (PGE_1)

PGE_1 (misoprostol) has been applied topically to the external os and within the cervical lumen to stimulate cervical relaxation. The clinical indication for the use of PGE_1 is in mares that fail to relax their cervix during estrus and retain inflammatory uterine fluid after breeding. Tablets of PGE_1 are crushed and the powder mixed into either dimethyl sulfoxide gel or sterile obstetrical lubricant prior to topical application onto and within the cervix. Alternatively, a gel or cream preparation of PGE_1 may be obtained through a compounding pharmacy.

Topical application by deep horn infusion of 200 μg of PGE_1 onto the utero-tubular junction (UTJ) of mares with a history infertility of unknown origin has been reported to result in an increased pregnancy rate (see Chapter 31). The hypothesis is that PGE_1 may dilate the UTJ and oviductal isthmus and "unblock" oviducts occluded with debris and allow for a resumption of fertility.

Prostaglandin E_2 (PGE_2)

PGE_2 is produced by the developing embryo and facilitates passage of the embryo through the isthmus of the oviduct and UTJ into the uterine lumen. Therapeutically, PGE_2 gel has been applied topically onto the serosal surface of the oviduct via a laparoscope in an attempt to cause dilation of the oviduct and resolution of suspected oviductal blockage in infertile mares (see Chapter 30).

Oxytocin

The most common clinical use of oxytocin in the non-pregnant mare is stimulation of uterine smooth muscle contractions for evacuation of uterine fluid. The administration of 10–20 units of oxytocin to a mare in estrus will stimulate uterine contractions for 30–45 minutes and hopefully expel retained uterine fluid through an open cervix. A slightly longer acting form of oxytocin (carbetocin) is available in Europe. The half-life of oxytocin is 6.8 minutes, while the half-life of carbetocin is 17.2 minutes in the mare.

Oxytocin has also been demonstrated to induce persistence of the corpus luteum (pseudopregnancy) when administered daily during mid-diestrus (days 8 to 14) and may therefore be used as a therapeutic regimen for estrus suppression. Additional clinical uses of oxytocin include induction of labor, treatment of a retained placenta, and milk letdown.

Dopamine Antagonists (Domperidone and Sulpiride)

Clinical uses of domperidone and sulpiride in equine reproduction include treatment of fescue toxicosis, stimulation of lactation in agalactic mares, induction of lactation in nurse mares, and induction of follicular development in transitional mares.

Dopamine antagonists bind to the dopamine receptor and block the binding of endogenous dopamine and/or the ergot alkaloid ergovaline, the agent of fescue toxicosis. The decrease in dopaminergic biological activity will result in an increase in prolactin secretion, as dopamine has a suppressive effect on prolactin secretion.

An increase in serum prolactin is thought to be responsible for the therapeutic activity of dopamine antagonists.

Further Reading

Alvarenga MA, Segabinazzi LG. 2018. Application of misoprostol as a treatment of unexplained infertility in mares. *J Eq Vet Sci* 71: 46–50.

Ferris RA, Hatzel JN, Lindholm ARG, Scofield DB, McCue PM. 2012. Efficacy of deslorelin acetate (SucroMate) on induction of ovulation in American Quarter Horse mares. *J Eq Vet Sci* 32: 285–8.

Gee EK, DeLuca C, Stylski JL, McCue PM. 2009. Efficacy of medroxyprogesterone acetate in suppression of estrus in cycling mares. *J Eq Vet Sci* 29: 140–5.

Lindholm ARG, Bloemen EHG, Brooks RM, Ferris RA, McCue PM. 2010. Comparison of deslorelin and buserelin in mares: LH response and induction of ovulation. *Anim Reprod Sci* 121S: 68–70.

Lindholm ARG, Ferris RA, Scofield DB, McCue PM. 2011. Comparison of deslorelin and histrelin for induction of ovulation in mares. *J Eq Vet Sci* 31: 312–13.

Ortis HA, Foss RR, McCue PM, Bradecamp EA, Ferris RA, Hendrickson DA. 2013. Laparoscopic application of PGE_2 to the oviductal surface enhances fertility in selected subfertile mares. *J Eq Vet Sci* 33: 896–900.

58

Estrus Suppression

Patrick M. McCue

Equine Reproduction Laboratory, Colorado State University, USA

Introduction

The expression of behavioral estrus can have a profound negative effect on training and performance. Owners and trainers report variations in performance and temperament of mares attributed to the estrous cycle. Clinical signs attributed to performance problems included attitude changes, tail swishing, difficulty in training, squealing, horsing, excessive urination, kicking, decrease in performance, and colic-like discomfort associated with ovulation. Mares may be in estrus approximately 20–30% of the normal 21-day estrous cycle during the physiological breeding season.

Numerous techniques to suppress or modify the estrous cycle or estrous behavior of the mare have been reported, including hormone administration, herbal supplements, non-steroidal anti-inflammatory drugs, acupuncture, intrauterine devices, and surgery.

Equipment and Supplies

Ultrasound unit, therapeutic agent (see text), delivery device (syringe and needle, etc.).

Technique

- *Altrenogest*. Daily oral administration of the synthetic progestin altrenogest at a dose of 0.044 mg/kg is very effective and is considered the "gold standard" for the suppression of estrus in mares. Treatment with altrenogest should be initiated 3–4 days prior to a show or event and must be continued daily in order to attain and maintain estrous suppression. Altrenogest may be administered for extended periods without adverse effects on future reproductive performance or fertility. There are currently three US Food and Drug Administration (FDA) approved altrenogest products available: the original Regu-Mate® (Merck Animal Health, Millsboro, DE, USA) and two generic altrenogest products called Altresyn® (Ceva Animal Health, Lenexa, KS, USA) and OvaMed® (Bimeda, Oakbrook Terrace, IL, USA).

Several compounding pharmacies produce an injectable (IM) altrenogest product. None of the injectable products are approved for use in the horse.

- *Progesterone-in-oil*. Administration of natural progesterone (P_4) is very effective in suppressing estrus in cycling mares. Natural progesterone in an oil base must be administered intramuscularly once daily at a dose of 100–150 mg to maintain blood progesterone levels high enough to suppress estrus. Local tissue swelling and pain may occur following a prolonged course of daily intramuscular administration.
- *Long-acting progesterone. Administration of* 1,500 mg of natural progesterone in a sustained release preparation (IM) may sustain blood levels high enough to suppress estrus for 7–10 days. Local swelling has been noted at the injection site in some mares.
- *Oxytocin*. Administration of 60 units of oxytocin (IM) once or twice daily from day 7 to 14 of the estrous cycle (ovulation = day 0) has been reported to result in prolongation of the corpus luteum or pseudopregnancy in approximately 60–70% of mares treated. An elevation in blood progesterone >1.0 ng/ml was detected for >50 days. The average duration of spontaneous prolongation of the corpus luteum in mares is approximately 60 days (range 35–95 days); 10 IU of oxytocin IV once daily from days 7 to 14 post-ovulation will also have a similar effect.
- *Intrauterine devices*. Insertion of a 35 mm sterilized glass marble into the uterus has been noted to cause

Equine Reproductive Procedures, Second Edition. Edited by John Dascanio and Patrick McCue.

prolongation of the corpus luteum in approximately 40% of mares treated (see Chapter 59). The cause of the persistent luteal activity has been hypothesized to be an alteration in prostaglandin secretion from the endometrium. Mares with a persistent corpus luteum maintained elevated progesterone levels for approximately 90 days. Spontaneous elimination of the marble, fragmentation of the marble within the uterus, and uterine infections have been reported. In addition, a novel triangular device, the iUPOD™, consists of three elliptically shaped units each with a magnetic core and coated with a polymer. Each magnetic unit is inserted independently from the other. Once inside the uterus, these magnetic elliptical units self-assemble and adapt the lower energy "ring" conformation. Mean duration of diestrus when iUPODs™ were inserted ranged from 51.3 ± 22.7 to 73.4 ± 36.6 days (mean $\pm$ SD).

- *Plant oils.* Intrauterine infusion of 1.0 ml of fractionated coconut or peanut oil on day 10 post-ovulation resulted in a prolongation of luteal function (pseudopregnancy) in approximately 90% of mares treated. The mechanism of action of plant oils in the inhibition of luteolysis is not known.
- *Gonadotropin-releasing hormone (GnRH) vaccine.* Vaccination against GnRH causes suppression of the synthesis and secretion of follicle-stimulating hormone (FSH) and luteinizing hormone (LH) from the anterior pituitary. As a consequence, ovarian follicular development is suppressed along with estrogen production and the stimulus for expression of estrus is removed. A GnRH vaccine (Equity®) is available in Australia (Zoetis, West Ryde NSW, Australia), but not in most other countries. The effect of the vaccine was reported to last a minimum of 3 months and was correlated with the level of antibody response. Caution should be taken with a GnRH vaccine as the duration of suppression of reproductive activity may not be as predictable or controllable as with other treatments. In addition, there are currently no commercial tests for the presence of anti-GnRH antibodies. Consequently, it is difficult to determine if a mare exhibiting inactive ovaries had been administered a GnRH vaccine.
- *Ovariectomy.* A last resort for behavioral modification is surgical removal of the ovaries. Ovariectomy would remove the source of hormones responsible for expression of estrus (estradiol) and the cause of periodic abdominal discomfort in some mares (ovulation). However, ovary removal would not be effective if the cause of the adverse or obnoxious behavior is something other than ovarian hormones.

Additional Comments

Implants used to promote weight gain and feed efficiency in cattle that contain progesterone and estradiol (Synovex®; Syntex Animal Health, Des Moines, IA, USA) have been administered to horses in an attempt to suppress heat. However, a clinical trial showed that administration of 8, 32, or 80 Synovex® pellets did not prevent ovarian follicular development or suppression of estrus. The low amount of progesterone in the implants and the designed slow release rate are responsible for the lack of efficacy. Consequently, the use of Synovex® pellets for suppression of estrus in mares is not supported or recommended.

Medroxyprogesterone acetate (MPA) (Depo-Provera®; Pfizer, New York, USA) has also been administered to mares as a monthly, every other week, or weekly intramuscular injection in an attempt to block estrus. A clinical trial showed that administration of MPA to mares, even in high doses, does not affect LH function, inhibit follicular development, or suppress estrus. The lack of efficacy is hypothesized to be an inability of this synthetic progestin to bind to the equine progesterone receptor. Consequently, although the supposed dosage regimen for MPA may appear to be convenient, it should not be used due to lack of efficacy. In addition, MPA is listed as a prohibited substance by the Fédération Équestre Internationale (FEI), the international governing body of equestrian sports.

Herbal supplements containing valerian root or chaste tree berries have been administered to mares in an attempt to calm the mare, modify an undesirable behavior, or alter ovarian function. However, the efficacy of herbal supplements has not been evaluated in controlled clinical trials and the use of herbal products is forbidden in performance horses.

Further Reading

Elhay M, Newbold A, Britton A, Turley P, Dowsett K, Walker J. 2007. Suppression of behavioural and physiological oestrus in the mare by vaccination against GnRH. *Aust Vet J* 85: 39–45.

McCue PM. 2003. Estrus suppression in performance horses. *J Eq Vet Sci* 23: 342–4.

Nie GJ, Johnson KE, Braden TD, Wenzel JGW. 2001. Use of a glass ball to suppress behavioral estrus in mares. *Proc Annu Conv Am Assoc Eq Pract* 47: 246–8.

Vanderwall DK, Rasmussen DM, Carnahan KG, Davis TL. 2012. Effect of administration of oxytocin during diestrus on corpus luteum function and endometrial oxytocin receptor concentration in cycling mares. *J Eq Vet Sci* 32: 536–41.

Vanderwall DK, Rasmussen DM, Woods GL. 2007. Effect of repeated administration of oxytocin during diestrus on duration of function of corpora lutea in mares *J Am Vet Med Assoc* 231: 1864–7.

Wilshire S, Allen WR. 2011. Intrauterine administration of plant oils inhibits luteolysis in the mare. *Eq Vet J* 43: 99–105.

59

Intrauterine Devices for Estrus Suppression

Carlos M. Gradil

Cummings School of Veterinary Medicine, University of Massachusetts Veterinary and Animal Sciences, USA

Introduction

Mares in estrus can behave in ways that can interfere with handling, training, and competition. Current methods to suppress estrus behavior include pharmacological treatments, glass/plastic/stainless steel balls/marbles, and negative reinforcement strategies.

Pharmacological therapy is a common strategy involving administration of a synthetic progesterone compound to a horse on a daily, weekly, or monthly basis. A popular synthetic progestin is altrenogest. The US Food and Drug Administration recently highlighted the potential health risks, including reproductive system disorders and other adverse effects, in people who are exposed to altrenogest through contact with skin or product residue on barn surfaces, equipment, or treated animals. Another pharmacological therapy includes injections of medroxyprogesterone acetate; however, this drug has limited efficacy in the horse and has been prohibited in Fédération Équestre Internationale (FEI) competitions. The administration of exogenous oxytocin during diestrus can disrupt luteolysis, but it requires intramuscular administration every 12 hours over specific days of the estrous cycle. All these treatments require frequent administration and generally only result in a short-term effect. Therefore, the use of these pharmacological therapies for behavioral control is limited.

Another protocol is the use of intrauterine devices, specifically 35 mm glass balls placed in the uterus of mares to extend the function of the corpus luteum. In general, approximately 40% of mares "treated" by insertion of a sterilized glass ball into their uterus exhibit a prolonged diestrus of approximately 90 days (Nie *et al.* 2003). Complications have been reported with the use of glass balls/marbles, including chronic endometritis, pyometra, and fragmentation of balls/marbles in the uterine lumen and glass shards becoming adhered to the endometrium.

A subsequent study used 20 mm plastic balls filled with water as the intra-uterine device (Rivera del Alamo *et al.* 2008). The study showed that 75% of mares experienced a prolonged diestrus period with an average length of 57 days.

A recent study evaluated a novel intrauterine device for its effect on estrus suppression (Gradil *et al.* 2019). The iUPOD™ consists of three elliptically shaped units each with a magnetic core and coated with a polymer. Each magnetic unit is inserted independently from the other. Once inside the uterus, these magnetic elliptical units self-assemble and adapt the lower energy "ring" conformation. In mares, the devices can be inserted using an applicator at any stage of the estrous cycle and retrieved using a magnetic retriever. Mean duration of diestrus when an iUPOD™ was inserted ranged from 51.3 ± 22.7 to 73.4 ± 36.6 days (mean $\pm$ SD). Endometrial biopsies showed no significant differences before and after iUPOD™ placement/retrieval with up to 18 months of uterine retention/presence. Fertility of eight mares bred the season after iUPOD™ removal was 100%.

The mechanism for altered reproductive physiology and behavior of mares treated with any type of intrauterine device is an alteration of endometrial prostaglandin secretion resulting in an extension of luteal function.

Equipment and Supplies

Tail wrap, non-irritant soap, betadine solution, chlorhexidine solution, isopropyl alcohol, roll cotton, stainless steel bucket with disposable liner, sterile obstetrical sleeves, sterile obstetrical lubricant, ultrasound with mid (5 MHz) frequency probe, paper towels, exam gloves, needles, syringes, either sterilized 35 mm glass/plastic/stainless steel intrauterine ball (IUB) or iUPOD™ devices, iUPOD™ applicator, iUPOD™ retriever, hand-held metal detector (optional), sedation, intrauterine antibiotics, *N*-butylscopolammonium bromide, prostaglandin, misoprostol (optional), needles, syringes.

Equine Reproductive Procedures, Second Edition. Edited by John Dascanio and Patrick McCue.

General Preparation

- Place a tail wrap and prepare the perineum (see Chapter 3)
- Tranquilization may be administered for restraint. Typically, a xylazine (0.33–0.44 mg/kg IV) and butorphanol (0.011–0.022 mg/kg IV) combination is used to provide sedation and a degree of immobility for the mare. Alternatively, detomidine (0.0088–0.011 mg/kg IV) may be used with butorphanol.
- A dose of *N*-butylscopolammonium bromide (0.1–0.2 mg/kg IV) may be administered to relax the smooth muscle of the rectum, diminish uterine contractions, and allow for easier transrectal palpation and manipulation.
- A double sterile obstetrical sleeve may be used to diminish vaginal contamination of the uterus during placement. Cut the end of an obstetrical sleeve at the wrist, fold it, and dress it over the working sleeve. When at the cervix, push through the fold of the outer sleeve. The device to be delivered is between the two obstetrical sleeves.
- It may be advisable to lavage the uterus after removal of an intrauterine device depending on the amount of manipulation required for removal, the presence of any uterine discharge or uterine fluid, or other uterine health concerns.
- Intrauterine antibiotics, such as 2 g of ampicillin or 3.1 g ticarcillin-clavulanate in 8–10 ml distilled water, may be administered at insertion and retrieval.
- Topical application of misoprostol (prostaglandin E_1; misoprostol 2,000 µg/3 g cervical cream) is an option to soften a tight cervix. Apply incremental amounts to effect.
- For retrieval of an intrauterine device, the mare should be administered prostaglandin to lyse any luteal tissue that may be present. Removal of an intrauterine device may be attempted 4–5 days after prostaglandin administration or when the mare is in good behavioral estrus and the cervix is relaxed. Some mares may pass the intrauterine device after prostaglandin administration.

Technique for Intrauterine Ball Placement

- The estrous cycle of the mare should be monitored. The ideal time for placement of the glass intrauterine ball (IUB) (Figure 59.1) is during behavioral estrus when the cervix is open. It may be best to insert the ball on the day ovulation is detected or the following day, since the subsequent rise in progesterone from the developing corpus luteum will begin to close the cervix and help with retention of the ball.

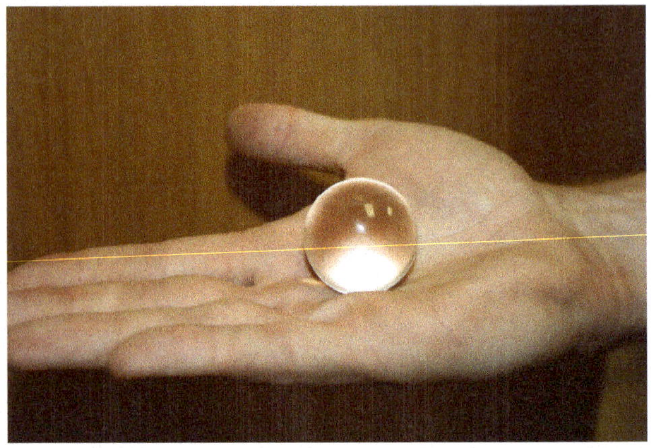

Figure 59.1 Unsterilized 35 mm glass ball.

- Place a previously sterilized IUB in the palm of the hand covered with a sterile obstetrical sleeve.
- Place sterile obstetrical lubricant on the back of the hand and down the sleeve arm.
- Introduce the sleeved arm into the vulva and proceed with the hand to the external cervical os.
- Introduce one and then two fingers into the cervical os to gently dilate the cervix to allow for insertion of the IUB.
- Gently push the IUB through the cervical canal and as deeply into the uterus as possible.
- Remove the arm from the vagina and place it per rectum to confirm the location of the IUB. Further manipulation may be performed per rectum to place the IUB into the base of one of the uterine horns.

Technique of IUB Removal

- The presence of an IUB should be confirmed through prior history of placement, palpation per rectum of the IUB, and/or ultrasonographic evidence of an IUB (Figure 59.2).
- It may be helpful to administer a low dose of *N*-butylscopolammonium bromide (3 ml IV) to facilitate relaxation of the rectal, uterine, and cervical smooth muscle immediately prior to the removal attempt.
- Remove feces from the rectum.
- Place a tail wrap and a tail rope.
- Clean and dry the perineum of the mare.
- On one arm don a sterile obstetrical sleeve and place sterile water-soluble lubricant on the outside of the hand and down the arm.
- On the other arm don a non-sterile obstetrical sleeve with applied non-sterile obstetrical lubricant.
- With one had per rectum (non-sterile sleeve), manipulate the IUB to enter the internal cervical os.

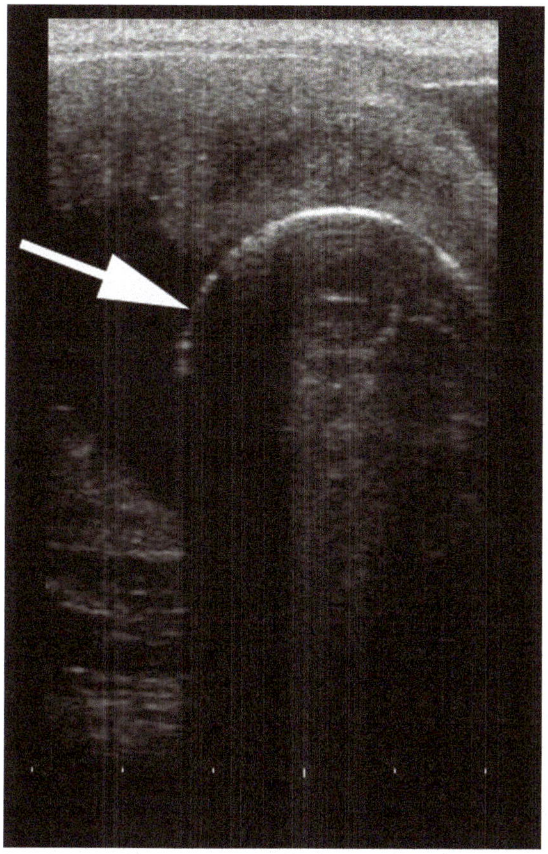

Figure 59.2 Ultrasound image of an intrauterine glass ball. The arrow points at the curved hyperechoic line depicting the edge of the glass ball.

- With the other hand per vagina (sterile sleeve), grasp the IUB within the cervical canal. Between pushing on the IUB per rectum and pulling on the IUB per vagina, remove the IUB from the reproductive tract.

Technique for iUPOD™ Placement

- Use a sterile iUPOD™ applicator and a sterile double obstetrical sleeve technique.
- The iUPOD™ (Figure 59.3), applicator, and retriever (Figure 59.4) cannot be steam sterilized. They are for one time use only, except for the retriever. The equipment can be sterilized by immersion in a chlorhexidine gluconate 4% solution for 20 minutes and rinsed with 70% isopropyl alcohol.
- The goal during manipulation should be minimal dilation of the cervix and distortion of the uterus.
- When using this device in mares with a pliable cervix (estrus), or within 48 hours post-ovulation, use either the iUPOD™ applicator with the three units loaded in tandem or manual insertion. For the manual technique, the three units are pushed through the cervix, one by one, until they just clear the internal cervical os. Check the location of the devices with ultrasound per rectum. The iUPOD™ will self-aggregate in the uterus in a "ring" configuration.

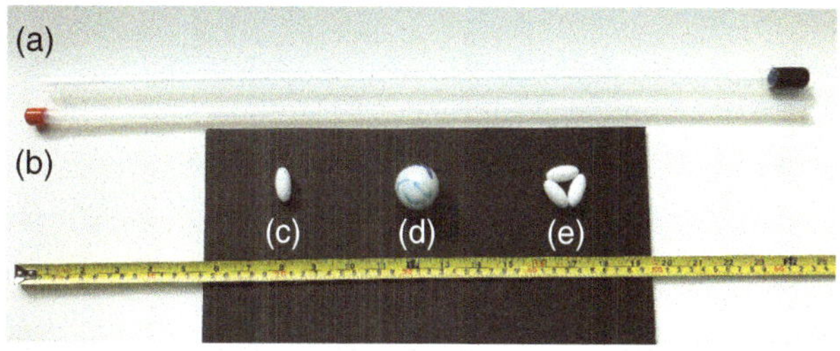

Figure 59.3 Disassembled iUPOD™ applicator: outer tube (A), applicator plunger (B), individual unit (10 g) (C), low quality 35 mm ball (~53 g) (D), and assembled units (~30 g) (E).

- When using this device in mares with a closed cervix (early estrus or diestrus and some mares (e.g., maiden) regardless of the stage of the estrous cycle), insert the individual units by hand. To do this, place the three units of the iUPOD™ in one's hand and push them all the way through the cervix one by one. One can confirm placement with the index finger or by using an AI pipette with a knobbed, non-blunt tip. Transrectal ultrasound will further pinpoint the exact location and self-assembling of the device.

Technique for iUPOD™ Retrieval

- The presence of an iUPOD™ should be confirmed through prior history of placement, palpation per rectum, and/or ultrasonographic evidence of devices (Figure 59.5).
- Remove feces from the rectum.
- Place a tail wrap and a tail rope.
- Clean and dry the perineum of the mare.
- When retrieving the iUPOD™ in mid-estrus use the retriever with the applicator (Figure 59.4). The retriever is attached to a fluorocarbon line and/or umbilical tape. Using a sterile obstetrical sleeve and sterile obstetrical lubricant, insert the applicator loaded with the retriever through the cervix. Push the retriever into the uterus. Make sure the retriever drops into the uterus.
- One can lift the cervix to allow the retriever to contact the iUPOD™. On occasion, in mares with a large uterus, one may facilitate the contact by manipulating the uterus per rectum. The applicator may remain in the cervix as the tag line is pulled. The device should be detected with the index finger at the end of the applicator. Alternatively, withdraw the applicator, first the plunger and then the outer tube, leaving and holding on to the tag line, before

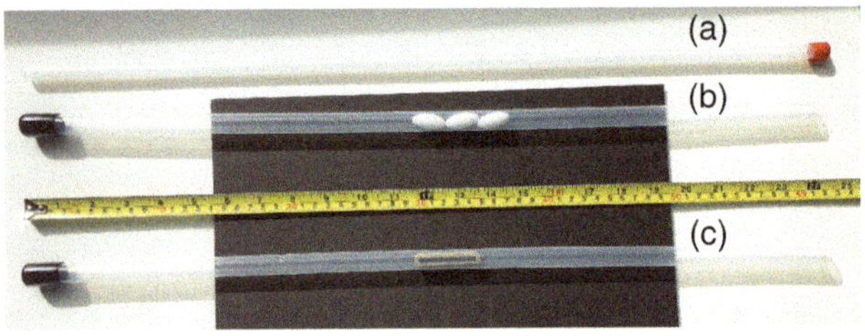

Figure 59.4 Disassembled iUPOD™ magnetic retriever and applicator: applicator plunger (A), applicator outer tube with three individual units loaded in tandem (B), and magnetic retriever loaded into the outer tube of the applicator (C).

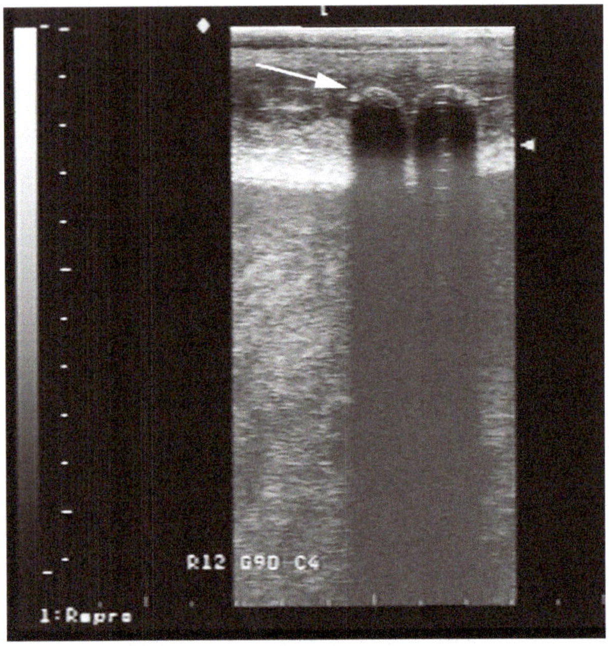

Figure 59.5 Ultrasound image of an iUPOD™ (arrow) in the uterus. Note the acoustic shadowing caused by the iUPOD™ that will aid in identification.

pulling and feeling the weight of the iUPOD™ attached to the retriever.
- It is recommended to keep the index finger inside the cervix as a fulcrum for the tag line to minimize tension of the tag line on the cervical tissues. This also guides the device and allows monitoring of the retrieval progress.

Interpretation

- A potential for a uterine infection exists if any intrauterine device is placed during diestrus and bacteria are introduced during insertion or if the device is not sterilized.
- Glass balls have been reported to fracture intrauterine, possibly due to improper autoclaving technique or due to the use of low quality glass marbles.
- Placement of a small (<25 mm) IUB may result in spontaneous expulsion and a return to estrus.
- The use of water-filled plastic balls may prevent untoward effects from glass fracture.
- Silicone 36 mm balls (veterinary ocular implant; Jardon Eye Prosthetics, Inc., Southfield, MI, USA), may be an alternative to glass balls.
- Biopsies conducted up to 2 years after the placement of a glass ball did not demonstrate significant uterine fibrosis.
- The placement of intrauterine devices should be documented and new owners informed that the device is present.
- Mares may cycle and become pregnant with a ball in place (Figure 59.6). There are also anecdotal reports of mares with a IUB carrying a foal to term and giving birth.
- The clinical use of balls for suppression of estrus has declined in recent years as the overall efficacy is not high, the efficacy in individual mares is not predictable, and the anecdotal reports of mares with uterine infections and fractured glass balls.
- Horses that are *not* candidates for intrauterine devices include:
  - Mares having a previous or current history of uterine inflammation or infection.
  - Mares with any uterine fluid during diestrus.
  - Mares with excessive uterine fluid during estrus (>10 mm).
  - Mares with history of pneumovagina or urine pooling.
  - Mares with granulosa cell tumor.

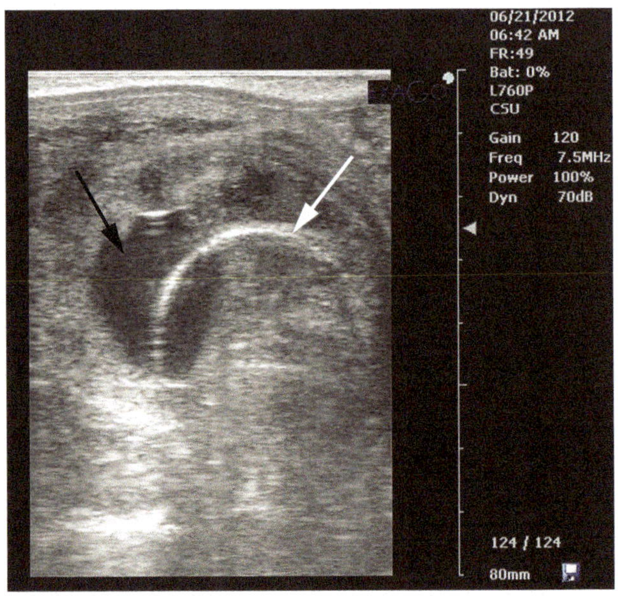

Figure 59.6 Ultrasound image of a 16-day embryonic vesicle (black arrow) adjacent to an intrauterine ball (white arrow).

- Mares that had more than 2 years of uninterrupted use of uterine glass balls.
- Mares with a dysfunctional/stenotic cervix (i.e., maiden mares ≥15 years of age).

- It is recommended that a intrauterine device is used for 5–7 months, at a time during the performance season, when mares are likely to be cycling and able to produce endogenous progesterone. Ultrasound the mare at least once during this time period, especially mares ≥15 years of age who may be predisposed to more uterine pathology. This will confirm the presence of the devices and any excessive accumulation of uterine fluid.
- The presence of an iUPOD™ within the uterus of a mare can also be confirmed by using a metal detector positioned along the external flank of the mare.

References

Gradil CM, Uricchio C, Schwarz A. 2019. Self-assembling intra-uterine device (Upod) modulation of the reproductive cycle in mares. *J Eq Vet Sci* 83: 102690.

Nie GJ, Johnson KE, Braden TD, Wenzel JW. 2003. Use of an intra-uterine glass ball protocol to extend luteal function in mare. *J Eq Vet Sci* 23: 266–73.

Rivera del Alamo MM, Reilas T, Kindahl H, Katila T. 2008. Mechanisms behind intra-uterine device-induced luteal persistence in mares. *Anim Reprod Sci* 107: 94–106.

Further Reading

Dascanio JJ, McCue PM. 2014. Use of an intra-uterine ball in estrus suppression. In: Dascanio JJ, McCue PM (eds). Equine Reproductive Procedures, 1st edn. Oxford: Wiley Blackwell, pp. 158–60.

McCue P. 2003. Estrus suppression in performance horses. *J Eq Vet Sci* 23: 342–4.

Squires EL. 1993. Progestin. In: McKinnon AO, Voss JL (eds). Equine Reproduction. Philadelphia: Lea and Febiger, pp. 311–18.

Vanderwall DK, Rasmussen DM, Woods GL. 2007. Effect of repeated administration of oxytocin during diestrus on duration of function of corpora lutea in mares. *J Am Vet Med Assoc* 231(12): 1864–7.

60

Immunocontraception

Patrick M. McCue

Equine Reproduction Laboratory, Colorado State University, US

Introduction

The term immunocontraception implies technology aimed at utilizing the immune system to prevent conception or pregnancy. The goals of immunocontraception in horses range from temporary blockage of behavioral estrus for mares in training to short-term, reversible contraception, or permanent sterilization for management of herds of feral horses.

There are two main types of immunocontraceptives currently in use in horses: vaccines against gonadotropin-releasing hormone (GnRH) and vaccines against porcine zona pellucida (PZP) antigens. Several other vaccines utilizing different antigens, such as growth differentiation factor 9 (GDF9) and bone morphogenic protein 15 (BMP15) are in development or are currently being tested. Most vaccine protocols are based on a primary immunization followed several weeks later by a booster immunization. This strategy may be manageable for domesticated mares, but is often not possible for feral horses, where the ultimate goal is a single immunization with prolonged efficacy.

GnRH is synthesized by neurons within the hypothalamus and regulates the production of follicle-stimulating hormone (FSH) and luteinizing hormone (LH) from the anterior pituitary gland. In return, FSH and LH regulate ovarian and testicular function. GnRH is a 10 amino acid peptide hormone that is highly conserved between mammalian species and is identical in males and females. The small size requires that the GnRH peptide be linked to a carrier protein to be immunogenic and utilized with an adjuvant to enhance the immune response. GnRH vaccines work on the principle that anti-GnRH antibodies bind to GnRH within the blood stream and prevent GnRH from linking to its receptor on pituitary gonadotroph cells. Lack of GnRH support results in decreased FSH and LH release and a subsequent decrease in ovarian or testicular function in mares and stallions, respectively. Theoretically, vaccinated mares will begin to exhibit normal estrous cycles when anti-GnRH antibody titers wane over time.

The zona pellucida is a glycoprotein investment surrounding the oocyte of mammals. Spermatozoa bind to a specific glycoprotein within the zona called ZP3, the structure of which is highly conserved across many species. Sperm binding to ZP3 initiates the acrosome reaction which allows the bound spermatozoon to penetrate the zona and fertilize the oocyte. Immunization of horses and other species with a vaccine containing zona pellucida proteins of porcine origin stimulates production of anti-zona pellucida antibodies. Anti-zona pellucida antibodies bind to the zona pellucida of ovulated oocytes and competitively inhibit sperm from binding, thus preventing fertilization. PZP vaccination protocols to prevent fertilization and pregnancy in horses and a wide variety of wildlife species have historically consisted of primary and booster immunizations followed by annual booster immunizations. However, as with GnRH vaccines, the ultimate goal of a PZP vaccine is single dose administration which would prevent pregnancy for multiple years.

Equipment and Supplies

Vaccine, syringe, needle.

Technique

Vaccination of domesticated horses with the GnRH vaccine Equity® is no different than administration of any other vaccine. The challenge is vaccination of feral horses with either a GnRH or PZP vaccine. Options include round-ups to capture horses for manual injections or the use of darts for remote delivery.

Equine Reproductive Procedures, Second Edition. Edited by John Dascanio and Patrick McCue.

Interpretation

At least three GnRH vaccines have been used in horses, including Equity® (Zoetis; approved for horses in Australia), Improvac® (Zoetis; approved for pigs in Europe) and GonaCon™-Equine (USDA National Wildlife Research Center; used in wildlife species). GnRH vaccines have an advantage as a contraceptive agent in being potentially applied to both stallions and mares. Vaccinated stallions with high anti-GnRH titers exhibit reduced libido, altered spermatogenesis, and decreased sperm output, while vaccinated mares with high titers do not exhibit behavioral estrus and do not develop large follicles or ovulate. Challenges with GnRH vaccines include variable efficacy in inducing an immune response in individual mares, requirement for a booster immunizations, and the need for either manual injection or darting for vaccine delivery.

The most common PZP vaccines used in horses are ZonaStat-H®, PZP-22®, and SpayVac® (ImmunoVaccine Technologies, Inc.). The latter vaccine incorporates liposome technology in a single dose vaccine with reported long-term efficacy. Zona pellucida vaccines can only be used as a contraceptive in mares (and not stallions) and the immune response of vaccinated mares varies widely. Additional challenges with zona pellucida vaccines are inconsistent results amongst various field trials, prolongation of reproductive cyclicity and reproductive behavior in vaccinated mares, decreased band fidelity in vaccinated mares, and decreased harem stability. In addition, limited data suggest that long-term repeated PZP vaccination may result in ovulation failure in some mares.

Depending on the adjuvant used, localized swellings or abscess at the injection site have been noted with some vaccines.

Further Reading

Davis KA, Klohonatz KM, Mora DS, *et al.* 2018. Effects of immunization against bone morphogenetic protein-15 and growth differentiation factor-9 on ovarian function in mares. *Anim Reprod Sci* 192: 69–77.

Hall SE, Nixon B, Aitken RJ. 2017. Non-surgical sterilisation methods may offer a sustainable solution to feral horse (Equus caballus) overpopulation. *Reprod Fertil Develop* 29: 1655–66.

Nolan MB, Bertschinger HJ, Roth R, *et al.* 2018. Ovarian function following immunocontraceptive vaccination of mares using native porcine and recombinant zona pellucida vaccines formulated with a non-Freund's adjuvant and anti-GnRH vaccines. *Theriogenology* 120: 111–16.

Roelle JE, Germaine SS, Kane AJ, Cade BS. 2017. Efficacy of SpayVac® as a contraceptive in feral horses. *Wildlife Soc Bull* 41: 107–15.

Swegen A, Aitken RJ. 2016. Prospects for immunocontraception in feral horse population control: exploring novel targets for an equine fertility vaccine. *Reprod Fertil Develop* 28853–63.

61

Harvesting and Shipping Ovaries for Oocyte Recovery

Patrick M. McCue

Equine Reproduction Laboratory, Colorado State University, USA

Introduction

Oocytes can be recovered from ovaries harvested from anesthetized or euthanized mares. The unexpected and often tragic loss of a valuable mare can be emotionally devastating to an owner. The opportunity to salvage genetic material and potentially generate one or more pregnancies can provide significant solace in an otherwise difficult situation.

Equipment and Supplies

Paper towels, surgery pack, plastic bags or obstetrical sleeves, sterile saline (0.9%) or lactated Ringer's solution, clean scissors, shipping container (e.g., Equitainer®).

Technique

- Ovaries are harvested either under general anesthesia prior to euthanasia or immediately after euthanasia, either via a flank or ventral midline approach.
- The ovaries are immediately and repeatedly rinsed with warm (37°C, 99°F) sterile saline or lactated Ringer's solution until clean.
- Excess tissue is trimmed off and the ovaries are placed in a plastic bag with approximately 60 ml of sterile saline or lactated Ringer's solution. Double bagging is recommended.
- The bagged ovaries are placed in a shipping container, surrounded by small saline bags *without ice packs*. The goal is to maintain temperature between 12 and 22°C (54–72°F) during shipment. Typically, if three small saline bags are shipped with the ovaries, then one bag that has been cooled to 5°C (40°F) is placed with two room temperature bags (20–22°C, 68–78°F) to provide the appropriate shipping temperature (Figure 61.1). Higher temperatures may result in increased cell apoptosis.
- The container should be sent to a referral center by counter to counter airline service. An overnight shipping service should not be used unless the ovaries are harvested late in the day. The ovaries should be harvested, if possible, in the morning so they can arrive at a processing facility the same day in the afternoon. The quicker the ovaries arrive at the processing facility, the better the results.
- Hairs, with intact roots, should be collected from the mare and stored for parentage testing, depending on requirements for individual breed associations.

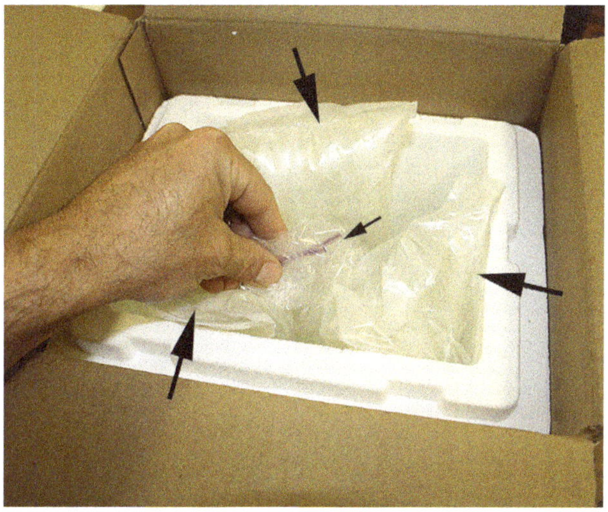

Figure 61.1 Ovaries (small arrow) in a plastic bag are placed into the center of three IV bags (large arrows). One IV bag was cooled to 5°C, while the other two are at room temperature. A Styrofoam lid is placed on the top of the box for shipment.

Equine Reproductive Procedures, Second Edition. Edited by John Dascanio and Patrick McCue.

- Once at the referral center, the ovaries are rinsed again with lactated Ringer's solution and the oocytes recovered by a combination of follicle aspiration and scraping.
- Oocytes are placed in maturation medium for 24 hours.
- Matured oocytes are utilized for either oocyte transfer or intracytoplasmic sperm injection.

Further Reading

Carnevale EM. 2004. Oocyte transfer and gamete intrafallopian transfer in the mare. *Anim Reprod Sci* 82: 617–24.

Love LB, Choi YH, Love CC, Varner DD, Hinrichs K. 2003. Effect of ovary storage and oocyte transport method on maturation rate of horse oocytes. *Theriogenology* 59: 765–74.

Preis KA, Carnevale EM, Coutinho da Silva MA, *et al*. 2004. In vitro maturation and transfer of equine oocytes after transport of ovaries at 12 or 22°C. *Theriogenology* 61: 1215–23.

Part II

Pregnant Mare

62

Embryo Collection

Patrick M. McCue

Equine Reproduction Laboratory, Colorado State University, USA

Introduction

Mares are typically flushed to recover embryos on day 7 or 8 post-ovulation. The collection procedure may be delayed by a half day for older mares and mares bred with frozen semen because of the possibility of a slight delay in embryonic development. Embryo collection attempts on day 9 after ovulation may result in the recovery of large embryos (i.e., >1–2 mm in diameter) that are easily damaged during handling and transfer.

Equipment and Supplies

Obstetrical sleeve, obstetrical lubricant, tail wrap, tail tie, examination gloves, bucket with liner, rolled cotton, mild detergent soap, catheter (80 cm, 36 Fr, 8 mm ID, 12 mm OD, 75 ml cuff), "Y" tubing or other tubing, embryo filter, embryo flush media, graduated cylinder(s), syringe (60 ml), stereomicroscope, search dish, 0.25 or 0.5 ml straw for general embryo handling, 1.0 ml syringe.

Flush Procedure

- Flush media options:
  - Commercially prepared "complete" flush media that contain a zwitterion-based buffer system, antibiotics, and purified albumin or polyvinyl alcohol (PVA) as a surfactant.
  - Lactated Ringer's solution or equivalent with or without the addition of a surfactant such as PVA, calf serum, or bovine serum albumen.
- Wrap the tail and tie it off to the side of the mare. Remove feces from the rectum (see Chapter 4).
- Wash the perineum with a mild detergent, rinsing well with clean water. Repeat the procedure until the perineum is clean. Dry the perineum with clean disposable paper towels (see Chapter 3).
- The standard method of embryo collection in the mare is a non-surgical, transcervical uterine lavage.
- All material should be sterilized prior to use.
- The spike on one end of the sterile "Y" tubing is connected into the bag of flush medium. The uterine catheter is subsequently attached to the "Y" tubing. The other arm of the "Y" tubing may be connected directly to a port on the embryo filter cap (closed system) or can be hand held within the embryo filter (open system).
  - The entire catheter–tubing system is primed or preloaded with flush medium to prevent air from entering the mare's uterus.
  - The catheter is then gently inserted through the cervix into the caudal uterine body and the cuff inflated with 60–75 ml of air (Figure 62.1).
- Approximately 1–2 liters of warmed flush medium is infused into the uterus by gravity flow (Figure 62.2). The amount of fluid used for each flush is dependent on the size of the uterus, parity of the mare, and preference of the clinician.
- The flush medium is allowed to flow back out of the catheter by gravity flow through the embryo filter. The outflow may be through an open system with the cap removed (Figure 62.3) or a closed air-free system with a cap on the filter (Figure 62.4).
- This process is repeated a total of three or four times using a total volume of 3–5 liters of flush medium.
- The uterus of the mare may be massaged per rectum during infusion and recovery of the media to ensure that fluid fills each uterine horn and to assist with recovery of the embryo.

Equine Reproductive Procedures, Second Edition. Edited by John Dascanio and Patrick McCue.

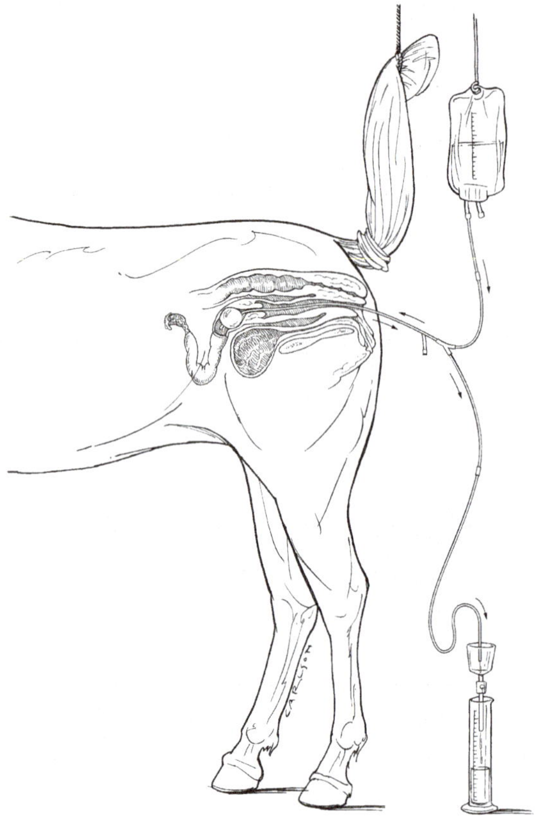

Figure 62.1 Non-surgical embryo collection procedure.

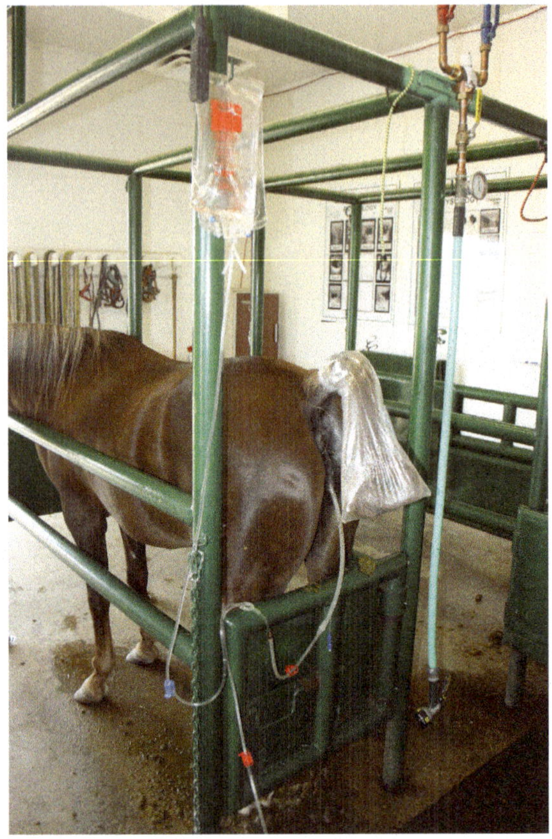

Figure 62.2 Embryo collection setup. The media bag is connected by "Y" tubing to a uterine lavage catheter.

- Oxytocin (20 IU IV) may be administered to stimulate uterine contractions and aid in fluid recovery.
- Examination of the uterus by transrectal ultrasonograpy may be indicated to document fluid retention and provide a visual assessment for manipulation of the uterus or redirection of the uterine catheter during recovery of fluid.
- Recovery of uterine lavage fluid may be monitored by collection of effluent into a graduated cylinder. One should recover >95% of the flush media infused into the uterus.
- At the conclusion of the flush procedure, the catheter may be temporarily left inside the mare while the fluid within the filter is examined for the presence of an embryo. If the embryo is not recovered on the initial attempt, a second flush procedure may be performed immediately.
- Once the lavage procedure is completed the cuff is deflated and the tubing gently removed from the mare's reproductive tract. All of the fluid within the catheter and tubing is allowed to flow through the embryo filter.

Embryo Search

- The contents of the filter are poured into a round, sterile, disposable, plastic search dish with a grid on the bottom to allow for a systematic search for the embryo. Alternatively, the filter may have a grid incorporated into it, allowing direct searching of the filter once the top is removed.
- The filter is then rinsed with 20–30 ml of flush medium.
- A gentle swirling motion may be used to move the embryo and cellular debris to the center of the search dish.
- The contents of the search dish are systematically examined using a stereomicroscope.

"Extra Flush" Procedure

- If an embryo is not recovered following the initial series of lavages, an additional 1–2 liters of media may be immediately infused into the uterus and 20 units of oxytocin administered intravenously. The media is allowed

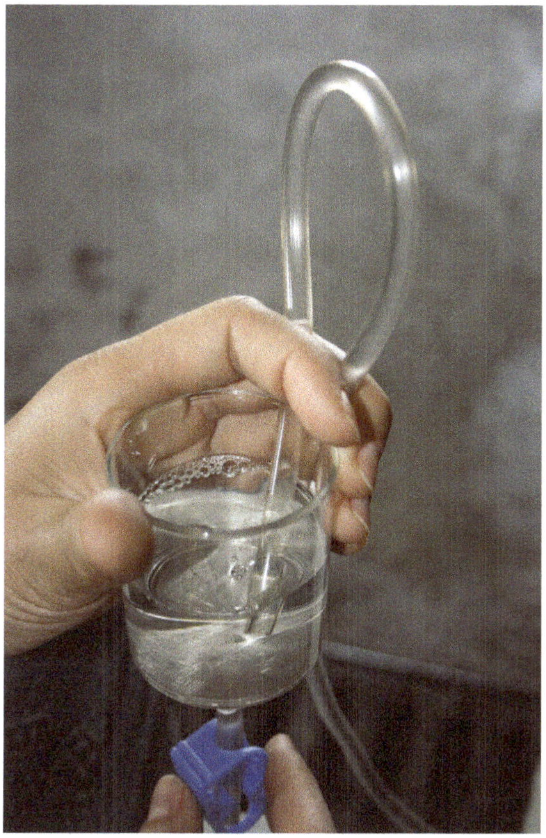

Figure 62.3 Flush media passing through an embryo filter (open system).

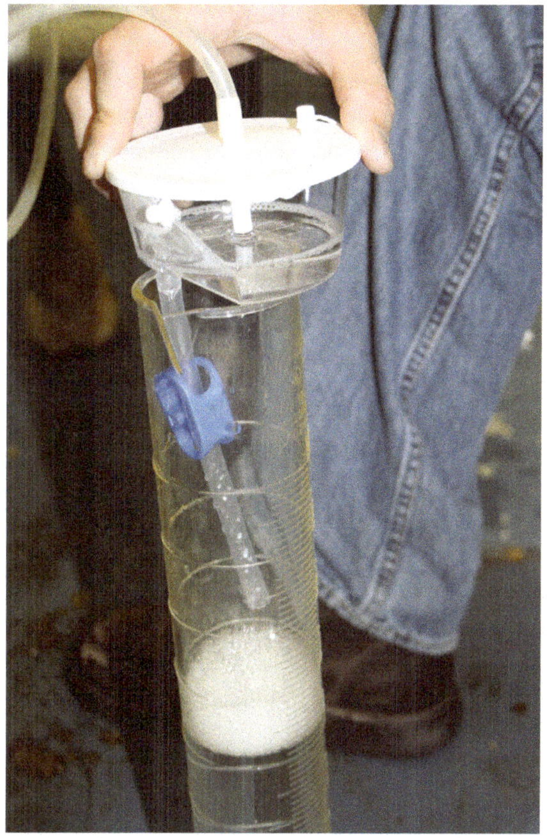

Figure 62.4 Flush media passing through an embryo filter (closed system).

to remain in the mare for approximately 3 minutes before being allowed to exit by gravity flow aided by uterine massage per rectum. The media is passed through an embryo filter, the content of which is subsequently examined under a microscope. This procedure will increase overall embryo recovery rate by 5–15%.

- Prostaglandins (e.g., cloprostenol sodium, 250 μg IM) should be administered after each embryo collection procedure. The goal is to facilitate evacuation of any fluid remaining in the uterus, to minimize the possibility of bacterial infection by lysing the corpus luteum and allowing the mare to return to estrus, and to eliminate the possibility that a pregnancy will continue in the donor mare if the embryo collection attempt was negative.

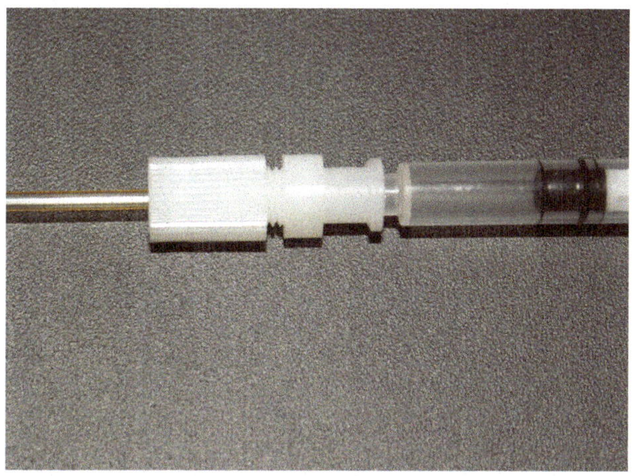

Figure 62.5 Straw (0.25 ml), connector and 1.0 ml syringe for handling small embryos.

Washing the Embryo

- Once the embryo has been identified in the search dish, it is removed using a 0.25 ml straw attached to a 1.0 ml syringe using a connector (Figure 62.5).
- The embryo is subsequently washed through 3–5 drops of embryo holding medium, changing straws after each transfer (Figure 62.6).

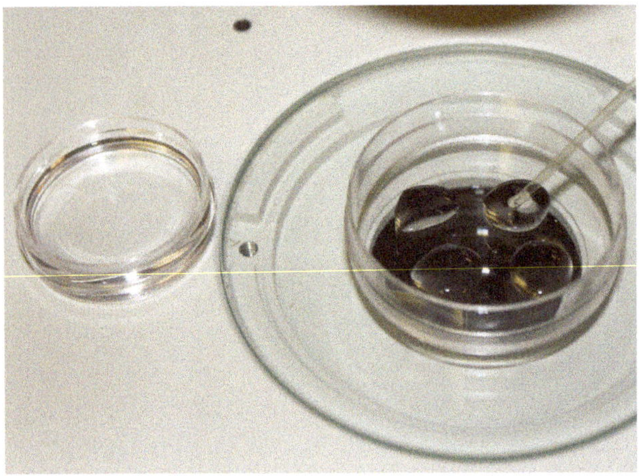

Figure 62.6 Petri dish (35 mm) with holding medium (left side). Washing an embryo through drops of holding medium (right side).

- The embryo is then placed into a small (i.e., 35 mm diameter) Petri dish containing holding medium to await transfer into a recipient mare.

Interpretation

It is normal to get some cellular debris in lavage fluid. However, if the flush media recovered from uterine lavage is cloudy or has excessive debris it may indicate that the mare has endometritis and the embryo recovery may be less successful. Embryos may still be present within fluid containing cellular debris, but it may be more difficult to locate the embryo.

Futher Reading

McCue PM, Ferris RA, Lindholm AR, DeLuca CA. 2010. Embryo recovery procedures and collection success: results of 492 embryo-flush attempts. *Proc Annu Conv Am Assoc Eq Pract* 56: 318–21.

Squires EL, Seidel GE. 1995. Collection and Transfer of Equine Embryos. Animal Reproduction and Biotechnology Laboratory Bulletin No. 11. Fort Collins, CO: Colorado State University.

Stout, TAE. 2006. Equine embryo transfer: review of developing potential. *Eq Vet J* 38: 467–78.

63

Embryo Evaluation

Patrick M. McCue

Equine Reproduction Laboratory, Colorado State University, USA

Introduction

An accurate evaluation of embryo size, grade, and developmental stage is important in a successful embryo transfer program. It is also critical that an embryo be differentiated from an unfertilized oocyte and non-embryonic structures.

Equipment and Supplies

Stereomicroscope with eye piece micrometer, Petri dish, embryo holding medium.

Developmental Stages

Morula stage embryos are 150–200 μm in diameter and have a thick zona pellucida and large distinct blastomeres that provide a scalloped or serrated appearance to the outer edge of the mass of cells (Figure 63.1). Further cleavage divisions and tight junctional complexes between blastomeres leads to the formation of a compact morula, with a perivitelline space visible between the embryo and zona pellucida.

Early blastocyst stage embryos are 150–250 μm in diameter or approximately the same overall size as a morula, have a slightly thinner zona pellucida, and are comprised of a larger number of smaller cells (Figure 63.2). Secretion of fluid produced by the blastomeres leads to the formation of the blastocoele cavity, a small fluid-filled pocket within the embryo, which is the hallmark of the blastocyst stage embryo.

Blastocyst stage embryos are 150–300 μm in diameter and develop following continued cellular division and fluid secretion, yielding a distinct trophoblast layer surrounding a blastocoele cavity (Figure 63.3). A cluster of cells that protrudes slightly into the blastocoele is the developing inner cell mass. An acellular capsule, unique to the horse, begins to form between the trophoblast layer and the thin zona pellucida 6–7 days after ovulation and disappears by day 23.

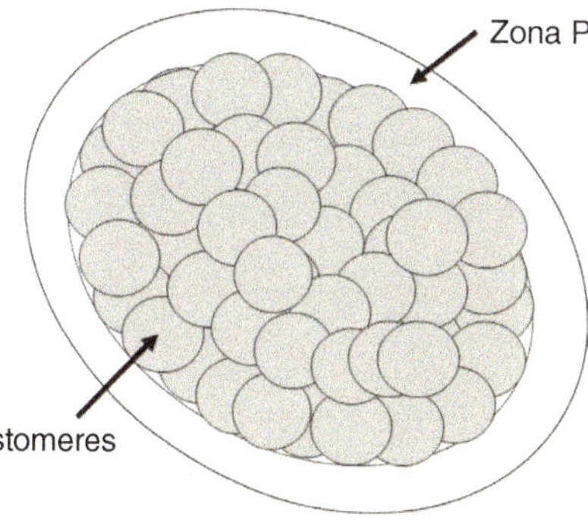

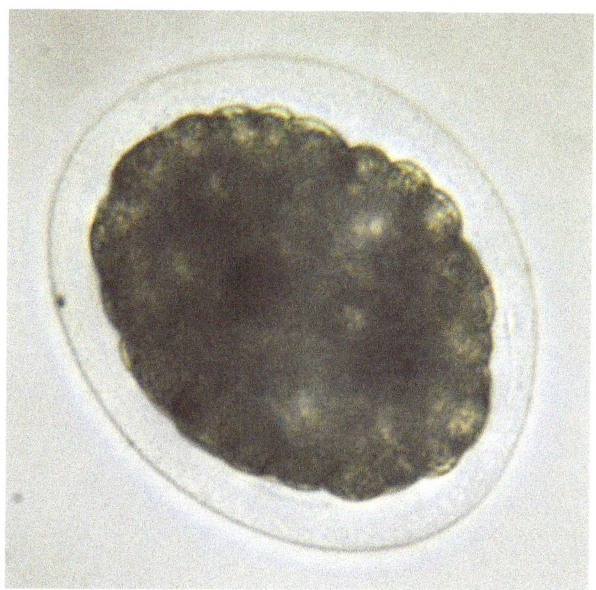

Figure 63.1 Morula stage embryo (grade 1). Note the thick zona pellucida and large blastomeres.

Equine Reproductive Procedures, Second Edition. Edited by John Dascanio and Patrick McCue.

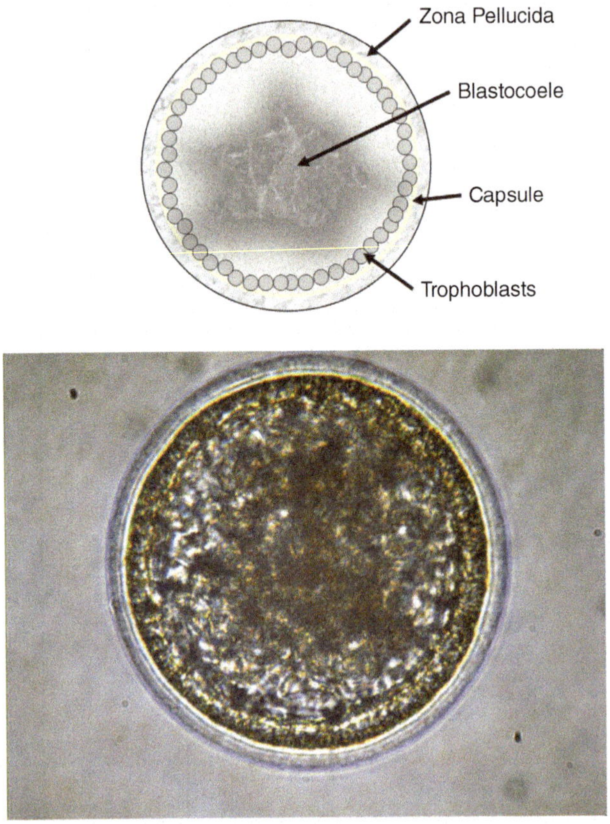

Figure 63.2 Early blastocyst stage embryo (grade 1). Note the thinner zona pellucida, capsule, and small blastocoele cavity.

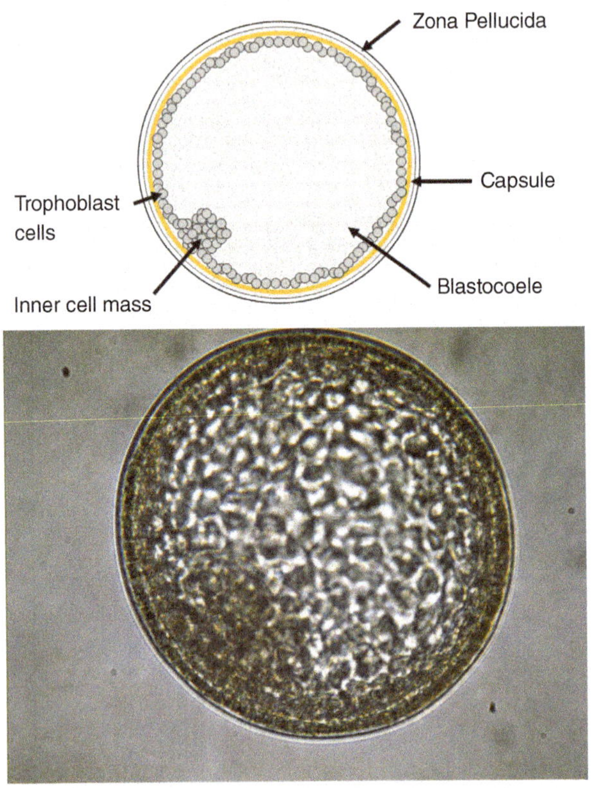

Figure 63.3 Blastocyst stage embryo (grade 1). Note the thin zona pellucida, blastocoele cavity, and distinct inner cell mass.

Expanded blastocyst stage embryos are 300 to >1,000 μm in diameter and result from the rapid expansion of the embryo beginning on day 7 post-ovulation (Figure 63.4). A large blastocoele cavity is surrounded by a thin layer of trophoblast cells which are small and uniform in appearance. The zona pellucida becomes progressively thinner as the embryo increases in diameter and is eventually shed.

Unfertilized oocytes are typically 125–150 μm in diameter and round or oval in shape, but are flat and do not roll when manipulated (Figure 63.5). The zona pellucida is thick and degeneration and fragmentation of the cytoplasm in this single cell structure may lead to a somewhat similar appearance as a morula stage embryo.

Embryo Grading

A four-point grading system may be used to evaluate equine embryos (Table 63.1). The vast majority of embryos collected from donor mares are good to excellent in quality

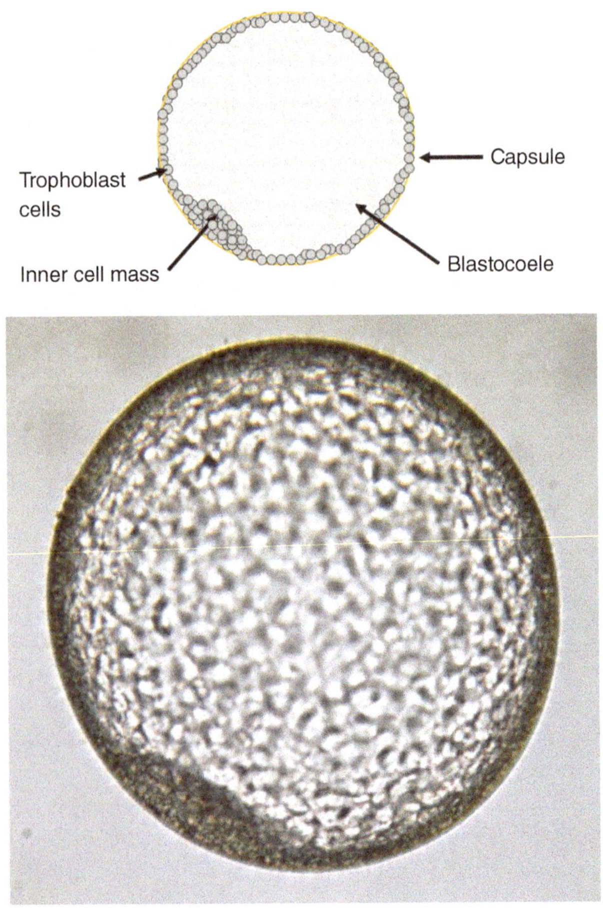

Figure 63.4 Expanded blastocyst stage embryo (grade 1). The zona pellucida has been shed and the capsule is tightly surrounding the embryo.

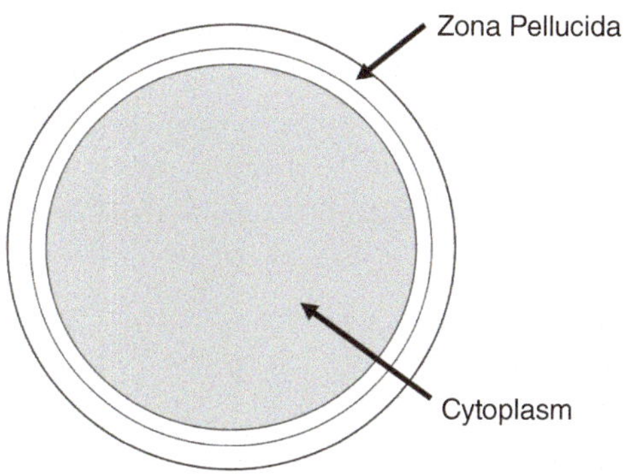

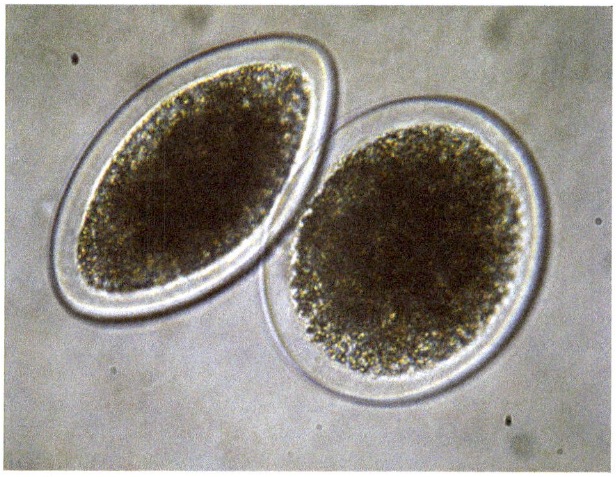

Figure 63.5 Unfertilized oocytes. Note the thick zona pellucida and lack of individual blastomeres. Two oocytes can be seen in the lower image.

Table 63.1 Embryo grade assignment based on a four-point system.

Grade	Comment	Description
1	Excellent	No significant abnormalities observed; symmetrical and spherical in shape; cells of uniform size, color, and texture; size and developmental stage appropriate for age post-ovulation
2	Good	Minor imperfections such as a few extruded blastomeres; slight irregularities in shape, size, color, or texture; limited separation between trophoblast layer and zona pellucida or capsule
3	Poor	Moderate level of imperfections such as a larger percentage of extruded or degenerated blastomeres; partial collapse of blastocoele; or moderate shrinkage of trophoblast from zona pellucida or capsule
4	Degenerate or dead	Severe problems easily identified, such as a high percentage of extruded blastomeres, complete collapse of blastocoele, rupture of zona pellucida, or complete degeneration and embryonic death

Adapted from the International Embryo Transfer Society (IETS) Manual.

(Figure 63.6). This is likely due to the selective transport of viable embryos through the oviduct. Poor quality embryos, dead embryos, and unfertilized oocytes are likely retained in the oviduct.

Determination of Embryo Size

Measurement of embryo size is used in conjunction with embryonic stage in evaluating development relative to age. Electronic calipers or a calibrated eye piece micrometer are the easiest ways to obtain an accurate measurement of embryo size (Figure 63.7).

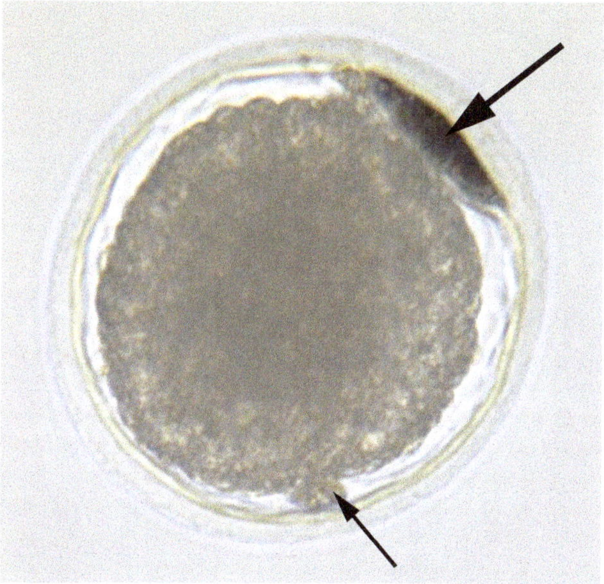

Figure 63.6 Grade 2 early blastocyst stage embryo. Note the extruded blastomeres (arrows).

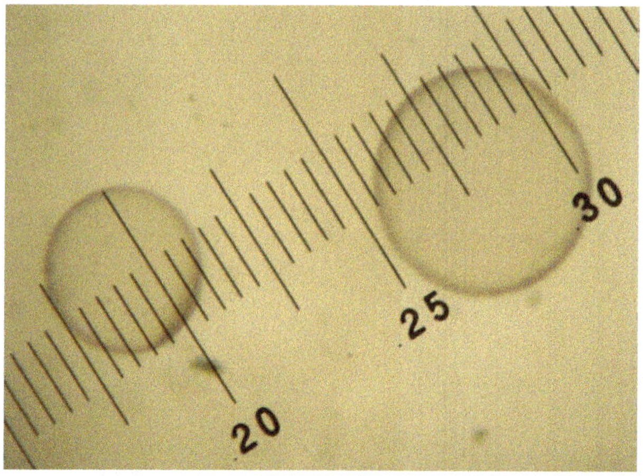

Figure 63.7 Measurement of embryo diameter using an eye piece micrometer.

Further Reading

McCue PM, DeLuca CA, Ferris RA, Wall JJ. 2009. How to evaluate equine embryos. *Proc Annu Conv Am Assoc Eq Pract* 55: 252–6.

McKinnon AO, Squires EL. 1988. Morphologic assessment of the equine embryo. *J Am Vet Med Assoc* 192: 401–6.

Squires EL, Seidel GE. 1995. Collection and Transfer of Equine Embryos. Animal Reproduction and Biotechnology Laboratory Bulletin No. 11. Fort Collins, CO: Colorado State University.

64

Embryo Biopsy

Patrick M. McCue

Equine Reproduction Laboratory, Colorado State University, USA

Introduction

Biopsy of an embryo after collection would allow for preimplantation genetic diagnosis (PGD). The potential goals of PGD include sex determination and the detection of genes associated with inheritable conditions, such as hereditary equine regional dermal asthenia (HERDA), hyperkalemic periodic paralysis (HYPP), cerebellar abiotrophy, and other genetic diseases. Biopsy samples can be collected using a microblade technique, but better results have been obtained by aspirating trophoblast cells after drilling through the zona pellucida. Biopsied embryos can be either transferred immediately into a recipient mare or can be cryopreserved and stored for future transfer.

Equipment and Supplies

Microscope, micromanipulator, microcentrifuge tubes, piezo drill, holding pipette, aspiration pipette, Petri dishes, embryo culture medium, Cassou gun.

Technique

- A morula, early blastocyst, or blastocyst stage embryo is collected 6.5–7 days after ovulation (see Chapter 62).
- The embryo is washed, evaluated, and maintained in holding medium in a small Petri dish.
- The Petri dish is placed on the working platform of a microscope equipped with a micromanipulator.
- A holding pipette is used to fix the embryo in position.
- A beveled glass aspiration pipette attached to a micromanipulator is used to drill a small hole in the zona pellucida and capsule (Figure 64.1).
- A piezo pulse may be used to facilitate penetration of the zona pellucida and capsule as well as to separate blastomeres or trophoblast cells for aspiration.
- A small number of blastomeres or trophoblast cells are removed by gentle aspiration and placed into a small container, such as a microcentrifuge tube, along with a minimal amount of holding medium.
- The cells are subsequently shipped to a genetics laboratory for analysis.
- The biopsied embryo can be loaded into a Cassou gun for immediate transfer into a synchronized recipient mare (see Chapter 67). The pregnancy can be allowed to proceed or terminated based on the genetic analysis.
- Alternatively, the biopsied embryo can be cryopreserved and stored in liquid nitrogen for later transfer into a recipient mare once the genetic analysis results are obtained (see Chapter 66).

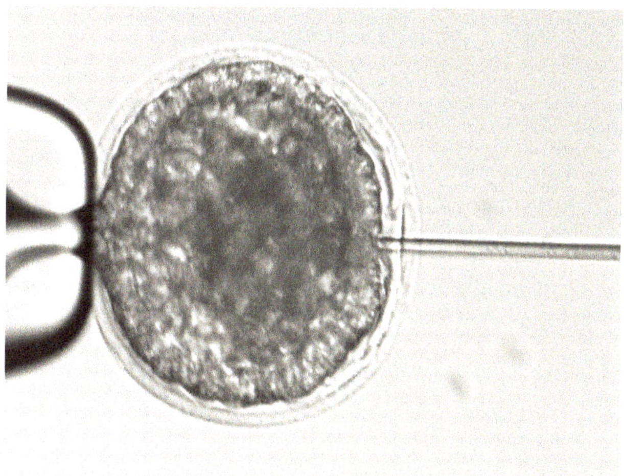

Figure 64.1 Aspiration biopsy of an equine blastocyst embryo.

Equine Reproductive Procedures, Second Edition. Edited by John Dascanio and Patrick McCue.

Further Reading

Hinrichs K. 2011. Biopsy and vitrification of equine expanded blastocysts. *Clin Theriogenol* 3: 314–17.

Peippo J, Huhtinen M, Kotilainen T. 1995. Sex diagnosis of equine preimplantation embryos using the polymerase chain reaction. *Theriogenology* 44: 619–27.

Seidel GE Jr, Cullingford EL, Stokes JE, Carnevale EM, McCue PM. 2010. Pregnancy rates following transfer of biopsied and/or vitrified equine embryos: evaluation of two biopsy techniques. *Anim Reprod Sci* 121S: 297–8.

65

Embryo Packaging for Cooled Transport

Patrick M. McCue

Equine Reproduction Laboratory, Colorado State University, USA

Introduction

Equine embryos are cooled for short-term storage to allow for shipment to another site for transfer into a recipient mare. A decrease in ambient temperature during short-term storage results in a slowing of embryo metabolism and embryos therefore do not advance in developmental stage or significantly increase in diameter during storage at 5°C (40°F).

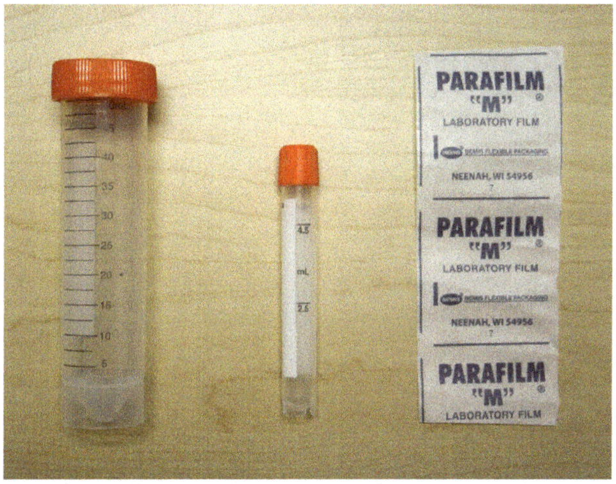

Figure 65.1 Left to right, 50 ml conical tube, 5 ml vial, and Parafilm® for cooled storage of equine embryos.

Equipment and Supplies

Commercial embryo holding medium, flush medium, 35 and 60 mm Petri dishes, 5 ml sterile plastic tube with screw or snap cap, 50 ml sterile centrifuge tube with screw cap, disposable pipettes, Parafilm® sealing film, passive cooling device (e.g., Equitainer®), embryo transfer device (straws and tuberculin syringe).

Technique for Packaging Embryos for Cooled Transport

The embryo should be washed through 3–5 drops of warmed holding medium after collection. The goal is to remove as much cellular debris and bacteria from the embryo as possible.

Place additional embryo holding medium on to a warming plate or in an incubator and allow time to warm to 37°C (99°F).

Fill the 5 ml plastic tube (Figure 65.1) with approximately 4.5 ml of warmed holding medium.

Carefully transfer the embryo into the plastic tube.

Rinse out the transfer straw and observe the rinse medium under a microscope to ensure that the embryo was properly transferred.

Slowly add more medium, drop by drop, into the 5 ml tube until it is full without overflowing the tube. This may be done with a disposable transfer pipette to carefully add the fluid. Fix the cap securely in place. Seal the tube with Parafilm® sealing film (Figure 65.2) by pulling the film so that it stretches as you wrap it around the screw top. The Parafilm® may be cut to an appropriate size for placement.

Place the 5 ml tube containing the embryo into the 50 ml centrifuge tube (Figure 65.3).

Fill the 50 ml centrifuge tube with flush medium.

Attach the cap of the 50 ml centrifuge tube securely in place and seal with Parafilm® (Figure 65.4).

Load the 50 ml tube containing the embryo into the passive cooling device (Figure 65.5). This is typically a semen shipment container that has frozen coolant cans/gel packs/gel bricks and will cool the embryo to 5°C after packaging.

Equine Reproductive Procedures, Second Edition. Edited by John Dascanio and Patrick McCue.

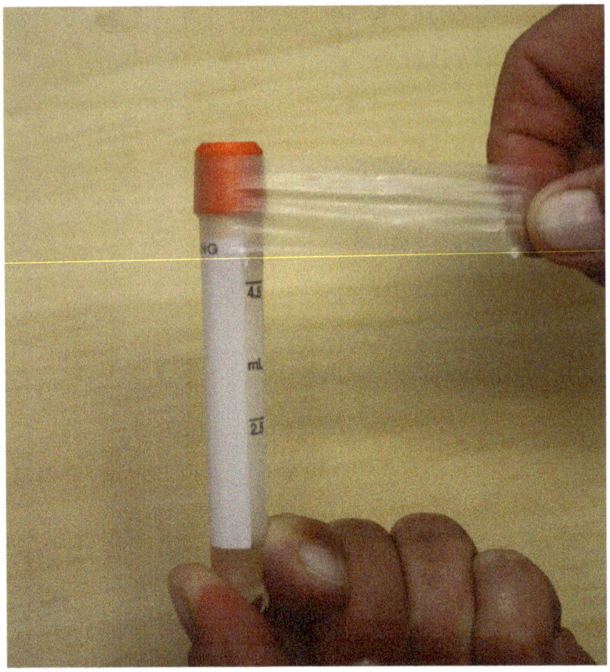

Figure 65.2 Sealing the 5 ml vial with Parafilm®. Pull the Parafilm® so that it stretches as it is applied around the screw top.

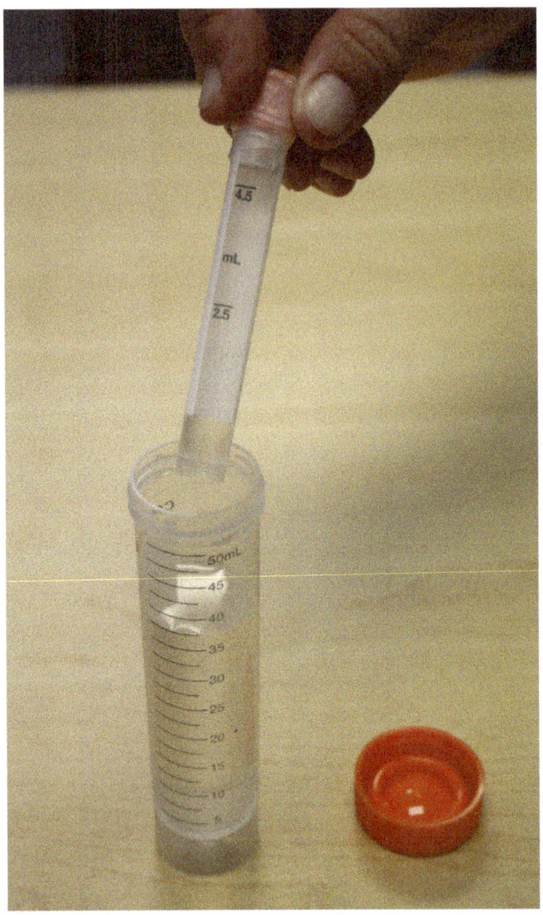

Figure 65.3 Placing the small 5 ml vial containing the embryo inside the larger 50 ml conical tube.

- Insert the appropriate documentation, including a description of the embryo (i.e., developmental stage, grade, and size), the donor mare, and flush date.
- Ship the container to the embryo transfer referral center by counter to counter airline delivery (preferred) or overnight courier service.

Technique for Receiving and Handling a Shipped Embryo

- Open the container in a clean laboratory space and review the documentation.
- Have embryo holding medium available to wash the embryo and rinse the plastic tube in the event that the embryo does not exit the small holding tube when the fluid is poured out.
- Open the centrifuge tube and remove the 5 ml tube containing the embryo.
- Gently invert the 5 ml tube several times to re-suspend the embryo as it has most likely settled onto the bottom of the tube.
- Remove the cap from the 5 ml tube, place the cap with the open end up on the counter top, and add several drops of holding medium into the cap in case the embryo is stuck to the cap.

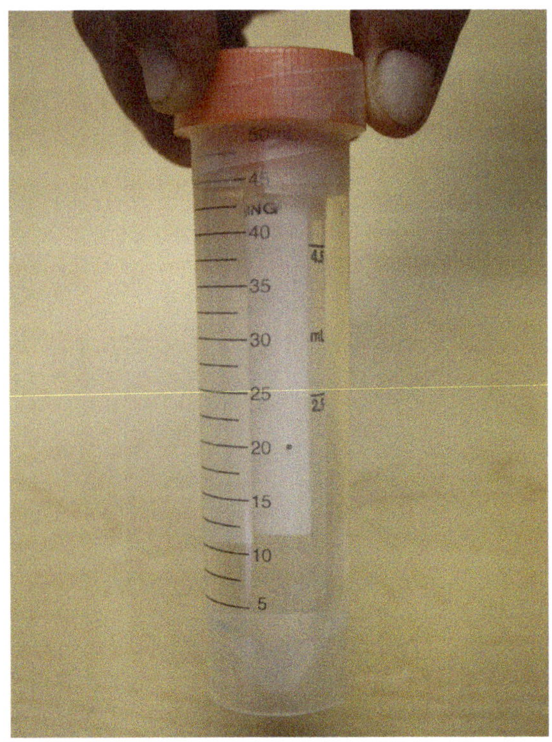

Figure 65.4 The 50 ml conical tube sealed with Parafilm® with a sealed 5 ml tube inside.

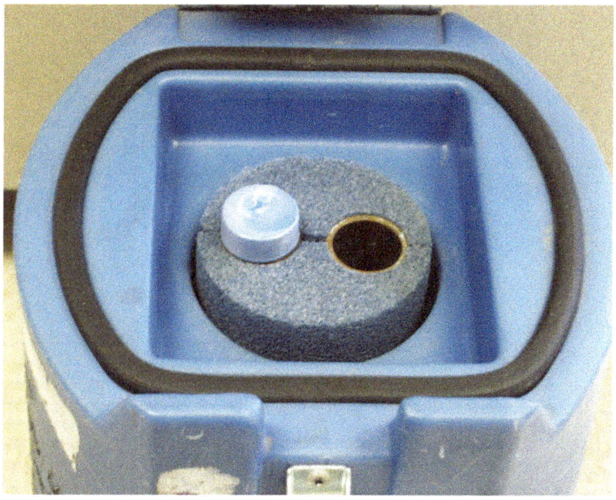

Figure 65.5 Loading the 50 ml conical tube into a passive cooling system for transport.

Pour the contents of the 5 ml tube into a sterile 60 mm Petri dish.

- Add several drops of holding medium into the empty 5 ml tube and set aside in case the embryo is still in the tube.
- Search the Petri dish for the embryo.
- If the embryo is not immediately visible, rinse the cap and the 5 ml tube several times with holding medium into the Petri dish. Embryos occasionally will stick to either the plastic tube or cap.
- Wash the embryo through a minimum of 3–4 aliquots of holding medium prior to transfer. Ideally, the medium used to wash the embryo should be the same as the medium used for cooled storage.
- The embryo is then loaded into a transfer device for transcervical deposition into a recipient mare.

Additional Comments

Transport of embryos from the site of collection to a referral center for transfer into a recipient mare is advantageous in that: (i) donor mares can be maintained and managed at home and transport is only necessary if an embryo is recovered; (ii) the cost of transport of an embryo is significantly less than transport of a mare; (iii) housing recipient mares at specialized centers eliminates the need to maintain a recipient herd at every breeding farm, and recipients are often best managed by experienced personnel; (iv) synchronization of a recipient with the donor is performed by the transfer center; (v) embryo transfer services are more widely available to mare owners; and (vi) pregnancy rates are usually better at dedicated embryo transfer facilities with more experienced personnel.

Cooled transport of equine embryos is now a routine procedure in the equine industry. Progress in the development of commercial complete holding media and passive cooling systems have simplified the process. Pregnancy rates following transfer of cooled transported embryos are similar to rates following the transfer of fresh embryos.

Further Reading

Carnevale EM, Squires EL, McKinnon AO. 1987. Comparison of Ham's F-10 with CO_2 or Hepes buffer for storage of equine embryos at 5°C for 24 h. *J Anim Sci* 65: 1775–81.

Clark KE, Squires EL, McKinnon AO, Seidel GE, Jr. 1987. Viability of stored equine embryos. *J Anim Sci* 65: 534–42.

McCue PM, DeLuca CA, Wall JJ. 2011. Cooled-transported embryo technology. In: McKinnon AO, Squires EL, Vaala WE, Varner DD (eds). Equine Reproduction, 2nd edn. Ames, IA: Wiley Blackwell, pp. 2880–6.

66

Embryo Cryopreservation

Patrick M. McCue

Equine Reproduction Laboratory, Colorado State University, USA

Introduction

Equine embryos are cryopreserved for long-term storage, import, or export, or to allow for collection of embryos late in the breeding season and transfer early the following breeding season for early foal production. Currently, the best pregnancy rates have been achieved following cryopreservation of embryos <300 μm in diameter. As a consequence, embryo recovery procedures are usually performed 6.5–7 days after ovulation in order to collect small embryos for cryopreservation.

The most common cryopreservation technique for equine embryos is vitrification. Vitrification is an ultrarapid freezing process for cryopreservation that does not require specialized equipment. The embryo is exposed to high concentrations of permeating cryoprotectants that prevent ice crystal formation and results in a "glass-like formation" within the embryo. Another advantage of vitrification is that the embryo can be rapidly warmed (thawed) within the straw and the straw loaded into a Cassou gun for direct transfer into a recipient mare.

Equipment and Supplies

Stereomicroscope, embryo holding medium, straws (0.25 ml for general embryo handling, 0.25 ml for vitrification, 0.5 ml for labeling), straw adaptor to connect a 0.25 ml straw to a 0.5 ml straw, syringes (1.0 ml), syringe straw connector to connect a 0.25 ml straw to a 1.0 ml syringe, embryo vitrification kit, Petri dishes (35 and 100 mm diameter), timers ×2, cane (for vitrification and storage), goblet (for vitrification and storage), tabs for labeling canes, Doyen forceps (straight, 25 cm (10 inches)), thermos (2 liters) or similar container for liquid nitrogen, marking pen(s), liquid nitrogen tank, mechanical pipetter (1.0–10 μl and 20–200 μl), pipette tips (0.1–10 μl and 0.5–200 μl), microcentrifuge tubes (1.5 ml) or nalgene cryogenic vials (1.2 ml each).

Initial Preparation Steps

Identify and wash the embryo through multiple aliquots of commercial holding medium.

Place the embryo in a small (35 mm diameter) Petri dish containing commercial holding medium. The embryo should be vitrified as soon as possible after collection.

Vitrification Technique

- Prepare a Petri dish (100 mm diameter) with five labeled areas for the vitrification solutions (Figure 66.1). One area for solution 1 (VS1), one area for solution 2 (VS2), one area for solution 3 (VS3), and two areas for galactose diluent (Gal). The bottom of the dish may be written on with a permanent marker to keep track of where each solution is placed.
- Set a countdown timer to 5 minutes, but do not start it yet.
- Move 200 μl of VS1 to the designated spot on the Petri dish.
- Transfer the embryo from the holding medium using a 10–20 μl mechanical pipetter with the smallest volume of holding medium possible (i.e., set the pipetter to 1 μl).
- Place a new tip on the pipetters after each use.
- Start the 5-minute countdown timer immediately. The embryo can only remain in solution 1 for 5 minutes.
- Label a 0.5 ml straw with information such as donor mare's name, embryo collection date, embryo size, grade, and morphology, stallion's name, and owner's name. This straw will be attached to the 0.25 ml straw with a plastic adapter and used as a label.
- With about 1 minute remaining on the timer, transfer 200 μl of VS2 into the appropriately labeled area of the Petri dish.

Equine Reproductive Procedures, Second Edition. Edited by John Dascanio and Patrick McCue.

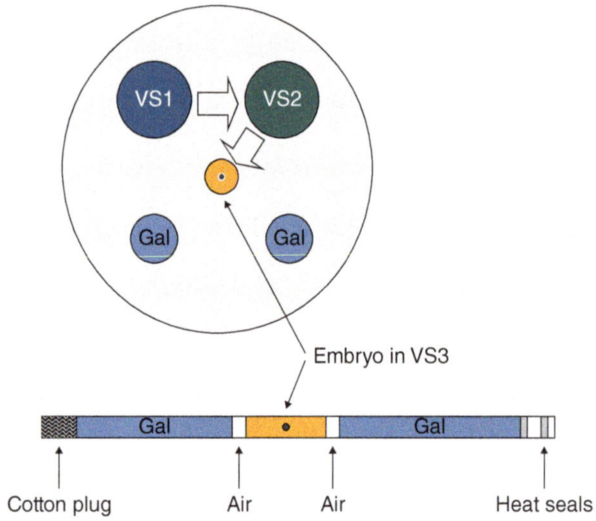

Figure 66.1 Petri dish prepared for vitrification of an embryo. VS1, solution 1; VS2, solution 2; center drop is VS3, solution 3; Gal, galactose diluent. From Carnevale (2006).

- After the 5-minute countdown timer ends, move the embryo from VS1 to VS2 with a minimum volume of solution (1 µl) using a 10–20 µl mechanical pipetter.
- Start the 5-minute countdown timer immediately again. The embryo can only remain in VS2 for 5 minutes.
- A 2 liter insulated fluid container with the top removed is filled with liquid nitrogen (Figure 66.2). A cane and goblet (10 mm diameter) is suspended vertically in the liquid nitrogen using forceps. The top of the goblet should be held just above the liquid level so that only liquid nitrogen vapor is within the goblet lumen. The straw will be placed into this goblet after filling and sealing.
- Transfer 90 µl of the diluent solution containing galactose into each of the two designated spots on the Petri dish and transfer 30 µl of VS3 into the designated spot.
- Draw up the entire first diluent solution drop (90 µl) into a 0.25 ml straw and then add an air gap (5–10 µl). Set the straw to the side.
- Set a second timer for 1 minute but do not start it yet. This will be used for VS3.
- After 5 minutes in VS2, move the embryo to VS3. The exposure time to VS3 is *extremely important*. Prolonged exposure to VS3 can be toxic to the embryo.
- Start the timer immediately (1-minute countdown). The next steps must be done within the 1-minute countdown (pull up the remaining solutions and attach the labeling straw).
- Using the straw that is already filled with the first diluent and air gap, immediately draw up the entire VS3 drop (30 µl) containing the embryo, then add a second air gap (5–10 µl), and finally draw up the remaining (second) diluent solution drop (90 µl) until the initial fluid contacts the straw's cotton sealing plug, thus sealing that end of the straw.
- Plug the open end of the 0.25 ml straw with a straw adaptor and attach the other end of the adaptor to the previously labeled 0.5 ml straw.
- Once the 1-minute countdown timer ends, place the 0.25 ml straw containing the embryo into the goblet attached to the cane that is suspended in liquid nitrogen vapor (Figure 66.3).
- Set the timer for 1 minute and start immediately.
- Plunge the entire cane into the liquid nitrogen at the end of the 1-minute period, immersing the goblet and straw containing the embryo (Figure 66.4).
- Transfer the cane into a liquid nitrogen tank for long-term storage and record the location on the semen tank inventory sheet.

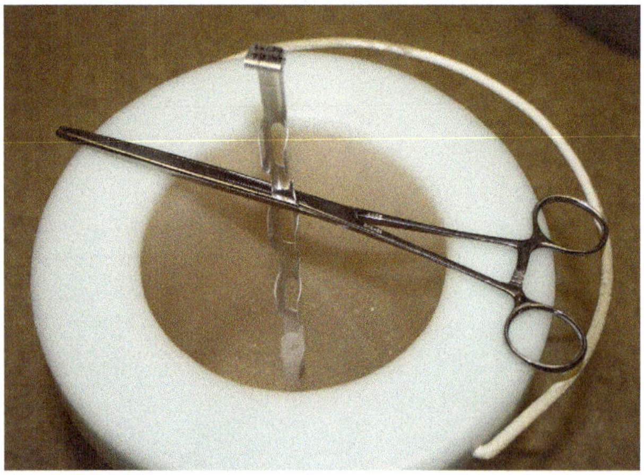

Figure 66.2 Thermos with a cane holding a goblet with the top suspended above liquid nitrogen.

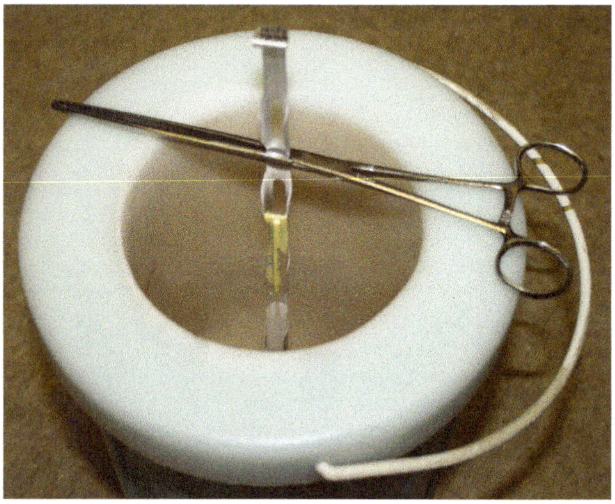

Figure 66.3 Straw placed into a goblet that is suspended above liquid nitrogen.

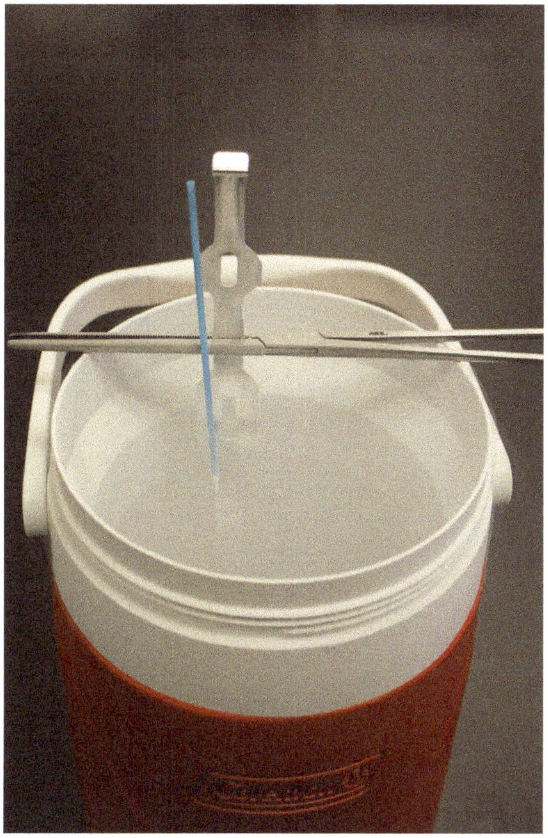

Figure 66.4 Embryo plunged into liquid nitrogen.

Warming (Thawing) and Transfer Technique

Establish a room temperature water bath (20–22°C, 68–72°F).

- The straw containing the correct embryo is identified and removed from long-term storage in the liquid nitrogen tank.
- The straw is held in room temperature air for 10 seconds.
- Next, the straw is placed in the room temperature (20–22°C, 68–72°F) water bath for an additional 10 seconds.
- The straw is removed from the water bath, wiped dry with a paper towel or Kimwipe™ and then "flicked" like a thermometer 5–7 times to mix the galactose dilution solution with the vitrification medium (VS3) containing the embryo.
- The straw is then placed in a horizontal position for 6–8 minutes. The embryo can be visualized in the straw (and potentially graded) through a microscope.
- The 0.5 ml straw (containing the label information) and plug are removed.
- The straw is loaded into a sterile sheath and a direct transfer to the recipient is performed using a Cassou gun.

Additional Comments

A technique has been described in which the blastocoele cavity of large equine embryos (i.e., ≥500 μm) was collapsed prior to cryopreservation. Pregnancy rates after transfer were reported to be good. This technique may allow for the successful cryopreservation of large expanded blastocyst stage equine embryos.

Reference

Carnevale EM. 2006. Vitrification of equine embryos. *Vet Clin North Am Eq* 22: 831–41.

Further Reading

Bruyas J-F. 2011. Freezing of embryos. In: McKinnon AO, Squires EL, Vaala WE, Varner DD (eds). Equine Reproduction, 2nd edn. Ames, IA: Wiley Blackwell, pp. 2887–920.

Carnevale EM, Eldridge-Panuska WD, di Brienza, VC. 2004. How to collect and vitrify equine embryos for direct transfer. *Proc Annu Conv Am Assoc Eq Pract* 50: 402–5.

Choi YH, Velez IC, Riera FL, *et al.* 2011. Successful cryopreservation of expanded equine blastocysts. *Theriogenology* 76: 143–52.

67

Non-Surgical Embryo Transfer

Patrick M. McCue

Equine Reproduction Laboratory, Colorado State University, USA

Introduction

Equine embryos can be transferred into a recipient mare using a non-surgical, transcervical procedure. Transfer rates are best if the recipient mare is synchronized with the donor and ovulates between 1 day before (+1) to 3 days after (–3) the donor.

If a cycling synchronized recipient is not available, a non-cycling hormone-treated mare may be utilized. Anestrus mares may be administered 5–10 mg of estradiol 17β once daily in the muscle for 2 days beginning the day the donor mare ovulates. Subsequently, the mare is administered 200 mg of short-acting progesterone in the muscle (or 0.044 mg/kg altrenogest orally) once daily for 5 or 6 days until the donor mare is flushed. If an embryo is collected and transferred, the recipient mare is maintained on progesterone or altrenogest until the pregnancy examination at 14–16 days of embryo age. Pregnant, non-cycling, hormone-treated recipient mares should be maintained on progesterone/progestin support until day 120 of gestation.

Equipment and Supplies

Option 1 (small embryos)
Cassou gun (0.25 ml, 53 cm (21 inches)), disposable sterile sheath, 0.25 ml straw.

Option 2 (large embryos)
Insemination pipette, syringe (1.0 ml), sterile chemise.

All transfers
Tail wrap, tail rope, non-irritant soap, roll cotton, stainless steel bucket, plastic bag/bucket liner, paper towels, examination gloves, sterile obstetrical sleeve, sterile obstetrical lube, equine embryo holding medium.

Transfer Technique

Preparation of the Recipient Mare

- Recipient mares are often sedated 5–10 minutes prior to the transfer procedure with either acepromazine maleate (0.02–0.04 mg/kg IV), xylazine hydrochloride (0.3–0.4 mg/kg IV) or detomidine hydrochloride (0.01–0.015 mg/kg IV).
- It is common practice to administer a single dose of a non-steroidal anti-inflammatory drug such as flunixin meglumine (1.0 mg/kg IV) prior to transfer.
- Other medications sometimes administered include corticosteroids, antibiotics, and tocolytic agents.

Transfer Procedure

- The tail of the recipient is wrapped and held away from the perineal area (see Chapter 4).
- Wearing examination gloves, the perineum is washed with a non-residual soap, rinsed with fresh water, and dried with paper towels (see Chapter 3).
- Embryos less than 1,000 μm in diameter may be transferred using a 0.25 ml straw, disposable sterile sheath, and stainless steel Cassou gun. The embryo is placed in the center of the straw within alternating columns of medium and air (Figure 67.1). The straw is loaded into the disposable sheath, which is then attached to the Cassou gun.
- Embryos greater than 1,000 μm in diameter are commonly transferred using a standard artificial insemination pipette, which is attached to a 1.0 or 3.0 ml syringe. The embryo is drawn up into the pipette in a small volume of medium between columns of medium and air. An outer sterile chemise should be used to protect the transfer gun or pipette from contamination with bacteria from the vulva, vestibule, or vagina. The transfer device should

Equine Reproductive Procedures, Second Edition. Edited by John Dascanio and Patrick McCue.

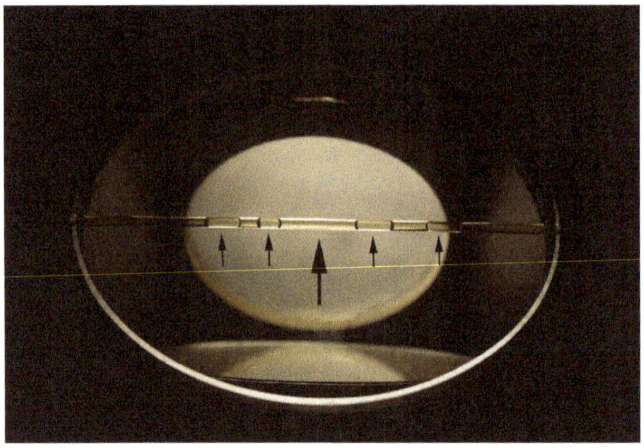

Figure 67.1 Embryo in a column of holding medium (large arrow) inside a 0.25 ml straw with two air gaps (small arrows) on either side of the column of fluid containing the embryo.

penetrate through the protective chemise within the external cervical os.

- Alternatively, a large embryo (i.e., >1,000 μm) may be transferred using a 0.5 ml straw and either a 0.5 ml sterile sheath and Cassou gun system or a 0.5 ml disposable embryo transfer gun.
- It is important to minimize manipulation of the cervix during the transfer procedure. The transfer instrument is gently maneuvered from the outside to place the tip of the instrument within the cervical lumen, and with a gentle, steady forward motion to facilitate passage of the instrument through the closed cervix into the uterine body. The embryo may be deposited into the uterine body or guided into a uterine horn via manipulation per rectum. The embryo should be gently deposited within the center of the uterine lumen as the transfer instrument is slowly withdrawn to lay the embryo in the space previously occupied by the transfer instrument. Consistent success is aided by attention to detail and a delicate transfer technique.

Examination of the Transfer Instrument After Transfer

Embryos are occasionally caught within the side ejecting stainless steel tip of the disposable sheath. Consequently, it is recommended that the tip of the sheath be rinsed after transfer and the rinse fluid examined under a dissecting microscope. Failure to examine the sheath after transfer may result in the inadvertent loss of an embryo.

Management of the Recipient Mare After Transfer

- Minimizing stress in the recipient mare after transfer is important to optimize pregnancy rates. Consequently, it may be beneficial to keep the recipient mare in her original herd after transfer as opposed to moving her immediately to a different herd of post-transfer mares.
- It is common practice, but possibly of limited benefit to a majority of recipient mares, to administer progesterone or progestins following embryo transfer. If progesterone supplementation is provided, recipient mares may receive either altrenogest (0.044 mg/kg PO, once daily), progesterone-in-oil (200 mg IM, once daily), or a long-acting progesterone preparation (1,500 mg IM, once every 7 days).
- Progesterone supplementation may be discontinued at any time provided that endogenous levels are measured and determined to be sufficient to maintain pregnancy (i.e., >4.0 ng/ml). Progesterone therapy in a recipient mare may be discontinued between 45 and 70 days of pregnancy if an ultrasound examination confirms the presence of secondary corpora lutea. Alternatively, progesterone or progestin therapy may be discontinued at approximately 100–120 days of gestation without testing to determine concentrations of endogenous progesterone. The placenta produces sufficient progesterone and other progestins by day 90 to maintain the pregnancy.

Additional Comments

Transfer of an equine embryo is both a clinical technique and an art. Attention to detail and a gentle consistent approach are important for success. Pregnancy rates (day 14) following non-surgical transfer in mares range from <70% to >90%. Initial pregnancy examination should be performed 4–7 days post-transfer.

An alternative transfer technique has been described in which a set of specialized forceps are used to grasp the external cervical os and retract it caudally. This was reported as allowing visualization of the cervical lumen and easier passage of the transfer pipette through the cervix for deposition of the embryo into the uterus.

Further Reading

Hartman DL. 2011. Embryo transfer. In: McKinnon AO, Squires EL, Vaala WE, Varner DD (eds). Equine Reproduction, 2nd edn. Ames, IA: Wiley Blackwell, pp. 2871–9.

Jasko DJ. 2002. Comparison of pregnancy rates following nonsurgical transfer of day 8 equine embryos using various transfer devices. *Theriogenology* 58: 713–15.

Wilsher S, Allen WR. 2004. An improved method for nonsurgical embryo transfer in the mare. *Eq Vet Educ* 16: 39–44.

68

Autogenous Transfer of ICSI-Derived Embryos

Jennifer N. Hatzel

Equine Reproduction Laboratory, Colorado State University, USA

Introduction

Intracytoplasmic sperm injection (ICSI) has provided a repeatable and effective method for creating *in vitro* equine embryos at multiple centers across the world. Although ICSI-derived embryos have gained in popularity over the past decade, the cost associated with production of these embryos is significant. Additionally, recipient mare lease and care throughout gestation is a substantial economic investment. Many of the oocyte donors presented to an ICSI program for stallion-related problems are capable of getting pregnant and carrying a foal to term themselves (Figure 68.1). With appropriate timing and management, a young reproductively sound mare can receive her own *in vitro* produced embryo, become pregnant, and carry that foal to term. Not only is this more financially appealing, it is also important for the overall reproductive health of that mare to carry a foal and experience successful parturition.

Equipment and Supplies

Halter and lead rope, nose twitch, non-steroidal anti-inflammatory drugs (flunixin meglumine), sedation (xylazine, acepromazine, detomidine), altrenogest, set of sturdy palpation stocks, tail wrap, exam gloves, betadine scrub, 10 × 10 cm (4 × 4 inch) gauze squares, palpation sleeves, non-sterile obstetrical lube, ultrasound unit with transrectal probe, sterile obstetrical sleeve, sterile obstetrical lubricant, embryo holding medium, small polystyrene Petri dish, dissecting microscope, warming plate, 0.25 ml sterile semen straw, urethral catheter adapter for a 1 ml tuberculin syringe, sterile embryo transfer pipette with chemise, embryo transfer Cassou gun.

Technique

- Managing a mare's reproductive cycle with the goal of receiving her own *in vitro* produced embryo during the same cycle is a hybrid of managing her for both transvaginal oocyte pickup (OPU) and as a recipient mare.
- The mare's reproductive cycle is followed via transrectal ultrasonography and the large pre-ovulatory follicle is aspirated as previously described (see Chapter 50).
- It is important to remember that the mare's endometrial tissue must be primed through the exposure to estrogen produced from a dominant follicle.
- If the mare does not have good uterine edema present for 2–3 days, she will not be a good candidate to receive an embryo back on the same cycle.
- If the ICSI process is successful and an early embryonic development has commenced, as evident upon the cleavage check, the next ultrasound evaluation of the donor/recipient mare should occur 5 days following the transvaginal OPU procedure. This is considered 4 days after ovulation, as she would have naturally ovulated the day after oocyte collection, or 36–40 hours following ovulation induction drug administration.
- This evaluation is intended to examine the quality of the developing corpus luteum, evaluate uterine and cervical tone, and ensure that there is no intrauterine fluid present.
- If the quality of the corpus luteum is poor and subsequently uterine and cervical tone are also poor, administration of a short-acting progesterone (200 mg IM, every 24 hours) or altrenogest (0.044 mg/kg PO, every 24 hours) is recommended in preparation for the embryo transfer.
- Another ultrasound evaluation will occur 6 days following the OPU procedure (5 days from ovulation) to evaluate the same parameters and effectiveness of treatment if implemented.
- Most *in vitro* produced embryos from a pre-ovulatory follicle are ready to be transferred 6 or 7 days following ICSI, which will be equivalent to day 6 or 7 post-ovulation in the donor/recipient mare.

Equine Reproductive Procedures, Second Edition. Edited by John Dascanio and Patrick McCue.

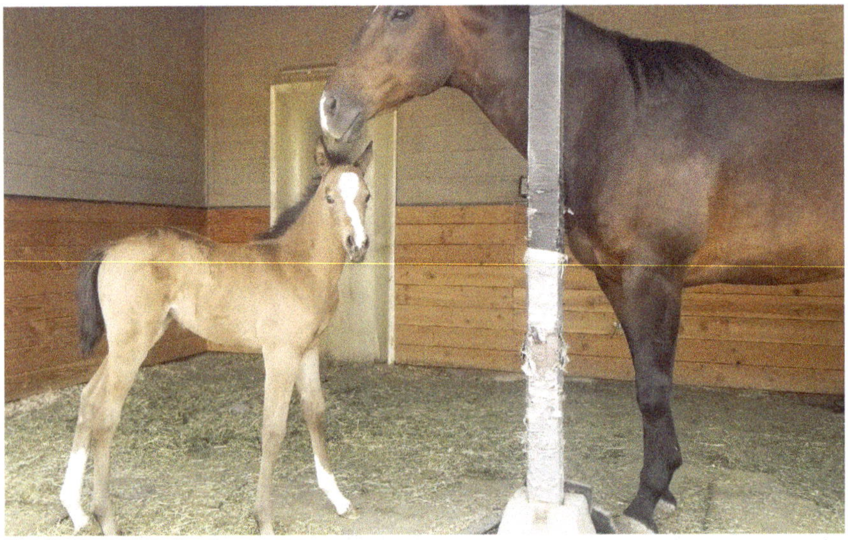

Figure 68.1 A filly successfully born from an *in vitro* produced embryo transferred back into her dam, in this case an older maiden mare.

- Upon confirmation of a good quality blastocyst, the donor/recipient mare is brought into the stocks and prepared for embryo transfer.
- The mare's tail is bagged/wrapped and secured to the side for the procedure.
- Manure is evacuated from the rectum as far cranial as possible and a final transrectal palpation and ultrasound examination of the ovaries and uterus is performed, as well as evaluation of uterine and cervical tone.
- Upon confirmation, flunixin meglumine (10 ml IV) and acepromazine (2–3 ml IV) are administered. If the mare is particularly nervous in the stocks, a dose of xylazine can be administered as well (1.5 ml IV).
- While waiting for the full effects of sedation, the perineum is thoroughly cleaned (see Chapter 3).
- To prepare the embryo for transfer, set a transfer sheath out, position a 0.25 ml straw into the urethral adapter of a 1 ml tuberculin syringe, and deposit at least half of the contents of a pre-warmed (37°C, 98.6°F) embryo holding medium into a small polystyrene dish on a warming plate (37°C, 98.6°F).
- Remove the embryo dish from the incubator, verify the name, and identify the embryo under the microscope.
- Pull up a small amount of embryo holding medium within the 0.25 ml straw and then the embryo, gently transferring it into the small dish filled with warm embryo holding medium.
- To position the embryo into the straw, begin by pulling up approximately half the length of the straw with embryo holding medium, add an air gap, pull up the embryo surrounded by media, add another air gap, and then continue to pull media until the cotton plug at the end of the straw begins to become saturated.
- Carefully remove the straw from the plug and slide it into the transfer pipette with the cotton plug on top.
- Slide the embryo transfer gun into the top of the pipette and gently move it down until it slips past the outer portion of the straw containing the embryo, being careful not to push the inner-most plunger down.
- Assertively, but gently, continue pushing the pipette until the scored plastic splits and enables the top of the pipette to reach the top of the transfer gun (this may vary with the type of transfer gun).
- Secure this junction with the plastic circular ring by sliding it to the top of the pipette, ensuring a tight fit.
- Gently push the plunger down until resistance is first felt indicating the cotton plug has just been contacted.
- Pick up the wrapped pipette, with transfer gun in place, and return to the sedated mare.
- With a sterile palpation sleeve in place, pull the embryo transfer pipette and gun out of the outer plastic wrapping, while ensuring the overlying sterile plastic chemise is still in place, and apply a small amount of sterile obstetrical lubricant to the back of the transfer hand.
  Confirm once again the name of the donor/recipient mare and the mare × sire of the embryo being transferred.
- Ensure that the mare is calm and adequately restrained and then swipe lubricant from the back of the hand onto the outer vulvar lips.
- Introduce the sleeved hand, with transfer pipette protected within the palm, through the vulva and towards the cranial vaginal vault.
- Identify the external cervical os and manipulate the tip of the transfer pipette into it without inserting a finger within the cervix.

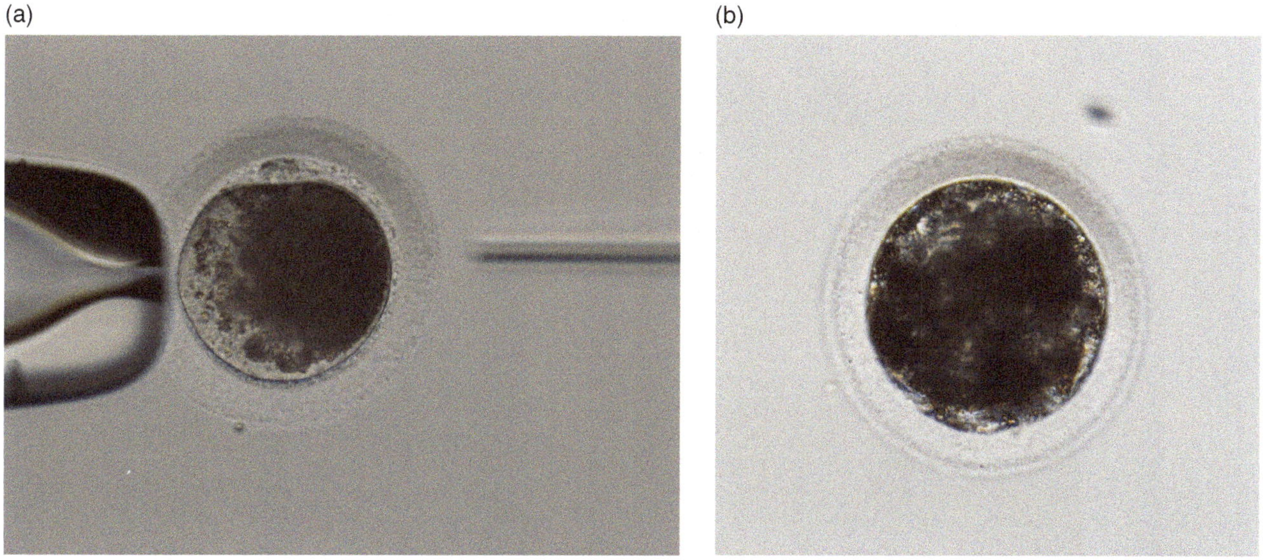

Figure 68.2 A mature oocyte from an autotransfer donor undergoing the ICSI procedure (a) and that same oocyte now a 6-day embryo ready for transfer back into the donor mare (b).

- Gently envelope the outer perimeter of the cervix by hand and pull it caudally to straighten any curvature within the lumen of the cervix, meanwhile gently advance the pipette through the cervix.
- While maneuvering the pipette within the cervix, pull back on the plastic chemise, effectively popping the tip of the transfer pipette through and advance the pipette through the internal cervical os into the uterine body, positioning it as far into the uterus as possible.
- Remove the hand from the vaginal vault, leaving the transfer pipette in place, apply non-sterile obstetrical lubricant, and introduce this hand rectally.
- Gently palpate the tip of the transfer pipette transrectally and guide it cranially into a uterine horn if possible.
- Once satisfied with its position, maneuver the tip of the pipette to rest within the center of the uterine lumen and begin gently pushing the plunger of the transfer gun.
- While plunging, slowly back the transfer pipette caudally to provide a gentle deposit of the embryo within the uterine lumen, being careful to not back too close to the internal cervical os.
- Once the plunger has completely been depressed, remove the entire embryo transfer pipette from the mare's reproductive tract, and your hand from the rectum.
- Return to the lab in order to gently flush the tip of the pipette used to transfer the embryo, ensuring the embryo did not stick within the lumen or tip. Examine the fluid under a stereomicroscope for the potential embryo if it was inadvertently retained within the tip of the transfer pipette.
- Once clear, relieve the mare's tail from positioning and remove the tail bag.
- Administer altrenogest (0.044 mg/kg PO, every 24 hours) and demarcate this mare as potentially pregnant (e.g., a red tag on her halter).
- All *in vitro* produced embryos are treated as day 6 in development (Figure 68.2) and the first pregnancy examination will take place 6 days following the embryo transfer (day 12 of gestation) (Figure 68.3).

Additional Comments

- Care is taken during the physical aspiration of the dominant follicle to not completely remove all granulosa cells, leaving behind a good population for luteal cell formation.
- If embryonic development is delayed during *in vitro* culture and the donor/recipient mare's cycle is beyond 7 days post-ovulation, alternative plans must be developed for that embryo, such as transfer to a different recipient mare or cryopreserve for later transfer.
- If immature oocytes are collected during this cycle as well, they will not typically line up to be transferred at the appropriate time and must be cryopreserved until a subsequent cycle or transferred fresh into an appropriately aligned recipient mare.
- Once an embryo is transferred, the donor/recipient mare is maintained on altrenogest through pregnancy confirmation and either continued on altrenogest or another progesterone supplementation through 120 days of gestation.

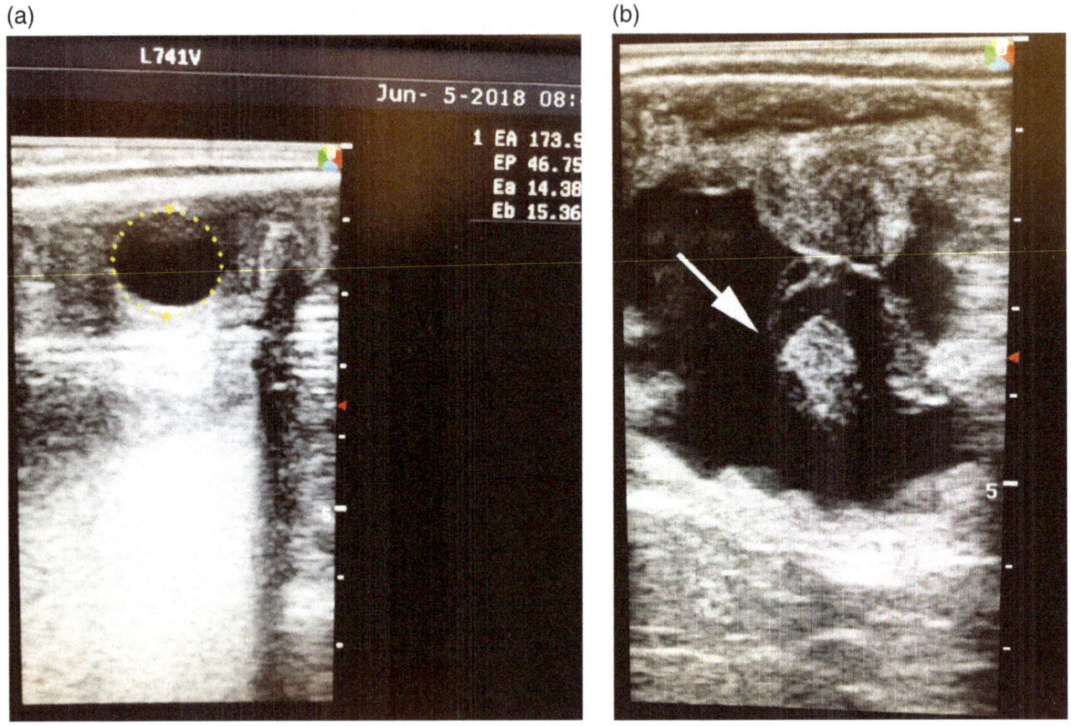

Figure 68.3 A 14-day embryonic vesicle (yellow dotted circle) (a) following transfer into the donor mare from the embryo pictured above (Figure 68.2a) and a 35-day image of that same pregnancy (white arrow pointing at the embryo proper) (b).

Further Reading

Carnevale EM, Rossini JB, Rodriguez JS, Sessions-Bresnahan DR, Stokes JE. 2013. Autogenous transfer of intracytoplasmic sperm injection-produced equine embryos into oocyte donor uteri. *Proc Annu Conv Am Assoc Eq Pract* 59: 526.

Hatzel JN, McCue PM, Ferris RA, Stokes JE, Carnevale EM. 2018. Clinical autogenous transfers into oocyte donor's uteri of embryos produced by intracytoplasmic sperm injection. *J Eq Vet Sci Suppl* 66: 195.

69

Palpation per Rectum of the Pregnant Reproductive Tract

Sofie Sitters

Amsterdam, The Netherlands

Introduction

Characteristic changes occur in the mare's reproductive tract during pregnancy. These changes are caused by the response of the genital organs to hormone stimulation, by increase in fetal fluid, and the growing conceptus. Many of these changes can be evaluated by palpation of the reproductive tract per rectum. Historically, palpation per rectum was the main technique for pregnancy determination before the advent and clinical use of ultrasonography. The accuracy of pregnancy diagnosis per rectum depends on the stage of gestation, individual mare characteristics (straining, peristalsis, rectal lumen diameter, etc.), and skill of the clinician.

Equipment and Supplies

Non-sterile obstetrical sleeve, non-sterile obstetrical lubricant. Optional: local anesthetic (2% lidocaine or mepivacaine), 60 ml catheter tip syringe, urinary catheter, step stand (step stool).

Technique

- The mare should be adequately restrained for safety of the mare, personnel, and equipment.
- If needed, the examiner can use a step stand (step stool) to obtain a better angle for palpation of mares with more advanced pregnancies.
- *Optional*: infusion of 50–60 ml of a local anesthetic (2% lidocaine or mepivacaine), into the lumen of the rectum via a urinary catheter attached to a 60 ml catheter tip syringe, may be indicated to induce relaxation of the smooth muscle of the rectum and facilitate a safe palpation of the reproductive tract. Please be aware that it is not advised to administer *N*-butylscopolammonium bromide to the pregnant mare since it may cause relaxation of the cervix.
- The reproductive tract should be examined in a systematic manner.
- Approximately 25–50 ml of obstetrical lubricant is applied to the obstetrical sleeve covering the hand and forearm.
- Fecal material in the rectum and distal small colon should be completely evacuated (as far as the palpating arm can comfortably reach) prior to manual palpation of the reproductive tract.
- The examiner should advance their hand cranially beyond the uterus (starting as far as almost shoulder length) and retract the cupped hand in a caudal–ventral direction to examine the uterus (generally at or slightly beyond elbow length).
- The uterus is identified and the cupped hand is gently moved along one uterine horn in a lateral, cranial, and dorsal direction until the horn tip is reached (Figure 69.1). The exam is repeated on the other horn.
- One should be able to discern uterine size, relative weight, and tone with the palm of the hand and fingertips. The

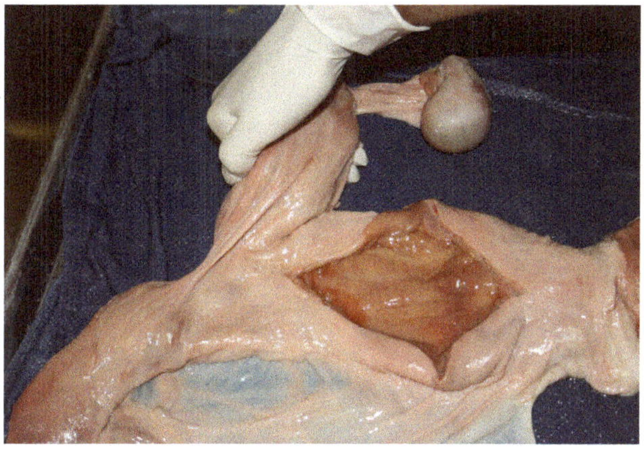

Figure 69.1 Palpation of a uterine specimen demonstrating the technique for palpation of the ventral aspect of the uterine horn for detecting early equine pregnancies.

Equine Reproductive Procedures, Second Edition. Edited by John Dascanio and Patrick McCue.

bulge of an early pregnancy is often best detected along the ventral aspect of the uterus due to the predominant dorsal attachment of the uterine broad ligament.

- In addition, the size, tone, and consistency of the cervix is evaluated. The cervix is located whilst slowly retracting the palpating arm back out of the rectum, moving the flat palm of the hand from left to right, whilst pushing down on the floor of the pelvis.

Interpretation

Progesterone and embryonic factors cause the pregnant uterus to become increasingly tubular and firm or toned. The increase in uterine tone in pregnant mares may be noted between 12 and 18 days after ovulation. The cervix of the pregnant mare closes tightly and becomes firm (toned) and elongated. Cervical relaxation takes place during the last 2 months of pregnancy, causing the cervix to soften and shorten. The cervix in a near-term mare may be difficult to distinguish from other soft tissue structures.

During the course of the pregnancy, the uterine wall gradually thins and loses tone over the developing conceptus. The pregnant uterus enlarges and changes in size, shape, and orientation as the pregnancy advances. The embryonic vesicle may be first detected as a 30–40 mm bulge ventrally at the base of a uterine horn as early as day 20 (Table 69.1). In early pregnancy, the pregnant uterus

Table 69.1 Characteristics of the equine pregnancy found on rectal palpation by day of gestation.

Day of Gestation	Palpable Characteristics
20	Embryonic vesicle: 30–40 mm in diameter (grape/walnut size) at the base of one horn Good overall uterine tone, slight decrease in tone over the embryonic bulge
30	Embryonic vesicle: 40–50 mm in diameter (walnut/lime size); noted as a discrete fluid swelling ventrally in the uterus More obvious decrease in uterine tone over the bulge
40	Fetal bulge: 65 mm in diameter (peach size) Decreased tone over the bulge and decreased tone of the pregnant horn Excellent tone of the cervix: rod-like consistency
50	Fetal bulge: at least 8 cm in diameter (orange size); the fluid-filled vesicle extends into the uterine body
60	Fetal bulge: 10–13 cm in diameter (grapefruit size); nearly the entire gravid horn and uterine body are filled, the non-gravid horn remains small More obvious loss of tone over the bulge Uterus starts to be pulled over the pelvic brim Ovaries are moving closer together Note: the urinary bladder may be mistaken for the conceptus
85	Fetus itself is palpable (chipmunk size) due to decreased turgidity of the conceptus
90	Conceptus fills the entire uterus Uterus is located further ventrally in the abdomen making direct palpation of the fetus more difficult Ovaries are pulled closed together in a more ventral position
90–150	Uterus in the abdominal position Fetus can usually be easily palpated (kitten/rabbit size) or balloted within the uterus
150–200	Uterus further ventrally in the abdomen Ovaries are pulled ventrally under the broad ligament and are not accessible Thorough evaluation of the fetus (cat/beagle size) is more difficult
200–270	Uterus expands further dorsally Fetus (lamb/German sheperd dog size) is more accessible
270 to parturition	Fetus is easily accessible and is usually in cranial presentation, dorsal recumbancy with head and forelimbs flexed, and hind limbs pointing towards the pelvis Note: several minutes might be needed for detection of fetal movements Cervical relaxation occurs causing the cervix to soften and shorten
Parturition	Increased uterine tone and myometrial contractions present Fetus extends the head, neck, and fore limbs and positions itself for parturition Cervical dilation will occur

bulges ventrally due to gravity and the presence of a dorsally attached broad ligament that initially prevents dorsal expansion. Thus it is important to palpate the ventral aspect of the uterus (Figure 69.1). It must be noted that an accurate early pregnancy diagnosis is easier in maiden and open mares compared with post-foaling mares.

The conceptus gradually increases in size while expanding into the rest of the uterus. As the gravid uterus enlarges it moves cranially and ventrally and is pulled over the pelvic brim by 2–3 months of gestation and descends into the abdominal cavity. Between 5 and 7 months the uterus is positioned ventrally in the abdomen, making palpation of the conceptus difficult. In the late-term mare, the fetus is again within reach of the examiner during palpation per rectum. The fetus is usually in cranial presentation in dorsal recumbency with a flexed head and fore limbs by 9 months of gestation. Movement of the fetus can readily be detected, although the normal fetus exhibits periods of inactivity.

Additional Comments

It should be noted that manual palpation per rectum is not an adequate technique for the early detection and management of twins, detection and characterization of uterine fluid, or evaluation of the corpus luteum. As a consequence, ultrasonography has become the preferred technique for detecting early pregnancy and monitoring ovarian and uterine function. Nonetheless, accurate palpation of the (tone of the) pregnant uterus and cervix is not to be neglected, as it provides important information on the (hormonal) status of the pregnancy. A regressing primary corpus luteum, causing a potentially dangerous decline in progesterone during early pregnancy, will initially not be detectable via ultrasonography; however, a decreased tone of the uterus and/or cervix may be noted on palpation enabling early intervention.

Further Reading

Bucca S. 2011. Ultrasonographic cervical parameters throughout gestation in the mare. *Proc Annu Conv Am Assoc Eq Pract* 57: 235–41.

Ginther OJ. 1998. Equine pregnancy: physical interactions between the uterus and conceptus. *Proc Annu Conv Am Assoc Eq Pract* 44: 73–104.

Jeffcott LB, Rossdale P. 1979. A radiographic study of the fetus in late pregnancy and during foaling. *J Reprod Fertil Suppl* 27: 563–9.

McCue PM, McKinnon AO. 2011. Pregnancy examination. In: McKinnon AO, Squires EL, Vaala WE, Varner DD (eds). Equine Reproduction, 2nd edn. Ames, IA: Wiley Blackwell, pp. 2245–61.

Solomon WJ. 1971. Rectal examination of the cervix and its significance in early pregnancy evaluation of the mare. *Proc Annu Conv Am Assoc Eq Pract* 17: 73–80.

van Niekerk CH. 1965. The early diagnosis of pregnancy, the development of foetal membranes and nidation in the mare. *J S Afr Vet Med Assoc* 36: 483–8.

Zemjanis R. 1961. Pregnancy diagnosis in the mare. *J Am Vet Med Assoc* 139: 543–7.

70

Ultrasound Examination of the Pregnant Reproductive Tract

Patrick M. McCue

Equine Reproduction Laboratory, Colorado State University, USA

Introduction

Ultrasound examination of the reproductive tract is the most reliable test for pregnancy diagnosis. In addition, ultrasound allows for early detection and management of twins, evaluation of the corpus luteum, assessment of the presence or absence of uterine edema, monitoring pregnancy viability, and detection of pregnancy loss.

A thorough, systematic approach to ultrasonographic pregnancy diagnosis is imperative in order to correctly diagnose pregnancy status and to detect twins. The entire uterus should be scanned in one continuous motion in order to avoid missing a section of the uterus. The most common locations for a single embryo or a twin embryo to be missed are the caudal uterine body adjacent to the cervix and the tip of a uterine horn.

A schedule of potential ultrasonographic examination dates is presented in Table 70.1. The frequency and schedule of initial and subsequent examinations are often dictated by factors such as availability of the mare or clinician, potential for twins, results of previous pregnancy examinations, a history of pregnancy loss in a particular mare, and economics. A common schedule may be initial pregnancy diagnosis at 14–16 days post-ovulation, confirmation of fetal heart beat at 25–35 days, and final confirmation of pregnancy at 45–60 days post-ovulation to monitor fetal viability after initial placental formation.

Equipment and Supplies

Ultrasound machine, obstetrical sleeves (non-sterile), obstetrical lubricant (carboxymethylcellulose).

Table 70.1 Schedule of potential ultrasonographic examinations in the early pregnant mare. Many modifications of this schedule are used in clinical practice.

Day of Gestation	Examination Procedure
12–15	Initial pregnancy examination; identification and management of twins; evaluation of the corpus luteum (CL), follicle status, and presence of endometrial edema
24–27	Examination for an embryo proper; detection of a heart beat; reconfirm the absence of twins
~35	Confirmation of pregnancy status at the stage of endometrial cup formation
~45	Initial development of supplemental CL; time service fees are often payable for pregnant mares
~60	Evaluation of pregnancy status and supplementary CL
60–90	Fetal sex determination
~150	Confirmation of pregnancy and administration of first equine herpesvirus 1 (EHV-1) vaccine
~300	Late-term fetal well-being assessment: monitoring of fetus, determination of fetal presentation (cranial versus caudal), and administration of preterm vaccinations

Technique

- The mare should be adequately restrained for safety of the mare, personnel, and equipment.
- Fecal material in the rectum should be completely evacuated.
- The reproductive tract should be examined by manual palpation for assessment of uterine size and tone as well as cervical tone (see Chapter 69).

Equine Reproductive Procedures, Second Edition. Edited by John Dascanio and Patrick McCue.

- The ultrasound exam should proceed in a systematic manner. The entire uterus should be carefully examined, as well as each ovary. It is important to scan from the tip of one uterine horn to the tip of the other horn and back across the uterine body without losing contact to make sure a small embryonic vesicle is not accidently missed.
- All significant structures and findings should be recorded. The interpretation should take into consideration any and all available information on the mare (last breeding date or ovulation date, number of ovulations, presence of endometrial cysts, etc.).

Interpretation and Additional Comments

An equine embryonic vesicle may be detected as early as day 10 or 11 after ovulation. Routine initial pregnancy examinations are typically performed 12–16 days post-ovulation (Figures 70.1 and 70.2). An ultrasonographic examination performed on or before day 16 is also beneficial for the identification and management of twin pregnancies, scheduling re-breeding in open mares, and early detection of problems associated with the pregnancy. Determination of the number of ovulations and a time course of ovulations is helpful in the subsequent detection and management of twins.

It is of great benefit to identify, measure, and map the location of uterine cysts prior to breeding a mare. The fact that "cysts do not grow (rapidly), do not move" within the uterus and do not possess a heart beat is beneficial in the differentiation of cysts from an embryonic vesicle. The equine embryo migrates throughout the uterus until day 16 or 17 (stage of fixation) and generally increases in diameter at a rate of approximately 3–5 mm per day.

Older broodmares may have a dependent uterus, hanging over the pelvic brim, making ultrasound examination more difficult. It is important to thoroughly ultrasonographically scan the most dependent aspects of the uterus to avoid missing an early pregnancy.

Examination of the ovaries for the presence and characteristics of a corpus luteum and the uterus for evidence of edema is valuable at the initial pregnancy examination. A corpus luteum should be present and there should not be uterine edema. The absence of a corpus luteum and the presence of uterine edema in a mare with a confirmed embryonic vesicle indicates that the mare is coming back into estrus and that the pregnancy is at risk. Pregnancies may be saved by initiating progesterone supplementation in cases of corpus luteum regression. Measurement of the blood progesterone level may be indicated to confirm the functional status of the corpus luteum.

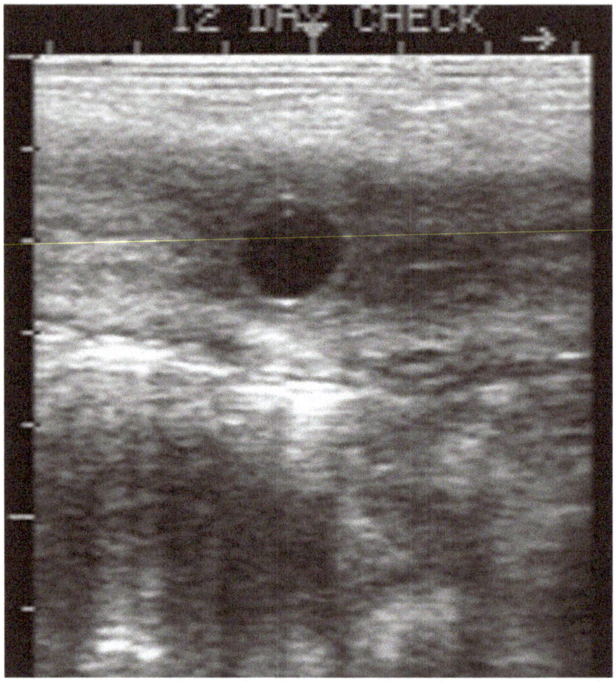

Figure 70.1 Ultrasonographic image of a 12-day pregnancy.

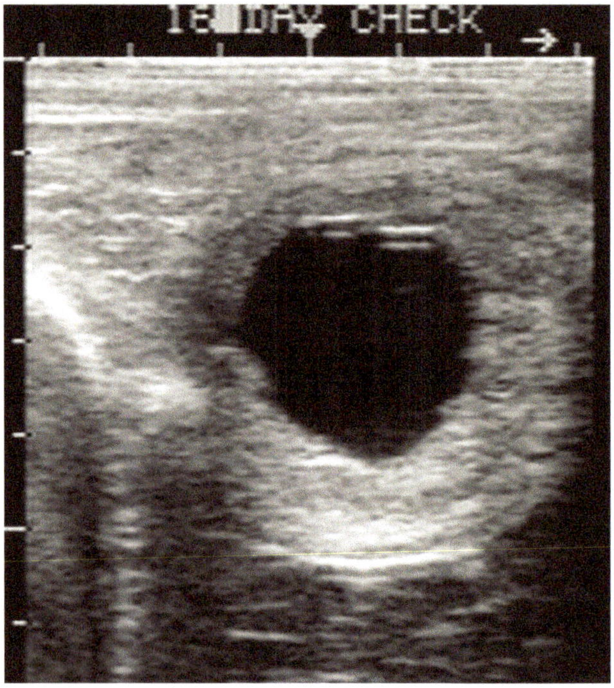

Figure 70.2 Ultrasonographic image of a 16-day pregnancy.

A routine follow-up examination by ultrasonography is generally recommended between 25 and 35 days post-ovulation to confirm that the pregnancy is ongoing and that a heart beat is present (Figures 70.3 and 70.4). It is also a useful time to reconfirm that twins are not present, as twin pregnancies or abortions have been reported in mares

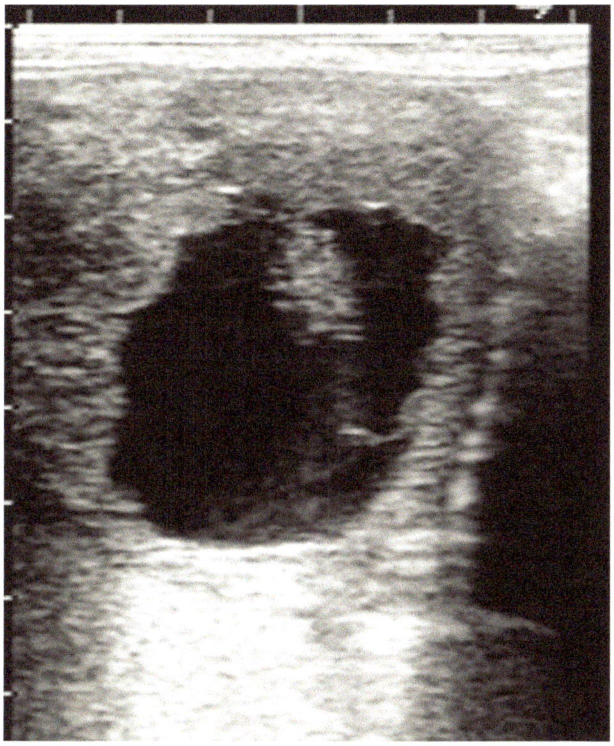

Figure 70.3 Ultrasonographic image of a 25-day pregnancy.

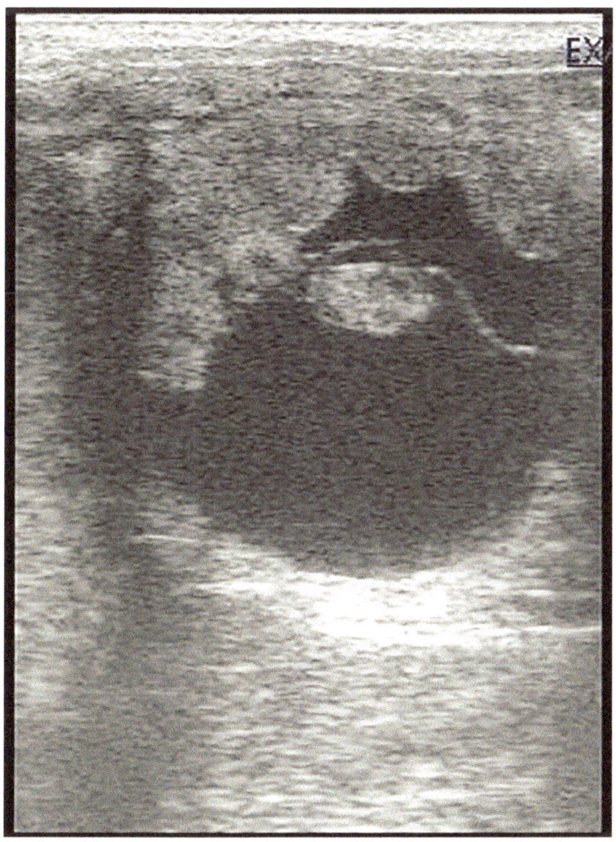

Figure 70.4 Ultrasonographic image of a 35-day pregnancy.

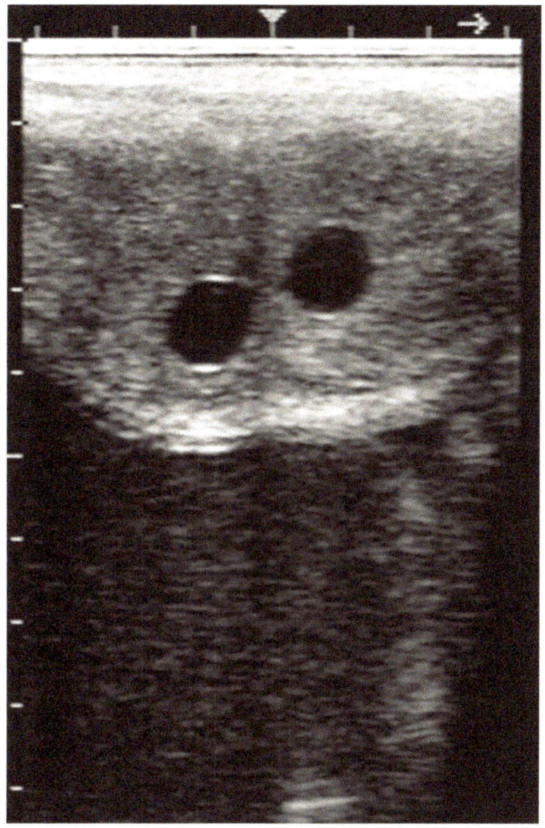

Figure 70.5 Ultrasonographic image of twin pregnancies, with the embryonic vesicles separated slightly.

where a single embryonic vesicle was observed during pregnancy examination at 14 days (Figures 70.5–70.7).

Rarely, a final diagnosis of pregnancy status may have to wait until after day 25 to determine if an embryonic vesicle, with an embryo proper and heart beat, is present amongst a cluster of cysts (Figure 70.8).

Empty trophoblastic vesicles (ETVs), defined as the presence of an embryonic (trophoblastic) vesicle without an embryo proper, have been identified in mares. An embryo destined to form an ETV often exhibits normal early growth (i.e., days 11 to 16). Ultrasonographically, an ETV is recognized as a static oval or irregular embryonic structure without an embryo proper after days 24–25 of gestation (Figure 70.9).

Supplementary corpora lutea may be identified in pregnant mares after 45–60 days of gestation. Ultrasonographic progression of accessory corpus luteum (CL) formation includes development of a large follicle, the presence of echogenic particles or strands within the follicular lumen, followed by infiltration of echogenic material within the follicular lumen (Figure 70.10). The mature secondary CL has similar ultrasonographic characteristics to the primary CL. Multiple supplementary CLs may be present on each

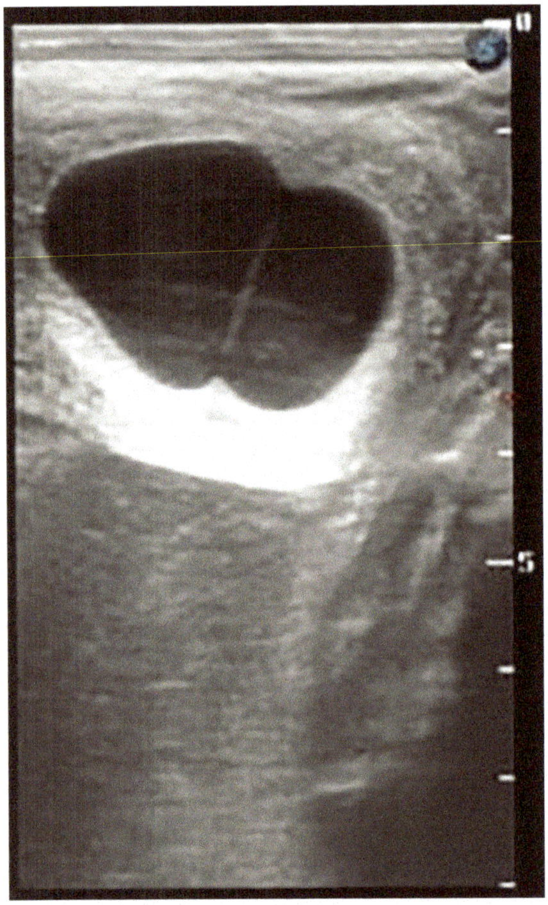

Figure 70.6 Ultrasonographic image of twin pregnancies, with the embryos touching each other.

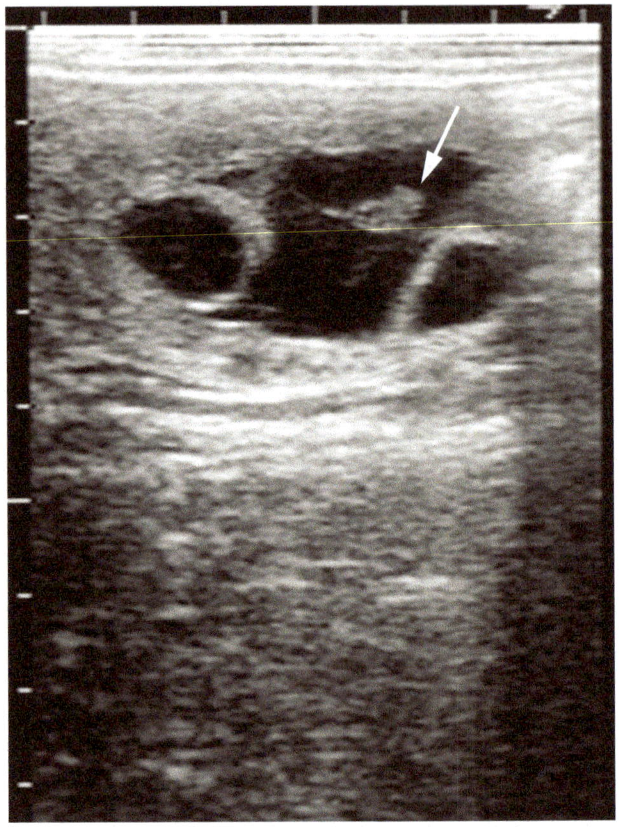

Figure 70.8 Ultrasonographic image of a 25-day pregnancy (arrow) and adjacent cysts.

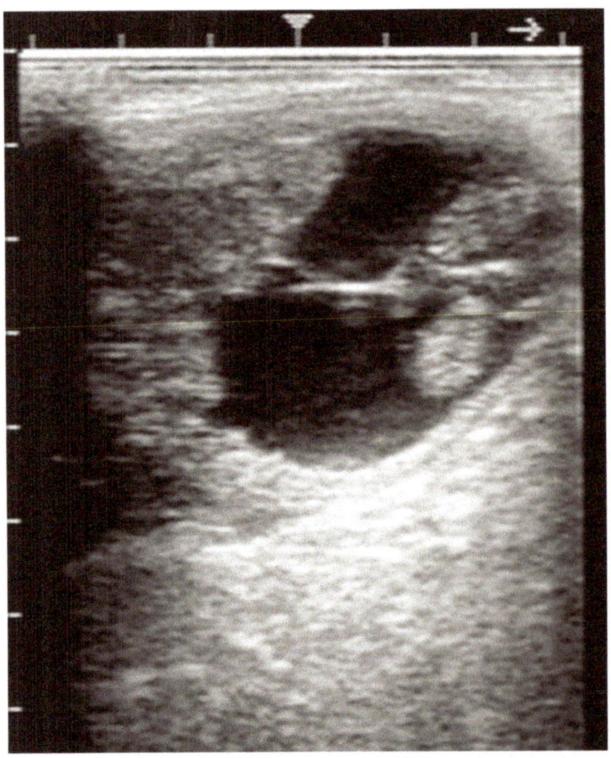

Figure 70.7 Ultrasonographic image of a 25-day pregnancy examination showing two embryo propers, each of which had a distinct heart beat, in a recipient mare following transfer of a single embryo. A single embryonic vesicle was observed during a routine 14-day pregnancy examination.

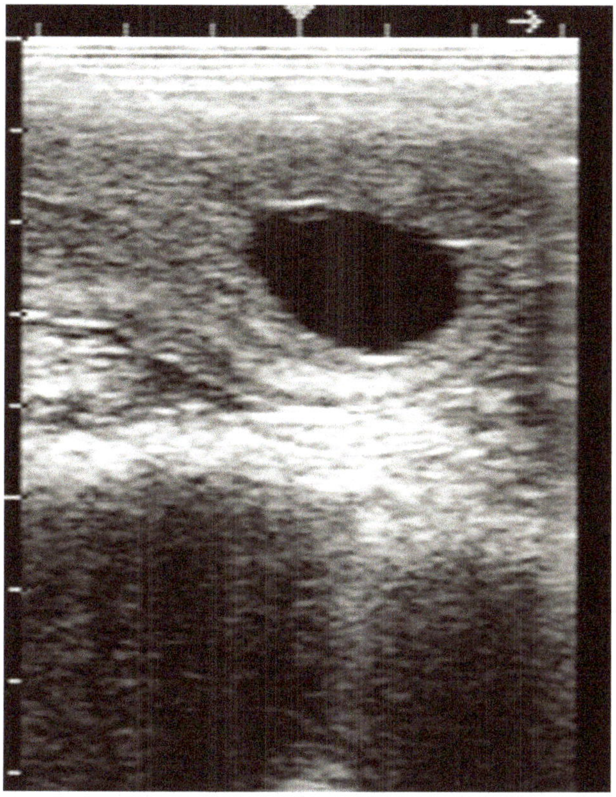

Figure 70.9 Ultrasonographic image of an empty trophoblastic vesicle 28 days after ovulation.

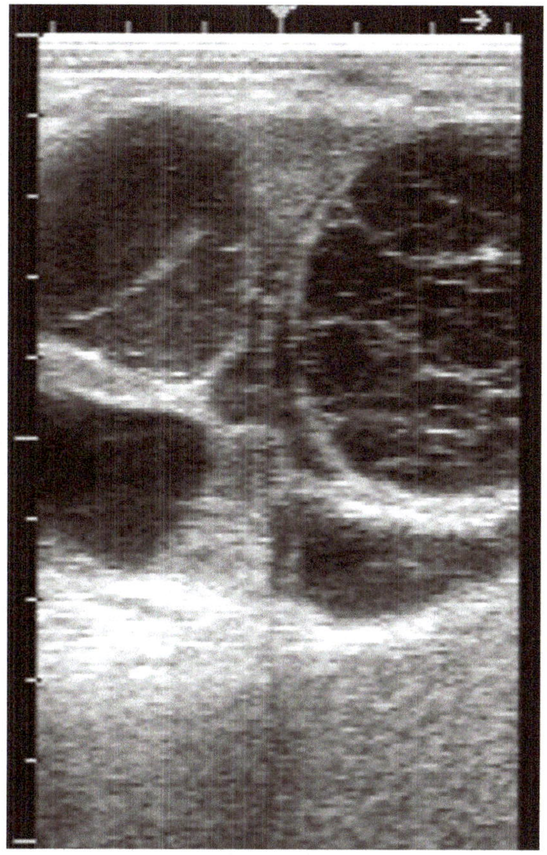

Figure 70.10 Ultrasonographic image of multiple supplementary (accessory) corpora lutea in a pregnant mare.

ovary and the size of the ovary is subsequently increased. Observation of supplementary CLs may be important for management decisions in mares being supplemented with exogenous progesterone or progestins. If supplementary CLs are present, progesterone levels are almost invariably elevated and progestin supplementation can be discontinued.

Further Reading

Allen WR, Goddard PJ. 1984. Serial investigations of early pregnancy in pony mares using real time ultrasound scanning. *Eq Vet J* 16: 509–14.

Ginther OJ. 1986. Ultrasonic Imaging and Reproductive Events in the Mare. Cross Plains, WI: Equiservices.

McCue PM, McKinnon AO. 2011. Pregnancy diagnosis. In: McKinnon AO, Squires EL, Vaala WE, Varner DD (eds). Equine Reproduction, 2nd edn. Ames, IA: Wiley Blackwell, pp. 2245–61.

71

Speculum Examination of the Pregnant Mare

Sofie Sitters

Amsterdam, The Netherlands

Introduction

Speculum examination of the internal genital tract of the mare during pregnancy is not entirely free of risk and should not be performed unless specifically indicated. The vagina in most pregnant mares has a thicker mucoid secretion, causing the vaginal walls to stick to each other thus forming a barrier to ascending infections. This mucoid barrier will become disrupted with a vaginal examination.

Direct visualization of the vaginal vault and cervix of a pregnant mare may be indicated when bleeding is evident at the vulva or when a vaginal discharge is noted in order to ascertain the origin.

Equipment and Supplies

Tail wrap, tail rope, non-irritant soap, roll cotton, stainless steel bucket, disposable liner bag for bucket, paper towels, exam gloves, sterilized glass speculum or disposable aluminum foil speculum or sterilized Polansky (Caslick) tri-valve speculum, sterile lubricant, light source.

Technique

- Remove feces from the rectum.
- Place a tail wrap and tie the tail out of the way (see Chapter 4).
- Clean and dry the perineum of the mare (see Chapter 3).
- Lubricate the end of the speculum with sterile lubricant. With the tube speculums, lubricant should not get into the lumen of the speculum so as to avoid obscuring visualization of the reproductive tract.
- Wearing exam gloves, separate the lips of the vulva and insert the speculum in an upward manner to pass over the ventral pelvic brim.
- Once over the brim, bring the speculum to a horizontal orientation. The tri-valve speculum is initially turned sideways to allow entry into the vulva and then turned 90 degrees once over the pelvic brim and past the vestibulo-vaginal fold. The tri-valve speculum is advanced into the vagina and opened by twisting the wing nut to extend the three arms outward.
- Some resistance will be encountered at the level of the vestibulo-vaginal fold. Slight forward pressure with some slight rotation will allow the speculum to enter the vagina. A slight sucking sound may be audible when the speculum passes through the vestibulo-vaginal fold caused by air being aspirated into the vagina.
- A light source is used to visualize the walls of the vagina and the cervix. The speculum may need to be moved in all directions and advanced inward or retracted outward to visualize all structures.
- Visualization should continue while the speculum is withdrawn from the vagina and vestibule.

Interpretation

- In a normal pregnant mare, progesterone causes the cervix to be tightly closed, dry, and pale white and to be located high on the wall of the cranial vaginal vault (Figure 71.1). A sticky vaginal secretion is often present, causing the vaginal walls to stick together. The cervix may contain a so-called "mucus plug," an accumulation of thick white mucus.
- During the last 2 months of pregnancy the cervix will soften and relax. During the first stage of labor the relaxed cervix will gradually dilate due to pressure of the chorioallantoic sac caused by coordinated uterine contractions.

Equine Reproductive Procedures, Second Edition. Edited by John Dascanio and Patrick McCue.

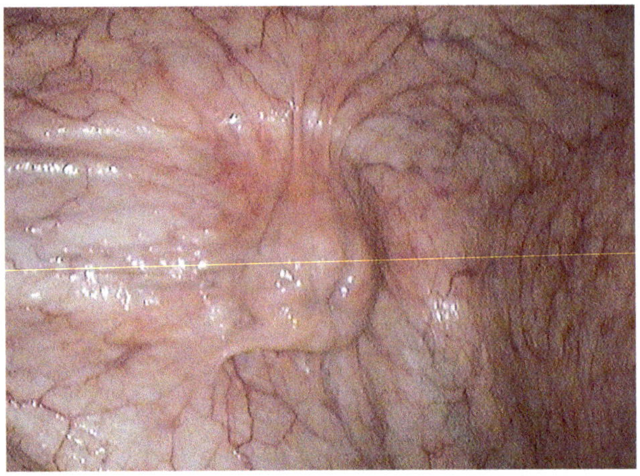

Figure 71.1 Cervix of a pregnant mare viewed through a speculum (day 45 of gestation).

- Varicose veins can develop in the vagina during pregnancy, especially in older mares (see Chapter 86). The etiology of these varicosities is unknown. On occasion, these veins can rupture and blood can be seen at the vulva lips. Vaginal varicose veins can be up to 5 mm in diameter and are most often located in the region of the vestibulo-vaginal fold. Because of their location they are easily missed during a speculum examination. Initial insertion of the speculum past the vestibulo-vaginal fold will bypass the varicose vein(s) and withdrawal of the speculum without continuous observation will also result in lack of visualization of the vein(s). Consequently, the recommended strategy is to very slowly withdraw the speculum while constantly observing the 360 degree region of the vestibulo-vaginal fold for varicose vein(s) or small areas of hemorrhage.

Additional Comments: Potential Risks

Initiation of an iatrogenic ascending infection is a potential risk when performing a speculum examination during pregnancy. Cleanliness is important in order to decrease the risk of infection. However, introduction of air through the speculum can not be avoided and this, on its own, could facilitate the introduction of microorganisms. Also, the air itself initiates an inflammatory response of the mucosal membranes of the vagina and cervix. In addition, pneumovagina may induce straining by the mare.

Finally, manipulation of the cervix should be avoided in the late-term pregnant mare due to the possibility of stimulating prostaglandin release and subsequent triggering of uterine contractions.

Further Reading

Bucca S. 2011. Ultrasonographic cervical parameters throughout gestation in the mare. *Proc Annu Conv Am Assoc Eq Pract* 57: 235–41.

Frazer GS. 2005. Differential diagnosis for vaginal haemmorrhage in the mare. *Eq Vet Educ* 17: 153–5.

McCue PM, McKinnon AO. 2011. Pregnancy examination. In: McKinnon AO, Squires EL, Vaala WE, Varner DD (eds). Equine Reproduction, 2nd edn. Ames, IA: Wiley Blackwell, pp. 2245–61.

72

Determination of Fetal Sex at 55–200 days

Richard D. Holder

Hagyard Equine Medical Institute, USA

Introduction

Ultrasonic determination of fetal sex is a useful management tool for the horse owner. The potential value of the offspring varies depending on the sex, the sire, and the dam. This affects the value of the pregnant mare, insurance coverage, sales appraisals, reserves, and the offspring value. Determination of fetal sex may assist the owner in determining the future direction for the mare or offspring in racing, sales, or breeding.

Equine fetal sex determination may be performed at three different periods of gestation. The earliest stage is the transrectal ultrasonographic evaluation of the fetal genital tubercle performed between 55 and 90 days of gestation. The genital tubercle becomes the penis in the male and the clitoris in the female. It is located between the hind legs at 52–53 days of gestation in both sexes. By 55 days the tubercle, which is a 2 mm bi-lobed hyperechoic structure, will move toward the base of the umbilical cord of the fetus in the male and toward the base of the tail in the female (Figures 72.1 and 72.2). The positioning of the ultrasound probe for fetal sexing is presented in Figure 72.3.

The optimal time to differentiate male and female fetuses using this technique is between 60 and 65 days of gestation. The technique is difficult to learn and a practitioner needs to be persistent and not be discouraged at first attempts.

The second stage at which fetal sex can be determined is at 90–150 days of gestation. At 80 days the uterus is pulled over the brim of the pelvis by the fluid of the pregnancy and is difficult to access per rectum. However, by 90 days the uterus elevates in the abdominal cavity and the fetus is again visible on transrectal ultrasound. The genital tubercle has evolved into the external genitalia, which is used to make the determination. At 90 days the genitalia is not well developed and it is often difficult to differentiate males from females (prepuce and mammary gland). The optimum time to examine the mare at this stage is between 110 and 125 days of gestation. The fetus is now easily accessible and the genitalia is adequately developed. At approximately 150 days of gestation, the fetus frequently assumes

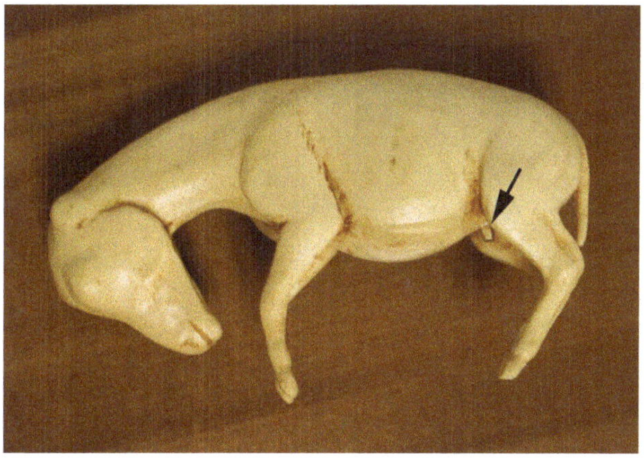

Figure 72.1 Location and appearance of the genital tubercle (arrow) in a male fetus at approximately 65 days of gestation.

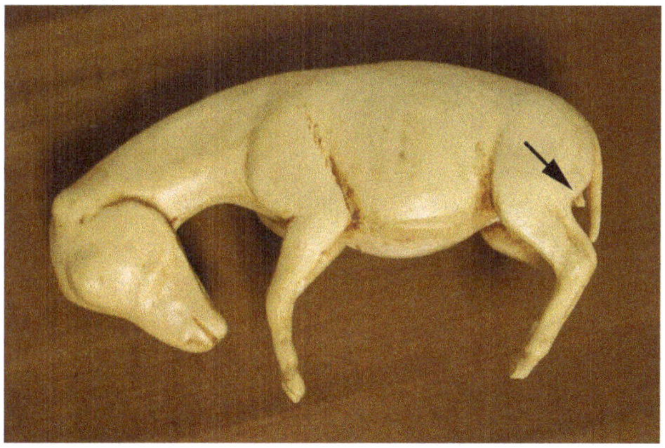

Figure 72.2 Location and appearance of the genital tubercle (arrow) in a female fetus at approximately 65 days of gestation.

Equine Reproductive Procedures, Second Edition. Edited by John Dascanio and Patrick McCue.

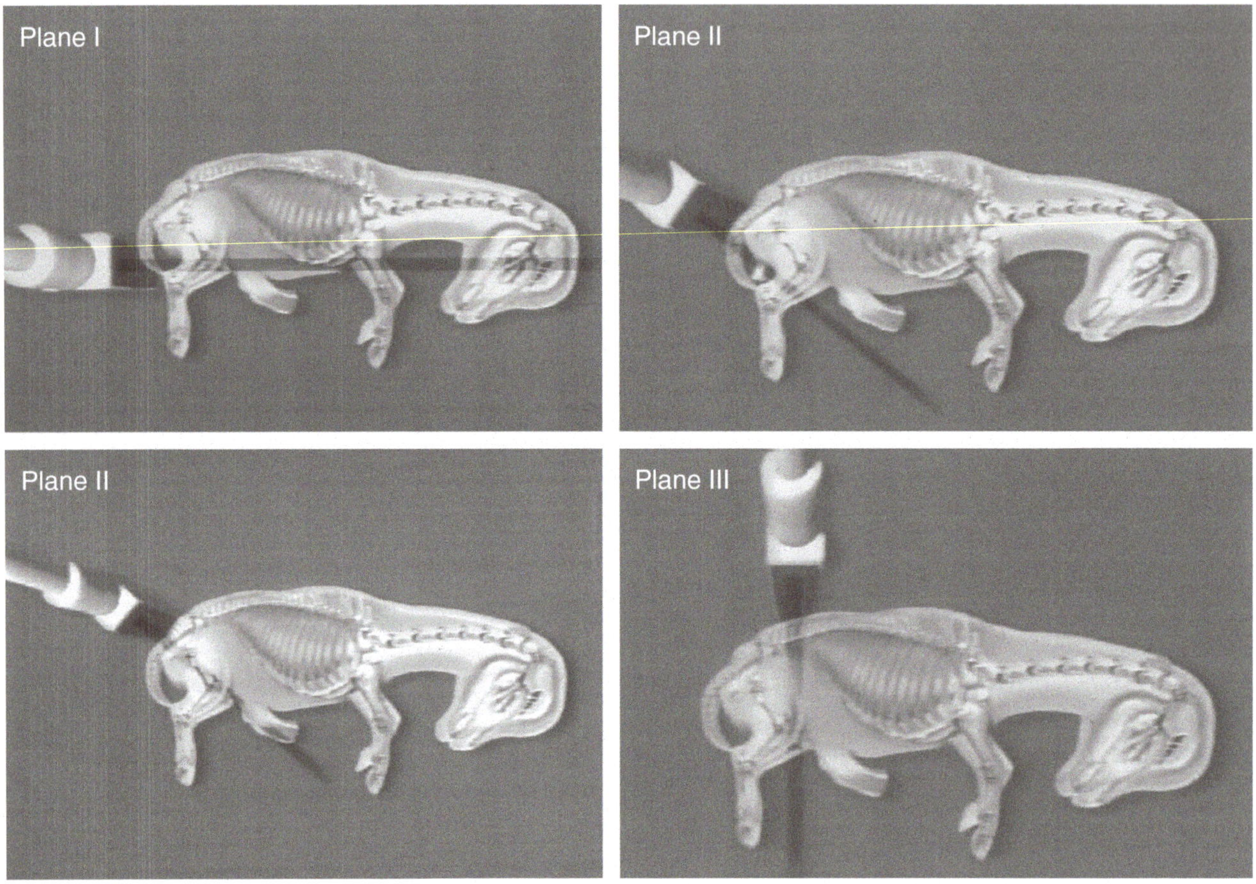

Figure 72.3 Directions of ultrasound imaging for fetal sexing (planes I, II, and III). From Holder (2011).

an anterior presentation, putting the posterior part of the fetus out of reach per rectum.

The third stage for sex determination is at 150 days and beyond and is performed using a transabdominal ultrasound approach. This stage is more difficult, takes longer to perform, and has a higher percentage of "no determination" than the other two stages. The procedure requires a quality ultrasound with a 2.0–4.0 MHz transducer. The mare is examined along the ventral midline from the udder to the sternum. The fetal genitalia are well developed, but the visual image is usually not quite as clear as a transrectal image at earlier stages. In addition, it is more difficult to obtain a proper plane of visualization than during a transrectal ultrasound examination as the probe angle and probe contact is limited by the external surface curvature of the abdomen. At this stage there is more crowding in the groin area of the fetus, an increase in the amount of placental tissue, and an increase in the overall size of the fetus. It is possible to do successful determination as early as 62 days transabdominally. Anytime the fetus becomes out of reach per rectum, the transabdominal approach is useful.

Equipment and Supplies

Ultrasound machine with 5 mHz linear array transrectal probe for 55–150 days or 2.0–4.0 MHz sector or curvilinear probe for transabdominal ultrasonography at 62 days or more; ultrasound cart on wheels, alcohol or contact lubricant for transabdominal scanning, obstetrical lubricant, obstetrical sleeve, examination stocks, twitch or lip chain, tranquilization medications (if needed, xylazine hydrochloride 200 mg plus butorphanol tartrate 5–10 mg IV or detomidine hydrochloride 5 mg IV for an adult light breed mare), medication to relax rectal musculature (propantheline bromide 30 mg IV or *N*-butylscopolammonium bromide 40 mg IV may be used in an adult light breed mare).

Technique: 55–90 Days of Gestation

- Place proper restraint on the mare and evacuate any feces as far anterior as possible. Many fetuses will be difficult to reach and the transducer will need to be extended in front of the hand. If the mare is straining, a smooth muscle relaxant such as propantheline or *N*-butylscopolammonium bromide may be administered.

- Determine the anterior–posterior positioning of the fetus. Locate the cranium (anterior marker). The heart and the umbilical entrance to the abdomen (which appears as a 3–4 mm dark hole on the posterior abdominal midline) are ventral markers. The ribs coming off the vertebrae and the spinal column are dorsal markers, and the tail head is a posterior and dorsal marker.
- Scan the posterior ventral area to see if an obvious genital tubercle is present. Next, try to obtain a transverse view of the thorax and abdomen where the plane of the ultrasound beam transects the fetus perpendicular to the axis of the fetal spine (plane III, Figure 72.3). It will be necessary to look for markers that identify the dorsal and ventral orientation on the fetus. The genital tubercle for the male will be on the ventral midline, just posterior to the umbilical entrance into the abdominal cavity (Figure 72.4). The genital tubercle for the female will be on the fetal ventral midline just under the tail head (Figure 72.5). A transverse ultrasound plane (plane III slightly perpendicular to the axis of the spine) will exhibit the ribs, which is the best dorsal marker (Figure 72.6). Continue with this plane until you move off the posterior part of the entire fetus. After there is no fetus in view, keeping this same plane II, ease back toward the fetus. The first hyperechoic area on the dorsal side (same side as the ribs) will be the tail head. The next hyperechoic areas will be the genital tubercle just under the tail (in a female), and then two hyperechoic areas (tibias, with no muscle mass around them) about 1–2 cm from the tail depending on the age of the fetus. The tubercle for a female is found within the triangle formed by the tail head and the two tibias.
- There should be either three or four hyperechoic areas in view. If it is a colt, there will be three hyperechoic areas forming a tail head–tibial triangle with no hyperechoic area below the tail within this triangle. If it is a filly, a bi-lobed hyperechoic "equal sign" will appear within the tail head–tibial triangle, slightly closer to the tail head. This view of plane II is a requirement for identifying a filly (Figure 72.5c).
- A colt tubercle can be visualized from many different angles, including a frontal plane that exhibits the front legs, ventral abdomen, and hind legs (plane I) (Figure 72.4a). The tubercle will appear on the ventral midline slightly anterior to a line drawn between the stifles and slightly posterior to the umbilical entrance into the abdominal cavity. If there is a negative filly view (nothing within the triangle), advance the probe anteriorly on the fetus. The male tubercle will appear just at the ventral edge of the abdominal wall as a hyperechoic bilobed "equal sign" (Figure 72.4b). The "equal sign" or a

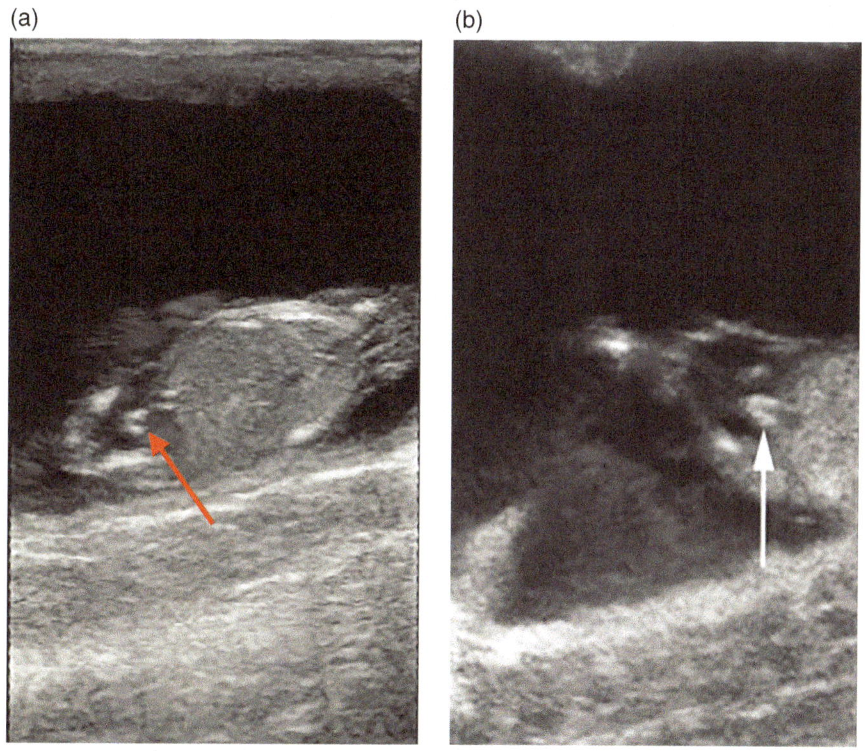

Figure 72.4 Genital tubercle (arrows) of a 68-day-old male equine fetus in plane I (a) and plane III (b).

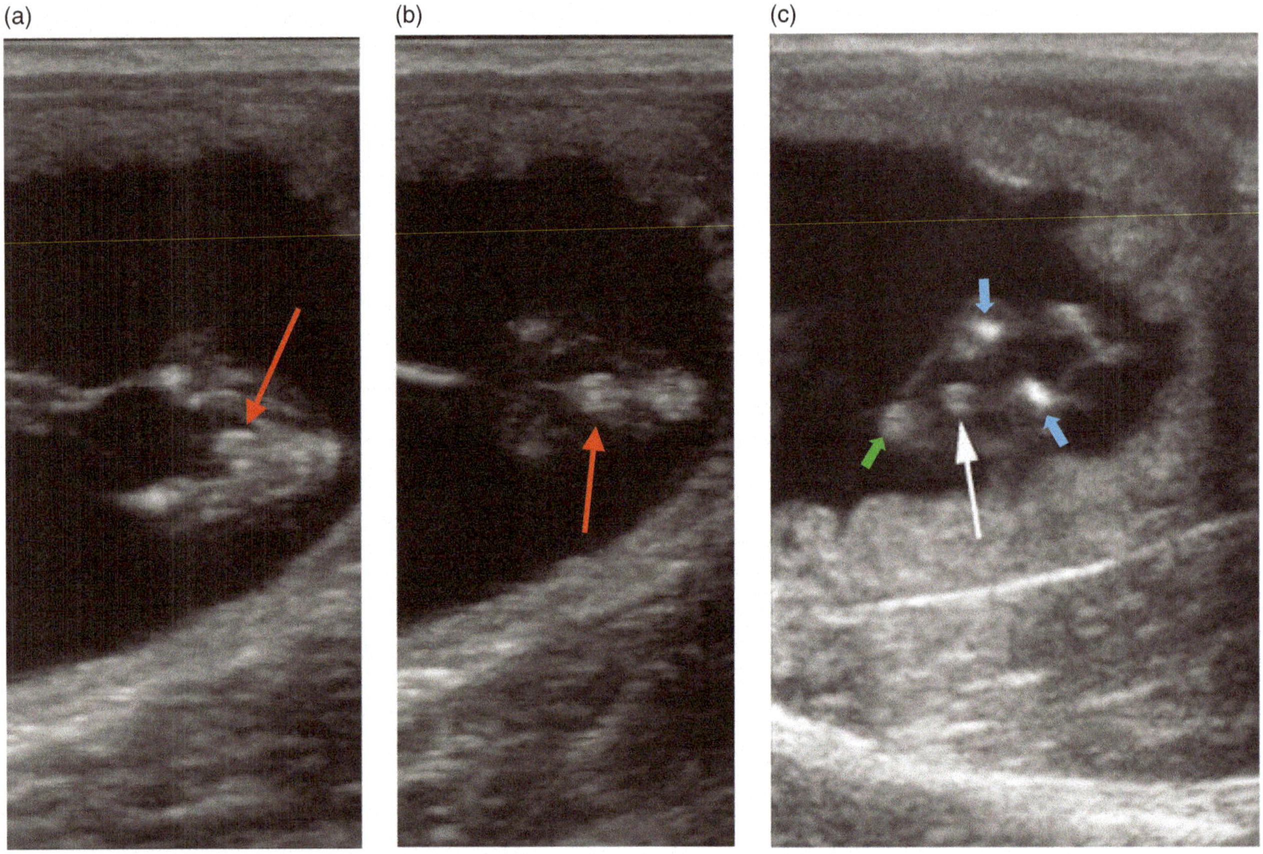

Figure 72.5 (a–c) Genital tubercle (arrows) of a 65-day-old female equine fetus in plane II. Note the tibias (blue arrows) and tail head (green arrow) in (c).

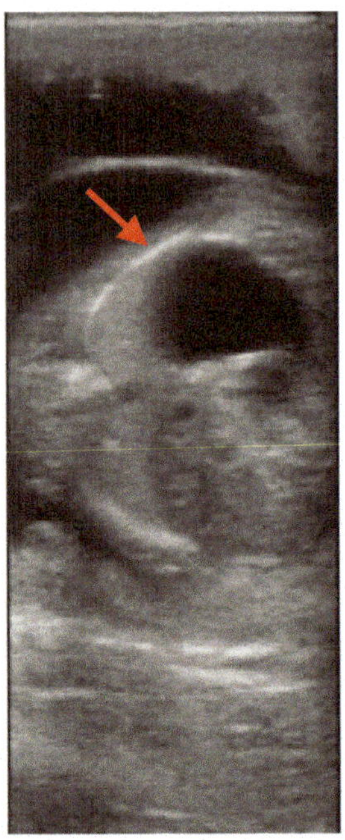

Figure 72.6 Ultrasound image of an equine fetus in plane III at day 100 of gestation showing the ribs (arrow) as a marker for the dorsum of the fetus.

small hyperechoic spot will be seen depending on the quality and focus of the ultrasound machine.

- Moving the ultrasound plane toward plane I, you will see the umbilical entrance to the abdominal cavity (appears as a small black hole). If you move the transducer to plane II you will see a tubercle between the hind legs. The tubercle should be anterior to a line drawn between the stifles if it is a colt (Figure 72.4a).
- Remember that at 52–53 days the tubercle is between the hind limbs in both the male and female. It is not until 55 days of gestation that it can be determined which direction the tubercle appears to be migrating. If the tubercle is anterior to a line drawn between the stifles it will be a colt (Figure 72.4a). If the tubercle is posterior to a line between the stifles it will be a filly (Figure 72.5a). If it is difficult to decide, wait 3 or 4 days and look again.
- Further along in gestation the shaft of the penis and glans penis of the male fetus may be visible (Figure 72.7).

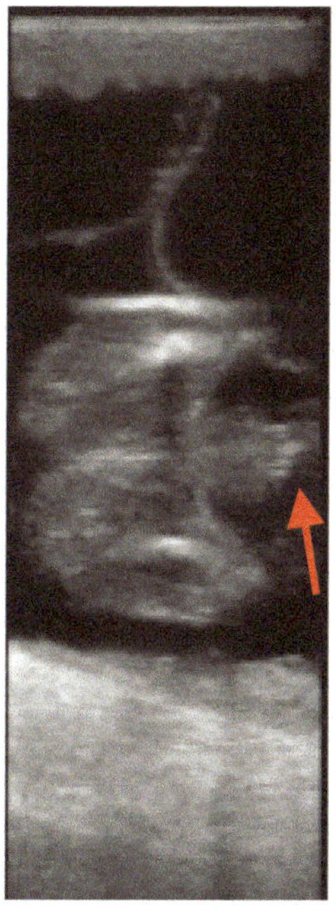

Figure 72.7 Ultrasound image of a male equine fetus in plane II at 95 days of gestation showing the shaft of the penis and glans penis (arrow), which is present anterior to a line drawn between the two stifles.

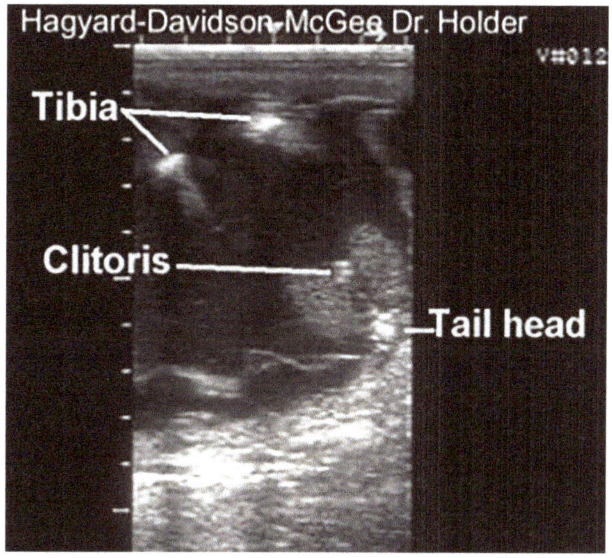

Figure 72.8 Female equine fetus at 112 days of gestation showing the hyperechoic clitoris located beneath the tail head.

Technique: 90–150 Days of Gestation

- Sex determination between 90 and 150 days of gestation involves assessment of the external genitalia of the fetus. After 90 days the fetus may be visible again on transrectal ultrasound examination.
- It is best to scan the entire fetus to become orientated anteriorly, posteriorly, dorsally, and ventrally. It is good to get a cross-sectional view of the abdomen and thorax and, keeping that plane, move off the fetus posteriorly. As you come back onto the fetus, it is possible to get the same tail head–tibial triangle with the clitoris showing up just under the tail head within the triangle (Figure 72.8). If the structure on the midline is too close to the tail, it could be the anus. The ventral midline will appear as a prominent white line running between the clitoris and tail head.
- In a filly, if you follow the prominent ventral midline posteriorly to the tail head, you will encounter the clitoris as asmall round hyperechoic mass or it may appear as two hyperechoic dots lying on each side of the ventral midline (Figure 72.9). If followed anteriorly, you will encounter the mammary gland.

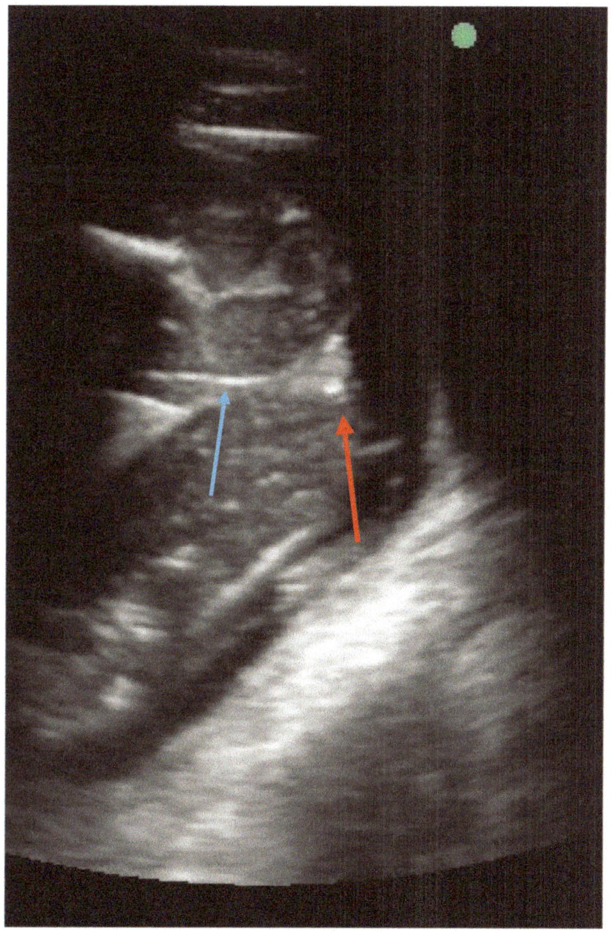

Figure 72.9 Ultrasound image of a female equine fetus at 125 days of gestation showing the clitoris (red arrow) and ventral midline (blue arrow)

- The mammary gland consists of three distinct parts; the bright small hyperechoic teats, on each lateral side of the gland, and two dense halves of the mammary gland separated by a translucent line between the two halves (Figures 72.10 and 72.11). It may be difficult to find all three characteristics of the mammary gland every time.
- Prepucial tissue is not as dense as a mammary gland, does not have a translucent line separating the halves, and obviously has no hyperechoic teats. The prepuce will usually have a hyperechoic glans penis.
- In a male, if you follow the ventral midline posteriorly using plane II, you will encounter nothing before you reach the tail head. If you follow it anteriorly, you will encounter the prepuce (a cone-shaped structure that comes to a point) (Figure 72.12).
- The penis can often readily be seen as a shaft-like structure with a bright hyperechoic mass on the end. This bright hyperechoic tip is the glans penis. A sagittal view through the flank may reveal the shaft of a penis with a hyperechoic tip.

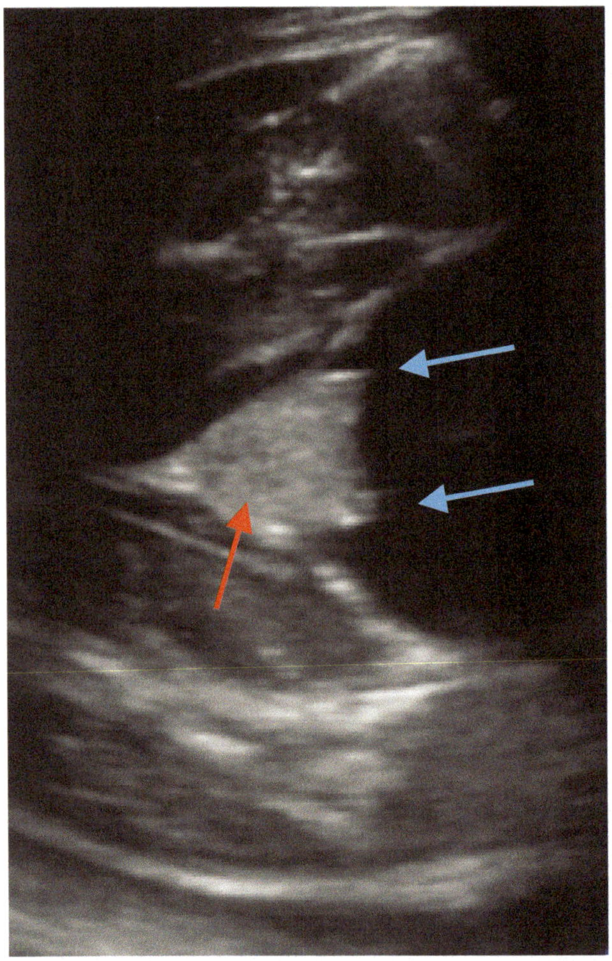

Figure 72.10 Ultrasound image of a mammary gland (red arrow) and teats (blue arrows) of a female equine fetus at 135 days of gestation.

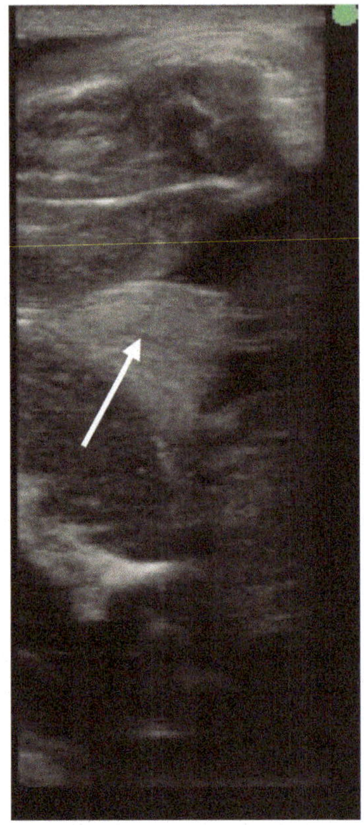

Figure 72.11 Ultrasound image of the mammary gland of a female equine fetus at 134 days of gestation showing a translucent line (arrow) separating the halves of the mammary gland.

- If you are using plane III view (a cross-section of the posterior abdomen), the prepuce will be seen as a cone-shaped structure off the ventral abdomen.
- Frequently, the hyperechoic mass of the glans penis will be seen within the prepuce. It is possible to get a plane III view of the glans penis with little of the prepuce in view as the glans penis frequently protrudes out of the front of the prepuce. This will appear as a hyperechoic mass off the ventral abdominal wall just posterior to the umbilical entrance into the abdominal cavity. The main marker to be utilized to find the external genitalia is the prominent ventral midline.
- The gonads can readily be seen, but in the author's opinion, should be used to support a diagnosis and not to make a diagnosis. The male gonads usually appear very homogeneous (Figure 17.13), whereas the female gonads have a dense central area surrounded by a more translucent peripheral oval ring (Figure 17.14). These can be difficult determinations and are not reliable for a diagnosis by themselves.

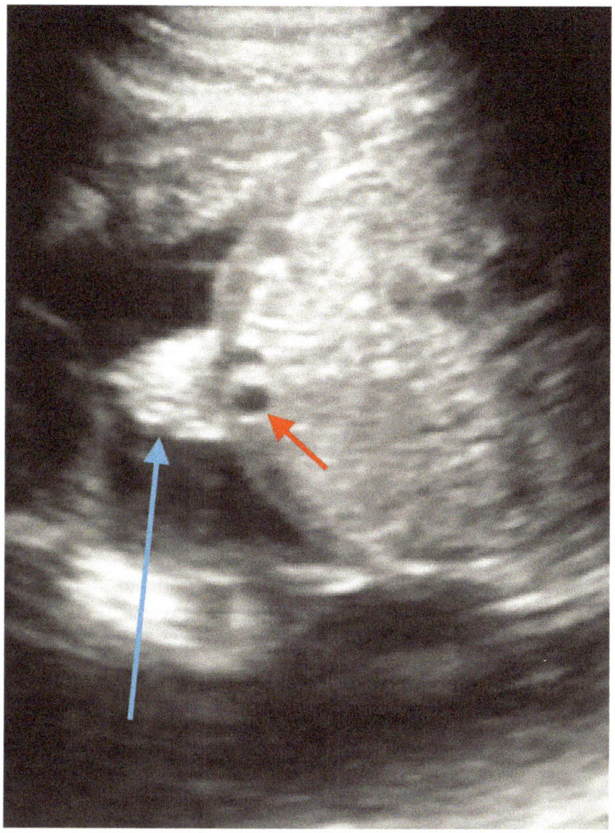

Figure 72.12 Glans penis (blue arrow) within the prepuce of a male equine fetus at 135 days of gestation. Note the urachus visible within the abdomen (red arrow).

- Color Doppler can be used to exhibit a central vein and pampiniform plexus in the male and a peripheral vascular component in the female,

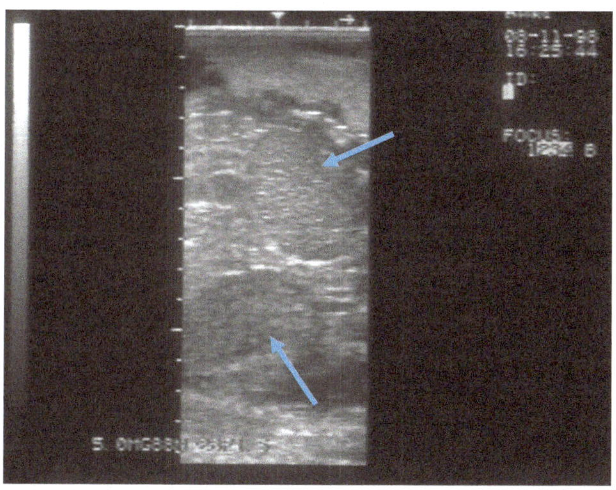

Figure 72.13 Gonads (testes) of a male equine fetus at 130 days of gestation (arrows).

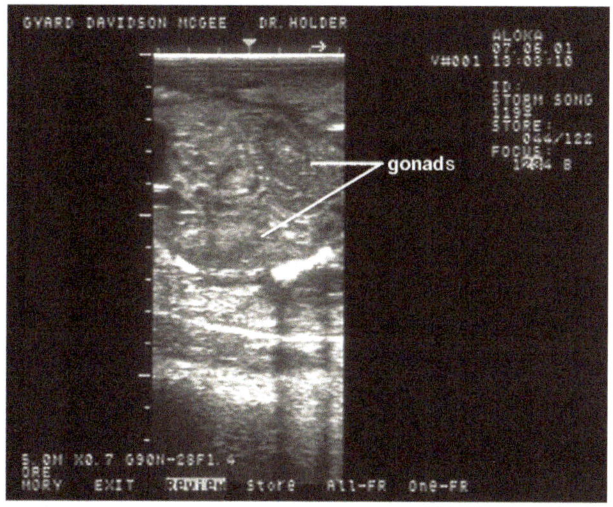

Figure 72.14 Gonads (ovaries) of a female equine fetus.

Technique: After 150 Days of Gestation

- Sex determination after 150 days of gestation is performed by transabdominal ultrasound examination. Around 200 days of gestation the posterior of the fetus is frequently in the area of the mare's sternum and is difficult to examine. The fetus is large and placental tissue is extensive. The fetal tissues are compressed in the groin area at this time making it more difficult to differentiate between tissues.
- Considering the position of the examiner under the mare, use caution. Sedation is frequently used, because a mare may stand quietly then become fractious.
- Alcohol is applied liberally over the ventral midline of the mare's abdomen. The abdomen may need to be clipped of long hair to achieve adequate ultrasound contact.
- Scan the entire ventral midline until the fetus is located. Subsequently locate the beating heart, ribs, and plane III view of the fetus, then proceed posteriorly. Locate the umbilical entrance to the abdominal wall. The transducer must be manipulated in many different directions to expose recognizable anatomic structures. If the mare is tranquilized, the fetus at 62 days can be seen transabdominally lateral to the udder (much higher in the abdomen). At 150 days, it will be near the ventral abdomen. Past 150 days, the posterior of the fetus can be near the sternum. The fetus can be seen transrectally at 150 days, but the posterior of the fetus is frequently out of reach.
- Moving very slowly, look for a hyperechoic mass (glans penis) just posterior to the umbilicus. If nothing is seen, slowly proceed posteriorly until the area of the posterior

abdominal midline and the hind legs converge at the perineal white line. A prepuce, glans, and penis in the male or the triangular mammary gland and teats in the female will be in this area. Caution: the male can exhibit a smaller, very hyperechoic triangular tissue in the groin area.

- If nothing is definitely identifiable, proceed on the ventral midline between the hind legs to the tail head. The clitoris can be seen on the midline in a female just before the tail head is reached. At this stage of gestation, the external genitalia is large and can be seen, but it is often difficult to distinguish between a mammary gland and a prepuce. The prepuce will have varying degrees of a hyperechoic glans and penis, whereas a triangular mammary gland will have no definite hyperechoic area except for two small hyperechoic teats laterally. The triangular mammary gland will be more dense and echoic than the surrounding tissue.
- These scans are difficult at first and may take considerable time. It is good to have a stool to sit on during the exam. Sedate the mare if you are working under her. Trying different sides of the mare sometimes gives better exposure if the posterior fetus is not on the midline.

Interpretation

- The most accurate and efficient time period in which to determine fetal sex is between days 60 and 70 of gestation.
- If the image is not clear at 55–90 days, push down gently on the uterus with the probe to bring the fetus closer to the probe. This changes the focal point for various areas of the fetus and creates movement of fluid in the allantoic fluid causing the fetus to change position slightly.
- If the view of fetus is not productive, turn the transducer 90 degrees to the left. If the view is still not productive, turn the transducer 180 degrees to the right. Somewhere in this 180-degree span is the proper scanning plane for viewing the tubercle.
- If the mare is straining, do not hesitate to use propantheline (30 mg IV) or *N*-butylscopolammonium bromide (40 mg IV) to lessen rectal straining. This enables one to easily move the probe to various positions to get different angles of view of the fetus.
- Do not make a diagnosis solely from a negative view. Always find the tubercle or genitalia to make a diagnosis.
- It may be necessary to extend the probe in front of the hand to reach older fetuses. This is difficult to do without a stiff probe cord.
- Evacuate fecal material as far anteriorly as possible to allow advancement of the probe in front of the hand.
- Get a cross-section of the abdominal cavity to identify the ribs. This will give you the dorso-ventral orientation (the dorso-ventral orientation is very critical in differentiating the hyperechoic tail head and tibias). Proceed posteriorly until you have moved off the fetus. The bright spot on the dorsal area of the posterior fetus as you move back on the fetus will be the tail head. The two bright spots on the ventral area of the posterior fetus will be the tibias. If there is nothing within the triangle formed by the tail head and two tibias, continue to move anteriorly observing the ventral midline.

Reference

Holder RD. 2011. Equine fetal sex determination between 55 and 150 days. In: McKinnon AO, Squires EL, Vaala WE, Varner DD (eds). Equine Reproduction, 2nd edn. Ames, IA: Wiley Blackwell, pp. 2080–93.

Further Reading

Bucca S. 2005. Equine fetal gender determination from mid-to advanced-gestation by ultrasound. *Theriogenology* 64: 568–71.

Curran S, Ginther OJ. 1993. Ultrasonic fetal gender diagnoses during months 5 to 11 in mares. *Theriogenology* 40: 1127–35.

Holder RD. 2001. Sex determination in the mare between 55–150 days gestation. *Proc Annu Am Assoc Eq Pract* 46: 321–4.

Holder RD. 2003. Determination of fetal gender. In: Robinson NE (ed.). Current Therapy in Equine Medicine, 5th edn. Philadelphia: Saunders, pp. 288–94.

Holder RD. 2007. Fetal sex determination. In: Samper JC, Pycock JF, McKinnon AO (eds). Current Therapy in Equine Reproduction. St Louis, NI: Saunders Elsevier, pp. 343–56.

Holder RD. 2014. Use of ultrasonography in equine fetal sex determination between 55 and 200 days of gestation. In: Kidd JA, Lu KG, Frazier M (eds). Atlas of Equine Ultrasonography, 1st edn, Oxford: John Wiley & Sons, pp. 329–40.

73

Assessment of Late-Term Fetal Well-Being

John J. Dascanio

School of Veterinary Medicine, Texas Tech University, USA

Introduction

Assessment of fetal well-being is usually performed by ultrasonographic examination of the uterus, placenta, and fetus in a mid- to late-term pregnant mare. The goal of the examination is to determine fetal and placental status related to gestational age and to identify pathology. The mare may also be examined for signs of premature labor such as an increase in mammary development, an increase in lactogenesis, the presence of vulvar discharge, and the relaxation of perineal ligaments/tissues. Measurement of progestin and total estrogen concentrations may be performed as indicators of premature delivery and fetal viability, respectively (see Chapter 85).

Transabdominal ultrasonography requires the use of a 2.0–4.0 MHz curvilinear array probe to allow for sufficient penetration to visualize structures within the pregnant uterus. A 5–7.5 MHz probe may be used either transabdominally or transrectally to assess more superficial structures, measure utero-placental thickness, and detect placental separation. Transrectal ultrasound examination provides an excellent means to examine the area proximal to the internal cervical os for ascending bacterial placentitis, for early placental detachment, or to detail the presence of fetal carotid/jugular blood flow.

Equipment and Supplies

Red top serum tube, Vacutainer® needles and Vacutainer®, clippers, clipper spray, ultrasound with low frequency probe (≤3.5 MHz), mid-frequency probe (5 MHz), ultrasound gel, obstetrical lubricant, obstetrical sleeves, alcohol, paper towels.

Technique

- Place the mare in stocks or provide sufficient restraint to allow for a safe ultrasonographic examination of her abdomen and to allow for palpation per rectum.
- Sedation is not usually required. If the mare is uncooperative, sedation may be given, but will cause a decrease in fetal viability parameters such as movement and heart rate and will cause extension of the uterus from myometrial relaxation.
- Place a tail wrap and tail rope.
- If the mare has a significantly long-haired coat, her ventral abdomen from the udder to the xyphoid process and laterally to an area level with the stifle may need to be clipped.
- Use an appropriate contact solution for the ultrasound probe such as ultrasound gel or alcohol. A small portable pump sprayer is a convenient way to apply 70% alcohol onto the abdomen or flank of the mare (Figure 73.1).
- Start with a general ultrasound examination to identify the location and orientation of the fetus (Figure 73.2). Fetal orientation does not change significantly after the 10th month of gestation.
- Once the fetus is located, measurements of fetal heart rate, using combined B-mode and M-mode ultrasonography, are made and recorded on a worksheet (Box 73.1). Fetal heart rate varies from about 60 to about 120 beats per minute (bpm) in the last few months of pregnancy. Specific heart rate values for each month of gestation from 6 months onward can be found in Bucca *et al.* (2007).
- Fetal movement should be noted during the examination and correlated with fetal heart rate accelerations/decelerations. An active fetus would be expected to have a higher heart rate.

Equine Reproductive Procedures, Second Edition. Edited by John Dascanio and Patrick McCue.

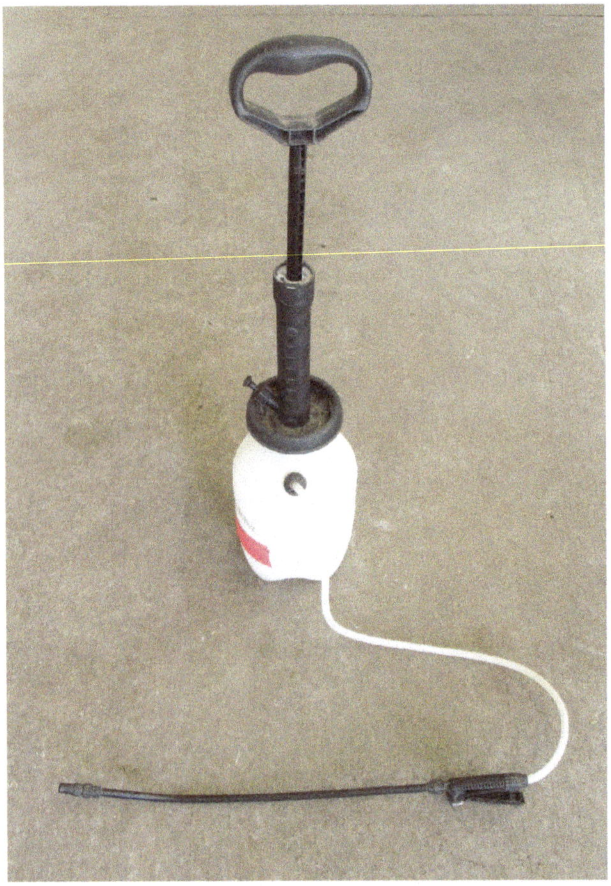

Figure 73.1 Portable pump sprayer for application of alcohol prior to ultrasound examination.

- The depth of allantoic and amniotic fluid compartments should be determined. This is often best done in the area of the uterus where the foal's legs are pushing the uterine wall away from the fetal core. Generally, a maximum value of approximately 14 cm for allantoic and approximately 7 cm for amniotic fluid depth is acceptable in a late-term fetus. An excessive depth of fluid may be associated with a placental hydrops condition. The allantoic and amniotic fluids usually have a small amount of echogenic particles visible, although with fetal movement the amniotic fluid may become slightly turbid.
- The placenta should be examined using transabdominal ultrasound to determine the thickness and to identify areas of separation. Generally, the utero-placental thickness is <20 mm and more commonly <16 mm when measured transabdominally. These measurements should be performed in separate quadrants of the abdomen. Past mid-gestation, the non-pregnant uterine horn often has folding of the placenta and appears to have a thicker measurement than the pregnant uterine horn.
- Transrectal ultrasonography should be performed to assess the utero-placental unit just in front of the internal cervical os (Figure 73.3). The thickness of the utero-placental unit (combined thickness of the uterus and placenta, CTUP) varies from a maximum thickness of ~8 mm at 270–300 days of gestation to ~10 mm at 300–330 days to ~12 mm at >330 days. An increased CTUP may indicate placentitis. Measurements are made over the left or right middle uterine artery.
- If the fetal heart rate was inaccessible via transabdominal ultrasound, then a fetal pulse rate may be obtained

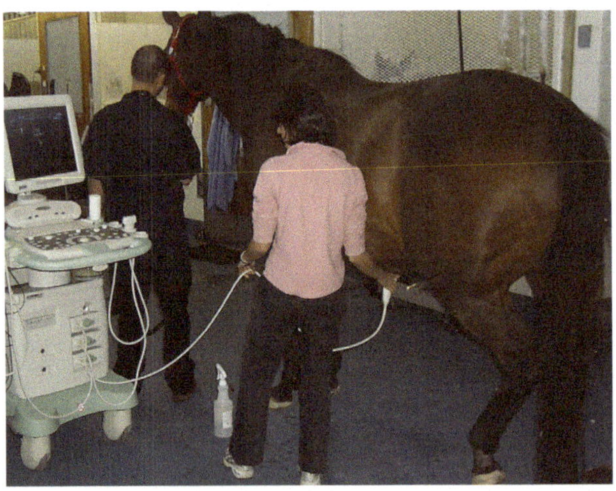

Figure 73.2 Transabdominal ultrasonography of a late-term pregnant mare.

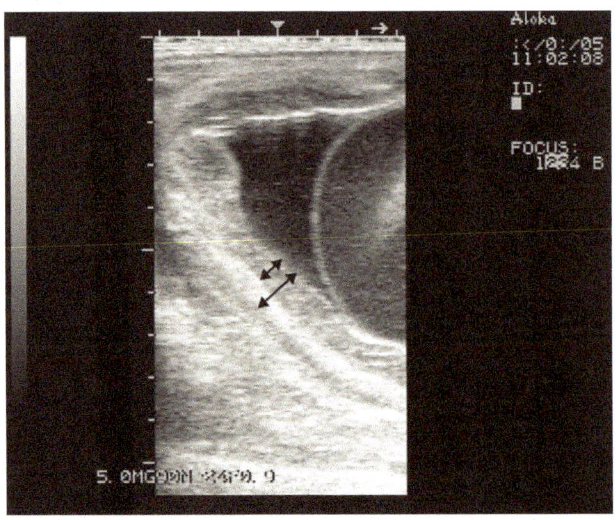

Figure 73.3 Transrectal ultrasonography of placental edema in a near-term normal mare, showing the placenta (short arrow) and utero-placental thickness or CTUP (combined thickness of the uterus and placenta) (long arrow).

Box 73.1 Late-Term Mare Ultrasound Worksheet

Date ____________________ Mare ____________________________ Clinician(s) ____________________

Combined Thickness of the Uterus and Placenta (CTUP): Taken over left and right middle uterine artery just cranial to cervix (normal ~8 mm <300 days, ~10 mm 300–330 days, ~12 mm >330 days)

Right CTUP ____ cm   Left CTUP ____cm

Utero-placental Thickness: Right cranial _____ cm   Left cranial _____ cm

(normal up to ~20 mm)   Right caudal _____ cm   Left caudal _____cm

Depth of Allantoic Fluid: Right cranial _____ cm   Left cranial _____ cm

(normal up to ~14 cm)   Right caudal _____ cm   Left caudal _____ cm

Quality of Allantoic Fluid: (circle one) – represents amount of echogenic debris (normal ~1.4)

0 = no particles   1 = small amount   2 = moderate   3 = very echogenic

Depth of Amnionic Fluid: Right   cranial _____ cm   Left cranial _____ cm

(normal up to ~7 cm) Right caudal _______ cm   Left caudal ______ cm

Quality of Amnionic Fluid: (circle one) – represents amount of echogenic debris (normal ~1.5)

0 = no particles   1 = small amount   2 = moderate   3 = very echogenic

Fetal Activity: (circle one) –% indicates time during exam that foal was active (normal ~1.5)

0 = no movement   1 = active <33%   2 = moderately active 33–66%   = very active >66%

Fetal Heart Rate (HR): Multiple measurements of HR over 30 minutes – average results from three measurements during same examination

____ bpm   ____ bpm   ____ bpm   ____ Average

Fetal Aortic Diameter: ____ cm   **Fetal Thoracic Diameter:** ____ cm

Fetal Orbital Measurements: Height ____ cm   Width ____ cm

Fetal Sex: Male   Female   **Fetal Presentation:** Anterior Posterior

Uterine Horn Fetus Occupying: Right   Left   **Mare Weight:** ____ lb

Comments: ____

____

____

transrectally by ultrasound examination of the carotid artery in the foal's neck.

- Other more specific measurements may also be taken including aortic root diameter, fetal eye width/height, and fetal breathing movements.
- Blood may be collected from the mare for progestin and total estrogen concentrations. This should be done every other day for three to four sampling periods to determine trends in hormone concentrations in mares at high risk of abortion.

Interpretation

- A change in progestin profile from that expected (increase or decrease) may signify a potential for premature delivery. A premature increase in progestin concentration prior to day 300 of gestation suggests fetal stress or accelerated maturation. A decrease in progestin, especially after an increase, may signify imminent parturition within a 7-day period. A consistently low concentration may signify exposure to fescue endophytes.
- A decrease in total estrogens from reference values over a number of days is potentially a negative indicator of fetal viability.
- Fetal movement may increase the echogenicity of allantoic or amniotic fluid. Highly echogenic fluid without fetal movement may indicate pathology.
- There should be no separation of the placenta from the endometrium. Separation of the chorioallantois from the uterus is highly suggestive of placentitis. Areas of separation should be monitored closely and treatment initiated, which may include systemic antibiotics, progestin administration, and anti-inflammatory medications.
- Any deviation of fetal heart rate values from normal should be correlated to fetal movement and should be checked again on secondary examinations. It is not uncommon for the heart rate to increase in an active fetus. Having a high heart rate in an inactive fetus may be a negative indicator.
- Large blood vessels in the uterine wall should be differentiated from areas of separation using Doppler ultrasonography (see Chapter 76).
- Placental edema may be present in a near-term fetus as seen with transrectal ultrasound assessment. In earlier stages of pregnancy it may indicate placental inflammation.

Reference

Bucca S, Carli A, Fogarty UMG. 2007. How to assess equine viability by transrectal ultrasound evaluation of fetal peripheral pulses. *Proc Annu Conv Am Assoc Eq Pract* 53: 335–8.

Further Reading

Bucca S, Fogarty U, Collins A, Small V. 2005. Assessment of feto-placental well-being in the mare from mid-gestation to term: transrectal and transabdominal ultrasonographic features. *Theriogenology* 64: 542–57.

Morris S, Kelleman AA, Stawicki RJ, *et al.* 2007. Transrectal ultrasonography and plasma progestin profiles identifies feto-placental compromise in mares with experimentally induced placentitis. *Theriogenology* 67: 681–91.

74

Combined Thickness of the Uterus and Placenta

Patrick M. McCue

Equine Reproduction Laboratory, Colorado State University, USA

Introduction

Bacterial and fungal infections of the pregnant mare's uterus and placenta are most commonly due to ascending infections through the cervix, which result in a localized thickening of the placenta in the area of the cervix. Measurement of the combined thickness of the uterus and placenta (CTUP) and evaluation of the relationship between the chorioallantoic membrane and uterus of the mare are used to screen for placentitis and placental separation.

Equipment and Supplies

Ultrasound machine, obstetrical sleeves, obstetrical lube.

Technique

- The CTUP measurement is obtained via ultrasonography per rectum. The chorioallantois and uterus may appear as one combined echogenic structure, although the echotexture between the two structures can be differentiated using a high detail ultrasound unit in mares and especially near parturition. There should not, however, be any separation between the chorioallantois and uterus.
- The optimal location for the CTUP measurement is the ventral aspect of the uterine body, below the cervical–placental junction and on either side just lateral to the midline. The landmarks for measurement are: (i) the hypoechoic uterine branch of the vaginal artery that courses along the outside of the uterus lateral to midline (Figure 74.1); (ii) the hyperechoic combined tissue of the uterine wall and the chorioallantois; and (iii) the hypoechoic allantoic cavity (Figure 74.2).
- The average CTUP measurements for normal mares are presented in Figure 74.3. In general, normal CTUP measurements are 8 mm or less from 270 to 300 days of gestation, 10 mm or less from 300 to 330 days of gestation, and 12 mm or less at 330+ days of gestation. Detection of a

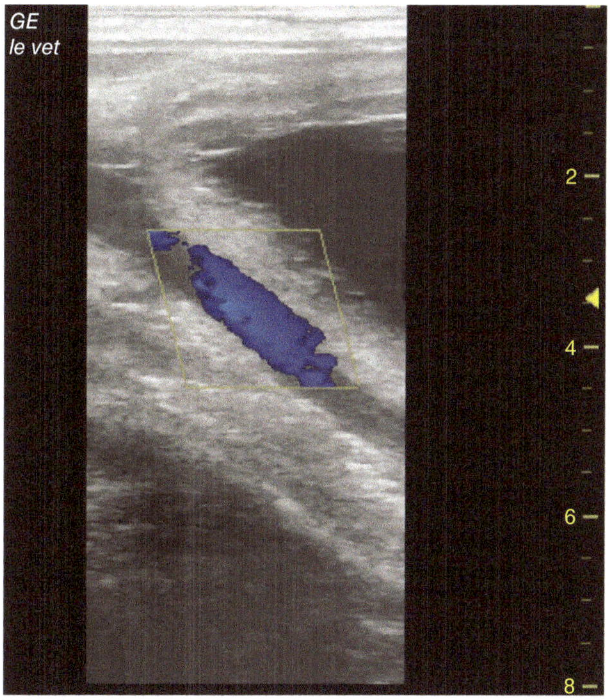

Figure 74.1 Color Doppler ultrasound image demonstrating the uterine branch of the vaginal artery vessel location next to the uterus.

Equine Reproductive Procedures, Second Edition. Edited by John Dascanio and Patrick McCue.

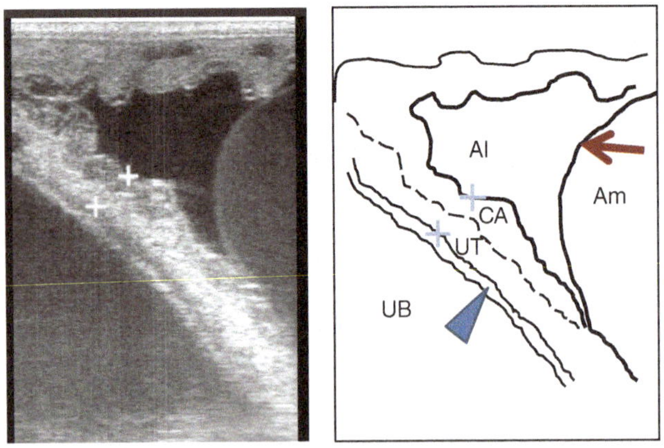

Figure 74.2 Ultrasound measurement of the combined thickness of the uterus and placenta (11.2 mm). The marker (+) on the left is along the outside of the uterus along the uterine branch of the vaginal artery. The marker (+) on the right is at the edge of the allantoic cavity. In the drawing on the right, Al is the allantoic cavity, Am is the amnionic cavity, CA is the chorioallantoic membrane, UT is the uterus, and UB is the urinary bladder; the red arrow points to the amnionic membrane, and the blue arrowhead points to the blood vessel outside the uterus.

CTUP value greater than that expected for the gestational age suggests ascending placentitis or another abnormality (Figure 74.4). Separation of the chorioallantois from the uterus is also likely due to placentitis (Figure 74.5).

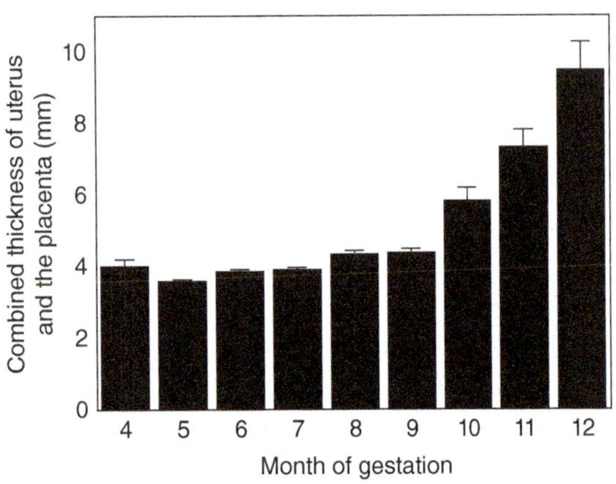

Figure 74.3 Average combined thickness of the uterus and placenta in normal mares. Source: From Renaudin CD, Troedsson MH, Gillis CL, King VL, Bodena A. 1997. Ultrasonographic evaluation of the equine placenta by transrectal and transabdominal approach in the normal pregnant mare. *Theriogenology* 47: 559–73. Reproduced with the permission of Elsevier.

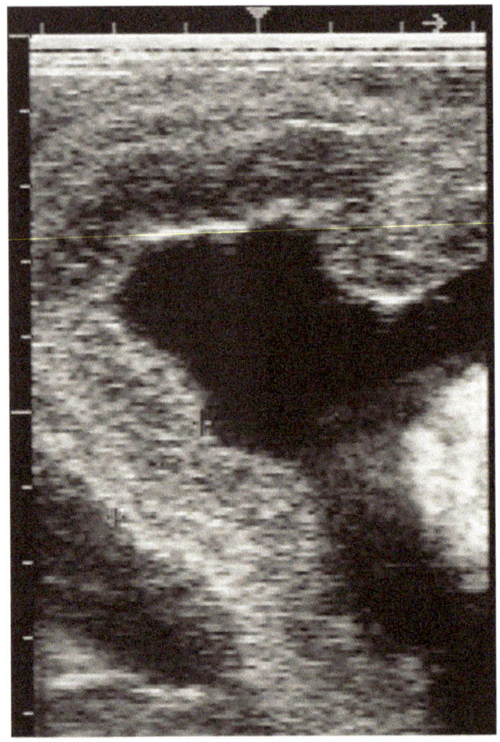

Figure 74.4 Ultrasound image of a placenta exhibiting increased thickness and a CTUP measurement of 17.5 mm.

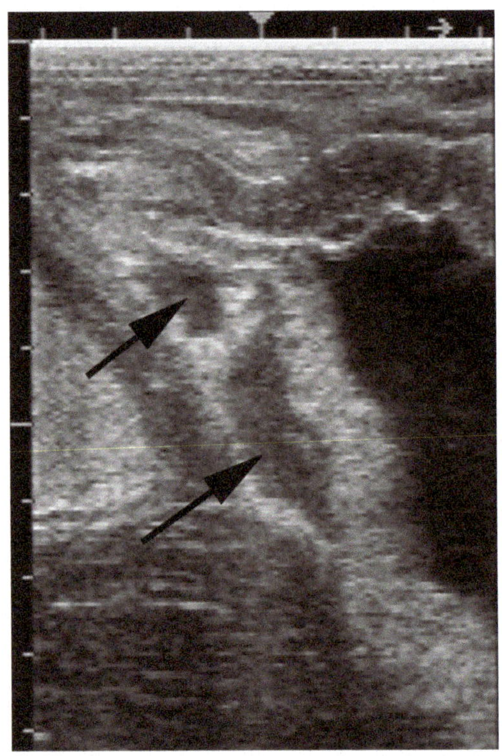

Figure 74.5 Ultrasound image showing separation (arrows) of the chorioallantois from the uterus. Echogenic fluid can be noted between the chorioallantois and the uterus.

Interpretation and Additional Comments

An increase in placental thickness, with or without evidence of separation from the uterus, may be due to placentitis. Other clinical signs associated with placentitis include mammary gland development, premature lactation, cervical discharge, and vaginal discharge. If untreated, placentitis may lead to abortion. Therapy usually consists of broad-spectrum antibiotics (i.e., either oral trimethoprim-sulfamethoxasole or a combination of penicillin and an aminoglycoside), progesterone or progestin (e.g., altrenogest), and a non-steroidal anti-inflammatory agent. Separation usually occurs ventral to the cervix, however cases have been documented where separation occurred on the dorsal uterus. Occasionally, a large blood vessel may be confused with a focal area of separation. Persistent ultrasonographic monitoring of the area in question may reveal turbulent blood flow through the vessel or the use of color flow Doppler ultrasound may distinguish these areas.

Reference

Renaudin CD, Troedsson MH, Gillis CL, King VL, Bodena A. 1997. Ultrasonographic evaluation of the equine placenta by transrectal and transabdominal approach in the normal pregnant mare. *Theriogenology* 47: 559–73.

Further Reading

Bucca S, Fogarty U, Collins A, Small V. 2005. Assessment of feto-placental well-being in the mare from mid-gestation to term: transrectal and transabdominal ultrasonographic features. *Theriogenology* 64: 542–57.

Troedsson MHT, Macpherson ML. 2011. Placentitis. In: McKinnon AO, Squires EL, Vaala WE, Varner DD (eds). Equine Reproduction, 2nd edn. Ames, IA: Wiley Blackwell, pp. 2359–67.

Troedsson MHT, Renaudin CD, Zent WW, Steiner JV. 1997. Transrectal ultrasonography of the placenta in normal mares and mares with pending abortion: a field study. *Proc Annu Conv Am Assoc Eq Pract* 43: 256–8.

75

Placentitis: Diagnosis and Treatment

Justin W. McNaughten[1] *and Margo L. Macpherson*[2]

[1]*Rhinebeck Equine LLP, USA*
[2]*College of Veterinary Medicine, University of Florida, USA*

Introduction

Placentitis, is an important cause of pregnancy loss in the mare. Placental infections occurring in late gestation may result in abortion, premature delivery, or increased neonatal morbidity and mortality. Bacterial infections are the most common cause of equine placentitis and include *Streptococcus equi* subspecies *zooepidemicus*, *Escherichia coli*, *Klebsiella* species, *Pseudomonas* species, *Staphylococcus aureus*, *Leptospira* species, and Nocardia-type (*Crossiella equi* and *Amycolatopsis* species) organisms. Fungal placentitis due to *Candida albicans* or *Aspergillus* species infections are less common.

Ascending infection is the most common route of placental infection in which bacteria invade the caudal reproductive tract and migrate proximally through the cervix to the placenta. Infective organisms colonize the caudal placenta at the cervical star and disrupt the intimate contact between the allantochorion and endometrium. Infection may spread to the fetus via the umbilical cord and amnion resulting in abortion. Secondary inflammation, placental thickening, separation, and compromise generally result in premature delivery of a non-viable foal. Mares affected with Nocardia-type placentitis often have significant placental compromise at the juncture of the uterine body and pregnant uterine horn, but the fetus itself is not infected. In some cases of placentitis, precocious maturation is induced and the foal survives early delivery. This scenario is particularly true in mares infected with Nocardia-type organisms.

Premature udder development and purulent vulvar discharge are clinical signs associated with placentitis. However, neither is pathognomonic for the condition. Premature mammary development might not be evident until placental lesions are well advanced. The presence of vulvar discharge is highly variable, as the discharge may be wiped away by the mare's tail and easily missed. Ultrasonography offers real-time information regarding placental integrity and fetal health. Transrectal ultrasonography is a useful tool for evaluating fetal viability, fetal activity, fetal fluid character, and placental integrity. The caudal aspect of the allantochorion at the cervical star is the most frequently affected area in mares with ascending placentitis. A thorough examination of this area using transrectal ultrasonography is critical when evaluating mares for the presence of placentitis. Values of the combined thickness of the uterus and placenta (CTUP) for normal pregnancies have been established (Renaudin *et al.* 1997). Mares with placental infection or inflammation usually have an increase in CTUP measurement and/or separation of the allantochorion from the uterus with purulent material. A thorough transabdominal ultrasonographic examination should be performed to establish a baseline information on placental integrity; placental fluid character; and fetal health including heart rate, activity, and size, as well as excluding the presence of twins (see Chapters 70 and 73).

Equipment and Supplies

Exam gloves, blood collection tubes and needles, ultrasound machine with linear (5–10 MHz) and curvilinear (2.5–3.5 MHz) ultrasound transducer, ultrasound lubricant, alcohol, obstetrical sleeves, obstetrical lubricant, clippers, tail wrap, tail rope, non-irritant soap, roll cotton, stainless steel bucket, disposable liner bag for bucket, paper towels, vaginal speculum, double-guarded swab, bacterial/fungal transport media, sterile lubricant, light source.

Equine Reproductive Procedures, Second Edition. Edited by John Dascanio and Patrick McCue.

Diagnosis

- The breeding records should be reviewed prior to the clinical examination. The mare's gestational length should be calculated based on the last breeding date or date of ovulation. A history of double ovulations or previous diagnosis of twins should be noted.
- The mare should be placed in stocks or have adequate restraint applied in order to perform a thorough clinical examination, transrectal palpation and ultrasonography, transabdominal ultrasonography, and vaginal exam/culture (if indicated) (see Chapter 10).
- Sedation should be avoided if possible so that fetal heart rate and fetal activity are not altered.
- A routine clinical examination should be performed, even though mares with placentitis are rarely systemically compromised.
- Baseline laboratory data obtained at admission may include a complete blood count, serum chemistry, and lactate. These data may help differentiate placentitis from conditions affecting the gastrointestinal or musculoskeletal systems.
- Additional tests that are often useful include blood progesterone and serum amyloid A levels. Serial measurements may be useful to assess initial condition and subsequent response to treatment.
- The mammary gland should be assessed for size, symmetry, and the presence of mammary secretions, milk, or wax (Figure 75.1). If mammary secretions can be readily expressed from the mare's teat, a sample should be collected to measure electrolytes and pH (see Chapters 89 and 90). Changes in mammary secretion electrolytes and pH can be monitored to predict impending parturition or response to treatment.

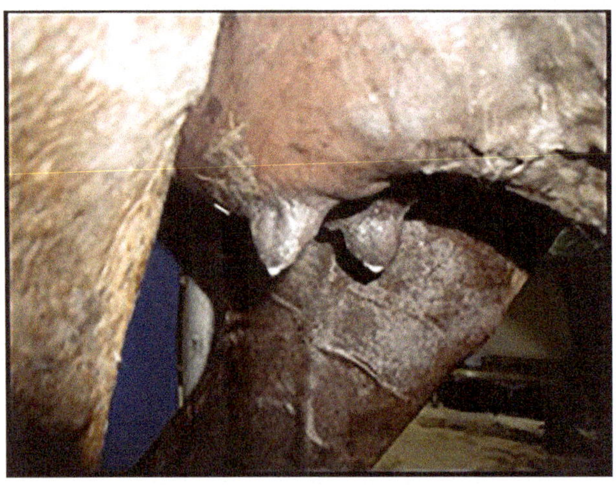

Figure 75.1 Milk secretions in a mare with precocious mammary development.

- The perineal conformation should be assessed. Mares with poor conformation are predisposed to an ascending bacterial infection and may benefit from a Caslick vulvoplasty (see Chapters 5 and 53).
- A visual inspection of the perineum, tail head, and hind quarters should be performed to identify presence of any discharge (Figures 75.2 and 75.3). If vulvar discharge is present, a sample of the discharge should be obtained for culture and cytology.
- Transrectal ultrasonographic examination should be performed prior to transabdominal examination so that the caudal placenta can be evaluated prior to fetal stimulation and movement into the pelvic canal.
- Prior to transrectal ultrasonography, the rectum should be evacuated of any fecal material. Care should be taken not to stimulate the fetus if possible. Increased fetal activity or presence of the fetal extremities in the area of the cervical star may impede the operator's ability to accurately measure the CTUP.
- A linear probe is introduced into the mare's rectum and advanced cranially beyond the urinary bladder and towards the caudal placenta (cervical star area). The transducer is placed slightly lateral to the cervix and cranial to the internal cervical os.

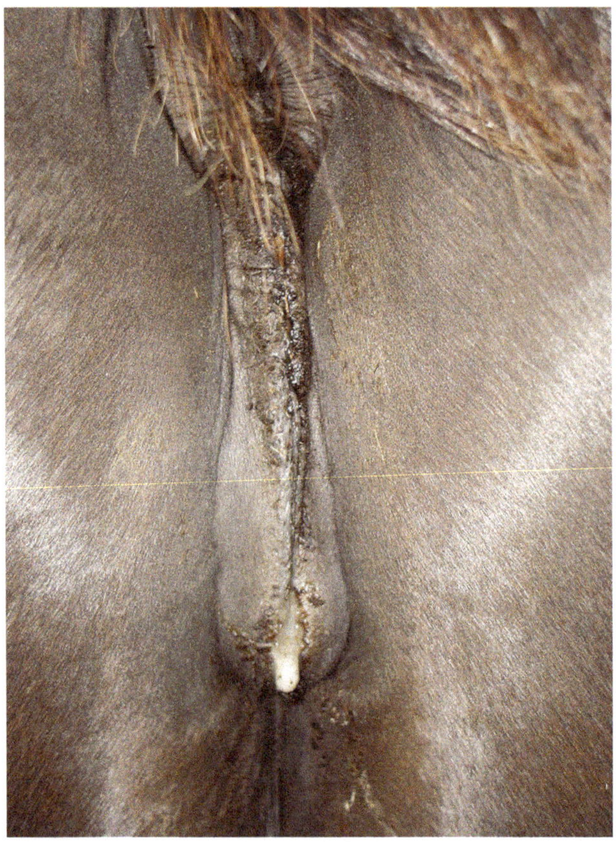

Figure 75.2 A late-term mare with purulent vaginal discharge.

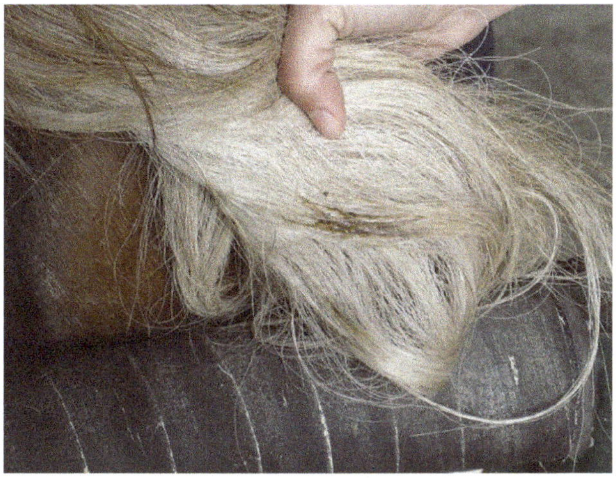

Figure 75.3 A late-term mare with purulent discharge in the ventral tail hairs. It is possible that this may be the only indication of a placentitis. The ventral tail should be examined with each reproductive examination.

- A large hypoechoic blood vessel below the uterus is used as a landmark to ensure uniform measurement of the CTUP.
- Digital calipers on the ultrasound machine are used to measure the CTUP. The points for measurement are: (i) the junction of the uterine branch of the vaginal arteries and the uterus; and (ii) the junction between the chorioallantois and the allantoic compartment (Figure 75.4). Three measurements should be taken and averaged. Values obtained can be compared with normal reference ranges (Table 75.1).
- The placenta is subsequently assessed for areas of placental separation and accumulation of hyperechogenic exudate near the area of the cervical star (Figure 75.5).
- Color Doppler is a useful tool to enable the operator to confidently differentiate areas of suspected placental separation from larger uterine vessels (see Chapter 76).
- The character of the fetal fluids is also evaluated with ultrasound examination. Allantoic fluid is generally anechoic (black) to slightly echogenic in the late-term mare. The amniotic fluid is mildly to moderately echogenic (light gray) in a normal pregnancy. A small amount of echogenic particles is normal with an active fetus.

Table 75.1 Normal values for ultrasound measurement of the combined thickness of the uterus and placenta (CTUP).

Gestational Day	CTUP (mm)
Day 271–300	<8 mm
Day 301–330	<10 mm
>Day 330	<12 mm

From Renaudin *et al.* (1997).

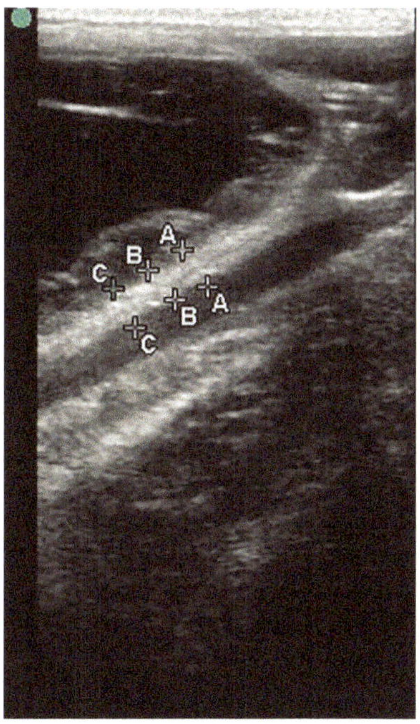

Figure 75.4 Measurement of the combined thickness of the uterus and placenta (CTUP). The span from A to A denotes the thickness of the placenta and uterus. Three measurements were taken in this examination as denoted by the letters (A-A, B-B, C-C).

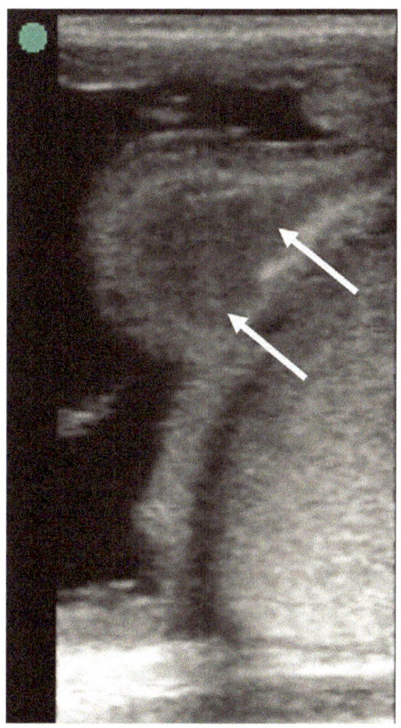

Figure 75.5 An area of separation of the chorioallantois from the uterine wall with accumulation of hyperechoic exudate (white arrows) near the cervical star.

- Fluids that are highly echogenic or consistently have flocculent material present may indicate infection.
- In mares with ascending bacterial placentitis, the echogenicity of the amniotic fluid often increases before echogenic changes occur in the allantoic compartment.
- Transabdominal ultrasonographic examination is performed, ideally, using a 2.5–3.5 MHz transducer. In some cases, evaluation of fetal heart rate and fetal fluid character can be accomplished with a linear ultrasound transducer.
- Contact solution (ultrasound gel or alcohol) should be applied liberally to the ventral abdomen. The abdominal area may require clipping to optimize evaluation.
- Transabdominal ultrasound examination often begins near the mammary gland and the transducer is moved cranial to the xiphoid, and caudal to the mammary gland, until the fetal thorax and heart are located. Serial fetal heart rate measures should be obtained as soon as possible in the event the fetus is stimulated and moves out of view.
- The fetal heart rate can be determined utilizing M-mode or by visual count. Minor adjustments or rotation of the transducer may improve the ability to clearly identify the chambers of the fetal heart. The average heart rate in a fetus greater than 300 days' gestation is approximately 75 ± 7 bpm, but there is significant individual variation in heart rates. Fetal heart rate decreases by approximately 10 bpm at greater than 330 days' gestation. Heart rates that are consistently low (less than 55 bpm) or high (greater than 120 bpm) are associated with fetal stress and warrant re-examination (Reef *et al.* 1996).
- In addition, color Doppler may be used to determine to confirm fetal viability by identifying blood flow within the fetal vessels and the umbilical cord.
- The placenta should be carefully evaluated during the transabdominal exam for any evidence of placental separation with hyperechoic exudate between the chorioallantois and the uterus which are suggestive of nocardioform placentitis.
- The entire abdomen should be sequentially examined for presence of twin fetuses as the transabdominal view is the only accurate way to identify late-term twins.
- A sample of cervical or vaginal discharge, if present, may be collected for microbial culture following ultrasound examinations. A vaginal speculum can be used to examine the vaginal vault and external cervical os for the presence of inflammation and exudate. A double-guarded uterine swab can be used to collect a sample of exudate from the external cervical os or cranial vagina. The cervix should not be penetrated to avoid possible stimulation of uterine contractions. Samples should be submitted for microbial culture and antibiotic sensitivity pattern.

Interpretation

A thorough physical examinations combined with reproductive history and advanced diagnostic tools are the most effective means of identifying mares with placentitis. The disease process is insidious and is often well advanced by the time clinical signs are identified. It may be beneficial to examine aged, multiparous mares and/or mares with a history of pregnancy loss as early as 5–6 months of gestation, followed by serial monitoring every 2–4 weeks thereafter in order to detect the onset of placentitis or to monitor response to treatment.

Therapy for Placentitis

Multiple components of placentitis must be addressed when considering therapeutic options. Therapies for treating mares with placentitis should be selected for efficacy, known pharmacokinetics in pregnant mares, and client compliance for administration. Drugs that are commonly used in mares with placentitis are listed in Table 75.2.

In most cases, bacterial infection is the cause of placentitis. Controlling bacterial infection through use of targeted antimicrobial treatment is a critical first step. Ideally, antimicrobial selection should be based on culture and sensitivity information obtained from a vulvar/cervical discharge sample. In the event of clinical signs (mammary development, placental thickening/separation) without vulvar discharge, antimicrobial therapies should be broad spectrum for Gram-positive and Gram-negative bacterial organisms. Prophylactic administration of antifungal agents is generally not recommended without evidence of fungal infection, such as identification of fungal organisms via culture and/or cytology.

Inflammation and prostaglandin production, as a result of bacterial infection, often persist after bacterial infection is cleared. Inflammatory processes are likely culprits in premature delivery of foals, therefore medications aimed at controlling inflammation and uterine contraction are an essential component of a therapeutic plan. Combined therapy, consisting of an effective antimicrobial agent, an anti-inflammatory agent, and supplemental progestins, have shown success in improving foal viability from mares with placentitis (Bailey *et al.* 2010).

It is recommended that mares diagnosed with placentitis be treated from the onset of clinical signs or detection of placentitis until the foal is born. Anecdotal reports have been made of recrudescence of clinical signs or active placentitis after shorter term (2–3 weeks) duration of treatment.

Table 75.2 Common therapies administered to pregnant mares.

Drug	Dosage	Mechanism of Action	Comments
Potassium penicillin	22,000 U/kg IV, q 6 hours	Antimicrobial	Identified in fetal fluids
Procaine penicillin	22,000 U/kg IM, q 12 hours	Antimicrobial	
Gentamicin sulfate	6.6 mg/kg IV or IM, q 24 hours	Antimicrobial	Identified in fetal fluids
Trimethoprim sulfamethoxazole	15–30 mg/kg PO, q 12 hours	Antimicrobial	Identified in fetal fluids, tissues, and placenta
Trimethoprim sulfadiazine		Antimicrobial	Not tested in placentitis; approved for horses
Ceftiofur sodium	4.4 mg/kg IM, q 24 hours	Antimicrobial	Does not pass placenta at therapeutic concentrations
Ceftiofur crystalline free acid	6.6 mg/kg IM, q 96 hours	Antimicrobial	Does not pass placenta at therapeutic concentrations
Doxycycline	10 mg/kg PO, q 12 hours	Antimicrobial	Identified in fetal fluids; safety for foals not established
Enrofloxacin	5 mg/kg IV 7.5 mg/kg PO q 24 hours	Antimicrobial	Effects on fetal cartilage unclear
Flunixin meglumine	1.1 mg/kg IV or PO, q 12–24 hours	Anti-inflammatory (mixed Cox-1 and -2 inhibition)	Not identified in fetal fluids
Phenylbutazone	2.2–4.4 mg/kg PO, q 12–24 hours	Anti-inflammatory	
Firocoxib	0.3 mg/kg PO, loading dose; 0.1 mg/kg PO, daily dose	Anti-inflammatory (Cox-2 selective)	Identified in fetal fluids, tissues, and placenta
Pentoxifylline	8.5 mg/kg PO, q 12 hours	Anticytokine/anti-inflammatory	Identified in fetal fluids and tissues
Altrenogest	0.088 mg/kg PO, q 24 hours	Anti-prostaglandin tocolytic	
Acetylsalicylic acid	50 mg/kg PO, q 12 hours	Anti-inflammatory antiplatelet	

References

Bailey CS, Macpherson ML, Pozor MA, *et al.* 2010. Treatment efficacy of trimethoprim sulfamethoxazole, pentoxifylline and altrenogest in experimentally induce placentitis. *Theriogenology* 74: 402–12.

Reef VB, Vaala WE, Worth LT, Sertich PL, Spencer PA. 1996. Ultrasonographic assessment of fetal well-being during late gestation: development of an equine biophysical profile. *Eq Vet J* 28(3): 200–8.

Renaudin CD, Troedsson MH, Gillis CL, King VL, Bodena A. 1997. Ultrasonographic evaluation of the equine placenta by transrectal and transabdominal approach in the normal pregnant mare. *Theriogenology* 47: 559–73.

Further Reading

Troedsson MHT, Macpherson ML. 2011. Placentitis. In: McKinnon AO, Squires EL, Vaala WE, Varner DD (eds). Equine Reproduction, 2nd edn. Ames, IA: Wiley Blackwell, pp. 2359–67.

76

Doppler Ultrasonography

John J. Dascanio

School of Veterinary Medicine, Texas Tech University, USA

Introduction

Doppler ultrasonography is an enhancement to regular ultrasound evaluations. Doppler may be used to detail blood flow within a mare's ovary and the testes in the stallion, and for assessing fetal viability. The pulsed wave Doppler form of spectral Doppler provides detailed information over a relatively small area whereas color Doppler and power Doppler provide limited information over a larger region. Depending on the reason for the examination, one or all modes may be used.

Pulsed wave Doppler will allow for specific measurement of blood flow, enabling the calculation of flow indices. The angle of the probe in relation to the vessel scanned will influence the velocity measurements obtained, but does not affect index measurements.

- Peak systolic velocity = PSV
- End diastolic velocity = EDV
- Mean velocity = MV
- Resistance index (RI) = (PSV – EDV)/PSV
- Pulsatility index (PI) = (PSV – EDV)/MV

With pulsed wave Doppler, as the probe becomes more perpendicular (90 degrees) to the vessel scanned, the amplitude of the waveforms obtained decreases. When measuring flow indexes, the angle of interrogation (ultrasound beam to vessel angle) should be <30 degrees and the gate (sample volume) should be minimized to be within the vessel scanned.

Color flow Doppler provides a colorized depiction of blood flow, providing a generalized idea of flow detail. Red colorization typically is blood flow toward the probe, while blue is blood flow away from the probe. This is currently the most common Doppler type used to determine fetal viability or the presence/absence of large blood vessels/areas of separation in the placenta. A higher gain setting on the ultrasound will tend to increase signals (artifacts) from the surrounding tissue. Too low a gain setting will not allow for the detection of vessels. Higher frequency probes tend to give more sensitivity to lower flow vessels. Decreasing the region of interest (width of the color flow area) should also enhance the examination area by improving frame rate and temporal resolution.

Power Doppler is similar to color Doppler, but there is only variation of one color (red). Power Doppler provides greater depiction of small blood vessels and lower flow rates than color Doppler and thus gives a better idea of total vascularity. Unlike color Doppler, power Doppler does not provide information about direction and velocity of flow.

Equipment and Supplies

Ultrasound machine with enabled Doppler functions and probes with Doppler abilities, ultrasound gel, clippers, clipper spray, obstetrical sleeve, obstetrical lubricant.

Technique for Assessing a Pregnant Mare and Fetus

- Items that may be assessed with Doppler include: fetal heart rate, umbilical blood flow, placental blood vessels, middle uterine artery blood flow, and blood flow in the area surrounding a developing embryo (Figure 76.1).
- Transabdominal ultrasound requires a lower frequency probe (2–4 MHz) to acquire enough penetration depth to adequately view mid- to late-term pregnancies. Most often transabdominal ultrasound examinations would be conducted after about 80 days of gestation. A mid-range probe (5–7.5 MHz) may be used to assess more superficial structures such as ventral placental wall blood flow.

Equine Reproductive Procedures, Second Edition. Edited by John Dascanio and Patrick McCue.

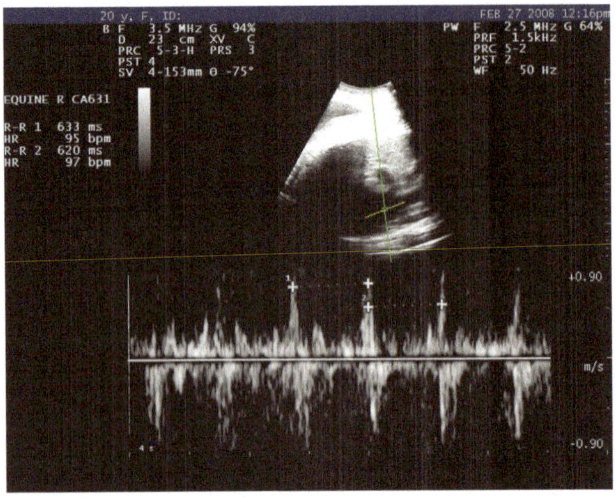

Figure 76.1 Pulsed Doppler used to obtain the heart rate during a transabdominal fetal well-being examination. The heart rate in this fetus on two measurements was 95 and 97 beats per minute.

- Transrectal ultrasound assessment may be performed throughout pregnancy. Early in pregnancy the ovaries, fetus, or uterus may be scanned. Later in pregnancy measurements for combined thickness of the uterus and placenta (CTUP) may be augmented by the use of color Doppler (Figure 76.2) (see Chapter 74). The viability of a late-term fetus may be detected by assessment of jugular/carotid blood flow.
- Doppler can be useful to distinguish areas of placental separation from large uterine vessels in pregnant mares when doing a fetal well-being assessment (Figure 76.3).

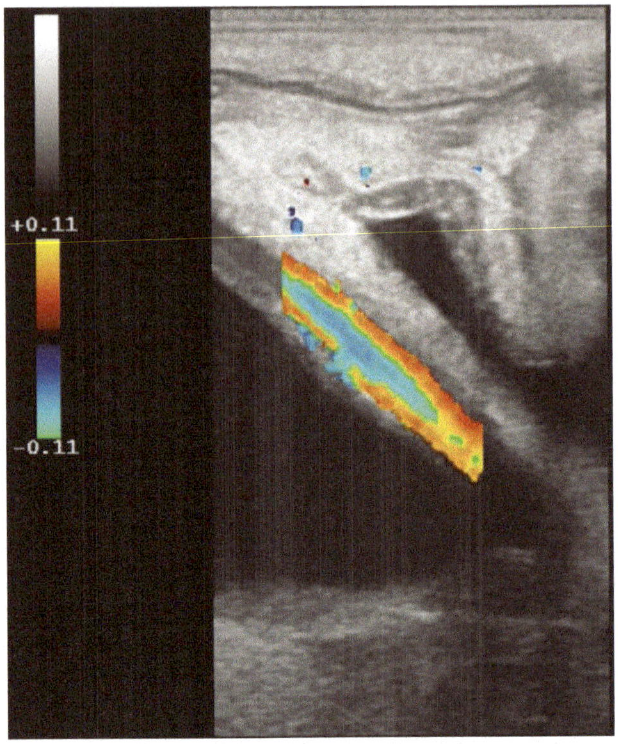

Figure 76.2 Color Doppler image of the cranial cervix and caudal uterus obtained per rectum, demonstrating the uterine branch of the vaginal artery used for combined thickness of uterus and placenta measurement.

- Normal resistance to blood flow in uterine arteries decreases with advancing pregnancy, thus providing more blood flow to the placenta and fetus. Future detail-

(a) (b)

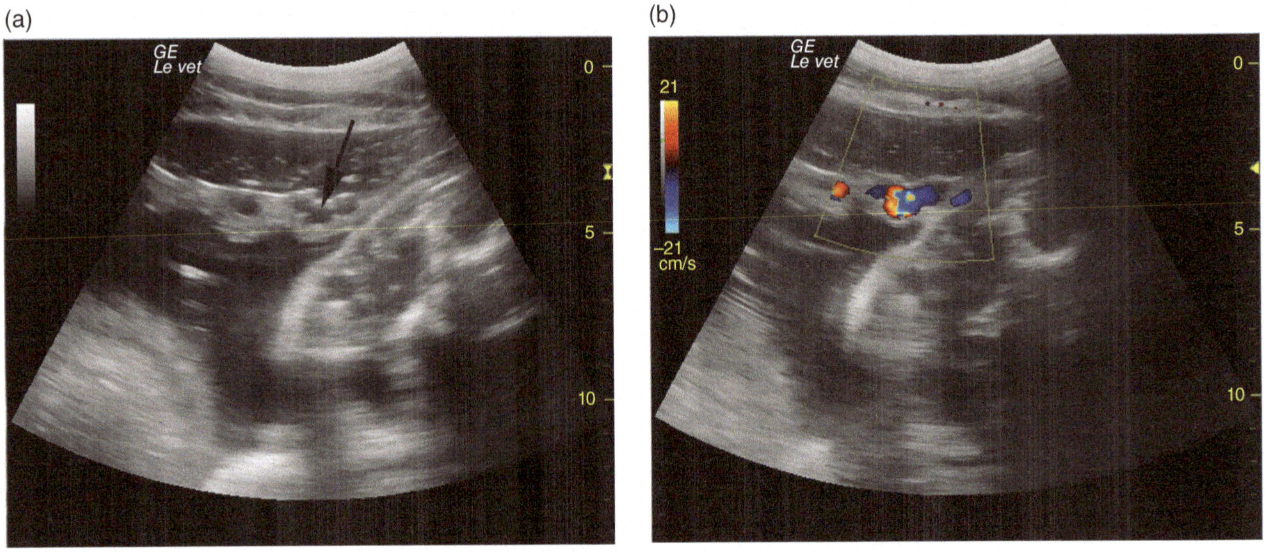

Figure 76.3 (a) Upper transabdominal image demonstrating potential placental separation or large blood vessels (arrow). (b) The color Doppler image confirms the presence of large vessels.

ing of flow indexes may aid with assessing high risk pregnancies where there may be decreased blood flow with pathologies.

- Color Doppler may be used to quickly evaluate fetal viability by imaging fetal vessels/heart or umbilical vessels for blood flow.

Technique for Assessing a Stallion

- A higher frequency probe (7.5+ MHz) should be used to scan the testes and spermatic cord.
- The stallion may be evaluated for blood flow in cases of testicular torsion, to help with the localization of a cryptorchid testis, and to look for enhanced or decreased blood flow in various pathologies such as testicular trauma, tumors, orchitis, or inguinal hernias. Determining the functionality of the testes is important for deciding on potential surgical removal.
- The presence of blood flow can be examined with color flow Doppler. Left and right testes and associated spermatic cords may be compared to determine relative blood flow patterns.
- Pulsed wave Doppler may be used to determine blood flow patterns within the convoluted testicular artery of the spermatic cord or the marginal artery of the testes (capsular artery). The normal resistance index in the convoluted testicular artery (spermatic cord) varies from 0.56 to 0.99. The normal resistance index in the marginal artery of the testes varies from 0.39 to 0.85.

Technique for Assessing Ovaries

- The mare's reproductive tract should be scanned with a 5–7.5 MHz probe.
- A developing antral follicle will have an increase in follicular wall blood flow. These blood vessels are within and outside the anechoic band surrounding a follicle in the 24–48 hours prior to ovulation. This flow pattern decreases within hours of ovulation and becomes less in the area where the follicle will rupture (follicle apex).
- A continued blood flow pattern circumferentially around a follicle near expected ovulation time may indicate the potential to form a hemorrhagic anovulatory follicle.
- Blood flow patterns around a corpus luteum (CL) may be examined to help determine the functionality of the CL. A CL may be followed over time, especially in a mare suspected to have luteal insufficiency, to see if blood flow patterns decrease, indicating the demise of the CL. During a regular cycle, the mare's CL will initially develop significant blood vessel patterns which will diminish closer to the end of diestrus. This may be used to help estimate the stage of diestrus.
- Color Doppler may assist with differentiating a CL (significant internal and circumferential blood flow) from a recent hemorrhagic anovulatory follicle (lack of internal blood flow).
- Vascular resistance patterns may have a future use in detailing vascular elastosis in uterine and/or ovarian blood vessels, especially in older mares and those with endometrosis. This could potentially be used to stage mares as to reproductive ability to support a pregnancy as is done with uterine biopsies.

Further Reading

Bollwein H, Weber F, Woschee I, Stolla R. 2004. Transrectal Doppler sonography of uterine and umbilical blood flow during pregnancy in mares. *Theriogenology* 61: 499–509.

Gastal EL, Gastal MO. 2011. Equine preovulatory follicle: blood flow changes, prediction of ovulation and fertility. *Bras Reprod Anim* 35: 239–52.

Ginther OJ, Utt M. 2004. Doppler ultrasound in equine reproduction: principles, techniques and potential. *J Eq Vet Sci* 24: 516–26.

Pozer MA, McDonnell SM. 2004. Color Doppler ultrasound evaluation of testicular blood flow in stallions. *Theriogenology* 61: 799–810.

Ousey JC, Kölling M, Newton R, Wright M, Allen WR. 2012. Uterine haemodynamics in young and aged pregnant mares measured using Doppler ultrasonography. *Eq Vet J* 44: 15–21.

Silva LA, Gastal EL, Beg MA, Ginther OJ. 2005. Changes in vascular perfusion of the endometrium in association with changes in location of the embryonic vesicle in mares. *Biol Reprod* 72: 755–61.

77

Prediction of Fetal Age

John J. Dascanio

School of Veterinary Medicine, Texas Tech University, USA

Introduction

Prediction of fetal age is best done within the first 40–60 days of gestation by the ultrasound characteristics of the developing embryo/fetus. After this time period, prediction of gestational age becomes less accurate. The growth or elongation of a variety of fetal body structures have been assessed in an attempt to determine fetal age, including eye diameter, biparietal diameter, aortic root diameter, femur length, thoracic diameter, and heart rate. Values listed are for light horse breeds unless noted otherwise.

Extrapolation to miniature horses or draft horses may lead to erroneous results. Some growth characteristics may also be influenced by the age of the mare and parity status within breeds, such that older mares (>15 years) may have smaller fetal aortic root diameter measurements than in young mares or that primiparous mares may have greater fetal eye measurements than in multiparous mares.

Equipment and Supplies

Ultrasound, variety of ultrasound probes, ultrasound acoustic gel, obstetrical sleeve, obstetrical lubricant, clippers, clipper spray.

Palpation Characteristics of the pregnant uterus

- See Chapter 69 on Palpation per Rectum of the Pregnant Reproductive Tract.

Embryo Characteristics

- Embryo characteristics are fairly uniform across horse types (miniature to draft).
- Gestational age is related to the size of the embryo (Figure 77.1). Gestational age charts have been developed along with tables that are incorporated into the measurement software with many veterinary ultrasounds.
- The relationship between the relative size of the fetal yolk sac and the developing allantoic cavity may be used to stage fetal development between 20 and 45 days of gestation:
- 20 days: the embryonic disk is visible at the edge of the embryo.
- 25 days: the yolk sac comprises ~75% of volume, the allantoic cavity is ~25% of volume, and the heart beat is visible.
- 30 days: the yolk sac and allantoic cavity are equal in size.
- 35 days: the yolk sac is ~25% and the allantoic cavity ~75% of volume.
- 40 days: the yolk sac disappears, and the fetus is at the top of the embryonic vesicle.
- 45 days: the umbilicus is elongating, and the fetus is at the bottom of the embryonic vesicle.

Aortic Root Diameter

- Aortic root diameter measurements are taken via transabdominal ultrasound using a ≤3.5 MHz transducer in pregnancies of more than 90 days. The aorta is measured during systole just prior to entering the ventricle (Figure 77.2).
- The aortic root enlarges from about 6 mm at 140 days of gestation to about 25 mm at term.
- Fetal aorta diameter (mm) = $-3.67 + 0.077x - 0.088z$; where x is the current gestational length in days and z is the age group (≥15 years = 0: <15 years = 1) (in Dutch Warmblood mares; Hendriks *et al.* 2009).
- Fetal aorta diameter (mm) = $-6.74 + 0.09x$; where x is the current gestational length in days (Renaudin *et al.* 2000).

Equine Reproductive Procedures, Second Edition. Edited by John Dascanio and Patrick McCue.

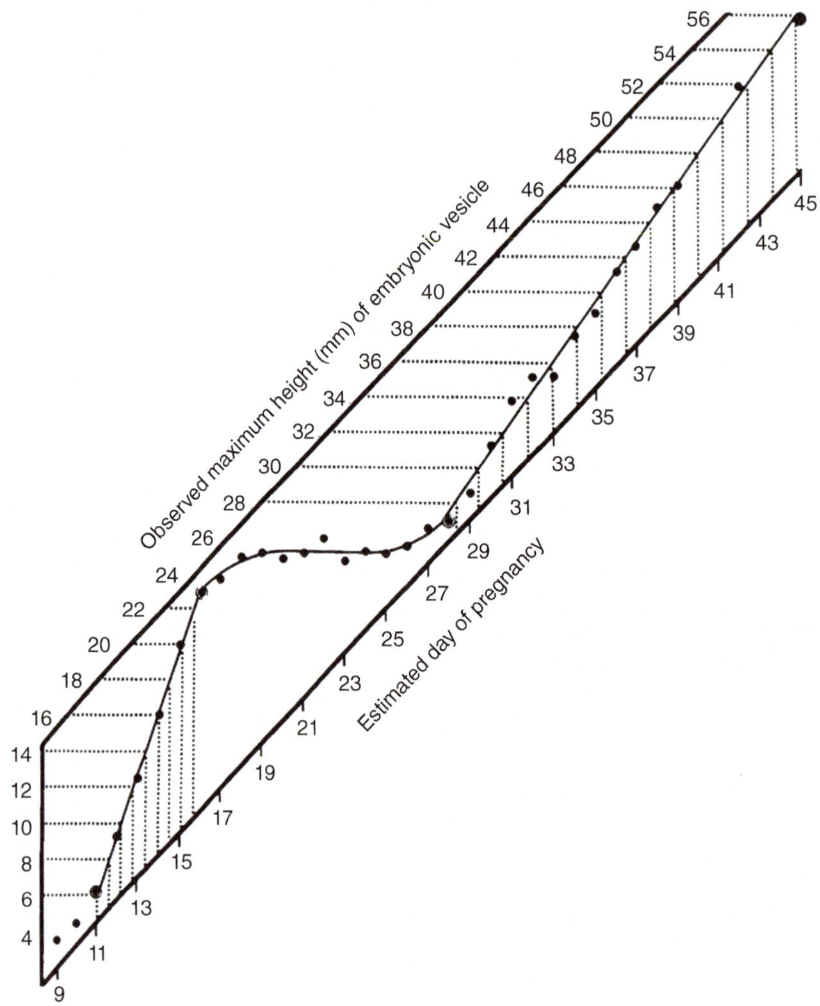

Figure 77.1 A graph of the maximum height (mm) of the embryonic vesicle versus the estimated day of pregnancy. Source: From Ginther. 1995. *Ultrasonic Imaging and Animal Reproduction: Horses. Book 2.* Equiservices Publishing, Cross Plains, WI by O.J. Ginther. Reproduced with the permission of Equiservices Publishing.

Fetal Biparietal Diameter

- Measurement of the width of the fetal head may be performed with an ultrasound either transrectally or transabdominally.
- Fetal biparietal diameter (mm) = $-26.64 + 0.597x - 0.0008x^2$; where x is the current gestational length in days (in Dutch Warmblood mares; Hendriks *et al.* 2009).
- Fetal biparietal diameter (mm) = $1.26 + 0.29x$; where x is the current gestational length in days (Renaudin *et al.* 2000).

Fetal Heart Rate

- A fetal heart rate is taken via transabdominal ultrasound using a ≤3.5 MHz transducer in pregnancies of more than 90 days.
- The fetal heart rate decreases with advancing gestational age and varies with fetal activity. An active fetus may range from ~145 beats per minute (bpm) at 6 months' gestation to ~105 bpm near term, while a resting fetus may range from a low of ~100 bpm at 6 months' gestation to ~55 bpm near term.
- Fetal heart rate (bpm) = $167.97 - 0.249x$; where x is the current gestational length in days (in Dutch Warmblood mares; Hendriks *et al.* 2009).

Fetal Eye Measurement

- Measurements of the fetal eye are best conducted per rectum using a 7.5 or 5 MHz transducer in a later term foal (7+ months), but may also be obtained transabdominally earlier in gestation (Figure 77.3; Tables 77.1 and Table 77.2).

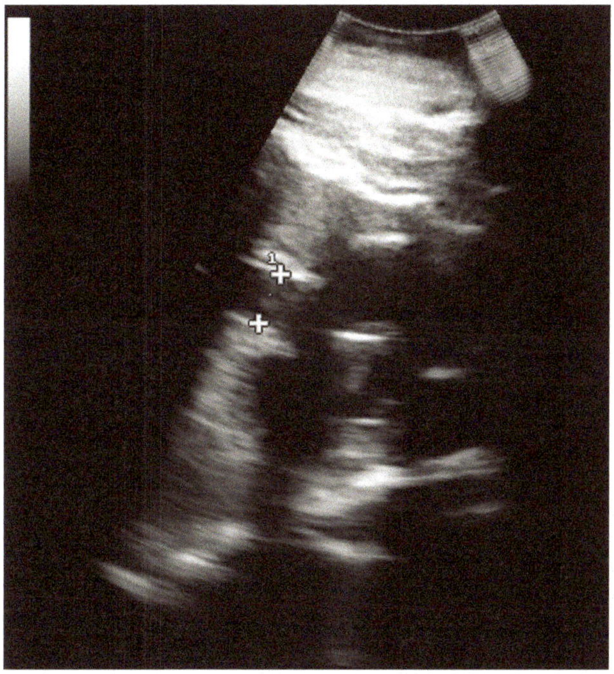

Figure 77.2 Aortic root diameter measurement of 22 mm in a mare 10 months' pregnant. The heart is located to the right of the cursors.

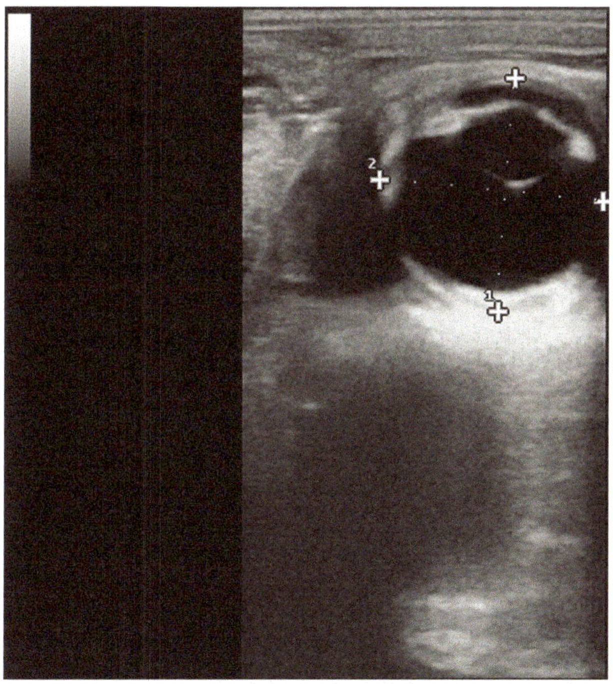

Figure 77.3 Per rectum measurement of fetal eye diameter showing a vertical measurement of 3.12 cm and horizontal measurement of 3.08 cm. The anterior chamber of the eye is orientated at the top of the picture, marked with the top cursor, with the fetal lens visible between the anterior chamber and posterior chamber.

- A pony eye regression equation was developed by Turner *et al.* (2006a). Days before parturition = 265.16 – (0.21 × vitreous body length in mm^2).
- Fetal eye orbit diameter (mm) = $-5.62 + 0.21x - 0.0003x^2$; where x is the current gestational length in days and fetal eye orbit diameter (mm) = (length + width)/2 (in Dutch Warmblood mares; Hendriks *et al.* 2009).
- Eye volume (mm^3) = $-8175.59 + 91.73x$; where x is the current gestational length in days (Renaudin *et al.* 2000).

Table 77.1 The relationship between eye length and days before parturition for pony mares (100–250 kg).

Eye Length (Vitreous Body Medial to Lateral, mm)	Days Before Parturition		
	Mean	75% PI	95% PI
15	209	184–251	160–275
16	203	177–245	153–269
17	197	170–238	146–262
18	190	153–230	140–254
19	183	155–223	131 -238
20	175	147–214	123–238
21	167	138–206	115 -230
22	158	129–197	106–220
23	150	120–187	96–211
24	140	110–177	86–201
25	131	100–167	76–191
26	121	89–156	65–180
27	110	78–145	54–169
28	99	66–133	43–157
29	88	54–121	31–145
30	77	42–109	18–133
31	65	29–96	5–120
32	52	16–83	0–107
33	39	2–69	0–93
34	26	0–55	0–79
35	13	0–41	0–64

Prediction mean with 75% and 95% prediction interval (PI) ranges of days before parturition. Source: From R.M. Turner, S.M. McDonnell, E.M. Feit, E.H. Grogan, R. Foglia. 2006a. Real-time ultrasound measure of the fetal eye (vitreous body) for prediction of parturition date in small ponies. *J Theriogenol* 2006; 66: 331–7. Elsevier © 2006. Reproduced with the permission of Elsevier.

Table 77.2 Relationship between eye length and days of gestation for light horses.

Eye Length (Vitreous Body Medial to Lateral, mm)	Day of Gestation		
	Mean	75% PI	95% PI
Kahn & Leidle (1987) (n = *77 TB and STB)*			
10	86	65–107	50–123
11	92	72–112	57–127
12	98	78–117	64–131
13	104	85–123	71–136
14	110	91–129	78–142
15	116	98–134	85–148
16	122	104–141	91–154
17	129	111–147	98–160
18	135	117–153	104–166
19	142	124–160	111–173
20	149	131–166	118–179
21	155	137–173	124–186
22	162	144–180	131–193
23	169	151–187	138–200
24	176	158–194	145–207
25	183	165–201	152–214
26	190	172–208	159–221
27	198	179–216	166–229
28	205	187–223	173–237
29	212	194–231	180–245
30	220	201–239	187–253
Turner et al. 2006b (n = *66 TB, STE, QH, Arabian, Warmblood)*			
30	284	247–321	220–348
31	291	254–328	227–355
32	298	261–335	234–361
33	303	266–340	239–367
34	308	271–345	244–372
35	312	275–349	248–376
36	315	278–353	251–380
37	318	280–356	252–384

Prediction mean with 75% and 95% prediction interval (PI) ranges for day of gestation.

QH, Quarter Horse; STB, Standardbred; TB, Thoroughbred. Source: From Turner RM *et al.* 2006b. How to determine gestational age of an equine pregnancy in the field using transrectal ultrasonographic measurement of the fetal eye. *Proc Annu Conv Am Assoc Eq Pract* 2006; 52: 250–5. Reproduced with the permission of American Association of Equine Practitioners.

References

Ginther OJ. 1995. Ultrasonic Imaging and Animal Reproduction: Horses, Book 2. Cross Plains, WI: *Equiservices*.

Hendriks WK, Colenbrander B, van der Weijden GC, Stout TAE. 2009. Maternal age and parity influence ultrasonographic measurements of fetal growth in Dutch Warm-blood mares. *Anim Reprod Sci* 115: 110–23.

Renaudin CD, Gillis CL, Tarantal AF, Coleman DA. 2000. Evaluation of equine fetal growth from day 100 of gestation to parturition by ultrasonography. *J Reprod Fertil Suppl* 56: 651–60.

Turner RM, McDonnell SM, Feit EM, Grogan EH, Foglia R. 2006a. Real-time ultrasound measure of the fetal eye (vitreous body) for prediction of parturition date in small ponies. *J Theriogenol* 66: 331–7.

Turner RM, McDonnell SM, Feit EM, Grogan EH, Foglia R. 2006b. How to determine gestational age of an equine pregnancy in the field using transrectal ultrasonographic measurement of the fetal eye. *Proc Annu Conv Am Assoc Eq Pract* 52: 250–5.

Further Reading

Bucca S, Fogarty U, Collins A, Small V. 2005. Assessment of feto-placental well-being in the mare from mid-gestation to term: transrectal and transabdominal ultrasonographic features. *Theriogenology* 64: 542–57.

Kahn W, Leidl W. 1987. Ultrasonic biometry of horse fetuses in utero and sonographic representation of their organs [in German]. *DTW Dtsch Tierarztl Wochenschr* 94: 509–15.

Pantaleon LG, Bain FT, Zent W, Powell DG. 2003. Equine fetal growth and development. *Comp Cont Educ Eq* 25: 470–7.

Reef VB, Vaala WE, Worth LT, *et al.* 1995. Ultrasonographic evaluation of the fetus and intrauterine environment in healthy mares during late gestation. *Vet Radiol Ultrasound* 36: 533–41.

78

Twin Reduction: Manual Technique

John J. Dascanio

School of Veterinary Medicine, Texas Tech University, USA

Introduction

It is undesirable for the mare to maintain twins throughout gestation, primarily due to the poor outcome obtained. There is a very small chance (approximately 1%) that multiple fetuses will be born alive and survive the neonatal period. A high percentage of mares with twins will abort the pregnancies by 7–9 months of gestation, due primarily to placental insufficiency. The first pregnancy examination should be performed at 14–16 days post-ovulation, while the embryonic vesicle is in the mobility phase. Around day 16 to 17 the vesicle becomes fixed in position at the base of one of the uterine horns.

If two embryonic vesicles are detected and they are not located adjacent to each other, the recommendation is to manually reduce one embryo immediately. Failure to eliminate one embryo may allow an opportunity for the two embryos to come into direct contact with each other and potentially make embryo reduction more difficult.

In contrast, if two embryonic vesicles are in close apposition, one option is to recheck the mare an hour or later in the day, providing an opportunity for the embryos to spontaneously move apart by natural uterine muscle contractions. In addition, there is a higher probability of natural reabsorption of one embryo if they are in close apposition than if they are located in opposite uterine horns. If the embryonic vesicles are located apart from each other, they may survive further into gestation and thus one should be immediately terminated.

Equipment and Supplies

Obstetrical lubricant, obstetrical sleeve, ultrasound with 7.5 or 5 MHz linear array transducer. Optional items include *N*-butylscopolammonium bromide (Buscopan®), flunixin meglumine, altrenogest, and sedation agents (e.g., xylazine, butorphanol, detomidine).

Technique

- Remove feces from the rectum.
- Identify and measure the embryonic vesicles within the uterine lumen.
- Typically, the smaller vesicle is chosen for manual reduction. However, if they are the same size, the more accessible vesicle is often selected for elimination (Figure 78.1).
- Optionally, prior to performing the reduction, flunixin meglumine (1.0 mg/kg IV) may be administered and/or a progesterone analog, such as altrenogest (0.044 mg/kg orally), as the reduction procedure may result in uterine prostaglandin release compromising the corpora lutea. With experience in performing the procedure quickly and with limited manipulation, there should be minimal need for drug therapy. A single dose of flunixin meglumine prior to reduction of one vesicle may be beneficial.

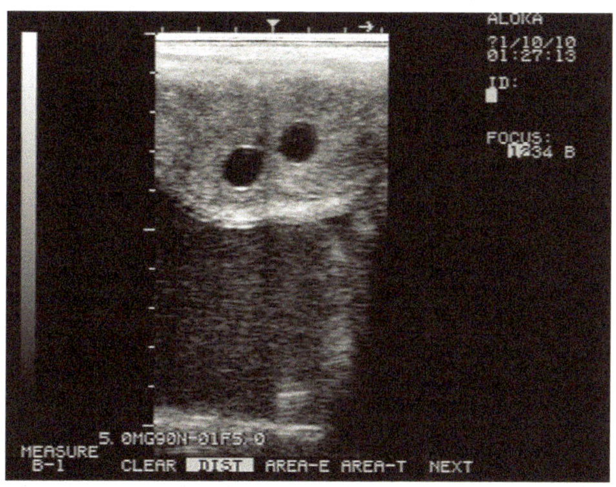

Figure 78.1 Two embryonic vesicles at 12 days post-ovulation located in close approximation. Note how circular the vesicles appear.

Equine Reproductive Procedures, Second Edition. Edited by John Dascanio and Patrick McCue.

- A dose of *N*-butylscopolammonium bromide (0.1–0.2 mg/kg IV) may be administered to relax the smooth muscle of the rectum and allow for easier transrectal palpation and manipulation. However, this will also cause some relaxation of the uterus, potentially making it more difficult to perform the manual reduction procedure.
- The vesicle to be crushed is gently moved toward the tip of the uterine horn opposite the remaining vesicle. This may be accomplished by massaging the uterus by hand or by using the ultrasound probe to exert ventral pressure from medial to lateral on the uterus. Once the vesicle is located near the tip of the uterine horn, pressure exerted by the ultrasound probe ventrally from medial to lateral will result in disruption of the embryonic membranes and the release of fluid from the vesicle. It is often possible to feel the capsule of the embryo rupture.
- Ultrasound of the vesicle immediately after manual rupture will reveal free fluid (yolk) within the uterine lumen and the absence of a discernible spherical vesicle (Figure 78.2). Initially, the fluid from the ruptured embryo will make the outline of the endometrial folds more evident and will then rapidly dissipate through the uterine horn, gravitating towards the uterine bifurcation (dependent part of uterus).
- The remaining vesicle should be re-examined to confirm that it is still present and intact.
- Progesterone administration, if utilized at all, should continue for 3–5 days at a minimum. An ultrasound examination can be used to verify the continued presence of a corpus luteum and a blood sample can be collected to evaluate endogenous progesterone concentrations, at which time progesterone administration may be terminated. A progesterone level of ≥4.0 ng/ml is considered adequate for maintenance of pregnancy.
- A recheck ultrasound examination is recommended in 2–4 days to confirm the continued survival of the remaining embryo.

Additional Comments

- Two embryos may also be reduced after fixation (days 16 to 17) up to approximately day 30 or more. However, aggressive uterine manipulation and/or the added fluid volume of the disrupted vesicle may result in increased loss of the remaining pregnancy.
- Twin embryos in direct contact (Figure 78.3) can be reduced after separation. The mare is administered sedation (xylazine and acepromazine) plus a dose of *N*-butylscopolammonium bromide (Buscopan®) to induce relaxation of the smooth muscle of the rectum and uterus. The ultrasound probe is positioned above the junction between the two embryos and a gentle vibration

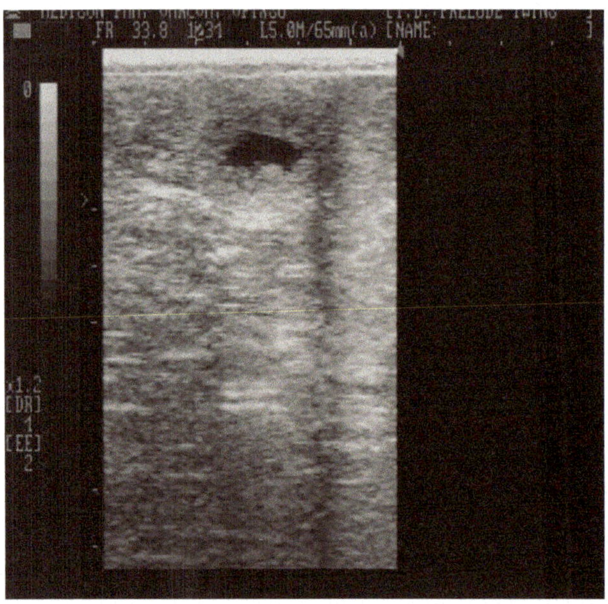

Figure 78.2 Irregular 14-day embryonic vesicle just after manual disruption. The fluid contents are leaking out, making the vesicle wall collapse.

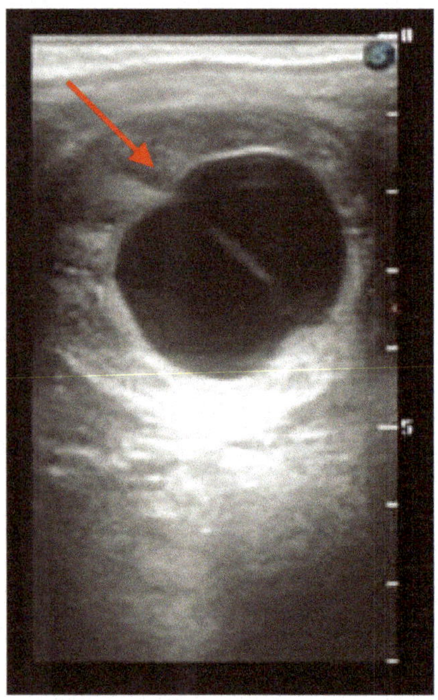

Figure 78.3 Two embryos adjacent to each other prior to separation and reduction of one embryo. The arrow denotes where the two embryos are in contact.

motion is applied to the probe along with continuous downward pressure. Eventually the probe will slip down between the embryos, allowing one embryo to be massaged away and disrupted.

- An alternative technique is to disrupt one embryonic vesicle by manual compression, not using the ultrasound probe. This could be considered if one embryo is in the tip of one horn and the other embryo is in the opposite horn. Ultrasound should be used to verify the position of the two embryos and, as needed, to move one embryo up a uterine horn.
- The quicker the procedure is performed, with the least amount of manipulation, the better the success in maintaining a singleton pregnancy.
- Success rate is dependent on practitioner experience, stage of gestation, and location of the embryos.

Further Reading

Ginther OJ. 1989. Twin embryos in mares. I: From ovulation to fixation. *Eq Vet J* 21:166–70.

Ginther OJ. 1989. Twin embryos in mares. II: Post fixation embryo reduction. *Eq Vet J* 21: 171–4.

MacPherson ML, Reimer JM. 2000. Twin reduction in the mare: current options. *Ann Reprod Sci* 60–1: 233–44.

Sheerin PC. 2010. Manual reduction of twins in the mare: effect of operator, mare age, and treatment. *Proc Annu Conv Am Assoc Eq Pract* 56: 322.

79

Twin Reduction: Transvaginal Aspiration

John J. Dascanio

School of Veterinary Medicine, Texas Tech University, USA

Introduction

Transvaginal aspiration of the allantoic fluid or yolk sac contents from a conceptus is one method of eliminating one conceptus in a twin pregnancy. This technique requires specialized equipment such as a transvaginal ultrasound unit (Figures 79.1 and 79.2) and the technical skill to safely and efficiently perform the procedure. The procedure is generally performed from day 20 to day 45 of the pregnancy, but may be attempted until the uterus is no longer able to be retracted into the pelvic inlet, which may extend to beyond day 60. This procedure is often best performed prior to day 35 of gestation.

The success rate in causing the demise of one pregnancy is very high with this technique, but there is a significant chance that the remaining conceptus will not survive after the procedure. Success rates for survival of the remaining twin vary from 20% to 70% and are largely dependent on the stage of gestation. The highest success rate occurs if the procedure is performed prior to day 25–35 of the gestation (70% with bilaterally fixed twins). The success rate is also higher if the twins are located in opposite uterine horns than if the twins are located within the same horn.

Alternative procedures utilizing the transvaginal probe to eliminate one conceptus include cardiac puncture without aspiration and injection of a substance such as potassium penicillin into one conceptus. Neither of these techniques provides any significant advantages over the aspiration of allantoic fluid or yolk sac contents.

Equipment and Supplies

Tail wrap, tail rope, non-irritant soap, roll cotton, stainless steel bucket, disposable liner for bucket, paper towels, exam gloves, obstetrical sleeves, obstetrical lubricant, twitch, lidocaine, 18 gauge 60 cm (24 inch) transvaginal ultrasound needle, ultrasound, 7.5 or 5 MHz convex or linear array ultrasound transducer, transvaginal case for transducer with needle guide, syringes, needles, extension tubing, sedation (optional), *N*-butylscopolammonium bromide (optional).

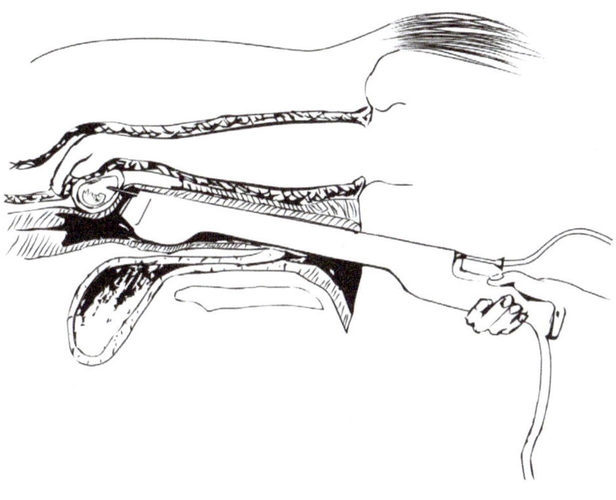

Figure 79.1 Hand, uterus, and transvaginal probe orientation for aspiration.

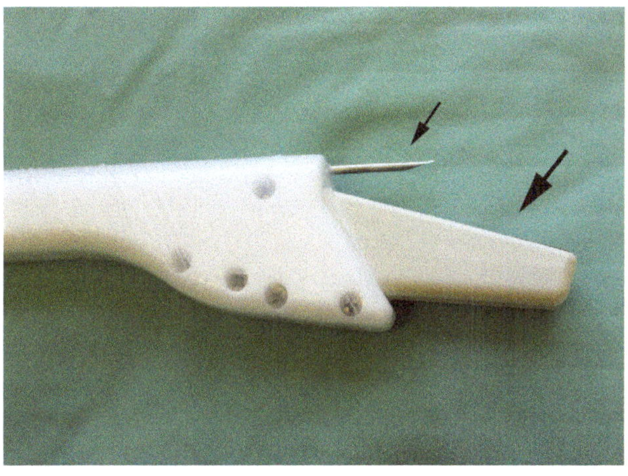

Figure 79.2 Needle extended from the needle guide (small arrow). Needle extension would only occur once the probe (large arrow) has been properly orientated on the uterus per vagina.

Equine Reproductive Procedures, Second Edition. Edited by John Dascanio and Patrick McCue.

Technique

- Remove feces from the rectum; 50 ml of 2% lidocaine may be infused into the rectum in an attempt to decrease rectal straining during manipulation of the uterus. Alternatively, *N*-butylscopolammonium bromide may be administered at a dose of 0.15 mg/kg slowly IV to decrease peristalsis, but this may also cause some uterine relaxation making manipulation of the uterus more difficult.
- Administer flunixin meglumine (1.1 mg/kg IV) to block prostaglandin release secondary to inflammation that may be associated with the procedure.
- Administer a progesterone analog, such as altrenogest (0.044 mg/kg orally), to provide a source of progesterone in the event that the corpus luteum is lysed due to inflammation.
- Place a tail wrap and tail rope (see Chapter 4).
- Clean and dry the perineum of mare (see Chapter 3).
- The plastic transvaginal housing into which the ultrasound transducer is placed should be gas sterilized or cold sterilized with a glutaraldehyde solution and rinsed with sterile saline. The 7.5 or 5 MHz ultrasound transducer should be cleansed with alcohol and rinsed with sterile water. A convex or linear array ultrasound transducer may be used, depending on user preference and availability. It is recommended that sterile gloves be worn while the ultrasound transducer is placed into the protective transvaginal case. The assembled probe may be inserted into a disposable sterile plastic cover such as an obstetrical sleeve that has been lubricated with sterile water-soluble lubricant or may be left as is for use. The sleeve may prevent contamination of the probe during placement, keeping the needle port cleaner.
- An extension set with a 60 ml syringe attached is placed onto an 18 gauge 60 cm single lumen, transvaginal needle with an echogenic ultrasound tip.
- The transvaginal probe is inserted through the vulvar lips and advanced cranially to the cranial vaginal fornix. The probe should be directed to the left or right of the cervix, corresponding to location of the embryo to be eliminated (Figure 79.1).
- The mare should be restrained with a twitch during penetration of the vaginal tissue with the aspiration needle. Alternatively, the mare may be sedated; however sedation may cause relaxation of the uterus, making it more difficult to grasp and hold the uterus in the correct position for aspiration. Typically a combination of detomidine (0.0088–0.011 mg/kg IV) or xylazine (0.33–0.44 mg/kg IV) plus butorphanol (0.011–0.022 mg/kg IV) is used for sedation.
- Place the transvaginal aspiration needle into the needle guide on the handle end of the transvaginal probe. Only insert the needle part way, so that the needle does not exit the port on the transducer end of the probe.
- With one hand per rectum, retract the uterine horn with the conceptus to be aspirated toward the vagina and the ultrasound probe. Line up the exit port of the needle guide with the allantoic cavity or yolk sac contents of the conceptus, using the ultrasound image for guidance.
- When properly aligned, advance the transvaginal needle in a quick, controlled motion, into the allantoic cavity or yolk sac contents.
- An assistant should then aspirate the allantoic contents or yolk sac contents by pulling back on the attached syringe plunger. The recovered fluid is often amber in color. Volume will vary depending on gestation length, but typically will only be a few milliliters.
- Only one puncture of the conceptus should be made. Multiple attempts will result in an increased risk of losing the second conceptus due to inflammation and prostaglandin release.
- Treatment with flunixin meglumine and a progesterone analog may be continued after the procedure. Typically, flunixin meglumine is administered twice a day for 2 days post-procedure and progesterone is administered for 10–14 days post-procedure. The concentration of serum progesterone may be measured prior to discontinuing altrenogest to determine endogenous levels. It is generally recommended that progesterone levels be at least 4.0 ng/ml for maintenance of the pregnancy.

Interpretation

- There is a slight risk for peritonitis or uterine infection due to needle penetration of the vagina, which has a normal resident bacterial flora.
- The second conceptus with a twin pregnancy may expire within days or a few weeks post-procedure due to inflammation, infection, or release of prostaglandin.
- The remaining conceptus should be examined for fetal heart beat and viability a few days post-procedure and again weekly for the first month post-procedure.
- Older mares (≥15 years of age) have a decreased success rate compared with younger mares (≤7 years of age).
- Antibiotics are not typically administered with this procedure. If desired, trimethoprim sulfamethoxazole could be administered at a dose of 30 mg/kg orally twice daily for 10–14 days.

Further Reading

Bracher V, Parlevliet JM, Pieterse MC, *et al.* 1993. Transvaginal ultrasound-guided twin reduction in the mare. *Vet Rec* 133: 478–9.

Govaere JLJ, Hoogewijs MK, deSchauwer C, Dewulf J, deKruif A. 2008. Transvaginal ultrasound-guided aspiration of unilateral twin gestation in the mare. *Eq Vet J* 40: 521–2.

Mari G, Iacono E, Merlo B, Castagnetti C. 2004. Reduction of twin pregnancy in the mare by transvaginal ultrasound-guided aspiration. *Reprod Domest Anim* 39: 434–7.

Rau J, Tiedemann D, Sielhorst J, *et al.* 2018. Effects of mares' age and day of gestation on efficacy of transvaginal ultrasound-guided twin reduction. *Tierarztl Prax Ausg G Grosstiere Nutztiere* 46(3):172–7.

Squires EL, Tarr SF, Shideler RK. 1994. Use of transvaginal ultrasound-guided puncture for elimination of equine pregnancies during days 50 to 65. *J Eq Vet Sci* 14: 203–6.

80

Twin Reduction: Cranio-Cervical Dislocation

Karen Wolfsdorf

Hagyard Equine Medical Institute, USA

Introduction

Cranio-cervical dislocation (CCD) is described as the dislocation of the first cervical vertebrae from the cranium, disrupting the ligamentous attachments and severing the spinal cord of the developing fetus. This procedure can be performed transrectally at 60–75 days, transabdominally at 70–110 days, or via a colpotomy at 60–95 days of gestation in order to produce a single foal. The basis for this procedure is to eliminate one twin before placental formation is complete, allowing the remaining fetus to utilize the entire endometrial surface for nutrient and oxygen exchange and grow to its full potential.

Technique

Transrectal Technique (Performed at 60–75 Days of Gestation)

- Restrain mare in stocks or twitched in a doorway.
- Sedate the mare using detomidine HCl, if needed, since relaxation of the uterus may result in the fetus moving cranially out of reach in abdomen.
- Administer *N*-butylscopolammonium bromide to relax the smooth muscle of the rectum and uterus. This will allow easier identification and manipulation of the fetuses.
- Administer flunixin meglumine prior to the procedure.
- Using ultrasound, identify both fetuses are viable and whether their location is bilateral or unilateral in the uterine horn.

Equipment and Supplies

Transrectal technique

Twitch, detomidine hydrochloride (0.0088–0.011 mg/kg IV), butorphanol tartrate (0.01–0.1 mg/kg), *N*-butylscopolammonium bromide (0.3 mg/kg IV), flunixin meglumine (1 mg/kg IV), altrenogest (0.088 mg/kg PO), obstetrical sleeve and lubricant, ultrasound with a 7.5 or 5 MHz linear array transducer, various needles and syringes, stocks.

Trans-abdominal technique

Twitch, detomidine hydrochloride (0.0088–0.011 mg/kg IV), butorphanol tartrate (0.01–0.1 mg/kg), *N*-butylscopolammonium bromide (0.3 mg/kg IV), flunixin meglumine (1 mg/kg IV), procaine penicillin (20,000–50,000 IU/kg IM, every 12–24 hours), gentamicin sulfate (6.6 mg/kg IV or IM, every 24 hours), trimethoprim-sulfamethoxazole (30 mg/kg PO, every 12 hours), altrenogest (0.088 mg/kg PO), local anesthetic, clippers, surgical scrub, surgical pack, sterile drape, suture material, sterile surgery gloves, fingerless sterile obstetrical sleeves, sterile lube, sterile saline, ultrasound with a 2.5 or 5 MHz linear or sector array transducer, stocks.

Colpotomy technique

Twitch and sedation; drugs: detomidine hydrochloride (0.0088–0.011 mg/kg IV), butorphanol tartrate (0.01–0.1 mg/kg), flunixin meglumine (1 mg/kg IV), trimethoprim-sulfamethoxazole (30 mg/kg PO, every 12 hours) or ceftiofur crystalline-free acid (6.6 mg/kg, two doses, 96 hours apart), local anesthetic for epidural, *N*-butylscopolammonium bromide (0.3 mg/kg IV), altrenogest (0.088 mg/kg PO); supplies: tail wrap, obstetrical sleeve and lubricant, sterile obstetrical sleeve, sterile lubricant, surgical scrub (perineum), povidone-iodine, sterile uterine lavage tubing, sterile saline, scalpel blade, sterile surgery pack, sterile drapes, urinary catheter (optional), 0 chromic cut on taper needle, various needles and syringes, stocks.

Equine Reproductive Procedures, Second Edition. Edited by John Dascanio and Patrick McCue.

- The smaller fetus or the fetus that has less contact with the endometrium and minimal space to grow is preferentially reduced.
- In unilateral twins, the fetus closest to the tip of the horn will be reduced, while in bilateral twins the smaller or more easily identified fetus will be reduced.
- Transrectally, isolate the chosen fetus and identify the head by its dome-shaped structure and the mandible or locate the cervical vertebrae. If the thorax is identified first work cranially to the cranial cervical vertebrae.
- Cranio-cervical dislocation is initiated by stabilizing the fetal head between the thumb and forefinger and bending the head from side to side. This will damage the ligaments attaching the head and neck (Figure 80.1).
- Dislocation is completed by placing the thumb at the base of the cranium and applying pressure proximal and dorsally. A distinctive pop is felt when dislocation is achieved, and the thumb and forefinger can be placed in the space created between the head and neck (Figure 80.2).
- Administer altrenogest for 1 month.

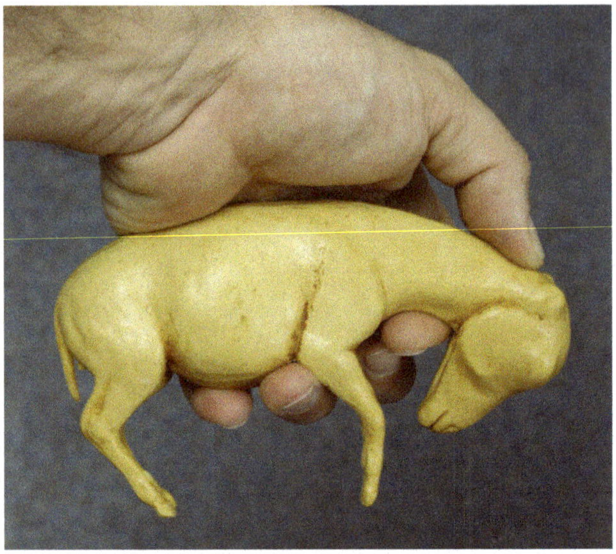

Figure 80.2 Position of fingers to cause dislocation of the cranium from the cervical vertebra.

Transabdominal Technique (Performed at 70–110 Days of Gestation)

- Restrain the mare in stocks.
- Identify two viable fetuses and the horn in which the most viable fetus is located by transabdominal ultrasound. Any flocculence in the fetal fluids, bradycardia, or abnormal fetal organ patterns should preclude CCD from being performed and continued monitoring should occur for death of that specific fetus. (See Chapter 73.)

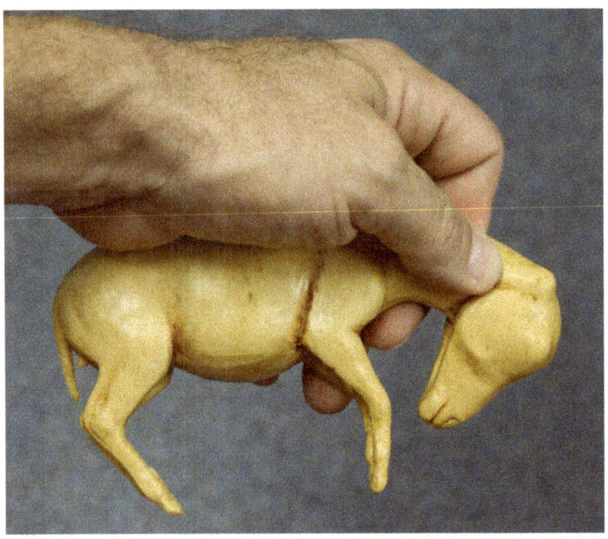

Figure 80.1 Position of fingers for side to side manipulation for the disruption of cranio-cervical ligaments.

- Give preoperative medications flunixin meglumine, procaine penicillin G, and gentamicin.
- The mare is sedated using detomidine HCl and butorphanol tartrate.
- The mare's right flank is clipped, scrubbed, and prepared for a surgical incision within the paralumbar fossa.
- A line block is performed where the incision will be made. This must be long enough to have a hand enter the abdomen.
- Administer *N*-butylscopalammonium bromide at the time of incision. This is essential for uterine relaxation and preventing uterine contraction while finding and manipulating the fetus.
- A standing flank laparotomy is performed using a grid approach on the right side of the abdomen. This eliminates the potential for splenic interference or damage.
- The uterus is located within the abdominal cavity with one arm by isolating the right ovary first. The ovary is located at the level of the incision as the hand enters the abdomen.
- Once the ovary is identified the uterine horn is followed ventrally towards the body. The relaxed uterus causes the twins to sit ventral at the base of the horns/body.
- The preferred twin is identified by manipulating one or the other towards the tip of a horn. The fetus that can be moved to the tip of a horn is the twin on which to perform the procedure.
- When twins are located in the left horn your arm can follow the uterus from the right horn to left across the abdomen. Care should be taken not to disrupt or tear the intestinal mesentery.

- The twin is isolated as described for transrectal dislocations.
- Cranio-cervical dislocation is performed, as described, by manipulating the fetus through the uterus, without incising or invading the uterine lumen.
- The flank incision is irrigated with sterile saline. The internal and external abdominal oblique muscles are sutured. The skin is sutured with a forward interlocking pattern leaving the bottom inch with simple interrupted in case drainage is required.
- Administer flunixin meglumine, procaine penicillin, and gentamicin for 2 days, then trimethoprim sulfamethoxazole for 1 week and double dose altrenogest for 1 month, followed by a single dose until the remaining pregnancy is stabilized.

Colpotomy Technique (Performed at 60–95 Days of Gestation)

- Identify two viable fetuses as described.
- Restrain the mare in standing stocks and sedate her with detomidine HCl and butorphanol tartrate.
- Administer preoperative medications flunixin meglumine, trimethoprim sulfamethoxazole, or ceftiofur crystalline-free acid.
- Administration of caudal epidural anesthesia may be used to help prevent the mare from straining during the procedure, if necessary (see Chapter 100).
- Wrap the tail and secure it away from the perineal region.
- Evacuate manure from the rectum to prevent contamination of the external genitalia.
- Routine aseptic preparation of the external genitalia and perineal region is performed (see Chapter 3).
- Lavage the vagina with 2 liters of povidone-iodine (5 ml/l) diluted in sterile saline solution using sterile uterine lavage tubing.
- In some mares, catheterization of a large urinary bladder will facilitate the procedure and may help reduce the risk of inadvertent injury during the procedure.
- Create a vaginal wall incision at either a cranio-dorsal (at 2 or 10 o'clock) or a cranio-ventral (at 4 or 8 o'clock) position using Mayo scissors as described in the next point. The 2 o'clock is preferred by the author. The incision should be started 3–5 cm caudal to the external os cervix to avoid disruption of the cervical musculature.
- Using the tip of 18 cm (7 inch) Mayo scissors, a small 1–2 cm vaginal incision is sharply/bluntly created in the vaginal wall. This initial incision should penetrate the full thickness of the vagina and peritoneum to prevent the peritoneum from lifting away from the underlying tissues during blunt dissection.
- Bluntly enlarge the incision digitally, as the peritoneum is perforated, to allow the surgeon's hand to enter the abdomen.
- Administer *N*-butylscopalammonium bromide (10 ml IV) for uterine relaxation once the uterus is located.
- The CCD is performed as described. Additional crushing of the thorax is optimal if possible.
- Close the incision with a one-hand cruciate suture pattern with 0 gut on a 5 cm (2 inch) curved taper-point needle.
- Continue postoperative antibiotics for 1 week. Altrenogest should be administered for 1 month.

Interpretation

- About 63% of mares deliver a single normal-sized fetus after transrectal reduction. This technique, however, necessitates multiple manipulations on multiple days, causing an increased chance of rectal tears; therefore, colpotomy and transabdominal approaches are preferred.
- CCD via the transabdominal approach produces a single, normal, healthy foal in 63% of mares. With this technique, death of the manipulated twin is evident from 24 hours to 8 weeks post-procedure.
- About 64% of mares have a single normal-sized foal with 36% aborting both when using the colpotomy approach (unpublished data from Dr Reed Holyoak).
- Re-evaluation of fetal viability is performed with transrectal or transabdominal ultrasonography every 2 weeks until demise of one twin is observed.
- Potential complications of a misplaced colpotomy incision include entering the rectum if the incision is placed too dorsal, injuring the urethra or bladder if placed too ventral, and incising the caudal uterine branch of the urogenital artery if too medial or lateral (at the 3 or 9 o'clock position).
- Signs of impending death of a fetus include: loss of thoracic shape, becoming more convex; loss of definition of abdominal organs; gas within the abdomen; and irregular, weak heart beat.
- The placenta from a mare delivering a singleton foal has a small sack attached to the allantoic surface. The reduced twin is marsupialized by the remaining twin's placenta, forming a pedunculated pouch off the allantoic surface (Figure 80.3). This pouch contains the mummified fetal bones. Examination of the chorionic surface reveals minimal evidence that a twin was present with microvilli present along the entire uterine attachment of the placenta.

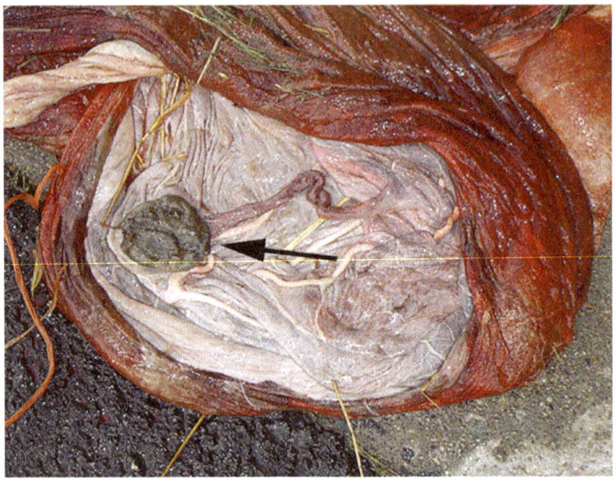

Figure 80.3 Placenta from a mare after cranio-cervical dislocation to eliminate one twin. The sac attached to the allantoic surface contains the remnants of the fetus that died after the dislocation.

Advantages of CCD

- Increased success rates for a normal-sized healthy foal.
- Earlier reduction allows full potential growth and use of placental function.
- An alternative procedure using transvaginal ultrasound-guided aspiration of the fetal fluid results in puncture of the uterus and release of fetal fluid from the reduced fetus. This procedure potentially disrupts the fetal membranes of the remaining fetus. Penetration of the abdomen and/or the uterine lumen with transvaginal ultrasound-guided aspiration also increases the chance of bacterial contamination and placentitis, thus making CCD a preferable procedure.

Disadvantages of CCD

- It may be difficult to isolate and identify the correct fetus within the uterus.
- If complete uterine relaxation is not produced prior to touching the uterus, identification of the desired fetus will not be possible due to uterine muscular tone.
- The extent of trauma or prostaglandin release that occurs with manipulation of the fetus through the uterus is unknown. The procedure is relatively rapid from isolation of the fetus to CCD; therefore, severe inflammation should not result, but proficiency and time of manipulations may affect the outcome.
- A seroma or cellulitis may develop at the incision site for the transabdominal technique. The incision can be opened ventrally and drained if this occurs. Scarring of the incision site is minimal, with the possibility of hair at the incision site becoming white.
- The duration of time that the manipulated fetus survives is inconsistent, and an explanation is unknown.
- The colopotomy technique has a slight risk for evisceration through the incision site. This is diminished by suturing of the vaginal wall.

Further Reading

Journee SJ, de Ruijter-Villani M, Hendriks WK, *et al.* 2013. Efficacy of transvaginal ultrasound guided twin reduction in the mare by embryonic or fetal stabbing compared with yolk sac or allantoic aspiration. *Theriogenology* 80: 346–9.

Klewitz JK, Krekeler N, Ortgles R, *et al.* 2013. Evaluation of pregnancy and foaling rates after reduction of twin pregnancies via transvaginal ultrasound-guided aspiration in mares. *J Am Vet Med Assoc* 242: 522–32.

Macpherson ML, Reimer JM. 2000. Twin reduction in the mare: current options. *Animal Reprod Sci* 60: 233–44.

Rantanen N. 1990. Ultrasound-guided fetal cardiac puncture for twin reduction in mares. *Proc Am Assoc Eq Prac* 36: 169–71.

Wolfsdorf K, Rodgerson DH, Holder R. 2005. How to manually reduce twins between 60–120 days gestation using cranio-cervical dislocation. *Proc Am Assoc Eq Prac* 51: 284–7.

81

Twin Reduction: Thoracic Compression

Patrick M. McCue

Equine Reproduction Laboratory, Colorado State University, USA

Introduction

Twins are a significant cause of decreased reproductive efficiency in the mare and if not managed often result in abortion, stillbirth, or early foal death. Good breeding management practices, anticipation of the potential for twins based on detection of multiple ovulations, and an early accurate pregnancy diagnosis are keys for successful prevention of twin issues. Management of twins is most successful between 13 and 15 days post-ovulation, while embryos are in their mobility phase.

The preferred technique for reduction of one twin in early gestation is manual disruption of one embryonic vesicle using an ultrasound probe or hand per rectum (see Chapter 78). Failure to perform an early pregnancy examination or failure to detect twins on an early pregnancy examination places the pregnancy at risk of subsequent embryonic or fetal loss. Options are limited and success rate lower for management of twin pregnancies that are first detected or if intervention is first attempted after day 35 of pregnancy. One potential option is to induce demise of one fetus by thoracic compression.

Equipment and Supplies

Ultrasound unit, obstetrical sleeve, obstetrical lubricant, sedation, *N*-butylscopolammonium bromide (Buscopan®).

Technique

- The procedure is most effective when the mare is 55–65 days in foal.
- The mare is placed in examination stocks or otherwise adequately restrained.
- The mare is sedated with a combination of detomidine hydrochloride (0.01 mg/kg) plus butorphanol tartrate (0.01 mg/kg) administered intravenously. A dose of *N*-butylscopolammonium bromide (Buscopan®, 0.1–0.2 mg/kg) is administered intravenously to relax the smooth muscle of the rectum and uterus and to allow for a safe transrectal examination and reduction procedure.A transrectal ultrasound examination is performed to confirm the presence of twins and to determine which fetus to reduce.
- Once identified, the ultrasound probe is removed and manual transrectal palpation is performed with the goal of grasping one fetus in the hand of the examiner. Once that is accomplished, the head and thorax are identified and the fetus is positioned between the thumb and finger(s). Significant constant pressure is applied to the thorax of the selected fetus for approximately one minute.
- A follow-up ultrasound examination is subsequently performed to evaluate the heart beat status of each fetus. The heart of the "treated" fetus may continue to beat slowly for a few hours. If successful, a subsequent ultrasound examination the following day will confirm that only one fetus is still alive with an active heart beat (Figure 81.1).
- The pregnant mare is administered a single dose of flunixin meglumine (1 mg/kg IV) prior to the procedure and maintained on altrenogest (Regu-Mate®, 0.044 mg/kg, orally once per day) for 1–2 months after the procedure.

Interpretation

Management of twin pregnancies becomes more complicated after day 35 due to the increased size of the fetus, amount of fetal fluids present, progressive development of

Equine Reproductive Procedures, Second Edition. Edited by John Dascanio and Patrick McCue.

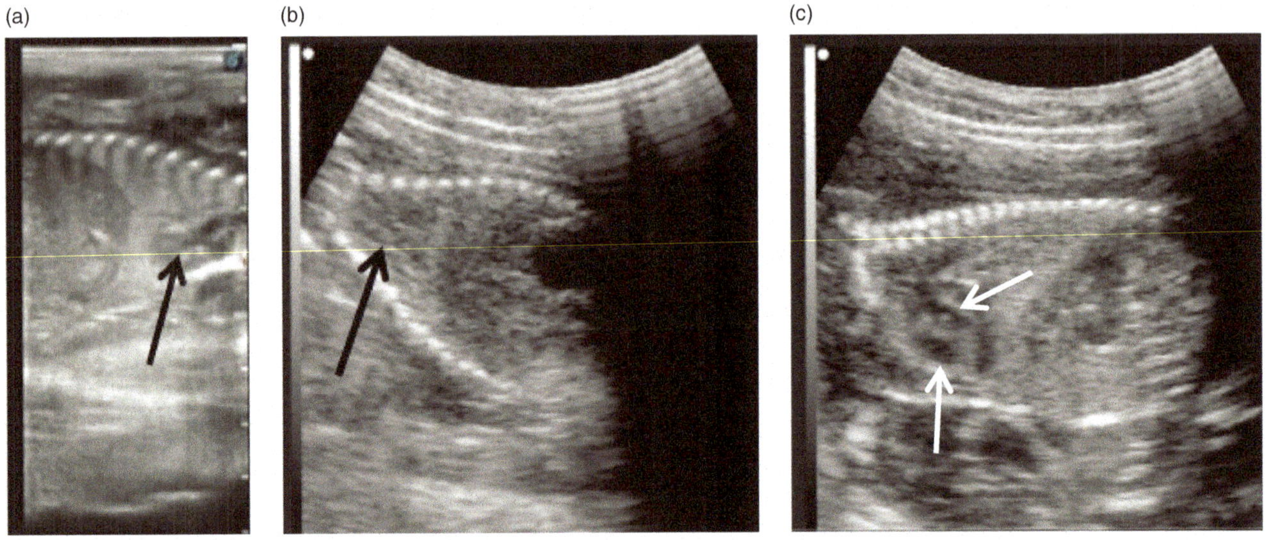

Figure 81.1 (a) Static image captured from a transrectal ultrasound video showing the heart of one fetus that had faint valve movements after thoracic compression. (b) Static image captured from a transabdominal ultrasound video showing an absence of heart function after thoracic compression in a second case. (c) Static image captured from an ultrasound video of the non-manipulated twin showing distended heart chambers (white arrows) associated with a normal heart rate and rhythm after conclusion of the thoracic compression procedure on the other twin. In each image the arrows show the location of the fetal heart. In (a) and (b) note the lack of normal hypoechoic cardiac chambers as compared with (c).

the placenta, and the fact that the mare may not return to a fertile estrus in the event that both twin pregnancies are lost during a reduction procedure.

Several procedures have been described for the reduction of one twin after day 35 of pregnancy including:

- Ultrasound-guided needle puncture and aspiration of amnionic or allantoic fluid from around one fetus (see Chapter 79).
- Ultrasound-guided cardiac puncture of one fetus with or without aspiration of fetal fluid.
- Transvaginal or transabdominal ultrasound-guided needle injection of potassium chloride or procaine penicillin into the heart, thorax, or abdomen of one fetus (see Chapter 82).
- Cranio-cervical dislocation of one fetus using either a transrectal or laparotomy approach (see Chapter 80).

Success rates for all fetal reduction techniques are highly variable between published reports and anecdotal statements. Another option is to terminate the twin pregnancy entirely with repeated doses of prostaglandins and rebreed the mare the next year (see Chapter 83).

In summary, thoracic compression can be successful in causing demise of one fetus in a set of twins. The technique is relatively easy to perform and fetal demise can be verified after the procedure with a follow-up ultrasound examination.

Further Reading

Mari G, Iacono E, Merlo B, *et al*. 2004. Reduction of twin pregnancy in the mare by transvaginal ultrasound-guided aspiration. *Reprod Domest Anim* 39: 434–7.

Rantanen N, Kincaid B. 1988. Ultrasound-guided fetal cardiac puncture: a method of twin reduction in the mare. *Proc Am Assoc Eq Pract* 34: 173–9.

Wolfsdorf KE, Rodgerson D, Schoergendorf A. 2009. Success rate of post-fixation twin reduction using cranio-cervical dislocation. *Proc Am Assoc Eq Pract* 55: 257–61.

82

Twin Reduction: Transabdominal Fetal Cardiac Puncture

John J. Dascanio

School of Veterinary Medicine, Texas Tech University, USA

Introduction

Twin reduction in the mare is usually performed in early gestation. However, circumstances may occur whereby termination of one foal in a twin pregnancy may need to be performed later in gestation. The best window of opportunity for transabdominal fetal cardiac injection is between days 100 and 120 of gestation. The uterus attains a ventral position within the abdomen of the mare by day 90 of gestation. Elimination of one fetus after day 150 may have an adverse effect on survival of the other fetus.

The first decision is to determine which fetus to terminate in a twin pregnancy. A complete ultrasonographic fetal well-being assessment should be performed to detail fetal sizes, heart rates, placental separation, echogenicity of allantoic and amniotic fluid compartments, and fetal movement. Generally, the fetus that is smaller in size, often determined by measuring the maximum fetal chest width, is marked for termination as it probably has the least amount of placental contact and the remaining fetus should have the greater chance of survival.

Equipment and Supplies

Tail wrap, tail rope, exam gloves, twitch, clippers, sedation, surgical scrub, local anesthetic, ultrasound, needle guide for ultrasound probe, needles, syringes, extension set, procaine penicillin, sterile surgery gloves, surgical pack, progesterone, systemic antibiotics, non-steroidal anti-inflammatory drug.

Technique

- Place a tail wrap and tail rope to keep the tail from interfering with the procedure.
- Perform a complete ultrasonographic fetal well-being assessment.
- Identify and confirm the presence of a twin pregnancy. Determine which foal has the narrowest chest width and select that one for termination if accessible.
- The administration of medications may vary amongst clinicians. Typically, antibiotics are administered to prevent infection with bacteria that may be introduced during placement of the transcutaneous needle. Trimethoprim sulfamethoxazole may be given at 30 mg/kg PO every 12 hours for 7–10 days. Exogenous progestin (altrenogest) is administered to keep the myometrium quiescent and to support pregnancy. Oral altrenogest may be administered at 0.044 mg/kg every 24 hours for 8 weeks. The longer duration is primarily due to experience with pregnancy loss occurring up to a least a month after completion of the procedure. It is during this time that the fetus that was terminated is undergoing resorption and mummification. Flunixin meglumine (1 mg/kg IV, every 12 hours for 2 days) is administered to limit inflammation from the procedure.
- Administer medications prior to preparation of the mare for fetal cardiac puncture.
- Sedate the mare. This is usually done with detomidine hydrochloride (0.0088–0.011 mg/kg IV) and butorphanol tartrate (0.011–0.022 mg/kg IV).
- Repeat the fetal heart rate assessment after sedation and relocate the foal to inject for termination. Sedation causes uterine relaxation and a reduction in fetal heart rate and movement.
- Clip and surgically scrub the ventral abdomen of the mare in an area that corresponds with the fetal heart to be injected.
- Inject a local anesthetic such as carbocaine into the subcutaneous tissue and ventral abdominal musculature of the mare in the area corresponding with injection of the fetus. Be careful to not enter the abdominal cavity.
- Complete a final surgical scrub.

Equine Reproductive Procedures, Second Edition. Edited by John Dascanio and Patrick McCue.

- Prepare a syringe with 35 ml procaine penicillin with a 76 cm (30 inch) extension set. Fill the extension set with penicillin.
- Disinfect the ultrasound probe with alcohol or place a sterile cover over the probe.
- Using sterile gloves, place a sterile water-soluble lubricant on the clipped skin and ultrasound probe transducer. Position the probe so that it overlies the fetal heart.
- Using a 9 cm (3.5 inch) 18 gauge spinal needle through a needle guide on the ultrasound probe (Figure 82.1), advance the spinal needle through the skin, muscle, and fat until it is easily identified on the ultrasound machine. Do not enter the peritoneal cavity yet. A 15 cm (6 inch) 18 gauge spinal needle may be needed for mares with significant abdominal fat.
- A needle guide may be created on an ultrasound probe by taping the cut end of a 14 gauge catheter onto the side of the probe (Figure 82.1). The inside of the 14 gauge catheter must be kept sterile.
- Make sure to practice needle placement with a balloon filled with lubricant so that you know which direction on the screen the needle will appear and how to direct the needle for placement into the heart.
- Make sure that the fetal heart is in line with the biopsy guide or path of the spinal needle. With a quick motion, push the spinal needle through the utero-placental tissue and into the chest and heart of the fetus. If the fetus is lying on its side within the mare's abdomen, be careful to avoid the fetal leg while placing the needle into the fetal chest (Figure 82.2).

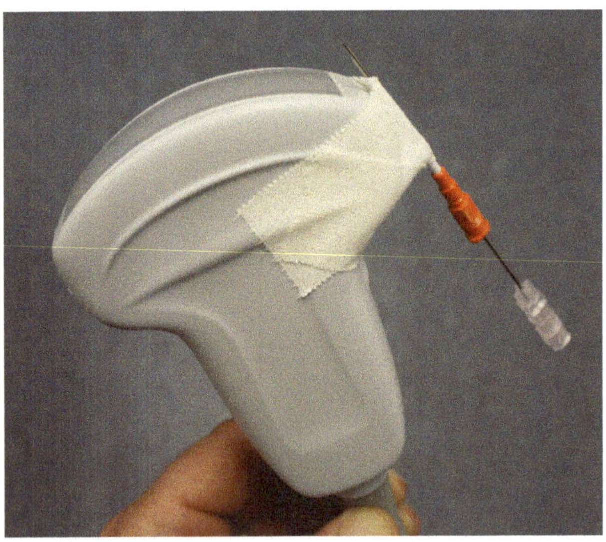

Figure 82.1 Ultrasound needle guide made with a shortened 14 gauge catheter and an 18 gauge spinal needle. Care must be taken to keep the inside of the 14 gauge catheter sterile.

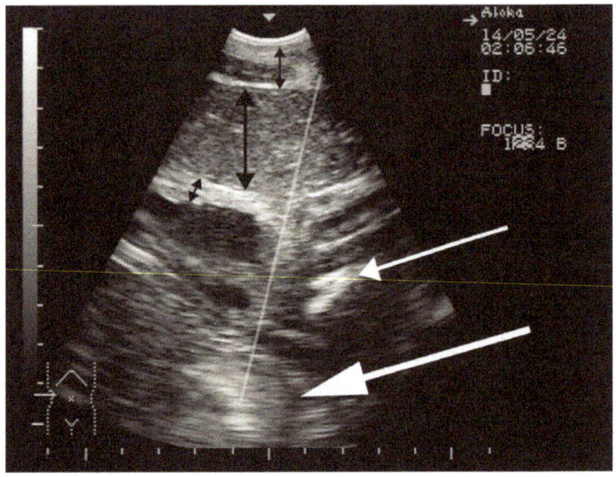

Figure 82.2 Transabdominal fetal cardiac puncture. The light white line depicts the needle entering the heart with an injection of procaine penicillin (white at the ventral end of the line). The large white arrow points to the fetal heart. The small white arrow points to the humerus (fetus lying on its side). The smallest black arrow is the width of the utero-placental tissue. The medium black arrow is the thickness of the abdominal musculature and skin. The large black arrow is a layer of abdominal fat.

- Inject 15–20 ml of procaine penicillin into the fetal heart chamber. This will be evident as a hyperechoic material flowing from the tip of the spinal needle on the ultrasound screen. Typically, if the procaine has been deposited into a heart chamber, the fetal heart rate will almost immediately decrease and/or stop.
- Pull the needle out of the fetus and the mare. Place a sterile 10 × 10 cm (4 × 4 inch) gauze over the needle hole on the mare's ventral abdomen to control hemorrhage. A light wrap may be placed around the abdomen to hold a sterile Telfa™ pad over the needle hole for 24 hours using an elastic adhesive bandage.

Interpretation

- The fetal heart rate should stop almost immediately after injection into one of the heart chambers.
- With successful injection of the heart, the heart chambers will be also be filled with the hyperechoic penicillin as evident on ultrasound. If the heart was not directly injected, the chambers will remain filled with hypoechoic blood (Figure 82.3). If the injection was made outside the heart chambers, such as into the chest cavity, the fetus may still die in the next 24-hour period. The heart chambers will then become filled with more hyperechoic clotted blood over time. A repeat ultrasound should be performed in 24–48 hours to document fetal death.

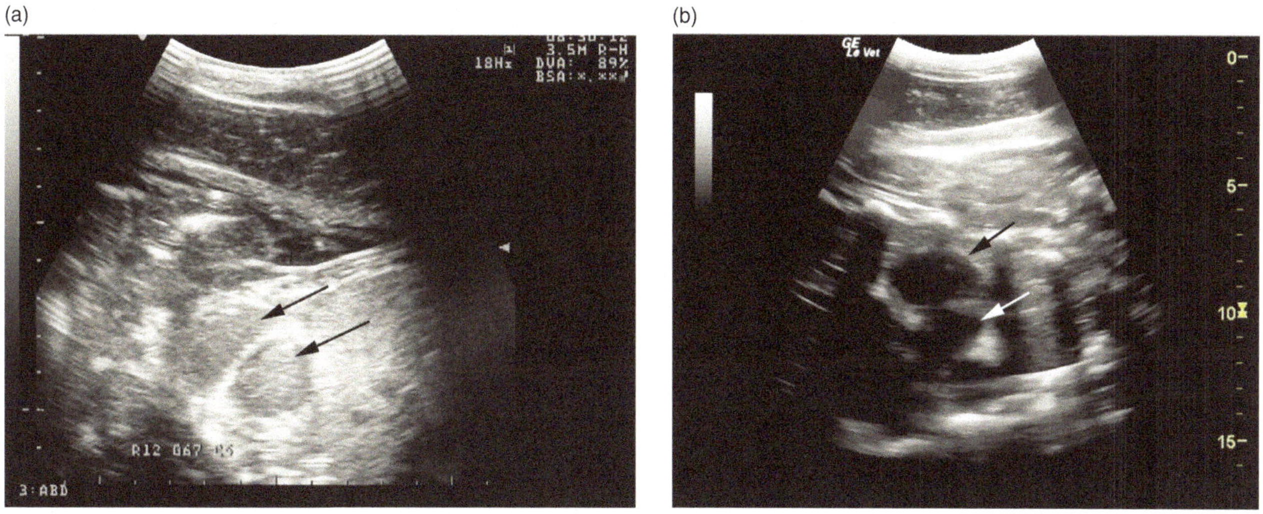

Figure 82.3 (a) Heart chambers (black arrows) filled with hyperechoic penicillin with successful intracardiac injection. (b) Heart chambers (black and white arrows) filled with hypoechoic blood with unsuccessful intracardiac injection of penicillin.

- If the targeted fetus did not die from the initial procedure, a second procedure may be attempted on the same fetus 4–7 days after the first attempt.
- The mare should be examined daily for any signs of potential abortion including premature udder formation, vulvar discharge, or expulsion of fetal membranes.
- The mare still has a chance of aborting both twins, especially in the first month post-procedure as the terminated foal is resorbed. Abortion may occur up to term due to placental insufficiency if the remaining fetus does not expand its placental contact area as it grows.

Further Reading

Hodder ADJ, Liu IKM, Ball BA. 2008. Current methods for the diagnosis and management of twin pregnancy in the mare. *Eq Vet Educ* 20: 493–502.

MacPherson ML, Reimer JM. 2000. Twin reduction in the mare: current options. *Ann Reprod Sci* 60–1: 233–44.

Rantanen NW, Kincaid B. 1989. Ultrasound guided fetal cardiac puncture: a method of twin reduction in the mare. *Proc Annu Conv Am Assoc Eq Pract* 34: 173–9.

83

Elective Termination of Pregnancy

John J. Dascanio

School of Veterinary Medicine, Texas Tech University, USA

Introduction

Elective termination of pregnancy may be necessary in the event of an accidental or undesired breeding or if the health status of a mare is compromised by pregnancy. Examples may include impending rupture of a pre-pubic tendon, a twin pregnancy, a hydrops condition, or a musculoskeletal issue such as advanced laminitis. Pregnancy may be terminated by pharmacological or manual techniques. There are usually few complications if pregnancy is terminated in the first trimester. Complications of later stage abortion may include retention of placental membranes, cervical trauma, dystocia, and uterine infection.

Equipment and Supplies

Tail wrap, non-irritant soap, roll cotton, stainless steel bucket, disposable liner for bucket, paper towels, examination gloves, sterile obstetrical sleeve, sterile obstetrical lubricant, prostaglandin E_1 or E_2, prostaglandin $F_{2\alpha}$, oxytocin, needles, syringe, uterine infusion pipette, sterile saline.

Technique

Confirm that the mare is currently pregnant and estimate the stage of pregnancy via transrectal palpation and ultrasonography.

Termination of an Early Pregnancy (Prior to Day 35)

- Pregnancy can be terminated in the event of an unwanted mating prior to day 35 of gestation by administration of a single intramuscular dose of prostaglandins (cloprostenol 250 μg or dinoprost tromethamine 2.5–10 mg).
- Lysis of the corpus luteum and the subsequent reduction in progesterone production will result in failure to maintain the pregnancy.
- The mare should return to estrus within approximately 4 days after prostaglandin administration.
- It would be appropriate to recheck the mare 4–7 days after prostaglandin administration to confirm that the pregnancy has been eliminated.
- Prostaglandin administration will not be effective if the mare has been mismated and has not yet ovulated or if ovulation has occurred within the previous 4–5 days. It is recommended that prostaglandins be administered at least 5 days after ovulation to result in complete luteolysis, and even then a single dose may not be sufficient.

Termination of Pregnancy Between Days 35 and 120

- Endometrial cups will begin to form at approximately day 35 of gestation. These fetal placental-origin cells invade into the endometrium of the mare and form discrete "islands" of cells that produce large quantities of equine chorionic gonadotropin (eCG). eCG will induce the formation of secondary or accessory corpora lutea within the ovary of the pregnant mare.
- It is recommended that prostaglandins (cloprostenol 250 μg or dinoprost tromethamine 2.5–10 mg) be administered once a day for 3–5 days to completely lyse the corpora lutea that are present or in development.
- In the absence of progesterone, the cervix will begin to relax. The ecbolic effect of the exogenous prostaglandins will cause sufficient uterine contractions to expel the fetus from the uterus.
- Endometrial cups will not be adversely affected (i.e., will not regress) as a consequence of prostaglandin administration. The cups will eventually regress due to immune rejection by the mare.

Equine Reproductive Procedures, Second Edition. Edited by John Dascanio and Patrick McCue.

- The mare may not return to normal cyclicity while the endometrial cups are functional.
- A uterine lavage may be warranted after the fetus is expelled to remove all fetal membranes and debris.

Termination of a Mid to Late Gestation Pregnancy

Pharmacological technique

- There are several techniques that may be used to pharmacologically induce a safe termination of a late-term pregnancy.

- *Option 1*:
  - Apply either prostaglandin E_1 (PGE_1) (misoprostol 1–2 mg or alprostadil 1 mg) or PGE_2 (dinoprostone 0.5 mg) topically to the external cervical os and cervical lumen to promote cervical relaxation. Allow 2–4 hours for the cervix to relax.
  - Administer a single intramuscular dose of a prostaglandin (cloprostenol 250 μg or dinoprost tromethamine 2.5–10 mg). Wait 1 hour before oxytocin administration.
  - Administer 5–10 IU of oxytocin intravenously or intramuscularly every 30 minutes until fetal expulsion. Two or three doses of oxytocin may be required. Manual dilation of the cervix may be beneficial if spontaneous passage of the fetus does not occur.
- *Option 2*:
  - Administer 5–10 mg of estradiol-17β as an intramuscular injection the day prior to induction of abortion. The goal is to promote relaxation of the cervix and potentially enhance the effect of prostaglandins.
  - Administer a single intramuscular dose of prostaglandins in the morning (cloprostenol 250 μg or dinoprost tromethamine 2.5–10 mg). Wait 1 hour before oxytocin administration.
  - Administer 5–10 IU of oxytocin intravenously or intramuscularly every 30 minutes until fetal expulsion. Manual dilation of the cervix may be beneficial if spontaneous passage of the fetus does not occur.
- *Option 3*:
  - Administer prostaglandins intramuscularly twice a day for 2–5 days. Usually a total of 2–4 daily doses are required to induce abortion.
  - Oxytocin may be administered to assist in expulsion of the fetus.

Manual technique

- Remove feces from the rectum.
- Place a tail wrap and tail rope on the mare (see Chapter 4).
- Wearing examination gloves, clean and dry the perineum of the mare (see Chapter 3).
- Don a sterile obstetrical sleeve and place sterile water-soluble lubricant on the outside of the hand and down the arm.
- The sleeved hand is inserted through the vulvar labia and advanced to the external cervical os. A slight rotational motion may be used to spread lubricant within the reproductive tract and aid in forward movement of the arm.
- The lumen of the external cervical os is located with the index finger. The os of the cervix may be directed slightly downward or to one side. Careful digital exploration will yield access to the cervical lumen.
- Place the index finger into the cervical canal, using a probing maneuver to locate the direction of the canal. The cervical canal is not always straight and may slightly curve, especially downward in a multiparous mare. The cervix is likely to be tight during pregnancy, and with constant light to firm pressure pushing forward, the cervix should gradually dilate.
- Once a single finger is advanced through the entire cervical canal, a second finger is slowly inserted into the cervical lumen. The two fingers may be slowly opened to further dilate the lumen. Additional fingers may be added as the cervix dilates.
- It may require up to an hour to adequately manually dilate the cervix for manual removal of the fetus.
- Topical administration of PGE_1 may make manual dilation of the cervix easier.

Other Methods to Terminate an Equine Pregnancy

- Infusion of the pregnant uterus with sterile saline, antibiotics, antiseptics, or other solutions may cause abortion. The technique is similar to that for uterine infusion in the non-pregnant mare, although the passage of the pipette is more difficult in the pregnant mare. Rupture of the placental membranes with the pipette may enhance the effect.
- Uterine biopsy forceps have been used to rupture placental membranes leading to abortion.

Interpretation

- An elective termination of pregnancy may lead to the passage of an intact chorioallantois with the fetus contained within the fetal membranes.
- In some instances the cervix may dilate, but the chorioallantoic membrane may fail to rupture. In this situation, it may be necessary to manually rupture the chorioallantoic

membrane to deliver the fetus and then facilitate removal of the fetal membranes.

- Trauma to the cervix may occur if the cervix is manually dilated too quickly or too aggressively.
- Administration of prostaglandins, especially in higher doses, may cause sweating and transient abdominal discomfort and diarrhea.

Further Reading

Card CE. 2011. Induction of abortion. In: McKinnon AO, Squires EL, Vaala WE, Varner DD (eds). Equine Reproduction, 2nd edn. Ames, IA: Wiley Blackwell, pp. 2320–4.

84

Abortion Diagnostic Evaluation: Sample Collection in the Field and Submission

Julie T. Cecere[1] *and John J. Dascanio*[2]

[1] *Virginia-Maryland College of Veterinary Medicine, USA*
[2] *School of Veterinary Medicine, Texas Tech University, USA*

Introduction

Approximately 10% of mares will lose their pregnancy between day 60 and term. All equine abortions should be investigated to determine the cause. The cause may be obvious in some cases, such as twins or a twisted umbilical cord. In other cases the cause may not be obvious and an accurate diagnosis may provide information for management changes or therapeutic interventions to prevent or minimize further pregnancy losses. Unfortunately, a definitive diagnosis is only obtained in approximately 50–60% of clinical cases evaluated.

Equine abortions may be categorized into infectious or non-infectious causes. The most common infectious causes of abortion in horses are ascending placentitis and equine herpesvirus type 1 (EHV-1) infection, while the most common non-infectious causes of abortion are twins and a twisted umbilical cord (Figures 84.1 and 84.2). Other less common or sporadic causes of abortion include equine viral arteritis, consumption of eastern tent caterpillars, leptospirosis, chronic nocardioform placentitis caused by *Crossiella equi*, and congenital abnormalities.

The objective of this chapter is to provide guidelines for a field evaluation of an equine abortion and outline samples to be collected and submitted to a diagnostic laboratory.

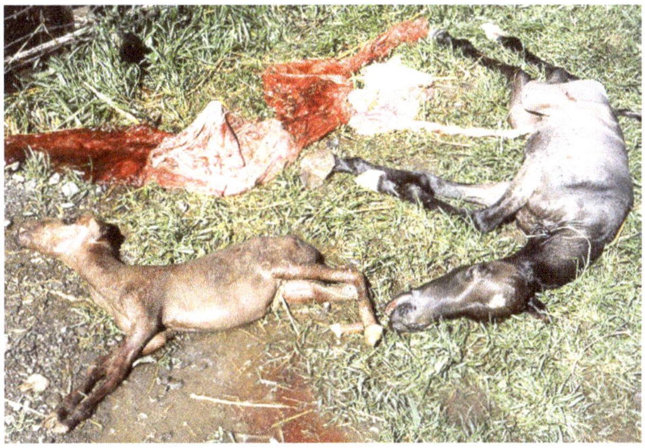

Figure 84.1 Abortion due to a twin pregnancy.

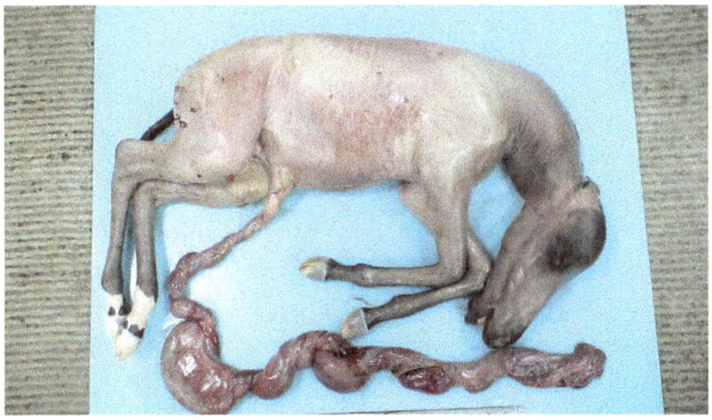

Figure 84.2 Twisted umbilical cord as a cause of abortion in a mare. Note edema in the umbilical cord.

Equipment and Supplies

Red top tubes, sterile containers or whirl packs, 10% formalin, culture swabs, surgical pack with sterile forceps and scissors, sterile gloves. In addition, a digital camera may be useful to document the condition of the fetus and placenta as well as to document gross pathology.

Technique

- The history, physical exam of the mare, and condition of the fetus should be carefully considered. For example, an autolysed fetus is more likely to have a bacterial origin of abortion.

Equine Reproductive Procedures, Second Edition. Edited by John Dascanio and Patrick McCue.

- Strict biosecurity protocols should be observed:
  - Washable footwear, disposable gloves, and washable or disposable coveralls should be used.
  - Foot baths should be placed outside the mare's stall door.
  - Feed the affected mare and clean her stall after all other horses. Care should be taken to wash all stall cleaning equipment between this mare and others on the farm or to dedicate equipment to this mare for the duration of any investigation.
  - Clothes should be changed after handling affected membranes or fetus.
- The mare should be isolated from other horses on the farm.
- The aborted fetus and associated membranes should be contained in plastic bags until examined to limit contamination of the premises. All tissues not submitted to a diagnostic laboratory should be burned or buried.
- The weight of the aborted fetus and placenta should be obtained.
- The length and characteristics of the umbilical cord should be noted.
- A state laboratory may supply veterinarians with an abortion kit that can be easily utilized in the field.

Submission Protocols

- The regional diagnostic laboratory should be contacted for specific submission guidelines.
- One half of each organ piece or tissue sampled should be placed in 10% buffered neutral formalin and the other half placed within a sterile container or whirl pack bag for culture, virus isolation, or fluorescent antibody tests.
- The tissue in formalin should be one part tissue to 10 parts formalin and the tissue thickness should not exceed 1 cm (0.4 inches) for proper fixation.
- Do not freeze any tissue as this will render it unusable.
- Tissues should be placed on ice or in a refrigerator until submission.
- A thorough history should accompany all samples.

Samples for Submission

Mare

- Place serum in two 10 ml red top tubes.
- Collect acute and convalescent samples 4–6 weeks apart.
- Take one uterine biopsy at the time of abortion.
- Submit the biopsy material for histology.
- Submit a uterine swab for virus isolation.

Foal

- The entire fetus should be submitted to the diagnostic laboratory, if possible. If not, samples should be collected from key organs, tissues, or anatomic sites as listed below:
  - Fetal sera and peritoneal fluid should be placed in a red top serum tube.
  - Tissue samples:
    - Spleen, liver, kidney, lung, heart, lymph nodes, adrenal glands, thymus and heart
    - Tissue should be approximately 1 cm (0.4 inches) thick by 3 cm square.
- Stomach contents should be put in a whirl pack bag. The fetus continually swallows amniotic fluid, so this sample can be highly diagnostic especially for bacterial etiologies.
- Aqueous humor should be placed in a red top tube and collected with a 6 ml syringe and 18 gauge needle, especially if a toxic insult is suspected.

Placenta

- The entire chorioallantois, amnion, and umbilical cord should be collected and submitted, if possible.
- If samples are to be collected for submission, at least four representative samples from multiple locations should be collected if the placenta is grossly normal. Full thickness biopsy samples should be collected from the cervical star region, body of the placenta, and each placental horn.
- Samples should be collected from the normal and abnormal areas in juxtaposition to any thickened, discolored, or abnormal regions.

Further Reading

Giles RC, Donahue JM, Hong CB, *et al.* 1993. Causes of abortion, stillbirth, and perinatal death in horses: 3,527 cases (1986–1991). *J Am Vet Med Assoc* 203: 1170–5.

Laugier C, Foucher N, Sevin C, Leon A, Tapprest J. 2011. A 24-year retrospective study of equine abortion in Normandy (France). *J Eq Vet Sci* 31: 116–23.

Ricketts, SW, Barrelet, A, Whitewell, KE. 2003. Equine abortion. *Eq Vet Educ* 6: 18–21.

Schlafer D, Foster R. 2015. Female genital system. In: Grant Maxie M (ed.). *Jubb, Kennedy and Palmer's Pathology of Domestic Animals*, Vol 3, 6th edn. pp. 358–464.

85

Endocrine Evaluation of Pregnancy

Patrick M. McCue

Equine Reproduction Laboratory, Colorado State University, USA

Introduction

Endocrine tests for pregnancy in mares may be used if palpation and ultrasound cannot be performed. Hormonal testing may also be used to look for trends in values for mares with high risk pregnancies or those with placentitis. Techniques used for pregnancy diagnosis and the timing of specific pregnancy tests are based on normal physiological events in the pregnant mare (Figure 85.1). Accurate breeding dates are consequently helpful when determining when to use an endocrine test for pregnancy. All methods of pregnancy examination have limitations and some may be associated with a false-positive or false-negative diagnosis.

Equipment and Supplies

Vacutainer® tubes and needles, endocrine diagnostic laboratory, centrifuge (optional).

Hormonal Tests for Pregnancy

Radioimmunoassay (RIA) and enzyme-linked immunoassay (ELISA) are the diagnostic procedures most commonly used for the measurement of hormone concentrations in blood to determine pregnancy status and to monitor fetal–placental health (Table 85.1). In many instances, an accurate diagnosis of true pregnancy status may be best determined by the evaluation of a combination of endocrine

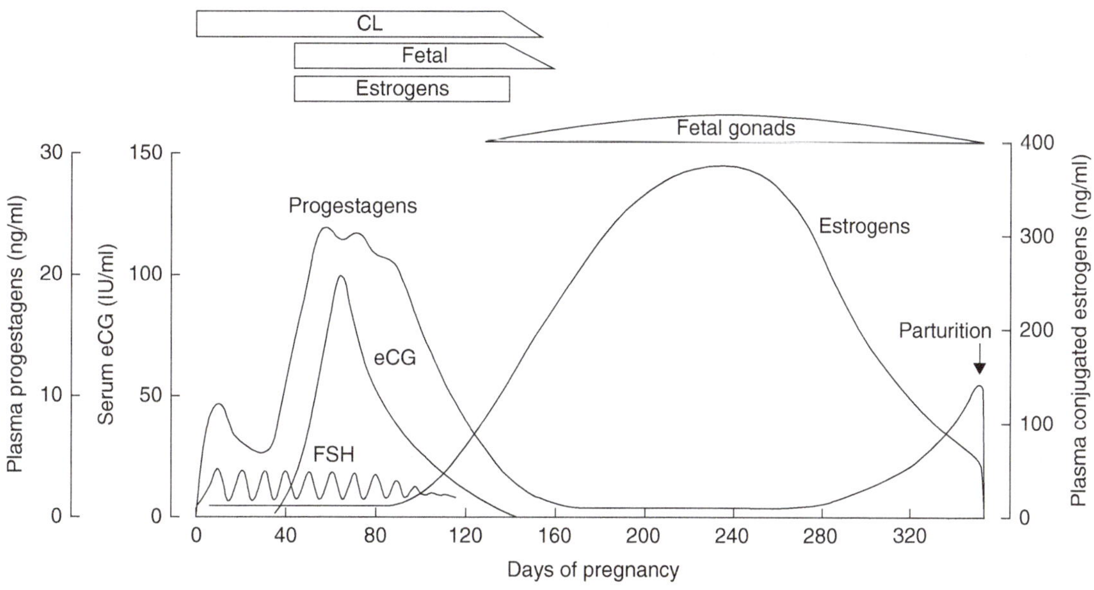

Figure 85.1 Reproductive physiology of the pregnant mare. CL, corpus luteum; eCG, equine chorionic gonadotropin; FSH, follicle-stimulating hormone. Source: From Allen WR, Short RV. 1997. Interspecific and extraspecific pregnancies in equids: anything goes. *J Heredity* 88: 384–92. Reproduced with the permission of Oxford University Press.

Equine Reproductive Procedures, Second Edition. Edited by John Dascanio and Patrick McCue.

Table 85.1 Endocrine tests for pregnancy diagnosis in the mare.

Hormone	Source	Time Course	Comments
Progesterone (P_4) and other progestogens	Corpus luteum (CL) and/or placenta	Initial elevation after primary ovulation; additional rise after formation of secondary corpora lutea begins on day 45–60	Not a direct indicator of pregnancy; levels >1.0 ng/ml are associated with the presence of luteal tissue in a non-pregnant or early pregnant mare; the placenta begins to produce progestins by day 70 that may be detected in a progesterone assay; levels <1.0 ng/ml are generally incompatible with pregnancy, in the absence of additional progestin support
Equine chorionic gonadotropin (eCG) or pregnant mare serum gonadotropin (PMSG)	Endometrial cups	Cup formation begins at approximately day 35 of pregnancy; eCG may be detected in the blood by day 35–42; maximum concentrations are reached by day 55–70; cups regress by day 100–140; eCG production and duration of secretion is highly variable between mares	Direct indicator of pregnancy; detection of eCG indicates the presence of endometrial cups; false negatives may occur if testing occurs before cup formation or after cup regression in a pregnant mare; false positives may occur following pregnancy loss after cup formation; some pregnant mares may not form endometrial cups
Estrone sulfate	Ovary (CL) and fetal–placental unit	Initial rise at day 35–45 of ovarian CL origin; substantial increase at day 90 of placental origin	Direct indicator of pregnancy after day 90; also useful in monitoring health status of the fetal–placental unit. Will decrease within 2–3 days of fetal demise
Relaxin	Placenta	Increased blood levels by day 80; levels remain elevated until foaling	Direct indicator of pregnancy in the mare; may be useful as a marker for placental health. Commercial testing not available
Testosterone	Fetal gonads	Increased blood levels in mare from first month of pregnancy; levels peak at 6–7 months and then decline	Not used as an indicator of pregnancy in the mare; levels increase in mares carrying either a male or female fetus

parameters. Individually, all endocrine tests have limitations associated with a false-positive or a false-negative diagnosis. A hormone or other factor may be considered a direct indicator of pregnancy if the source is limited to the fetus and/or placenta.

Progesterone

Pregnant mares should have a continued secretion of progesterone from the ovarian corpus luteum beyond the period of maternal recognition of pregnancy (MRP) (days 12 to 14), whereas non-pregnant mares should experience a rapid decline in progesterone following the release of prostaglandins from the endometrium. However, some non-pregnant mares have elevated progesterone beyond the time of MRP (i.e., mares with a persistent corpus luteum, luteinized anovulatory follicle, or diestral ovulation). Consequently, measurement of progesterone in the blood of mares is of limited value for an accurate pregnancy diagnosis.

Detection of a progesterone concentration less than 1 ng/ml usually indicates the absence of a pregnancy, unless the mare is being supplemented with a synthetic progestin. However, occasionally a 16-day ultrasound pregnancy examination will reveal an embryo in the presence of mild uterine edema and a regressing corpus luteum. Low plasma progesterone in these cases suggests failure of MRP and progesterone supplementation would be indicated.

Progesterone measurement is valuable in determining if a pregnant mare is producing sufficient progesterone to maintain her pregnancy. Generally, a serum concentration of ≥4 ng/ml is considered adequate to maintain the pregnancy when measured during the first 2–3 months of gestation when the ovary is the primary source of progesterone.

Progesterone levels may rise substantially by day 60 in mares that form supplementary corpora lutea. The evaluation and interpretation of progesterone levels in samples collected after day 100 are more complicated. Most progesterone assays utilize an antibody specific for natural progesterone (P_4), with some potential cross-reactivity with other progestins.

Placental production of other progestins, such as dihydroprogesterone (DHP), begins at approximately 70–80 days of gestation. DHP and other progestins are not detected by a standard progesterone assay or have limited cross-reactivity in the assay. Consequently, it is not unusual to detect a "progesterone" level of 2.5–4.0 ng/ml in a normal pregnant mare in the second half of gestation, even though the overall "progestin profile" of a mid- to late-term pregnant mare would consist of high levels of various progestins. Consequently, the interpretation of progesterone values must be based on the stage of pregnancy.

Altrenogest, a synthetic progestin commonly used to supplement endogenous progesterone, is not detected in commercial progesterone assays.

Equine Chorionic Gonadotropin

The detection of elevated levels of equine chorionic gonadotropin (eCG), formerly called pregnant mare serum gonadotropin (PMSG), in the blood of mares may be used as a direct positive indicator of pregnancy. eCG is produced by specialized placental cells called endometrial cups that begin to form from the invasion of trophoblast cells into the maternal endometrium at approximately day 35 of gestation. An increase in blood eCG levels can be detected by days 35–42, with maximum concentrations achieved by days 55–70. Complete regression of the cups and an absence of eCG occurs by day 100 to 140.

Concentrations of eCG are higher in horse or hinny pregnancies than in mule or donkey pregnancies (Figure 85.2).

Two major problems exist using eCG levels for pregnancy diagnosis. First, a false-negative diagnosis (i.e., no eCG detected in a mare that is truly pregnant) can occur if a blood sample is collected prior to day 35, before the endometrial cups form, or after day 120 of pregnancy after regression of the cups. Second, a false-positive pregnancy diagnosis (i.e., elevated eCG detected in a mare that is truly not pregnant) can occur if a blood sample is collected from a mare that lost her pregnancy after endometrial cup formation. Mares that experience pregnancy loss after day 40 of gestation will usually not return to estrus until cup degeneration is complete and after all luteal tissue has regressed. Therefore, detection of elevated eCG in the blood of a mare will only confirm that endometrial cups are present and does not indicate current pregnancy status or fetal health. Persistence of endometrial cups with prolonged secretion of eCG well beyond the expected time period has been reported following abortion and following a full-term pregnancy.

Estrogens

Conjugated estrogens (e.g., estrone sulfate) and total estrogens (conjugated plus unconjugated estrogens) in blood, milk, urine, or feces have been used for the diagnosis of pregnancy and as an indicator of fetal viability in domestic and feral horses. Total estrogen and conjugated estrogen levels initially increase between days 35 and 40 of pregnancy. This first increase in estrogens is due to production by the corpus luteum in response to eCG stimulation. This early rise in estrogens cannot be used as a direct indicator of pregnancy in mares.

A second larger increase in estrogens begins after day 55 of pregnancy. The source of estrogen production at this stage of

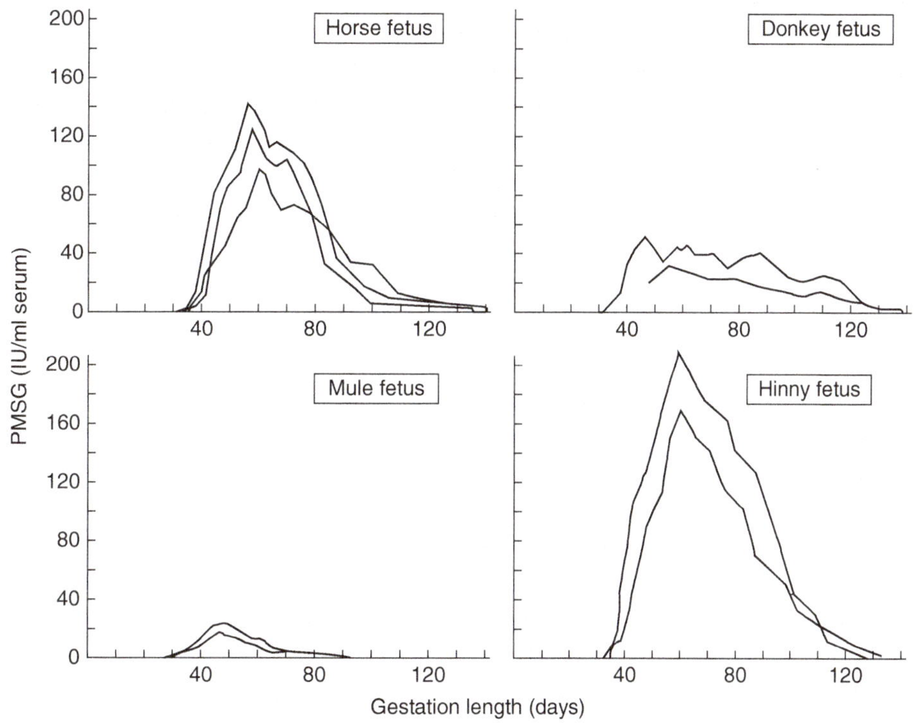

Figure 85.2 Concentrations of equine chorionic gonadotropin (pregnant mare serum gonadotropin or PMSG) in various horse × donkey crosses. Source: From Allen WR, Short RV. 1997. Interspecific and extraspecific pregnancies in equids: anything goes. *J Heredity* 88: 384–92. Reproduced with the permission of Oxford University Press.

gestation is the fetal–placental unit. The pattern of estrogen secretion during gestation mirrors the pattern of fetal gonad development. Estrogen concentrations increase by the end of the first trimester, reach peak concentrations by days 210 to 240, and then gradually decline over the remainder of gestation. Consequently, an increase in total estrogens or conjugated estrogens after day 70 to 80 of gestation can be used as a direct indicator of pregnancy. Measurement of estrogen levels after the third month of pregnancy can also be used to evaluate fetal viability. Fetal death leads to a rapid decline in total estrogen and conjugated estrogen levels within a few days. Determination of estrone sulfate levels in urine or serum is the basis of several stall-side pregnancy tests.

Relaxin

Relaxin is a protein hormone produced primarily by the placenta in the mare. Production of relaxin by the placenta begins at approximately 80 days of gestation. Concentrations peak between days 176 and 200 and remain elevated to term. Relaxin concentrations decrease rapidly following foaling and expulsion of the placenta. The measurement of relaxin has been used as an indicator of pregnancy and as a biomarker for placental function in the mare.

Testosterone

Concentrations of testosterone in maternal blood increase from the first month of pregnancy and reach peak concentrations at approximately 6–7 months of gestation and subsequently decline. The pattern of testosterone during pregnancy follows a similar pattern to that of estrogens. The early rise of testosterone in pregnancy may be from the maternal ovaries, while the much larger later rise and fall is due to development and regression of the fetal gonads. Elevated testosterone levels in mid-gestation is associated with behavioral changes (i.e., masculine or aggressive behavior) in some pregnant mares.

Additional Comments

A combination of serum progesterone, eCG, and total estrogens (or conjugated estrogens) may be used to assess whether or not a mare is pregnant, if that mare cannot be examined by ultrasonography. Examples may include miniature horses, wild or feral horses, fractious horses, and horses with a previous history of a rectal tear. Endocrine tests can be strongly suggestive of the presence of a pregnancy, but false positives can occur. The optimal technique for pregnancy diagnosis is a combination of transrectal palpation and ultrasonography.

Mares with high risk pregnancies or those with current health issues, especially placentitis, may be monitored for progestogen and estrone sulfate concentrations as an indication of the maintenance of pregnancy and inflammation. Conclusions should not be based on a single point in time measurement, but should be based on trends from sampling every other day for three to four sampling periods. A premature rise in progestogens (primarily progesterone) or a decrease in estrone sulfate from reference ranges or in trends may indicate a negative outcome, such as abortion or fetal demise, and may be the basis for interventional therapy.

Reference

Allen WR, Short RV. 1997. Interspecific and extraspecific pregnancies in equids: anything goes. *J Heredity* 88: 384–92.

Further Reading

Allen WR. 2001. Fetomaternal interactions and influences during equine pregnancy. *Reproduction* 121: 513–27.

Allen WR, Wilsher S, Stewart F, Ousey J, Fowden A. 2002. The influence of maternal size on placental, fetal and postnatal growth in the horse. II. Endocrinology of pregnancy. *J Endocrinol* 172: 237–46.

Cole HH, Hart GH. 1930. Properties of gonad-stimulating principle of mares' serum. *Am J Physiol* 93: 57.

Conley AJ. 2016. Review of the reproductive endocrinology of the pregnant and parturient mare. *Theriogenology* 86: 355–65.

Daels PF, Shideler S, Lasley BL, Hughes JP, Stabenfeldt GH. 1990. Source of oestrogen in early pregnancy in the mare. *J Reprod Fertil* 90: 55–61.

McCue PM, McKinnon AO. 2011. Pregnancy diagnosis. In: McKinnon AO, Squires EL, Vaala WE, Varner DD (eds). Equine Reproduction, 2nd edn. Ames, IA: Wiley Blackwell, pp. 2245–61.

Nett TM, Holtan DW, Estergreen VL. 1973. Plasma estrogen in pregnant and postpartum mares. *J Anim Sci* 37: 962–70.

Stewart DR, Addiego LA, Pascoe DR, Haluska GJ, Pashen R. 1992. Breed differences in circulating equine relaxin. *Biol Reprod* 46: 648–52.

86

Treatment of Vaginal Varicosities

John J. Dascanio

School of Veterinary Medicine, Texas Tech University, USA

Introduction

Vaginal varicosities are superficial blood vessels that are often located just cranial to the vestibulo-vaginal fold (remnant of the hymen). The vessels may spontaneously rupture causing blood to exit from the vulva. Mares that are pregnant, especially in the last trimester, may have more prominent vascularity, causing the potential for more bleeding of varicosities. Most bleeding varicosities are small and non-life-threatening and pose no immediate health risk. The treatment of varicosities includes benign neglect, topical treatment with astringent creams (phenylephrine hydrochloride cream), ligation of vessels, cautery of vessels, and laser photocoagulation of vessels. If bleeding from the vulva is present, the source of the bleeding should be determined by the use of a vaginal speculum (Figure 86.1) or an endoscope (Figure 86.2) passed into the vagina. The endoscope may be retroflexed back toward the vulva to examine the inner aspect of the vestibulo-vaginal fold for varicosities.

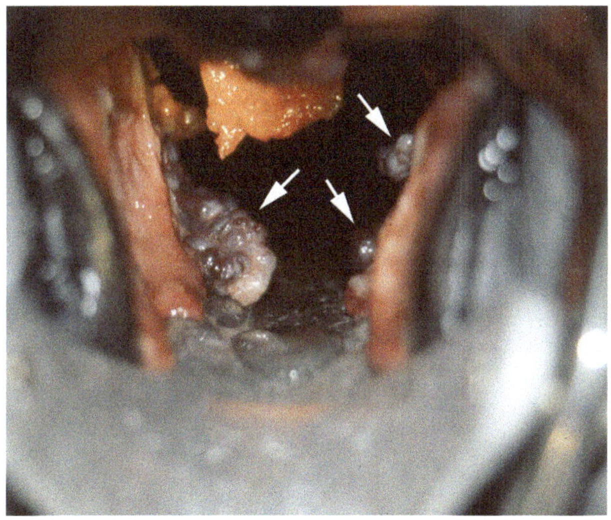

Figure 86.1 Mare with numerous varicose veins (arrows) near the vestibulo-vaginal fold as viewed through a vaginal speculum.

Equipment and Supplies

Tail wrap, non-irritant soap, roll cotton, stainless steel bucket, disposable liner for bucket, paper towels, exam gloves, sterile obstetrical sleeve, sterile lubricant, sterilized videoendoscope, sterile saline, flunixin meglumine, altrenogest (optional), laser (optional).

Technique for Endoscopic Examination

- Remove feces from the rectum.
- Place a tail wrap and tie the tail out of the way (see Chapter 4).
- Wash and dry the perineum of the mare (see Chapter 3). Cold sterilize a 1 m long, 11 mm diameter endoscope in an activated solution of 2.4% glutaraldehyde (Cidex®; Johnson & Johnson Co., Irvine, CA, USA) and rinse thoroughly with sterile saline, making sure to properly clean and rinse the accessory channel.
- Place a sterile obstetrical sleeve on one arm and hold the end of the endoscope in this gloved hand.
- Place sterile lubricant on the back of the gloved hand and down the sleeve, being careful to not get lubricant on the camera end of the endoscope.
- Separate the vulvar labia and introduce the gloved hand/endoscope into the vestibule, through the vestibulo-vaginal fold and into the vagina.

Equine Reproductive Procedures, Second Edition. Edited by John Dascanio and Patrick McCue.

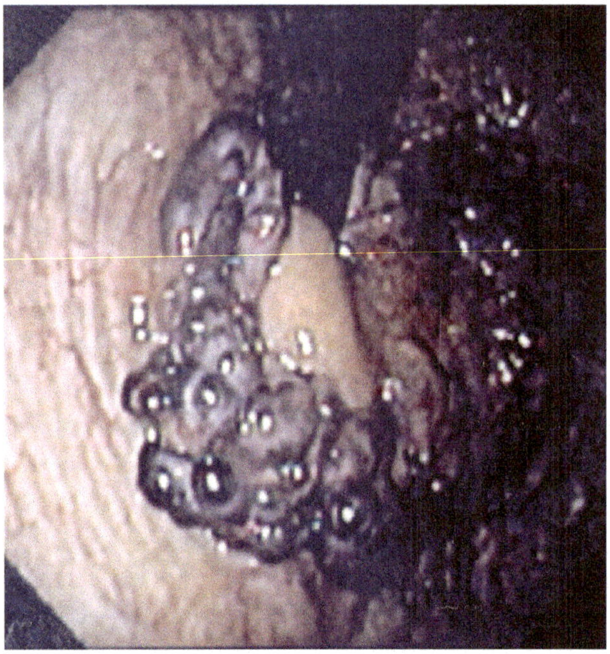

Figure 86.2 Mare with numerous varicose veins in the inner aspect of the vestibulo-vaginal fold as viewed with a retroflexed endoscope. Reproduced with permission from: DeLuca C, Dascanio JJ, Berry DB. 2007. Nd:YAG laser treatment of a vestibulovaginal varicosity in a 15-year-old pregnant mare. *J Eq Vet Sci* 2007; 27: 217–20.

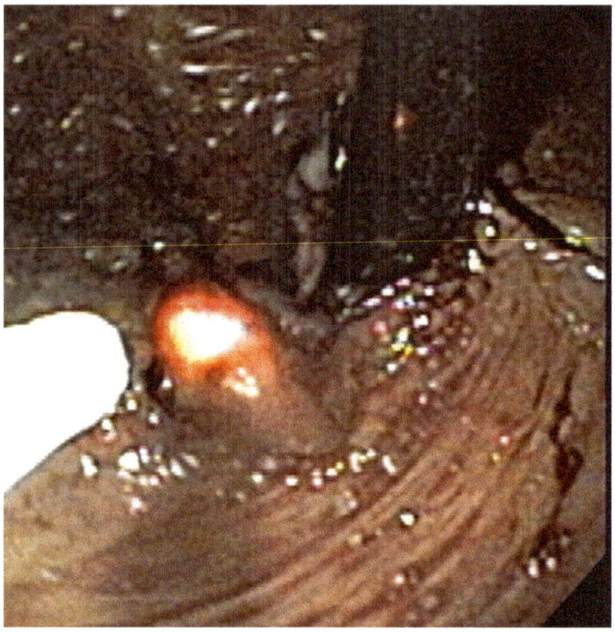

Figure 86.3 Laser endoscopic ablation of varicose veins surrounding the vestibulo-vaginal fold. Reproduced with permission from: DeLuca C, Dascanio JJ, Berry DB. 2007. Nd:YAG laser treatment of a vestibulovaginal varicosity in a 15-year-old pregnant mare. *J Eq Vet Sci* 2007; 27: 217–20.

- Visually examine the vagina for any varicosities. The endoscope should be retroflexed back towards the vestibule to examine the inner aspect of the vestibulo-vaginal fold (Figure 86.2). Air may need to be insufflated into the vagina to allow visualization, but usually enough air enters with the passage of the endoscope.
- The cervical canal should be examined for any hemorrhagic discharge. It could be possible that a uterine tumor could be the source of the hemorrhage.

Technique for Laser Photocoagulation of Varicosities Using an Nd:YAG Laser

- Position the endoscope directly in front of the vessel to be coagulated.
- Advance a 2.1 mm diameter coaxial transmitting tube (600 µm diameter non-contact glass laser fiber) through the accessory channel of the endoscope. Carbon dioxide is then passed through the tubing surrounding the laser fiber to insufflate the uterus.
- Extend the fiber beyond the end of the tip of the endoscope, being careful to not touch the tissue (non-contact mode).
- Deliver 600 J of energy at 10 W/cm^2 in non-contact mode for a maximum of 5-second continuous bursts. This mode provides coagulation of the vessel without rupturing it (Figure 86.3).
- Apply this setting along the vessel(s) until the dilated vessels are no longer visibly distended with blood.
- Administer flunixin meglumine (1.1 mg/kg PO or IM, twice a day) for 3 days for inflammation.
- If the mare was pregnant at the time of photocoagulation, give altrenogest (0.044–0.088 mg/kg PO, once per day) or an exogenous progesterone alternative may be administered to support the pregnancy for a minimum of 2 weeks.

Interpretation

- After Nd:YAG photocoagulation, the mare should have a repeat vaginal endoscopic examination in about 3 weeks to detail the presence of any remaining varicosities that need to be re-treated (Figure 86.4).
- If the mare was placed on altrenogest, a serum progesterone concentration may be assessed and if it is greater than 4 ng/ml the mare may be weaned off the altrenogest.

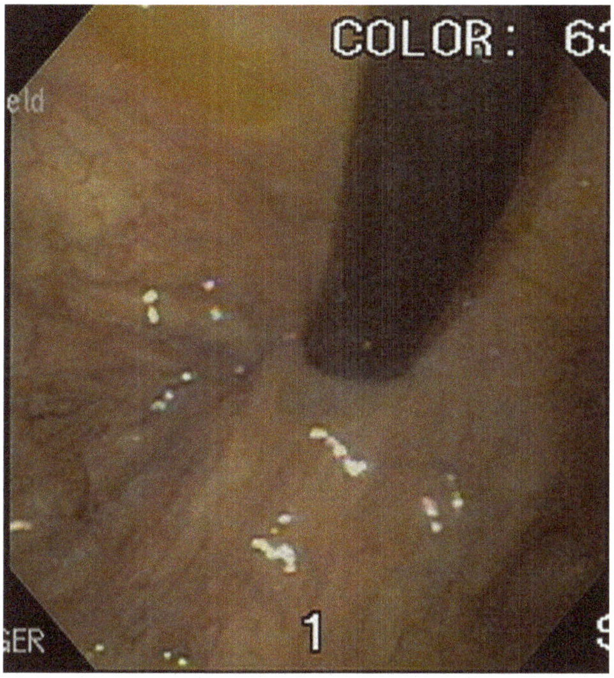

Figure 86.4 The same mare shown in Figures 86.3 and 86.4, 1.5 years after laser ablation as viewed through a retroflexed endoscope. Reproduced with permission from: DeLuca C, Dascanio JJ, Berry DB. 2007. Nd:YAG laser treatment of a vestibulovaginal varicosity in a 15-year-old pregnant mare. *J Eq Vet Sci* 2007; 27: 217–20.

- It has been suggested that pneumovagina may predispose an already formed varicosity to bleed after the blood vessel(s) becomes dry. Completing a vulvoplasty (Caslick operation) may prevent air introduction and subsequent bleeding.

Reference

DeLuca C, Dascanio JJ, Berry DB. 2007. Nd:YAG laser treatment of a vestibulovaginal varicosity in a 15-year-old pregnant mare. *J Eq Vet Sci* 27: 217–20.

Further Reading

Frazer ES. 2005. Differential diagnosis for vaginal haemorrhage in the mare. *Eq Vet Educ* 17: 153–5.

White RA, Gerring EL, Jackson PG, Noakes DE. 1984. Persistent vaginal haemorrhage in five mares caused by varicose veins of the vaginal wall. *Vet Rec* 115: 263–4.

87

Manual Correction of Uterine Torsion

John J. Dascanio

School of Veterinary Medicine, Texas Tech University, USA

Introduction

Uterine torsion refers to a twisting or rotation of the uterus on its long axis. Uterine torsion in mares may occur from 5 months to term, but is most commonly diagnosed at 7–9 months of pregnancy. Mares may present with signs of mild, recurrent, or intermittent colic, acute unrelenting colic, restlessness, sweating, frequent urination, or dystocia. Anorexia, fever, and depression have also been noted in some mares with chronic uterine torsions. The uterus is most commonly twisted 180–360 degrees, but occasionally the rotation may be greater than 540 degrees.

Diagnosis of a uterine torsion is primarily based on palpation of the broad ligaments per rectum for location and tension. The broad ligaments in a normal pregnancy suspend the uterus relatively symmetrically within the abdomen. In a clockwise uterine torsion (as described from a position behind the mare), the left broad ligament passes dorsally over the top of the uterus and the right broad ligament passes ventrally as it goes under the uterus. The opposite is true for a counterclockwise torsion, with the left broad ligament going under and the right broad ligament going over the uterus. In most instances, the torsion does not involve the cervix or vagina. The right broad ligament tends to be in a more cranial position compared with the left broad ligament. Methods of correction include standing flank laparotomy, ventral midline laparotomy, manual rotation through the cervix, and rolling the mare.

Equipment and Supplies

Obstetrical sleeve, obstetrical lubricant, anesthesia drugs, 3 m (10 foot) long, 20–30 cm (8–12 inch) wide wooden board.

Technique for Manual Rotation of the Uterus Through the Cervix

- Correction through the cervix may be attempted if the mare is at full term and the cervix already dilated. This procedure is most successful with a torsion of less than 270 degrees.
- The procedure must be done with the mare in a standing position. If the mare is lying down, the pressure of the intestinal contents on the uterus will prevent the required motion of the uterus. It could be possible to perform this procedure in an anesthetized mare if her rear legs were elevated sufficiently.
- Sedation of the mare should be avoided if possible as the mare may become recumbent with the manipulations. An epidural may help the mare to remain standing.
- The mare's perineum is washed and her tail completely wrapped.
- Using a sterile obstetrical sleeve and sterile lubricant, the arm is introduced into the uterus.
- If not already ruptured, the fetal membranes are manually ruptured and allantoic and amnionic fluids are released to decrease the weight within the uterus.
- An upper leg or part of the body of the fetus is grasped.
- The fetus (and uterus) is gently rocked back and forth in an arc to create momentum until the uterus can be rotated in the opposite direction of the initial torsion. The procedure may be repeated if the detorsion is not complete.
- This technique requires coordination, strength, and a long arm.
- *Detorsion rod.* If the cervix is open and the fetal limbs are accessible, a Cornell detorsion rod (or similar instrument) may aid in rotating the uterus. Caution should be used to avoid uterine rupture with excessive pressure.

Equine Reproductive Procedures, Second Edition. Edited by John Dascanio and Patrick McCue.

- Individual chain loops are placed on the limbs as far proximal as possible. The end of these chains are placed through one end of the detorsion rod ring.
- This end of the detorsion rod is then placed close to the limbs where the chains are looped around the limbs.
- The remaining chains are wrapped a few times around the detorsion rod in the same direction as the detorsion rod is to be turned (rod to be turned in the opposite direction as the uterine torsion so as to untwist the uterus).
- A round wooden stick, or similar, is placed through the unused outer end of the detorsion rod to act as a handle.
- The detorsion rod is turned using the wooden handle in a direction to untwist the uterus.
- A hand may be placed *in utero* to monitor progress, to aid in detorsing the uterus, and to direct amount of pressure to exert.

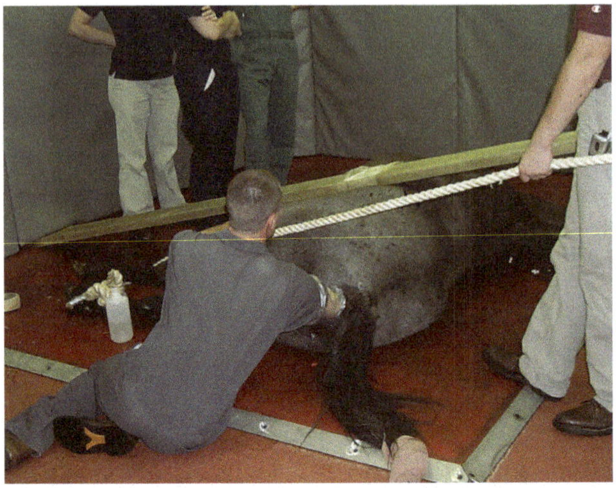

Figure 87.1 Palpation of the mare once recumbent to reorientate the location of the broad ligaments. This mare has a clockwise uterine torsion (as viewed from behind the mare).

Technique for Rolling ("Plank in the Flank")

- The mare should initially be palpated while standing to determine the presence and direction of the torsion (i.e., clockwise or counterclockwise).
- The mare is anesthetized and placed in lateral recumbency. The mare should be rolled in the same direction as the uterine torsion while fixing the uterus in position. For example, with a clockwise uterine torsion, the mare should be placed in right lateral recumbency and subsequently rolled over into left lateral recumbency.
- The mare should be re-palpated per rectum, with the mare in recumbency, to confirm the location and position of the broad ligaments (Figure 87.1).
- Ropes should be placed on the most ventral front and rear legs.
- *Rolling without a plank*:
  - The mare is rolled quickly in the direction of the torsion. If initially unsuccessful, the mare may be rolled again and this time held in dorsal recumbency and rocked back and forth to help with correction before finishing the rolling procedure.
  - To reposition the mare for a second attempt, the mare should first be rolled into a sternal position and then into lateral recumbency in the same direction as the torsion.
  - The mare should not be rolled opposite to the direction of the torsion as this may exacerbate the condition.
- *Rolling with a plank:*
  - A wooden board (plank) approximately 3 m (10 foot) long, and approximately 20–30 cm (10 inch) wide, is placed into the paralumbar fossa of the mare (Figure 87.2).

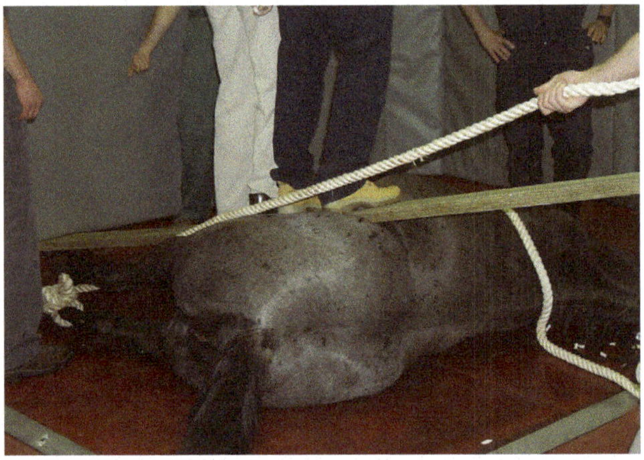

Figure 87.2 Start of the rolling procedure with one or two people standing on the plank.

  - The purpose of the plank is to place pressure on the torsed uterus to hold it stationary while the mare is rotated around the uterus, thus correcting the torsion.
  - Pressure is placed on the plank by having one or two people (approximately 110 kg (~250 lb) total weight) either kneel or stand on the plank while the mare is slowly rolled in the direction of the torsion (Figure 87.3).
  - If the foal can be palpated through the abdominal wall, the plank should be placed over the foal to increase the likelihood that the foal/uterus is held stationary.
  - Once the mare is rotated, the broad ligaments are once again palpated per rectum to determine if relief of the torsion was successful.
  - The procedure may need to be repeated to completely detorse the uterus.

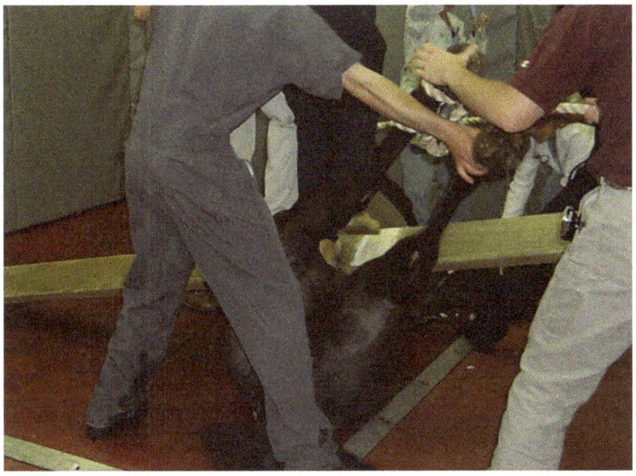

Figure 87.3 Rolling of the mare from right lateral recumbency to left lateral recumbency with plank pressure on her abdomen.

Interpretation

- "Plank in the flank" correction is less successful with a full-term fetus as the foal's body is further from the paralumbar area, making this correction difficult. Complications of the plank procedure may include uterine rupture and premature placental separation with subsequent fetal hypoxia.
- Even with successful resolution of the torsion, the mare may still abort the fetus in the next few days or weeks possibly due to placental or fetal compromise from inflammation or blood flow alterations.
- If manual correction is not successful, surgical correction is required.
- The prognosis for foal and mare survival is better if the uterine torsion occurs at less than 320 days of gestation. Non-steroidal anti-inflammatory drugs should be administered to reduce inflammation and provide analgesia. Other medications may be considered depending on the stage of gestation and suspected fetal compromise and may include drugs such as exogenous progesterone and pentoxifylline.

Further Reading

Chaney KP, Holcombe SJ, LeBlanc MM, Hauptman JG, Embertson RM, Mueller POE, Beard WL. 2006. Effect of uterine torsion on mare and foal survival: a retrospective study 1985–2005. *Proc Annu Conv Am Assoc Eq Pract* 52: 402–3.

Martens KA, Govaere JLJ, Hoogewijs MK, *et al.* 2008. Uterine torsion in the mare: a review and three case reports. *Vlaams Diergen Tijds* 77: 397–405.

Riggs LM. 2006. How to perform non-surgical correction of acute uterine torsion in the mare. *Proc Annu Conv Am Assoc Eq Pract* 52: 256–8.

88

Preparation for Foaling

John J. Dascanio

School of Veterinary Medicine, Texas Tech University, USA

Introduction

Preparation of the mare for foaling takes place months in advance of the predicted due date and includes planning for a foaling location, administering vaccinations, and reviewing potential foaling complications and developing an emergency plan. Depending on racing incentives, availability of help, or the need for veterinary intervention, the mare may need to be moved to a different location prior to foaling. Ideally, a pregnant mare should be moved to the foaling location at least a month prior to her due date so that she can develop colostral antibodies against local pathogenic organisms.

Mares are usually bedded on straw for foaling within a large stall. Sawdust bedding or shavings are usually avoided as they have a greater chance of contaminating the reproductive tract due to their small particle size and ability to harbor pathogens such as *Klebsiella* species if they have not been cured. If sawdust or shavings must be used, they may be top dressed with a layer of straw to decrease adherence to the mare.

The mare should have an adequate flat area for foaling with good drainage and footing so that with the expulsion of fetal fluids, the floor does not become slippery. A large stall or small paddock is recommended to allow the mare to easily get up and lie down in preparation for foaling. All bedding should be changed and the area disinfected between foaling mares. Spraying the walls with a dilute chlorine solution and using lime on dirt flooring may be adequate as a routine management procedure.

Equipment and Supplies

Tail wrap, non-irritant soap, roll cotton, stainless steel bucket, disposable liner for bucket, paper towels, exam gloves, basic surgery pack, pre-foaling vaccinations, milk calcium test kit, foaling kit.

Technique

- Move the mare to the final location for foaling 4–6 weeks prior to the due date so that she can acquire colostral immunity to local pathogens.
- Vaccinations to increase colostral immunity should be given 4–6 weeks prior to foaling. Typical pre-foaling vaccines may include tetanus toxoid, eastern and western equine encephalomyelitis virus, West Nile virus, rabies, and influenza virus. The mare may have also received vaccination against equine herpesvirus type 1 (rhinopneumonitis) at 5, 7, and 9 months of pregnancy.
- Any increase in nutritional demands for late pregnancy and lactation should be gradually introduced over 1–2 weeks.
- Remove the vulvoplasty (Caslick), if present, 1–2 weeks prior to the due date. Place the mare in stocks and wash the perineum. Place a twitch on the mare and use sharp, straight Metzenbaum scissors to fully open the Caslick to the normal dorsal commissure of the vulva (Figures 88.1 and 88.2). Local anesthesia and sedation can be utilized as needed.
- The stall size should be adequate for the mare to get up/down and to allow for potential intervention. A typical size for a foaling stall would be at least 3.5 by 5 m (12 by 16 feet).
- If a large stall is not available, a level pen/paddock with good footing may be used. The fencing around the pen/paddock should not allow a newborn foal to slip underneath, thus separating the foal from the mare.
- Udder development usually begins 2–4 weeks prior to parturition depending on parity. Concentration of calcium in the mammary secretions can be monitored once mammary fluid can be obtained. Measure the calcium concentration once a day until the value reaches 100 parts per million (ppm) and then one can perform the

Equine Reproductive Procedures, Second Edition. Edited by John Dascanio and Patrick McCue.

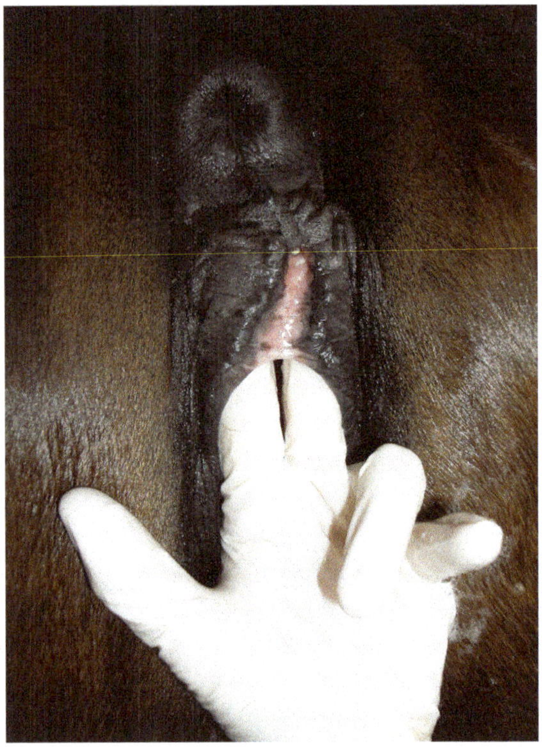

Figure 88.1 Two fingers placed inside the vulva to separate the labia in preparation for the removal of vulvoplasty.

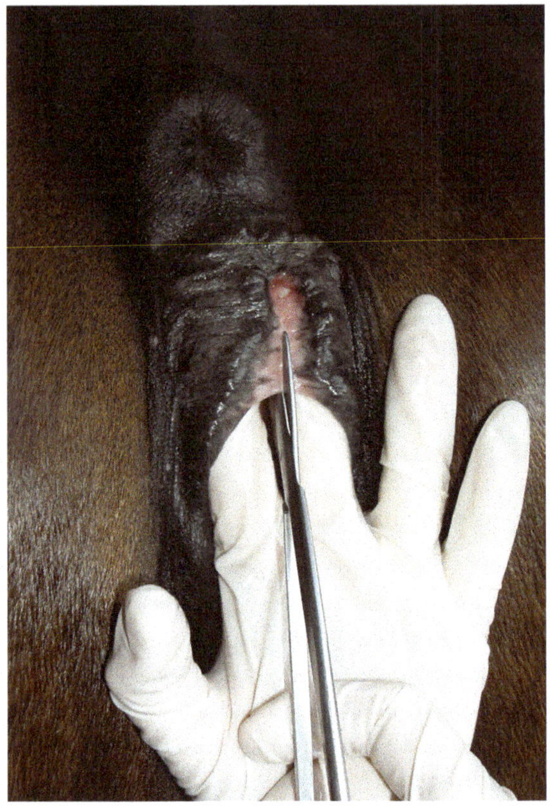

Figure 88.2 Metzenbaum scissors can be used to open a Caslick vulvoplasty.

test twice a day, if desired, to detect when levels first rise above 200 ppm (see Chapter 89). The pH of mammary secretions may also be measured to indicate readiness for birth (see Chapter 90).

- Once milk calcium reaches 100 ppm, place the mare in a foaling stall or paddock and have her monitored by experienced personnel for parturition. A majority of mares foal after milk calcium levels are greater than 200 ppm. However, approximately one third of mares give birth with a milk calcium of less than 200 ppm (Figure 88.3).
- When foaling is imminent, place a tail wrap that encompasses the entire tail so that no tail hair is visible. This will keep the hairs out of the way during foaling and make any interventions quicker and cleaner to perform.
- Wash the perineum, udder, and stifle area where the foal is likely to first suckle. Place the Foalert® transmitter (if one is to be used) (see Chapter 92). The labor alert device may be very helpful for mares that foal out during the day; however, most mares will foal out at night (Figure 88.4).
- Develop an emergency plan in the event of a dystocia, premature placental separation, or neonatal emergency.

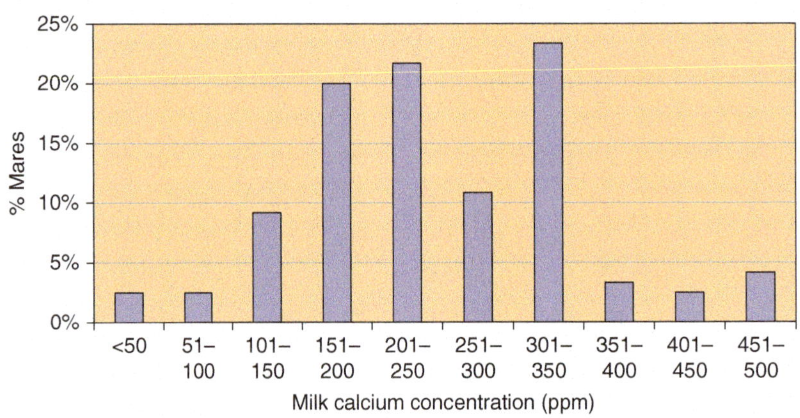

Figure 88.3 Final milk calcium levels in 120 mares prior to foaling.

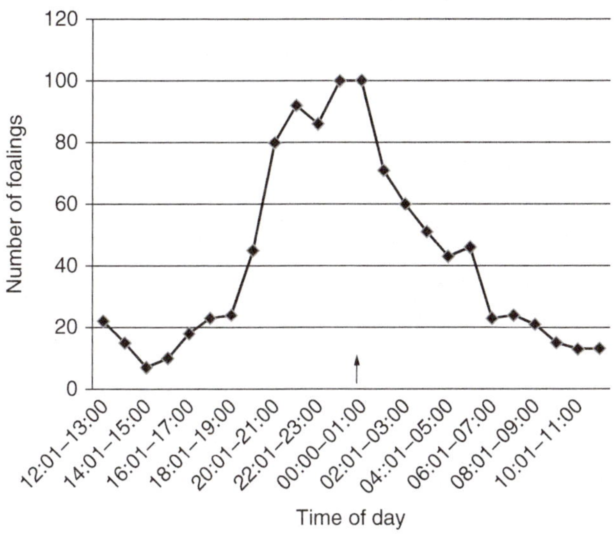

Figure 88.4 Relationship between the number of foalings and time of day. Most mares foal out between 9:00 pm and 6:00 am. Arrow indicates midnight (00:00 hours).

- Prepare an owner's foaling kit (see Appendix 4), which may include: veterinarian's telephone number, examination gloves, umbilical tape or umbilical clamp, navel disinfectant (iodine or chlorhexidine based), towels to dry the foal, trash bag to store the placenta until examined for completeness and pathology, scissors to potentially open thickened placental membranes or a 'red bag', flashlight, and watch. Other items such as obstetrical sleeves, sterile lubricant, and obstetrical chains/straps/handles may be included if the owner has been trained as to when and how to use them.

Interpretation

- It is not uncommon for late-term multiparous mares to acquire ventral abdominal edema that may extend from the udder cranially to the front legs. The mare should receive regular exercise to control the edema and decrease the risk of rupture of the pre-pubic tendon or abdominal musculature.
- Maiden mares may not have much udder development or milk secretion prior to foaling.
- A lack of udder development may also be caused by exposure to endophyte-infected fescue grass or hay. If this is the case, the D2 dopamine receptor antagonist domperidone may be administered to block the effects of the ergovaline toxin.

Further Reading

Frazer GS, Perkins NR, Embertson RM. 1999. Normal parturition and evaluation of the mare in dystocia. *Eq Vet Educ* 11: 41–6.

89

Assessment of Mammary Gland Secretions to Predict Foaling

John J. Dascanio

School of Veterinary Medicine, Texas Tech University, USA

Introduction

Serial monitoring of electrolyte concentrations of calcium, sodium, and/or potassium in pre-foaling mammary secretions can help assess fetal maturation and a mare's readiness to foal in normal pregnancies. The mare should be adequately restrained to allow for sampling of secretions from her udder. Sampling usually begins once the mare is within 2 weeks of her foaling date, which is calculated as 340 days from ovulation, and has secretions in her teat cistern.

There are several commercial kits available for on-farm or in-clinic use to measure the calcium content of the milk. These systems are essentially water hardness test kits that have been adapted for use in measuring calcium levels in equine milk. Commercial kits consist of either test strips with a series of precalibrated squares that change color depending on the calcium level or a quantitative system that titrates the calcium level in a sample. A milk sample must be sent to a diagnostic laboratory for the measurement of sodium and potassium content.

The units of assessment may vary between test kits or systems. The most common units for calcium are mmol/l and parts per million (ppm). The conversion from mmol/l to ppm is expressed as mmol/l = ppm/atomic mass of the ion, so for calcium mmol/l = ppm/44.078. One ppm is equal to 1 mg/l.

Equipment and Supplies

Distilled water, distilled rinsed and dried containers, syringes, commercial test kit, mammary gland secretions, alcohol swab.

Technique

- Wipe the teat end with an alcohol swab to remove debris and to disinfect the teat end.
- The first milk discharged from the teat should be discarded to remove the dried secretions/bacteria from the teat canal.
- Collect equally from both teats a total of approximately 2 ml of mammary secretions in a small, clean, dry container (Figure 89.1).

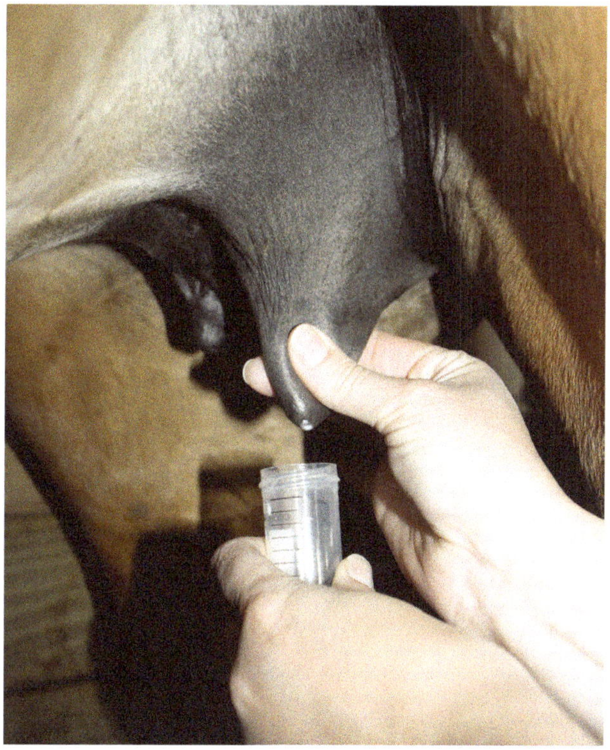

Figure 89.1 Collection of mammary secretions.

Equine Reproductive Procedures, Second Edition. Edited by John Dascanio and Patrick McCue.

Calcium Testing of Milk

Milk titration test kit

- A milk titration test kit such as FoalWatch™ test kit (Chemetrics, Midland, VA, USA) is used.
- Using a syringe, measure 1.5 ml of milk and dispense into a 25 ml sample cup.
- Add 9 ml of distilled water and gently mix.
- Add 1 drop of indicator dye solution to the milk/distilled water and gently mix.
- Assemble the titration device by pushing a valve assembly onto a glass ampule and then cracking the tip of the glass ampule. The ampule is then inserted into the titrettor.
- Insert the valve assembly into the prepared milk solution and gently push the control bar very briefly to allow a small quantity of the milk solution to enter the glass ampule (Figure 89.2). It is important that only a very small amount of milk enters the ampule at one time in order to be accurate in the titration.
- Once milk has entered the ampule, invert the ampule and note the color of the mixed liquid in the ampule. The color will change to blue when the titration is complete. Repeat small aspirations of the milk solution into the glass ampule until a color change is noted. Stop aspiration once a color change is detected and turn the glass ampule right side up to read the liquid level (Figures 89.3 and 89.4). This number corresponds to the parts per million of calcium in the milk sample.
- The glass ampule is discarded; all sample containers may be reused after rinsing with distilled water and drying.

Interpretation of titration

- If the sampling equipment has been washed with tap water it must be rinsed with distilled water to remove any calcium residue to avoid a false-positive test result.
- According to the manufacturer:
  - There is a 54% probability that the mare will foal within 24 hours of the milk calcium first reaching 200 ppm.
  - There is an 84% probability that the mare will foal within 48 hours of the milk calcium first reaching 200 ppm.

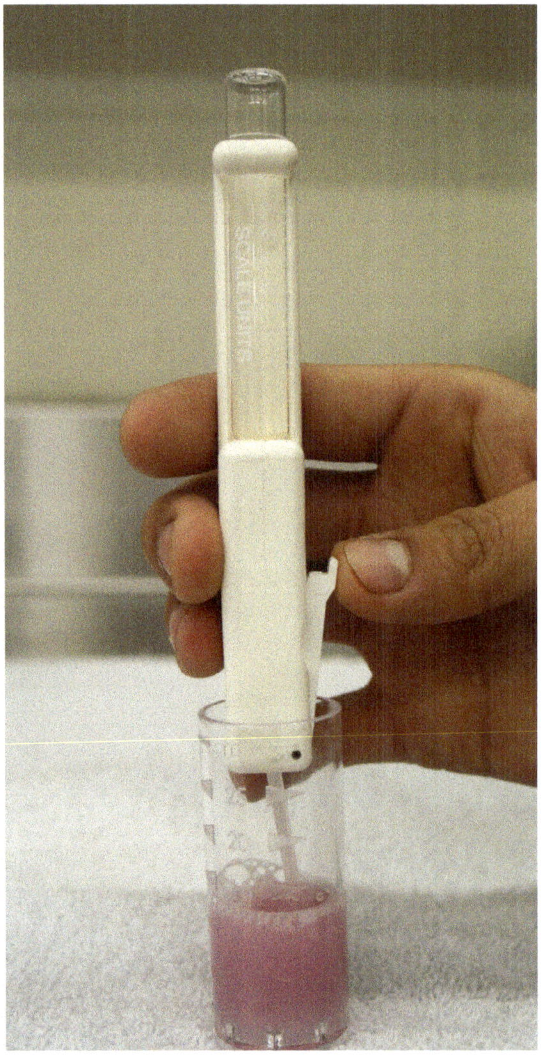

Figure 89.2 Titration instrument immersed in milk with dye. Gentle pushing of the lever allows milk to enter the device.

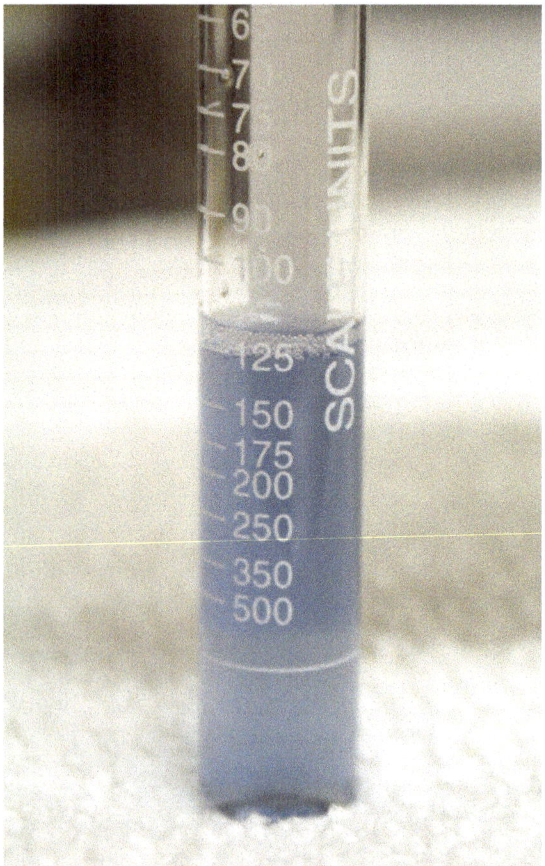

Figure 89.3 Milk calcium content of 125 ppm using a milk titration test kit.

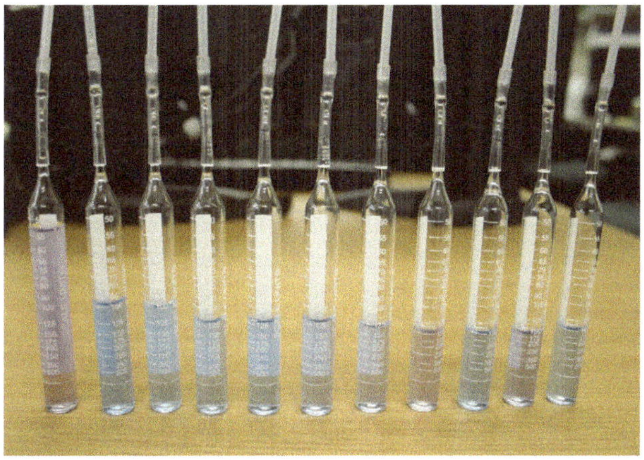

Figure 89.4 Milk titration test kit results from a mare over 11 days starting on the left progressing toward the right. The sample on the left did not register, while the sample on the right had approximately 150 ppm calcium.

- There is a 98% probability that the mare will foal within 72 hours of the milk calcium first reaching 200 ppm.
- There is a 98% probability that foaling will not occur in the next 24 hours if the milk calcium is less than 200 ppm.

- In clinical practice it is recognized that many mares give birth without milk calcium reaching a level of 200 ppm.
- Note: the FoalWatch™ test measures uncorrected calcium carbonate ($CaCO_3$) levels. To convert a $CaCO_3$ value in ppm to a calcium value in ppm, multiply the $CaCO_3$ value by 0.4. For example, a $CaCO_3$ value of 250 ppm would be the equivalent of a calcium value of 100 ppm, as the calcium in $CaCO_3$ is 40% of the total molecular weight. This would be important if comparing test kit results with a laboratory analysis of secretions for calcium.

Milk test strips ("Predict-A-Foal")

- Commercial water hardness test strips or strips marketed for testing pre-foaling milk secretions from mares may be used. Water hardness test strips can be obtained from scientific supply companies such as Fisher Scientific (Pittsburg, PA, USA; Catalog no. M1100250001). It is important that there be a scale with multiple indicator levels corresponding to calcium content. Some farms use the milk test strips until the milk calcium concentration is around 100 ppm and then switch to the titration method to increase accuracy.
- Obtain about 2 ml of milk secretions from the mare.
- Using a syringe measure 1 ml of milk into a 10 ml sample container.
- Add 6 ml of distilled water into the milk in the 10 ml container and gently mix.
- Dip the test strip into the milk/distilled water for a few seconds and then remove, shake off excess fluid and wait approximately 15 seconds to read. These time frames may change depending on the manufacturer's instructions and may go up to 1 minute prior to reading.
- Compare the colors on the test strip with the supplied chart colors to estimate milk calcium concentration (Figures 89.5 and 89.6).

Interpretation of test strips

- Once the calcium content has exceeded 200 ppm or the test reads "very hard water," the mare should foal within a few days.

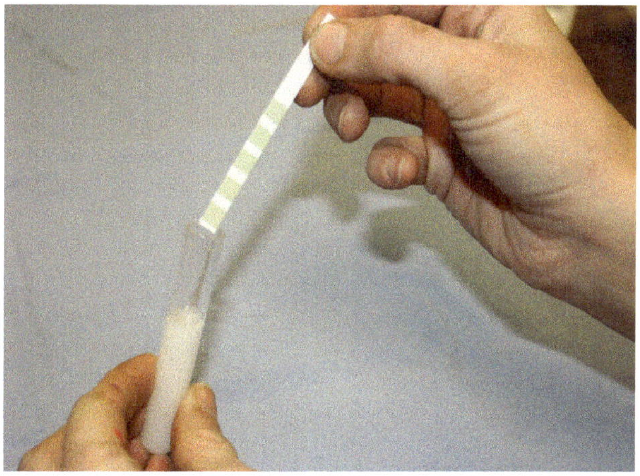

Figure 89.5 Dipping a test strip into a glass vial of diluted milk to evaluate the calcium level.

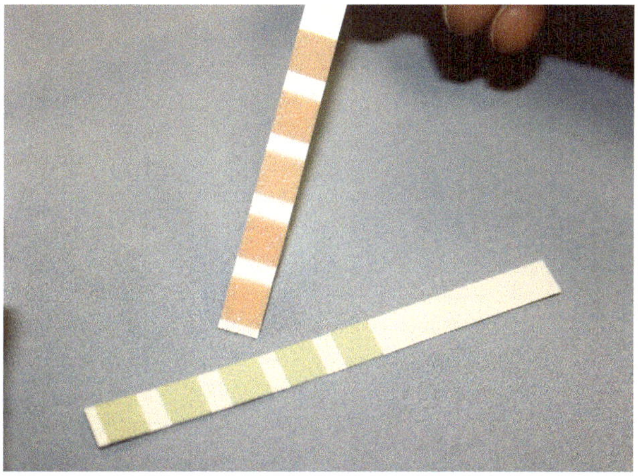

Figure 89.6 All five boxes have changed color (upper strip) indicating a high milk calcium level and a high probability of foaling.

Comments

- Maiden mares may not produce adequate milk to sample properly.
- Mares with placentitis may prematurely have an increased milk calcium.
- It is recommended to measure the milk calcium twice a day after the mare exceeds 125 ppm calcium to increase the accuracy of determining when the concentration exceeds 200 ppm.

Sodium/Potassium Testing of Milk

- When the mare is within a few days of parturition the sodium and potassium concentrations invert: the potassium concentration becomes higher than the sodium (sodium decreases and potassium rises).
- This test is not commonly used as it requires samples to be run at a diagnostic laboratory.
- Obtain 2 ml of milk in a sterile container such as a red top blood tube.
- Instruct the laboratory to centrifuge the sample to remove the fat which will potentially clog automatic diagnostic machinery.
- Also instruct the laboratory to run the sample using the urine chemistry settings as the potassium may be too high when using blood chemistry settings.

Further Reading

Ley WB. 1994. The use of a pre-foaling milk calcium test kit in the foaling management of mares. *Eq Pract* 16(6): 15–22.

Ley WB, Hoffman JL, Meacham TN, Sullivan TL, Kiracofe RL, Wilson ML. 1989. Daytime foaling management of the mare: 1. Pre-foaling mammary secretions testing. *J Eq Vet Sci* 9: 88–94.

Ousey JC, Dudan F, Rossdale PD. 1984. Preliminary studies on mammary secretions in the mare to assess fetal readiness for birth. *Eq Vet J* 16: 259–63.

90

Assessment of pH of Mammary Gland Secretions to Predict Foaling

Patrick M. McCue

Equine Reproduction Laboratory, Colorado State University, USA

Introduction

Laboratory techniques to predict foaling include the measurement of calcium carbonate, electrolytes (sodium, potassium, chloride), and pH in mammary secretions and potentially progesterone in the peripheral blood of the mare.

A decrease in pH has been reported in the milk of women and mares prior to giving birth. In mares, the positive predictive value (PPV) or the likelihood of an individual mare foaling within 24, 48, or 72 hours after the milk pH first decreases to ≤6.4 was 54.2%, 85.4%, and 97.9%, respectively. The negative predictive value (NPV) or the likelihood of a mare *not* foaling within 24, 48, or 72 hours when the pH is >6.4 was 99.4%, 97.5%, and 81.6%.

Equipment and Supplies

Disposable collection cup; alcohol swabs; option 1: pH indicator strips (Fisher Scientific, Catalog no. 13640517), pH detection range of 5.5–8.0 in 0.2 increments; option 2: pH meter; pH standards for calibration; distilled or deionized water in rinse bottle; pipettes for sample transfer when using the pH meter.

Technique

- Milk sampling should begin as the mare approaches her due date, or in the event of premature udder development and impending early foaling or abortion (see Chapter 106).
- The mare's teat end should be wiped clean with an alcohol swab.
- The first milk discharged from the teat should be discarded to remove the dried secretions/bacteria from the teat canal.
- Approximately 0.5–1.0 ml of mammary secretion is collected equally from each teat from the pregnant mare into a small disposable cup.

pH Indicator Strip Testing

- The test box at the end of the plastic pH indicator strip is immersed directly into the milk sample within the collection cup.
- The color of the box is immediately evaluated and compared with the colors on a standard chart provided by the manufacturer to determine the pH score (Figure 90.1).

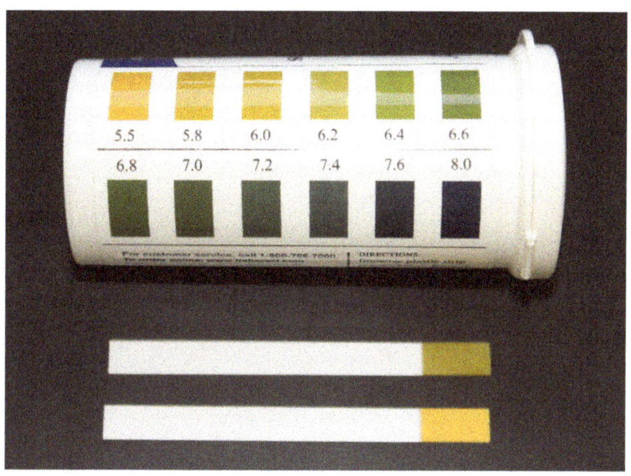

Figure 90.1 pH indicator strips (range 5.5 to 8.0) that may be used to determine the pH of a milk sample (bottom strip prior to dipping in milk; top strip after dipping in milk).

Equine Reproductive Procedures, Second Edition. Edited by John Dascanio and Patrick McCue.

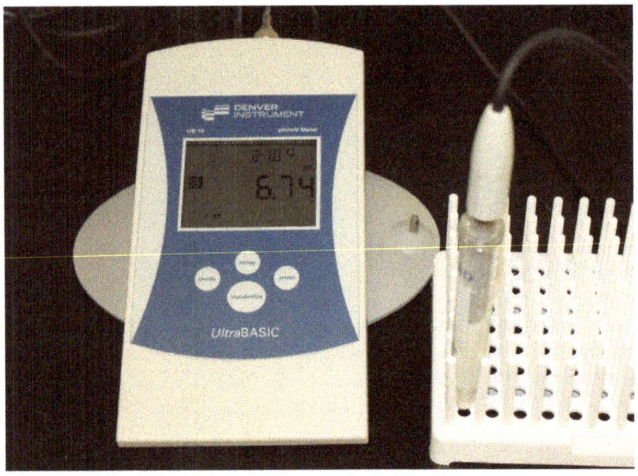

Figure 90.2 pH meter being used to determine the pH of a milk sample.

pH Meter Testing

- The pH meter should be standardized prior to use to obtain an accurate reading using the instructions that come with the meter.
- The electrode is rinsed with distilled or deionized water prior to evaluation of the test sample and blotted to remove excess water.
- The electrode is placed down into the sample until the pH is determined by the meter (Figure 90.2).

Additional Comments

Mammary fluid pH can be used in conjunction with clinical signs and other laboratory tests to predict foaling. A pH value of 6.4 has been suggested as a standard value for assessment of impending parturition in mares. Unfortunately, the PPV to estimate the likelihood of an individual mare foaling within 24 hours when her milk pH first decreases to ≤6.4 is only 54.2%.

Perhaps the best clinical use of the milk pH test is to predict when a mare is *not* ready to foal. The NPV of an individual mare not foaling within 24 hours if the pH is >6.4 is 99.4%.

Measurement of pH with a meter is more accurate than estimation with pH paper. The type of pH paper may be critical as some cannot detect a small change in pH. It is recommended that pH paper that detects pH in a range of 5.5–8.0 in increments of 0.2 be used to evaluate mare mammary fluid. Performing the test with pH paper is rapid, easy to perform, and inexpensive. In addition, no sample dilution or other equipment/supplies are needed.

The relationship between mammary fluid pH and calcium carbonate levels relative to the day of foaling for an individual mare is presented in Figure 90.3.

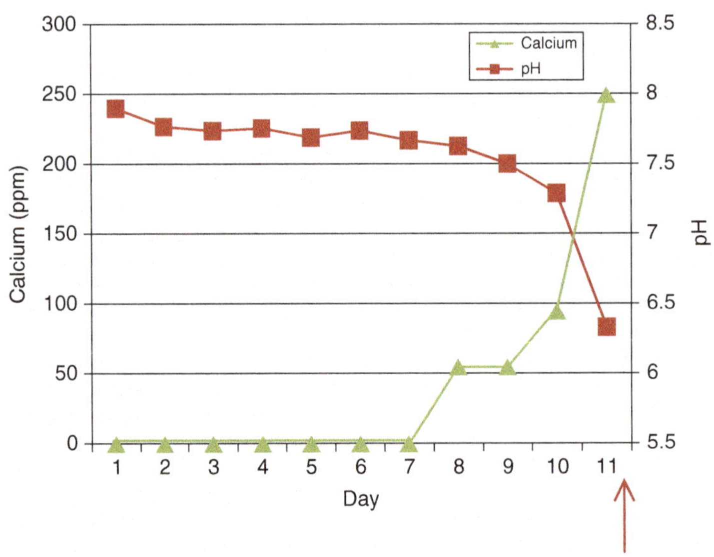

Figure 90.3 Comparison of pH and calcium carbonate levels in the mammary fluid of a mare relative to day of foaling. Arrow indicates foaling at day 11 of testing.

Further Reading

Canisso IF, Ball BA, Troedsson MH, Silva ESM, Davolli GM. 2013. Decreasing pH of mammary gland secretions is associated with parturition and is correlated with electrolyte concentrations in prefoaling mares. *Vet Record* 173: 218–22.

Korosue K, Murase H, Sato F, Ishimaru M, Kotoyori Y, Tsujimura T, Nambo Y. 2013. Comparison of pH and refractometry index with calcium concentrations in preparturient mammary gland secretions of mares. *J Am Vet Med Assoc* 242: 242–8.

91

Monitoring of Peri-Parturient Mares Using Video and Web Cameras

Ryan A. Ferris

Summit, Equine, USA

Introduction

The majority of mares foal at night. A number of video monitoring systems have been developed to monitor late-term mares. Barn camera systems are modifications of standard video security systems and are available in wired, wireless, and internet/web-based formats. In general, black and white cameras are capable of displaying more detail in a low light environment as compared with color camera systems. Infrared cameras are available that can monitor foaling stalls with no external light.

Cameras located in the barn should be waterproof with a proper connection to electrical sources. Less expensive security cameras may be used or direct marketed equine foaling cameras are available. Wireless systems will require adequate Wi-Fi upload speeds are available through an internet service provider to stream video to devices. A camera will generally require an internet upload speed of around 2.5 Mbps for high definition video streaming.

Lux rating or minimum illumination rating specifications will determine if a camera can function in low ambient light conditions. The lower the number, the better the camera will perform in a low light environment. Infrared or night vision cameras have a lux rating of 0, meaning that an image can be obtained in complete darkness. Infrared cameras that display a clear image are more expensive than black and white or color cameras.

Equipment and Supplies

Cameras; video, audio, power cable from camera to transmitter; receiver; quad processor and TV monitor; internet connection; proprietary software for internet access.

Wired Camera Systems

- Hard-wired systems require one or more cameras, a coaxial cable, and a monitor (Figure 91.1). A splitter can be used to view multiple cameras on one screen (e.g., side by side) or a switching unit can be used to select cameras, alternate between cameras, and determine camera dwell time.
- The advantages of a wired system are a consistent signal from the camera and low cost. The primary disadvantage is the need for a long coaxial cable to connect the camera to the monitor and having to have a fixed location for viewing.

Wireless Camera Systems

- Wireless systems require one or more cameras, cables from the camera to the transmitter, a transmitter

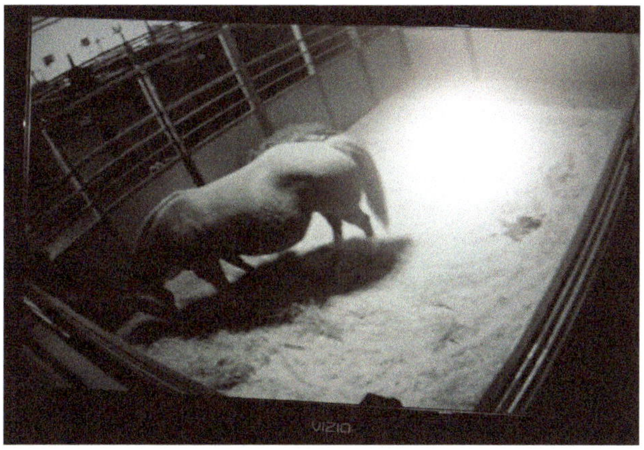

Figure 91.1 Hard-wired black and white camera monitoring a foaling stall.

Equine Reproductive Procedures, Second Edition. Edited by John Dascanio and Patrick McCue.

(e.g., 2.4 GHz), a receiver, and a monitor. Options include a switching unit to utilize multiple cameras and extended range transmitters and receivers. Many systems are based on "line of sight" distances, while others can transmit through barriers (e.g., barn walls). It may be advantageous to mount the transmitter on the outside of the foaling barn for better signal strength.

- The primary advantage of a wireless system is elimination of the requirement for a coaxial cable between the camera and monitor. Disadvantages include disruption of the video stream by objects within the "line of sight," adverse weather, and long distance or occasionally other transmission signal interference.
- If only one camera is being installed, the camera is connected to the transmitter directly by an audio/video power cable. If two or more cameras are being installed, the cameras are connected via a cable to a quad processor that is in turn connected via a cable to a transmitter.
- The transmitter should be installed in a location that minimizes the number of barriers/obstacles that the signal must pass through to reach the receiver.
- The receiver is connected to a monitor in the residence, office, or other station and must be within the distance allowed by the transmission capability of the transmitter, which is typically less than 1.6 km (1 mile).

Internet/Web-Based Camera Systems

- Internet or web-based systems require one or more cameras, an internet connection (wireless, hardwired, or cellular), and a device to connect to the internet.
- The advantages are easy setup, no installation of cables (if wireless or cellular internet is available), and access from any device with internet access (computer, tablet, smartphone, etc.) (Figure 91.2). In addition, many systems can incorporate zoom and pan features and battery backup. The cost is comparable or less than wireless systems and cable-based systems. The primary disadvantage is lack of function if the internet connection is unavailable or if the internet service provider upload speeds vary.
- There are many different types of web cameras available (Figure 91.3). The cameras have to be connected to a computer hooked up to an internet service provider or are streamed to a service provider (such as a security company) so that the image may be transmitted through the internet.
- The real-time image may then be viewed using a software package on remote computers anywhere in the world that internet service is available. Multiple cameras may be viewed from different locations on the same computer.

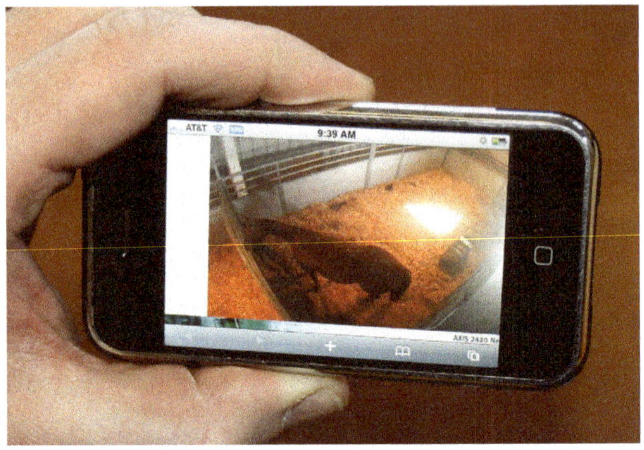

Figure 91.2 Web-cam on a foaling stall as viewed on a smart phone.

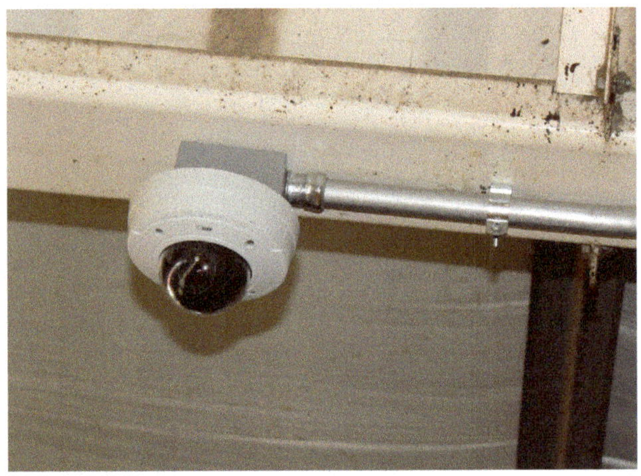

Figure 91.3 Mounted video camera.

Interpretation

- As with any system, cameras are not 100% foolproof. They are only useful if the person monitoring the mares is awake and paying attention to the video display.
- In most stalls there are blind spots that the camera image does not reach. If the mare is standing in such a blind spot, it may be difficult to determine exactly what she is doing.
- Cameras are often utilized in conjunction with a second form of labor alert device, thereby providing two methods of surveillance in case one system fails.

92

Foaling Alert: Vulvar Device

John J. Dascanio

School of Veterinary Medicine, Texas Tech University, USA

Introduction

Ideally a foaling attendant should be present during stage 2 of labor when the fetus is expelled. Several commercial devices are available which are designed to warn the attendant that parturition is imminent. These range from positional switches on halters or girth straps to devices attached to the labia of the vulva. The labia transmitter devices span the vulvar opening. When the foal passes through the vulva, the labia separate and the transmitter is activated. An audible signal is produced from a base station receiver and additional telecommunication devices such as pagers or phones can also be programmed to be activated by an autodialer (Figure 92.1). The vulvar transmitter device is generally attached 1–2 weeks prior to the anticipated foaling date. The device may also be used to monitor pregnant mares with precocious mammary development and possible premature foaling.

Equipment and Supplies

Obstetrical sleeve, obstetrical lubricant, tail wrap, tail rope, non-irritant soap, roll cotton, stainless steel bucket, disposable liner for bucket, paper towels, examination gloves, twitch, local anesthetic, sterile surgery gloves, surgical pack, sedation and/or twitch, 2-0 nylon suture, Foalert® device.

Technique

- Remove feces from the rectum.
- Place a tail wrap and tail rope (see Chapter 4).
- Clean and dry the perineum of the mare (see Chapter 3).
- Place a twitch on the mare or provide adequate sedation.
- Wearing examination gloves grasp the vulvar lips and instill 2–5 ml of local anesthetic (lidocaine or carbocaine) within the subcutaneous tissue using a 22 gauge 2.5 cm (1 inch) needle in the areas for suture placement. Sutures are placed about midway between the dorsal and ventral commissures of the vulva, about 1 cm laterally from the vulvar opening.
- A final wash of the perineum may be performed prior to suturing the device onto the labia.
- The Foalert® transmitter is attached to the left labia using two sutures.
- The magnet is attached to the right labia using a single suture (Figure 92.2).
- The device is typically removed immediately after the birth of the foal.
- The transmitter can be used again depending on the model purchased and battery life. The blue transmitter has a few hours of battery life and can be used up to 10 times while the less expensive red transmitter is for single use.

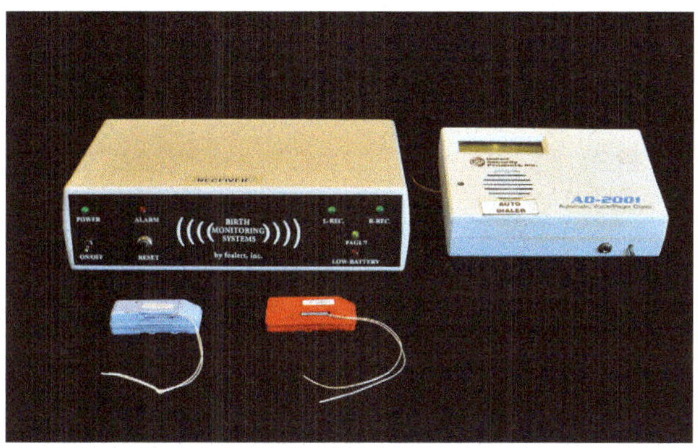

Figure 92.1 Base receiver (left) and auto dialer (right) along with blue and red Foalert® transmitters. The blue transmitter (left) has a longer battery life and is meant for multiple uses while the red transmitter (right) is for a single use. Used with permission from Foalert®.

Equine Reproductive Procedures, Second Edition. Edited by John Dascanio and Patrick McCue.

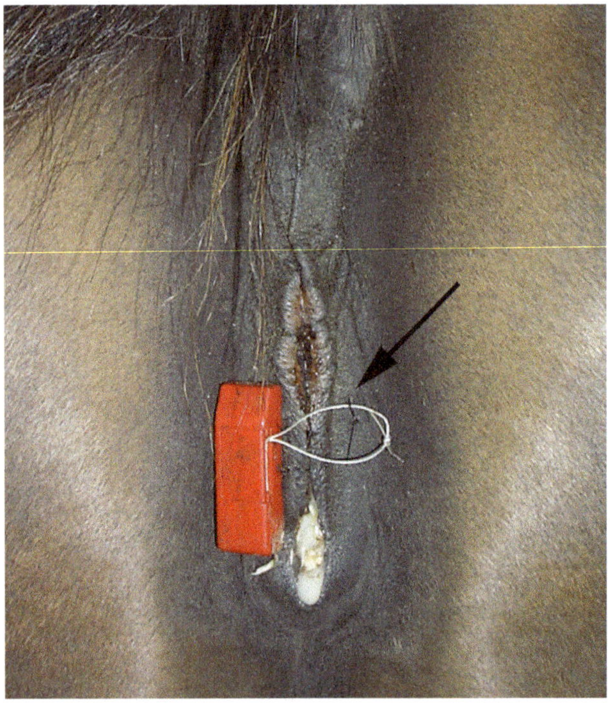

Figure 92.2 Foalert® device in a mare at 300 days' gestation with a purulent vaginal discharge and precocious mammary development. The arrow is pointing to small black suture in the skin that is holding the larger white loop attached to the Foalert® magnet.

Interpretation

- The labor alert device is especially helpful in alerting farm or ranch personnel in the event of a daytime foaling.
- Occasionally the alarm may be triggered if the mare strains to urinate, separating the vulvar lips. This occurs especially when the sutures spanning the vulvar opening are too tight.

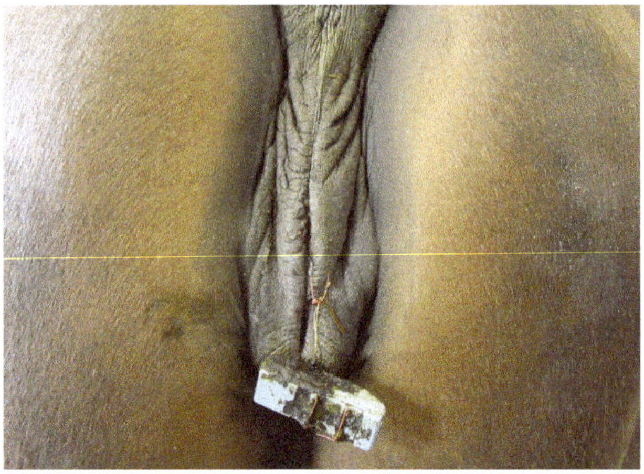

Figure 92.3 Foalert® device; the pregnant mare partially rubbed out the unit, which is hanging from the magnet.

- Individual mares may rub their perineal area against a stall wall or other objects and remove or activate the transmitter (Figure 92.3).
- If left in place over a long period of time, feces may accumulate on the sutures and lead to possible increased bacterial numbers or may pull on the sutures, setting off the alarm. Make sure that the sutures stay free of fecal material.
- With a multiparous mare, the birth may occur so quickly that the foal is delivered soon after the alarm sounds, not providing the attendant time to attend the birth.
- If a dystocia occurs whereby the vulvar labia are not separated, such as with a breach presentation, the alarm will not sound. Consequently, it is important to continue to regularly monitor the mare for other signs of parturition such as discharge of allantoic/amniotic fluid, straining, or passage of placental membranes.

Further Reading

Frazer GS, Perkins NR, Embertson RM. 1999. Normal parturition and evaluation of the mare in dystocia. *Eq Vet Educ* 11: 41–6.

93

Positional Labor Alert Devices

Ryan A. Ferris

Summit, Equine, USA

Introduction

Due to the rapid nature of parturition, mares require almost continuous observation to ensure that an attendant is on hand at the onset of delivery in the event assistance is needed. A number of systems have been developed to detect labor and send a signal to alert foaling attendants that a mare is starting to deliver a foal. These systems decrease the number of hours spent directly observing each mare and allow the foaling attendants to be alerted to a foaling even if they are not in the same facility as the mare.

Equipment and Supplies

Halter or girth strap, transmitter, repeater, pager and/or auto telephone dialer, pager and/or telephone, telephone jack, source of electricity.

Halter Devices

One type of system that has been developed utilizes a transmitter that is attached to the mare's halter. There are several different systems available commercially that utilize this technology (Figures 93.1–93.3) (Breeder Alert®, Allsman Enterprises, LLC, Rogue River, OR, USA; Magic Breed (AUST) PTY Ltd, Cairnes, Australia; EquiPage, Kee-Port, Inc., Arlington, WA, USA).

This transmitter is designed to detect when the mare is lying in lateral recumbency (i.e., during labor) since a majority of mares in late gestation do not sleep lying on their sides. Once the mare has been lying laterally for 7–9 seconds the transmitter sends a signal to a main unit that is installed in close proximity (up to approximately 150 m (165 yards)) to where the mare is housed. The signal is then sent via a repeater or antenna to the programmed telephone or pager number(s), thereby alerting the appropriate individuals to the pending parturition.

Halter Device Technique

- Since several different commercial systems are available, the directions for the specific system should be used to ensure that it is installed correctly.
- The main unit is installed on a shelf 1–2 m (3–6.5 feet) above the ground in an indoor area that is within no more than approximately 150 m (164 yards), clear line of sight, from where the mare is housed. Walls and other obstacles may affect the signal range. The main unit is plugged into a standard electrical outlet. Some systems have the ability to connect the main unit to a 12 V battery source if the power fails or if an electrical source is not available.

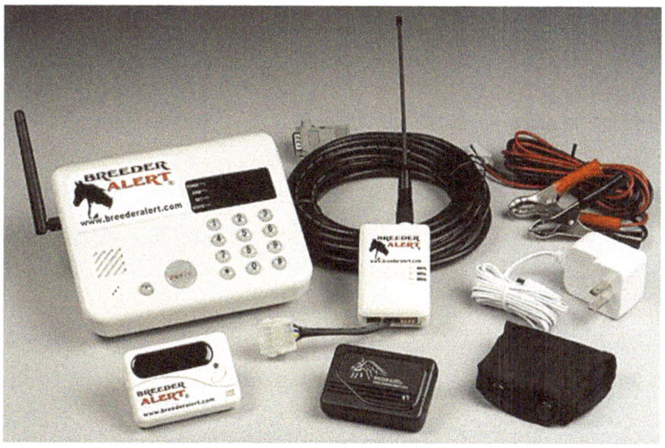

Figure 93.1 Breeder Alert® system with a main unit and autodialer, repeater, transmitter, and pouch, and pager. Photo courtesy of Breeder Alert®.

Equine Reproductive Procedures, Second Edition. Edited by John Dascanio and Patrick McCue.

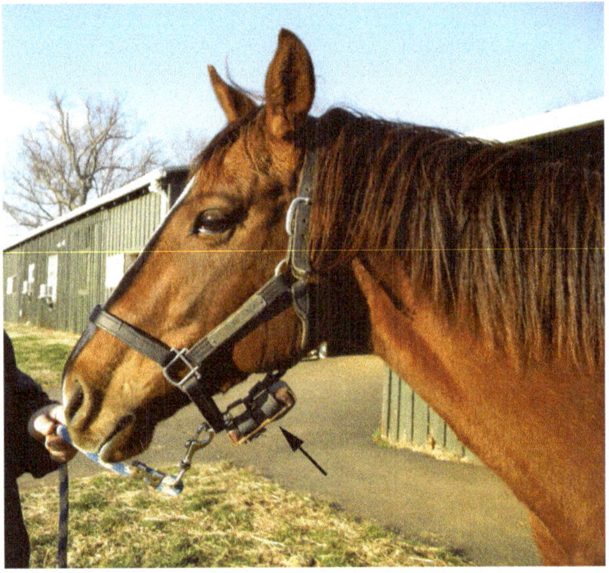

Figure 93.2 Mare wearing a Breeder Alert® transmitter (arrow).

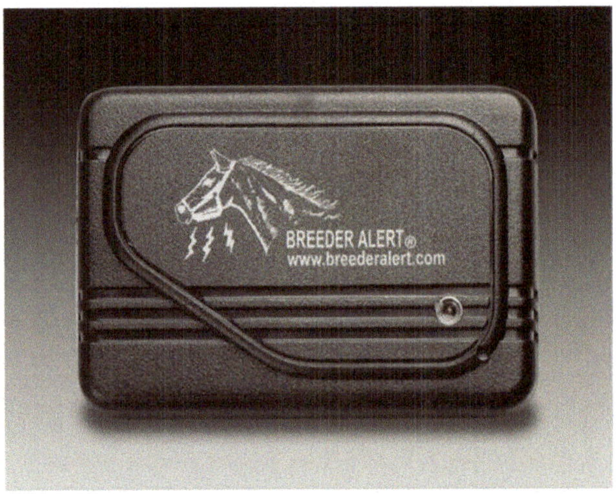

Figure 93.3 Breeder Alert® transmitter. Photo courtesy of Breeder Alert®.

- Some systems have the option of attendants being alerted via a telephone or pager while others just use a pager. To be called by telephone an autodialer is programmed with the desired numbers and connected to a phone jack. These systems require two numbers/lines, the one that the system dials out on and a different one to receive the call. If a pager is being used, the main unit is connected to a repeater with an antenna. The repeater needs to be placed near a window or door to ensure that the signal can reach the pager outside the barn. The range for the pager is approximately 1.6 km (1 mile).
- Once the system is installed and the mare is approaching her due date and exhibits normal udder development, the transmitter should be secured to her halter on the strap that runs ventrally from the chin to the throatlatch (Figure 93.2). Depending on the system, it may be recommended that the transmitter be placed in a plastic bag for extra protection against moisture before being placed in a pouch and attached to the halter.

Girth Device Technique

- The Birth Alarm® system (http://www.birthalarmusa.com, last accessed October 2020) utilizes a positional switch attached to a specialized girth strap as a labor alert device.
- As with the halter systems, the device is in the off position when the mare is standing. The device is activated when the mare lies down to foal.
- The Birth Alarm® system has a setting for mares that lie down in lateral recumbency frequently. The theory is that a foaling mare will be in lateral recumbency only when uterine contractions occur that last for less than 2.5 minutes.
- The system measures the duration of time the mare is in lateral recumbency and the alarm is triggered only if the mare is in this position for less than 3 minutes before returning to an upright position. This function assumes that most mares will stand up or roll to sternal recumbency between uterine contractions.

Biometric Technique

- These systems utilize measurements every few seconds of the mare's position, heart rate, respiratory rate, movement, and other factors to determine if the mare is in distress.
- While these systems have primarily been used to monitor horses for colic signs, they also can be used to predict foaling. These systems typically require a wireless internet and/or cellular data connection and can call, text, and/or email staff that the mare is starting to show signs of labor.
- The advantage of these systems is that they may be able to pick up on subtle changes in your mare's behavior before the actual start of stage 2 of labor with the mare breaking her water. One system that is currently available is NightWatch®. At the time of writing this chapter additional validation is required to determine, with this system, what percentage of mares can be predicted to foal within so many hours of the alert. These type of systems are more expensive, as compared with the systems already discussed, and require a wireless/cellular data connection, but offer the strong potential of being

notified prior to the mare breaking her water. The author has utilized these systems with good results if the system has several days to "learn" the mare's normal behavior prior to the foaling event. However, if the halter is placed on the mare and she foals that night, the reliability is low of predicting when the mare will foal. The NightWatch® system has gone through numerous updates and this may improve functionality in the future.

Interpretation

- No labor alert system is 100% reliable and it is important to remember the limitations of each system.
- Some mares will foal standing up and therefore may not trigger the transmitter.
- A small percentage of mares will sleep in a lateral "foaling position" even in late gestation and will trigger a false alarm. Close attention should be made to ensure that the system is set up properly and is working correctly.
- Establish a backup plan or system in case of system failure. The installation of cameras or visual inspections by an attendant in combination with a transmitter system can provide a facility with two methods to monitor mares, thus avoiding the pitfalls associated with an individual system.

Further Reading

Wessel M. 2005. Staging and prediction of parturition in the mare. *Clin Tech Eq Pract* 4: 219–27.

94

Induction of Parturition

John J. Dascanio

School of Veterinary Medicine, Texas Tech University, USA

Introduction

Elective induction of labor in the mare for non-medical reasons is generally not recommended and under most circumstances it is advised that the mare be allowed to carry her foal to term and give birth without hormonal intervention. The induction of labor does allow for the opportunity to have professional assistance available to assist with foaling and care of the newborn foal following a high risk pregnancy.

Clinical reasons for a controlled induction of labor in a mare include management of high risk pregnancies, monitoring of labor in mares that have had a history of dystocia, premature separation of the placenta ("red bag"), or other foaling complications. Late-term pregnant mares with a ruptured pre-pubic tendon, placental hydrops, or life-threatening medical conditions may require foaling assistance. In addition, induction of labor may make it easier to prevent a newborn foal from nursing from its dam when neonatal isoerythrolysis (jaundice foal syndrome) is expected.

Criteria have been established for the elective induction of labor. The mare should be more than 330 days into the gestation, have a well-developed udder, have a milk calcium carbonate content greater than 200 parts per million, and (optional) have a relaxed cervix as determined by palpation per rectum. Failure to follow these guidelines may result in initiation of parturition in a mare not ready for delivery, which could possibly lead to placental detachment and fetal hypoxia. Ultimately, the goal is to induce a controlled delivery, with personnel available to monitor and assist as needed, within just a few hours or days before the mare would normally give birth.

Equipment and Supplies

Tail wrap, non-irritant soap, roll cotton, stainless steel bucket, disposable liner for bucket, obstetrical sleeves, obstetrical lubricant, ultrasound with low (3.5 MHz) and mid (5 MHz) frequency probes, paper towels, exam gloves, oxytocin, needles, syringe, obstetrical equipment.

Technique

- Locate a level area free of obstructions, with good footing. An example may be a movable round pen on short grass or a large foaling stall.
- Place a tail wrap so that the entire tail is encompassed (see Chapter 3). Folding the tail and placing a self-adhering bandage tape over the entirety works well.
- Clean and dry the perineum of the mare. This will limit the necessity to perform a more involved scrub later, if intervention is required. Ensure that if a vulvoplasty (Caslick) is present, that it has been opened prior to induction.
- Repeat a milk calcium test to confirm that the concentration is greater than 200 parts per million.
- Re-confirm the breeding date of the mare to make sure that her gestational length has been calculated correctly.
- Palpate the cervix per rectum. The cervix should be flaccid and almost undistinguishable from the surrounding soft tissue in a term mare. This procedure is considered to be optional by some veterinarians in certain clinical situations, as the cervix of a mare will relax dramatically once labor is induced.
- Perform an ultrasound examination per abdomen and per rectum to determine fetal well-being and to document any placental detachment (see Chapter 73).
- Administer a dose of oxytocin. There are several protocols that vary in the initial dose and in the timing of

Equine Reproductive Procedures, Second Edition. Edited by John Dascanio and Patrick McCue.

Table 94.1 Dosage protocols for the administration of oxytocin to induce labor.

Oxytocin Protocols	Comments
10–20 units IM, once	Delivery usually occurs within 60 minutes
5 units IV, as an initial dose, followed by 10 units IV, 15 minutes later	Mare usually "breaks her water" and enters stage 2 of labor 10–15 minutes after the second dose
100 units in 1 liter of 0.9% sterile saline, administered by slow IV infusion over 1 hour	Mare usually foals by the time the infusion is completed

subsequent doses or the use of a constant rate infusion of oxytocin (Table 94.1). The protocol described herein uses an initial 10–20 IU intramuscularly.

- Record the time of oxytocin administration. Depending on the induction protocol selected, the induction may be successful with one dose of oxytocin or a second dose may be indicated.
- The mare should show progressive signs of parturition such as tail flagging (Figure 94.1), defecation, lying down/getting up, and sweating (Figure 94.2) with eventually rupture of the chorioallantois and expulsion of the allantoic fluid (i.e., "breaks her water"). The amnion should be the first placental membrane that is visible passing through the vulvar labia (Figure 94.3).
- If after 20–30 minutes there has not been adequate progression, perform ultrasound examinations per abdomen and per rectum to determine fetal well-being and placental contact and compare these results with those of the previous examination.
- Palpate the mare per rectum to determine if the foal is within the pelvic canal. Occasionally, parturition is delayed due to the need for the foal to reposition itself or the cervix to dilate further.

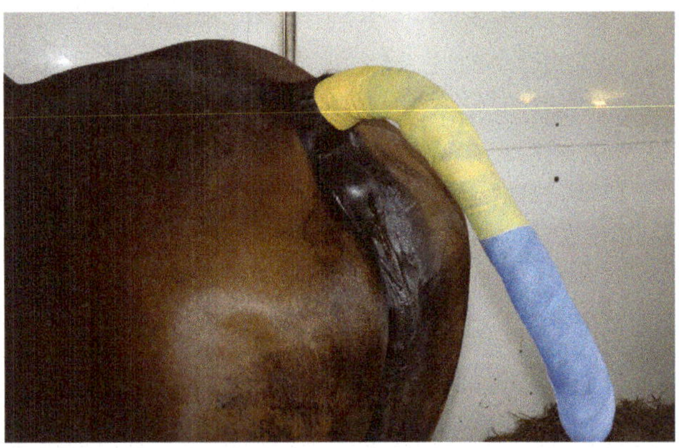

Figure 94.1 Mare lifting her tail after the administration of oxytocin to induce labor. This is usually an indication of stage 1 of parturition.

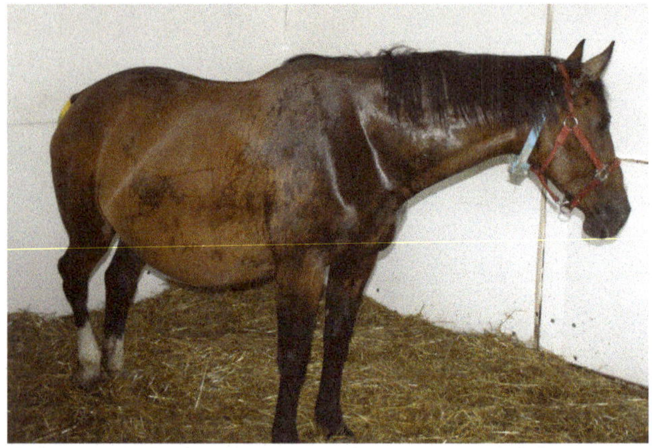

Figure 94.2 Mare sweating after the administration of oxytocin to induce labor. This is also an indication of stage 1 of parturition.

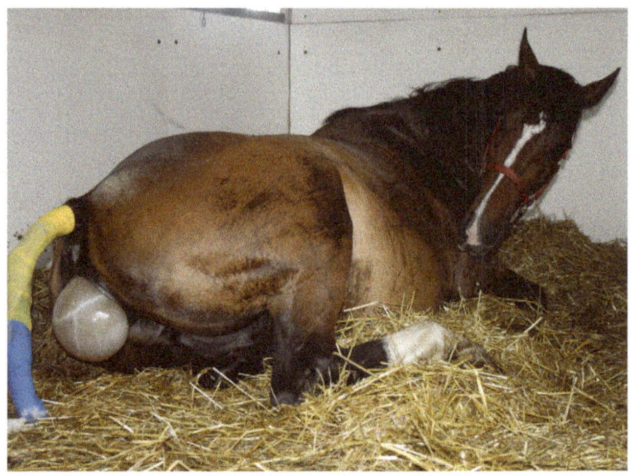

Figure 94.3 Mare in stage 2 of parturition with the amnion presented at the vulva.

- At this point, some clinicians will opt to perform a vaginal/cervical examination to determine the extent of cervical dilation, evaluate the possibility of premature separation of the placenta and protrusion of the intact chorioallantois through an open cervix, and evaluate the presentation, position, and posture of the fetus (if possible).
- A second dose of oxytocin may be administered if the mare has not delivered by 30–60 minutes and no complications are noted.
- If after two doses, parturition has not occurred, no further oxytocin should be administered. The mare should be examined per rectum for fetal orientation. The mare should have another ultrasound examination per abdomen and per rectum to determine fetal well-being and placental contact and these results compared with

previous examinations. It may be necessary to manually dilate the mare's cervix and manually rupture the chorio-allantois to initiate parturition, although this is not generally recommended. Alternatively, the mare could be placed under constant supervision and re-examined periodically for progression toward delivery.

- Obstetrical equipment should be immediately available to address potential foaling complications.

Interpretation

- With the proper selection of mares (i.e., full term with imminent parturition), foaling occurs with a single dose of oxytocin and complications rarely occur.
- Mares that do not have cervical relaxation will take longer to foal and placental detachment may occur, placing the fetus at risk of hypoxia.
- Potential complications may include premature placental separation, fetal hypoxia, abnormal orientation of the fetus in the birth canal, most commonly involving the front leg(s) or head, and retained fetal membranes.
- Alternative methods for the administration of oxytocin involve more frequent low dose bolus injections (every 10–30 minutes), administration of a single larger dose, or slow administration of a larger dose diluted in 1 liter of saline in a constant rate infusion through an intravenous catheter. The latter is not common in clinical practice due to the constant movement of the mare in the foaling stall or paddock.

Further Reading

Ley WB, Parker NA, Bowen JM, Digrassie WA, Jack NE. 1998. How we induce the normal mare to foal. *Proc Annu Conv Am Assoc Eq Pract* 44: 194–7.

Macpherson ML, Chaffin KM, Carroll GL, *et al.* 1996. Three methods for oxytocin-induced parturition: effects on the neonatal foal. *Proc Annu Conv Am Assoc Eq Pract* 42: 150–1.

Ousey J. 2003. Induction of parturition in the healthy mare. *Eq Vet Educ* 15: 164–8.

95

Normal Foaling

John J. Dascanio

School of Veterinary Medicine, Texas Tech University, USA

Introduction

In order to determine issues surrounding foaling, it is important to recognize normal parturition events. Since the consequences of a dystocia may lead to the death of the foal or mare, or severe pathologic damage, the foaling event should be attended by experienced personnel.

The mare should be properly prepared and monitored for foaling (see Chapters 88–93). The personnel monitoring the mare must be able to recognize the signs of dystocia so that an intervention plan can be implemented quickly (see Chapter 97).

The mare should develop impending signs of parturition in accordance with her expected due date (Table 95.1). Premature sign development may indicate an impending abortion or premature delivery. The gestation period for a mare is approximately 340 days, with a range of 320–360 days. Most mares will foal during the night with a peak around midnight.

Equipment and Supplies

Tail wrap, non-irritant soap, roll cotton, stainless steel bucket, disposable liner for bucket, foaling supplies (see Appendix 4).

Technique

- Locate a level area free of obstructions, with good footing for foaling. An example may be a movable round pen on short grass or a large foaling stall (3.5 × 5 m (12 × 14 feet) or larger).
- Place a tail wrap so that the entire tail is encompassed. Folding the tail and placing a self-adhering bandage tape over the entirety works well.
- Clean and dry the perineum of the mare, udder, and flank. This will limit the necessity to perform a more involved scrub later, if intervention is required and will ensure that the foal has a clean area to suckle. If a vulvoplasty (Caslick) is present, it should be opened (see Chapter 88).
- A foaling kit should be available to handle foaling and post-foaling procedures (see Appendix 4).
- Stage 1 of labor is marked by the repositioning of the foal in preparation for delivery. Stage 1 ends with the rupture

Table 95.1 Relative timeline of events leading up to, during, and after normal foaling. Note that there is individual mare variation in the events, especially in maiden mares.

Parturition sign	Timeline
Ventral edema (Figure 95.1)	Some weeks prior to foaling. Edema will be more pronounced with a decrease in activity and an increase in parity
Udder formation	2–6 weeks prior to foaling. Maiden mares may not develop a significant udder
Relaxation of the perineal ligaments	1–3 weeks prior to foaling
Relaxation, elongation, and edema of the vulva	A day or two prior to foaling
Cervical relaxation	A few days prior to foaling, although in some mares it may not occur until stage 1 labor is initiated
Milk within the gland	4–6 days prior to foaling. Maiden mares may not develop a significant secretion until after foaling
"Waxing" of teat ends	24–48 hours prior to foaling
Increased milk calcium	Within 96 hours of foaling
Decreased milk pH	Within 24 hours of foaling
Stage 1 of labor	1–2 hours in duration
Stage 2 of labor	20–30 minutes in duration
Stage 3 of labor	Up to 3 hours post-foaling

Equine Reproductive Procedures, Second Edition. Edited by John Dascanio and Patrick McCue.

of the chorioallantois and expulsion of allantoic fluid ("water breaking").

- The mare should show progressive signs of parturition including lying down/getting up, defecation, urination, stretching out (Figure 95.2), sweating, pawing, curling of upper lip, looking at her abdomen, appearing slightly colicy, kicking at her abdomen, biting at her flanks, tail swishing, and/or flagging her tail (Figure 95.3). These signs are an outward display of uterine contractions and fetal reorientation. They should be differentiated from colic of intestinal origin.
- A yellow-tinged fluid (allantoic fluid), discharged from the vulva, marks rupture of the chorioallantois (Figure 95.4).

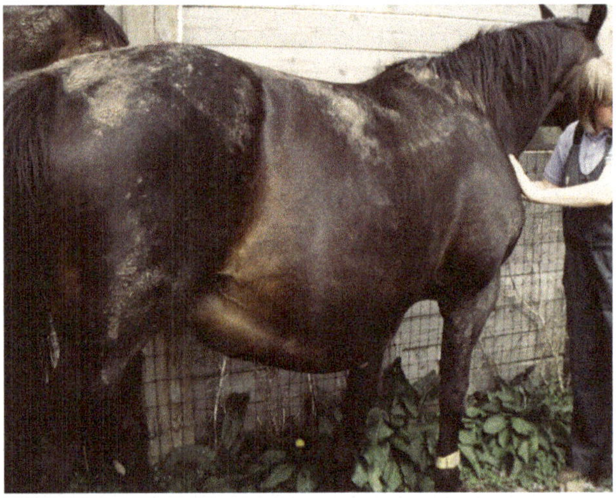

Figure 95.1 Ventral edema plaque in a later term pregnant mare.

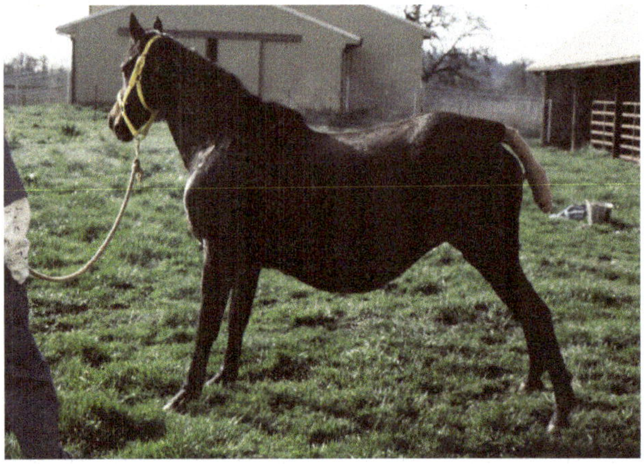

Figure 95.2 Mare in stage 1 of labor. Note the extended stance and steam rising from her back due to sweating in a cold environment.

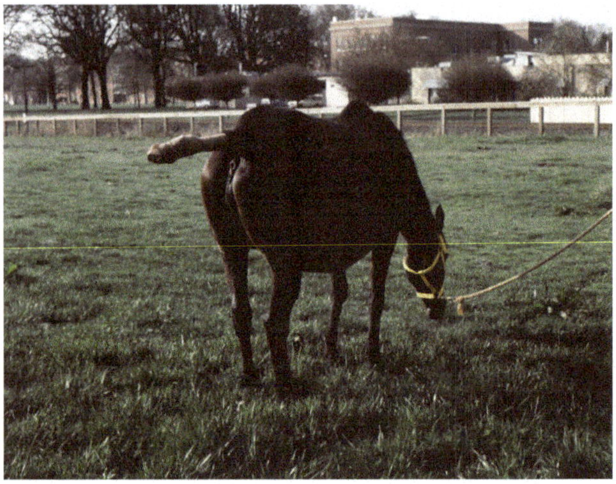

Figure 95.3 Mare in stage 1 labor. The mare is flagging her tail up and down with her head in a downward position. The mare was positioning herself to lie down.

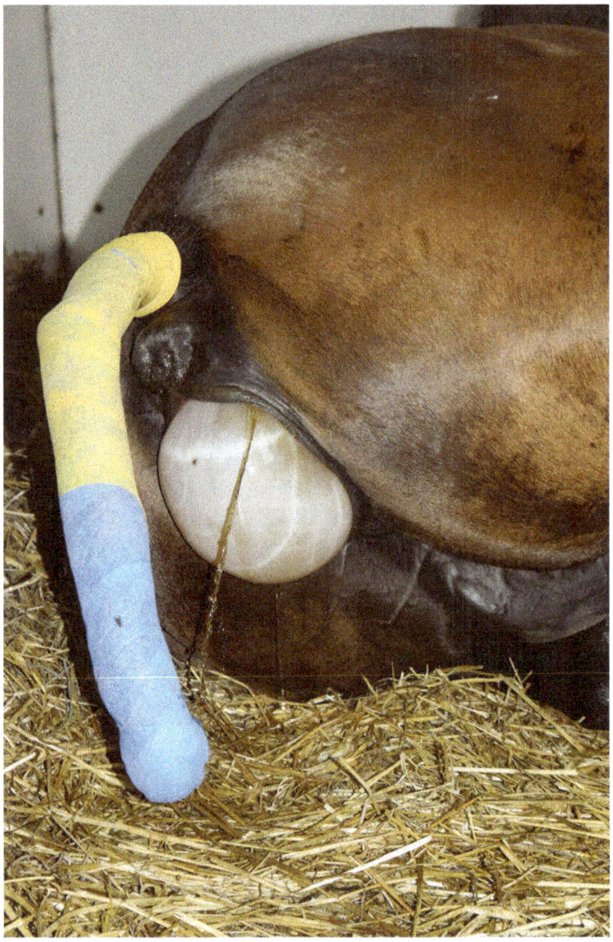

Figure 95.4 Mare in stage 2 of parturition with the amnion presented at the vulva. Note the normal yellow-tinged allantoic fluid discharge.

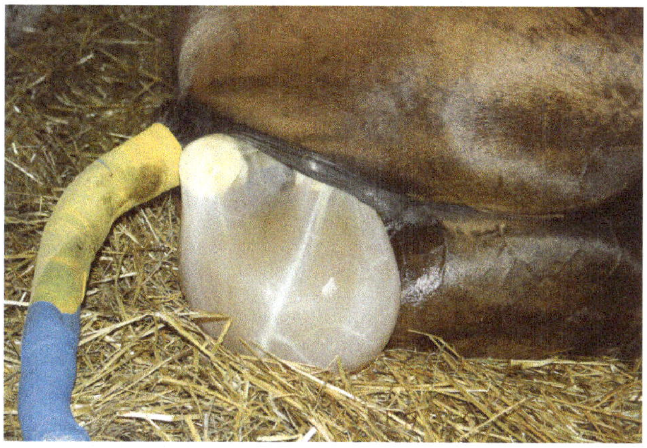

Figure 95.5 Mare in stage 2 labor. The first foot appears covered by amnion.

- A hippomane(s) may be discharged in the fluid or may be delivered with the foal.
- Stage 2 of labor is the delivery of the foal through the pelvic canal.
  - The white to grayish, opaque amnion should appear through the vulva first (Figure 95.4).
  - Two feet should be visible next through the vulva with the solar surface of the foal's feet orientated toward the mare's ventrum (Figure 95.5). Often one foot will be slightly ahead of the other foot, allowing the shoulders an angled delivery through the pelvic canal. It is not uncommon for a mare to stand and lay down again once the foal's feet are present at the vulva.
  - The fetlocks should bend in the same direction as the next most proximal joint (carpus). If it bends in the opposite direction (hock), the foal is being delivered posteriorly.
  - By the delivery of the foal's carpus through the vulva, the foal's nose/head should be visible. Typically, by the time the mid-cannon of the foal is evident, the foal's nose should be evident (Figures 95.6 and 95.7)
  - The top of the foal's head and back should be orientated toward the mare's back.
  - The vulva will initially prevent the crown of the foal's head from being delivered until it is properly dilated. Once the entire head is out, the delivery should progress within a few minutes to deliver the foal's chest until the foal's pelvis engages the mare's pelvic canal (Figure 95.8).
  - Once the foal's head is outside the vulva, the foal's chest and umbilical cord may be compromised by pressure within the pelvic canal. It is important that parturition progress and that the foal's chest exit the pelvic canal to allow for lung insufflation.

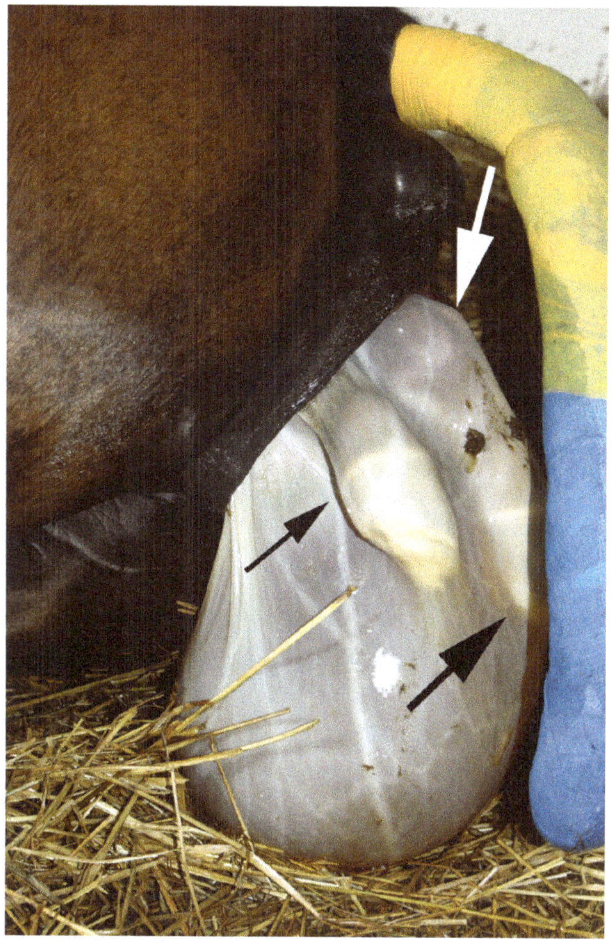

Figure 95.6 Mare in stage 2 labor. The foal's right front foot (small black arrow), left front foot (large black arrow), and nose (white arrow) are presented.

  - The delivery of the foal may pause slightly as the foal's hips pass through the pelvic canal. Once the foal's pelvis clears the pelvic canal, the foal's feet often remain within the vestibule/vagina until the mare stands or the foal attempts to orientate itself (Figure 95.9).
  - The umbilical cord will generally break once the mare stands up. There is no appreciable blood flow through the umbilicus at this point.
  - If intervention occurs, the foal should be placed in sternal recumbency so that both lung fields aerate.
  - Refer to Chapter 193 for immediate post-foaling care of the foal.
- Stage 3 of labor involves the delivery of the placenta. The placenta should be expelled by 3 hours post-foaling. Failure of delivery may predispose the mare to uterine infection.

(a) (b)

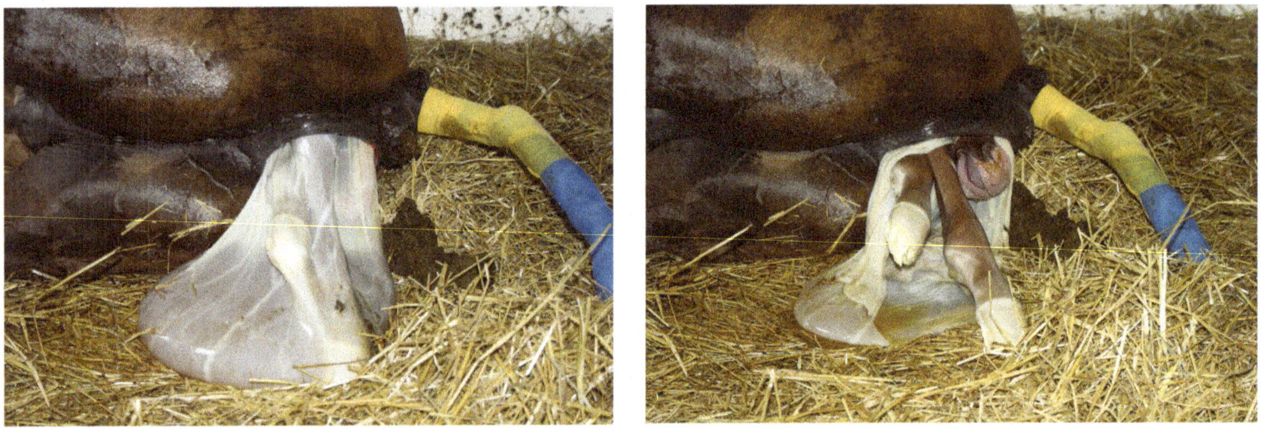

Figure 95.7 Mare in stage 2 labor. (a) The foal's nose is about even with the mid-cannon of the right front limb. It is normal for the mare to defecate during contractions. (b) The amnion was torn free from the foal's nose which facilitates visualization of the foal's position. The amnion normally remains over the foal until the majority of the foal has been delivered, at which time it is tears on its own.

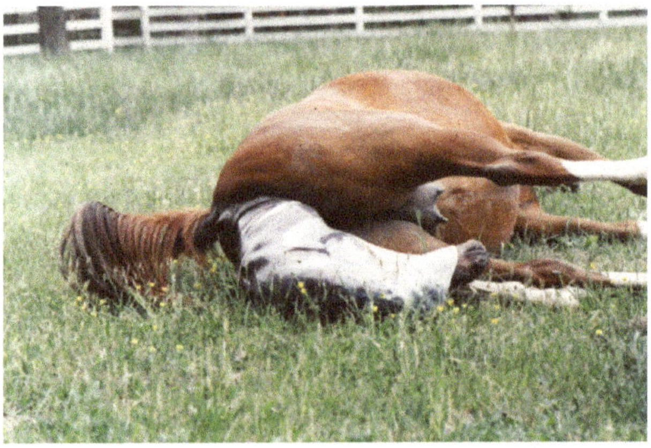

Figure 95.8 Mare in stage 2 labor. Note that the foal's chest has passed the vulva and the foal's hips are within the mare's pelvis. This is the position where the amnion normally tears free from the foal's nose.

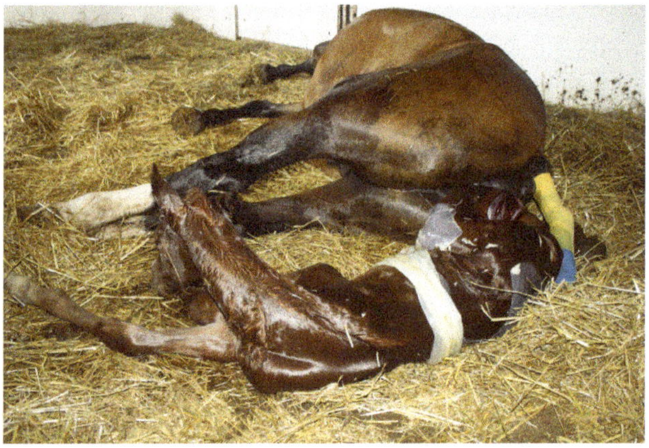

Figure 95.9 Mare in stage 2 labor. The foal is completely delivered with the exception of its hind feet which may remain within the mare until she stands or the foal orientates itself.

Interpretation

- Significant ventral edema may lead to complications such as pre-pubic tendon rupture or hernia formation. Controlled exercise may limit edema formation.
- If after 20 minutes of stage 2 labor there has not been adequate progression, the mare should be examined by experienced personnel. A duration of stage 2 labor over 30–40 minutes has an increased in foal morbidity and mortality.
- A reddish, velvety membrane presented at the vulva may indicate premature placental separation and an emergency situation (see Chapter 96).
- If the foal's nose is encased in amnion by the time the entire chest is delivered, it should be removed to allow normal respiration.
- The most difficult part of attending a foaling is knowing when to intervene. All too often personnel enter the foaling stall and assist in the delivery when all is normal. Care must be exercised to not tear or damage the mare's reproductive tract or injure the foal from overzealous intervention. As long as progression is made in the delivery of the foal, and the total foaling time for stage 2 is within 20–30 minutes, intervention should be cautiously restrained so that proper dilation of the vulva may occur to accommodate exit of the foal.
- Allow time post-foaling for the mare and foal to bond. Mares will often change their behavior and become very protective of their foal, so caution should be used when entering a stall with a newborn foal.
- Maiden mares may have a delayed onset of impending parturition signs.
- Mares that have had multiple foals may have a decreased duration for parturition.

- Mares that foal in the early spring will generally have a longer gestation period by 5–10 days than mares who foal in the summer.
- Failure to develop impending signs of parturition may be associated with incorrect breeding dates, an erroneous determination of pregnancy, a natural delay in expected due date, or as a result of fescue toxicosis.
- Potential complications may include premature placental separation, fetal hypoxia, abnormal orientation of the fetus in the birth canal, damage to the mare's reproductive tract, foal injuries (broken ribs), uterine prolapse, and retained fetal membranes.
- Additional guidelines may be found in Chapter 97.

Further Reading

American Association of Equine Practitioners. 2020. Foaling mare and newborn: preparing for a safe and successful foal delivery. https://aaep.org/horsehealth/foaling-mare-newborn-preparing-safe-successful-foal-delivery.

McCue PM, Ferris RA. 2012. Parturition, dystocia and foal survival: a retrospective study of 1047 births. *Eq Vet J* 44: 22–5.

96

Premature Separation of the Placenta

Patrick M. McCue

Equine Reproduction Laboratory, Colorado State University, USA

Introduction

The equine placenta consists of a co-joined outer membrane called the chorioallantois, which is attached to the uterus, an inner membrane called the amnion, which surrounds the foal, and the umbilical cord. The chorionic surface of the chorioallantois is connected to the uterine wall by millions of microscopic attachments called microcotyledons, except for the area of the placenta that is in contact with the cervix, the oviducts, where the endometrial cups form, where uterine cysts may be present, and where twin placentas touch each other. The absence of uterine glands on various structures leads to a failure of microcotyledon development on the adjacent part of the placenta. Consequently, whereas a majority of the outer chorionic surface of the placenta has a brick-red velvety appearance due to the presence of the microcotyledons, the region of placenta abutting the cervix lacks microcotyledons and has a smooth, white, star-like appearance, known as the cervical star. Attachment of the placenta to the uterus via the microcotyledons is critical for the transfer of nutrients and oxygen from the mare across the placenta to the fetus.

With the onset of labor, the cervix starts to relax and the uterus begins to contract. Increased pressure from the uterus causes the chorioallantois to bulge into the open cervix. In the normal progression of foaling, the chorioallantois ruptures at the cervical star and results in the release of a large quantity of allantoic fluid (i.e., the "water breaks"). The amnion, a thin, transparent, grayish-white membrane should begin protruding through the vulva within 2–5 minutes after the mare breaks her water (Figure 96.1). As the mare continues to push, the foal's front legs and then a nose should appear inside the amnionic sac. The foal is usually delivered within 5–20 minutes after the mare breaks her water.

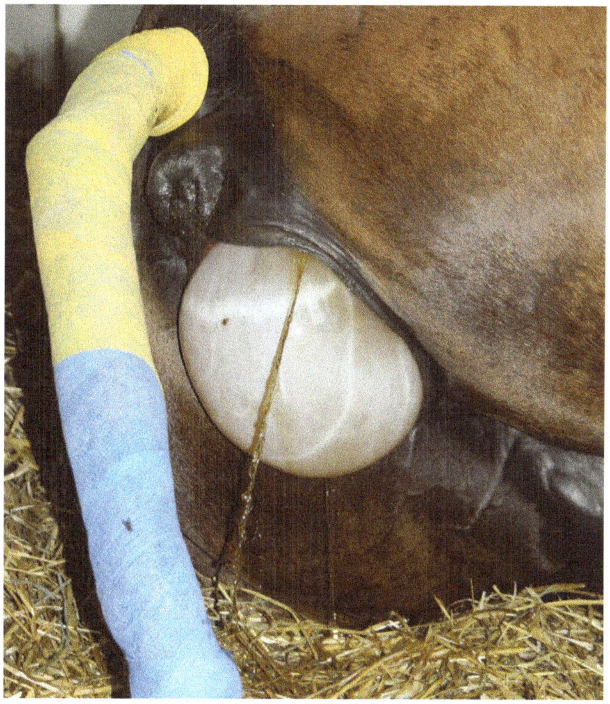

Figure 96.1 Amnion protruding through the vulva during a normal foaling.

Occasionally, premature separation of the outer placental membrane from the uterine wall may lead to protrusion of the intact fluid-filled chorioallantois through the vulva (Figures 96.2 and 96.3). The dark red color of the outer surface of the chorioallantois gives rise to the common term for premature separation of the placenta – "red bag." Confirmation of the condition may be made by observing the cervical star on the chorionic surface.

Equine Reproductive Procedures, Second Edition. Edited by John Dascanio and Patrick McCue.

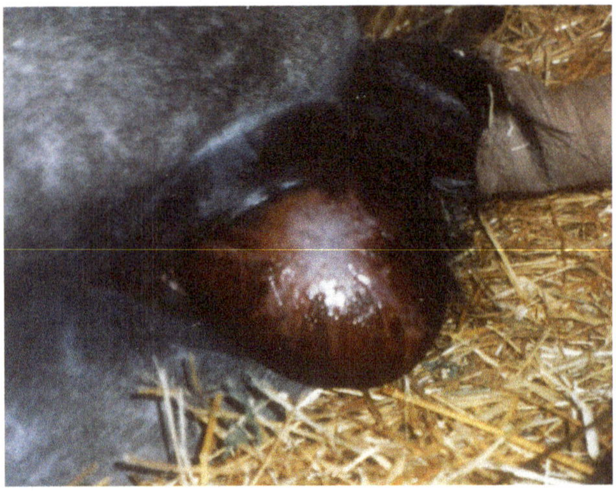

Figure 96.2 Intact chorioallantoic membrane protruding through the vulva, indicative of premature separation of the placenta. Note the prominent white cervical star.

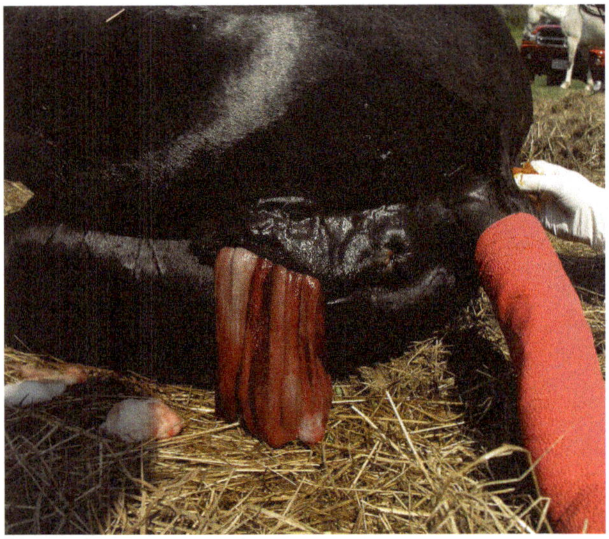

Figure 96.3 Another example of premature placental separation. The brick-red velvety chorionic surface of the intact chorioallantois is plainly visible.

Equipment and Supplies

Sharp instrument (scissors or knife).

Technique

- Owners or foaling personnel must quickly recognize the red bag condition and intervene immediately. The protruding tissue should be felt for an underlying presence of the fetal limbs/head. A careful decision must be made as other structures that may protrude through the vulva of a mare in labor include a bladder prolapse, vaginal prolapse, or eviscerating intestinal loops.
- An intact chorioallantoic membrane is thin walled. Fetal extremities should be palpable through the membrane.
- The placental membrane should immediately be opened with a sharp instrument such as a knife or scissors. This will result in a release of allantoic fluid and a transient delay in uterine contractions.
- Appropriate traction should be applied to the foal in unison with uterine contractions of the mare to expedite a delivery.
- It is warranted to immediately summon additional assistance to help with delivery of the foal and subsequent care of the newborn foal.
- Oxygen should be administered to the newborn foal if available. Foals may develop problems associated with hypoxia even though they may appear to be normal at birth. The foal should be considered at a high risk of developing hypoxic ischemic encephalopathy and

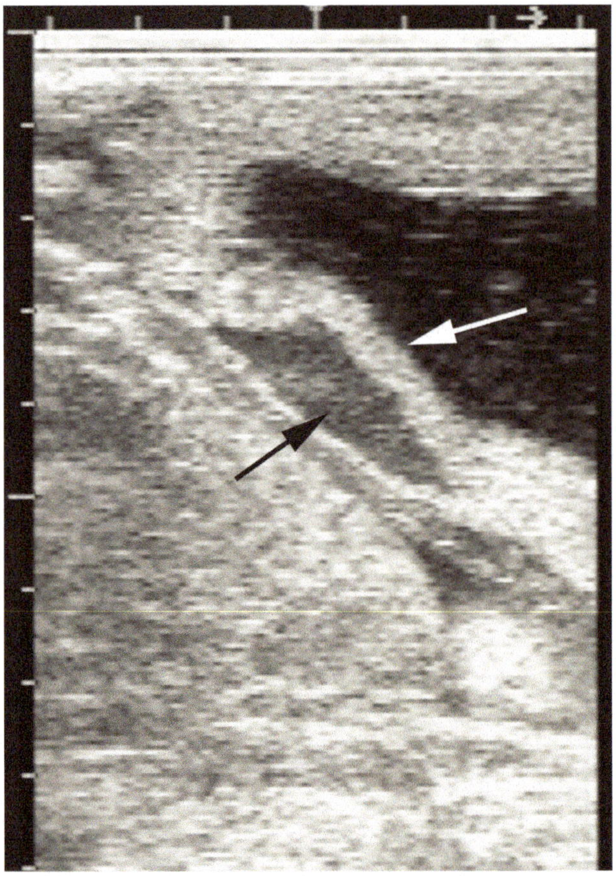

Figure 96.4 Ultrasound showing slight separation of the chorioallantoic membrane (white arrow) from the uterus (black arrow pointing to the area of separation).

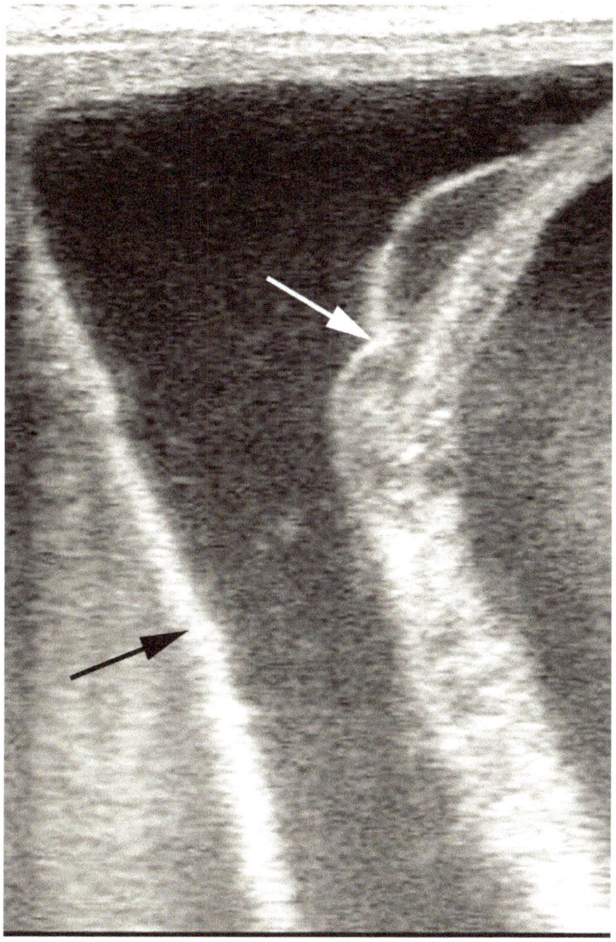

Figure 96.5 Ultrasound showing massive separation of the chorioallantoic membrane (white arrow) from the uterus (black arrow). This mare aborted 2 days later.

appropriate preventative care/observation should be administered.

Additional Comments

Premature separation of the placenta accounts for up to 5–10% of all cases of abortion, stillbirth, and perinatal death. The most common causes of red bag are placental infections, fescue toxicosis, and stress. Chronic placental separation from the uterus may occur over a period of several days or weeks during late gestation as a consequence of placentitis. The condition may be associated with a cervical discharge or mild blood loss out the vulva. A diagnosis of placental separation may be possible by ultrasound examination of the pregnant uterus (Figures 96.4 and 96.5). If separation of the chorioallantois from the uterus is noted in a late-term pregnant mare, emergency therapy should be immediately instituted, including altrenogest (double dose), broad-spectrum antibiotics, a non-steroidal anti-inflammatory medication (e.g., firocoxib) and, potentially, pentoxifylline if available.

Failure of the outer placental membrane to rupture during labor and the subsequent separation of the attachments between the uterus and placenta lead to a rapid decrease in oxygen transport to the fetus. An intact cervical star region of the placenta after parturition should be considered a predisposing factor for neonatal hypoxia since the placenta did not open in its normal location or time frame. As a consequence, the fetus may suffer from lack of oxygen (hypoxia) or may die of asphyxiation if the condition is prolonged or progresses.

Recognition of premature placental separation and appropriate intervention are the key factors for survival of the foal.

Further Reading

Frazer GS, Perkins NR, Embertson RM. 1999. Normal parturition and evaluation of the mare in dystocia. *Eq Vet Educ* 11: 41–6.

Rossdale PD, Ricketts SW. 2002. Evaluation of the fetal membranes at foaling. *Eq Vet Educ* 14: 78–82.

97

Dystocia Management

Patrick M. McCue[1] and Sofie Sitters[2]

[1]*Equine Reproduction Laboratory, Colorado State University, USA*
[2]*Amsterdam, The Netherlands*

Introduction

The term dystocia refers to an abnormal or difficult birth and is a medical emergency. Dystocia occurs in approximately 10% of foalings and is more common in mares during their first foaling (i.e., maiden mares) than in mares that have previously given birth to one or more foals. Active (stage 2) labor is usually completed within 10–20 minutes. An owner or foaling attendant should be concerned if a foal has not been born within 20 minutes after a mare "breaks her water" or releases allantoic fluid.

The most common cause of dystocia in the mare is malposture, especially retention of the front legs and/or head. Failure of the foal to be properly orientated (cranial presentation, dorsal–sacral position with head and front limbs extended (posture)) will prevent normal passage through the birth canal.

Intervention is often required in a dystocia to assist with delivery of the foal. The ultimate goals are to save the life of the foal, save the life of the mare, and to preserve the future fertility of the mare. Time is critical during an equine dystocia as placental separation may rapidly lead to fetal hypoxia. It has been estimated that for each 10-minute increase in duration of labor beyond 30 minutes, there is a 10% increased risk of the foal failing to survive.

Repeated non-productive in and out movements of the examiner's arm into the reproductive tract of the mare should be avoided to prevent damage to the mucosa, which could lead to vaginal adhesions, tears associated with delivery, or abrasions susceptible to infection. Investigation or intervention may be indicated under the following circumstances:

- If there has been no progress toward delivery after 10–20 minutes:
  - Failure of the amnionic membrane to appear at the vulva within 10 minutes after rupture of the chorioallantoic membrane (mare "breaks her water").
  - Failure of fetal parts to appear within 15 minutes after rupture of the chorioallantois.
- Lack of uterine contractions after rupture of the chorioallantois
- Premature placental separation is noted (i.e., "red bag" delivery).
- If delivery progress abruptly stops.
- If the mare becomes acutely painful or shocky.
- If a moderate to severe dystocia is suspected.

The most common causes of dystocia in the mare, categorized by management difficulty, are presented in Table 97.1. Mild dystocias are commonly managed on the farm by foaling personnel. More complicated dystocias may require advanced training or experience and often need veterinary intervention.

Equipment and Supplies

Dystocia kit including (minimally) a naso-gastric tube, pump, bucket, obstetrical lubricant, obstetrical sleeves, non-residual soap, towels, tail wrap, obstetrical chains or straps, obstetrical handles and nylon ropes; medications may include sedation drugs, tocolytic agents, oxytocin, local anesthetic agents, non-steroidal anti-inflammatory drugs, antibiotics.

Technique

- In the event of a dystocia on a breeding farm, the owner or foaling attendant should keep the mare standing and walking to minimize non-productive straining.

Equine Reproductive Procedures, Second Edition. Edited by John Dascanio and Patrick McCue.

Table 97.1 Common causes of dystocia in mares arranged by degree of difficulty in correction.

Correction Difficulty	Foaling Complication or Issue
Mild	Elbow lock
	Upside-down foal
	Backwards foal
	Uterine inertia
	"Red bag" (premature placental separation)
Moderate	Front leg(s) flexed at the knee (carpus)
	Neck flexed ventrally; muzzle below pelvic brim
	"Hip lock"
	Feto-maternal disproportion
Difficult	Congenital abnormalities (e.g., contracted tendons)
	Front leg(s) flexed at shoulder
	Neck flexed to side; muzzle not reachable
	"Breech" presentation (posterior presentation with both hind limbs flexed at the hip)
	Transverse presentation
	Twins (when both entering birth canal simultaneously)

- The reproductive history of the mare should be quickly obtained, including mare age, breeding/due date, previous foaling history, pertinent medical conditions, duration of labor, and attempts at relieving the dystocia.
- The mare should be placed in an area that is safe for her and for all personnel. Stocks with fixed posts and sides should be avoided as mares in labor tend to lie down quickly when examined or when a fetus is manipulated or pulled.
- A brief physical examination should be performed of the mare to determine her health status, as subsequent decisions may be based on this critical information. Clinical signs of hemorrhage (i.e., pale mucous membranes), dehydration, or shock should be noted.
- The chorioallantoic membrane should be ruptured immediately and the fetus delivered as soon as possible if there is evidence of premature placental separation (i.e., a "red bag" delivery) (Figure 97.1).
- If time permits, the tail of the mare should be wrapped and the perineum washed to minimize contamination of the reproductive tract during obstetrical examination or manipulations.
- An efficient evaluation of her reproductive tract should follow to identify the obstetrical problem, to determine if the fetus is alive, and to formulate a plan. This exam may begin with a transrectal palpation to determine if the foal is alive and its position, to evaluate the broad ligaments for uterine torsion, and to determine if parturition has truly started.

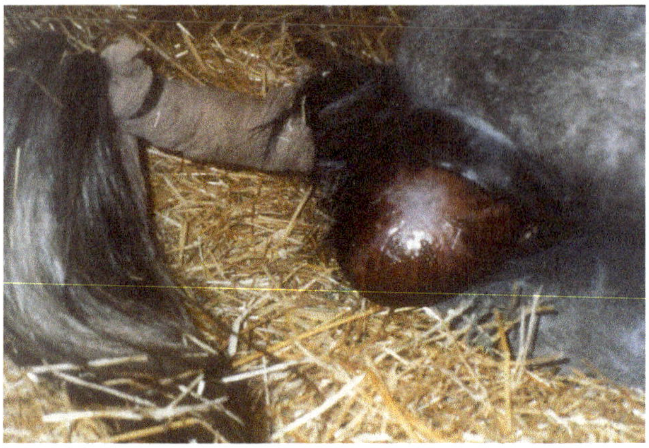

Figure 97.1 Premature placental separation ("red bag") with the intact chorioallantoic membrane protruding through the vulva and the white cervical star visible.

- In some instances, sedation of the mare, placement of an epidural anesthetic (see Chapter 100) to decrease pain and straining, and/or general anesthesia may be necessary to facilitate safe evaluation of the mare, to reposition the fetus if necessary, and to allow for a controlled vaginal delivery.
- A vaginal exam should be performed next to determine the presentation, position, and posture of the fetus and to assess whether or not the fetus is already engaged in the pelvis. The Ferguson reflex, a neuroendocrine reflex activated when fetal body parts are engaged within the vagina/cervix, will induce release of oxytocin from the posterior pituitary. This will in turn stimulate uterine contractions and increase the impaction of the fetus into the birth canal.
- An assessment of fetal viability should be made by noting fetal movements and response to stimulation of the eye, tongue, coronary band, or anus, or by detection of a fetal heart beat on transabdominal ultrasound or a jugular/carotid pulse on transvaginal or transrectal ultrasound.
- Choices for resolving an equine dystocia include vaginal delivery, cesarean section surgery, or fetotomy. The final decision may depend on the status of the fetus, duration and severity of the dystocia, economic value of the mare and fetus, clinician expertise, client preference, facilities available, and other considerations.
- The first option for delivery (on a farm or at a referral center) is a vaginal delivery with the mare awake and either standing or lying down. If significant progress is not made in 15–20 minutes, the strategy for relieving the dystocia should be changed.
- Sedation may be indicated and may include acepromazine, xylazine (alone), or a combination of xylazine and butorphanol tartrate.

- A tocolytic agent may be administered in an attempt to control myometrial contractions and induce uterine relaxation. Potential options include clenbuterol, isoxsuprine, or *N*-butylscopolammonium bromide. Efficacy at inducing uterine relaxation with clenbuterol or isoxsuprine in a late-term mare is controversial.
- A copious amount of obstetrical lubricant should be infused into the uterus along all sides of the fetus to facilitate safe repositioning and extraction of the fetus (see Chapter 98). Often the uterine lumen will be devoid of allantoic and amnionic fluid in a prolonged dystocia. Caution should be exercised when infusing polyethylene polymer obstetrical lubricants into the uterus as fatal peritonitis has been reported following leakage of this polymer into the peritoneal cavity (e.g., in a uterine tear or subsequent cesarean surgery). A methylcellulose-based lubricant is a better choice for a general obstetrical lubricant.
- Repulsion of the fetus into the uterus may be required to gain sufficient space to mutate a fetal body part into proper orientation. Repulsion and other obstetrical manipulations may be easiest with the mare standing as gravity will keep the abdominal contents out of the way and allow for more space to maneuver the fetal body parts.
- A judicious amount of traction may be applied to the fetus once it has been confirmed that the limbs and head are correctly aligned within the birth canal. It is recommended that the amount of traction used to pull an equine fetus should not exceed that provided by two people (Figure 97.2). A fetal extractor (calf jack) is generally not recommended, but may be used with extreme caution in certain circumstances, with clinician guidance, as a mare's reproductive tract is more susceptible to trauma than that of a cow.
- Traction should be performed in conjunction with the mare's contractions. A set of obstetrical chains or wide-webbed nylon obstetrical straps, applied correctly by trained personnel, may be used in the assisted delivery of a fetus. It is important that the chains be placed above and below the fetlock of the fetus prior to applying traction so that the forces are distributed over a wider area. It is critical that chains are not placed near the coronary band, as severe trauma may result during traction.
- "Hip lock" is very uncommon in the horse due to the more circular pelvic opening; once the shoulders are through the pelvic canal, the remainder of the fetus should also pass. A 0.8% incidence of hip lock has been reported in a retrospective study of 1,047 equine births.
- Pull in an outward (initially) and then in a slightly downward direction to correspond to the spinal curvature of the foal.

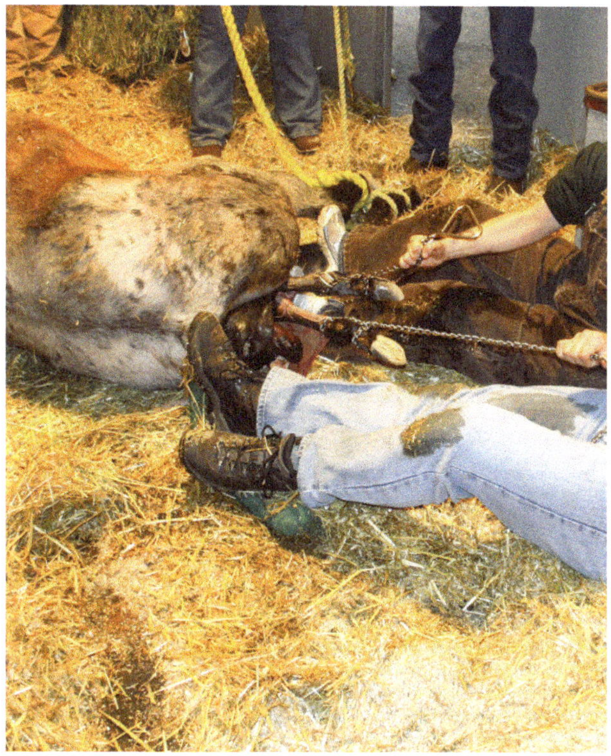

Figure 97.2 Applying traction to a fetus in a mare exhibiting uterine inertia.

- "Walk" the shoulders of the fetus through the pelvic canal one at a time. Pull on one front leg and then the other to advance the shoulders diagonally through the pelvis.
- Option 2 for delivery is to put the mare under general anesthesia for a controlled vaginal delivery. This may be the optimal strategy to obtain a live foal at a referral hospital if previous attempts at a vaginal delivery have already been performed on the breeding farm.
- Elevation of the hindquarters of an anesthetized mare may be beneficial to increase space in the caudal abdominal cavity. This will make it easier to repel the fetus into the uterus and reposition fetal body parts that are not aligned properly in the birth canal (Figure 97.3).
- If the dystocia is prolonged and the foal's nose is accessible, EXIT (*ex utero,* intrapartum treatment) may be used whereby the foal is intubated via a naso-tracheal tube and is actively ventilated with an Ambu bag. This may alleviate some hypoxia and allow for a longer time to correct the dystocia.
- Traction will be necessary to extract a fetus from a mare under general anesthesia due to a lack of spontaneous uterine contractions.
- Option 3 is cesarean surgery. A cesarean is indicated if the fetus is alive and cannot be delivered vaginally.

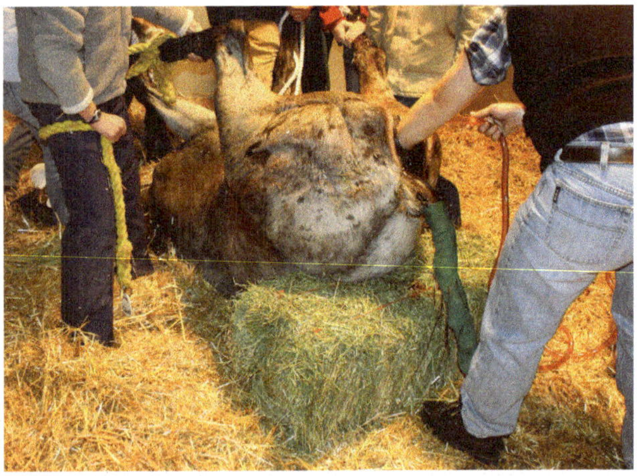

Figure 97.3 Elevation of the hind end of a mare to facilitate examination and mutation of the fetus.

- Option 4 is a fetotomy. A fetotomy may be indicated if the fetus is dead and cannot be delivered intact through the birth canal and if cesarean surgery is not an option (see Chapter 99).
- Resuscitation equipment should be available on farms that foal out a lot of mares and farm personnel should be trained in the proper care and use of the equipment. A resuscitation bag attached to a face mask is a simple to use device that can be safely applied to foals by farm personnel to help stimulate breathing in a newborn foal.
- Immediate attention must be given to the foal following a dystocia. The foal is at high risk of many neonatal diseases including hypoxia, neonatal maladjustment syndrome (hypoxic ischemic encephalopathy), failure of passive transfer, a ruptured bladder, and trauma such as rib fractures.
- The mare should also be examined in due course following resolution of a dystocia. It is common for the placenta to be retained following a dystocia and preventative treatments are often instituted after a dystocia has been relieved. The mare's udder should be examined for the presence of colostrum and absence of mastitis.
- Finally, the reproductive tract of the mare (i.e., perineum, vagina, cervix, uterus) should be carefully examined for trauma that may be life threatening (e.g., a uterine tear or rupture) or limit her future reproductive performance.

Additional Comments

It is strongly recommended that an emergency plan be formulated prior to the foaling season to prepare for a difficult birth or a medical problem with a newborn foal. The plan should be the result of a conversation between the mare owner, farm manager, foaling attendant, and farm veterinarian. All personnel involved with foaling should be trained, able to recognize normal foaling patterns and a dystocia, instructed to call for assistance early in the course of a difficult birth, and be ready to assist if needed. In addition, a foaling kit (see Appendix 4) should be available near the foaling stall.

Further Reading

Frazer GS, Perkins NR, Embertson RM. 1999. Normal parturition and evaluation of the mare in dystocia. *Eq Vet Educ* 11: 41–6.

McCue PM, Ferris RA. 2012. Parturition, dystocia and foal survival – a retrospective study of 1,047 births. *Eq Vet J* 44(suppl. 41): 22–5.

Norton JL, Dallap BL, Johnston JK, Palmer JE, Sertich PL, Boston R, Wilkins PA. 2007. Retrospective stud of dystocia in mares at a referral hospital. *Eq Vet J* 39: 37–41.

98

Dystocia Correction

John J. Dascanio

School of Veterinary Medicine, Texas Tech University, USA

Introduction

Safe and expedient correction of a dystocia requires the optimal use of techniques, equipment, personnel, and facilities. The reproductive tract of the mare should be protected from damage due to pressure points created during manipulation of the fetus and equipment used in the correction of a dystocia. Manipulations of the fetus such as repulsion, mutation, and version and equipment such as ropes, chains, and snares are commonly used to correct a dystocia. *Repulsion* refers to pushing the fetus back into the uterus to gain additional room for manipulations. *Mutation* refers to the manipulation of the fetus to return it to a normal presentation, posture, and position. *Version* refers to changes in the longitudinal axis such as moving the foal from a transverse to anterior presentation. A veterinarian should be able to use either arm, as needed, to reach and manipulate fetal body parts to correct a dystocia.

Key elements to resolving a dystocia are adequate lubrication, time management, and obtaining sufficient room in the pelvic inlet and caudal abdomen for manipulation of the fetus. The latter is often accomplished by getting a prone mare to temporarily stand or raising the posterior end of a mare under general anesthesia. It should be recognized that time is critical to the survival of a fetus, as each 10-minute delay in stage 2 of labor beyond 30 minutes is associated with a 10% increased risk of the fetus being born dead.

Equipment and Supplies

Dystocia kit including (minimally) a naso-gastric tube, pump, bucket, obstetrical lubricant, clean water, obstetrical sleeves, non-residual soap, towels, tail wrap, obstetrical chains or straps, obstetrical handles and nylon ropes. In addition, a Kuhn crutch may be of assistance; this is basically a long metal rod with a "U"-shaped blunt end that allows the operator to repel a fetus while his/her arm is still in the mare. Care should be taken to maintain the crutch on the fetus to avoid trauma to the uterus. Medications may include sedation drugs, tocolytic agents, oxytocin, local anesthetic agents, non-steroidal anti-inflammatory drugs, antibiotics. Equipment for fetal resuscitation and fetal care should also be available.

Technique

This chapter describes the fetal orientation (presentation, position, and/or posture) and correction of common causes of equine dystocia. A majority of equine dystocias are caused by abnormalities of fetal posture (orientation of the fetal limbs and head relative to the fetus itself). The basic corrections of major malpostures are presented here.

Elbow Lock

- *Fetal orientation.* The foal is in an anterior presentation, in a dorso-sacral position, with the head extended. One or both front limbs are not fully extended. The hallmark of elbow lock is the location of the fetal hoof or hooves even with its nose (Figure 98.1). In a normal delivery, the fetal nose should be at the level of the mid-cannon bone region.
- *Correction.* Manually extend the retained limb when the mare is relaxed in between uterine contractions. One can often feel a "pop" when the fetal elbow is dislodged from the maternal pelvis. If both limbs are retained in an elbow lock, extend one limb at a time. Occasionally, the foal may need to be repulsed to aid in the correction.

Head and Neck Flexion

- *Fetal orientation.* The fetus is in an anterior presentation, in a dorso-sacral position, with the front legs extended

Equine Reproductive Procedures, Second Edition. Edited by John Dascanio and Patrick McCue.

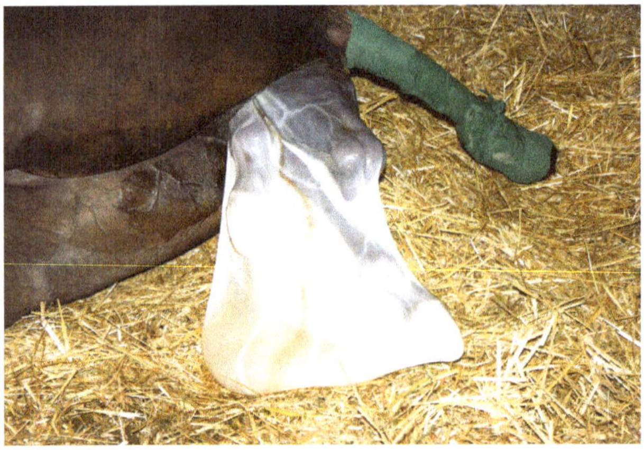

Figure 98.1 Elbow lock. Note the retained right front leg of the foal with the hoof adjacent to the nose of the foal.

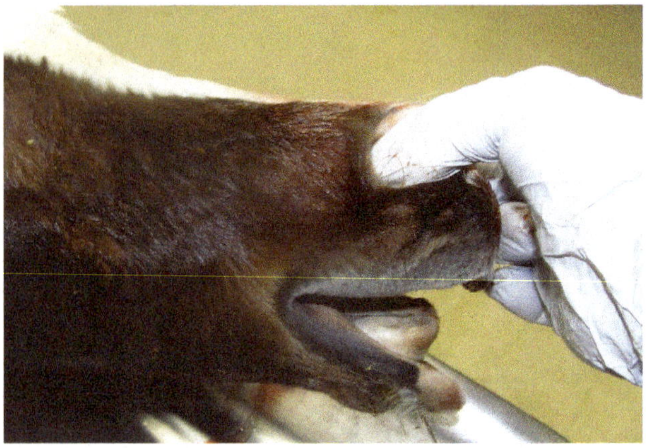

Figure 98.3 Grasping the foal by the nostrils using the thumb and middle finger.

but the fetal head/neck flexed laterally or ventrally. Protrusion of two feet out of the vulva without a head is obviously normal in a posterior presentation. Differentiation of the front feet from the hind feet is best and unequivocally accomplished by determination of the direction of flexion of the first two major distal limb joints. The joints both flex in the same direction with the front legs (fetlock and carpus) and flex in opposite directions in the rear limbs (fetlock and hock).

- *Correction*. The key to correction is to gain access to the end of the muzzle in order to turn the head.
- The long length of the foal's neck may preclude access to the foal's head, making correction extremely difficult, especially with lateral deviations.
- Structures to grasp for head manipulation include the orbital rims (Figure 98.2), nostrils (Figure 98.3), an ear, or the inter-mandibular space (Figure 98.4).
- Any part of the bony structure of the head can be grasped and the head rotated and extended. The ears should not have excessive force applied to prevent nerve damage. The muzzle should be brought close to mid-line during correction to minimize the space required to extend the head.

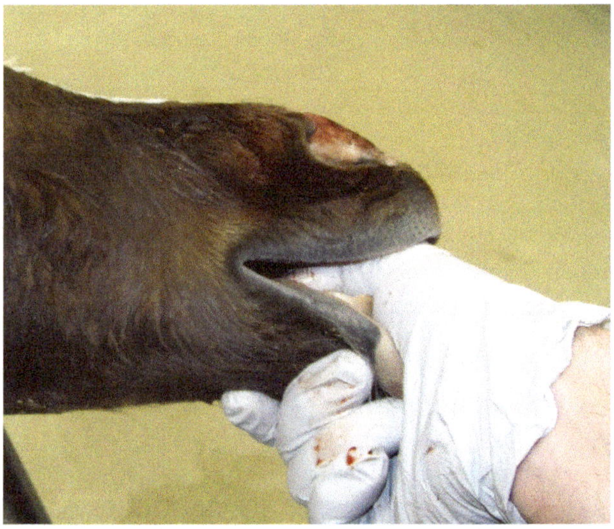

Figure 98.4 Grasping the inter-mandibular space behind the incisors to hold onto the foal's head.

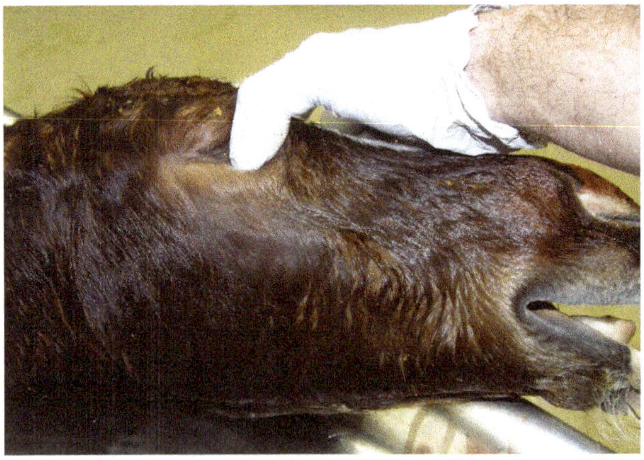

Figure 98.2 Grasping the foal by the orbital rims using the thumb and middle finger.

- A head snare or nylon rope may be used if hand gripping pressure is inadequate for correction. Typically a head snare is placed over the ears and poll and brought through the foal's mouth (Figure 98.5). Alternatively, the snare or a soft nylon rope may also be looped around the lower jaw to help gently pull the foal's muzzle medially and caudally while applying repulsion pressure to the lower neck or chest to aid in correction (Figure 98.6).
- A "wry neck" or fused neck vertebrae should be considered in situations where the correction of a deviated head does not progress normally.

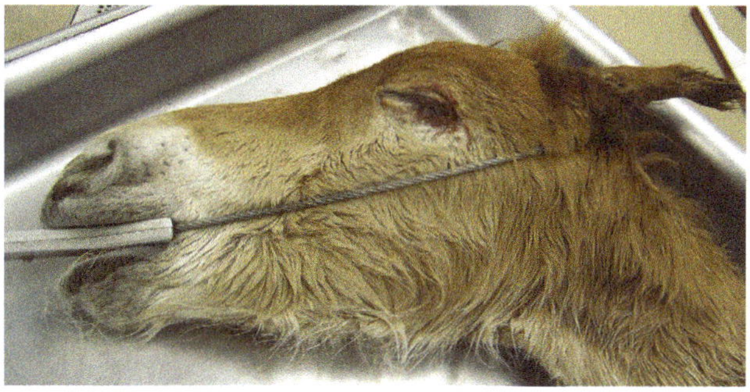

Figure 98.5 Proper placement of a head snare over the poll, behind the ears, and in the mouth.

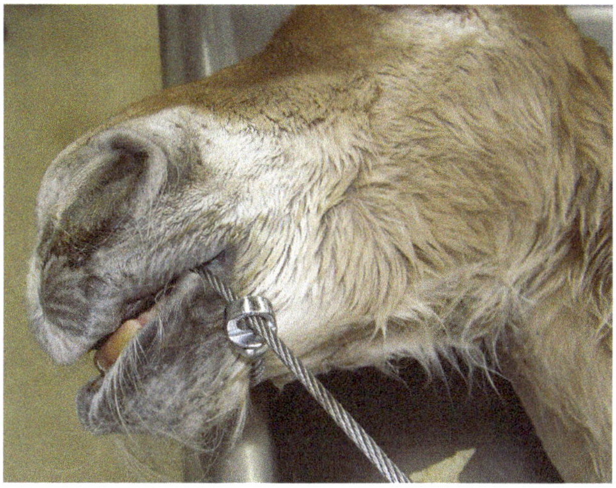

Figure 98.6 Placement of a snare over the lower jaw.

Foot Nape

- *Fetal orientation.* The term "foot nape" refers to an abnormal fetal posture in which one or both front limbs are located over the head or neck. This may result in recto-vaginal trauma with the possibility of a third degree perineal laceration if it is not corrected and the foal is delivered by forced extraction in this manner.
- *Correction.* The fetus should be repulsed into the abdomen and the limbs moved to their correct location under the head. Normal spontaneous delivery should allow the subsequent passage of the fetus, or a controlled vaginal delivery may be required.

Carpal Flexion

- *Fetal orientation.* Typically, the fetus will be in anterior presentation, in a dorso-sacral position, with the head extended and one or both front limbs flexed at the carpus.
- *Correction.* If enough space is present within the pelvic canal and uterus, the hoof of the retained limb is covered by the veterinarian's hand and the hoof is first pulled medially and then pulled toward the pelvis to extend the limb.
- If it is not possible to grasp the hoof or easily extend the limb, the cannon bone or fetlock may be grasped and the carpus repulsed dorsally into the uterus while simultaneously pulling the fetlock medially and then toward the pelvic opening. Once the hoof is within reach, it should be cupped with the hand to protect the uterus before the limb is fully extended.
- If it is not possible to fully extend the fore limbs, contracture of the flexure tendons may be present (Figure 98.7).

Shoulder Flexion

- *Fetal orientation.* The fetus is typically in an anterior presentation, in a dorso-sacral position, with the head extended and one or both front legs retained or flexed at the shoulder. Bilateral shoulder flexion with an extended head will result in only the foal's head being presented through the vulva (Figure 98.8). The foal may be deceased, especially if the duration of the dystocia is prolonged due to compression of the chest/umbilical cord within the pelvic canal.
- *Correction.* If the fetus is dead, a fetotomy may be performed and the head/neck cut off and removed (see Chapter 99). This may allow for additional room to manipulate the retained limbs into normal extension. If the fetus is alive, a cesarean section would provide the best chance of delivering a live foal versus extensive and prolonged manipulation to correct both limbs. With this dystocia it may be exceedingly difficult to repulse the fetus into the abdomen for proper manipulations.

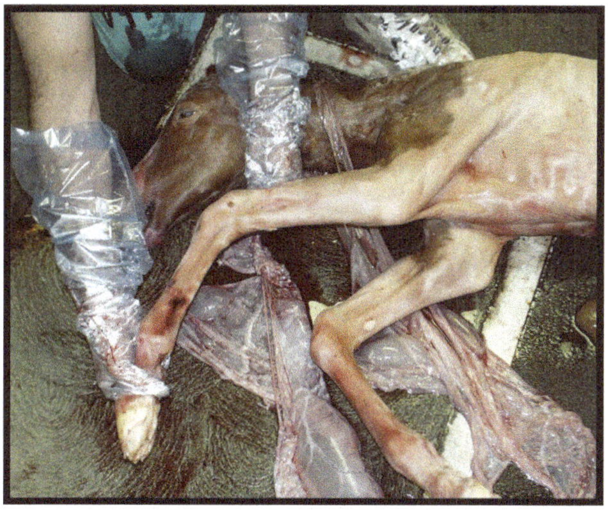

Figure 98.7 Congenital contracted tendons leading to dystocia in a mare.

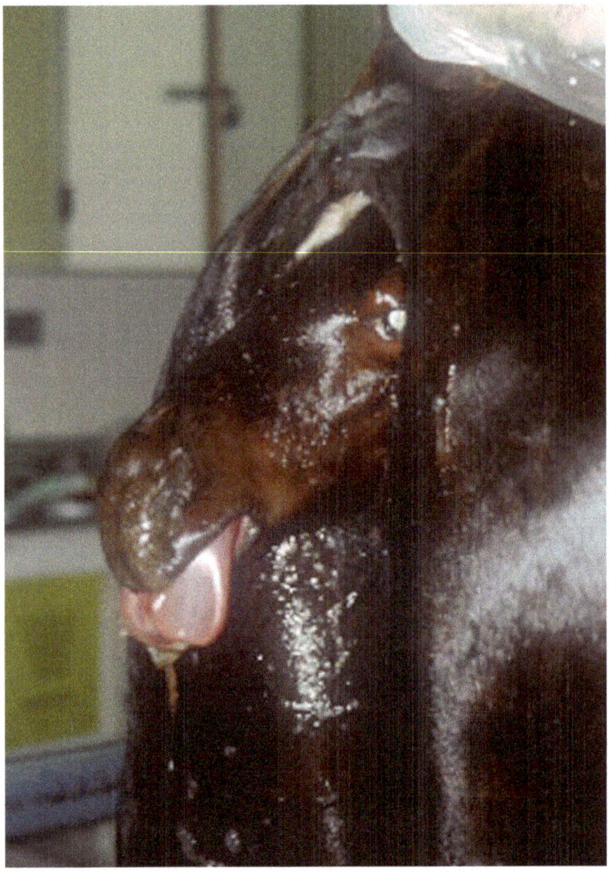

Figure 98.8 Retention of both fore limbs in an equine dystocia.

- If a vaginal delivery is attempted, one front limb should be initially manipulated into carpal flexion. The fetal forearm is grasped and the proximal portion of the limb (and fetus) is repulsed while the distal portion is pulled medially and toward the pelvic canal to place the limb into carpal flexion. The limb is then manipulated to full extension as described previously.

Posterior Presentation

- *Fetal orientation.* The fetus is in a dorso-sacral position, and both hind limbs are extended.
- In most instances the fetus should be delivered spontaneously or is deliverable with mild to moderate traction. It is important that once delivery of the fetus commences, it should proceed without delay as the umbilicus may be occluded against the ventral pelvis and oxygen delivery compromised.
- If the position of the foal is dorso-ventral (dorso-pubic), there is a potential for development of a recto-vaginal fistula or a third degree perineal laceration due to trauma from the hind hooves.
- *Correction.* The fetus may be rotated by crossing the hind legs while applying traction to mutate the foal into a more traditional and safe dorso-sacral position.

Hock Flexion

- *Fetal orientation.* The fetus is in a posterior presentation, in a dorso-sacral or dorso-ileal position, with one or both hind limbs flexed at the hock.
- *Correction.* Attention should be paid to prevent excessive pressure and trauma to the uterus by the retained hoof.
- If the hoof is within reach, the foot may be cupped in the hand and pulled medially to extend the limb while repelling the fetus.
- If the hoof is not within reach, the cannon bone should be grasped and the point of the hock repulsed dorsally and inward while traction is placed on the fetlock to pull it closer to the pelvic canal. The foot should be cupped once within reach to prevent it from damaging the uterine wall. The foot is subsequently pulled medially and caudally to correct the malposture.
- A loop of soft rope or a nylon strap may be placed near the fetlock or around the pastern so that one hand may repulse the point of the hock while the other hand provides gentle firm traction on the loop to extend the limb.

Hip Flexion

- *Fetal orientation.* The fetus is in a posterior presentation, in a dorso-sacral position, with one or both hind legs flexed at the hip. Hip flexion is a difficult dystocia to correct as it may not be easily possible to grasp the lower part of the hind leg. Bilateral hip flexion is commonly referred to as a "true breech" presentation.
- *Correction.* A cesarean surgery should be considered with bilateral hip flexion. If a vaginal delivery is attempted, the initial goal is to manipulate each limb into hock flexion and subsequently extend the leg as previously described.

Transverse Presentation

- *Fetal orientation.* The back (dorso-transverse) or abdomen (ventro-transverse) of the fetus is presented to the pelvic canal.
- *Correction.* Dorso-transverse presentations are very difficult to correct as there are no fetal structures within reach. Consequently, it may be more prudent to immediately refer the case or perform a cesarean section if the fetus is alive.

- In a ventro-transverse presentation the fetus may present with all four limbs coming into the pelvic canal. In some of these cases it is easier and quicker to deliver the fetus posteriorly to avoid having to correct the head and neck. This malposture should be differentiated from a twin pregnancy with multiple legs from two fetuses presented within the pelvic canal. Trace the limbs back to the foal's body to identify if one or two fetuses are present.

Further Reading

Frazer GS, Perkins NR, Embertson RM. 1999. Normal parturition and evaluation of the mare in dystocia. *Eq Vet Educ* 11: 41–6.

McCue PM, Ferris RA. 2012. Parturition, dystocia and foal survival – a retrospective study of 1,047 births. *Eq Vet Educ* 44(suppl. 41): 22–5.

Norton JL, Dallap BL, Johnston JK, Palmer JE, Sertich PL, Boston R, Wilkins PA. 2007. Retrospective stud of dystocia in mares at a referral hospital. *Eq Vet Educ* 39: 37–41.

99

Fetotomy

John J. Dascanio

School of Veterinary Medicine, Texas Tech University, USA

Introduction

Fetotomy involves the dissection of the fetus inside the mare's reproductive tract. The mare should be placed in a large stall with good drainage and footing as the mare will often become recumbent during the procedure. The ideal fetotomy in the mare should only require one or two cuts, such as to remove a head or single limb in order to deliver a fetus. If a whole body fetotomy is required (5–6 cuts), the mare's reproductive tract may become damaged during the procedure, resulting in a decrease in future fertility.

The mare's reproductive tract mucosa may become irritated, edematous, and/or ulcerated from repetitive movements and continuous exposure to the fetotomy instruments and veterinarian's arm. Make sure that each movement is purposeful and efficient and utilize a sufficient amount of lubricant. An epidural may be administered to provide analgesia, but may not eliminate abdominal contractions. A fetotomy should only be performed on a dead fetus. If the fetus is alive, other methods of delivery such as cesarean section should be considered.

Equipment and Supplies

Tail wrap, non-irritant soap, roll cotton, stainless steel bucket, disposable liner for bucket, paper towels, examination gloves, sterile obstetrical sleeves, fetotomy instruments (Figure 99.1), fetotome with wire threader, wire cutters, lubricant, sterile stomach tube, pump, obstetrical chains, obstetrical handles.

Fetotomy Instruments

Fetotome – used to protect the mare's reproductive tract from the obstetrical wire and to guide the wire for cutting the fetus. The fetotome, made of high strength stainless steel, has two channels so the wire does not cross, preventing the wire from breaking during cutting (Figures 99.2 and 99.3).

Fetotome wire threader – used to thread the obstetrical wire through the fetotome. The threader is introduced into the handle end of the fetotome and passed through to exit at the fetotome head.

Obstetrical wire – attached to the threader and pulled back through the fetotome (Figures 99.2 and 99.3). It is easier to pull the wire through the fetotome than to try to push it through. The opposite end of the threader often has a brush used to clean the fetotome channels out after completion of the fetotomy.

Curved wire introducer – used to pass obstetrical wire around limbs or retained heads. The wire is attached to the introducer and the introducer is passed around the extremity, pulling the wire along (Figure 99.4).

Wire handles – used to hold the obstetrical wire while making a cut (Figure 99.5). The handles protect the veteri-

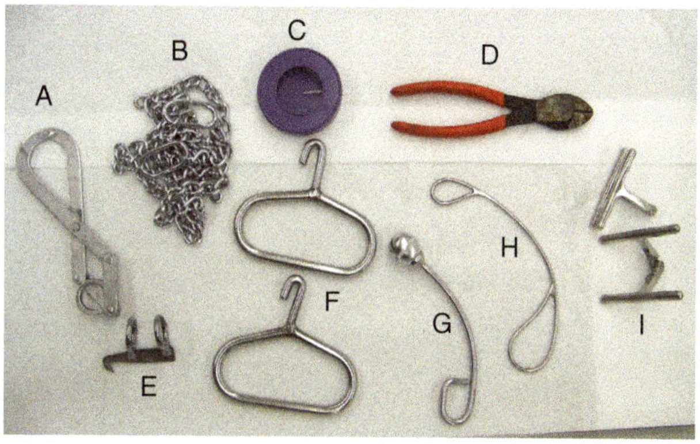

Figure 99.1 Fetotomy equipment: A, Krey hook; B, dystocia chains; C, obstetrical fetotomy wire; D, wire cutters; E, Guenther embryotomy knife; F, Moore chain handles; G, Hauptner wire introducer; H, wire introducer; I, Lyss wire handles.

Equine Reproductive Procedures, Second Edition. Edited by John Dascanio and Patrick McCue.

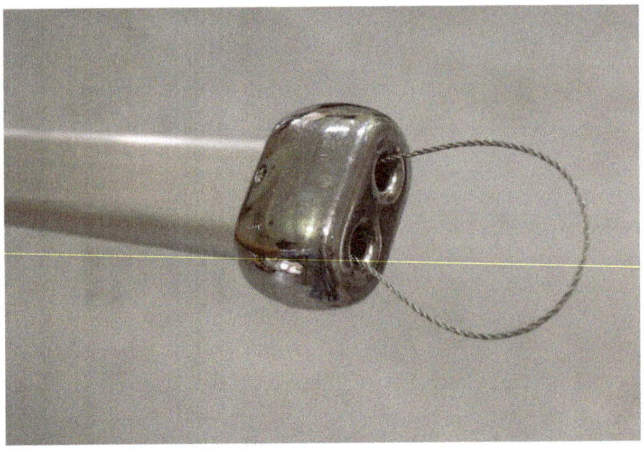

Figure 99.2 Head of a fetotome demonstrating a loop of fetotomy wire passed through both channels of the fetotome.

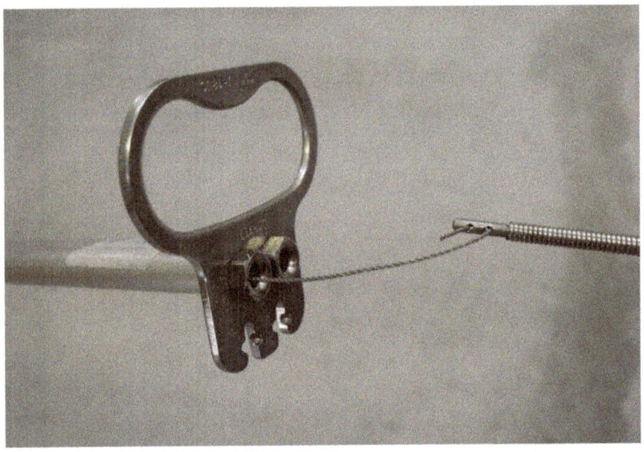

Figure 99.3 Handle end of the fetotome with a wire threader pulling the fetotomy wire through one channel of the fetotome. The slots on the bottom of the handle are for chains to be placed to keep the fetotome secured to the fetus.

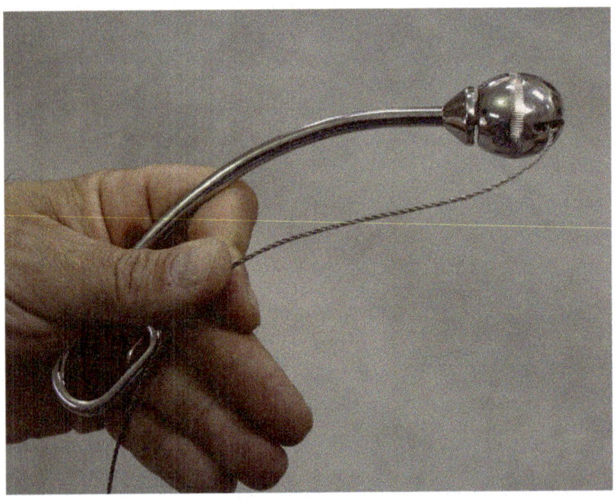

Figure 99.4 Curved wire introducer. This model has a weighted head that screws onto the shaft allowing placement of the wire end into the weighted head for protection of the uterus from the sharp end of the wire.

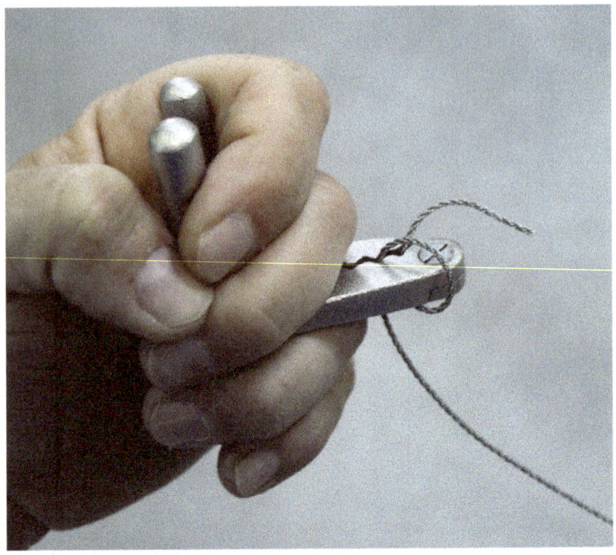

Figure 99.5 Wire handles in a closed position holding a fetotomy wire in between the hinged handles. The wire is wrapped around the handles in an open position and closed to grip the wire.

narian's hands from the wire and provide a means to hold onto the wire.

Embryotomy knife (fetotomy knife) – used to cut the skin or muscle of the fetus (Figure 99.6). This may be done to help seat the obstetrical wire for a cut, to eviscerate a dead fetus to help with delivery, or to cut skin or other tissue to remove gas in an emphysematous fetus. The knife may be used to pierce the thin skull of a hydrocephalic foal to help deflate the head for delivery.

Krey hook – used to hold onto the fetal spinal column after removal of the head/neck or to grasp a disarticulated bone. The Krey hook should be attached to bone as it will tear loose from muscle. An obstetrical chain and handle is attached to the Krey hook so that tension may be placed on the instrument to close the two opposing hooks into the bone (Figure 99.7).

Technique

- Remove feces from the rectum.
- Place a tail wrap and tie the tail out of the way (see Chapter 4).
- Clean and dry the perineum of the mare (see Chapter 3).
- Organize the equipment needed for the fetotomy (see Figure 99.1).
- Place a sterile obstetrical sleeve on the arm and perform a manual examination to determine the location of any extremities to remove.
- Infuse obstetrical lubricant into the uterus, if needed.
- Place an obstetrical chain on an extended limb to anchor the fetotome head.

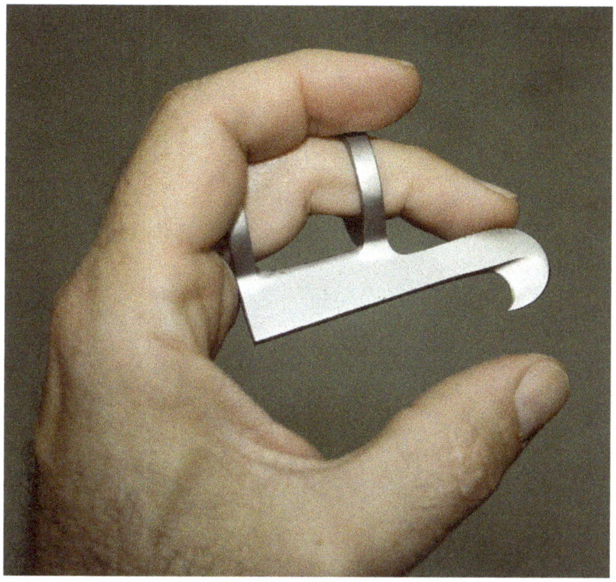

Figure 99.6 Embryotomy knife held in an open position. The thumb would be placed over the sharp point of the knife during placement. The knife cuts when pulled (blade on concave aspect of tip).

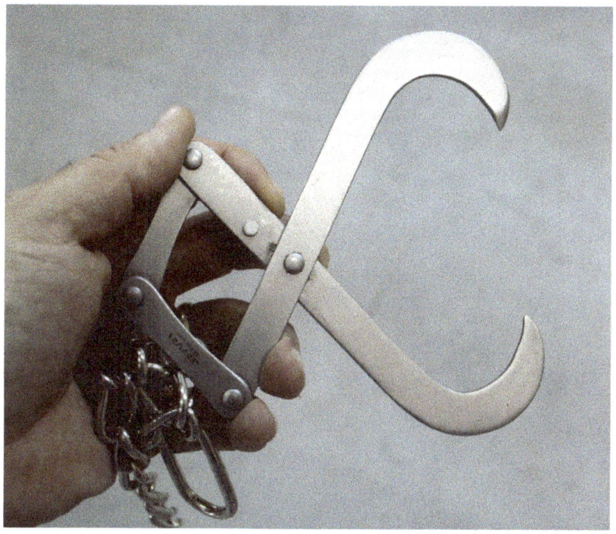

Figure 99.7 Krey hook in an open position with an obstetrical chain attached. The Krey hook would be in this position to grip a bone on the fetus and in a closed position for introduction into the reproductive tract.

- Either place a loop of obstetrical wire over the extremity or use a wire introducer to place the wire over a limb.
- Thread the wire through the fetotome channels and wrap the wire around the wire saw handles.
- Place the head of the fetotome in the proper location for the cut. The angle of the cut should be made to decrease any sharp protuberances on remaining bony structures.
- Tighten the obstetrical chain on the previously placed extremity and hook it to the outer end of the fetotome to hold the fetotome in location. This may be the limb to remove or it may be another extremity. Securing the chain to the fetus and the fetotome will prevent the head of the fetotome from moving caudally and helps to stabilize the location for the cut.
- One hand is placed over the end of the fetotome (the end with the loop around the extremity) and the other hand on the outer end handle of the fetotome to hold it in place. By pulling outward on the fetotome handle, the chain attached to the fetus comes under tension thus helping to stabilize the fetotome head for the cut.
- Ensure that the wire is not twisted as it comes out of the fetotome head prior to making a cut. If it is twisted, then rotate the fetotome along its long axis to untwist. A twist in the wire will cause the wire to break.
- With the veterinarian's hands on the fetotome, a second operator uses long strokes to make the cut through the extremity. Long strokes allow for the distribution of heat along the wire and make for a more efficient cut. Initially, short strokes may be used to get the cut started, but should then be integrated into longer strokes. The operator making the cut should brace their body position in case the wire breaks so that they do not fall and injury themselves.
- The detached fetal piece should be removed from the mare prior to delivery of the fetus. This will prevent the fetal piece from getting stuck in the pelvic canal thus inhibiting delivery of the remaining fetus and potentially contributing to trauma to the mare's reproductive tract.
- The site of the fetotomy cut should be examined for any sharp protuberances on the remaining fetus. If sharp bone fragments are present, they should be covered by the veterinarian's hand during delivery of the fetus or, if needed, removed with a fetotomy knife.
- The mare's reproductive tract should be examined manually for any trauma from the dystocia or fetotomy procedure.

Specific Fetotomy Cuts

- *Removal of the head and neck.* The head of the fetotome is placed between the shoulder blades on the dorsal midline so that the neck is taken off at the base and so that the spinal column has a tapered edge on its dorsal aspect (obtuse cut) (Figure 99.8).
- *Removal of the lower limbs.* With a folded front or rear limb, the fetotomy cut may be made through the joint (carpus (Figure 99.9) or tarsus (Figure 99.10)). If the cut was made above the joint, the tapered leg would not retain chains placed on it to remove the fetus.

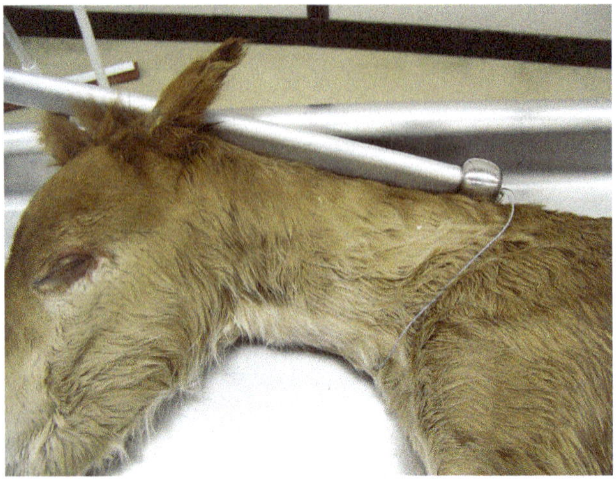

Figure 99.8 Placement of the fetotome for removal of the head and neck. The head of the fetotome should be between the shoulder blades so that an obtuse angle cut of the vertebral column will be made.

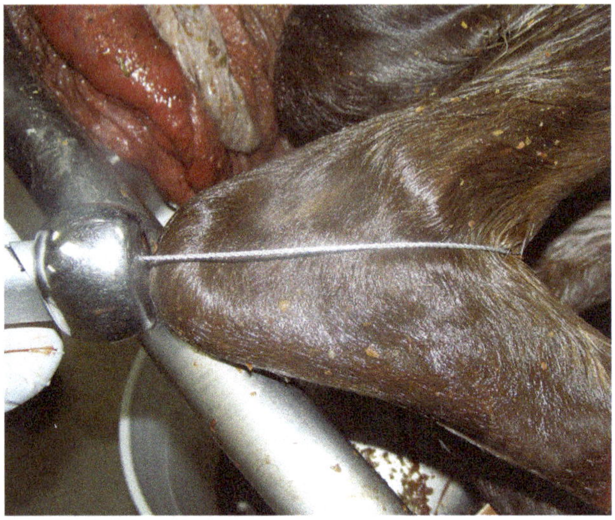

Figure 99.10 Fetotomy cut through the mid-tarsal region.

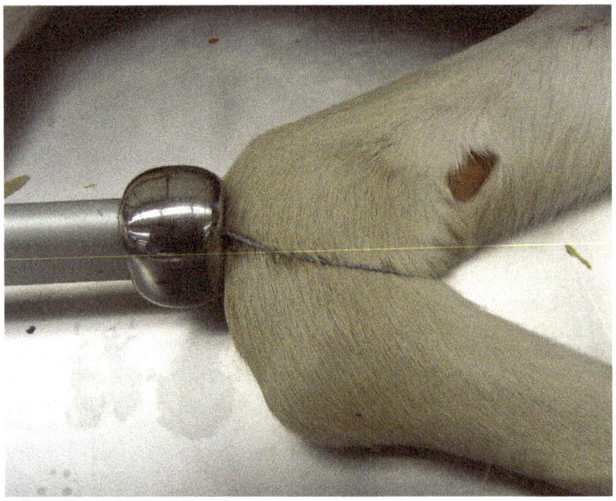

Figure 99.9 Fetotomy cut through the mid-carpal region.

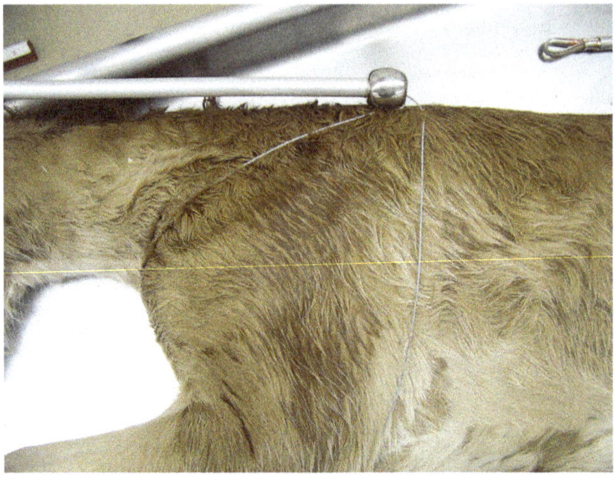

Figure 99.11 Placement of the fetotome for removal of the front limb. The head of the fetotome should be placed at the dorso-caudal aspect of the scapula.

- *Removal of the front limb.* The head of the fetotome is placed at the dorso-caudal edge of the scapula (Figure 99.11). It is not easy to completely remove the entire scapula, so care should be taken to examine the fetus for sharp fragments of any remaining scapula prior to delivery.
- *Removal of the entire hind limb.* The head of the fetotome is placed on the opposite side of the tail head from the limb to be removed (Figure 99.12). This will help to keep the fetotome at an angle so that the cut will remove the head of the femur and acetabulum. Occasionally, even with this placement, the cut goes through the femur, resulting in a sharp protuberance that must be protected from lacerating the reproductive tract on removal of the remaining fetus. The wire may be place over the tuber coxae to help keep the wire forward to aid in removing more of the pelvis.
- *Removal of the pelvis and back legs.* Alternatively, the entire pelvis may be removed by placing the wire cranially to both tuber coxae with the head of the fetotome along the spine cranial to the sacrum. This would make a transverse cut through the fetal abdomen and lumbar spinal column. The remaining pelvis and hind legs may

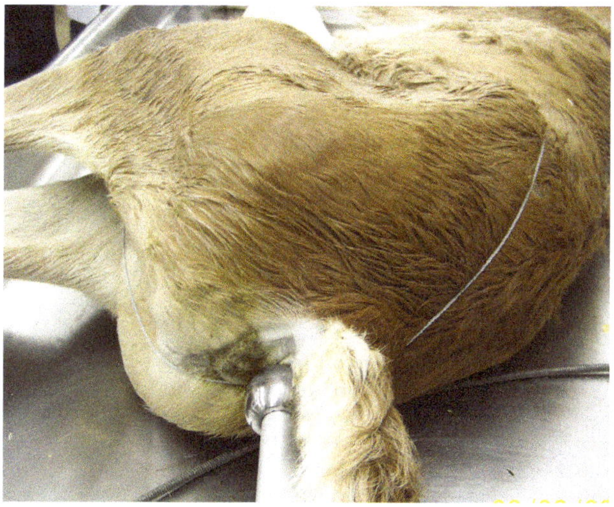

Figure 99.12 Placement of the fetotome for removal of a hind limb. The head of the fetotome is on the opposite side of the tail head from the limb to be removed. The wire may be placed over the tuber coxae if the width of the hip is preventing delivery.

then be cut in half longitudinally, separating the pelvis into two pieces, each with an attached hind leg if necessary.

Additional Comments

- Aftercare should include examination of the reproductive tract for tears, abrasions, or retained fetal pieces.
- Potential sequelae after prolonged dystocia and fetotomy may include reproductive tract trauma, retained placenta, metritis, and/or laminitis. The incidence of metritis and laminitis may be abated with prophylactic use of antibiotics, non-steroidal anti-inflammatory drugs, ecbolic drugs such as oxytocin, and uterine lavage. A tetanus booster should also be considered.
- With a skilled clinician performing the fetotomy and a minimum number of cuts and manipulations, fertility after fetotomy should not decrease significantly.

Further Reading

Carluccio A, Contri A, Tosi U, De Amicis I, De Fanti C. 2007. Survival rate and short-term fertility rate associated with the use of fetotomy for resolution of dystocia in mares: 72 cases (1991–2005). *J Am Vet Med Assoc* 230: 1502–5.

Frazer GS. 2001. Fetotomy technique in the mare. *Eq Vet Educ* 13: 151–9.

100

Epidural

John J. Dascanio

School of Veterinary Medicine, Texas Tech University, USA

Introduction

An epidural is performed to provide anesthesia and/or analgesia to the anus/rectum, perineum, vulva, and vagina without loss of motor function to the rear limbs. Epidurals are performed to aid with surgery of the perineum, to assist with dystocia correction, or to provide pain relief. An epidural may not totally ablate the ability of a mare to strain during delivery, but should decrease her effort sufficiently to allow the mutation of a fetus in the event of a dystocia.

Although a local anesthetic such as lidocaine may be used alone, it is common to combine lidocaine with xylazine to achieve a quick onset (lidocaine: 5 minutes) and longer duration (xylazine: 4–6 hours) of effect. A common dosage for the lidocaine and xylazine combination is 0.22 mg/kg lidocaine plus 0.17 mg/kg xylazine. This equates to approximately 5 ml of 2% lidocaine and 0.75 ml of xylazine (100 mg/ml) for a 450 kg mare.

Equipment and Supplies

Clippers, surgical scrub on gauze sponges, alcohol swabs, exam gloves, sedation, lidocaine or carbocaine, xylazine, 18 or 20 gauge 7.5 cm (3 inch) spinal needle or 20 gauge 4 cm (1.5 inch) needle, assorted needles, assorted syringes, sterile surgical gloves, twitch (optional).

Technique

- Place the mare into stocks or on a level surface with good footing. Care should be exercised to avoid being kicked during preparation and needle placement. Sedation may be administered or a twitch placed to facilitate these procedures.
- While raising and lowering the tail with one hand, the other hand is used to palpate the most cranial coccygeal space that borders a moveable and non-moveable vertebra. This is most often the first intercoccygeal space (Figure 100.1).
- Clip the hair from an 8 × 8 cm (3 x 3 inch) area centered over that space.
- Perform a surgical scrub of the clipped area.
- Using a small gauge needle, such as a 25 gauge needle, administer 1–2 ml of a local anesthetic into the skin and subcutaneous tissues over the intercoccygeal space. This will facilitate placement of a large diameter needle into the epidural space.
- Using either a 7.5 cm (3 inch), 18 or 20 gauge spinal needle (for a large body frame or higher body condition score) or a 4 cm (1.5 inch), 20 gauge needle (for a small body frame or lower body condition score), place the needle with the bevel pointed cranial at a 45-degree angle with the hub of

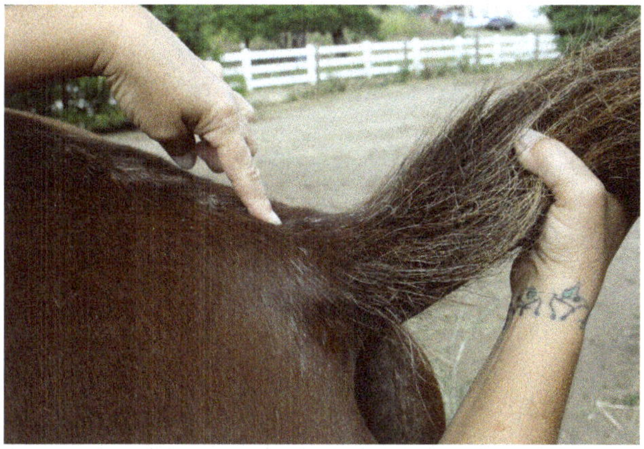

Figure 100.1 Location for the placement of an epidural. While raising and lowering the tail with one hand, the other hand is used to palpate the most cranial coccygeal space that borders a moveable and non-moveable vertebra.

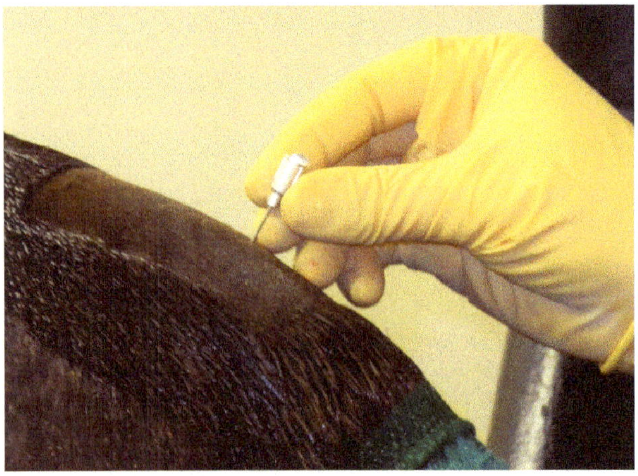

Figure 100.2 Hanging drop technique – notice the drop in the hub of the needle.

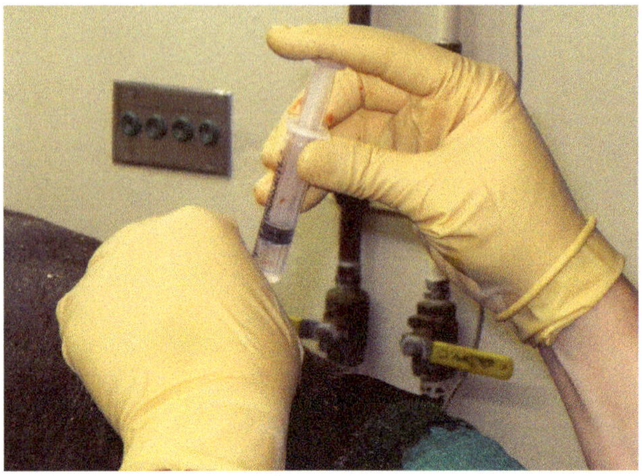

Figure 100.3 Administration of the epidural.

the needle more caudal and the needle tip more cranial through the skin and into the subcutaneous tissue on the midline directly over the moveable coccygeal space.

- If a spinal needle is used, then remove the stylet after placement through the skin and into the subcutaneous tissue.
- Once into the subcutaneous tissue, stop advancement of the needle and place a drop of anesthetic/analgesic into the hub of the needle – this is called the "hanging drop technique." The drop should be visible in the hub of the needle or slightly protruding from the hub (Figure 100.2).
- Continue to advance the needle ventrally making sure that the needle stays on a vertical plane and does not tilt left or right from midline. Be careful to not displace the drop within the hub.
- When the needle enters the epidural space a feeling of the needle entering less tissue resistance is encountered, or a feeling of penetration of the ligament between two vertebrae is felt, and the drop of liquid within the needle hub is pulled down the needle into the epidural space. Stop advancement of the needle when this occurs.
- Attach the syringe with the anesthetic/analgesic and inject slowly (Figure 100.3). There should be no significant resistance to injection if the tip of the needle is in the epidural space. If significant resistance is detected, such as is encountered with an intramuscular injection, the needle may need to be repositioned. Be careful to hold the needle so that it does not advance further with depression of the syringe plunger.
- Once the injection is complete, remove the needle and apply a disinfectant to the needle entry site on the skin.

Interpretation

- Within 5 minutes the perineum should become desensitized and the ability of the tail to move should decrease.
- Lifting the tail up and down should meet with very little resistance from the horse. Digital pressure on the anus should not elicit a response.
- Using a blunt-tipped instrument, such as a pair of hemostats, and exercising caution so as to not be kicked, the skin may be gently tested to delineate the area of skin anesthesia achieved by the epidural.
- Generally avoid greater than 10 ml of total fluid volume for injection as this may cause the drug to travel cranially within the epidural space, affecting innervation to the hind limbs.
- If removing a horse from stocks after an epidural, exercise caution as the horse may experience ataxia that was not previously observed.
- Avoid multiple epidurals as ataxia may occur as well as an increased risk of infection. Use less volume with subsequent epidurals in the same procedure.
- Turn the horse out into a small flat area with good footing until the effects of the epidural have worn off.
- Do not transport the horse until the epidural has worn off.

Further Reading

Ball MA, Cable CS, Kirker EJ. 1998. How to place an epidural catheter and indications for its use. *Proc Annu Conv Am Assoc Eq Pract* 44: 182–5.

Natalini CC, Driessen B. 2007. Epidural and spinal anesthesia and analgesia in the equine. *Clin Tech Eq Pract* 6: 145–53.

101

Induction of Lactation to Create a Nurse Mare

Pouya Dini[1] *and Peter F. Daels*[2]

[1] *School of Veterinary Medicine, University of California-Davis, USA*
[2] *Faculty of Veterinary Medicine, University of Gent, Belgium*

Introduction

The induction of lactation has been successfully done in non-pregnant mares, sheep, goat, and cattle. The primary reason for the induction of lactation in a mare is to provide a nurse mare to an orphan foal for nutrition, equine companionship, and protection in a herd. The ideal nurse mare for an induced lactation would be a calm, halter-broke, gentle, non-pregnant mare, that has given birth at least once previously, successfully raised a foal, and is preferably cycling and not in seasonal anestrus or ovariectomized.

Milk production is induced by stimulation of pituitary secretion of prolactin. Prolactin secretion is under tonic inhibition by the neurotransmitter dopamine. Blocking the inhibitory action of dopamine by administration of a dopamine antagonist results in an increase in prolactin secretion. Estradiol (at physiological concentrations) has a priming effect and administration of estradiol is advantageous for the successful induction of lactation. Ovariectomized or anestrous mares do not produce milk when treated only with a dopamine antagonist. Pre-treatment or simultaneous supplementation of estradiol during dopamine antagonist treatment significantly increases prolactin secretion, which stimulates lactation.

Standard treatment for induction of lactation in mares is to administer a luteolytic dose of prostaglandin $F_{2\alpha}$ on the first day, which may bring the mare into estrus and thus increase endogenous estradiol production. At the same time, daily dopamine antagonist treatment is started (optionally combined with estradiol). On average, about 5–7 days of treatment are required to generate enough milk production for the adoption. After the adoption, dopamine antagonist treatment is continued for up to 1 week, which in combination with the frequent suckling by the foal will further increase milk production.

The strongest stimulus for lactation is the frequent nursing by the foal and this will stimulate adequate lactation until weaning of the foal. Prolonged dopamine antagonist administration after adoption does not appear to be beneficial and has no effect on the quantity of milk. It should be noted that mares with induced lactation will not produce any significant amount of IgG antibodies (colostrum) in their milk.

Equipment and Supplies

Dopamine D2 antagonist available as domperidone (Equidone® Gel, Motilium®) or sulpiride (Dogmatil®, Dolmatil®, and others), estradiol-17ß or estradiol benzoate, prostaglandin $F_{2\alpha}$, syringes and needles, wipes for cleaning the teat, container to collect and measure the volume of milk, equine hand milking pump (Ultimate Ez Milker™).

Technique

- Administer estradiol benzoate (50 mg) intramuscularly once on the first day of the treatment protocol or estradiol-17β (3–5 mg) intramuscularly once daily for 5–7 days during the dopamine antagonist treatment period. In countries where estradiol administration is prohibited for use in horses (i.e., Europe), dopamine antagonist treatment without estradiol supplementation appears equally effective if the mare is cycling or in transition with significant ovarian activity (i.e., uterine edema is present).
- Administer a luteolytic dose of prostaglandin $F_{2\alpha}$ (mostly done when estradiol treatment is not an option). This may induce estrus in cyclic mares and further increase endogenous estradiol production.

Equine Reproductive Procedures, Second Edition. Edited by John Dascanio and Patrick McCue.

- Initiate dopamine antagonist therapy:
  - Domperidone (1.1 mg/kg PO, twice daily) or
  - Sulpiride (0.5–0.7 mg/kg IM, twice daily) or
  - Sulpiride oral (1.5–2 mg/kg PO, twice daily).
- After 4–5 days of dopamine antagonist treatment, when an increase in the size of the mammary gland is observed, start milking 5–6 times per day.
  - Hand milking can be facilitated by administering 1–5 IU oxytocin 2–5 minutes before milking (optional). Gentle and careful milking is advised to avoid adverse reaction to the touching of the mammary gland by the handler and/or foal.
  - A hand-held manual milking device for mares (Ultimate Ez Milker™, Lexington, KY, USA) is recommended as it is an efficient and easy to handle device (Figure 101.1). This device significantly reduces discomfort in the mare and stress in both mare and handler, assures that the udder is sufficiently emptied and also shortens the milking time (see Chapter 106).
  - Alternatively, a milking machine (goat-type milking machine) can also be used. The machine should be set at 120 aspirations per minute, a vacuum of 22–37 cmHg, and an alternation of suction: relaxation ratio of 50:50.
  - Care needs to be taken to verify that both quarters of each side are effectively milked. If milk starts to accumulate for longer periods (>3–5 hours) this may result in an irreversible drying-up reaction (pressure atrophy) that cannot be overcome by treatment.
- Introduce the foal after 3–5 days of milking, when milk production has increased to >3 liters per day.
- Continue dopamine antagonist treatment (not estradiol supplementation) for up to 1 week after adoption. In general, a total of 1–2 weeks of dopamine antagonist treatment is needed. Treatment for longer than 2 weeks is ineffective as the stimulatory effect of dopamine antagonist treatment on prolactin secretion seems to gradually decrease.
- During the first days after adoption, when the milk production is still increasing as a result of the frequent nursing of the foal, the foal can be supplemented with milk replacer. The supplementation is given at intervals of >3 hours to assure that the foal will continue to nurse frequently from the mare and thereby stimulate milk production. In general, foals either do not take the bottle any more immediately after adoption or gradually show less interest in the days following adoption.

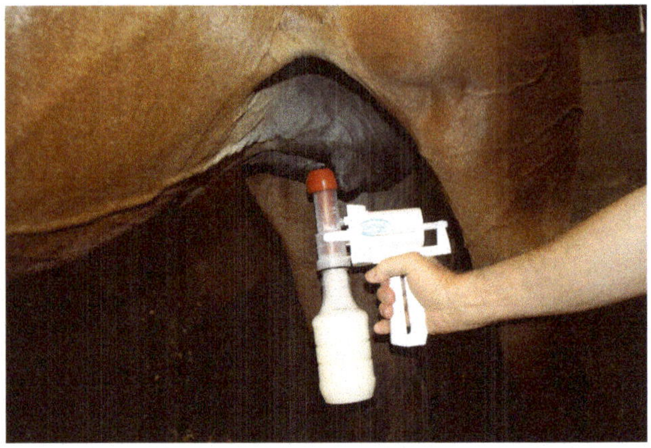

Figure 101.1 A hand-held manual milking device for mares (Ultimate Ez Milker™, Lexington, KY, USA).

Additional Comments

The introduction of a foal to a nurse mare should be done under strict supervision. Maternal behavior is induced using a high dose of prostaglandin $F_{2\alpha}$ and results in the majority of cases in a smooth, peaceful, and rapid adoption of the foal (<15 minutes).

Further Reading

Chavatte-Palmer P, Arnaud G, Duvaux-Ponter C, *et al.* 2002. Quantitative and qualitative assessment of milk production after pharmaceutical induction of lactation in the mare. *J Vet Intern Med* 16: 472–7.

Daels P. 2018. Induction of lactation. *In: Proceedings of British Equine Veterinary Association BEVA Congress* 66.

Kelley KK, Thompson DL, Jr, Storer WA, Mitcham PB, Gilley RM, Burns PJ. 2006. Estradiol interactions with dopamine antagonists in mares: prolactin secretion and reproductive traits. *J Eq Vet Sci* 26: 517–28.

102

Screening to Prevent Neonatal Isoerythrolysis

Patrick M. McCue

Equine Reproduction Laboratory, Colorado State University, USA

Introduction

Neonatal isoerythrolysis (NI) or jaundice foal syndrome is an uncommon but potentially life-threatening alloimmune disease of newborn foals that is characterized by hemolytic anemia. It has been estimated to occur in 1–2% of equine births. The condition occurs when a foal ingests colostrum containing antibodies directed against antigens on the surface of its red blood cells (RBCs). The most common antigens associated with NI in the horse are Aa and Qa, which account for approximately 90% of clinical cases. Other blood group antigens that are occasionally associated with NI include Ab, Pa, Dc, and Ua.

The possibility that a foal may develop NI early in the neonatal period can be evaluated by screening blood of the late-term pregnant mare for antibodies against equine RBC antigens. It is suggested that the screening take place within the last 2–4 weeks prior to her due date.

A newborn foal will be at significant medical risk if the mare has antibodies in her blood directed against antigens present on the RBCs of the foal. The foal will not be at risk if the mare is either negative for anti-RBC antibodies or if the mare has antibodies directed against RBC antigens that the foal does not possess.

Unfortunately, the blood type of the foal cannot be determined prior to birth. In addition, most equine breeding farms do not have the ability to determine the blood type of the foal immediately after birth or to 'cross-match' colostrum of the mare with blood of the foal immediately after birth (jaundiced foal agglutination or JFA test). As a consequence, screening for the potential for NI to occur involves testing the late-term pregnant mare's blood for anti-RBC antibodies.

Equipment and Supplies

Vacutainer® tube (without anticoagulant), Vacutainer® needle, plastic tube with cap (sterile), mailing box.

Technique

- A blood sample is collected from the mare 2–4 weeks prior to her due date into a Vacutainer® tube (red top tube without anticoagulant).
- The blood is allowed to clot and the serum transferred into a sterile plastic tube, and the tube securely capped.
- The tube is then packed into a shipping container and sent to a diagnostic laboratory for testing.
- The laboratory will evaluate the serum for the presence of anti-RBC antibodies.
  - Contact the diagnostic laboratory in advance of the foaling season to confirm that the test will be performed on a routine basis, determine the cost of the test and sample shipment recommendations, and obtain the proper submission forms.
  - In addition, the laboratory should indicate how test results will be sent (email, fax, phone, etc.) and how to interpret the test results.

Additional Comments

Exposure of the mare during pregnancy or at foaling to RBC antigens other than her own will cause her immune system to develop antibodies against the "foreign" RBCs. Typically only a limited amount of antibodies are produced during the first exposure to a foreign RBC group and consequently the syndrome is rare in maiden mares.

However, if the mare is exposed a second time, a far greater quantity of antibodies may be produced. The

Equine Reproductive Procedures, Second Edition. Edited by John Dascanio and Patrick McCue.

antibodies are concentrated in the colostrum over the last 2–3 weeks of pregnancy. Unfortunately, in most instances the presence of anti-RBC antibodies in a mare goes unnoticed and her foal is allowed to nurse colostrum. Colostral antibodies are absorbed into the blood stream of the foal, where they attack the RBCs of the foal. Clinical signs can range from mild to severe depending on the amount of antibodies ingested and absorbed.

Affected foals usually begin to show clinical signs between 24 and 72 hours of life. Signs may include jaundice, weakness, lethargy, decreased nursing vigor, increased respiratory and heart rate, recumbency, passage of red-colored urine, and possibly death. Icterus of mucous membranes is due to release of bilirubin following the destruction of RBCs.

If a mare has had a foal affected by NI in the past, or if she is found to have antibodies in her blood against other equine blood groups, a critical decision has to be made before the newborn foal is allowed to nurse. If a JFA test can be accurately performed (often in the middle of the night) by trained personnel, the test will determine whether or not an agglutination reaction occurs between colostrum from the mare and RBCs of the foal. If the JFA test is positive at a titer of 1:16 or greater, colostrum should be withheld and an alternative source of antibodies provided to the foal. If the test is negative, the foal may be allowed to nurse from the mare.

If the JFA test is not available, the newborn foal should not be allowed to nurse from her dam and should be provided colostrum or antibodies from another known safe source. The foal can be muzzled to prevent nursing and yet still allowed to remain with the mare (Figure 102.1). The colostrum of the mare should be stripped out every few hours and discarded. After approximately 12–24 hours, the mammary gland of the mare will no longer be producing colostrum and the foal can no longer absorb antibodies across the intestine. The muzzle can then be safely removed and the foal allowed to nurse milk from the dam.

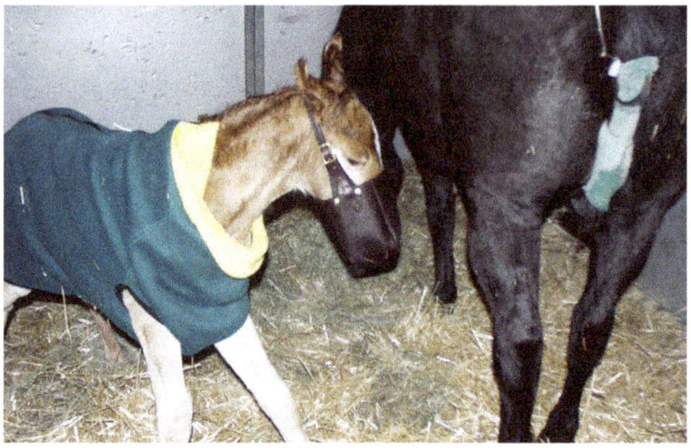

Figure 102.1 Foal wearing a muzzle to prevent nursing. The mare was positive for anti-RBC antibodies prior to foaling.

Evaluation of the mare's mammary fluid with a Brix refractometer every time an NI positive mare is milked out can help determine when the fluid is no longer antibody-laden colostrum (Brix score of ≥15%), but is instead low-antibody-containing milk with a Brix score of <15%. This generally occurs at approximately 12 hours post-foaling if the mare is stripped out every 2 hours.

Further Reading

Bailey E, Conboy S, McCarthy PF. 1987. Neonatal isoerythrolysis of foals: an update on testing. *Proc Annu Conv Am Assoc Eq Pract* 33: 341–53.

Boyle AG, Magdesian KG, Ruby RE. 2005. Neonatal isoerythrolysis in horse foals and a mule foal: 18 cases (1988–2003). *J Am Vet Med Assoc* 227: 1276–83.

McClure JJ. 1997. Strategies for prevention of neonatal isoerythrolysis in horses and mules. *Eq Vet Educ* 9: 118–22.

Part III

Postpartum Mare

103

Evaluation of Colostrum Specific Gravity

Patrick M. McCue

Equine Reproduction Laboratory, Colorado State University, USA

Introduction

Successful passive transfer of antibodies from the mare to her foal depends on many factors, including quality and quantity of colostrum, timing of the ingestion of colostrum, health status of the foal, and absorption of antibodies by the small intestine. Assessment of colostrum quality prior to nursing can be important in predicting passive transfer outcome. The incidence of passive transfer failure is increased in mares with premature leakage of colostrum, if colostrum quality is poor, or if limited mammary development is present at foaling. The evaluation of colostrum quality is also valuable in determining if colostrum should be harvested and stored in a colostrum bank.

Quantitative measurement of IgG levels in colostrum can be obtained by a radial immunodiffusion (RID) assay. Unfortunately, the RID technique cannot be performed easily on a farm and takes approximately 24 hours to obtain results. Colostrum quality can be estimated by the measurement of specific gravity, which is correlated with antibody (IgG) content of the colostrum. The specific gravity or density of equine colostrum can be determined by use of a colostrometer. Colostrum with high IgG levels has a greater density and therefore a higher specific gravity.

Equipment and Supplies

Alcohol swab, collection cup, colostrometer, 20 ml syringe, distilled water, graduated cylinder (300 ml).

Technique

- The teats of the mare should be cleaned to avoid the introduction of bacteria. An alcohol swab works well for this. One or two squirts of milk should be voided from each teat prior to sampling to clear the teat orifice of dried secretions and bacteria.
- Samples should be collected immediately after foaling and prior to the foal nursing.

Colostrometer Design 1

- Approximately 6 ml of colostrum should be obtained equally from both teats. The chamber in this colostrometer holds about 5 ml of colostrum (Figure 103.1).
- The large chamber of the colostrometer is filled with distilled water to approximately two thirds of the total volume.
- The smaller chamber in the floating measuring device is also filled with distilled water to zero the reading. This

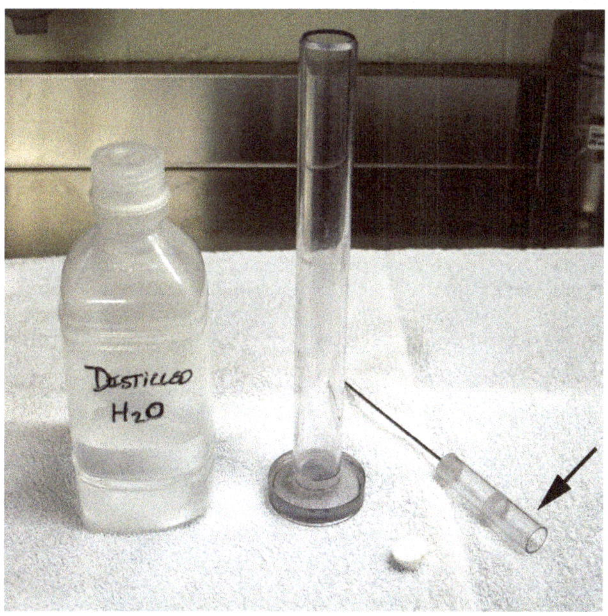

Figure 103.1 Components of the colostrometer design 1. The arrow is pointing at the chamber to fill with colostrum.

Equine Reproductive Procedures, Second Edition. Edited by John Dascanio and Patrick McCue.

device is then placed inside the graduated cylinder and floated to obtain a reading on the graduated metal stick where it meets the water line. Whatever is read is recorded and subsequently subtracted from the colostral measurement. To fill the small chamber properly a slight excess of liquid is poured into the chamber to form an upward meniscus. When the cap is placed on the chamber, the excess liquid will squirt out a slit in the cap, thus ensuring that no air is present.

- The smaller chamber in the floating measuring device is emptied of distilled water and refilled with the colostral sample in the same manner as stated above.
- The floating measuring device is once again placed inside the graduated cylinder (Figure 103.2) and floated to obtain a reading (Figure 103.3).
- The first reading with distilled water is subtracted from the second reading with colostrum to determine the corrected specific gravity.

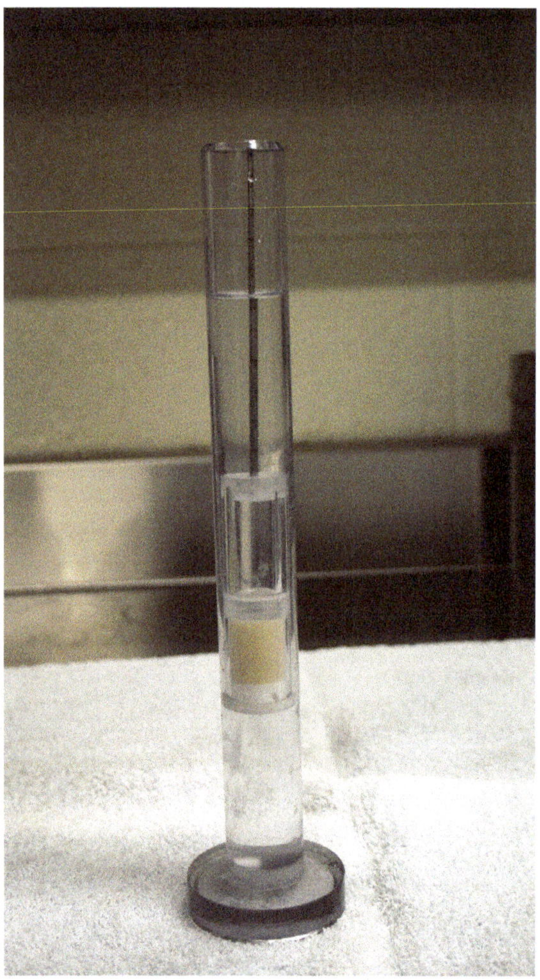

Figure 103.2 Floating the colostrometer design 1 inside a graduated cylinder.

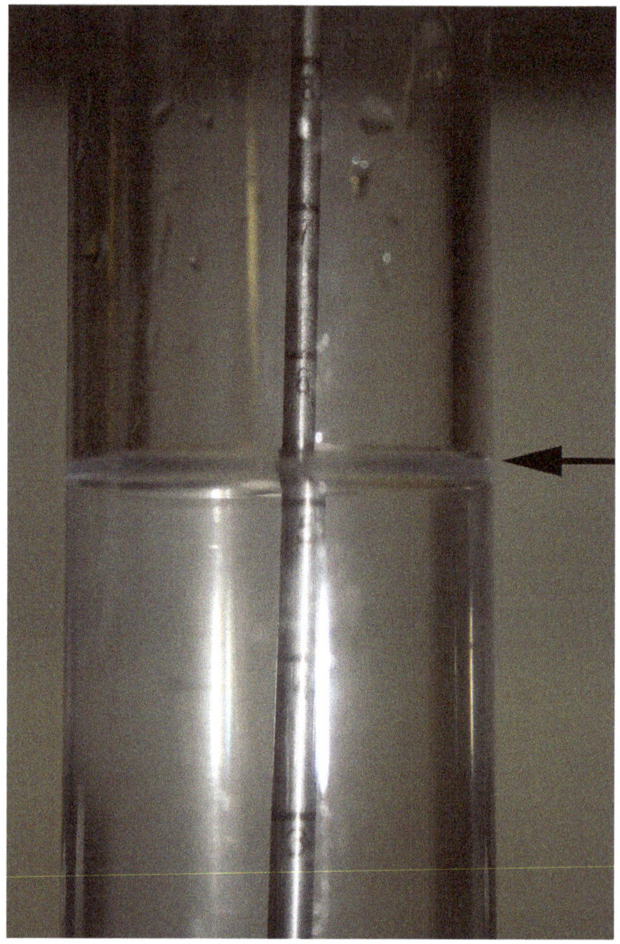

Figure 103.3 Reading the specific gravity of the colostrum using the colostrometer design 1. The specific gravity of this sample is just above 1.05 (arrow).

Colostrometer Design 2

- A 20 ml sample of colostrum is collected equally from the teats.
- A volume of exactly 15 ml, measured in a syringe, is added to the calibrated glass chamber.
- A graduated cylinder (300 ml) is filled with approximately 275 ml of distilled water.
- The colostrum-filled chamber is then gently placed into a graduated cylinder containing distilled water and allowed to float (Figure 103.4).
- The specific gravity of the colostrum is determined by reading the scale on the glass cylinder (Figure 103.5).

Interpretation

- A volume of 15 ml of distilled water added to the colostrometer design 2 chamber should yield a specific gravity

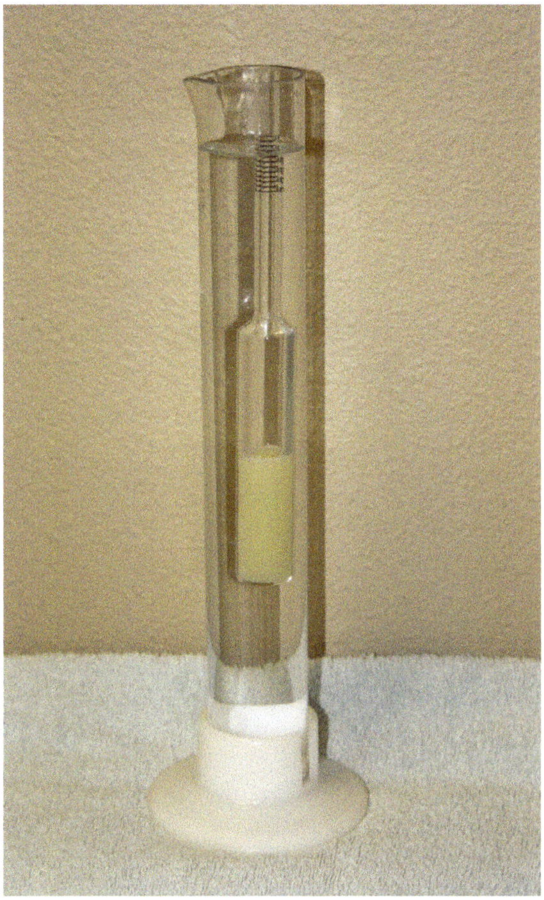

Figure 103.4 Colostrometer design 2 floating in a graduated cylinder full of distilled water.

of 1.00 when placed into a graduated cylinder also containing distilled water.

- Density of equine colostrum (i.e., specific gravity) is positively correlated with antibody content. Determination of the specific gravity of equine colostrum is dependent on accurate measurement of an exact volume (15 ml) of colostrum. Small errors in volume measurement lead to inaccuracy of specific gravity determination.
- Colostrum with a specific gravity of >1.08 is considered good quality, while colostrum with a specific gravity level of <1.06 is considered poor (Table 103.1). Detection

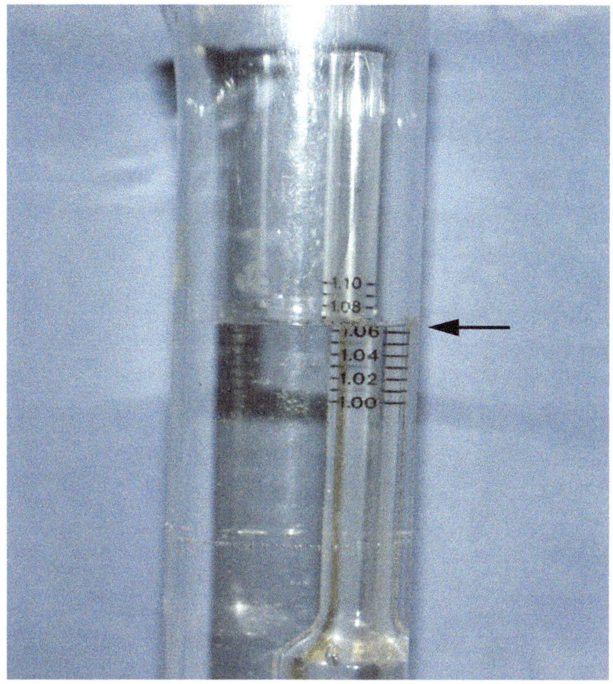

Figure 103.5 Detailed view of the colostrometer design 2 floating in distilled water. The specific gravity of this colostrum sample is 1.07 (arrow).

Table 103.1 Relationship between colostrum quality, IgG concentration measured by radial immunodiffusion assay, and specific gravity.

Colostrum Quality	IgG Concentration (mg/dl)	Specific Gravity
Very good	>8,000	≥1.10
Good	5,000–8,000	1.08–1.09
Fair	2,800–5,000	1.06–1.07
Poor	<2,800	<1.06

of poor quality colostrum in a postpartum mare would indicate a need for antibody supplementation for the newborn foal, either through the administration of frozen-thawed colostrum from a colostrum bank, intravenous plasma, or other sources of equine antibodies.

Further Reading

Dascanio JJ, Ley WB, Warnick LD, Austin SM. 1997. Use of a new colostrometer to predict equine colostral immunoglobulin from specific gravity. *Eq Pract* 19(5): 23–9.

LeBlanc MM, McLaurin BI, Boswell R. 1986. Relationships among serum immunoglobulin concentration in foals, colostral specific gravity, and colostral immunoglobulin concentration. *J Am Vet Med Assoc* 189: 57–60.

Lester GD. 2011. Colostrum: assessment of quality and artificial supplementation. In: McKinnon AO, Squires EL, Vaala WE, Varner DD (eds). Equine Reproduction, 2nd edn. Ames, IA: Wiley Blackwell, pp. 99–110.

104

Evaluation of Colostrum Quality: Brix Refractometry

Patrick M. McCue

Equine Reproduction Laboratory, Colorado State University, USA

Introduction

The evaluation of mare colostrum immediately after foaling and prior to nursing can be helpful in predicting if adequate passive transfer or failure of passive transfer is likely to occur. This is especially important in situations in which colostrum has been lost due to premature leakage from the mammary gland. The evaluation of colostrum is also valuable in determining the quality of colostrum to be harvested and stored in a colostrum bank.

Quantitative measurement of IgG levels in colostrum can be obtained by a radial immunodiffusion (RID) assay at a diagnostic laboratory. Unfortunately, the time period required to obtain RID results (≥24 hours) is too long for practical clinical use. Qualitative assessment of colostrum can be performed using a sugar (Brix) refractometer (Figure 104.1), which measures the concentration of dissolved solids in a solution. Optical density is correlated with antibody (IgG) content of the colostrum. The test is rapid (less than 1 minute), repeatable, and uses a very small volume of colostrum (1–2 drops).

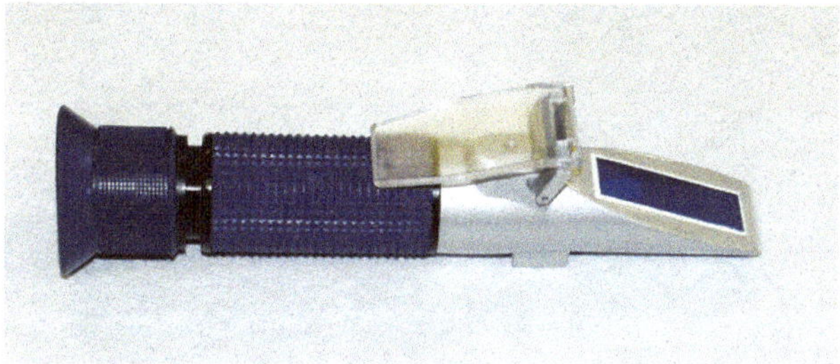

Figure 104.1 Brix refractometer.

Equipment and Supplies

Disposable pipette, disposable tissue wipes, distilled water to rinse, Brix refractometer.

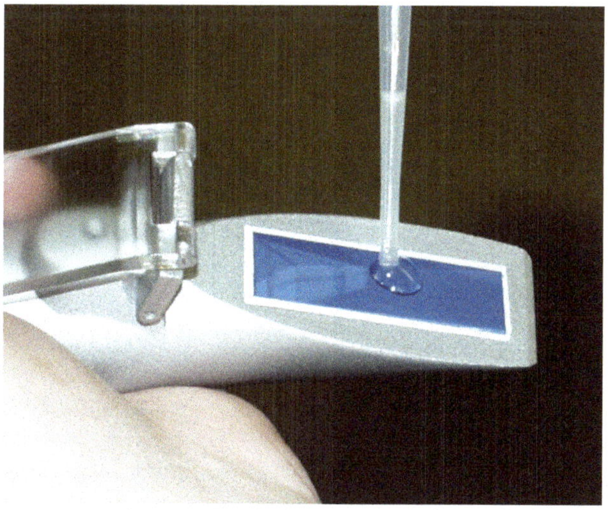

Figure 104.2 Placing a drop of colostrum on the prism of a Brix refractometer.

Technique

- The teats of the mare should be cleaned to avoid the introduction of bacteria. An alchohol swab works well for this. One or two squirts of milk should be voided from each teat prior to sampling to clear the teat orifice of dried secretions and bacteria.
- A small amount (<1 ml) of colostrum is collected equally from each teat from the mare and 1–2 drops are placed on the prism of the refractometer after mixing (Figure 104.2).
- The light plate is subsequently closed, which spreads the colostrum evenly across the prism.

Equine Reproductive Procedures, Second Edition. Edited by John Dascanio and Patrick McCue.

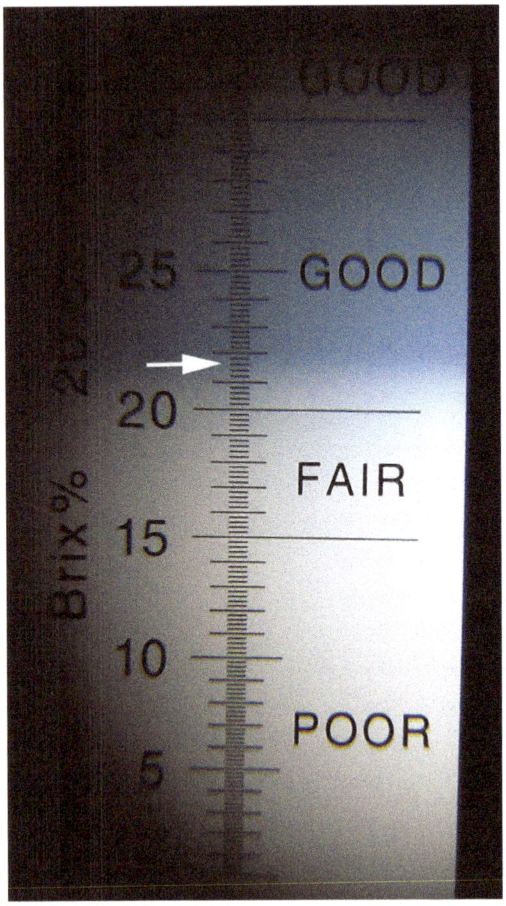

Figure 104.3 View through the refractometer. The Brix score for this colostrum sample is 21.6% (the arrow marks where the darker and lighter areas meet), which is in the lower part of the good category.

- The refractometer is held in the direction of a light source and the deviation or refraction of light is evaluated on a scale as a percentage score (Figure 104.3).

Table 104.1 Relationship between colostrum quality, IgG concentration measured by radial immunodiffusion assay (RID) and Brix refractometry score.

Colostrum Quality	IgG Concentration (mg/dl)	Brix Score (%)
Very good	>8,000	>30
Good	5,000–8,000	20–30
Fair	2,800–5,000	15–20
Poor	<2,800	<15

- After recording the result, the refractometer should be rinsed with distilled water and wiped clean with a soft disposable tissue.

Interpretation and Additional Comments

Distilled water will have a Brix score of zero (0%). Colostrum with a low amount of dissolved solids (i.e., low IgG level) will have a low amount of light scatter and subsequently a low percentage score. Colostrum with a high amount of dissolved solids (i.e., high IgG level) will cause increased light scatter and therefore a higher percentage score.

Brix refractometer evaluation of equine colostrum has been shown to be highly repeatable and highly correlated with IgG levels as measured by RID assay. Brix refractometers designed specifically for the evaluation of equine colostrum are commercially available and contain a scale with graduations (%) and a quality assessment score for clinical interpretation. The relationship between refractometry percentage, IgG content as determined by RID assay, and overall colostrum quality assessment is presented in Table 104.1.

Further Reading

Cash RSG. 1999. Colostral quality determined by refractometry. *Eq Vet Educ* 11: 36–8.

Chavatte P, Clement F, Cash R, Grongnet JF. 1998. Field determination of colostral quality by using a novel, practical method. *Proc Annu Conv Am Assoc Eq Pract* 44: 206–9.

Lester GD. 2011. Colostrum: assessment of quality and artificial supplementation. In: McKinnon AO, Squires EL, Vaala WE, Varner DD (eds). Equine Reproduction, 2nd edn. Ames, IA: Wiley Blackwell, pp. 99–110.

105

Colostrum Banking

Patrick M. McCue

Equine Reproduction Laboratory, Colorado State University, USA

Introduction

Colostrum is the thick, sticky yellow fluid produced by the mammary gland of the mare during the last 1–2 weeks of pregnancy. It is comprised of carbohydrates, fats, proteins, and electrolytes. Colostrum is rich in antibodies or immunoglobulins that are critically important for immune protection of the newborn foal. The process by which foals acquire antibodies from the colostrum of their dam is called passive transfer of immunity. The epitheliochorial-type placenta of the horse prevents *in utero* transfer of antibodies from the mare to the fetus. As a consequence, foals are born without antibody protection. The newborn foal is thus entirely dependent on antibodies from colostrum for protection against infection during the early neonatal period.

Foals need to ingest approximately 2–3 liters of good quality colostrum within the first few hours of life to acquire sufficient antibodies to protect against infectious diseases. If the quality of colostrum produced by a mare is inadequate, the foal can be supplemented with additional frozen-thawed colostrum of good quality within the first 12 (preferably) to 24 hours of life. An owner or farm manager generally does not know in advance which newborn foal will need supplemental colostrum. An on-site supply of frozen colostrum can be critical for the health of a valuable neonate.

Equipment and Supplies

Warm water, non-irritant soap, alcohol swab, collection cup (i.e., plastic measuring cup), cotton gauze or cheesecloth as a filter, plastic storage bottle (labeled), colostrum collection device (optional).

Technique

- The udder of the mare should be washed with warm water and soap to remove debris and bacteria. The teat end should be disinfected with an alcohol swab and the first secretions discarded to flush the teat end of bacteria/debris.
- It is recommended that colostrum be collected from the mammary gland from a donor mare in the first hour after foaling before her foal has nursed.
- Colostrum should be evaluated for quality using a Brix refractometer (see Chapter 104) or colostrometer (see Chapter 103) to determine if it is of adequate quality for banking and subsequent administration.
- A total of 240–475 ml (8–16 oz) may be safely harvested from the mare without adversely affecting the ability of her newborn foal to acquire sufficient colostrum for adequate passive transfer of antibodies.
- Options for collecting colostrum include hand milking (Figure 105.1), using an inverted syringe

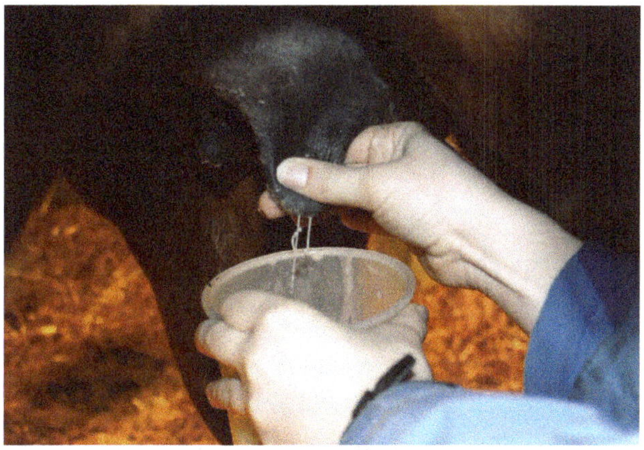

Figure 105.1 Manual collection of colostrum into a plastic measuring cup. Note milk obtained from both teat orifices.

Equine Reproductive Procedures, Second Edition. Edited by John Dascanio and Patrick McCue.

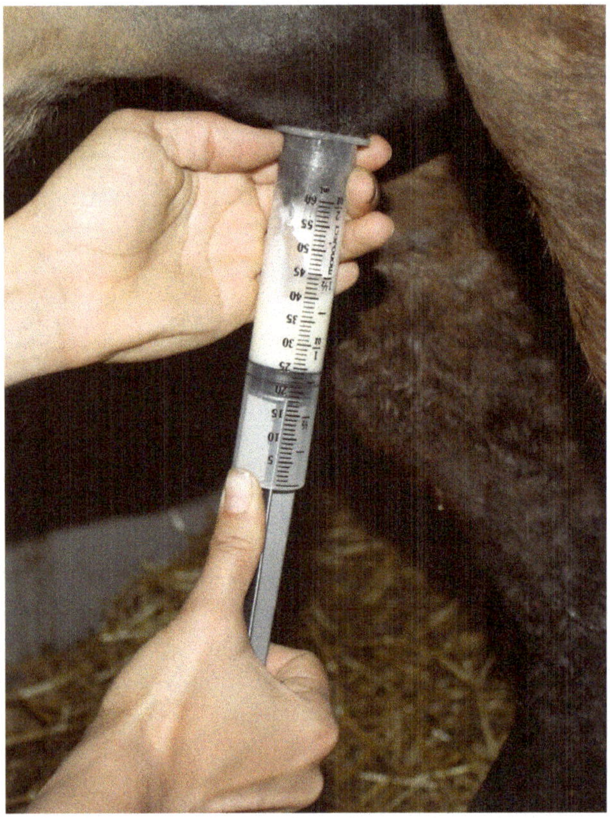

Figure 105.2 Collection of colostrum using an inverted 60 ml syringe.

(Figure 105.2), or using a commercial milking device (see Chapter 106).

- Stripping or milking colostrum by hand directly into a clean glass or plastic measuring cup of 475–950 ml (16–32 oz) capacity will make it easy to evaluate the volume that has been collected (Figure 105.1).
- Harvested colostrum should be passed through a gauze filter or new cheesecloth into a storage container (Figure 105.3) to remove any gross debris.
- Colostrum should be stored in 240–475 ml (8–16 oz) plastic bottles labeled with the donor mare's name, collection date, colostrum quality, and other pertinent information. Glass bottles or plastic freezer bags are not recommended for storage of frozen colostrum because glass bottles may break when the liquid colostrum freezes and plastic bags may tear easily.

Interpretation and Additional Comments

Mares produce colostrum only once during the course of a pregnancy. Antibody-rich colostrum is rapidly depleted as a foal nurses throughout the first day of life, so colostrum

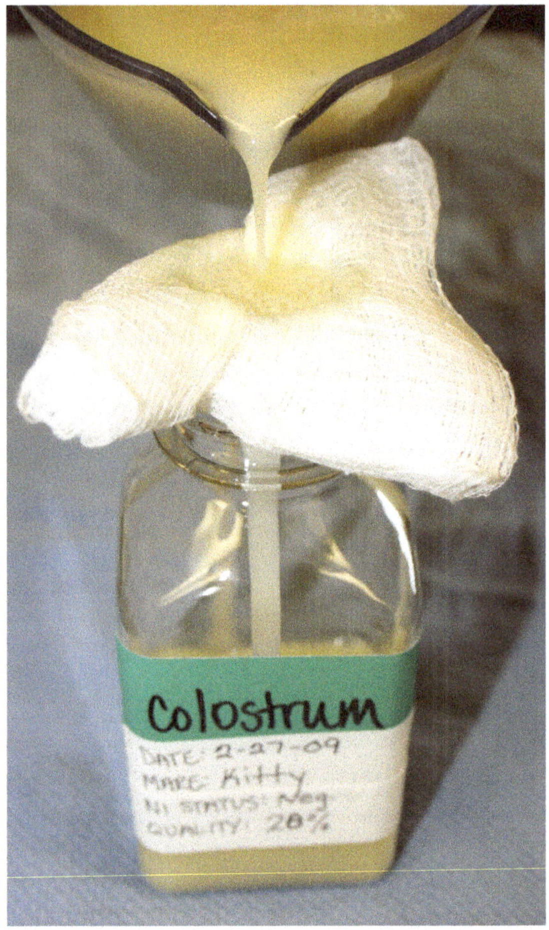

Figure 105.3 Straining colostrum through a cotton gauze filter.

for banking should be harvested soon after birth. Colostrum should be evaluated and determined to be of good quality (Brix score of >20 or a specific gravity of 1.08 or greater) before a decision is made to collect for a colostrum bank (Table 105.1). In addition to the evaluation of antibody level by Brix refractometry or specific gravity, it would be ideal to screen the donor for antibodies against equine red blood cell (RBC) antibodies 2–4 weeks prior to the mare's due date (see Chapter 102). Anti-RBC antibodies in colostrum may induce a clinical case of neonatal isoerythrolysis (jaundice foal syndrome) if administered to a foal with that specific RBC type.

The best colostrum donors are mares that have had one or more foals and are 4–15 years of age as they will have more colostrum potentially available and possibly better immunoglobulin content. Vaccination 4–6 weeks prior to foaling will increase the antibody content of the colostrum and consequently increase the quality of the colostrum to be collected for storage. Colostrum volume and quality are not as good from young maiden mares or old mares. Mares that have dripped milk for several hours prior to foaling

Table 105.1 Comparison of the Brix refractometer score and specific gravity of colostrum.

Colostrum Quality	IgG Concentration (mg/dl)	Brix Score (%)	Specific Gravity
Very good	>8,000	>30	≥1.10
Good	5,000–8,000	20–30	1.08–1.09
Fair	2,800–5,000	15–20	1.06–1.07
Poor	<2,800	<15	<1.06

may not have a large volume of good quality colostrum remaining in their udder and may not make suitable donors for a colostrum bank.

Frozen equine colostrum can be safely stored for 1–2 years in a standard −20°C (−4°F) freezer. Once thawed, any remaining colostrum should not be refrozen. Colostrum should be harvested each breeding season to replenish the colostrum bank with a fresh supply.

Frozen colostrum should be thawed in a water bath at room temperature. Thawing in hot water or in a microwave may destroy the antibodies and render the colostrum useless. It is recommended that colostrum be administered immediately after thawing (see Chapter 188). Foals can be administered 300–400 ml of colostrum at one time via a nasogastric tube, depending on the size of the foal. It is recommended that IgG levels be measured again the following day after colostrum supplementation to determine the final antibody concentration. Once the foal is greater than 24 hours of age, the only way to supplement antibodies is through a plasma transfusion (see Chapter 191).

Further Reading

Massey RE, LeBlanc MM, Klapstein EF. 1991. Colostrum feeding of foals and colostrum banking. *Proc Annu Conv Am Assoc Eq Pract* 37: 1–8.

Nath LC, Anderson GA, Savage CJ, McKinnon AO. 2010. Use of stored equine colostrum for the treatment of foals perceived to be at risk or failure to transfer of passive immunity. *J Am Vet Med Assoc* 235: 1085–90.

Vivrette SL. 2011. Assessment and modification of passive transfer. In: McKinnon AO, Squires EL, Vaala WE, Varner DD (eds). Equine Reproduction, 2nd edn. Ames, IA: Wiley Blackwell, pp. 346–52.

106

Obtaining Milk from the Mare

John J. Dascanio

School of Veterinary Medicine, Texas Tech University, USA

Introduction

The mammary gland of the mare has four quarters completely separated by fibrous connective tissue. A left and right teat each contain two teat orifices, one orifice serves the cranial quarter on that side while the other orifice serves the caudal quarter. When collecting milk from a mare's teat one can usually obtain a stream from both the cranial and caudal quarters simultaneously.

Obtaining milk from the mare is primarily performed for assessment of pre-mammary electrolyte concentrations as a predictor of readiness for birth, to obtain samples for bacterial culture for mastitis, and to obtain milk/colostrum for feeding a foal unable to nurse on its own. Udder secretions may also be obtained to help in the diagnosis of trauma, where the secretion may be bloody, or rarely with tumors, where the secretion could be black in color from a melanoma. Mammary fluid secretions may also be used for culture or cytology. Both hand milking and the use of a milk pump will be described. Milk collection is easiest if the mammary gland is gently massaged for a few minutes prior to performing the collection procedure to stimulate endogenous oxytocin release.

Equipment and Supplies

Alcohol swab, sterile 15 ml tube, 60 ml syringe.

Hand Milking Technique

- Stand bent with your head near the mare's stifle facing toward her hind end. This keeps most of your body well away from the mare's hind legs and allows visualization of the mare's udder.
- Gently place the index finger and thumb on either side of the mare's teat and press together and take apart to see if there is fluid within the teat proper. If no fluid is felt within the teat cistern then no secretions will be obtained.
- Wipe each teat end with an alcohol swab to remove debris and to disinfect the teat end.
- Strip a few milliliters of secretions from each teat to clear the teat orifice of dried secretions and bacteria within the teat canal.
- Occlude the proximal teat near its connection with the main udder with the thumb and index finger and then use the remaining fingers to gently but firmly squeeze the teat against the palm of the hand from proximal to distal to eject milk from the teat orifice.
- Alternatively, the teat may be occluded proximally and, with the fingers held closed, they are pulled gently downward to discharge milk (Figure 106.1). The key is to occlude milk from traveling proximally back into the gland cistern while causing enough distal pressure to open the teat canal to ensure milk flow.
- Collect milk equally from each teat into a sterile disposable container (culture) or a container that has been rinsed with distilled water and dried (milk calcium testing). Tap water may leave residues, which is especially important if measuring milk electrolytes.

Milk Pump Technique

- Remove the plunger from a 60 ml syringe.
- Cut off the closed end of the syringe.
- Push the plunger into the cut-off end so that the plunger is in the syringe in the opposite direction from normal.
- Place the open end of the syringe over the teat and firmly against the udder (Figure 106.2). A seal needs to be established between the udder skin and the end of the syringe.

Equine Reproductive Procedures, Second Edition. Edited by John Dascanio and Patrick McCue.

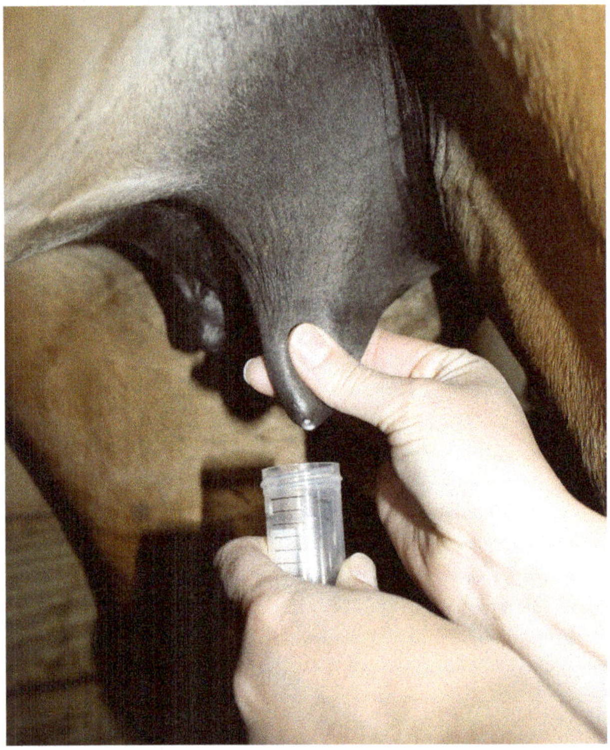

Figure 106.1 Hand milking a mare.

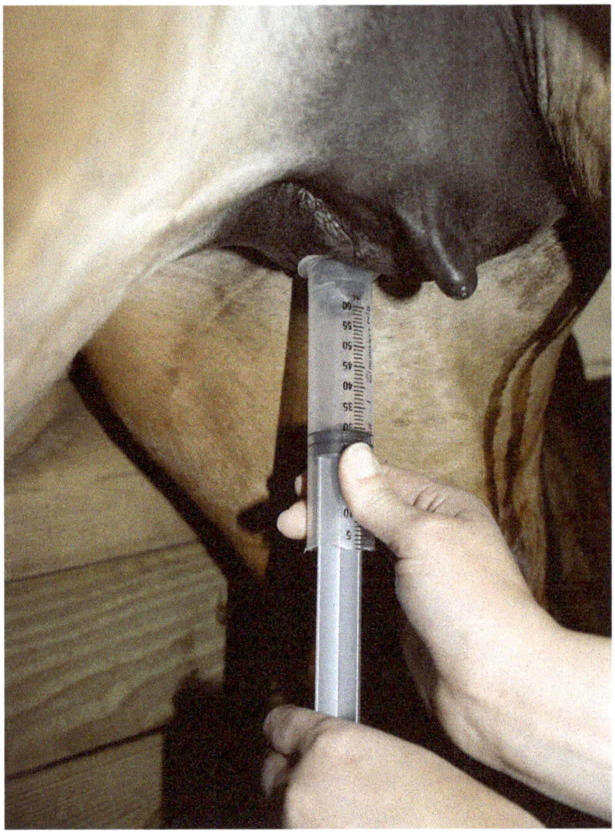

Figure 106.2 Use of a hand-made milk pump.

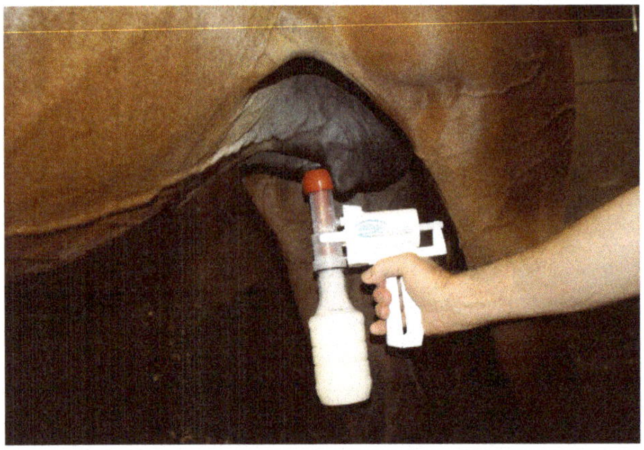

Figure 106.3 A hand-held manual milking device for mares (Ultimate Ez Milker™, Lexington, KY, USA).

- Slowly pull on the plunger of the syringe to provide negative suction on the teat. Milk will start to flow into the syringe barrel.
- Pour the contents of the syringe through a gauze sponge into a sterile container for collection.
- Repeat the procedure until sufficient milk has been collected or until milk is no longer obtained.

Additional Comments

- In hand milking, excessive pulling on the teat should not occur. Care should be exercised to not cause any skin abrasions from repeatedly pulling downward on the teat skin. Pulling downward on the teat excessively may also cause discomfort to the mare and possible reaction with her hind legs.
- Commercial equine milk pumps are also available (Ultimate Ez Milker™; Lexington, KY, USA, see Figure 106.3).
- When using a milk pump, be careful to not exert excessive suction on the teat end. This could cause blood vessels to rupture or cause the teat canal to evert. Continued trauma to the teat canal may increase the incidence of mastitis.

Further Reading

Ley WB, Hoffman JL, Meacham TN, Sullivan TL, Kiracofe RL, Wilson ML. 1989. Daytime foaling management of the mare: 1. Pre-foaling mammary secretions testing. *J Eq Vet Sci* 9: 88–94.

107

Placental Evaluation

Patrick M. McCue

Equine Reproduction Laboratory, Colorado State University, USA

Introduction

The fetal membranes, commonly called the placenta, are the connection between the developing fetus and the uterus of the mare. A healthy functional placenta is critical for fetal nutrition and gas exchange. Examination of the placenta after foaling can offer valuable insight into the *in utero* health of the newborn foal. Consequently, it is recommended that owners, farm managers, foaling attendants, or veterinarians perform an evaluation of each placenta.

The examination of a normal placenta should only take a few minutes and should be accomplished as soon after foaling as possible. If the placenta is determined to be abnormal, representative samples or the entire placenta may be submitted to a diagnostic laboratory for further evaluation. The information gained may be critical for early medical management of the foal.

Equipment and Supplies

Disposable exam gloves, bucket, scales.

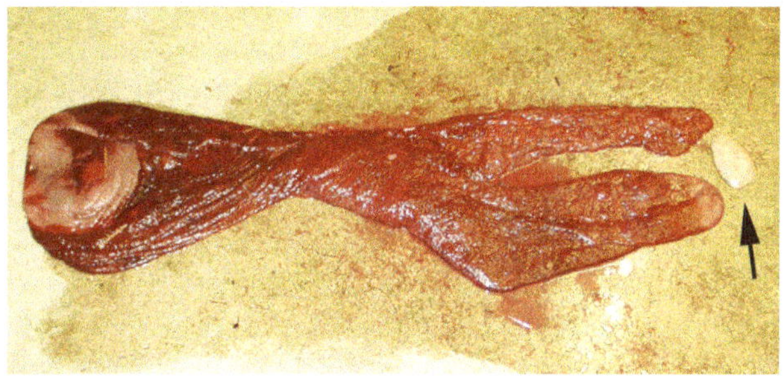

Figure 107.1 Placenta with the chorionic surface visible. A hippomane (arrow) is visible adjacent to the horn tips.

Technique

- Rinse the placenta free of gross debris.
- Weigh the placenta. The weight of the placenta should be approximately 11% of the body weight of the foal.
- The placenta usually inverts during passage out of the mare (i.e., it is passed with the allantoic surface exposed). Turn the placenta "right side out" so that the chorionic surface is exposed. The chorionic surface has a brick-red, velvet-like appearance due to the presence of microcotyledons (Figure 107.1). The allantoic surface, which is the side toward the foal, is smooth and a light pink-purple color and blood vessels are visible coursing along its surface (Figure 107.2).
- A hippomane, also called an "allantoic calculi," which is a soft, flat, oval mass tan to brown in color and about 10–16 cm (4-6 inches) in diameter is commonly passed as the mare gives birth. The hippomane consists of a mass of lipids, placental cells, and debris that aggregates in the allantoic cavity of the placenta. Typically one large hippomane is present, but multiple small hippomanes may be present in some cases.
- Spread the placenta out on a clean flat surface in an "F" or "Y" shape, with the two horns of the placenta forming the arms of the "F" or "Y" and the body of the placenta forming the base. There should only be one opening in the placenta corresponding with the region of the cervical star through which the fetus passed during delivery.
- Examine the tips of the placental horns. The "pregnant horn" is larger and thicker, while the "non-pregnant horn" is thinner and has a corrugated appearance (Figure 107.3). The tip or the entire non-pregnant horn can tear off and be retained inside the uterus (Figure 107.4).
- Examine the area around the cervical star. The portion of chorionic surface in direct contact with the cervix will

Equine Reproductive Procedures, Second Edition. Edited by John Dascanio and Patrick McCue.

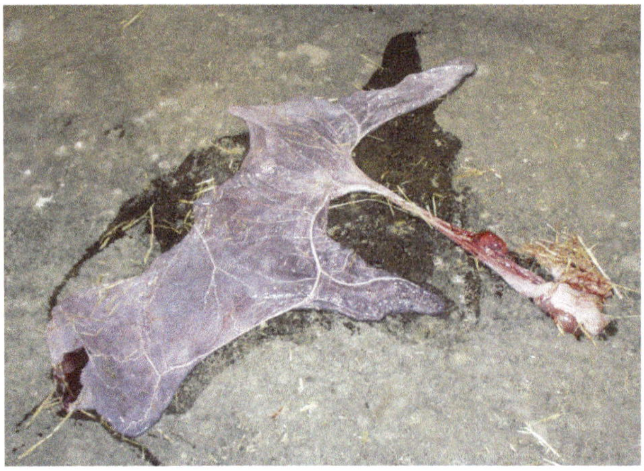

Figure 107.2 Placenta with the allantoic surface visible.

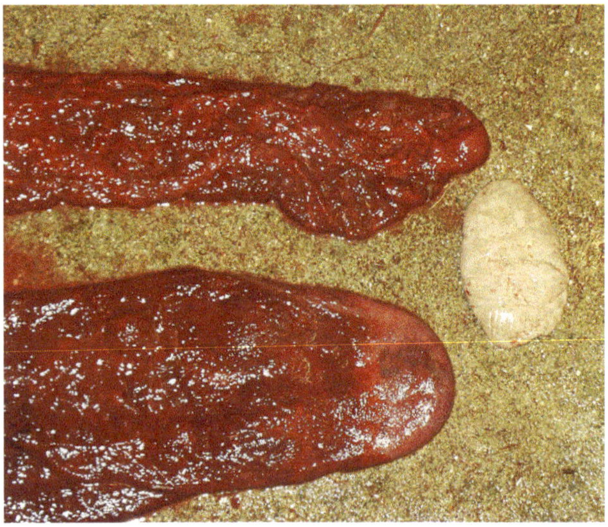

Figure 107.3 Close-up showing the difference in thickness between the "pregnant" and "non-pregnant" horn tips (the pregnant horn is at the bottom of the picture); the hippomane is also visible.

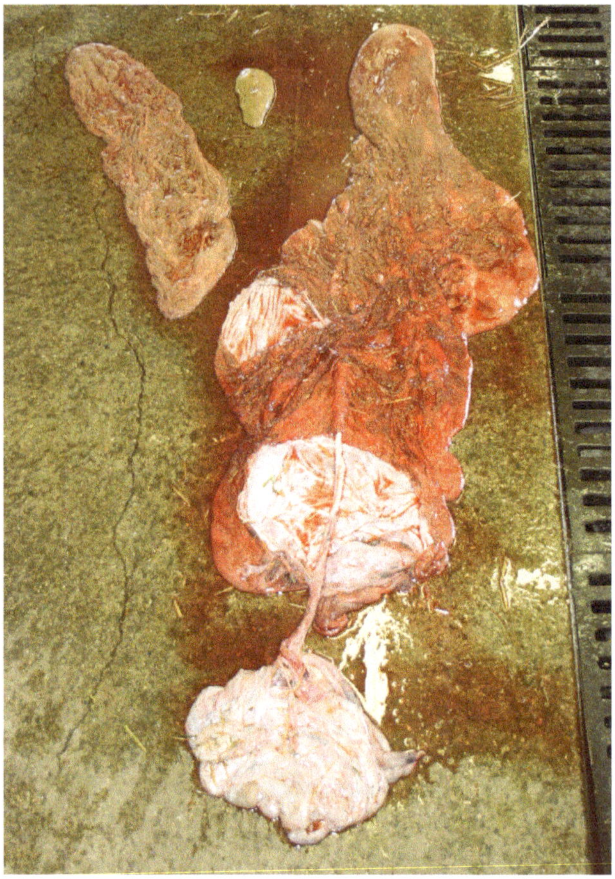

Figure 107.4 Equine placenta in which the entire "non-pregnant" horn (upper left) had detached from the remainder of the placenta and was retained in the mare for several hours. A hippomane is present between the two placental horns.

have white radiating bands devoid of microcotyledons (the "cervical star") (Figure 107.5). The chorioallantois ruptures at the cervical star when a mare "breaks her water" or releases allantoic fluid at the end of stage 1 of labor.

- Examine the entire chorionic surface of the placenta. The chorionic surface may have several small white areas devoid of microcotyledons. A single small (0.5 cm, 0.2 inch) circular avillous area is often visible near the tip of each horn and represents the area of placenta opposite the utero-tubular (oviductal) junction. A ring of disconnected avillous areas may be present at the base of the pregnant uterine horn where the endometrial cups formed. Other small scattered avillous areas may also be randomly distributed on the chorionic surface and may be caused by a fold of placenta, an opposing endometrial cyst, or may overlay a blood vessel on the allantoic surface. Microcotyledons should be relatively evenly or diffusely distributed on the chorionic surface yielding a uniform, red, velvety appearance.

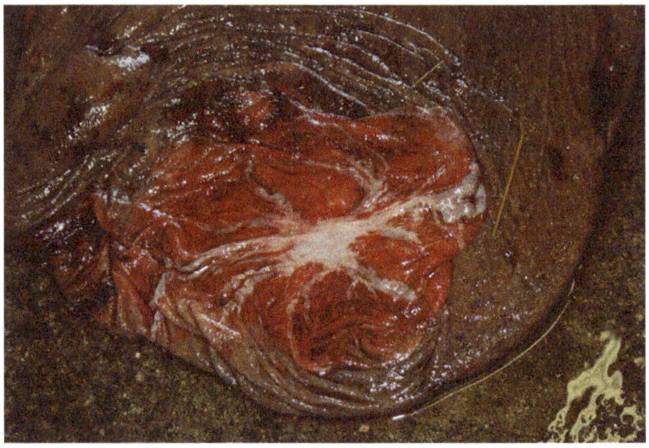

Figure 107.5 Cervical star area of the chorionic surface.

- Examine the allantoic surface of the chorioallantoic membrane. Pathologic lesions are less common on this surface. Allantoic pouches may be present, but are not of clinical significance (Figure 107.6).
- Examine the amnion. An uncommon but significant finding is yellow-orange discoloration due to meconium staining. Occasionally, scattered small, white, raised areas called amnionic plaques are visible on the inner surface of the amnion. These plaques are clusters of amnionic epithelium that have undergone squamous metaplasia and are not considered to be a significant abnormality (Figure 107.7).
- Examine the umbilical cord. The normal equine umbilical cord may have a mild to moderate degree of gently spiraling present. Excessive twisting of the cord can restrict blood flow from the placenta to the fetus, prevent urine flow through the urachus from the fetus to the allantoic cavity, and lead to fetal compromise or death (Figure 107.8). Complications are more common in umbilical cords of excessive length (i.e., >85 cm (33.4 inches) in length in a full-term fetus) than normal or shorter cords.
- An interesting but relatively uncommon finding associated with the umbilical cord is a yolk sac remnant. These are identified as a single, round, fluid-filled sac with a lining that may be ossified (i.e., consist of a round, bony outer shell), connected to the umbilical cord by a small membraneous stalk. A yolk sac remnant (Figure 107.9) may occasionally wrap around the umbilical cord and constrict blood flow to or from the fetus.

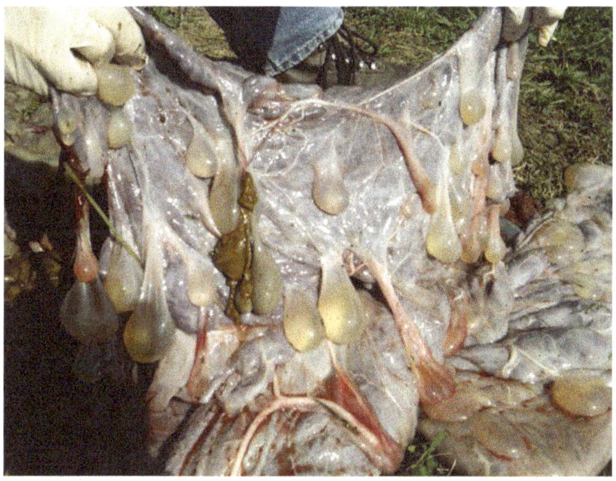

Figure 107.6 Allantoic pouches from an equine placenta. Photo courtesy of Dr Valerie J. Linse.

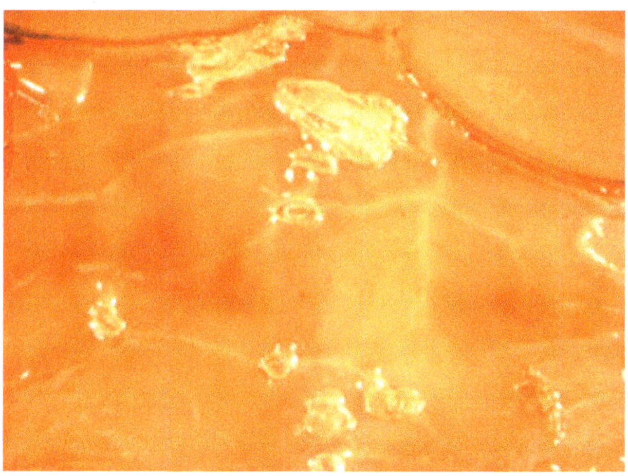

Figure 107.7 Amnionic plaques from an equine placenta.

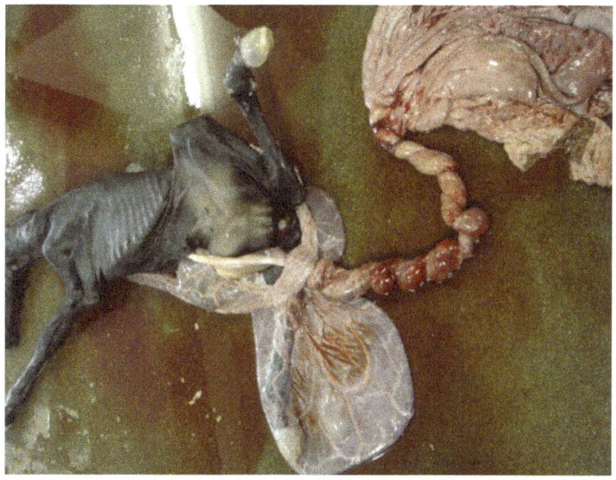

Figure 107.8 Twisted umbilical cord from an aborted fetus.

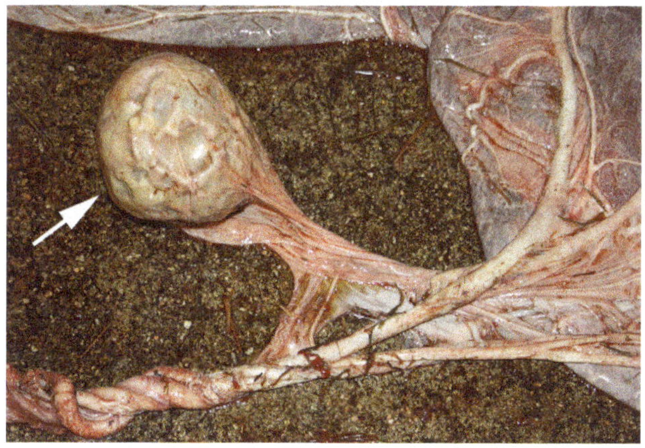

Figure 107.9 An ossified yolk sac remnant (arrow) from an equine placenta.

Interpretation and Additional Comments

The vast majority of equine placentas examined will be normal. However, occasionally a significant abnormality will be detected that may be associated with medical issues of the mare or newborn foal. It is not uncommon to see lighter and darker areas on the chorionic surface due to some areas of the placenta separating from the endometrium sooner (darker) than other areas (lighter). The placenta in these lighter and darker areas is of normal thickness and without abnormal discharges.

Prolonged retention of all or part of the chorioallantoic membrane may result in a rapid growth of bacteria and ultimately systemic illness. A placenta is considered retained in a mare after 3 hours. Medical intervention is warranted to remove the placenta and prevent untoward sequelae such as metritis, endotoxemia, and laminitis.

Ascending bacterial infections usually result in discoloration (i.e., tan to brown) and thickening of the chorionic surface of the placenta near the cervical star (Figure 107.10). In addition, a thick fibrin necrotic exudate may be present on the chorionic surface of the cervical star region. A dry, leather-like appearance in the cervical star region may be indicative of ascending fungal placentitis. Nocardioform placentitis is characterized by the accumulation of inflammatory debris on the chorionic surface at the base of a uterine horn. If placentitis is identified, the foal may have been exposed to pathogenic microorganisms *in utero* and should be considered high risk for medical complications.

An increased placental weight may be the result of edema associated with factors such as fescue toxicosis or may be due to an infectious condition such as placentitis. In some mares with fescue toxicosis, the cervical star may not rupture properly due to thickening and edema in the placenta. The placenta may rupture in a different location during labor in affected mares. Foals born to mares with an intact cervical star region should be examined for possible fetal hypoxia. Mares with heavy placentas due to fescue toxicosis may also demonstrate fluid accumulation (sacculations) along the allantoic vessels on examination.

A decreased concentration or uneven distribution of microcotyledons (i.e., chorionic villus hypoplasia) may be associated with advanced uterine pathology. Twin pregnancies result in a large avillous area where the placenta of one fetus was in contact with the placenta of the other fetus. If such a placenta is passed, the uterus of the mare should be examined for the presence of a second fetus.

Stress to the fetus prior to birth may result in the premature passage of fecal material (meconium). Meconium staining may be an early warning sign that the foal is compromised. In addition, affected foals may aspirate meconium into their lungs and develop serious respiratory complications.

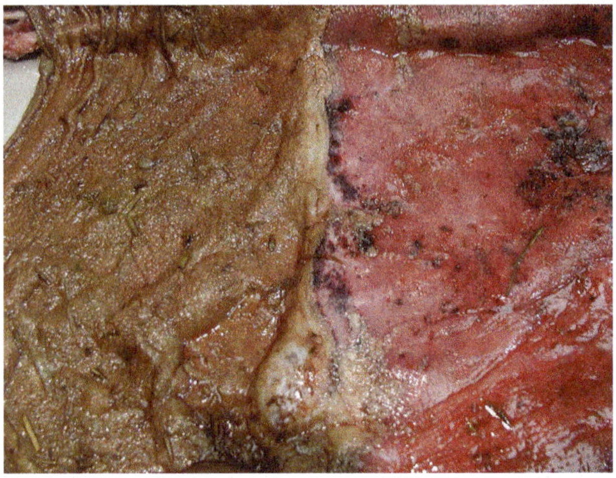

Figure 107.10 Infected region of the chorionic surface in a mare with ascending placentitis.

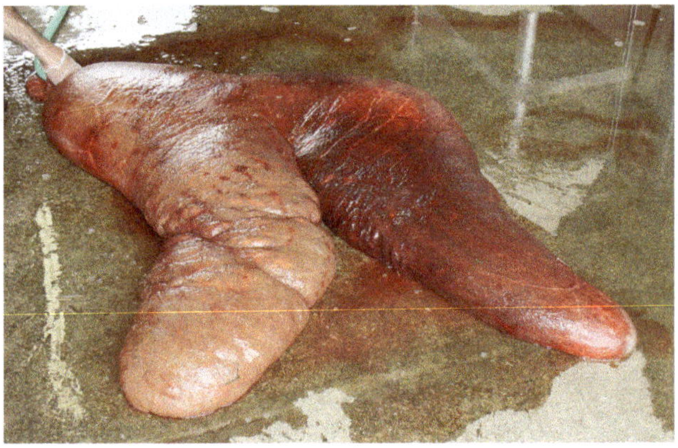

Figure 107.11 Placenta inflated with water.

An alternative technique for examination of the placenta is to inflate the chorioallantois with water (Figure 107.11). The placenta should be rinsed off and turned right-side out as previously described. A hose is passed through the ruptured cervical star area and the chorioallantois is inflated with water as the cervical area of the placenta is clamped by hand around the hose to prevent leakage. This technique will allow one to rapidly determine if the placenta is intact and will provide an excellent view of the chorionic surface. If an opening is present in the placenta it should be determined if a piece of the placenta is missing and possibly retained in the mare or if the placenta is simply torn. Turning the placenta inside out so that the allantoic surface is visible will allow one to match blood vessels along the tear, thus putting "puzzle pieces" together to see if the tissue is continuous or if a piece of tissue is missing.

Further Reading

Cassar TIY, Fallon LH, Martinez EH, Schlafer DH. 2006. Segmental ossification of involuted yolk sacs in equine umbilical cords. Ninth International Symposium on Equine Reproduction. Kerkrade, the Netherlands, August 7–11, 2006. *Anim Reprod Sci* 94: 439–42.

Schlafer DH. 2004a. The umbilical cord – lifeline to the outside world: structure, function, and pathology of the equine umbilical cord. In: Powell DG, Furry D, Hale G (eds). Proceedings of the Workshop on the Equine Placenta. Lexington, KY: University of Kentucky, pp. 92–8.

Schlafer DH. 2004b. Postmortem examination of the equine placenta, fetus, and neonate: methods and interpretaton of finding. *Proc Annu Conv Am Assoc Eq Pract* 50: 1–19.

Schlafer DH. 2011. Examination of the placenta. In: McKinnon AO, Squires EL, Vaala WE, Varner DD (eds). Equine Reproduction, 2nd edn. Ames, IA: Wiley Blackwell, pp. 99–110.

108

Removal of Retained Placenta

John J. Dascanio

School of Veterinary Medicine, Texas Tech University, USA

Introduction

During stage 3 of parturition, the fetal membranes or placenta should be expelled. In the horse, the placenta is considered to be abnormally retained beyond 3 hours post-foaling. A retained placenta may predispose a mare to metritis with subsequent laminitis and thus should be removed in a timely fashion. Retained placentas are more common with dystocias, abortions, and after induction of labor. The incidence of retained placenta in the general horse population is 2–10% of foalings with higher rates reported in draft horses (up to 50% reported in Friesian horses).

Equipment and Supplies

Tail wrap, tail rope, non-irritant soap, roll cotton, stainless steel bucket, disposable liner for bucket, paper towels, examination gloves, obstetrical sleeve, sterile water-soluble lubricant, oxytocin, uterine lavage tubing, lavage fluids, garden hose, hose flow control valve, hose connector (sweeper nozzle), stallion urinary catheter, scalpel blade.

Technique

- Perform a physical examination on the mare:
- Confirm that the mare has foaled; occasionally a mare that is still pregnant is presented to a clinic that "presumably foaled or aborted" in pasture and has fetal membranes visible at the vulva.
- Confirm that a second fetus is not present.
- Administer 10–20 IU oxytocin intramuscularly. Doses of oxytocin may be repeated at 1-2 hour intervals to promote uterine contractions. In a hospital situation a constant rate infusion of 100 IU oxytocin in 1,000 ml saline delivered over a 1-hour period through an intravenous jugular catheter may be used. Often one or two doses of oxytocin are all that is needed to relieve a retained placenta.
- Calcium gluconate may be given intravenously to assist with uterine contractions. A solution of 100–150 ml of 23% calcium gluconate is added to 1 liter of lactated Ringer's solution and administered intravenously over 45–60 minutes while occasionally monitoring heart rate/rhythm.
- Remove feces from the mare's rectum.
- Place a tail wrap and tail rope on the mare (see Chapter 4).
- Wearing examination gloves, clean and dry the perineum of the mare and as much of any exposed placental tissues as possible (see Chapter 3).
- Don a sterile obstetrical sleeve and place a sterile water-soluble lubricant on the outside of the hand and down the arm.
- Insert a gloved hand through the vulvar labia and reach as far forward in the vagina as possible. Gently, but firmly, grasp placental tissue and apply mild traction to determine if the membranes can be delivered manually. Gentle, constant traction over a few minutes of time may result in disengagement of the microcotyledons of the fetal membranes from the endometrium (Figure 108.1). The traction should not result in tearing of the placental tissue. Occasionally, a placenta may be already detached from the endometrium and merely sitting within the uterus. This is most common when the amnion and umbilical cord have been detached and the chorioallantoic membrane is retained within the uterus.
- It is not recommended to manually separate the chorion from the endometrium as this may result in shearing of microvilli or tearing off a piece of placenta, or lead to intramural uterine hemorrhage. However, skilled experienced veterinary practitioners commonly perform

Equine Reproductive Procedures, Second Edition. Edited by John Dascanio and Patrick McCue.

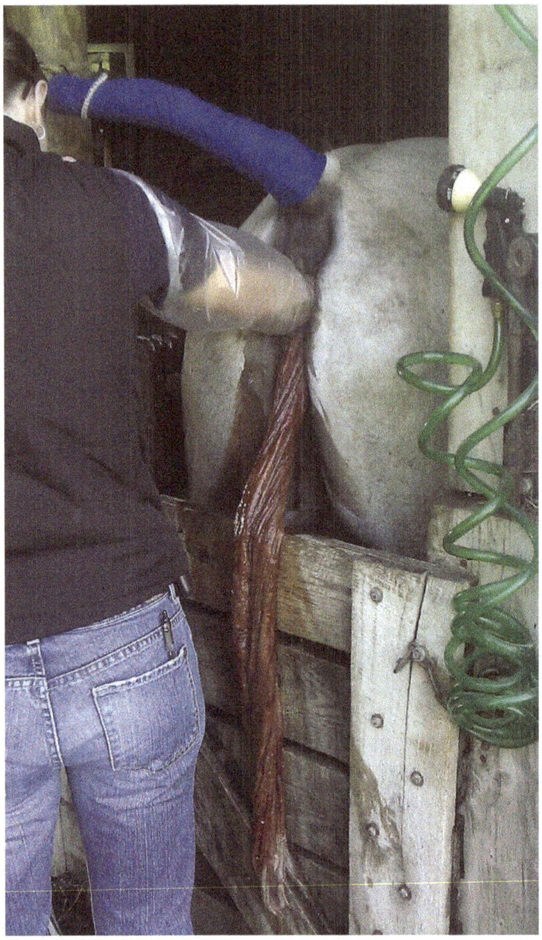

Figure 108.1 Most of the chorioallantois can be delivered from the uterus with gentle traction.

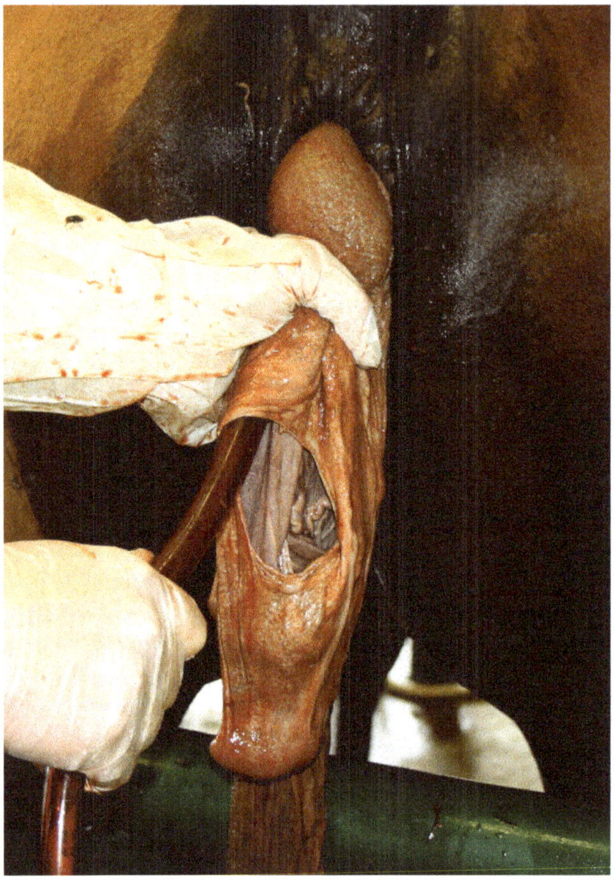

Figure 108.2 'Burns technique' – pumping water into the allantoic cavity of a retained placenta.

manual removal of the fetal membranes without untoward issues.

- Use of excessive traction on the placenta may induce uterine contractions and result in either inversion of a uterine horn or uterine prolapse.
- If the placenta does not become detached with gentle traction, alternative methods may be attempted such as twisting the placenta, infusing fluids within the allantoic cavity, infusing a placental blood vessel with fluids, administration of oxytocin, or repeating the attempt several hours later.
- *Twisting method.* One method used to release the microcotyledons attaching the chorion to the endometrium is to gently and very slowly twist the placenta in one direction while applying gentle traction. The constant twisting pressure will often allow a slow methodical detachment of the microcotyledons from the chorion. The placenta is grasped as far forward within the vaginal canal as possible and is twisted, hand over hand, in one direction to minimize the diameter of the placental mass, potentially allowing egress from the cervix/uterus. The procedure may be repeated in the opposite direction. Care should be taken to not tear the placenta or cause the microcotyledonary tissue to tear from its uterine attachment.
- *Burns technique.* A second technique is to infuse a large volume of fluid into the allantoic cavity. The cervical star area is identified and a large bore tube, such as a clean stomach tube, is passed along the umbilical cord into the allantoic cavity (Figure 108.2). The caudal chorioallantoic membrane is held tightly closed around the tube. A large volume (8–10 liters) of warm fluids, such as sterile saline or tap water with a small amount of povidone-iodine solution added (10 ml of 1% solution per liter) are pumped into the allantoic space, distending the placenta and any folds in the uterine horns. The fluid is held in the allantoic space for several minutes and then allowed to drain out by gravity flow. The procedure may be repeated, and in many cases, refilling the allantoic cavity results in disassociation of chorionic membranes. This procedure may have multiple positive effects including stimulation of uterine contractions, expansion of the

closed uterine horns, and detachment of microvilli from the endometrium. The "water technique" will not be effective if the chorioallantois is torn, which would allow the infused fluid to escape into the uterine lumen.

- *Dutch technique*. A third technique is to slowly infuse an umbilical blood vessel (vein or artery) with tap water. Infusion of water is thought to expand capillary beds, causing edema of the chorion, leading to microcotyledonary separation. In addition, weight from tissue fluid or any fluid that leaks into the uterine space may also augment detachment. A stallion urinary catheter (maximum of 9 mm diameter) is attached to a water hose using a flow control valve and a hose connector (Figures 108.3 and 108.4). A small incision is made into one umbilical vessel with a scalpel blade (Figure 108.5). The end of the stallion catheter is threaded proximally into the umbilical vessel (Figure 108.6). Water is slowly infused into the umbilical vessel for 3–5 minutes while grasping around the umbilical vessel/stallion catheter to prevent flow out the incision (Figure 108.7). Flow may need to be started and stopped occasionally depending on the response of the mare, who may demonstrate discomfort. The water is held within the placental tissues for an additional 5 minutes. Gentle traction is then applied to the retained placenta to augment removal. The procedure may be repeated in other umbilical vessels as needed.
- If the placenta is not delivered, the amnion should be elevated to the level of the mare's hocks and tied at that level to provide some weight and constant mild traction on the umbilical cord which is attached to the chorioallantoic membrane. This is often sufficient to facilitate separation of the chorioallantoic membrane from the endometrium and will also prevent the mare from stepping on the exposed amnion and causing excessive pull-

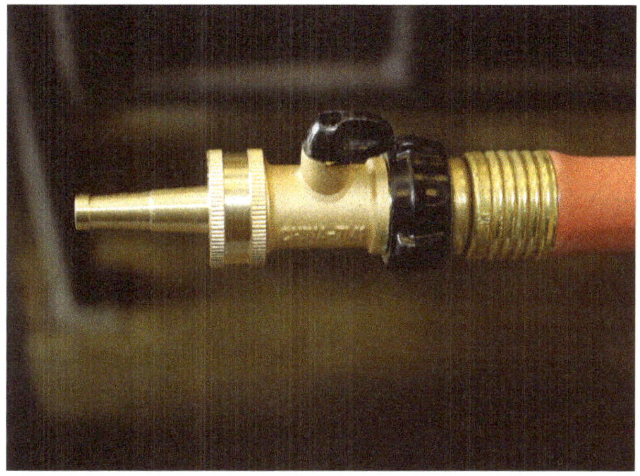

Figure 108.4 Assembled hose connector, hose flow control valve, and hose.

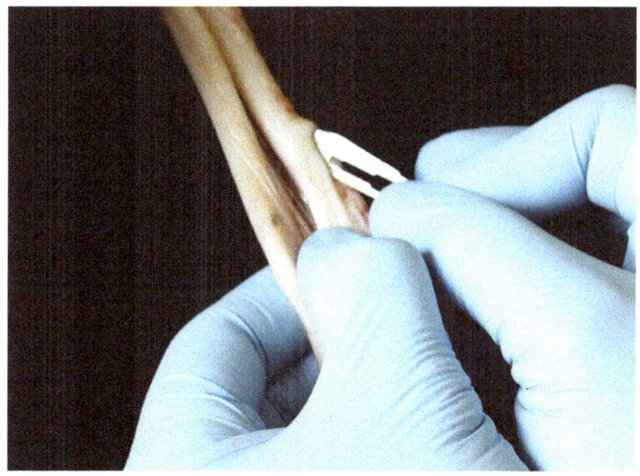

Figure 108.5 A small incision is made into an umbilical vein or artery using a scalpel blade.

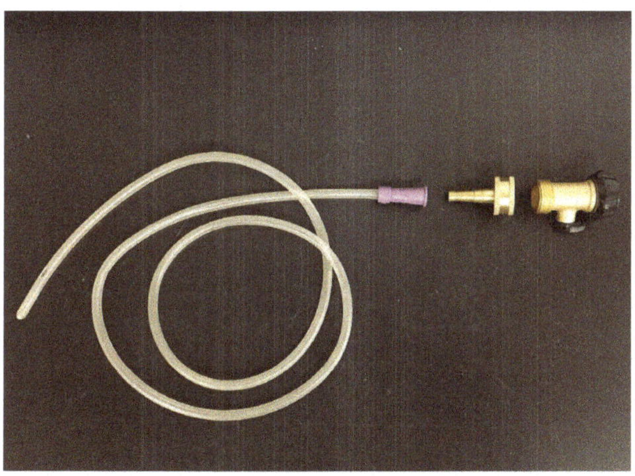

Figure 108.3 Stallion catheter, hose connector (sweeper nozzle), and hose flow control valve.

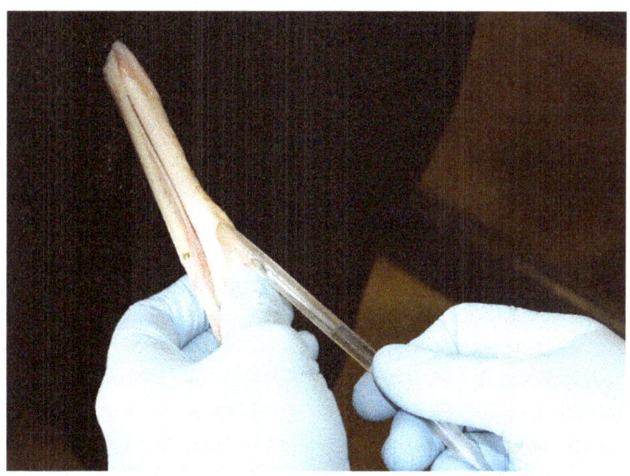

Figure 108.6 A stallion catheter is threaded up the umbilical vessel until resistence is encountered.

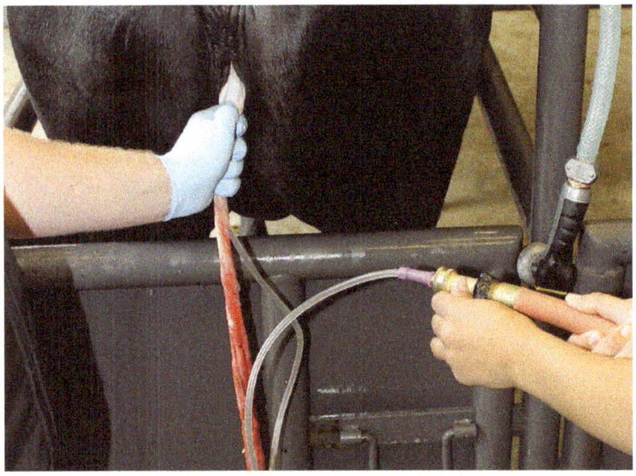

Figure 108.7 Water is slowly infused into the umbilical vessel using the flow control valve while the catheter is held in place to prevent water outflow.

ing on the placenta. It is not recommended to attach extra weights (such as bricks, water jugs, towels, etc.) as the procedure may lead to tearing of the placenta and retention of small placental tags. However, attachment of a jug containing a small volume of water may be appropriate to attach to an umbilical cord if the amnion has been torn off and no longer providing weight to naturally disengage the chorioallantois from the uterus (Figure 108.8).

- The mare should be started on systemic medical therapy including broad-spectrum antibiotics and a non-steroidal anti-inflammatory drug if the placenta is retained more than 3 hours post-foaling or if there was significant contamination of the placental membranes or uterus.
- Oxytocin therapy may be continued to encourage uterine evacuation and placental expulsion.
- Laminitis prophylaxis may also be instituted depending on the clinical circumstances. This may include non-steroidal anti-inflammatory drugs, ice boots, digit or frog support, pentoxifylline, acepromazine, or other measures.
- Large volume uterine lavage may be performed as needed to remove tissue debris, retained fluids, and bacteria from the uterus.
- In addition, the mare should be updated on tetanus prophylaxis.

Interpretation

- Attempts to manually remove the placenta should not be performed within 1–2 hours after foaling so as to not predispose to intramural hemorrhage from pulling on the endometrium or to tear the microcotelydonary attachment.
- Mares with a retained placenta should be monitored for signs of metritis and systemic illness, such as fever,

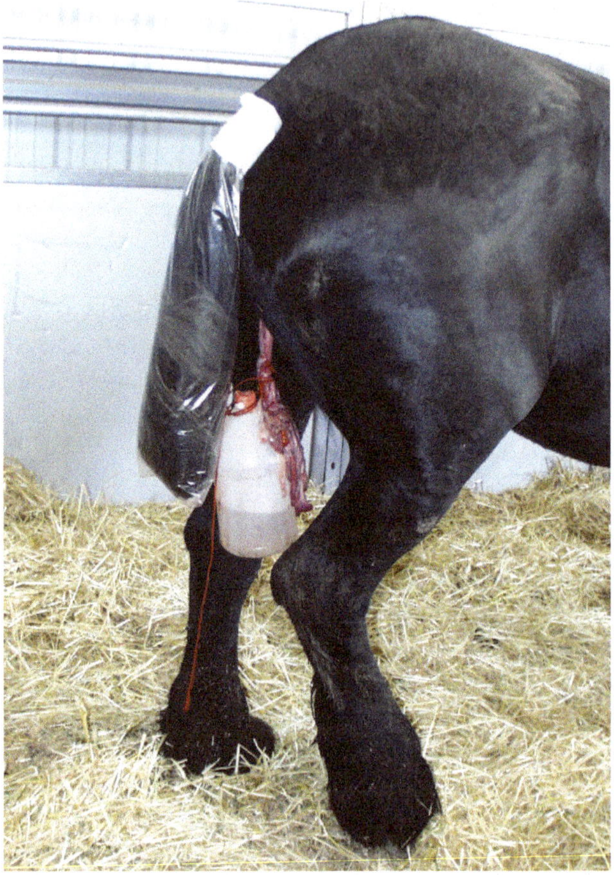

Figure 108.8 Plastic jug containing approximately 1 liter of water attached to the umbilical cord of a Friesian mare with a retained placenta.

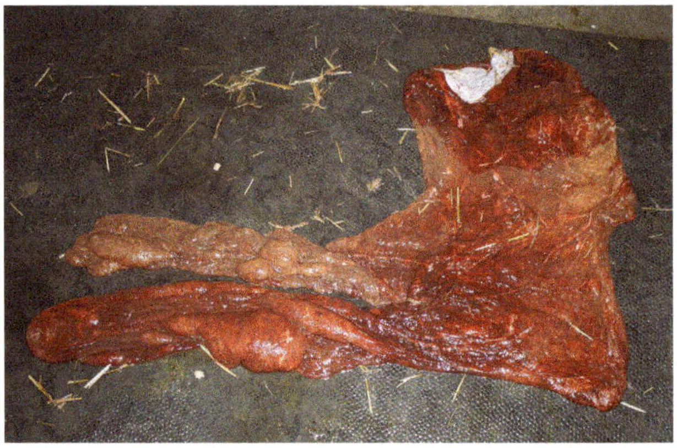

Figure 108.9 Placenta laid out in an "F" shape demonstrating that both uterine horns are intact and that the only opening in the chorioallantois is where the placenta ruptured at the cervical star during parturition.

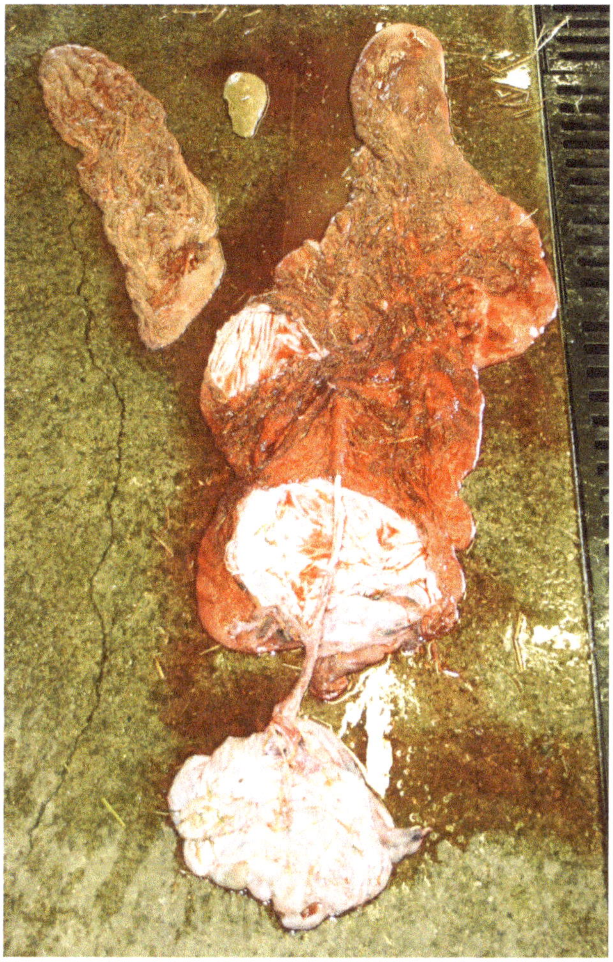

Figure 108.10 Chorioallantois in which the entire non-pregnant horn had been torn off and retained in the uterus (upper left).

anorexia, and a malordorous reddish-brown vaginal discharge.

- Laminitis may occur secondary to metritis. Affected mares demonstrate a reluctance to walk, a variable front leg lameness, increased digital pulses, and possible rotation of the third phalanx.
- The entire placenta should be examined after passage to determine if it is complete or if a section of the placenta still remains within the mare (Figures 108.9 and 108.10) (see Chapter 107). If a piece is missing, the placenta should be turned inside-out and the vessel pattern on the allantoic side matched to determine if a piece is missing or if the placenta is just torn (Figure 108.11). If a piece is missing, a manual examination of the uterine lumen may be performed to identify any remaining fragments. Ultrasound of the uterus per rectum may also identify placental remnants as hyperechoic tissue suspended in hypoechoic fluid.
- Uterine prolapse is a concern in post-partum mares following obstetrical intervention or manipulations to remove a retained placenta.

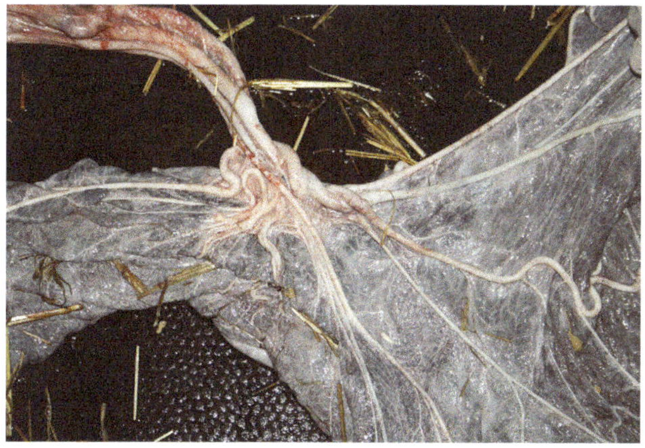

Figure 108.11 Allantoic surface of the placenta. Matching vessels on the allantoic surface across placental tears may allow determination of any missing placental tissue (uterine remnants).

Further Reading

Meijer M, Macpherson ML, Dijkman R. 2015. How to use umbilical vessel water infusion to treat retained fetal membranes in mares. *Proc Annu Conv Am Assoc Eq Pract* 61: 478–84.

Provencher R, Threlfall WR, Murdick PW, Wearly WK. 1988. Retained fetal membranes in the mare: a retrospective study. *Can Vet J* 29: 903–10.

Sevingaa M, Barkemab HW, Stryhnb H, Hesselink JW. 2004. Retained placenta in Friesian mares: incidence, and potential risk factors with special emphasis on gestational length. *Theriogenology* 61: 851–9.

Vandeplassche M, Spincemaille J, Bouters R. 1971. Aetiology, pathogenesis and treatment of retained placenta in the mare. *Eq Vet J* 3: 144–7.

109

Abdominocentesis

John J. Dascanio

School of Veterinary Medicine, Texas Tech University, USA

Introduction

Abdominocentesis is a diagnostic technique commonly used in horses with abdominal pain (colic). Abdominal discomfort can occur in the post-foaling mare for a number of reasons including a primary gastrointestinal issue, uterine or broad ligament hematoma, secondary gastrointestinal issue, peritonitis due to vaginal, cervical, or uterine tear, urinary bladder rupture, or lesions in other abdominal organs.

Ultrasound should be used to guide abdominal paracentesis to locate fluid in the ventral abdomen. In addition, the characteristics and amount of peritoneal fluid should be noted. Hyperechoic fluid may indicate free blood within the abdomen or a hypercellular inflammatory fluid. Hypoechoic fluid usually indicates a non-cellular fluid.

Fluid obtained from abdominocentesis should be submitted to a diagnostic laboratory for gross, biochemical, and microscopic analysis.

Equipment and Supplies

Ultrasound, clippers, surgical scrub, alcohol soaked gauze, lidocaine or carbocaine, needles, syringes, sterile stainless steel teat cannula, EDTA blood tube (purple top), serum tube (red top), sterile telfa pad, conform bandage wrap, 15 cm (6 inch) elastic adhesive tape.

Technique

- Perform transcutaneous ultrasound on the ventral abdomen to locate any accumulations of peritoneal fluid that would make a good site for abdominocentesis.
- Clip the hair on the ventral abdomen in a small area overlying an area of peritoneal fluid accumulation. If there is no fluid detected on ultrasound, then the most ventral aspect of the abdomen just to the right of midline should be clipped in a small area. The left abdomen is avoided to prevent puncture of the spleen.
- Perform a surgical scrub of the clipped area.
- Fluid is collected into an EDTA blood tube (purple top) and a serum tube (red top). The rubber stoppers of the tubes are removed to allow fluid to drip from the cannula/needle into the tubes. The tops are replaced immediately after sample collection for laboratory submission. Insertion of a needle through the top will relieve air pressure within the tube, preventing the top from being forced off.

Teat Cannula Technique

- Using a 22 gauge 2.5 cm (1 inch) needle, place 1–2 ml of lidocaine or carbocaine into the skin and ventral abdominal muscles in the area to perform the abdominocentesis.
- A sterile scalpel blade is used to make a 1 cm (0.4 inches) incision in the skin over the desensitized area. This will allow the teat cannula to be introduced through the skin. Any blood should be wiped away with a sterile gauze sponge. If bleeding persists, then a piece of gauze is held over the incision and the teat cannula introduced through the gauze and then into the incision.
- Don surgical gloves and insert a sterile 5 cm (2 inch) stainless steel teat cannula through the cut skin and advance it through the abdominal muscles and fascia bluntly until it enters the peritoneal cavity. Hold the teat cannula close to the closed end to prevent the teat cannula from bending. A slight decrease in resistance to advancement is felt when the teat cannula punctures the peritoneal lining. If no fluid spontaneously runs out of the teat cannula, the teat cannula may be gently rotated

Equine Reproductive Procedures, Second Edition. Edited by John Dascanio and Patrick McCue.

and/or advanced in small increments until fluid is recovered.

- One to 2 ml of air may be pushed through the needle to facilitate a return of peritoneal fluid if it is determined that the teat cannula is obstructed.

Needle Technique

- An 18 gauge 4 cm (1.5 inch) needle is slowly inserted through the skin, subcutaneous tissue, and ventral abdominal musculature. A decrease in resistance to advancement is felt when the needle enters the peritoneal cavity. Care should be exercised to avoid large movements of the needle so as to avoid puncture or laceration of the abdominal contents. Advancement should stop when the tip of the needle is just within the peritoneal cavity. If there is no spontaneous outflow of peritoneal fluid, the needle may be rotated along its long axis. The needle may be advanced further in small increments with twisting in an attempt to locate peritoneal fluid.
- One to 2 ml of air may be pushed through the needle to facilitate a return of peritoneal fluid if it is determined that the needle is obstructed.
- If the mare is significantly overweight, an 18 gauge, 9 cm (3.5 inch) spinal needle may be substituted.

Interpretation

- The normal values for equine peritoneal fluid should be a total protein of <2.5 g/dl, a total nucleated cell count of <5,000 cells/μl, and <70% neutrophils.
- Mares with a total protein of >3.0 g/dl, total nucleated cell count of >15,000 cells/μl, and >80% neutrophils would be considered to have a significant abdominal lesion that would require further diagnostics and/or treatment. Variations in these numbers may occur depending on the stage of disease. Mares with an elevation of two of the three indices above have a higher probability of systemic illness.
- Repeated abdominocentesis at 24-hour intervals should not result in an increase in normal values.
- A normal delivery, dystocia, or fetotomy, in the absence of a reproductive tract tear, should not significantly elevate peritoneal fluid values.
- Mares with a cranial vaginal, cervical, or uterine tear may have an increased protein and cell count. The fluid may appear cloudy and red tinged from increased red blood cell numbers.
- A second abdominocentesis is indicated in mares that continue to be ill, especially if previous results are normal. Occasionally, reproductive tract trauma may result in necrosis of the wall over time, resulting in peritonitis.

Further Reading

Frazer G, Burba D, Paccamonti D, Blouin D, LeBlanc M, Embertson R, Hance S. 1997. The effects of parturition and peripartum complications on the peritoneal fluid composition in mares. *Theriogenology* 48: 919–31.

110

Uterine Prolapse Treatment

John J. Dascanio

School of Veterinary Medicine, Texas Tech University, USA

Introduction

Uterine prolapse may occur early in the post-partum period after a normal delivery, after an assisted delivery, or after an abortion. A complicating factor may be a retained placenta that starts the inversion of a uterine horn. When a mare lies down, the push of the abdominal contents on the uterus, the downward slope of the pelvic canal, the action of gravity on the flaccid uterus, the potential pull of a retained placenta, and possible abdominal contractions once the uterus has contacted the vaginal wall may all contribute to prolapse of the uterus.

Excessive straining secondary to obstetrical manipulations or aggressive traction applied to a retained placenta during a manual removal attempt may trigger uterine and abdominal contractions that lead to a uterine prolapse.

Uterine prolapse requires immediate emergency treatment. Damage to blood vessels and nerves may lead to necrosis of the uterine tissue. Pulling on the uterus from a prolapse may result in rupture of the uterine blood vessels resulting in fatal hemorrhage. Trauma to the uterine tissue may result in subsequent metritis or peritonitis. In addition, a tear in the prolapsed uterus may lead to evisceration. A complete uterine prolapse is more likely to result in a fatal outcome than a partial prolapse due to the pull on vascular structures.

Equipment and Supplies

Tail wrap, non-irritant soap, roll cotton, stainless steel bucket, disposable liner for bucket, paper towels, exam gloves, obstetrical sleeves, sterile lubricant, oxytocin, antibiotics, needles, syringes, non-steroidal anti-inflammatory drugs, Buhner needle, umbilical tape, lidocaine, sedatives, large garbage bag.

Immediate Prolapse Treatment

- The prolapsed uterus (Figure 110.1) should be kept wet to prevent desiccation of the tissue. Warm, clean tap water can be poured over the prolapse or clean wet towels may be placed over the prolapse.
- The uterus should be kept clean. A plastic garbage bag may be placed by the owner over the prolapse to keep it clean until veterinary care arrives.
- The mare should be kept quiet and her movements limited. Excessive movement could result in tearing of the blood vessels and a subsequent fatal hemorrhage from the swinging weight of the exposed uterus.

Technique for Replacing a Uterine Prolapse

- The mare should be adequately restrained to prevent movement. The mare should not be placed in stocks as she may lie down during the prolapse correction.
- A physical examination is performed. Intravenous fluids should be administered via a jugular catheter if the mare is in shock or cardiovascularly compromised.
- The mare may be administered appropriate antibiotics (trimethoprim-sulfamethoxazole 30 mg/kg PO, b.i.d. for 7–10 days or another antibiotic combination) and a non-steroidal anti-inflammatory drug (flunixin meglumine 1 mg/kg IV, b.i.d. for 3 days). Tetanus prophylaxis should be updated.
- An epidural should be administered to decrease straining (see Chapter 100). Additional sedation and/or pain medication such as butorphanol tartrate should be administered as needed for restraint and pain relief pending

Equine Reproductive Procedures, Second Edition. Edited by John Dascanio and Patrick McCue.

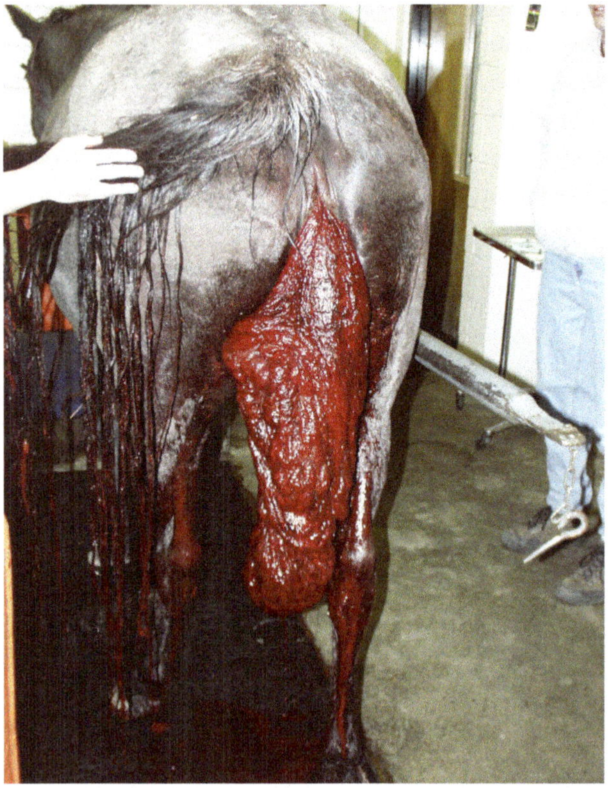

Figure 110.1 Uterine prolapse.

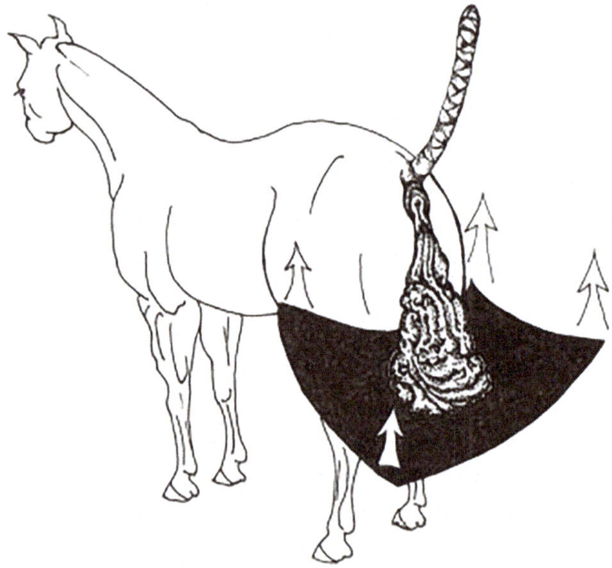

Figure 110.2 Elevation of a prolapsed uterus with a thick plastic garbage bag.

cardiovascular assessment and ability of the mare to stand.

- The tail should be folded and wrapped in its entirety so that no tail hairs are visible, using an elastic disposable wrap (see Chapter 3).
- Gross debris may be manually removed and the uterus inspected for signs of trauma or tears. The perineum and prolapsed uterus should be washed with a mild non-residual soap and copiously rinsed with tap water. A povidone-iodine scrub or chlorhexidine scrub may be used as long as the endometrial surface is rinsed thoroughly.
- Small tears involving only the endometrium may be left to heal by second intention. Full thickness tears should be sutured using absorbable monofilament suture prior to replacement of the prolapsed uterus.
- To aid in replacement, the prolapsed uterus should be elevated so that it is even with or slightly above the level of the pelvic canal (Figure 110.2). This may be accomplished by placing a large, clean garbage bag over a wide wooden board and having two assistants hold the board under the prolapse. It may also be achieved with a thick plastic garbage bag alone. Elevation of the prolapsed uterus will also help by relieving the weight and consequent discomfort and reduce the risk of further damage.
- The uterus should be covered with sterile lubricant, and with gloved hands the prolapse massaged toward its center and toward the pelvic opening. Work on the uterine segment closest to the body, returning that section first and then as the uterus telescopes back inward, continue to work the next portion closest to the body.
- Only flat hands or rolled fists should be used. Direct individual digital pressure should be avoided to prevent accidental puncture of the uterus.
- The uterine horns should be extended into the abdomen as far as possible once the uterus has been pushed completely back into the mare. The goal is complete eversion of both uterine horns. This can be accomplished by reaching up into the uterus as far as possible with a closed hand (i.e., fist) to evert the horns or using the blunt end of a clean, empty wine bottle as an extension of the arm. Care should be taken to not accidently puncture or tear the uterus while extending the horns.
- A purse-string suture using a Buhner needle may be placed around the vulvar opening to prevent re-prolapse of the uterus (see Chapter 111). This suture may be removed in a couple of days once the uterus has slightly involuted.
- The mare may be administered small doses of oxytocin (5–20 IU IM) to stimulate uterine contractions and seal small tears.

Interpretation

- The horse owner should be warned that upon replacement of the uterine prolapse, the mare may experience fatal hemorrhage from large uterine blood vessels that may have been damaged while the uterus was prolapsed, but had been compressed due to the prolapsed tissue. Upon replacement and removal of tissue compression, the blood vessels may now leak blood into the abdomen or broad ligament, or intramurally.

- If it is not possible to replace the uterus in the standing mare or in a mare in recumbency, the mare may be anesthetized and her hind end elevated by hoisting her hind legs upward to obtain the downward pelvic angle needed to replace the uterus and to decrease straining.
- If the placenta is still attached to the uterus it may be removed if it will come off with very gentle traction. Otherwise, the placenta should be cleaned and as much as possible removed before replacing the prolapsed uterus. Appropriate therapy for a retained placenta should subsequently be performed (see Chapter 108).
- The mare may develop metritis secondary to uterine contamination. Uterine lavage may be performed in the ensuing days, being careful to not distend the uterus very much as the uterine wall may have devitalized tissue.
- The mare may experience peritonitis up to a week post-prolapse replacement due to necrosis of the uterine wall from trauma.
- Differential diagnoses would include bladder prolapse, vaginal prolapse, evisceration, or rectal prolapse.
- It is generally not advisable to transport a mare with a uterine prolapse due to the pull on the uterine vasculature, possible resulting in fatal hemorrhage. If transport is necessary, the uterus should be supported.
- A mare with an uncomplicated uterine prolapse should have a fair to good prognosis for future fertility.
- There is a minimal risk of a recurrence of a uterine prolapse with a subsequent parturition.
- If a uterine tear or other trauma is identified, the edges should be debrided and sutured with absorbable suture material in an inverting pattern.
- A complete hysterectomy of the exposed uterus may be attempted if the structure is devitalized, but control of hemorrhage may be especially difficult in a field situation.
- Euthanasia may be considered for a mare with a severely traumatized prolapsed uterus.

Further Reading

Spirito MA, Sprayberry KA. 2011. Uterine prolapse. In: McKinnon AO, Squires EL, Vaala WE, Varner DD (eds). Equine Reproduction, 2nd edn. Ames, IA: Wiley Blackwell, pp. 2431–4.

111

Buhner Needle Placement of a Perivulvar Suture

John J. Dascanio

School of Veterinary Medicine, Texas Tech University, USA

Introduction

The placement of a perivulvar subcutaneous suture using a Buhner needle is performed primarily to aid in the retention of a prolapsed uterus or vaginal tissue. The suture is generally placed immediately after the replacement of prolapsed tissue. It is uncommon to have a uterine prolapse in the horse and a vaginal prolapse is even rarer. The Buhner needle suture constricts the opening of the vulva making it less possible for the reproductive tissue to prolapse again.

Equipment and Supplies

Tail wrap, non-irritant soap, roll cotton, stainless steel bucket, disposable liner for bucket, paper towels, exam gloves, clippers, lidocaine, needles, syringes, surgical scrub, alcohol swabs, No. 10 scalpel blade, umbilical tape or Buhner tape, Buhner needle, povidone-iodine.

Technique

- Administer an epidural (see Chapter 100).
- Remove feces from the rectum.
- Place a tail wrap and tail rope on the mare (see Chapter 4).
- Wearing examination gloves, clean and dry the perineum of the mare (see Chapter 3).
- Make a 0.5 cm (0.2 inch) skin incision about 2 cm (0.75 inch) ventral to the ventral commissure of the vulva.
- Make a 0.5 cm skin incision about 2 cm above the dorsal commissure of the vulva.
- Cut a length of umbilical tape (or Buhner tape) 3 times the length of the Buhner needle length.
- Soak the umbilical tape in dilute (0.05%) povidone-iodine.
- Place the Buhner needle into the ventral incision and push the needle through the subcutaneous tissue so that the needle passes laterally to the vulva and exits at the dorsal incision. Placement of a hand into the vulva will aid in keeping the needle at the appropriate depth and to keep it from entering the vestibule. Care should be taken to not inadvertently pierce the hand with the Buhner needle.
- Thread one end of the tape into the eyelet on the Buhner needle (Figures 111.1 and 111.2) and pull the needle

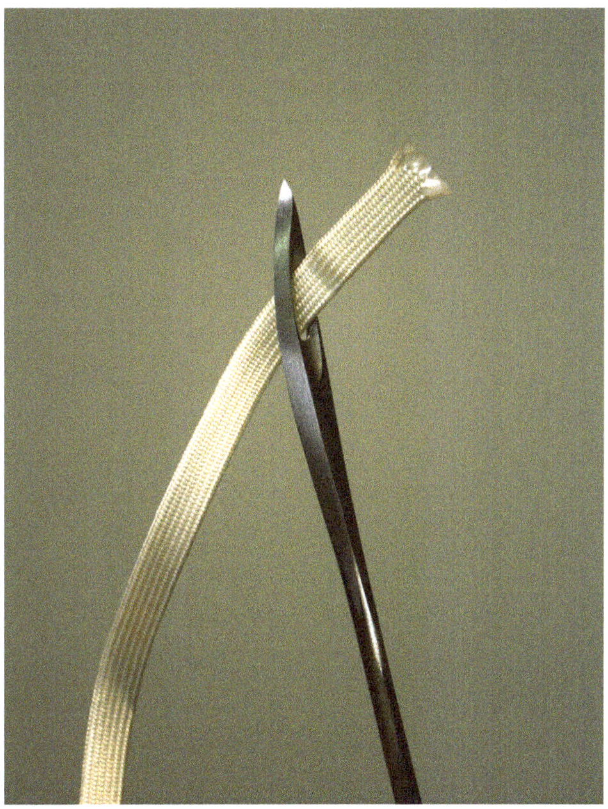

Figure 111.1 End of a Buhner needle with Buhner tape threaded through the eyelet.

Equine Reproductive Procedures, Second Edition. Edited by John Dascanio and Patrick McCue.

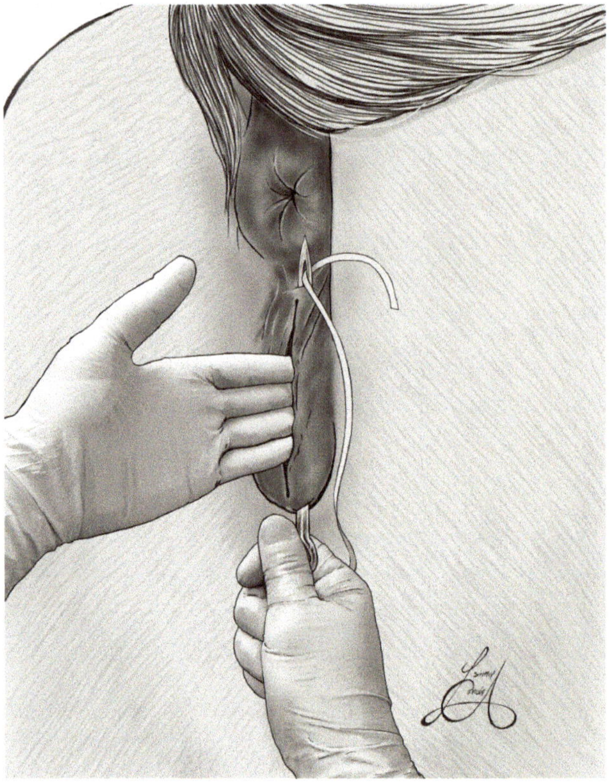

Figure 111.2 Buhner needle exited through dorsal incision, threaded, and about to be pulled downward to place the Buhner tape lateral to the right vulvar lip. Drawing courtesy of Dr Ismael Concha-Albornoz DVM, MVSc (www.anato.cl).

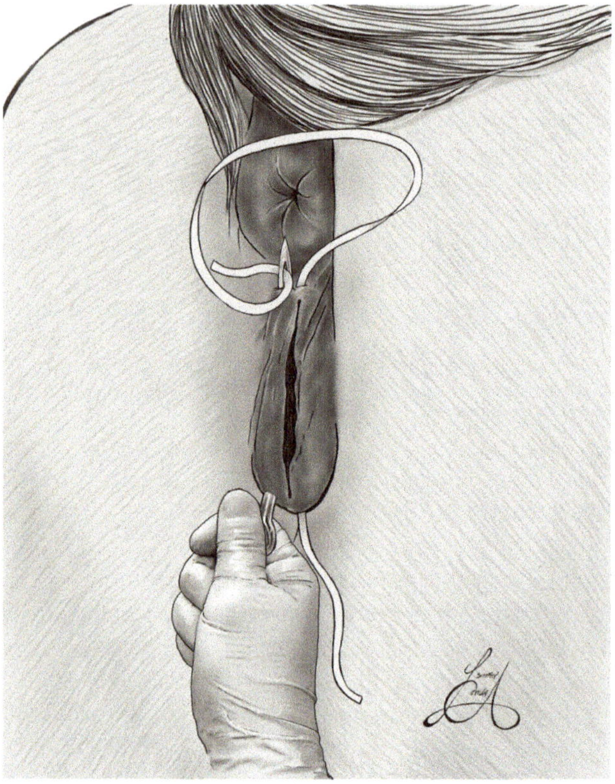

Figure 111.3 Buhner needle exited through same dorsal incision, threaded, and about to be pulled downward to place the Buhner tape lateral to the left vulvar lip. Drawing courtesy of Dr Ismael Concha-Albornoz DVM,MVSc (www.anato.cl).

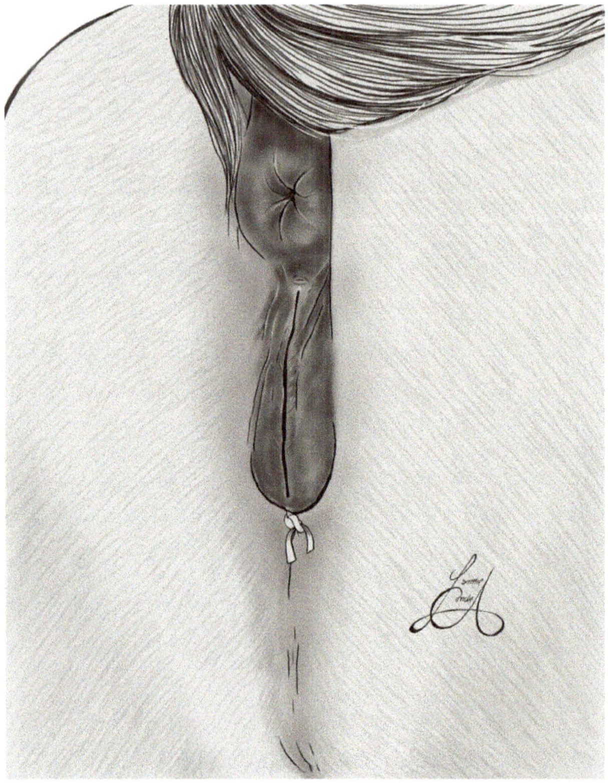

Figure 111.4 Buhner tape tied ventral to the vulva. Drawing courtesy of Dr Ismael Concha-Albornoz DVM,MVSc (www.anato.cl).

back through the subcutaneous tissue to exit the ventral incision.

- Remove the tape from the eyelet in the Buhner needle and repeat the procedure with the opposite side of the vulva (Figure 111.3). There should be two ends of the tape exiting the ventral incision with the middle of the tape loop present within the dorsal incision and the loop surrounding the vulvar opening.
- Tie a single throw with the tape ends (Figure 111.4). Pull this throw tight until the vulvar opening has about a 6 cm (2.4 inch) opening remaining to allow for urination (about three fingers wide).
- Tie a bow knot or double-slip knot to complete the peri-vulvar suture placement.

Interpretation

- The tape may be loosened in 3 days by untying the knot. The mare should be observed for any propensity to re-prolapse any reproductive tissue. If this appears imminent, then the tape should be re-tied. If everything appears normal, the tape may be cut at the dorsal aspect and both ends pulled through the subcutaneous tissue to remove the suture from the ventral end.
- There may be a slight discharge from the incisions where the tape was placed, but this should resolve over the next few days. There should be no evidence of a subcutaneous infection from the tape placement.
- Buhner tape is slightly different from umbilical tape. Umbilical tape will degrade over time if the tape is accidently left without removal, while the Buhner tape will remain indefinitely. In addition, umbilical tape will wick liquid and potentially bacteria, whereas Buhner tape is less likely to do this due to its construction and the material from which it is made.
- Two incisions may be made ventral to the vulva rather than one to pass each arm of the tape through. After placement through the subcutaneous tissue, the tape may then be threaded through a needle cap with the closed end removed to act as a stent preventing the knot from becoming buried in the soft tissue ventral to the vulva.

Part IV

Stallion

112

Breeding Soundness Evaluation

Patrick M. McCue

Equine Reproduction Laboratory, Colorado State University, USA

Introduction

A reproductive evaluation, often termed a breeding soundness examination (BSE), may be performed to: (i) estimate the future reproductive potential of a stallion; (ii) provide a routine evaluation prior to purchase; or (iii) determine the cause(s) of poor reproductive performance. The BSE should encompass the general health of the horse, behavior, mating ability, genital examination, semen evaluation, and other parameters. This chapter outlines the components of a BSE; details on specific aspects are presented in other chapters. A standardized stallion BSE form is available through the Society for Theriogenology (see Appendix A).

Examination Technique

Identification

Each stallion should be properly and positively identified prior to evaluation; registration name and number, age, and breed are recorded. Coat color and markings, lip tattoos, microchip information (if used), body brands, hair whorls, permanent scars, and any other identifying features should all be noted. A digital photograph may be valuable as part of the permanent medical record. The goal is to be able to accurately connect the results of a BSE to a specific stallion at a later date if necessary.

Reproductive History

A complete breeding history should be obtained as past breeding results (conception and foaling rates) are the best indicators of a stallion's previous fertility level. The number and type of mares bred per season (i.e., maiden, open, barren, and foaling mares) and the breeding method used (i.e., hand breeding, pasture breeding, or artificial insemination with fresh, cooled, or frozen semen) are recorded. The results of previous reproductive evaluations, medical conditions, vaccination history (especially vaccination against equine arteritis virus), and other significant information are noted. It is also important to record the intended future use of the stallion and the number of mares anticipated for the next season, as it will be important for breeding management recommendations.

Physical Examination

A general physical examination should be performed on each stallion. To be considered fertile, a stallion must be able to mount a mare in estrus, insert his penis into the vagina, thrust appropriately, and ejaculate completely. Musculoskeletal abnormalities that may interfere with mating ability, such as back, hock, or lameness issues, or neurologic problems should be identified along with other medical conditions. Any evidence of heritable or congenital conditions should be reported. The serum of stallions should be tested for the presence of antibodies against equine arteritis virus, the agent that causes equine viral arteritis. The current status for equine infectious anemia titers and contagious equine metritis cultures should be noted.

Examination of External Genitalia

The penis, prepuce, sheath, scrotum, and scrotal contents are routinely evaluated during a BSE. Inspection of the penis and prepuce is often performed after the stallion has either "dropped" his penis or gained an erection after teasing a mare in estrus. The penis should be of normal size and shape and be free of lesions. Palpation of the testes and

Equine Reproductive Procedures, Second Edition. Edited by John Dascanio and Patrick McCue.

epididymides are often performed after semen collection, as the stallion will be less excited and this will allow for a more complete and safe examination. There should be two testes fully descended into the scrotum. Each testis should be smooth, slightly turgid, and resilient on palpation, and freely movable within the scrotum. The tail of the epididymis should be easily palpated at the caudal pole of each testis. The spermatic cord should be identified on the cranial dorsal aspect of each testis.

Total scrotal width can be determined with scrotal calipers. Testicular volume is determined after measuring the length, width, and height of each individual testis with an ultrasound machine. Testicular volume can be used to estimate potential daily sperm production.

Ultrasound examination of the testes and other scrotal contents may also be performed in stallions to identify lesions within the testes or to characterize fluid within the scrotum.

Examination of Internal Genitalia

Examination of the internal genitalia of a stallion per rectum is not always performed as part of a reproductive evaluation, unless indicated by an abnormal history, physical examination findings, or abnormal semen parameters. This is performed, most commonly, after semen collection.

Evaluation for Venereal Disease

Microbiological aerobic culture swabs are routinely collected as part of a complete BSE. Swab samples to be collected prior to washing the stallion and collection of semen include the urethral fossa, urethra, shaft of the penis, and prepuce. A culture of the urethra should be done after sexual arousal so that pre-ejaculatory seminal fluid is present at the distal urethra. After semen collection, a second swab from the urethra is obtained and the semen itself is often cultured. The post-ejaculate urethral swab is considered to be similar to a culture of the semen. A positive post-ejaculate urethral culture suggests an infection of the urethra, accessory sex glands, or epididymis.

Libido and Mating Ability

A stallion's libido when teased to a mare in estrus and ability to gain and maintain an erection are recorded. Subsequently, the ability to mount a mare or breeding phantom, insert the penis into the mare or artificial vagina, thrust, and ability to ejaculate completely are all noted.

Semen Evaluation

Semen is often collected in an artificial vagina twice, 1 hour apart, as part of a BSE. Assessment of each ejaculate should include: (i) a gross evaluation of semen quality; (ii) determination of semen pH; (iii) determination of the volume of gel-free semen; (iv) determination of sperm concentration; (v) calculation of the total number of sperm in the ejaculate; (vi) estimation of the percentage of sperm that are progressively motile; (vii) determination of the percentage of morphologically normal spermatozoa in the ejaculate; and, finally (viii) calculation of the number of progressively motile, morphologically normal sperm in the ejaculate.

It is anticipated that: (i) the total number of spermatozoa on the second ejaculate of most horses will be approximately one half that of the first ejaculate; (ii) the volume of the two ejaculates will be approximately equal; (iii) the pH should remain the same or go up slightly; and (iv) the spermatozoal motility should stay the same or increase. Semen parameters of the second ejaculate are used as an estimate of daily sperm output. True daily sperm output is determined after collection from the stallion once per day for 5–7 days.

Gross evaluation of semen quality

The gel fraction of the semen, produced by the seminal vesicles, is removed using an in-line filter or by aspiration into a syringe, and is discarded without further evaluation. The gel-free semen is transferred into a warm, graduated cylinder and initially evaluated for color and consistency. Color changes may be associated with the presence of debris, blood, urine, or purulent material (i.e., infection of the reproductive tract).

pH

A pH meter should ideally be used to determine the pH of raw semen (see Chapter 140). The normal pH of equine semen ranges from 7.2 to 7.7. The pH of normal stallion semen can be affected by season, frequency of ejaculation, and sperm concentration. Inflammation of the reproductive tract or contamination of the ejaculate with soap or urine can lead to an abnormally high pH.

Volume

The volume (in milliliters) of gel-free semen is determined using a graduated cylinder. An accurate assessment of volume is critical for the determination of total number of spermatozoa in an ejaculate. Volume of the ejaculate may be increased following excessive teasing of a stallion to a mare in estrus prior to collection. However, the concentration of sperm per milliliter is reduced, and as a consequence the overall number of sperm in the ejaculate is not affected. Concentration and volume are thus inversely related: the higher the concentration, the lower the volume, and vice versa.

Concentration

Concentration of spermatozoa per milliliter in the ejaculate may be manually counted using a hemocytometer or estimated using a commercial calibrated spectrophotometer or cell counter (see Chapters 127-129).

Motility

An accurate evaluation of sperm motility is an important component of the BSE. The motility of raw, gel-free semen may be difficult to evaluate accurately since the concentration is often too high to examine individual cells, and sperm cells in raw semen tend to clump or agglutinate. Consequently, raw semen is usually diluted to a concentration of 25 million sperm per milliliter with warm semen extender to aid in the evaluation of total and progressive sperm motility (see Chapter 130-131).

Longevity of sperm motility is used as an indicator of ejaculate quality. Longevity can be determined by the evaluation of motion characteristics over time for raw and extended semen samples maintained at either room temperature (20–25°C, 68–77°F) (see Chapter 147) or cooled to refrigerator temperature (4–6°C, 39–43°F).

Morphology

Sperm morphology can be determined after staining with an eosin-nigrosin stain, which has also been used as a "live-dead" stain. An alternative is to preserve semen in buffered formol-saline, prepare a wet mount slide, and examine the semen sample using a phase-contrast microscope or a differential interference contrast (DIC) microscope (see Chapters 132-133 and 136-138).

Other Tests

The presence of an adequate number of motile spermatozoa in an ejaculate is no guarantee of fertility. If the results of a standard BSE do not identify a cause of subfertility or infertility, additional diagnostic tests may be indicated (Table 112.1).

Daily Sperm Output

Daily sperm output is determined after sperm collection from a stallion once per day for a minimum of 5–7 days to deplete the extragonadal sperm reserves (epididymis and

Table 112.1 Diagnostic tests that may be performed in addition to the standard tests in a stallion breeding soundness evaluation.

Test	Indication
Sperm chromatin structure assay	To evaluate the structural integrity of sperm chromatin by determining the susceptibility of sperm DNA to denaturation *in vitro*
Fluorescent stains	Evaluation of plasma membrane integrity (5-CFDA and PI), viability (SYBR-14), acrosomal integrity (PSA), or mitochondrial function (JC-1 and rhodamine 123)
Hypo-osmotic swelling test	Evaluation to determine if the sperm plasma membrane is intact and osmotically active
Sperm capacitation test	To determine the percentage of sperm that are capacitated and able to undergo the acrosome reaction (CTC assay and merocyanine 540)
Acrosome reaction tests	To determine the percentage of acrosome-intact and acrosome-reacted sperm in untreated semen (FITC-PNA) and to evaluate the ability of spermatozoa to undergo the acrosome reaction *in vitro* (calcium ionophore A23187)
Transmission electron microscopy	Evaluation of ultrastructure detail of spermatozoa and to evaluate the acrosome status of the sperm
Chromosome analysis	To evaluate numeric or structural changes in chromosomes
Testicular biopsy	Histologic evaluation of the testicular parenchyma
Hormone analysis (baseline and provocative endocrine tests)	To evaluate pituitary and gonadal endocrine function
Ultrasound	Evaluation of the accessory sex glands, penis, testes, and scrotum
Alkaline phosphatase test	Evaluation of ejaculatory function in azoospermic stallions
Urethral endoscopy	To evaluate urethral integrity in stallions with hemospermia

CFDA, 5-carboxyfluorescein diacetate; CTC, chlortetracycline; FITC, fluorescein isothiocyanate; JC-1, tetraethylbenzimidazolylcarbocyanine iodide; PI, propidium iodide; PNA, peanut agglutinin; PSA, plant agglutinin; SYBR-14, permeable DNA-binding dye.

ductus deferens) (see Chapter 134). Thereafter, the total number of sperm collected each day will be relatively constant and represents the number of sperm produced each day. The determination of daily sperm output can be used to estimate the number of mares that may be bred per day and therefore the number of mares that may be booked to a stallion for a season.

Interpretation and Additional Comments

Interpretation of the results of a stallion BSE should take into account the number of mares to be bred and the type of breeding program to be utilized (i.e., live cover or insemination with fresh, cooled, or frozen semen). Accepted values for semen analysis are: (i) a minimum of 60% progressively motile spermatozoa and 60% morphologically normal spermatozoa in each ejaculate collected; and (ii) a minimum of 1.0 billion progressively motile, morphologically normal spermatozoa in the second of two ejaculates collected 1 hour apart after sexual rest for 1 week at any time of the year.

Based on the overall results of the reproductive evaluation, stallions are classified as satisfactory, questionable, or unsatisfactory breeding prospects. The original guidelines for the BSE suggested that a satisfactory prospective breeder could expect a minimum pregnancy rate of 75% if booked to breed 40 mares by natural service or 120 mares by artificial insemination. It is well recognized that current book sizes for many stallions are well above the original "40/120" guideline. With these stallions, it may be advantageous to evaluate semen quality at daily sperm output to determine if there are sufficient progressively motile, morphologically normal sperm available for the anticipated book size. If the stallion has had a significant medical condition (i.e., fever or colic) recently, it may be recommended to re-evaluate him in 60–70 days before a final classification is assigned after the next spermatogenic wave has matured.

If the BSE identifies a stallion with a potential reproductive problem, management or therapeutic programs can be instituted to optimize future fertility. It is important to emphasize that the final criteria upon which to assess stallion fertility are ultimately the conception and foaling rates in mares bred.

113

Training the Stallion to Use a Phantom

John J. Dascanio

School of Veterinary Medicine, Texas Tech University, USA

Introduction

Training a stallion to use a phantom, breeding dummy, or breeding mount can take just a couple of training sessions or may require many sessions over several days or weeks depending on the nature of a particular stallion. It is difficult to predict which stallions will fall into each category until the training sessions start. Typically, a stallion that has had semen collected using a jump mare with an artificial vagina (AV) is the easiest to train to a phantom. A stallion that has never been allowed to interact with a mare or has never bred a mare previously may be more challenging to train. The key to training a stallion is to have excellent assistants, a mare in good estrus, proper facilities, and to titrate the exposure to stimuli properly.

Equipment and Supplies

Phantom, proper padded teasing wall, mare in good heat or an estrogen-treated ovariectomized mare, artificial vagina, experienced assistants, wash bucket or bottle to wash stallion's penis, examination gloves, paper towels, urine from mare in estrus (optional).

Technique

- The area used for training the stallion should be free of visual or auditory distractors.
- The ground behind the phantom should be level and provide adequate traction so that the stallion's hind feet will not slip during mounting and thrusting. Slippery or unsure footing will inhibit some stallions from mounting the phantom.
- The stallion should be handled with a chain over the nose or a lead line with a bit in the mouth. In Europe, it is common to lead the stallion from the left side of the horse and to collect semen from the right side of the horse. In many other parts of the world, including North America, the handler and semen collector are both on the left side of the stallion. More severe restraints such as a chain in the mouth or over the gums may inhibit some novice stallions from achieving adequate sexual responses. Sometimes having two lead lines, one over the nose or hooked to the halter and a second in the mouth, can allow guidance for direction and correction of behavior separately, but may make the stallion handler's job more difficult in manipulating two lead lines simultaneously.
- If the stallion has never been near a phantom, walking him up to it and allowing him to smell and interact with the phantom should be undertaken prior to any training session, so that he is not apprehensive of approaching the equipment.
- Caution and safety precautions should be exercised when attempting to wash the penis of a novice stallion. The novice stallion may kick out if his ventral abdomen is touched, when his penis is first touched, or when warm water is first applied. If there are too many stimuli for the stallion (i.e., the jump mare is too close), there is more propensity for a stallion to kick out or rear from washing as he desires contact with the mare.
- Stimuli that may be used to achieve/maintain a stallion's erection are the visual, auditory, and olfactory stimuli from direct interaction with a mare in estrus (Figure 113.1), use of urine collected from a mare in estrus, massage of the prepuce (to entice the stallion to drop his penis and gain an erection), cupping of the glans penis with the hand, massage of the glans penis with the fingers, manual pressure on the base of the penis, and

Equine Reproductive Procedures, Second Edition. Edited by John Dascanio and Patrick McCue.

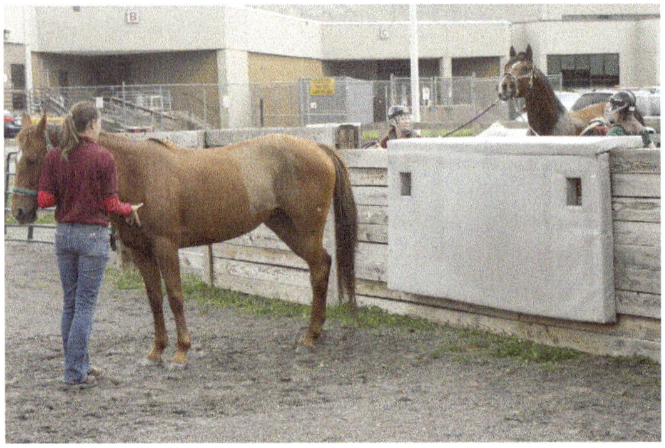

Figure 113.1 Mare positioned in front of a phantom across a teasing wall to provide visual stimulation for the stallion during semen collection.

washing of the penis with warm water (see Chapter 123). The stallion may tease an estral mare across a phantom, using teasing stocks (Figure 113.2), with the mare in a stall or across a fence.

- There should be a plan as to how a stallion is routinely led from his stall or paddock to the collection area. This should include an area where the stallion is routinely stopped prior to entering the collection area.
- The stimuli provided to the stallion may be titrated to enhance or remove stimulation. This would depend on the stallion-handling facilities, personnel, and the individual stallion. An example would be in an open paddock where the mare may be positioned further from the stallion or the stallion turned away from the mare to decrease visualization. In an enclosed collection shed, either the stallion or the mare may be removed from the collection area to quiet the stallion if he becomes too excited by the collection procedure.
- The mare used to provide visual stimulation may be placed at some distance from the stallion. The mare may be brought closer to the stallion as needed to enhance his interest and libido. The mare should be kept as far away from the stallion as possible while still maintaining his interest, so that he does not become too aggressive in attempting to interact with the mare. With some stallions, as long as they are well behaved and controllable, the mare may be placed adjacent to the phantom, on the side opposite to his approach, to enhance his interest (Figure 113.3). Typically, the stallion would approach the left rear corner of the phantom with a mare positioned on the right side of the phantom. Otherwise, it may be prudent to keep the stallion and mare separated with a teasing wall.

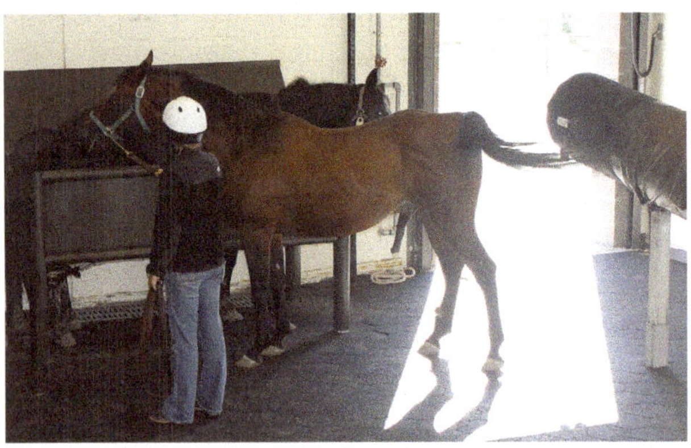

Figure 113.2 Stallion teasing an estral mare in stocks in close approximation to a phantom.

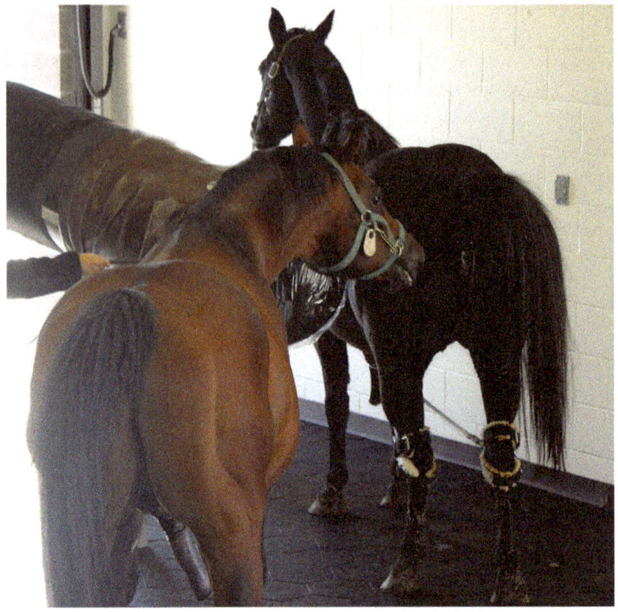

Figure 113.3 Estral mare in hobbles positioned on the opposite side of a phantom. The stallion is approaching at a 45-degree angle to the phantom.

- The stallion should be directed toward the phantom using a large circular pattern. Approximately 9–12 m (30–40 feet) from the phantom, the stallion should be stopped and the penis washed and dried to remove debris and to stimulate his erection. This also teaches the stallion to not always go directly to the phantom. Cupping of the hand over the end of the glans penis may be done to maintain the stallion's erection and to encourage thrusting activity during washing (see Chapter 123). This will be helpful once the stallion is near the phantom to encourage mounting activity.
- During the approach to the phantom, the stallion should be stopped or alternatively backed up to ensure his attention and compliance. This should be unpredicted by the stallion so that he does not know what command may come next to ensure his attention.

- The stallion must be well halter broken and must follow commands from the stallion handler. In the last 6 m (20 feet) or so to the phantom, the stallion should be allowed to approach the phantom under control, but without undue impedance so that he may position himself for mounting. He should not rush the phantom, but should be allowed to walk at a brisk pace.
- The stallion must not circle around the handler on the way to the phantom. This presents the stallion's hind end to others and demonstrates a lack of stallion control. If it is impossible to prevent the stallion from circling, a second lead line may be placed on the side opposite the first so that two handlers may be used to keep the stallion walking straight.
- A paper towel soaked in urine from a mare in heat may be used to provide pheromones for enhancing stimulation. It is common to present this towel to the stallion prior to washing the penis to encourage erection of the penis. Rubbing this towel on the phantom may make the phantom more attractive to the stallion. During actual placement of the AV on the stallion's penis during mounting, the towel may be presented to the stallion to smell during thrusting. Some stallions that rear or climb up the phantom during thrusting may be inhibited from that activity by the presentation of an estral towel to refocus their attention.
- The stallion should be orientated with his chest against the back part of the phantom. Sometimes bouncing his chest against the back of the phantom may stimulate the stallion to mount the phantom. If this does not occur, or the stallion does not freely mount the phantom, some stimuli to the glans penis may encourage mounting. The hand may be cupped and pressure applied directly to the glans penis or the AV may be slid onto the distal penis to cause a reflex mounting activity (Figure 113.4).
- If the mare is positioned next to the phantom, usually on the right side of the phantom, the stallion should approach the phantom from the left hind corner in order to keep the phantom between the mare and the stallion. If the stallion desires to mount the mare, he may be directed toward the phantom with a lead attached to his halter as he is mounting. The lead should not be disciplinary, as would occur with a chain shank, as this would decrease his desire to service the AV.
- The phantom may need to be adjusted for the height of the stallion, so that the top of the rear of the phantom is about the height of the thoracic inlet of the stallion or the height of the mares the stallion would normally service. The angle of the phantom should be such that the front of the phantom is higher than the rear by about 15 cm.
- The stallion handler should communicate freely with the semen collector to alert them as to the stallion's position on the phantom and any need to move if the stallion dismounts expectantly or inappropriately.

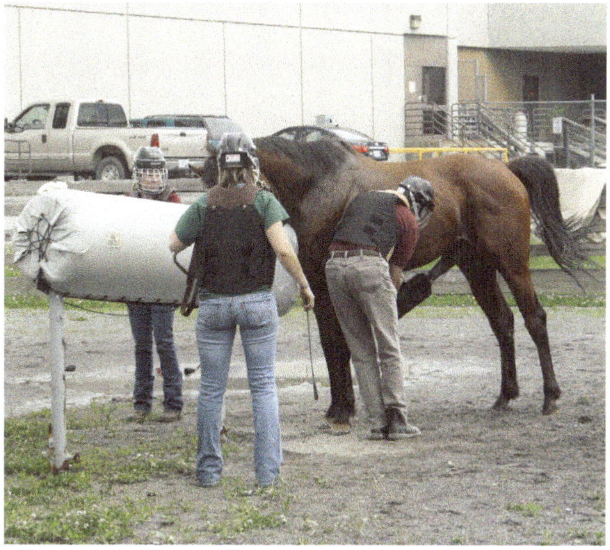

Figure 113.4 Placement of an artificial vagina on the glans penis to stimulate mounting activity by a stallion.

Interpretation

- If a stallion does not ejaculate during multiple mount attempts on the phantom, the training session should be terminated for that day and all procedures evaluated to determine any improvements in technique.
- The stallion may acquire rub sores on the inside of the forearms from gripping the phantom, or may get rub sores on the penis from hitting the phantom with an erect penis or multiple intromissions into an AV. Sometimes training sessions need to be suspended if this occurs. Alternatively, the stallion's front legs or the phantom may be wrapped to prevent injury or to prevent further irritation.
- A different type of AV may be tried to provide alternative stimulation if the stallion refuses to ejaculate with the use of a phantom.
- A low dose tranquilizer such as 100 mg of xylazine for a 450 kg horse may lower their ejaculatory threshold.
- A reluctant stallion may also be allowed to mount a mare in estrus for a semen collection with an AV in order to get him used to the AV. The stallion could then be transitioned back to the phantom with the mare next to the phantom.
- A biting strap or grip rope wrapped around the phantom may make the stallion more comfortable about holding onto the phantom (Figure 113.5).
- It is not uncommon for a novice stallion to mount the phantom, have the AV placed on the penis, thrust, and not ejaculate. Ejaculation may be stimulated by increasing the pressure and temperature of the AV.

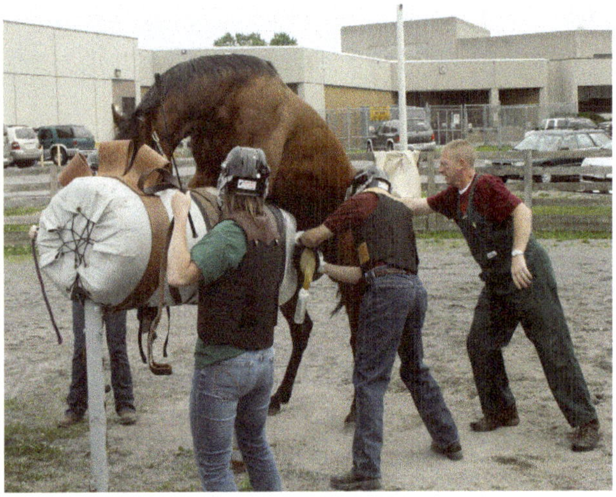

Figure 113.5 Stallion mounted on a phantom with an extra person pushing the stallion's hip to keep him aligned with the phantom. Note the bite bar and leather forearm grip on the phantom.

- If a disposable liner is used in the AV and the stallion will not ejaculate, remove the disposable liner and use a rubber or latex liner to change the feel of the AV to the stallion.
- Massaging of the glans penis through the AV or manual hand pressure on the base of the penis may enhance ejaculation.
- An extra person may be needed to keep the stallion from working his way up the side of the phantom during thrusting into the AV. The role of this person is to push against the point of the hip (tuber coxae) to keep the stallion in line with the long axis of the phantom (Figure 113.5). If the stallion comes around the side of the phantom and works his way forward, his front feet may come off the front of the phantom or he could turn sideways on the phantom.
- Once ejaculation has occurred, a subsequent training session may be conducted with the mare or other stimulus further removed from the stallion.
- Typically, once ejaculation occurs with a training session, further training sessions are more successful and require less time.
- Training sessions (once successful) should be repeated every other day for 1 week and then weekly to reinforce the collection process.
- If the stallion goes around the phantom to get to a mare near the phantom, the mare handler should move the mare to try to keep the phantom between the stallion and the mare to prevent the stallion from mounting the mare.
- The phantom should be disinfected between stallions to avoid transmission of contagious diseases Wrapping the back half of the phantom with disposable clear 45–50 cm (18–20 inch) wide stretch film wrap between stallions may also be used to prevent transmission of pathogenic organisms.

Further Reading

Crump J, Crump J. 1989. Stallion ejaculation induced by manual stimulation of the penis. *Theriogenology* 31: 341–6.

McDonnell SM. 2007. Starting a novice breeding stallion. *Clin Tech Eq Pract* 6: 232–8.

114

Missouri Artificial Vagina

John J. Dascanio[1] and Lynda M. J. Miller[2]

[1] *School of Veterinary Medicine, Texas Tech University, USA*
[2] *College of Veterinary Medicine, Lincoln Memorial University, USA*

Introduction

The Missouri artificial vagina (AV) consists of an outer leather jacket and a double-walled rubber liner. The liner has an attached cone on one end that is made of a single layer of rubber. The Missouri AV is one of two main AVs used in North America, the other being the Colorado AV. In Europe, the Hannover AV is the predominant AV used.

The Missouri AV has some advantages in that it is easy to fill, allows some external manipulation of the stallion's penis through the AV, heats up relatively quickly, allows semen to be deposited in the cone end past the warm water bladder, and is intermediate in weight (the Colorado AV is the heaviest). The Missouri AV may be used with or without an inner disposable plastic liner. The liner allows for easier clean-up and better control of infectious disease transmission, but some stallions may not like the feel of the plastic over the rubber liner.

Equipment and Supplies

Missouri artificial vagina, optional plastic disposable liner, baby bottle, in-line filter, disposable baby bottle liners, 2.5 cm (1 inch) white dressing tape, non-spermicidal lubricant, sterile obstetrical sleeve, warm water to fill the AV, thermometer, pump with hose or faucet adapter with hose for filling the AV, optional weight scale, insulated cover for baby bottle.

Technique

- A warm water source is needed to fill the AV. This may be accomplished by a bucket heater or increasing the temperature of a piped hot water heater. The filling temperature should be around 52°C (125°F).
- If using a disposable AV liner, it should be inserted prior to attachment of the collection bottle. The disposable liner is everted over each end of the AV and secured with 2.5 cm (1 inch) white dressing or medical tape.
- An in-line semen filter is placed inside a new plastic bag or liner (i.e., baby bottle liner bag or Whirl-Pak® bag), which will remove gel and debris. The plastic liner bag is subsequently inserted into the collection bottle (i.e., baby bottle). The tops of the filter and baby bottle liner are everted over the top of the collection bottle.
- An adapter cap previously fixed onto the coned end of the AV is screwed onto the collection bottle. This cap will go over the filter/bag and secure them to the bottle (Figures 114.1–114.3).
- Optionally, 2.5 cm white dressing or medical tape may be wound in a spiral fashion from the baby bottle, over the adapter, and up onto the cone end of the AV to help

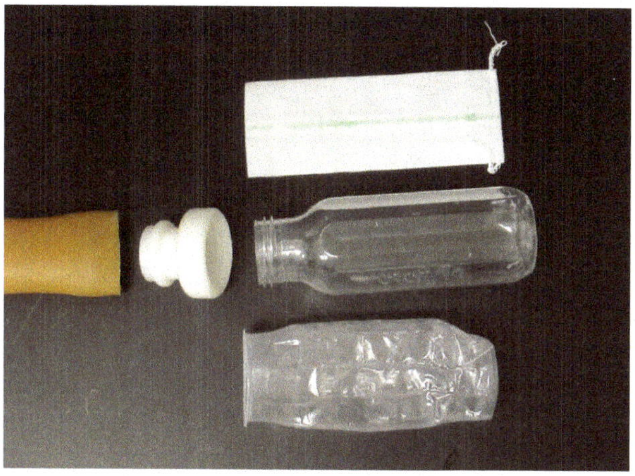

Figure 114.1 Adapter cap, collection bottle (center), baby bottle liner (below), and filter (above) adjacent to the cone end of a Missouri artificial vagina.

Equine Reproductive Procedures, Second Edition. Edited by John Dascanio and Patrick McCue.

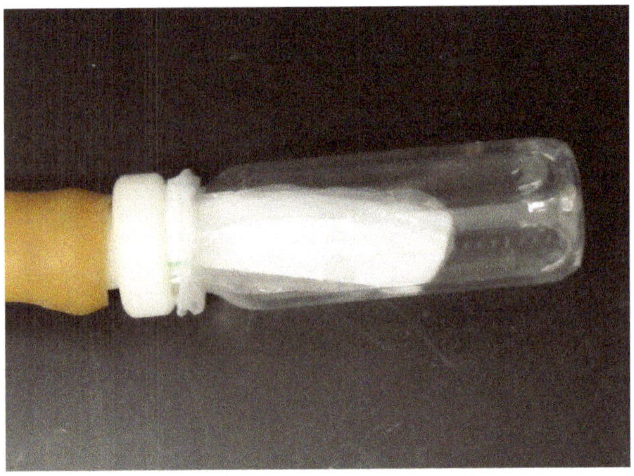

Figure 114.2 Components put together and attached to the cone end of a Missouri artificial vagina.

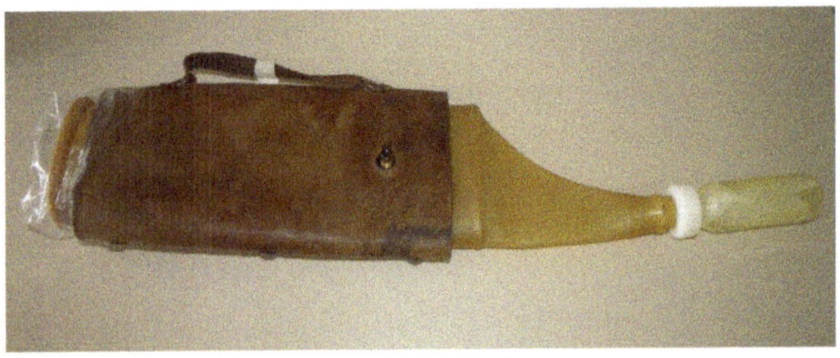

Figure 114.3 Fully assembled Missouri artificial vagina.

secure the bottle to the AV (Figure 114.4). If this is not done, the bottle may become detached during collection due to stallion movement.

- Remove the valve stem from the water port on the AV and set aside to use later.
- If the ambient temperature in the area to collect the stallion is cold, the AV may be prefilled with warm water to warm up the rubber liner. The water is then removed and the AV refilled with hot water of the correct temperature prior to collection. As noted above, the filling temperature of the AV should be around 52°C (125°F). Pre-warming the AV prevents the temperature in the AV from decreasing too quickly prior to collection.
- Fill the AV through the water port using a direct sink/faucet connection or a pump with appropriate hosing (if filling from a bucket), until the AV becomes distended with water. Quickly remove the hose attached to the filling port and insert the valve stem to seal the port.
- Don a sterile obstetrical sleeve and place non-spermicidal lubricant in the palm of the hand in the sleeve. Insert the gloved hand into the large open end of the AV and distribute lubricant circumferentially around the inside of the AV to about halfway down its length.
- The pressure within the lumen of the AV may be adjusted depending on the needs of the stallion by adding or

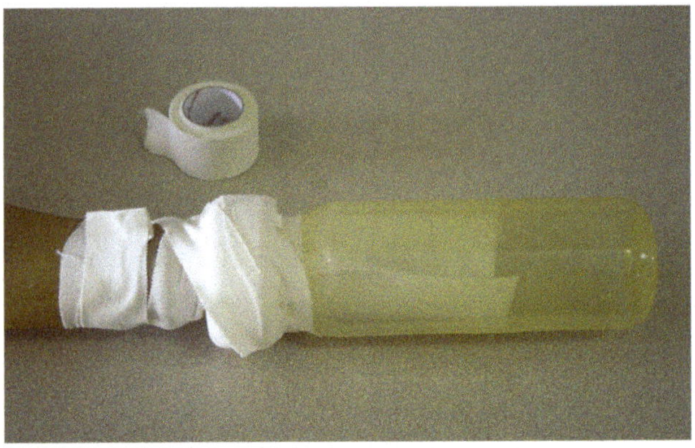

Figure 114.4 White dressing tape on the bottle and liner.

removing water from the AV. Typically, a balled-up fist should be able to be inserted one half to three fourths of the way through the AV.

- The sleeve should be taken off the arm and left inserted in the AV until the time of collection. This will prevent the lubricant from drying out.
- The temperature of the water within the AV should be at approximately 48°C (118°F) at the time of collection or slightly lower to prevent thermal damage to spermatozoa if the semen comes into contact with the water-filled liner. A thermometer inserted into the AV lumen may be used to monitor the temperature. Occasionally, a higher temperature in the AV may be required for a stallion being trained to collect. If a particular stallion requires an AV warmer than 48°C (118°F), the Missouri AV allows for the semen to be deposited past the warm water bladder, preventing thermal damage as long as the semen is deposited into the cone end. If the ambient temperature in the area used to collect the stallion's semen is cool, an insulated cover may be fitted over the baby bottle to prevent temperature shock to the semen. A wool sock over the bottle or a commercial cover over the bottle and AV cone may be used.
- Just prior to collection, as the stallion is mounting the mare or phantom, the obstetrical sleeve is removed from the AV and may be retained for possible reuse if the first collection attempt is not successful.
- Once the AV is placed on the stallion's penis, it is held even with the mare's hind end or the end of the phantom.
- Additional stimulation may be provided by massaging the stallion's glans penis through the cone end of the Missouri AV (Figure 114.5). Typically the stallion's penis will contact the cone if properly fitted.
- Ejaculation can be confirmed by detection of pulses in the urethra near the base of the penis or observing characteristic flagging of the tail. Visualization of the ejaculate will not be possible if an insulating cover has been placed over the collection bottle.

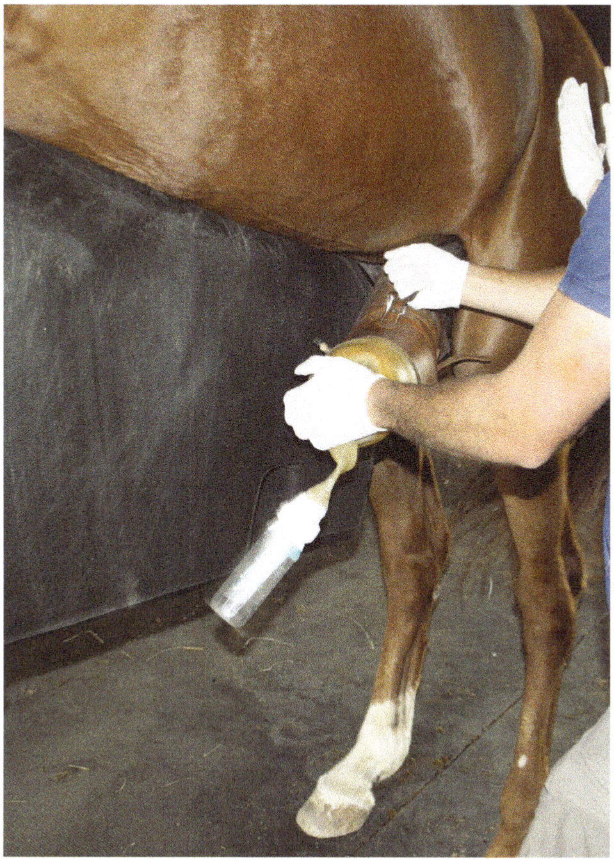

Figure 114.5 Massage of the glans penis through the rubber cone to enhance stallion stimulation.

- Following removal of the AV from the penis, it should be held in a vertical position to prevent semen from spilling outward. The valve stem in the water fill port should be removed to allow water to drain out. Deflating the AV will also allow any semen trapped in the water jacket to flow into the collection bottle. Care should be taken so that water does not enter the AV and negatively affect spermatozoal function.
- The collection bottle is removed from the AV and the filter is removed from the plastic liner and discarded. The liner is removed from the bottle and the semen processed.
- The AV should be cleaned, disinfected, and dried prior to reuse:
- Disposable gloved/sleeves should be worn to clean the AV and the gloves should be changed between each cleaning procedure.
- Rinse the AV liner, inside and outside, thoroughly in hot (>50°C (122°F)) running tap water. Use a clean large bottle, flask, beaker, or brush to aid in the removal of any particulate matter that is adhered to the latex rubber. The brush should be cleaned with hot water and 70% isopropyl alcohol between uses. Since soaps or disinfectants may permeate the latex rubber and subsequently leach into semen, their use is not recommended.
- Rinse the AV with 70% isopropyl or ethyl alcohol in its entirety. Rinsing can be done by dipping the AV into a large vat of alcohol or by using a squirt or spray bottle designed for this purpose.
- Hang the AV in a clean, covered cabinet for drying and storage. The storage area should be protected from UV rays and natural sunlight to avoid drying and cracking of the latex rubber over time.
- Thoroughly rinse the sink used for cleaning the AV with tap water followed by 70% alcohol after each use.
- The case/cover of the AV should also be thoroughly cleaned with hot water, sprayed or rinsed with 70% isopropyl alcohol, and allowed to air dry.

Interpretation

- If the stallion will not ejaculate into the Missouri AV a number of possible actions may be attempted:
  - Remove the disposable AV liner if present.
  - Increase the water volume and thus AV pressure.
  - Increase the water temperature. Occasionally, if the outside temperature is very low, a lowering of the AV temperature may be successful to limit the temperature differential to the stallion's penis.
- Stallions will generally prefer a specific combination of pressure and temperature. The amount of pressure can be determined by adding the same volume of water each time, which can be determined by weight.
- In some breeding farms, each stallion will have a specific AV dedicated to that individual horse for repeatability of AV preparation and biosecurity.

Further Reading

American Association of Equine Practitioners. 2019. Biosecurity Guidelines for Control of Venereally Transmitted Diseases. https://aaep.org/guidelines/infectious-disease-control/biosecurity-guidelines-control-venereally-transmitted-diseases (last accessed October 2020).

Love CC. 1992. Semen collection techniques. *Vet Clin North Am Eq Pract* 8: 111–28.

115

Colorado Model Artificial Vagina

Patrick M. McCue

Equine Reproduction Laboratory, Colorado State University, USA

Introduction

The Colorado model artificial vagina (AV) consists of a rigid plastic case with a handle and a port for filling the system with water (Figure 115.1). A straight, latex rubber tube is used to create a "bladder" within the plastic case that can be filled with warm water. A second latex rubber tube with a coned end serves as a reusable liner during semen collection. The liner is removed and washed in between uses. Other components of the AV include a disposable collection bottle, disposable nylon mesh gel filter, and an insulated cover to protect the collection bottle from sunlight and temperature fluctuations.

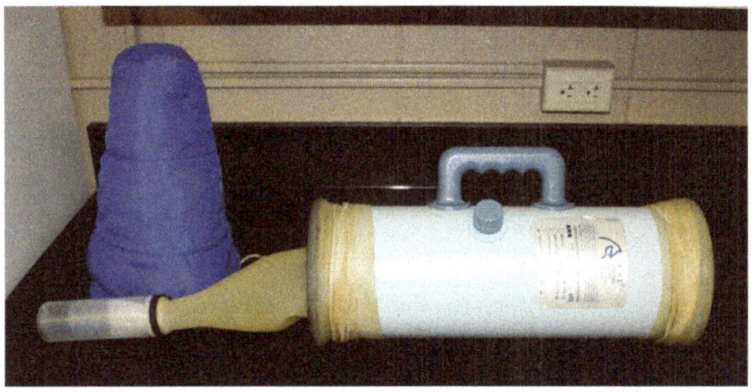

Figure 115.1 Colorado model artificial vagina and collection cover.

Equipment and Supplies

Artificial vagina case, rubber bands (large), round reusable latex collection liner, disposable plastic collection liner, 165 mm (6.5 inch) large clamp, disposable collection bottle (200 ml) with disposable coupling nut, disposable nylon mesh gel filter, small clamp, disposable coupling nut, obstetrical lubricant (sterile, non-spermicidal), collection bottle cover, collection bottle cover warmer, thermometer.

Technique for Assembly of the Colorado Model Artificial Vagina

- The Colorado model AV is easiest to assemble if an assembly stand is used (Figure 115.2). The plastic AV case is placed on the assembly stand (handle down) and the tubular latex bladder is passed down the center of the case.
- The latex bladder is first reflected over the rubber collar of the *posterior* end of the AV case (the end the penis of the stallion will enter). A rubber band should be placed snugly (two or three wraps) over the reflected bladder to hold it in place to prevent slippage and leakage of water. By stretching the rubber band to its maximum possible length, it is possible to get several wraps around the bladder and AV case. It is essential that this junction be tight, since the tubular latex bladder is not removed routinely, but cleaned while in the AV case.
- The next step is to reflect the other end of the tubular latex bladder over the anterior end of the AV case. This is the first point in assembling the AV in which it is possible to adjust the internal diameter, and ultimately internal pressure. Increasing the tautness, that is, the amount that the latex bladder is stretched before it is reflected over the anterior end of the AV case, reduces the amount of water that can be added. Conversely, a loose bladder will allow more water to be added and permits an increase in internal pressure.
- Once the bladder is appropriately positioned, a rubber band is also used on the anterior end. When the bladder is in place, the inside should resemble a smooth tube with the rubber stretched equally all the way around the inside of the AV case.

Equine Reproductive Procedures, Second Edition. Edited by John Dascanio and Patrick McCue.

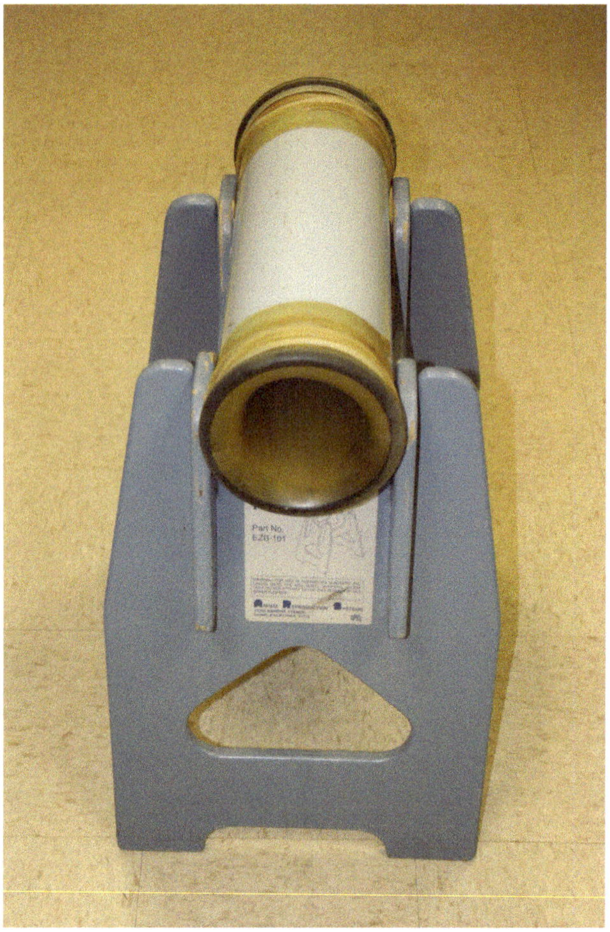

Figure 115.2 Assembly stand with a Colorado model artificial vagina after insertion of the latex bladder.

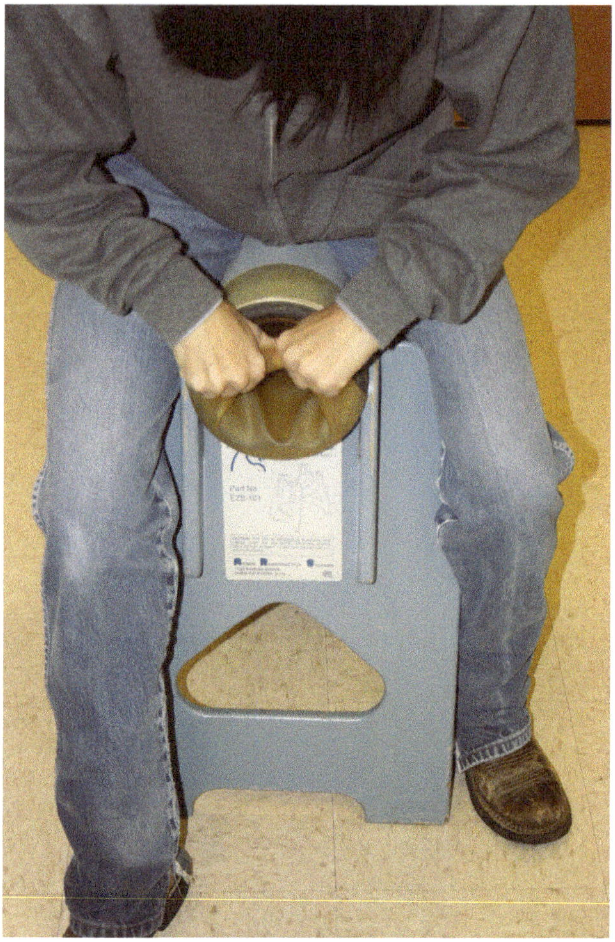

Figure 115.3 Insertion of the latex liner into the artificial vagina case; note that the bladder is already attached.

- A collection liner is inserted through the center of the AV case, and reflected over the posterior end of the AV case and tubular latex bladder (Figure 115.3).
- The collection liner must be free of twists, folds, or wrinkles and be reflected completely over the rubber collar to prevent it slipping during collection. Stretching the reusable latex collection liner over the posterior end of the AV case is an art. The rubber is relatively thick and is smaller in diameter than the flared, posterior end of the AV case. Consequently, considerable stretching is necessary to reflect the rubber over the posterior end. A rubber band is therefore not needed to hold this liner in place. Unfortunately, if the stretching and reflecting is not done in one smooth, fluid movement, the rubber may tear, especially if brute force is used. This should be avoided as reusable latex collection liners are relatively expensive, and it is time consuming to start over.
- Disposable liners can be convenient and effective. However, a disposable plastic collection liner is more likely to become twisted or wrinkled within the AV than a latex collection liner. Therefore, more precautions are necessary to position a disposable plastic liner properly than for a reusable latex collection liner. Stallions generally object to creases and wrinkles in a collection liner, particularly with a disposable plastic liner. Once the disposable plastic collection liner is appropriately positioned, the flared end is reflected over the posterior end of the AV case. Since the plastic has little or no stretch, a large clamp (165 mm (6.5 inch diameter)) or second large rubber band must be used to hold the disposable plastic collection liner in place. It is advisable to pull on the tapered end of the liner during filling to ensure that wrinkles and twists do not develop, particularly when a disposable liner is being used. Some stallions may not respond favorably to the feel of the plastic disposable liner against their penis, and prefer the feel of the latex collection liner.
- After the AV is filled with water, a thermometer is placed inside to monitor the temperature. When the internal temperature has stabilized at 48–50°C (approximately 118–122°F), the AV ready for lubrication and use.

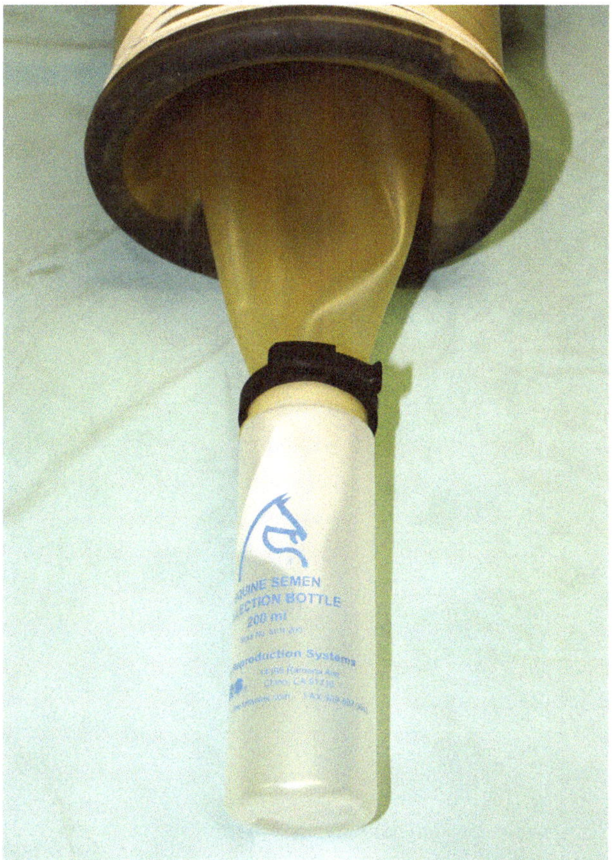

Figure 115.4 Collection bottle attached to the latex liner.

- A disposable collection bottle is fitted with a disposable nylon mesh gel filter. The collection bottle, with gel filter assembly, is placed into the tapered end of the latex collection liner, and held in place with a small clamp (45 mm (1.8 inches)) (Figure 115.4).
- When a disposable plastic collection liner is to be used, the tapered end is attached to the collection bottle with a disposable coupling nut (Figure 115.5). The tapered end of the disposable plastic liner is threaded through the hole in the center of the coupling nut, and then the coupling nut is screwed onto the collection bottle, attaching the tapered end of the plastic liner to the collection bottle.
- An insulted protective cover can be placed over the end of the AV once the AV has been fully assembled. The cover helps maintain optimal temperature and protects the semen from heat and/or cold and light.

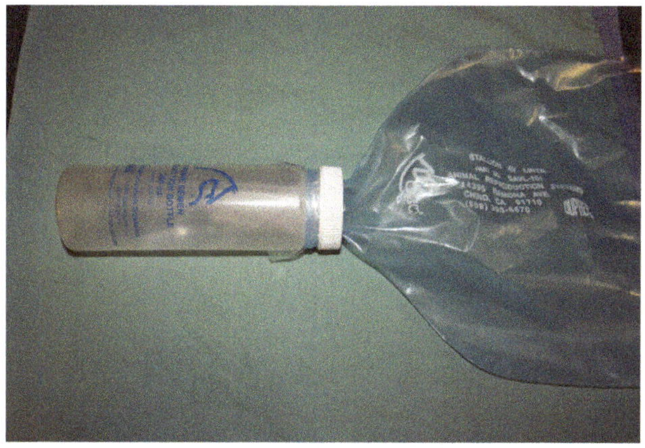

Figure 115.5 Collection bottle attached to a disposable collection liner with a coupling nut.

- A water-soluble, non-spermicidal lubricant is used to lubricate the posterior two thirds of the AV. The obstetrical sleeve is left inside the AV after the hand is withdrawn to prevent entry of foreign material, to prevent the lubricant from drying out, and to aid in the maintenance of temperature. A thermometer is placed within the obstetrical sleeve in the lumen of the AV to monitor temperature. The thermometer and sleeve are removed prior to semen collection.

Additional Comments

The primary advantage of the Colorado model AV over other types of artificial vaginas is that the Colorado model maintains its temperature for an extended period of time during cold weather due to a large water reservoir. In addition, the rigidity of the plastic AV case permits the collector an opportunity to manipulate the AV, which can provide additional stimulation for the stallion. The rigid AV case of the Colorado AV may also allow placement of the AV into some types of phantoms, allowing hands-free collection of stallions.

Further Reading

Boyle MS. 1993. Collection of stallion semen. *Eq Vet Educ* 5: 245–9.

Brinsko SP. 2011. Semen collection techniques and insemination procedures. In: McKinnon AO, Squires EL, Vaala WE, Varner DD (eds). Equine Reproduction, 2nd edn. Ames, IA: Wiley Blackwell, pp. 1268–77.

Pickett BW, Squires EL, McKinnon AO. 1987. Procedures for Collection, Evaluation and Utilization of Stallion Semen for Artificial Insemination. Animal Reproduction Laboratory General Series Bulletin 03. Fort Collins, CO: Colorado State University.

116

Roanoke Artificial Vagina

John J. Dascanio

School of Veterinary Medicine, Texas Tech University, USA

Introduction

The Roanoke artificial vagina (AV) provides a unique stimulation unlike the Missouri or Colorado model AVs. The Roanoke AV provides circumferential pressure and end pressure primarily on the distal penis and the glans penis, respectively, somewhat similar in manner to a Japanese model AV. The glans penis will bell or flower within the enclosed end of the expanded part of the AV providing increased stimulation to the stallion (Figure 116.1).

Initially the AV is filled with a standardized volume of water, independent of stallion penis size. The water fill port contains a pop-off valve that will open at a pressure of approximately 2.3 kPa (0.33 lb/sq. inch). Consequently, upon entry of a stallion's penis, the AV self-adjusts to the size of the stallion's penis.

The Roanoke AV is relatively short and extends only about half way down the penile shaft, thus extra stimulation may need to be provided by grasping the base of the penis with a gloved hand (Figure 116.2). This is thought to simulate contractions of the vulva on the penile shaft, providing stimulation for ejaculation.

External manipulation of the stallion's penis through the AV is not possible due to its hard case. The Roanoke AV does not have a handle on it, so it takes some training to become comfortable in supporting its weight during placement and semen collection. The disposable liner allows for easy clean-up and prevention of transmission of pathogenic organisms, but some stallions may not like the feel of the plastic over a rubber-type liner.

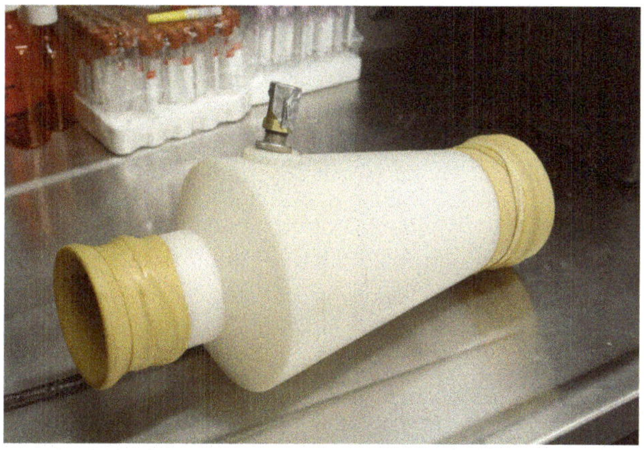

Figure 116.1 Roanoke artificial vagina with a rubber liner. Note the large rubber bands holding the liner to the plastic case on either end. Also note the one-way pressure release valve/water filling port on top. The end that will accept the semen collection bag is to the left and the end that the penis will enter is to the right.

Equipment and Supplies

Roanoke artificial vagina (Roanoke A. I. Laboratories, Inc., Roanoke, VA, USA), 2 mm thick 18 × 60 cm (7 × 24 inch) polyethylene disposable liner, 15 × 25 cm (6 × 10 inch) polyethylene collection bag, in-line filter, disposable baby bottle liners, 2.5 cm (1 inch) white dressing tape, non-spermicidal lubricant, sterile obstetrical sleeve, warm water to fill the AV, thermometer, pump with hose or faucet adapter with hose for filling the AV, insulated cover for baby bottle.

Technique

- Prepare a warm water source to fill the AV. This may be accomplished by a bucket heater or increasing the temperature of a piped hot water heater. The filling temperature should be around 52°C (125°F).
- Remove the valve from the water port on the AV and set aside to use later.
- With the yellow rubber liner inserted and held in place with large rubber bands, fold a 2 mm thick 18 × 60 cm

Equine Reproductive Procedures, Second Edition. Edited by John Dascanio and Patrick McCue.

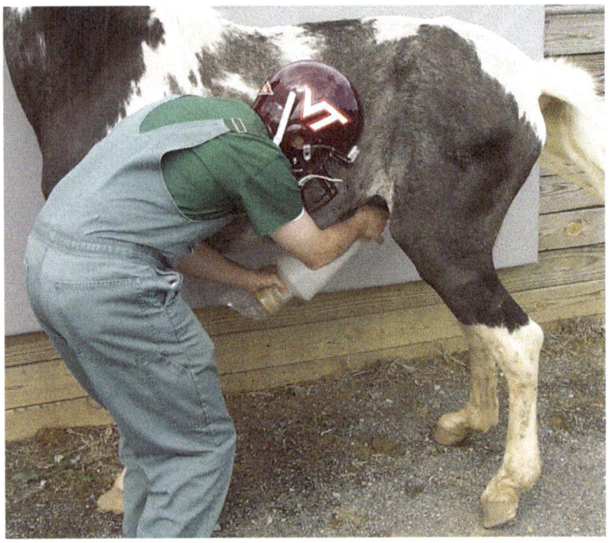

Figure 116.2 Hand position for holding the Roanoke artificial vagina during semen collection. The right hand is gripping the base of the penis for enhanced stimulation. This stallion was ground-collected using the Roanoke AV.

(7 x 24 inch) disposable polyethylene liner in half down its longitudinal axis and insert it into the Roanoke AV, unfolding it after insertion. Evert the two ends of the disposable liner over each end of the AV and secure them with 2.5 cm white dressing tape or large rubber bands. Make sure that the disposable liner is not twisted along its axis, preventing penile entry. If rubber bands are used to hold the disposable liner, it is extremely important to count the number used prior to and after semen collection as the rubber bands could come off onto the stallion's penis during vigorous collection, leading to significant penile damage. The liner material may be purchased in large rolls and cut to length. An alternative is to use sterile obstetrical sleeves with the hand portion cut out, but some of these tend to tear more easily as the material is thinner (<2 mm).

- Don a sterile obstetrical sleeve and place non-spermicidal lubricant in the palm of the hand in the sleeve. Insert the gloved hand into the large open end of the AV and distribute lubricant circumferentially around the inside of the AV to about halfway down its length. It is important to lubricate the Roanoke AV prior to filling with water.
- The sleeve should be taken off the arm and left inserted into the AV until the time of collection. This will keep the lubricant from drying out.
- Place a 15 × 25 cm (6 x 10 inch) semen collection bag onto the smaller open end of the Roanoke AV. Collection bags can be made from Layflat 2 mil (0.05 mm) polyethylene tubing (Associated Bag, Harrisburg, PA, USA) that has been heat sealed on one end. This bag is secured with 2.5 cm white dressing tape or large rubber bands. The collection bag will be orientated 90 degrees to the water fill port on the AV.
- Hold the Roanoke AV in front of the operator with the smaller end to the left and larger open end to the right and the water fill port directed 180 degrees away. The collection bag should be rotated so that the flat aspect of the bag is toward the operator, thus the corners of the bag are located in a vertical line. Cut a 1.5 cm (0.6 inch) air vent hole in the collection bag on the upper aspect near the smaller open end of the AV (Figure 116.3). This will allow air to escape during penile insertion, preventing the collection bag from rupturing. The hole must be located in this fashion, on the upper aspect of the collection bag, to prevent semen from spilling out the cut hole.
- Using a stomach pump with attached tubing, fill the Roanoke AV to approximately two thirds full with warm water at approximately 52°C (125°F). A thermometer inserted into the water port on the AV may be used to monitor the internal water temperature of the AV until collection of the stallion is attempted. The temperature within the AV will cool from the time of filling until the time for collection. Temperatures above 48°C (118°F) should be avoided at the time of collection so that high water temperature will not affect spermatozoal function.
- Since the stallion will self-adjust the AV to his penile size by water exiting the water fill valve, the Roanoke AV is filled to a similar degree for all stallions.
- If the ambient temperature in the area to collect the stallion is cold, the AV may be prefilled with warm water to warm the rubber liner and case. The water is then removed and the AV refilled with warmer water prior to collection. This prevents the temperature in the AV from decreasing too much prior to collection.

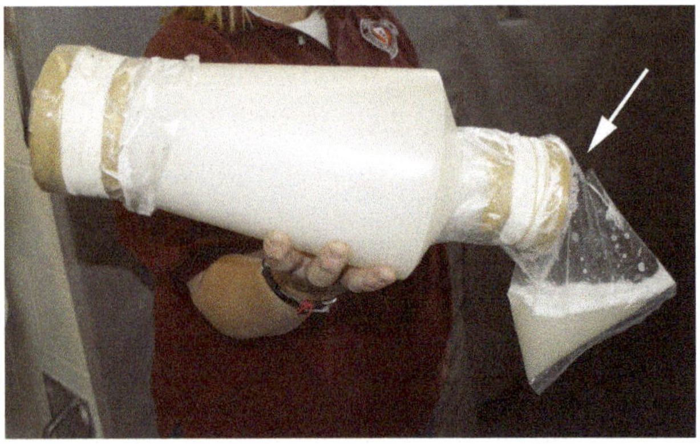

Figure 116.3 Roanoke artificial vagina with a disposable liner and collection bag. Semen is present within the collection bag. The water port is 180 degrees away from the camera. The arrow is pointing at the cut air vent hole in the collection bag.

- Holding the AV with the water fill port upward, remove the filling hose and reinsert the one-way valve.
- If the ambient temperature in the area to collect the stallion is cool, an insulated cover may be fitted over the collection bag to prevent temperature shock to the semen.
- Just prior to collection, as the stallion is mounting the mare or phantom, the sleeve used to lubricate the AV is removed.
- For collection from the left side of the stallion, the collection bag is orientated toward the operator's left and the one-way valve directed away. After the stallion has been properly teased and/or washed, the Roanoke AV is held with the left hand, palm up, at the narrow neck near the collection bag, while the operator's right hand is used to guide the penis into the AV. This is for an approach on the left side of the stallion with a right-handed operator. There is no handle on the AV, so persons with small hands may find this slightly awkward.
- Once the penis is inserted into the AV, the AV may be slid onto the penis until the glans penis contacts the front of the AV. The operator's hands may be repositioned so that the right hand is palm up, holding the large bore end of the AV. The left hand may be repositioned so that it is now palm down on the narrow neck near the collection bag. The AV is held stationary on the stallion's penis. With this type of AV there is not the thrusting to stimulate ejaculation typical of other AVs. The stallion will still thrust, but the AV does not slide back and forth on the penile shaft to a large degree since the "belled" glans becomes trapped inside the AV. The AV may be pushed so that the glans contacts the case to provide extra stimulation and the penile base may be grasped intermittently with a gloved hand.
- Water should be ejected from the AV, 180 degrees away from the operator, outward toward the right side of the stallion, as the penis equalizes with the internal water volume.
- Ejaculation may be confirmed by pulsations of the urethra near the base of the penis, noting ejaculation into the collection bag, or flagging of the tail (up and downward motion). Visualization of the ejaculate will not be possible if an insulating cover has been placed over the collection bag.
- After collection, the valve stem in the water fill port may be removed to allow water to exit. This will allow semen trapped in the water jacket to flow into the collection bag. Care should be taken so that water does not enter the AV or collection bag and negatively affect spermatozoal function. The AV should be held to prevent semen from spilling outward. Care should be taken to avoid accidently pouring the ejaculate through the previously cut air vent.
- Remove the tape or rubber bands off the collection bag, being careful to not spill the semen. The semen should be passed through a semen filter to remove gel and gross debris prior to further processing. A disposable piece of gauze may be placed between the collection bag and the AV prior to collection to serve as an in-line filter.
- The disposable liner should be removed and discarded.
- The AV should be cleaned, disinfected, and dried prior to reuse:
  - Disposable gloved/sleeves should be worn to clean the AV and the gloves should be changed between each cleaning procedure.
  - Rinse the AV liner, inside and outside, thoroughly in hot (>50°C (122°F)) running tap water. Use a clean large bottle, flask, beaker, or brush to aid in the removal of any particulate matter that is adhered to the latex rubber. The brush should be cleaned with hot water and 70% isopropyl alcohol between uses. Since soaps or disinfectants may permeate the latex rubber and subsequently leach into semen, their use is not recommended.
  - Rinse the AV with 70% isopropyl or ethyl alcohol in its entirety. Rinsing can be done by dipping the AV into a large vat of alcohol or by using a squirt or spray bottle designed for this purpose.
  - Hang the AV in a clean, covered cabinet for drying and storage. The storage area should be protected from UV rays and natural sunlight to avoid drying and cracking of the latex rubber over time.
  - Thoroughly rinse the sink used for cleaning the AV with tap water followed by 70% alcohol after each use.
  - The case/cover of the AV should also be thoroughly cleaned with hot water, sprayed or rinsed with 70% isopropyl alcohol, and allowed to air dry.
  - Optionally, the AV may be gas sterilized after use.
- The remaining water is drained from the AV and the water port valve is left off so that the space between the plastic AV wall and the rubber liner will dry.
- In cold weather, a large wool sock or similar insulator may be placed over the collection bag to prevent cold shock to the semen.

Interpretation

- Since the Roanoke AV provides a unique feel for a stallion, stallions who have not previously used this AV may demonstrate behavior uncharacteristic of previous semen collections.
- If the stallion will not ejaculate into the Roanoke AV, a number of possible actions may be attempted:
  - Remove a disposable AV liner if present.
  - Increase the water temperature. Occasionally, if the outside temperature is very low, a lowering of the AV

temperature may be successful to limit the temperature differential to the stallion's penis.
  - Alter the contact of the glans penis with the closed end of the AV to enhance stimulation.
- The Roanoke AV may also trap the tumescent penis within the AV after the stallion "bells" or "flowers," making it difficult to remove the AV from the stallion if he does not ejaculate and becomes frustrated with the collection. The AV may be carefully directed downward between the stallion's hind legs and he will lose his erection making removal possible. Care should be taken to not be kicked during this procedure.
- If the Roanoke AV is pushed onto the semi-erect penis too far, the glans penis may protrude through the small open end of the AV that has the collection bag and the penis may become trapped. Make sure the penis is fully erect prior to AV placement.

Further Reading

American Association of Equine Practitioners. 2019. Biosecurity Guidelines for Control of Venereally Transmitted Diseases. https://aaep.org/guidelines/infectious-disease-control/biosecurity-guidelines-control-venereally-transmitted-diseases (last accessed October 2020).

Love CC. 1992. Semen collection techniques. *Vet Clin North Am Eq Pract* 8: 111–28.

117

Hannover Artificial Vagina

Sofie Sitters

Amsterdam, The Netherlands

Introduction

The Hannover artificial vagina (AV) is the most commonly used model in Europe (Figure 117.1). This model AV holds approximately 1–3 liters of water and is considerably lighter than the Colorado model, which holds 6–8 liters of water.

The Hannover model is composed of a plastic case with a leather handle and a single rubber liner. The hard case has a large circular opening on one end through which the stallion's penis will enter and a smaller circular opening on the other end. The smaller opening is off-centered, forming a dead end that will create pressure on the erect penis.

A rubber liner holds the water and is held to the plastic case on either end by a double set of extra wide rubber bands. The liner may be first attached to the AV by tightly applying 2.5 cm (1 inch) surgical tape before applying the rubber bands. An inner disposable plastic liner is attached to a semen collection bottle. The disposable liner allows for easy clean-up and better prevention of transmission of venereal pathogens. However, some stallions may not like the feel of the plastic over the rubber liner. The disposable liner may be removed, allowing the stallion to contact the inner rubber liner directly. In this case the plastic collection bottle is replaced by a glass collection bottle (Figure 117.2).

Equipment and Supplies

Hannover artificial vagina, leather handle, 2.5 cm (1 inch) surgical tape, rubber liner, large rubber bands, plastic disposable polyethylene liner, plastic semen collection bottle, coupling nut for the collection bottle, optional semen filter and semen bottle liner, optional non-spermicidal lubricant, sterile obstetrical sleeve, warm water to fill the AV, funnel for filling of the AV, thermometer, insulated cover for semen collection bottle, optional glass semen collection bottle.

Technique

- Remove the valve from the water port on the AV and set aside to use later. A cork can also be used in the water port.
- Fold a disposable polyethylene liner in half along its longitudinal axis and insert it into the AV and unfold after insertion. Evert one end of the disposable liner over the larger opening of the AV and secure it with a large rubber band. Make sure that the disposable liner is not twisted along its axis.
- Place a coupling nut over the loose end of the disposable liner.
- Fold the open end of the disposable liner over the opening of the collection bottle and then screw the coupling nut onto the collection bottle.
- An insulated cover may be fitted over the collection bottle if the ambient temperature is low to prevent temperature shock to the semen.

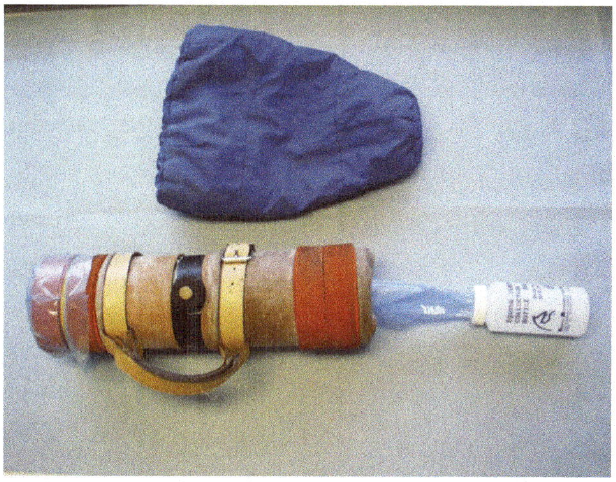

Figure 117.1 Hannover artificial vagina assembled with an inner disposable liner and collection bottle along with an insulated cover.

Equine Reproductive Procedures, Second Edition. Edited by John Dascanio and Patrick McCue.

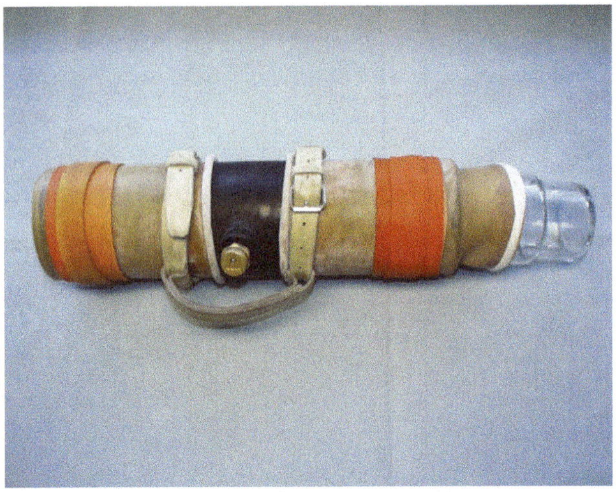

Figure 117.2 Hannover artificial vagina assembled with only an inner rubber liner and glass semen collection bottle.

- Fill the AV with hot water at 60–80°C (140–176°F) through the water port with the help of a funnel and then insert the valve stem to seal the port.
- The pressure of the AV may be adjusted depending on the size and preference of the stallion. The valve is opened by twisting the top part of the water port.
- The use of a lubricant is optional if a disposable liner is used and required if only the rubber liner is used. Apply a small volume of non-spermicidal lubricant in the palm of the hand in the obstetrical sleeve. Insert the gloved hand into the large open end of the AV and apply lubricant circumferentially around the inside of the AV about halfway down its length.
- The sleeve can be taken off the arm and left inserted into the AV until the time of collection to keep the lubricant from drying out.
- A thermometer should be inserted into the AV lumen to monitor the temperature. The temperature of the contact surface of the AV should be a maximum of 45–50°C (113–122°F) at the time of collection to prevent thermal damage to the spermatozoa.
- The thermometer and lubricated sleeve are removed prior to semen collection.
- The stallion is allowed to mount the breeding phantom or jump mare and the AV is placed over the stallion's penis and held in position.
- Ejaculation should be noted by palpation of the urethra near the base of the penis or can be noted by a flagging motion of the tail. Visualization of the ejaculate will not be possible if an insulating cover has been placed over the collection bottle.
- If the stallion does not ejaculate, the AV pressure can be increased or decreased, the water temperature adjusted, or the disposable plastic liner removed.
- After collection, the AV should be held vertically and the valve stem in the water fill port removed to allow water to drain, allowing any semen trapped in the water jacket to flow into the collection bottle.
- The collection bottle is removed from the AV for processing and the filter, if present, is removed and discarded.
- The AV should be cleaned, disinfected, and dried prior to reuse. Remove the disposable liner by pulling it through the AV from "front to back," preventing semen that might be attached to the disposable liner from leaking onto the inner rubber liner. Cleaning should be performed with a mild detergent to remove all smegma and secretions. Copious amounts of warm water should be used to remove any soap residue. The AV may be immersed in an alcohol bath or alcohol may be poured into the inner lumen of the AV to disinfect the liner. The AV should be suspended vertically to dry before reuse.

Additional Comments

- It is important to carefully select an appropriate lubricant for semen collection in stallions. Some lubricants may adversely affect sperm viability.
- Prolonged contact of a lubricant within a warm AV, prior to semen collection, may result in liquefaction of the gel and subsequent passage into the semen receptacle. Exposure of stallion sperm to certain types of rubber and cleaning solutions can be detrimental to sperm quality and leaching of toxicants from rubber can be enhanced by elevated temperature.

References

Hillman RB, Olar TT, Squires EL, *et al.* 1980. Temperature of the artificial vagina and its effect on seminal quality and behavioral characteristics of stallions. *J Am Vet Med Assoc* 177: 720.

Hohertz WW, Duarte JM, LaCaze KA, Teague SR, Varner DD, Love CC. 2018. Toxicity of latex rubber in artificial vaginas on equine sperm. *J Eq Vet Sci* 66: 69.

Love CC. 1992. Semen collection techniques. *Vet Clin North Am Eq Pract* 8: 111–28.

Serafini R, Ghosh S, Love CC, Medrano JMR, Teague SR, LaCaze KA, Varner DD. 2019. Effect of artificial vagina lubricants on stallion sperm quality. *Theriogenology* 139: 121–5.

118

Teaser Stallions

Charles F. Scoggin

Rood and Riddle Equine Hospital, USA

Introduction

Teaser stallions are an essential part of commercial live-cover operations using planned in-hand matings. A teaser stallion is used at the breeding shed to determine if arriving mares are in estrus and receptive to a stallion. The teaser initially interacts with the mare through a partition prior to washing her. In certain instances, the teaser will also be asked to simulate the act of mating (i.e., "test jump") prior to the actual breeding by the covering stallion. Test jumps are routinely performed on maiden mares being bred for the first time and done to gauge the temperament and behavior of the mare, as well as to avoid undue harm to the standing stallion. Because the act of breeding is new to maiden mares, they can become anxious, fractious, or even aggressive during the breeding process. Test jumps can thus desensitize and condition the mare to the process of mating. They may also be performed on any mare that fails to display adequate signs of estrus when initially exposed to the teaser but is deemed otherwise suitable for mating.

Teaser stallions are also routinely used on broodmare farms for estrus detection in resident mares, traveling from barn to barn via trailering, walking, or riding. They can also be used to test jump maiden mares prior to their departure to the breeding shed to prepare them for the act of mating. Most commercial sheds have this requirement, and it serves as an added level of safety for the covering sire.

Essential characteristics of teaser stallions include soundness of hoof, a good libido, and even temperament. Bonus qualities include tractability, perseverance, tenacity, and courage – useful merits when either test jumping or teasing mares.

Equipment and Supplies

Lead shank, helmet, leather apron.

Technique

- A large, leather "apron" or "shield" may be secured around the ventral abdomen of the teaser stallion to prevent accidental intromission during a test jump (Figure 118.1).
- Test jumps are performed as many times as needed until the stallion foreman is satisfied that the mare will not harm the stallion to which she will ultimately be mated.
- Resident maiden mares are also "test jumped" prior to departing for the breeding shed to ensure they are receptive.

Additional Comments

Teaser stallions are allowed to breed nurse mares that were purchased to raise orphan foals. While they may only breed one to two mares a year, it does appear to maintain their interest and dampen any perceived sexual frustration.

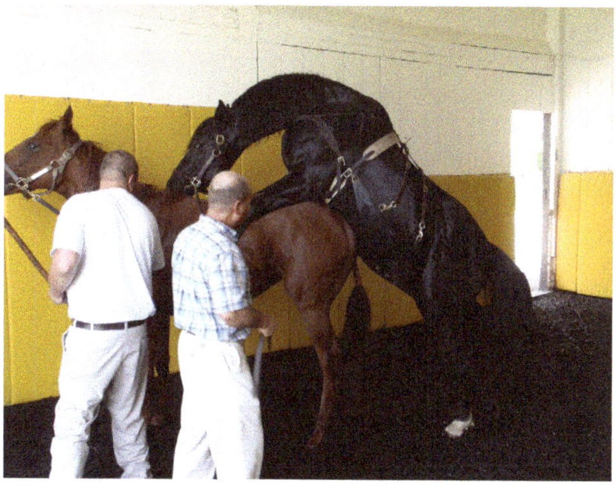

Figure 118.1 Teaser stallion wearing a leather apron during a test jump.

Equine Reproductive Procedures, Second Edition. Edited by John Dascanio and Patrick McCue.

Further Reading

McCue PM, Scoggin CF, Lindholm ARG. 2011. Estrus. In: McKinnon AO, Squires EL, Vaala WE, Varner DD (eds). Equine Reproduction, 2nd edn. Ames, IA: Wiley Blackwell, pp. 1716–27.

Umphenour NW, McCarthy P, Blanchard TL. 2011. Management of stallions in natural-service programs. In: McKinnon AO, Squires EL, Vaala WE, Varner DD (eds). Equine Reproduction, 2nd edn. Ames, IA: Wiley Blackwell, pp. 1208–27.

119

Standing Semen Collection

John J. Dascanio

School of Veterinary Medicine, Texas Tech University, USA

Introduction

Collection of semen from the stallion may be performed by use of an artificial vagina (AV) with the stallion mounting a jump mare, mounting a phantom, or by having him stand on all four limbs on the ground (also called ground collection). Ground collection is advantageous for stallions that have musculoskeletal or neurologic issues that prevent them from mounting a mare or phantom. In addition, stallions without any medical issues may be taught to ground collect so as to avoid the cost associated with purchasing a phantom or to remove issues with having to find a proper jump mare. Most stallions can be trained for ground collection, but it requires multiple training sessions and repetition to reinforce the behavior. Clients may be hesitant to pay for the number of initial sessions or the reinforcement training if their stallion is only collected a few times each breeding season.

Equipment and Supplies

Artificial vagina, non-spermicidal lubricant, sterile obstetrical sleeve, warm water to fill the AV, thermometer, pump with hose or faucet adapter with hose for filling the AV, warm wash water for cleaning the penis prior to collection, paper towels, examination gloves, pheromone towel, estral mare.

Technique

- To train a stallion for ground collection it helps if the stallion is already being successfully collected with an AV. An area should be chosen that allows the placement of the stallion's right side against a solid wall, ideally one that is padded. The wall in front of the stallion should be a padded half wall that allows for visualization of a mare, but not for him to gain access to her for mounting. A regular horse stall may work for this with appropriate precautions to prevent injury to the stallion from bucket hooks and feeders attached to the wall. Alternatively, the stallion may be held in an alleyway with a mare in the stall. If this is used, selecting a stall at the end of the barn with a wall will help to keep the stallion focused and directed toward the stall window. The stallion should only be taken to the area chosen for collection for actual semen collections and not as part of any other routine so that he associates it with semen collection.
- Care should be constantly exercised to prevent injury to handlers and the semen collector by the stallion, especially in enclosed spaces. Appropriate protective gear should be worn, including helmets.

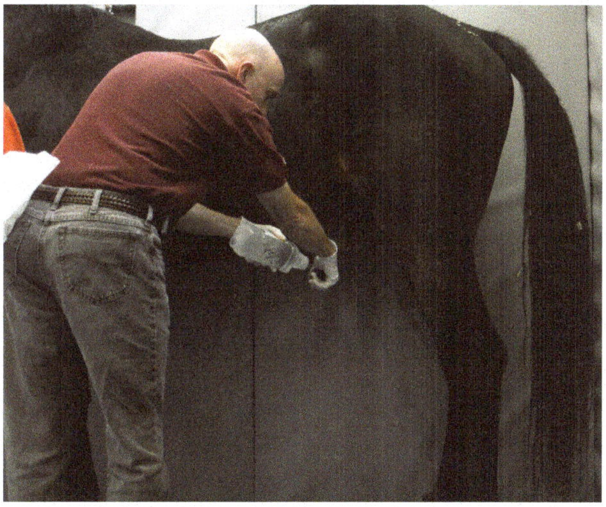

Figure 119.1 Washing a stallion's penis with warm water and gloved hands to stimulate an erection and to cleanse the penis.

Equine Reproductive Procedures, Second Edition. Edited by John Dascanio and Patrick McCue.

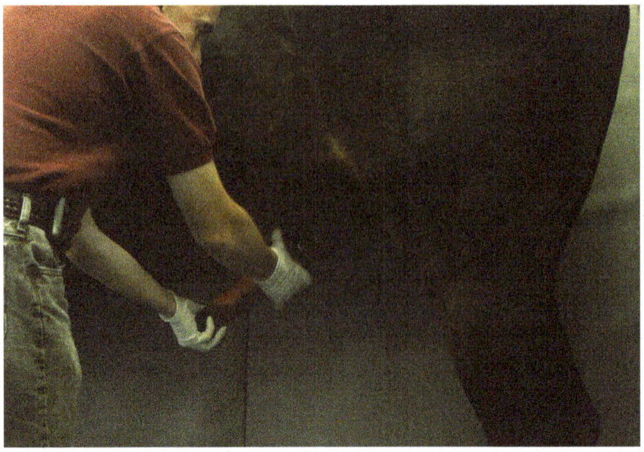

Figure 119.2 Hand position to stimulate the stallion's penis. One hand is cupping the glans penis and the other grips the shaft. The hand gripping the shaft may be closer to the base of the penis to simulate vulvar contractions.

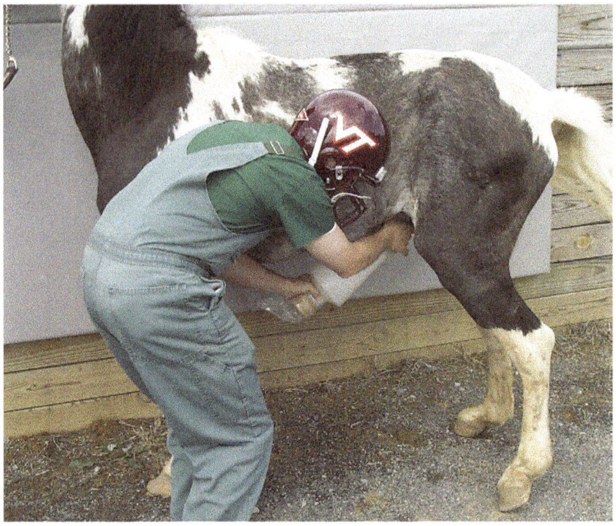

Figure 119.3 Proper body position for standing semen collection. A Roanoke model artificial vagina is used with this stallion.

- Stimulation should be provided to the stallion to achieve an erection and interest in servicing the AV. Overstimulation may cause the stallion to become aggressive or fixated on mounting the mare, making him difficult to handle, especially in a stall.
- Titrate the stallion's exposure to stimuli by providing penile stimulus first with warm water washes (Figure 119.1) and manual compression of his glans penis and penile shaft. The penis should be dried before placing the AV. Placing a gloved cupped hand over the glans with slight pressure and grasping the penile shaft will often excite a stallion (Figure 119.2). Circling the penis just behind the glans with the thumb and forefinger and using the remaining fingers to massage the glans can also result in a positive response. Secondly, a urine-soaked pheromone paper towel may be offered to the stallion. Lastly, a mare may be brought into his distant visual field and brought closer to the stall, as needed, to obtain increasing stimulation. Placement of the mare's hind end just on the outside of the stall from the stallion would be the last option.
- With the stallion's penis fully erect, an AV is placed just over the glans penis to entice the stallion to further thrust into the AV. If required to augment acceptance of the AV, it may be slid further onto the shaft of the penis or moved slightly forward and backward to elicit a positive response from the stallion. It is best if the stallion performs thrusting actions rather than the handler with the AV as the stallion may lose interest.
- Gripping of the penile shaft with a gloved hand near the base with firm pressure may simulate vulvar contractions around the penile shaft and enhance the stallion's response (Figure 119.3).
- Each stallion responds to different stimuli. Sometimes hand pressure over the glans penis through an AV (such as with a Missouri AV) may excite a stallion. Alternatively, an AV with a closed front end, such as a Roanoke AV, will provide extra glans pressure. Once the stimulus is identified that the stallion likes, further collections will be more productive.
- Often as a stallion approaches ejaculation, he will have significant pelvic drop and will thrust forward. His head may lower to counterbalance his pelvis. At this time, the stallion may raise his front feet off the ground slightly. The stallion handler should be aware of this. The stallion must learn to become comfortable without a support during ejaculation.
- As the stallion ejaculates, he sometimes requires some support by pressure against his shoulder or hip to provide a secure feeling and to keep him from circling toward the person holding the AV (Figure 119.4).

Interpretation

- If the stallion will not ejaculate a number of possible actions may be attempted:
  - Remove the disposable AV liner if present.
  - Increase the water volume and thus AV pressure.
  - Increase the water temperature.
- Multiple attempts may be made at each training session. The penile shaft should not become irritated by

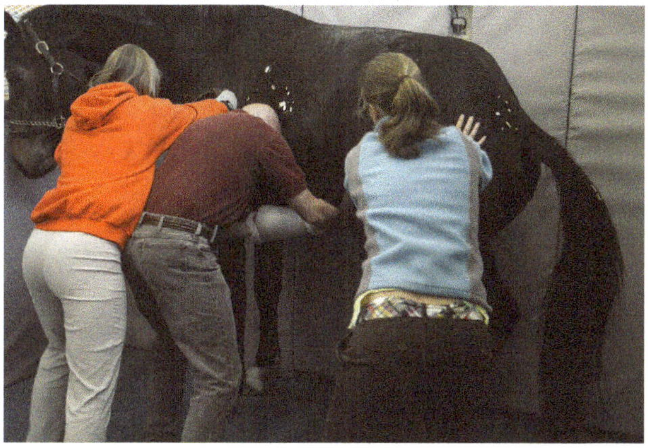

Figure 119.4 Stallion thrusting into a Roanoke model artificial vagina. A handler is pushing on the stallion's hip to keep his body straight and along the wall. Note that the stallion is postured for ejaculation.

multiple AV placements and thrusting. If the stallion still will not ejaculate, either the session should end for that day or he may be collected off a jump mare or phantom to provide a positive release. The training sessions should then recommence later that day or the next morning.

- It may require 3–5 training sessions for the average stallion that is already in a collection program with 2–3 reinforcements per week. Ideally the stallion would then go into a regular collection program to continue to reinforce this collection technique.

Further Reading

Crump J, Crump J. 1989. Stallion ejaculation induced by manual stimulation of the penis. *Theriogenology* 31: 341–6.

Forney BD, McDonnell SM. 1999. How to collect semen from stallions while they are standing on the ground. *Proc Annu Conv Am Assoc Eq Pract* 45: 142–4.

McDonnell SM, Love CC. 1990. Manual stimulation collection of semen from stallions: training time, sexual behavior and semen. *Theriogenology* 33: 1201–10.

120

Collection of Semen Using an Open-Ended Artificial Vagina

Patrick M. McCue

Equine Reproduction Laboratory, Colorado State University, USA

Introduction

Semen collection from stallions is most commonly performed using an artificial vagina with a collection cup, bag, or other device attached to catch the ejaculated semen. However, in some circumstances collection of semen using an open-ended artificial vagina may be indicated. Potential reasons include:

- Collection of only the sperm-rich fraction of the ejaculate and avoidance of gel contamination.
- Avoidance of urine contamination in stallions with urospermia.
- Isolation of the sperm-rich fraction from the gel fraction in stallions with hemospermia secondary to seminal vesiculitis.
- Avoidance of blood contamination in stallions with hemospermia.
- Avoidance of microbial contamination of semen by the bacteria on the surface of the penis.
- Diagnostic visualization of the engorged glans penis for pathology, such as determining a source of blood in the ejaculate.

Equipment and Supplies

Artificial vagina, sterile obstetrical lubricant, plastic cup or other clean disposable container.

Technique

A stallion typically ejaculates 6–9 "jets" of semen with approximately 80% of the spermatozoa present in the first three jets (i.e., the sperm-rich fraction). The gel fraction, if present at all, exits in the last three jets. An open-ended artificial vagina can be used to selectively capture the first few jets of sperm-rich semen into a hand-held cup.

An artificial vagina without a collection device attached (Figure 120.1), the stallion, tease mare (if needed), and/or breeding phantom are prepared as for a traditional semen collection. The stallion is allowed to mount the breeding phantom or tease mare. The penis of the stallion is diverted into the artificial vagina and the stallion is allowed to work the artificial vagina as normal. A small to moderate volume of clear pre-seminal fluid of prostate or bulbo-urethral gland origin may be passed out from the urethra prior to ejaculation. Collection of this fluid should be avoided if possible. When the stallion begins to ejaculate, a second person holds the disposable collection cup against the open end of the artificial vagina. It is easy to miss the first jet of semen (Figure 120.2). After the first three jets of semen are ejaculated, the cup is removed and a second cup can be quickly placed into position if additional semen is to be collected or the gel fraction is to be evaluated.

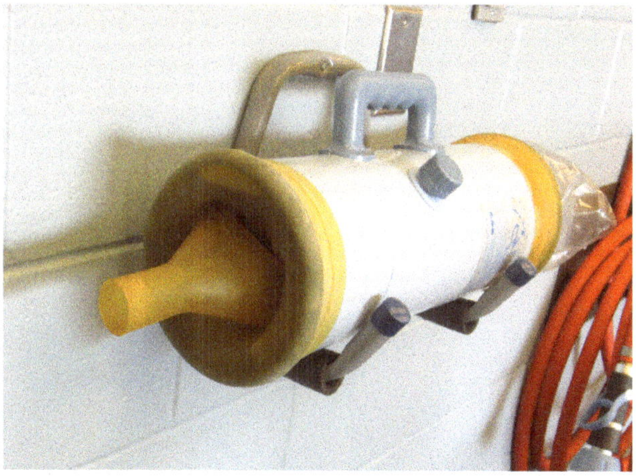

Figure 120.1 An open-ended artificial vagina prior to semen collection.

Equine Reproductive Procedures, Second Edition. Edited by John Dascanio and Patrick McCue.

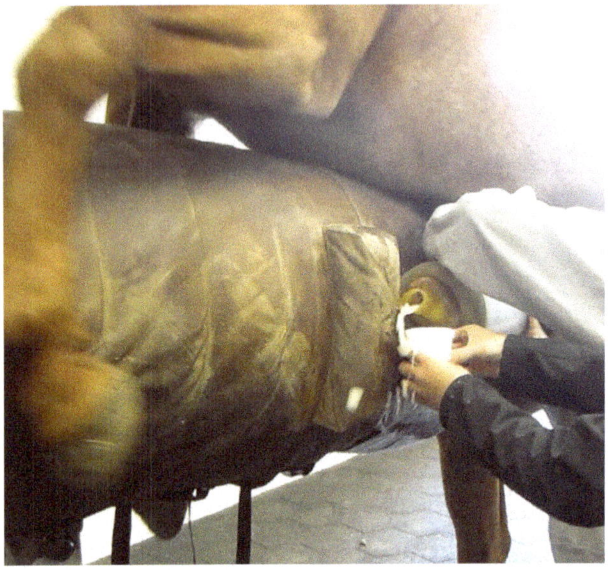

Figure 120.2 Attempting to place a disposable cup against the open end of the artificial vagina during the initial phase of ejaculation. A small volume of semen was lost during this attempt.

The first collection cup should contain most of the sperm-rich fraction of the ejaculate. The second cup, if used, will likely contain sperm as well as the gel fraction of the ejaculate. The cups should be transported directly into a laboratory for evaluation of the semen contents.

Interpretation

The primary clinical reasons to utilize an open-ended artificial vagina are to separate the sperm-rich fraction from the gel fraction and/or to avoid contamination of the semen with blood, urine, or bacteria. The technique is easy to perform, but does require one additional person to manage the collection cup and enhanced attentiveness during the collection process. However, there is no great advantage to routinely using the open-ended artificial vagina technique over traditional semen collection using a standard in-line collection device.

For diagnostic visualization of the engorged glans penis, the artificial vagina inner liner/sleeve will need to be removed. The artificial vagina water liner is still present.

Further Reading

Hurtgen JP. 2009. Semen collection in stallions. In: Samper JC (ed.). Equine Breeding Management and Artificial Insemination, 2nd edn. Philadelphia: Saunders Elsevier, pp. 33–9.

Katila T, Kareskoski M. 2006. Components of stallion seminal plasma and their influence on spermatozoa. *Pferdeheilkunde* 22: 193–200.

Love CC. 1992. Semen collection techniques. *Vet Clin North Am Eq Pract* 8: 111–28.

121

Chemical Ejaculation

Patrick M. McCue

Equine Reproduction Laboratory, Colorado State University, USA

Introduction

Semen may be collected from stallions with physical disabilities or ejaculatory dysfunction by a procedure known as "pharmacologically induced *ex copula* ejaculation" or more commonly referred to as "chemical ejaculation." Stallions for which this procedure may be beneficial include horses with severe musculoskeletal issues, neurologic defects, penile paralysis, ejaculatory failure, or other physiological, pathologic, or behavioral problems.

Chemical ejaculation may be accomplished by the administration of a pair of medications in sequential order. Imipramine hydrochloride, a tricyclic antidepressant medication, is used in an attempt to lower the ejaculation threshold. As ejaculation is mediated by an α-adrenergic mechanism, xylazine hydrochloride – an α_2-adrenergic agonist – has proven successful in various protocols, usually in combination with imipramine.

Equipment and Supplies

Medications: imipramine, molasses, xylazine hydrochloride or detomidine hydrochloride; collection device: harness with collection cup or a pole with collection funnel and cup.

Technique

- Maintain the stallion in a quiet place (i.e., the stallion's regular stall). Distractions should be minimized or eliminated (noise, foot traffic, etc.).
- The stallion is administered imipramine at a dose of 2.2 mg/kg orally. Imipramine tables are crushed and mixed with molasses or other suitable syrup for oral administration (Figure 121.1).
- Approximately 1–2 hours later, xylazine hydrochloride is administered at a dose of 0.3–0.4 mg/kg intravenously to induce emission of semen; detomidine hydrochloride at a dose of 0.01 mg/kg intravenously can be substituted for xylaxine hydrochloride.
- Passive emission of semen usually occurs within 3–5 minutes after administration of xylazine as the stallion is becoming sedated, or as the sedation is wearing off approximately 12–15 minutes after administration. It is common for the testes within the scrotum to have some upward movement at the time of ejaculation (cremaster and tunica dartos contraction). This may be monitored to know when to expect ejaculation will occur.

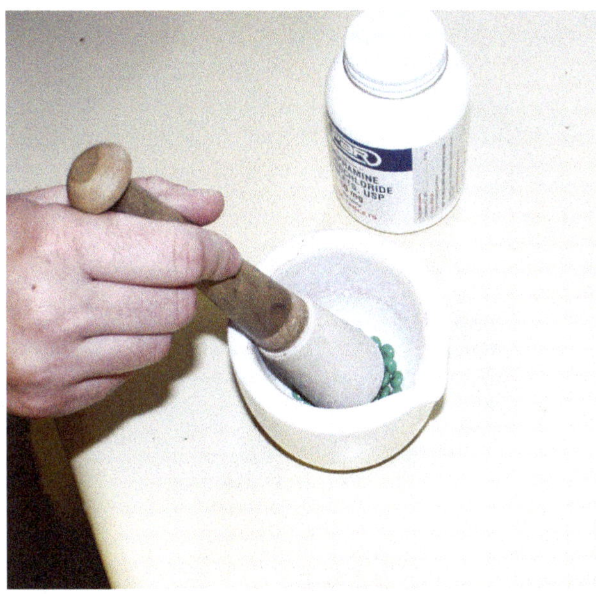

Figure 121.1 Crushing imipramine tablets prior to oral administration.

Equine Reproductive Procedures, Second Edition. Edited by John Dascanio and Patrick McCue.

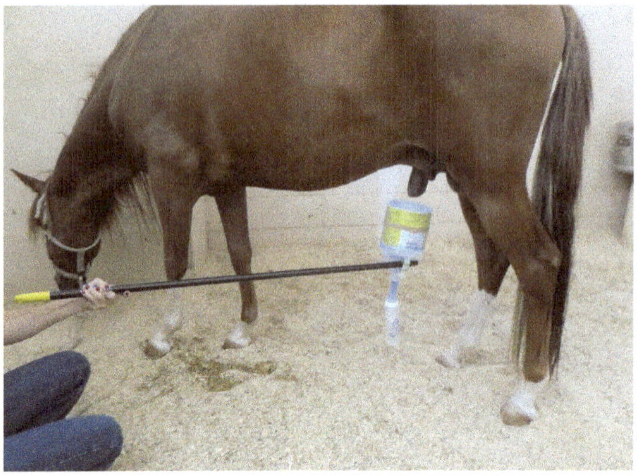

Figure 121.2 Collection of chemically ejaculated semen using a pole and attached cup.

- Semen can be captured using a hand-held cup on a long pole (Figure 121.2) or via a collection device placed over the prepuce and tied over the back of the horse (Figure 121.3).

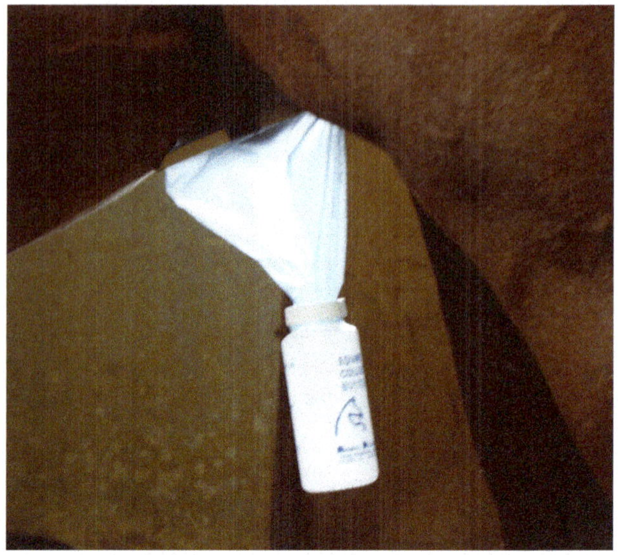

Figure 121.3 Collection of chemically ejaculated semen using a collection cup attached to the horse.

Additional Comments

Approximately 30–75% of treated horses ejaculate in response to imipramine xylazine treatment. Ejaculates obtained are typically low in volume and high in sperm concentration. Semen collected by chemical ejaculation can be used to inseminate mares immediately, processed for cooled semen shipment, or can be cryopreserved for future use.

Further Reading

McDonnell SM. 2011. Pharmacological manipulation of ejaculation. In: McKinnon AO, Squires EL, Vaala WE, Varner DD (eds). Equine Reproduction, 2nd edn. Ames, IA: Wiley Blackwell, pp. 1413–14.

122

Preparation of a Jump Mare or a Mare for Natural Cover

John J. Dascanio

School of Veterinary Medicine, Texas Tech University, USA

Introduction

Preparation of a mare for natural cover or preparation to serve as a jump mare for semen collection are similar. The main goals are to ensure that the mare tolerates mounting by the stallion without harm to the mare, the stallion, or the handlers and that the possibility of venereal disease transmission is minimized.

Equipment and Supplies

Tail wrap, non-irritant soap, roll cotton, stainless steel bucket, disposable liner for bucket, paper towels, exam gloves, twitch, hobbles, rope, sedation, protective neck pad, padded protective rear foot boots.

Technique

- The area for the stallion to mount the mare should provide good footing, be free from obstructions, and be level. A stallion may fall and be injured if attempting to mount a mare on an incline. Grass areas that are wet and slippery should also be avoided.
- A temporary tail wrap should be placed on the mare's tail (Figure 122.1) (see Chapter 3). The tail may be wrapped entirely with the tail hair folded at the level of the last coccygeal vertebra or the tail may be wrapped so that the wrap extends below the level of the ventral vulvar commissure. The purpose of wrapping the tail is to keep the perineal area clean, to avoid contamination, and to prevent the stallion's penis from getting tangled in the tail hairs of the mare.
- A broad region of the mare's hind end should be washed and dried in an area that may contact the stallion's penis (Figure 122.2).
- The mare may have soft leather or felt boots placed on the rear feet so that if she were to kick the mounting stallion, the blow would be softened. Alternatively, bandage material may be wrapped on the rear hooves in a similar manner. Care should be taken when applying boots to

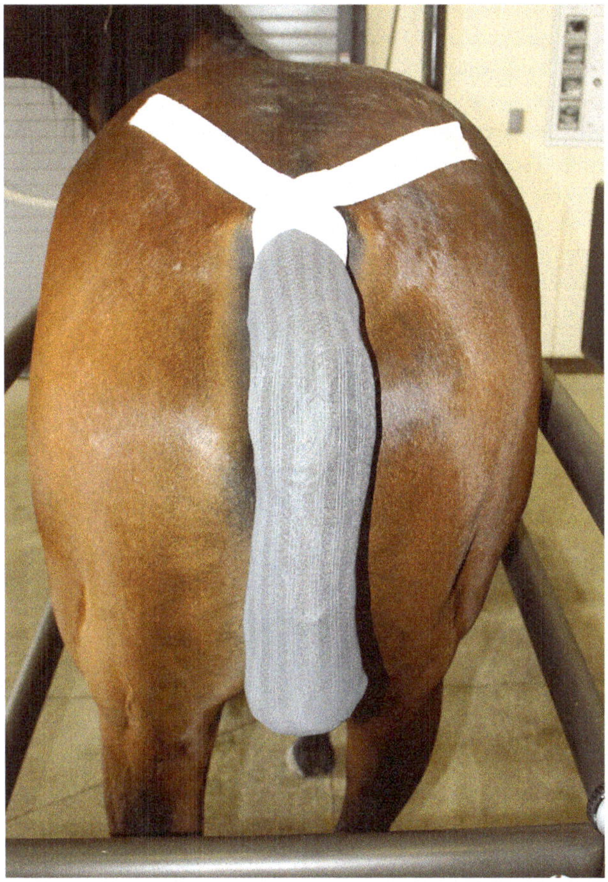

Figure 122.1 Tail wrap prior to live cover or semen collection.

Equine Reproductive Procedures, Second Edition. Edited by John Dascanio and Patrick McCue.

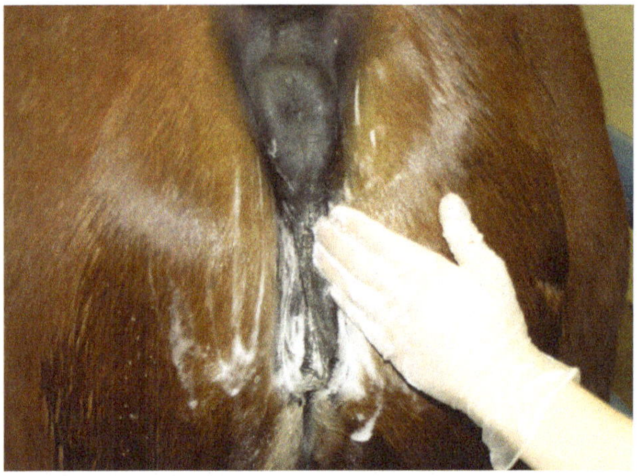

Figure 122.2 Washing the perineum of a mare prior to live cover or semen collection.

the rear feet, especially if the mare has not had them on before.

- A piece of leather attached to a washable cover may be placed over the mare's neck to provide a safe spot for a stallion to grip with his teeth during mating (Figure 122.3). These covers typically hook into the halter with a strap under the neck and girth to keep them from flipping upwards.
- The mare may also be sedated, placed in breeding hobbles, or twitched during the procedure (see Chapter 40).

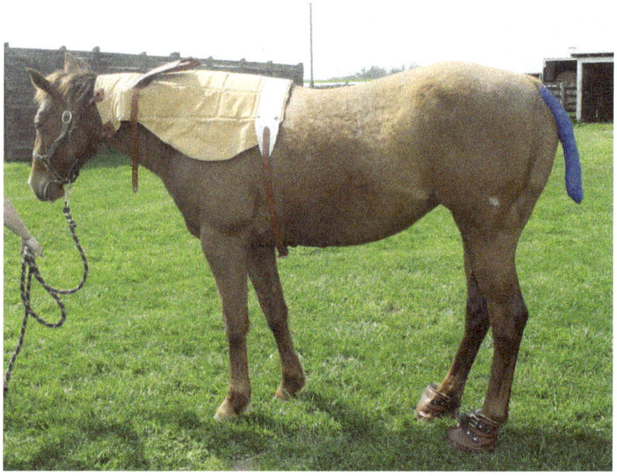

Figure 122.3 Mare prepared for natural cover, with protective boots on the rear feet, her tail wrapped, and a bite cover over the neck.

Additional Comments

- The mare may high step or kick after the application of boots on her rear feet. The mare should be walked after application to familiarize her with their feel.

123

Washing the Penis

John J. Dascanio

School of Veterinary Medicine, Texas Tech University, USA

Introduction

The penis of a stallion or gelding is washed to remove smegma and other dirt or debris. With a stallion this may occur prior to and/or after breeding, while with a gelding it generally occurs during preventative health care visits. Generally, a gelding would have his penis and prepuce cleaned once or twice a year. Smegma is an accumulation of skin cells, glandular secretions, and environmental debris.

The normal penile skin harbors a number of commensal bacteria which are considered non-pathogenic. Overgrowth of specific organisms such as *Pseudomonas aeruginosa* or *Klebsiella pneumoniae* on the male external genitalia may result in venereal transmission of the organisms to mares. Routine washing of the stallion's penis with antiseptic soaps should be avoided as it may remove normal non-pathogenic microbial flora which could be replaced by other more pathogenic bacteria. Warm clean water should be used for routine cleansing of the penis. A non-irritant mild soap may be used occasionally if smegma accumulation is significant. All soap residues must be thoroughly rinsed from the penis so as to not have an effect on ejaculated spermatozoa.

Equipment and Supplies

Non-irritant soap, plastic 1 liter bottle, roll cotton, stainless steel bucket, disposable liner for bucket, paper towels, roll cotton, exam gloves, sedation, water-soluble lubricant.

Technique

- The penis of a stallion can be washed after he has dropped his penis or gained an erection by teasing mares.
- Some stallions will extend the penis from the prepuce with gentle massage of the penis through the prepuce.
- The penis of a gelding may have to be gently manually exteriorized from the sheath, or the penis of the horse may drop after the horse is sedated. If needed, a short-acting tranquilizer such as xylazine hydrochloride with or without butorphanol may be used for sedation. Administration of phenothiazine-type tranquilizers, such as acepromazine, should be avoided due to the possibility of paraphimosis.
- Care should be exercised to avoid being kicked as some horses may not be accustomed to the procedure.
- The stallion should be properly restrained.
- The person washing the penis should stand with their body alongside the left side of the horse facing toward the tail, with their body approximately even with the front legs.
- Use the back of a hand (so as to not contaminate the palm) to contact the horse's back, side, and ventrum, carefully working to a position to where the hand may be placed on the prepuce. With horses less accepting of the procedure, a handful of mane may be grasped in the left hand while the right hand attempts to contact the prepuce to prevent the horse from moving forward and away from the veterinarian.
- Disposable examination gloves should be used to limit contamination and spread of disease.
- Once extended, the penis should be examined for any pathology such as ulceration, infection, tumors, abrasions, or lacerations.
- The penis should be washed with warm water (40°C, 105°F) from the base (near the prepuce) toward the glans penis so as to prevent contaminated water from running from the prepuce toward the glans penis (Figure 123.1). Thus the glans is the last structure to be rinsed. The washing procedure should be stimulatory to the stallion or gelding.

Equine Reproductive Procedures, Second Edition. Edited by John Dascanio and Patrick McCue.

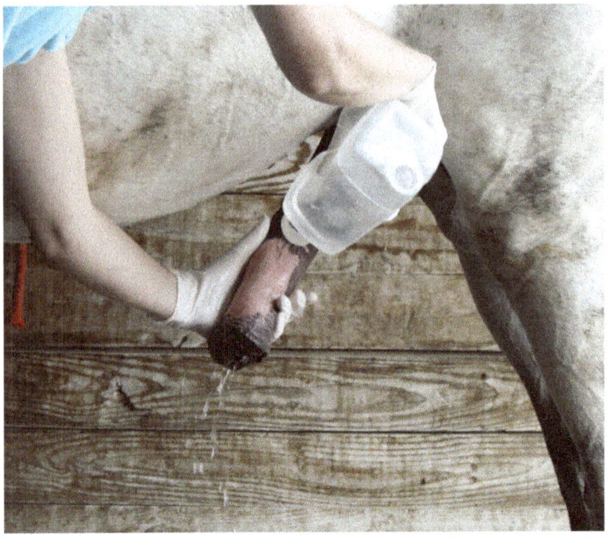

Figure 123.1 The penis is cleaned from the base towards the glans using water squirted from a plastic bottle.

- Excessive water should be wiped from the surface of the penis or the penis may be dried with clean disposable paper towels. The glans penis is dried first and then the penile shaft, progressing towards the prepuce (Figure 123.2).
- Thus the penis is washed from proximal to distal and dried from distal to proximal.
- One method of washing the penis utilizes a plastic 1 liter bottle (such as a 1 liter saline bottle) that has holes cut into the top lid with a 14 gauge needle to form a sprinkler. One hand holds the penis while the other hand rinses it or squirts warm tap water over the penis (Figure 123.1).
- A second method of washing the penis uses a stainless steel bucket with a disposable liner with handfuls of roll cotton soaked in warm water. Using the classic "clean hand, dirty hand" technique, one hand (clean) reaches into the bucket to retrieve a piece of cotton. This is held over the other hand to rinse any dirt or debris off and then dropped into the palm (dirty). The dirty hand washes the penis. The procedure is then repeated until the penis is clean. Using this technique maintains clean wash/rinse water. If a second person is available, they may serve as the "clean" hand, allowing the person cleaning the stallion to use two hands on the penis.
- A third method utilizes a disposable cup, dipped into a bucket of warm water, to thoroughly rinse off the penis distally from the prepucial ring to the glans penis. A gloved hand may be used to strip off (i.e., "squeegee") any residual water on the penis distal to the prepucial ring (Figure 123.3).

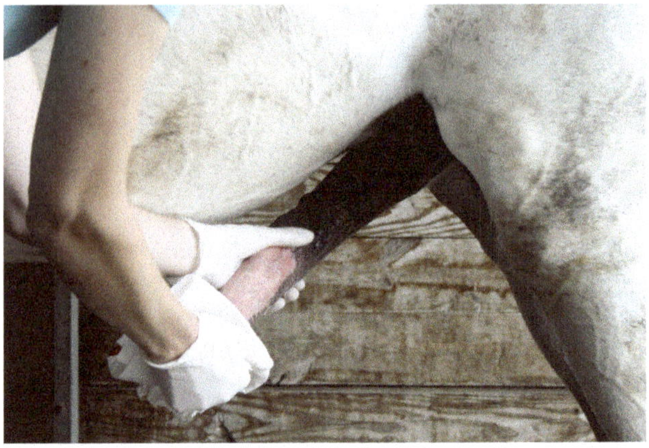

Figure 123.2 The penis is dried from the glans toward the base using disposable paper towels.

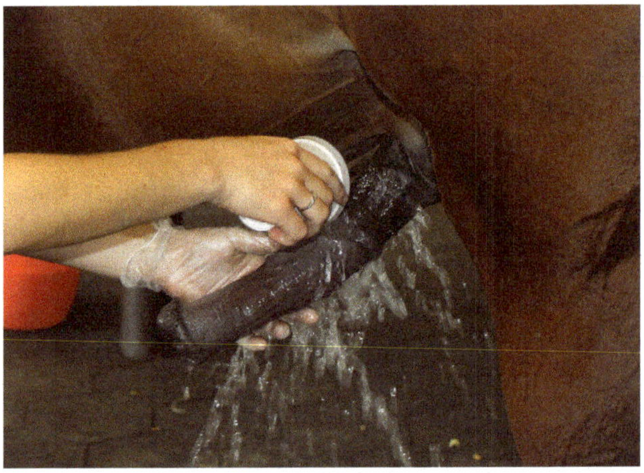

Figure 123.3 The penis is washed/rinsed using a disposable cup.

- A rinse with warm tap water should be sufficient for a stallion that has been breeding regularly or has been washed recently. A mild non-residual soap may be used if smegma has built up on the penis.
- Prior to the regular breeding/collection season, the urethral fossa should be digitally examined for the presence of a concretion of smegma commonly referred to as a "bean." The bean may be detected and removed by sweeping the fossa with a finger.
- Cupping of the hand over the glans penis with the application of light pressure should enhance penile tumescence. In addition, gripping the penile base in a handshaking-type grip, with cupping of the glans, should further stimulate a stallion (Figure 123.4). Stimulation of the stallion may aid in maintaining tumescence and increase libido for semen collection.

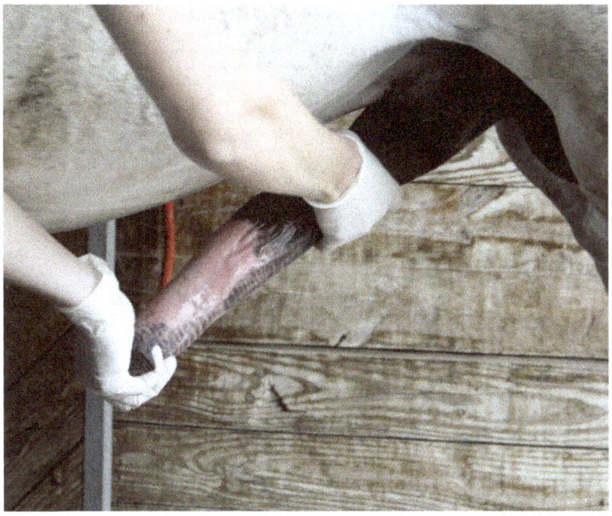

Figure 123.4 Manual stimulation with one hand cupped over the glans penis and the other applying circumferential pressure on the upper penile shaft.

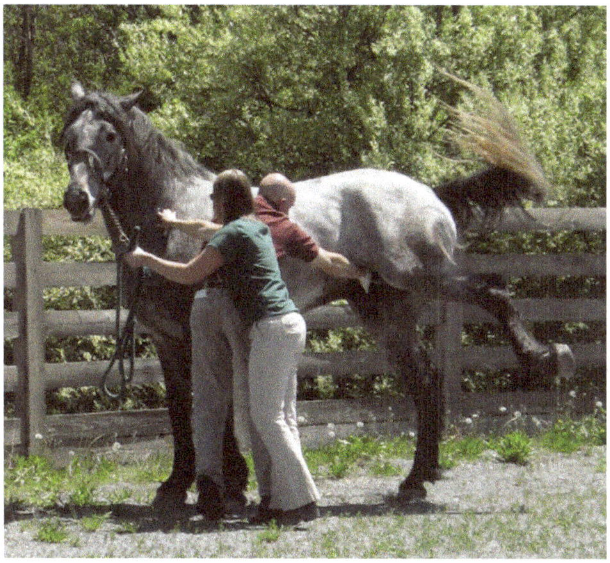

Figure 123.5 Stallion kicking in response to washing of the penis with warm water. Note body position to avoid back leg.

Interpretation

- Cleaning of the penis should be stimulating for a stallion.
- Males with pigmented skin on the penis will have black-colored smegma. Males with primarily unpigmented penile skin will have a slightly yellow-colored smegma.
- There should not be an appreciable odor to the smegma.
- Excessive accumulation of smegma, excessive odor, or wetness may be indications of abnormal bacterial flora or the presence of pre-cancerous lesions.
- Some stallions may kick out to the side when the penis is grasped or when it is washed (Figure 123.5).
- The ventral abdomen should be free of loose hair and debris so that the cleaned, erect penis does not become contaminated.

Further Reading

Bowen JM, Tobin N, Simpson RB, Ley WB, Ansari MM. 1982. Effects of washing on the bacterial flora of the stallion's penis. *J Reprod Fertil Suppl* 32: 41–5.

Crump J, Crump J. 1989. Stallion ejaculation induced by manual stimulation of the penis. *Theriogenology* 31: 341–6.

Madsen M, Christensen P. 1995. Bacterial flora of semen collected from Danish Warmblood stallions by artificial vagina. *Acta Vet Scand* 36: 1–7.

Varner DD. 1998. External and internal genital infections of stallions. In: *Proceedings of the Society for Theriogenology Stallion Reproduction Symposium*, pp. 84–94.

124

Evaluation of Sexual Behavior

John J. Dascanio[1] *and Sue M. McDonnell*[2]

[1]*School of Veterinary Medicine, Texas Tech University, USA*
[2]*New Boton Center, School of Veterinary Medicine, University of Pennsylvania, USA*

Introduction

Sexual arousal and response (often referred to in animal breeding as *libido*) may vary quite a bit among stallions and may reflect the training level and past experiences for that stallion. Stallions that are not well halter-trained may not be as controllable when handling for natural cover or semen collection with an artificial vagina. Stallions that have bred in a pasture situation with no handling and then are transitioned to a supervised breeding situation often appear more cautious in their approach. Inexperienced stallions may initially be either shy or aggressive towards mares or difficult to guide in their initial sessions in the breeding shed.

The history of the stallion may help determine in advance factors that that may influence or adversely affect his breeding behavior. For example, if a stallion has had a performance career where he was actively discouraged from responding sexually to mares, or having a sexual or spontaneous erection, he may appear hesitant to respond in a breeding situation, as if having difficulty understanding what he is allowed to do.

It is important for a stallion to have good libido and be able to express it in an appropriate manner and environment. Stallions have been known to rear in the air, strike down their handlers, or jump fences in order to get to a mare in estrus (Figure 124.1). Arousal of any particular stallion and the handlers' skills can often be managed at a safe, efficient level by titrating the level of stimulation.

Evaluation of Sexual Behavior

Stimuli

With experience, stallions typically learn the various particular environmental conditions associated with opportunities to breed. Examples of these inadvertently *conditioned stimuli* that can evoke sexual arousal and response include a particular handler, equipment used specifically for breeding, such as a breeding halter or leg wraps, movement to the breeding area, and preparation once there. A routine of cleansing of the penis with warm water and gently drying with hand pressure on the glans penis and penile shaft may further stimulate most stallions. Olfactory stimuli may be used to augment the stallion's arousal in the form of a urine-soaked paper towel if needed. Paper towels may be soaked in urine from a mare in estrus and frozen in plastic bags until needed.

The next stimulus would be the sight of another horse. The teaser mare may be kept at a distance or placed on the opposite side of a teasing wall or rail as needed to stimulate

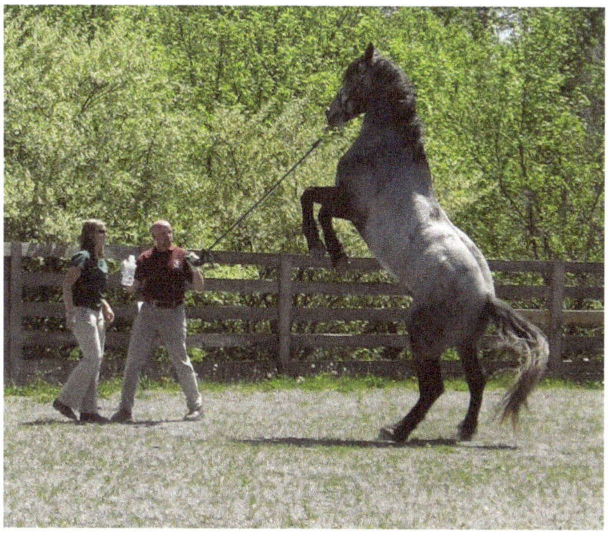

Figure 124.1 Stallion rearing in response to being stopped on the way to the teasing wall. Restraint at the head and mouth is often the trigger for rearing in this context.

Equine Reproductive Procedures, Second Edition. Edited by John Dascanio and Patrick McCue.

sexual response. If this is not sufficient, direct contact with the mare in the breeding shed or collection area may be helpful. In most instances, even a novice breeding stallion will interact sexually and mount the mare and his penis can be diverted into an artificial vagina (AV) for collection. However, in some cases it may be beneficial to allow a novice breeder to cover a mare naturally and ejaculate and then transition him to an AV.

For stallions that have achieved an erection and are positioned behind the mare or mount, but appear hesitant to mount, an AV may be gently slid onto the stallion's glans penis to evoke a reflexive mount. The glans penis may be further stimulated by gentle massage through the AV end while the stallion is servicing the AV to stimulate thrusting activity and ejaculation. Some stallions, however, react negatively to manipulation of the penis, and may squeal and dismount. It is helpful to understand the specific needs and quirks of individual stallions in order to be successful on a routine basis.

Behavior Training

Effective stallion handling for breeding requires respectfully guiding the stallion without discouraging sexual arousal or inciting the stallion's normal aggressive response to a thwarted goal situation. Punishment, whether purposeful or inadvertent, of normal sexual response is typically counterproductive. Most normal sexual interactive behaviors are appropriate for in-hand breeding. Examples of normal behavior that are not necessarily associated with reduced efficiency or increased risk to the safety of animals or personnel include vocalization, olfactory investigation, and flehmen response, and other behaviors associated with the stallion "acting like a male," including body position changes and arching the neck and prancing in response to a mare's presence. Interruption or punishment of these normal behaviors can lead to problem behavior in various directions. For some stallions, punishment of natural responses will result in general sexual inhibition. For others, attempts to punish these behaviors may provoke a natural but nonetheless dangerous aggressive response toward the handler and/or the mare.

Ideally, a stallion with a sexual behavior problem should be examined on the farm of origin and not at a referral center. Each aspect of the breeding program should be examined. If the problem occurs after a successful breeding career, the stallion should be examined for lameness or neurologic issues prior to extensive behavior modification. In addition, a complete breeding soundness examination should be performed to assess the stallion specifically for age-related testicular degeneration or other pathologies.

Pre-breeding activities such as turnout and exercise may affect a stallion's behavior. An example would be excessive exercise for an older arthritic stallion just prior to live cover or semen collection. In contrast, some stallions require significant exercise to tone down their more aggressive nature prior to breeding or collection.

The handling of the stallion from the stall or paddock to the breeding shed and during the live cover or collection should be evaluated. Randomly stopping a stallion on the approach to the breeding area or mount and sometimes calmly backing up, and then moving on, can be helpful in teaching a stallion to follow the handler's lead. Excessive restraint may inhibit expression of normal behavior. In some situations, the person training the stallion for performance may not be the ideal person to handle the horse in the breeding shed.

It is common to use a chain lead shank for handling a stallion for breeding. Opinions vary widely, but for a well-behaved stallion a chain shank over the bridge of the nose or even a simple cotton lead shank may be sufficient for judicious guidance. If more restraint is required, there are other arrangements that may be more effective, for example a driving bridle, gum chain, or chain over the tongue like a flexible bit, but these typically require greater skill maintain comfortable, effective, non-confrontational guidance. Placing a chain shank in the mouth of some stallions may result in too much pressure on the angle of the mouth. Additionally, care must be taken to use hardware on the halter that allows for smooth application and release of pressure. A chain over the gums is common on some breeding farms, but too firm pressure or jerking on the chain, whether deliberate or accidental, may sexually inhibit some stallions, or incite defensive aggression. The best results can be expected when handlers consider how much and what type of restraint works best for each individual stallion for their skill level.

The ambient environment of the breeding shed should be evaluated. Are there extraneous distractions such as delivery trucks going by or train tracks with passing trains? Are other horses being walked nearby to distract him? Having the stallion's attention focused on the job at hand is best. If possible, the breeding shed area should be enclosed to prevent distractions, especially with stallions in breeding training.

The equipment used in the breeding/collection process may also influence behavior. The dummy mount may have a surface that results in abrasions to the stallion's inner forearms. The AV may have a plastic liner that results in a different feel than a latex liner or the type of AV may offer different pressure points to either stimulate or inhibit different stallions.

The footing near the dummy mount may not be adequate. Gravel, or any other loose material, may become scooped out by mounting activities resulting in a deeper or uneven hole that does not allow the stallion to have secure rear leg footing when mounted or results in the stallion reaching for solid footing when mounted. The flooring material such as wet grass or a wet floor could be slippery and cause the stallion to be inhibited from mounting. Individual stallions may prefer a particular height to feel comfortable and secure when mounted.

Certain characteristics of a stimulus mare may influence stallion behavior. A chestnut mare may have kicked the stallion in the past and thus now he is not as stimulated by a chestnut mare, but responds well to gray mares. Some stallions respond well when a mare vocalizes while others may not. Reluctant stallions may also demonstrate enhanced libido if allowed to follow the tease mare in a slow walk around the collection shed. Also, a stallion hesitating to mount a phantom may be stimulated by positioning the tease mare against the opposite side of the phantom and directing the head of the tease mare back toward the stallion.

With stallions that are in initial training programs for artificial insemination or natural cover, the handlers may tolerate less desirable behaviors by the stallion until an ejaculation is achieved so that the stallion learns the eventual outcome of the session. Once the stallion has ejaculated on a few occasions, the undesirable behaviors usually diminish with judicious guidance. An AV may also be filled with warmer water than desired in order to stimulate ejaculation.

Especially highly aroused stallions that are urgent to breed may rear or lunge when approaching to mount. Under natural herd breeding conditions, rearing is not usually an element of the pre-copulatory interaction. It does occur when the approach is thwarted or interrupted, often by a competing stallion. Hand breeding can represent a similar thwarted goal situation, inadvertently evoking inter-male interactive responses toward the handler. Additionally, restraint of the head and mouth can easily provoke rearing in an animated stallion. Stallions that are new to manipulation of the penis or have had previous difficulties abiding preparation, may kick out, rear, strike, bite the handler, or move away during washing of their penis (Figure 124.2). Decreasing the stimulation by taking the stimulus mare from view or orientating the stallion away from the mount, may help. Preparing the stallion just outside the breeding area, even with only a partial erection, may reduce the sensitivity of the genital tissues, allowing the stallion to be more comfortable with manipulation. Creative adjustments to the protocol, such as backing an enthusiastic, urgent stallion up to the mount until almost in contact before turning, for some stallions, may reduce the tendency to rear or to charge the mount. Acclimating a stallion to genital manipulation and washing of their prepuce and penis in a non-sexual situation before introduction of these procedures is recommended. Some stallions may be a danger to handlers and should not be used for breeding purposes until they have been well trained for basic ground handling. Some horses may benefit from turnout with mares in a natural pasture breeding environment to become better organized with their pre-copulatory and copulatory behavior.

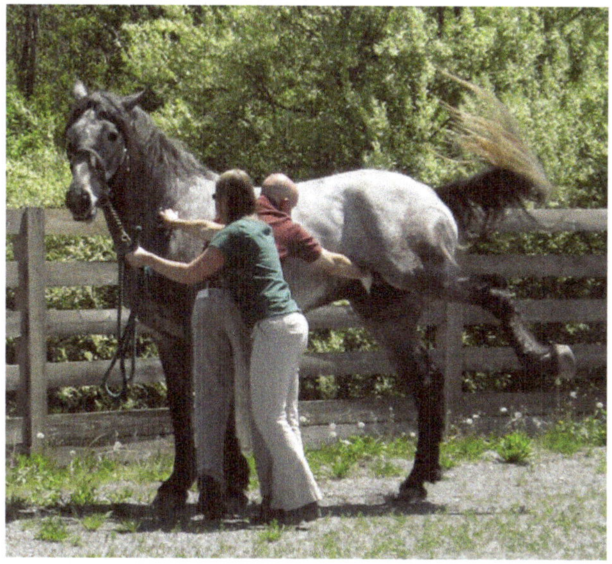

Figure 124.2 Stallion kicking in response to washing of the penis with warm water.

If the experience level of the current personnel does not result in the expected results, consultation with a stallion behavior specialist is recommended. This can be especially effective for actual hands-on training of the handlers for the needs of the particular stallions in their care. For inhibited or low interest or slow response stallions, the use of anti-anxiety medications such as diazepam or midazolam may effectively reduce anxiety and release innate goal-directed sexual behavior. Various behavioral and medication approaches to improve sexual interest by increasing testosterone, may also be useful.

Further Reading

McDonnell SM. 2009. Stallion sexual behavior. In: Samper JC (ed.). Equine Breeding Management and Artificial Insemination. St Louis, MI: Saunders Elsevier, pp. 41–6.

McDonnell SM, Hinze AL. 2005. Aversive conditioning of periodic spontaneous erection adversely affects sexual behavior and semen in stallions. *Anim Reprod Sci* 89: 77–92.

125

Enhancement of Sexual Interest and Response

Sue M. McDonnell

New Bolton Center, School of Veterinary Medicine, University of Pennsylvania, USA

Introduction

There are a number of management and therapeutic interventions that typically can improve sexual arousal, response, breeding efficiency, and/or endurance of breeding stallions. The following outlines a variety of management factors and interventions to be considered for stallions presenting for inadequate interest in breeding.

General Health and Fitness

Poor health, regardless the cause, can affect a stallion's interest in breeding, sexual arousal, and response. The impact of discomfort of various common conditions tends to vary widely among individual stallions. Relief from the discomfort of any health conditions, including such common problems as gastric ulcers, dental conditions, lameness, foot soreness, back or neck discomfort, airway compromise, muscle disease, and arthritis, even when minor, can improve sexual interest and response.

Poor nutrition, whether resulting in obesity or extremely thin condition, can impact a stallion's interest, enthusiasm, and comfort for breeding. In general, the preferred body condition for most busy breeding stallions is slightly thin (i.e., 4 on the Henneke scale), but well muscled and physically fit, much like a horse in athletic work. Exercise to maintain a reasonable level of cardiovascular and muscular fitness not only enhances physical comfort for breeding, but also appears to benefit temperament and behavior relative to handling.

For horses with potentially painful conditions, pain management can be challenging. For back and hind limb discomfort, weight reduction can be especially helpful. Oral phenylbutazone has been consistently effective to alleviate discomfort. It also should be noted that it is not uncommon, when evaluating low interest or response, to identify several minor potential sources of discomfort, any one of which may not be judged sufficient to adversely affect breeding response. Every identifiable health issue or potential source of discomfort should be simultaneously addressed, no matter how minor. This typically results in considerable improvement. A reasonable interpretation is that multiple minor discomforts can be additive.

Housing and Breeding Environment

Stallion behavior clearly can be affected, positively or negatively, by the social environment provided. For the majority of stallions, sexual interest and response will be greatest when housed away from other, particularly more dominant, stallions, along with visual and olfactory exposure to one or more mares. This best simulates the natural social environment of a harem breeding stallion. If housing with mares is not an option, exposure to olfactory stimulation, for example mare urine, feces, or soiled bedding, appears to aid in building stallion confidence. Similarly, some stallions do much better when breeding or when semen collection is done in a "private" area, as in their own paddock or in a breeding area used by no other stallions, and out of sight, smell, or sound of other stallions.

Handling for Breeding

Sexual arousal is greatly affected by the handling style and breeding environment. For most horses, respectful, encouraging guidance and team work will promote and maintain the most efficient breeding behavior. The goal should be for the stallion to abide certain necessary limitations and direction, while being allowed focused attention

Equine Reproductive Procedures, Second Edition. Edited by John Dascanio and Patrick McCue.

on the mare. The minimum effective restraint arrangement is least likely to adversely affect the stallion's focus on the mare. The all too common handling habits or actions deliberately aimed at keeping the horse's attention on the handler, for example routine rhythmic jerking on the lead, are best avoided. Some horses more or less habituate to these handler habits. Nonetheless, the result for most stallions is unnecessary distraction. Similarly, confining headgear with severe bits that can easily inadvertently inflict discomfort or which keep the horse in dramatic collection with the head at or behind vertical, is often counterproductive. This can lead to a variety of behavior problems, including reluctance to mount, failure to ejaculate, and in some cases eventually breaking away, savaging the handler or mare. Occasionally, we have encountered stallions routinely exposed to this type of handling where the rhythmic jerking of the lead or extreme "collection" at particular junctures of the breeding process, for example, just at the moment of decision to allow mounting, has become a conditioned stimulus for mounting. In other words, the jerking on the lead becomes a safety signal for the stallion that it is time to proceed. Until that occurs, the stallion's arousal diminishes as if waiting for "permission." Unfortunately, some handlers interpret this phenomenon as a positive relationship, perpetuating the practices.

Some horses appear to tire of a rigid "one size fits all" breeding routine. This is more commonly the case for semen collection where clearly suboptimal stimulus mares and/or less than ideal mount characteristics and artificial vagina conditions occur, and because they work for some or most stallions, they are accepted as adequate for all stallions. For many stallions, carefully considered changes, particularly relaxation of rigidity of the breeding routine and/or improvements in stimulus mares, and how they are handled, can refresh sexual interest. Careful consideration and ongoing evaluation of such changes for the particular stallion cannot be overemphasized.

Certain individuals do appear to be ritual bound, in that sexual response may be adversely affected, at least temporarily, by changes in breeding conditions. Other important aspects of the breeding environment include distractions in or near the breeding area, for example the vocalizations of other horses, particularly stallions.

Stimulus Mare

The stimulus mare, and the manner in which she is presented, can greatly affect sexual interest and response. In general, positive natural movement of the mare, as opposed to tightly restrained immobility, is most effective at stimulating arousal and response (Figure 125.1). Handling in a manner that facilitates natural pre-copulatory postures and interactive responses are typically quite effective at stimulating or increasing stallion arousal. The general rule is to present the mare as naturally as possible, including an intact mare in natural estrus (without cycle manipulation), with an unwashed perineum with tail naturally exposed, and with no potentially off-putting odors such as residues from other stallions, fly sprays, perineal wash, or tail covers. Lip twitches and hobbles in particular not only inhibit natural behavior, but also provoke ambiguous unnatural postures with hints of aggressive postures that tend to be off-putting to most stallions, and particularly to hesitant stallions. Occasionally, it appears that certain individual mares or particular characteristics of mares are more or less arousing to an individual stallion. Accommodating these apparent preferences and respecting apparent aversions can be a useful strategy for maintaining adequate response. In spite of apparent preferences, some stallions also benefit from having some variety in mares.

Endocrine Strategies for Boosting Stallion Sexual Interest and Arousal

A number of endocrine approaches have been useful for boosting stallion sexual arousal and response. In general the aim is to increase androgens within safe limits so as to avoid downregulation of gonadotropins. Gonadotropin-releasing hormone (GnRH), the native decapeptide, 50 μg administered subcutaneously 2 hours, and again 1 hour, before breeding, should temporarily elevate circulating testosterone to roughly double baseline concentrations. Human chorionic gonadotropin (hCG; 5,000–10,000 IU administered intravenously once) typically results in a prolonged elevation of gonadal steroids, for as long as a week or more, and reaching greater circulating concentrations than with the GnRH regimen described. There is concern for potential adverse reaction with repeated hCG treatments.

Administration of testosterone can be useful, but very careful monitoring of circulating levels is recommended to ensure circulating levels remain within a range that is unlikely to adversely affect spermatogenesis. Individual blood levels response to various testosterone preparations and routes of administration make management tedious and expensive. Exogenous testosterone, using particular preparations, can also lead to increased aggressive tendencies. Nonetheless, in certain circumstances, particularly near the end of a breeding

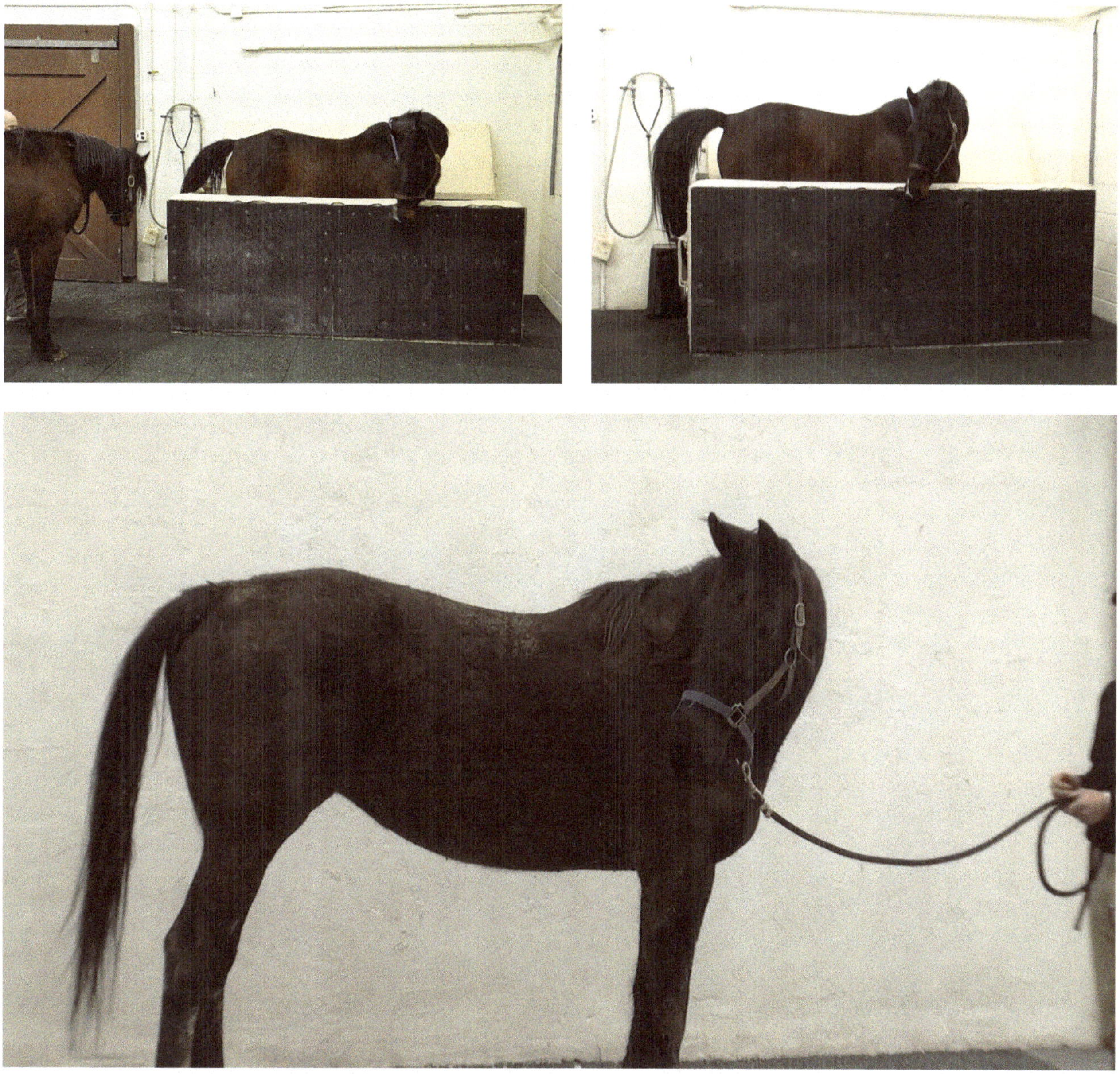

Figure 125.1 Allowing the mare to express natural receptive behavior, especially turning the head back toward the stallion while lifting the tail in response to the stallion's approach. The mare may also simultaneously lift one foreleg. This interactive response represents the natural mount invitation gesture, as if communicating to the stallion "I am not going to move forward or kick."

season, if all parties involved understand the risks, testosterone supplementation can be helpful.

Psychotropics/Anxiolytics

Anxiolytics can also be helpful in improving sexual arousal and response for stallions with naturally low confidence, social inhibition, or conditioned suppression of sexual response. Both diazepam and midazolam have been used at low doses of 0.05 mg/kg, not to exceed a total of 20 mg per horse, administered intravenously slowly, 7 minutes before breeding. An estimated one third of stallions that appear to lack confidence or show signs of inhibition respond well when administered this regimen. Another third appear quieter, in which case repeating the treatment on another occasion with a lower dose may be effective. The remaining third appear to have no change in behavior. This regimen is most often employed with young novice breeders. Once they breed successfully, it is usually not necessary to repeat.

Further Reading

McDonnell SM. 2009. Stallion sexual behavior. In: Samper JC (ed.). Equine Breeding Management and Artificial Insemination, 2nd edn. St Louis, MI: Saunders Elsevier, pp. 41–6.

McDonnell SM. 2016. Revisiting stallion sexual behavior: ethology in the breeding shed. *J Eq Vet Sci* 43: 18–22.

126

Management of Ejaculation Difficulty

Sue M. McDonnell

New Bolton Center, School of Veterinary Medicine, University of Pennsylvania, USA

Introduction

Ejaculation failure in stallions, consistently or intermittently, can result from a variety of factors. These include inadequate arousal due to, for example, immaturity and lack of experience, social insecurity due to intimidation by other stallions, conditioned suppression of sexual response, handling style, health, discomfort, suboptimal stimulus, and breeding environment conditions. Discomfort of any type can also result in failure to ejaculate. In addition, dysfunction can result from disruption of the neurovascular control or other conditions specific to the ejaculatory apparatus. Other more simple physical conditions, such as occluded ampullae, cysts in the seminal colliculus, or bladder neck dysfunction, can result in ejaculation difficulties.

In managing stallions with ejaculation failure, it is helpful to consider possibilities for maximizing sexual interest, arousal, and response (see Chapter 125). This chapter describes additional methods that can be considered for stallions with ejaculation difficulty, including for stallions where the known contributing conditions cannot be sufficiently relieved or where the cause of dysfunction is uncertain.

Equipment and Supplies

Video camera and tripod, phantom or jump mare, phantom leather aids, artificial vagina, small bottle for warm water, sponge for hot compress, disposable examination gloves, needles and syringes.

Handling for Breeding

In addition to the handling discussed in Chapters 124 and 125, it is not unusual to find that the ejaculation dysfunction results from a simple, easily corrected handling mistake, resulting in conditioned interruption of emission. For example, particularly for natural cover, sometimes a handler has the habit of inadvertently increasing tension on the stallion's head restraint just at the moment of the final committed thrust. This habit develops in anticipation of the need to quickly dismount the stallion in order to obtain a dismount semen sample. The tension on the lead becomes a conditioned stimulus for the imminent forced dismount. The distraction can interrupt the fine sympathetic/parasympathetic tone required for emission. Some stallions tend to anticipate the tension, and so dismount before it occurs.

Similar disruption of ejaculation may develop for horses breeding on unsure footing, again the stallion appearing to become anxious in anticipation of dismount. This has been seen in horses breeding by natural cover where mats are used to elevate the stallion and, as the mare moves forward, the stallion steps off the mat, getting the hind limbs trapped between the mare's hind limbs and the mat. Another quite common, similar example involves horses with tender forelegs or carpal rub sores that appear reluctant to grasp firmly for the final committed thrust preceding emission. They often appear anxious and/or distracted, groping for a comfortable position. Some stallions with sore forelegs sometimes hop up to stand with their hooves on the back of the mount, or slide back off the mare or dummy during emission. For semen collection, they may also swing around with both forelegs over the back of the mount.

Equine Reproductive Procedures, Second Edition. Edited by John Dascanio and Patrick McCue.

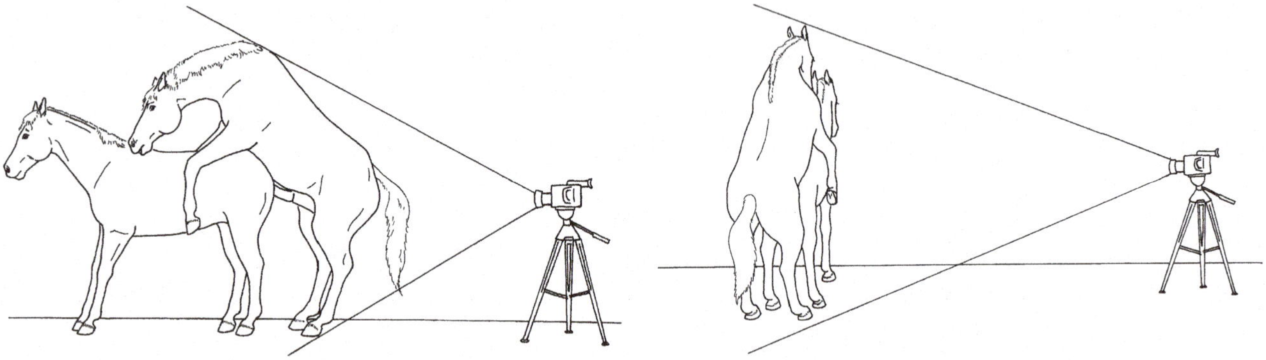

Figure 126.1 Preferred full side and rear video views for evaluating ejaculation failure. In the case of in-hand breeding or semen collection, the view should include the personnel.

Often the best way to evaluate these potential inadvertent conditioning scenerios is to obtain video footage for frame by frame review. The two simultaneous views shown in Figure 126.1 are recommended for this purpose.

Techniques for Enhancing Ejaculation

For semen collection, there are several factors to consider for facilitating efficient ejaculation, in terms of fewer mounts and fewer thrusts required on the ejaculatory mount. Mount height and fit, particularly for disabled stallions, can make a considerable difference. Generally a higher mount, where the stallion's forelegs and chest land just cranial to the "tail" is most helpful for accommodating back or hind limb discomfort or instability. That is especially helpful for dismounting. Well positioned "hips" and bite leathers on a dummy mount can help the stallion stabilize himself as he would on a live mount. A warmer artificial vagina (AV; lumen surface up to 50°C (122°F)) is generally helpful. Firm circumferential pressure applied to the base of the penis generally stimulates more vigorous committed thrusting. The addition of hot compresses (dipped in 50–55°C (122–131°F)) or a warmed hand (using a small bottle filled with similarly hot water in a pocket) can enhance the thrusting response. Holding the distal end of the AV right up against the stallion's ventral midline, as opposed to horizontal or angled below horizontal and/or laterally off the midline, helps many stallions ejaculate with fewer thrusts. While generally not as efficient as an AV, in rare instances in our experience, manual stimulation using hot compresses on the glans and base of the penis has yielded more organized committed thrusting and more consistent ejaculation.

Pharmacological Aids

In addition to the endocrine, analgesic, and anxiolytic agents previously outlined for maximizing arousal and breeding behavior, various neuroactive agents can be useful aids to managing ejaculation difficulties or failure. Alpha-adrenergics, such as xylazine and detomidine, at certain doses can result in ejaculation *ex copula*, in the absence of sexual stimulation. The tricyclic antidepressant benzodiazepines, imipramine, and clomipramine, can similarly induce ejaculation in the absence of sexual arousal. Ejaculation can also occur in stallions treated with prostaglandin $F_{2\alpha}$. A few different protocols have been reported using various combinations of these agents. Semen characteristics (volume, concentration, and total sperm numbers) vary with the agent and particular protocol used. There is a certain art to gauging doses, and the best results and safety levels can be expected when (i) full reports of the various protocols are carefully considered, (ii) the weight of the stallion is measured rather than estimated, and (iii) in the case of α-adrenergics, the stallion is calm and in a quiet environment at the time of administration. These induced ejaculation methods can be particularly useful in disabled or recovering stallions unable to mount or exert for ground semen collection. Imipramine can also be used to reduce the ejaculatory threshold *in copula*, thus reducing the amount of work and potential risks for injury.

In instances where neurogenic discomfort is suspected or known, gabapentin treatment may be helpful. In some cases, a combination of phenylbutazone and gabapentin may be considered.

Ground Semen Collection

For certain stallions with ejaculation failure related to mounting or dismounting difficulties due to discomfort or incoordination, semen collection can be done with the stallion standing (see Chapter 119). Coordinated thrusting can be stimulated with application of an AV or with manual stimulation. Disabled stallions can be stabilized against a padded wall. As with application of an AV for a mounted horse, stabilization of the AV against the ventral midline appears most effective for efficient ejaculation.

Additional Comments

Modifications in breeding schedule or semen collection and processing, as well as upgraded mare management modifications, can often help prolong the breeding career of stallions with chronic ejaculatory difficulty. For horses breeding small books by natural cover, mares can be managed to reduce the total number of covers, and the interval that favors consistent ejaculation. For horses breeding by semen collection, the following can reduce the pressure on the stallion and staff: cryopreserved semen available as a backup, synchronizing mares for maximum use of each ejaculate, and any other semen processing methods that prolong the fertile life of fresh semen.

Further Reading

Forney BD, McDonnell SM. 1999. How to collect semen from stallions while they are standing on the ground. *Proc Annu Conv Am Assoc Eq Pract* 45: 142–4.

Martin BB, McDonnell SM, Love CC. 1998. Effects of musculoskeletal and neurologic disease on breeding performance in stallions. *Compendium* 20: 1159–69.

McDonnell SM. 2001. Oral imipramine and intravenous xylazine for pharmacologically-induced *ex copula* ejaculation in stallions. *Anim Reprod Sci* 68: 153–9.

McDonnell SM. 2001. How to select and fit a breeding dummy mount for stallions. *Proc Annu Conv Am Assoc Eq Pract* 47: 417–19.

127

Calibrated Spectrophotometer Evaluation of Sperm Concentration

John J. Dascanio

School of Veterinary Medicine, Texas Tech University, USA

Introduction

Determination of spermatozoal concentration is required for the accurate calculation of a breeding dose and subsequent dilution of semen for cooled semen transport. Sperm concentration should also be determined as part of a routine stallion breeding soundness examination. Sperm concentration may be determined via a number of methods including manual counting with a hemocytometer, spectrophotometer, computer aided microscopy, and fluorescent assay techniques.

Calibrated spectrophotometers dedicated to estimating stallion sperm concentration are commercially available. The principle by which spectrophotometers estimate sperm concentration is based on measuring the transmission of light of a known wavelength directly through a semen sample or through a suspension of sperm in a known volume of media. The amount of light transmission is inversely correlated with the concentration of sperm. Most dedicated spectrophotometers automatically convert the percent light transmission to sperm concentration in millions of sperm per milliliter.

Equipment and Supplies

Spectrophotometer system, cuvettes, pipettes, paper towel, formalin-saline solution (if needed).

Technique Using a Cuvette

- Collect a semen sample.
- Filter the semen to remove gel and debris.
- Gently mix the semen sample to ensure that a uniform sample is obtained and that spermatozoa have not settled to the bottom of the sample container.
- Spectrophotometer systems available for use include the 590B or 591B Densimeter (Animal Reproduction Systems (ARS), Chino, CA, USA), Quick Check™ Sperm Counting System (Exodus Breeders, York, PA, USA), Accucell or Accuread Equine Photometer (IMV Technologies USA, Maple Grove, MN, USA), Photometer SDM 6 (Minitube USA, Verona, WI, USA), and the iSperm® (Breeder's Choice, Detroit, MI, USA)
- Most of these spectrophotometer systems use a cuvette (Figure 127.1) into which a specific volume of diluent is added, the machine is zeroed, and then a specific volume of semen is added into the diluent. Instructions on the screen or that come with the machine will detail the volume of diluent and semen to add to the cuvette (e.g.,

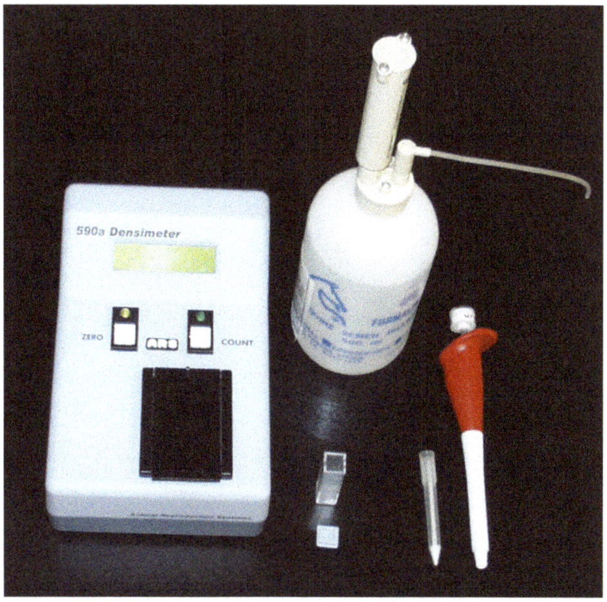

Figure 127.1 The 590B Densimeter model with a dispensing bottle of formalin-saline solution, a cuvette with cap, and a pipette and tip.

Equine Reproductive Procedures, Second Edition. Edited by John Dascanio and Patrick McCue.

3.42 ml of diluent and 0.18 ml semen for the ARS Densimeter).
- The cuvette is gently mixed to evenly distribute the spermatozoa throughout the diluent.
- The cuvette is placed into the unit and the percent light transmission is determined and automatically converted to sperm concentration.
- Care should be exercised to not place fingerprints on the sides through which light transmission will occur to help insure an accurate reading. A soft cloth may be used to wipe the plastic to clean it if needed.
- There are both portable and desktop models available (Figure 127.2). The desktop models may interface with computers to upload results.

Technique Using a Microcuvette

- Collect a semen sample.
- Filter the semen to remove gel and debris.
- Gently mix the semen sample to ensure that a uniform sample is obtained and that spermatozoa have not settled to the bottom of the sample container.
- The Minitube Photometer SDM 1 device does not require semen dilution for measurement (Figure 127.3).
- The tip of the microcuvette may be placed into the semen sample or a disposable pipette may be used to load the microcuvette.
- The outer surface of the microcuvette should be wiped clean of any excess semen prior to placement into the device (Figures 127.4 and 127.5).
- The cuvette is placed into the device and the drawer closed to activate the reading and calculation of spermatozoal concentration.

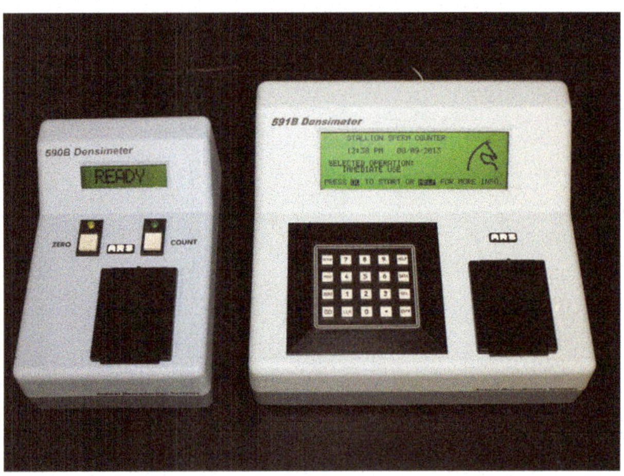

Figure 127.2 The 590B and 591B Densimeter models.

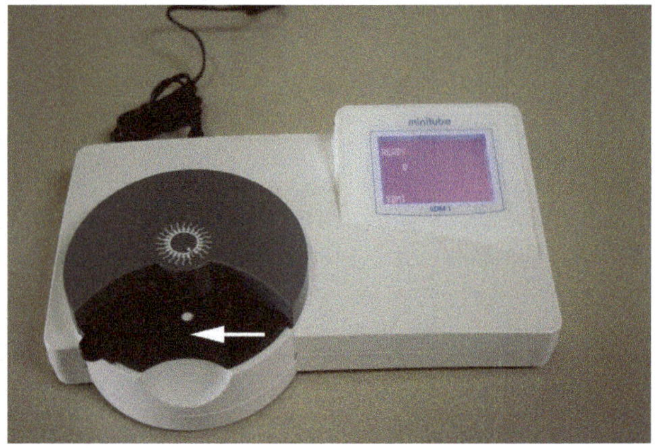

Figure 127.3 Minitube photometer. The arrow is pointing at the tray that the cuvette will lie in once loaded with a semen sample. The drawer is rotated closed and the machine will then automatically read the concentration and display the results in the window.

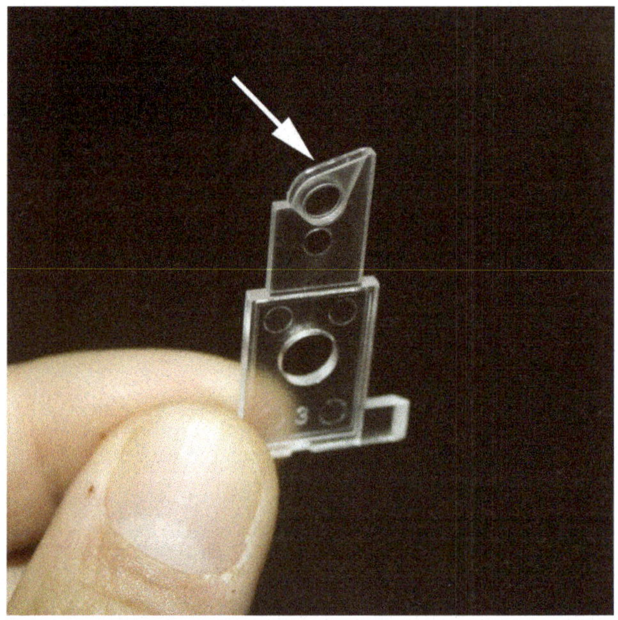

Figure 127.4 Minitube Photometer SDM 1 microcuvette. Semen is loaded into the slot (arrow) on the cuvette either with a disposable pipette or by dipping the end of the cuvette in the semen. Make sure there is no semen on the outside of the cuvette before placement in the device.

Technique Using a Chip

- Collect a semen sample.
- Filter the semen to remove gel and debris.
- Gently mix the semen sample to ensure that a uniform sample is obtained and that spermatozoa have not settled to the bottom of the sample container.
- The iSperm® can be used with raw or extended semen and does not require dilution.

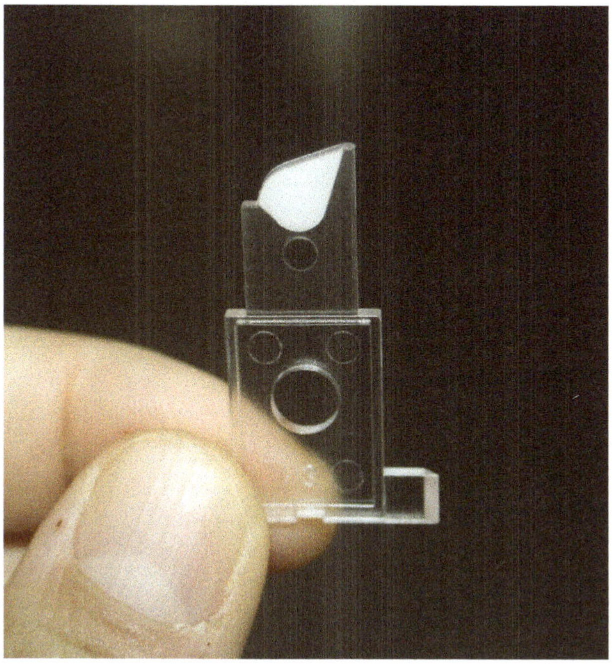

Figure 127.5 Minitube Photometer SDM 1 microcuvette showing the cuvette properly loaded with semen.

- Attach a chip onto the sample collector.
- Dip the chip into the semen sample.
- Cap the cover chip.
- Screw the sample collector into the lens which is attached to an iPad.
- Using proprietary software, an analysis of concentration and motility is performed.
- An optional heating stage is available.

Interpretation

- Any substance that increases optical density will artificially increase the densimeter readings. This includes urine, blood, cellular material, and organic matter. Stallions that have not been washed adequately may have debris in their semen, which can lead to an inaccurate determination of sperm concentration.
- Spectrophotometric estimation of sperm concentration can only be done using raw semen as opaque extenders used for cooled transport or cryopreservation will alter light transmission.
- Erroneous measurements may be obtained if the semen sample is not mixed evenly prior to sampling. Spermatozoa will gradually settle to the bottom of the holding container unless remixed.
- Densimeters tend to be less accurate with very low (<50 million spermatozoa/ml) or very high (>500 million spermatozoa/ml) sperm concentrations.
- A manual hemocytometer count can be performed in the event that a spectrophotometric determination of sperm concentration is in question (see Chapter 128).

Further Reading

Baumber-Skaife J. 2011. Evaluation of semen. In: McKinnon AO, Squires EL, Vaala WE, Varner DD (eds). Equine Reproduction, 2nd edn. Ames, IA: Wiley Blackwell, pp. 1278–91.

Pickett BW, Squires EL, McKinnon AO. 1987. Procedures for Collection, Evaluation and Utilization of Stallion Semen for Artificial Insemination. Animal Reproduction Laboratory General Series Bulletin 03. Fort Collins, CO: Colorado State University.

Rigby SL, Varner DD, Thompson JA, Love CC, Brinsko SP, Blanchard TL. 2001. Measurement of sperm concentration in stallion ejaculates using photometric or direct sperm enumeration techniques. *Proc Annu Conv Am Assoc Eq Pract* 47: 236–8.

128

Hemocytometer Evaluation of Sperm Concentration

John J. Dascanio

School of Veterinary Medicine, Texas Tech University, USA

Introduction

There are several methods used to determine spermatozoal concentration in semen samples, including the use of a hemocytometer, spectrophotometer, computerized microscopy, or fluorescent assay techniques. The hemocytometer is the least expensive method, but is more time consuming than other techniques. The hemocytometer has two individual sides that are counted independently. Results from each side are then averaged to determine the total number of spermatozoa per milliliter. There are a number of mixing, loading, and reading steps that may be affected by human error when performing hemocytometer counts. Multiple studies have shown that the hemocytometer has a high variation and is prone to imprecision, so care must be taken in sample preparation and the counting procedure.

Equipment and Supplies

Microscope, hemocytometer, disposable micropipettes or mechanical pipettes, manual cell counter, distilled water or formal buffered saline, humidified chamber, Thrombo-TIC® kit (Bioanalytic, Germany) (optional).

Technique

- Collect a semen sample.
- Filter the semen to remove gel and debris.
- Gently mix the semen sample to ensure that a uniform sample is obtained and that spermatozoa have not settled to the bottom of the sample container.
- Dilute the raw semen 1:100 in 10% formal buffered saline, distilled water, or other appropriate solution. The goal is to obtain the correct dilution and to immobilize spermatozoa for counting. Options include:
  - *Method 1.* Add 0.1 ml raw semen to 0.9 ml formal buffered saline (or distilled water) using a calibrated pipette. Gently mix the diluted semen sample. Remove 0.1 ml of the mixture and combine with another 0.9 ml of formal buffered saline (or distilled water). This will yield two 1:9 dilutions (10× dilution) and result in an overall dilution of 100×.
  - *Method 2.* Add 20 μl raw semen to 1.98 ml formal buffered saline and gently mix.
  - *Method 3.* Add 10 μl raw semen to 990 μl formal buffered saline and gently mix.
  - *Method 4.* Utilize a commercial kit to achieve a 1:100 dilution. The Thrombo-TIC® kit consists of a prefilled 990 μl reservoir (microcentrifuge tube) and a 10 μl capillary tube (Figure 128.1). The capillary tube is filled completely with raw semen and dropped into the reservoir. The reservoir is gently inverted several times to mix.
- Center a hemocytometer coverslip on the rails of the hemocytometer. Wetting the rails with a minimal amount of water will hold the coverslip in place and make loading the hemocytometer with a semen sample easier. Do not wet the counting grid.
- Gently mix the diluted (100×) semen sample to obtain a uniform solution.
- Using a disposable micropipette or mechanical pipette, load the hemocytometer with 10–15 μl of the diluted semen sample, carefully watching that the chamber under the coverslip is not over- or underfilled. The hemocytometer chamber is filled by placing the pipette tip in the groove on the hemocytometer near the placed coverslip at a 45-degree angle to horizontal (Figure 128.2). A meniscus of fluid may be seen traversing the chamber as

Equine Reproductive Procedures, Second Edition. Edited by John Dascanio and Patrick McCue.

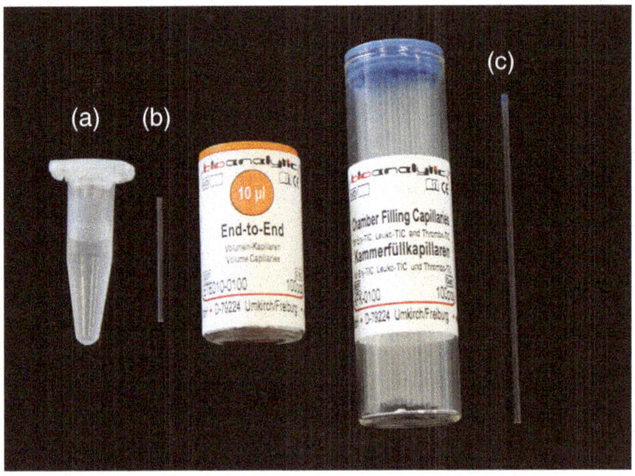

Figure 128.1 Thrombo-TIC® kit used to achieve a 1:100 dilution: prefilled microcentrifuge tube with 990 μl (A), 10 μl capillary tube (B), and 100 μl capillary tube (C). Only the 10 μl capillary tube is used with the prefilled microcentrifuge tube.

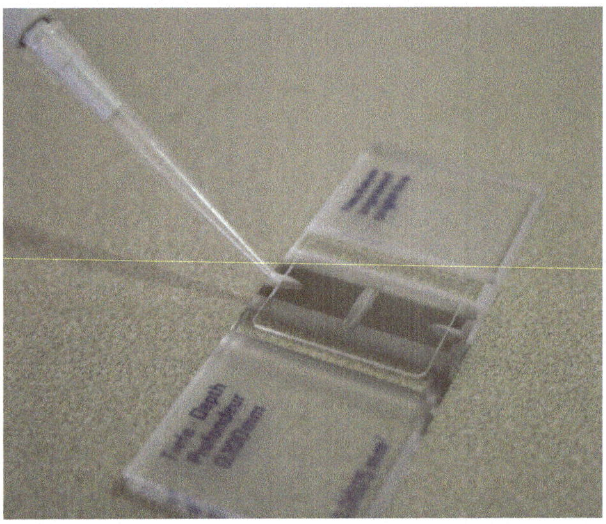

Figure 128.2 Hemocytometer being filled with a mechanical pipette.

it fills. Stop filling the chamber when the meniscus reaches the far side of the chamber. The coverslip should not move during filling and no air bubbles should be present under the coverslip.

- Both sides of the hemocytometer should be filled or loaded.
- The hemocytometer should sit for approximately 5 minutes before counting spermatozoa so that the spermatozoa can settle onto the hemocytometer counting grid from the fluid volume within the hemocytometer chamber. The hemocytometer should be maintained in a humid environment during the 5-minute period to prevent the chamber from drying out. Placement of the hemocytometer within a closed Petri dish, suspended on small straws, overlying wet filter paper or paper towel, will prevent drying. Another practical method would be to cover the hemocytometer with a plastic cup with a slightly damp paper towel underneath.
- Any residual water on the bottom of the hemocytometer slide from the humidity chamber should be removed with a dry wipe. The hemocytometer is then placed on the microscope stage and the central grid of the hemocytometer is located while under a 10× power objective (100× magnification).
- The microscope is then brought to the 40× objective (400× magnification) to count the spermatozoa in the central grid. If spermatozoa are difficult to visualize, the condenser is lowered to increase the contrast.
- If a low number of spermatozoa appear on the large central grid, all spermatozoa in that grid are counted. If the number of spermatozoa is high, then five out of the 25 medium-sized grids in the large central grid are counted and the number multiplied by 5 to obtain the number of spermatozoa in the large central grid (Figure 128.3). A

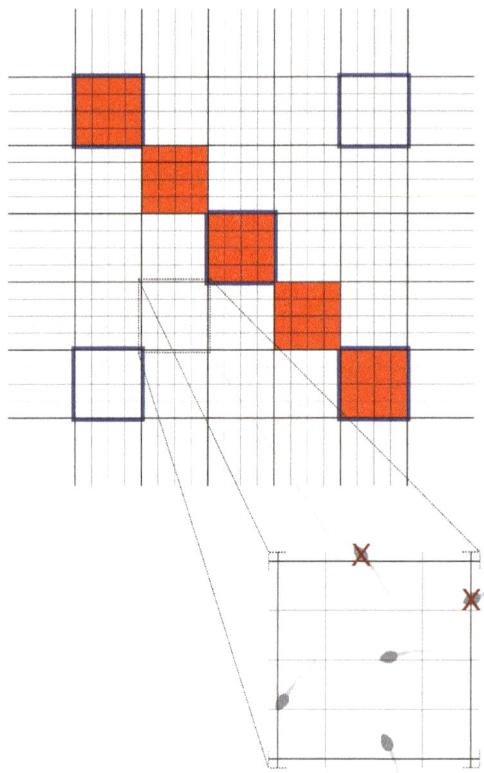

Figure 128.3 Central hemocytometer grid. All spermatozoa within the 25 medium-sized grids (each having 4 × 4 small squares) should be counted. Alternatively, with high concentration samples, five diagonal squares (shaded) or four corner and one central square (darker outline) may be counted and then multiplied by 5. Sperm heads that cross a neighboring upper or right hand line should not be counted (insert).

manual cell counter is used to keep track of counted spermatozoa.

- Only spermatozoal heads are counted, not tails, so that double counting of spermatozoa does not occur.
- If spermatozoal heads are lying on a bordering line, only count those spermatozoal heads on the lower or left lines. This will prevent counting spermatozoa twice once moving to the next square grid (Figure 128.3 insert).
- The volume of liquid under the hemocytometer coverslip is 0.1 mm^3 or 0.1 µl. Thus to get back to 1 ml, multiple by 10,000. The dilution ratio also needs to be factored in, so the final number also needs to be multiplied by 100 (100×). This correlates to a total multiplication factor of 1 million (100 × 10,000); consequently, the total number of spermatozoa in the large central grid of the hemocytometer is equal to that number of millions of spermatozoa per milliliter. As an example, if 430 spermatozoa are counted in the central large grid, then the concentration of spermatozoa is 430 million spermatozoa/ml.
- Ideally 100 spermatozoa or more should be counted in the large central grid for accuracy. Counting less than 100 spermatozoa may result in an error in calculation of the concentration since the sample is too dilute. If less sperm are present, then the dilution factor and multiplication factor need to be altered. As an example, if only a 1:9 dilution is used (10× rather than 100×), then if 305 spermatozoa are counted, the calculation would be 30.5 million spermatozoa/ml (multiplication of 10,000 for volume and 10 for dilution).

Interpretation

- If the results from each side of the hemocytometer are greater than 10% different, the test should be performed again, assuming errors in processing or counting.
- Failure to mix samples at each stage will result in erroneous results.
- When working with small volumes (i.e., 10–20 µl), errors in pipetting can add significant error.
- Over- or underfilling of the hemocytometer chambers will result in erroneous results.
- Use the provided coverslip for the hemocytometer. A disposable coverslip is thinner and may deform, changing the volume in the hemocytometer chamber.
- Read the directions included with the hemocytometer to make sure it is a standard hemocytometer and follows the instructions presented here.

Further Reading

Prathalingam NS, Holt WW, Revell SG, Jones S, Watson PF. 2006. The precision and accuracy of six different methods to determine sperm concentration. *J Androl* 27: 257–62.

Rigby SL, Varner DD, Thompson JA, Love CC, Brinsko SP, Blanchard TL. 2001. Measurement of sperm concentration in stallion ejaculates using photometric or direct sperm enumeration techniques. *Proc Annu Conv Am Assoc Eq Pract* 47: 236–8.

129

NucleoCounter® Evaluation of Sperm Concentration and Viability

Patrick M. McCue

Equine Reproduction Laboratory, Colorado State University, USA

Introduction

An accurate measurement of sperm concentration is an integral part of the determination of the total number of spermatozoa in an ejaculate. Techniques available for the evaluation of sperm concentration include a manual hemocytometer count, spectrophotometric analysis, flow cytometry, and fluorescent microscopy. "Viability" of spermatozoa is typically an evaluation of sperm plasma membrane integrity and may not be related to true live-dead status.

The NucleoCounter® is an automated cell counter that may be used to determine the concentration of spermatozoa in equine semen. The unit uses fluorescent microscopy to objectively count cells (i.e., spermatozoa) containing DNA. A specific volume of semen is added to a specific volume of reagent that disrupts the sperm plasma membrane and dilutes the semen sample. Sperm cells in this lysate mixture are subsequently exposed to a fluorescent dye (propidium iodide, PI) which binds to the DNA within the sperm nuclei. The suspension of diluted semen is then exposed to a green light, which elicits a red fluorescence from the packets of DNA (nuclei) stained with PI. A camera records the image and the unit converts the photon signals into electrical signals. Image analysis software counts the number of nuclei and displays the results as number of spermatozoa (millions) per milliliter.

The NucleoCounter® is also designed to estimate the viability of spermatozoa in a semen sample by assessing the concentration of non-viable sperm cells. A different dilution reagent and possibly a different dilution factor is used in the analysis. The dilution reagent (i.e., phosphate buffered saline, PBS) for non-viable cell analysis does not contain any detergent or other substances designed to disrupt cell membranes. Therefore the NucleoCounter® should only detect sperm cells with already damaged cell membranes (i.e., dead spermatozoa) when performing the analysis of non-viable cells. The viable count can be determined by subtracting the number of non-viable cells from the total number of cells and expressing the result as a percentage of the total number of cells using the following formula (Box 129.1):

$$\text{Viability}\left(\%\right) = 100 \times \left(\text{Total cell count} - \text{Non-viable cell count}\right) / \text{Total cell count}$$

The primary advantages of the NucleoCounter® are that it is rapid, repeatable, and can determine sperm concentration in either raw or extended semen. The latter function makes it different from spectrophotometer-based systems, which cannot determine sperm concentration in solutions with increased optical density such as semen extended with opaque extenders or semen contaminated with urine or non-cellular debris. In addition, the accuracy of sperm concentration determination is greater when using a DNA-binding stain than in a spectrophotometric system looking at semen samples with low sperm concentrations.

The main disadvantages are the initial cost of the system and cost for each measurement of sperm concentration. In addition, the viability assessment of the NucleoCounter® does not always correlate highly with other measures of sperm viability, such as flow cytometry or eosin-nigrosin (EN) staining.

Equipment and Supplies

NucleoCounter® SP-100 (ChemoMetic A/S, Allerod, Denmark), SP1 cassettes (single use, disposable), lysis/dilution buffer (reagent S100) and dispenser, phosphate buffered saline (dilution buffer) and dispenser, pipette and disposable tips, sample cup.

Equine Reproductive Procedures, Second Edition. Edited by John Dascanio and Patrick McCue.

Box 129.1 Calculation of Percent Viability for a Semen Sample

Example:

- Total cell count = 375 million sperm/ml
- Non-viable cell count = 125 million sperm/ml
- Insert the values for the Total cell count and Non-viable cell count into the formula:
  Viability (%) = 100 × (Total cell count − Non-viable cell count)/Total cell count
  Viability (%) = 100 × (375 − 125)/375
  Viability (%) = 100 × (250)/375
  Viability (%) = 100 × (0.667)
  Viability (%) = 66.7%

Technique

Total Cell Count

- Six options are available for semen dilution prior to the total cell count; selection of the optimal semen dilution should be based on an estimation of the sperm concentration in the original ejaculate. The most commonly used is dilution factor (DF) = 201, which is optimal for semen samples with a sperm concentration of 250 million to 1.0 billion sperm/ml (outer range 100 million to 1.4 billion sperm/ml) (Figure 129.1)
- For DF = 201, a 50 μl sample of raw semen is placed in the bottom of a 20 ml sample cup (Figure 129.2).
- 10.0 ml of reagent S100 is added to the sample cup.
- The sample is thoroughly mixed.
- A small volume (approximately 60 μl) of the lysate mixture is loaded into a SP1 casette by pressing on the cassette piston while the cassette tip is immersed in the mixture (Figure 129.3).
- The cassette is inserted into the NucleoCounter® set to DF = 201 and the lid is closed (Figure 129.4).
- The analysis is initiated by pressing the "Run" button and takes approximately 30 seconds to complete.
- The concentration of spermatozoa in the original sample of raw semen is displayed and presented as millions of sperm per milliliter (Figure 129.5).
- Other semen : reagent dilutions may also be used and are selected based on the estimated sperm concentration in the initial semen sample. Note that other dilutions require different dilution factors to be selected on the NucleoCounter® (see manufacturer instructions for details).

Viability Count

- Note that the semen sample should be diluted in PBS not reagent S100.
- The DF used for viability can either be the same as used for the total cell count or the next lower DF; for example, if DF 201 is used for the total cell count (DF1), then the viability count (DF2) should either be 201 or 101.
- As an example, using DF 201 for the viability count, a 50 μl sample of raw semen is placed in the bottom of a 20 ml sample cup.
- 10.0 ml of PBS is added to the sample cup.
- The sample is thoroughly mixed.
- A small volume (approximately 60 μl) of the semen/PBS mixture is loaded into a SP1 cassette by pressing on the cassette piston while the cassette tip is immersed in the mixture.
- The cassette is inserted into the NucleoCounter® set to DF2 (viability mode) and the lid is closed.
- The analysis is initiated by pressing the "Run" button and takes approximately 80 seconds to complete.
- The concentration of non-viable (i.e., membrane damaged) spermatozoa in the original sample of raw semen is displayed and presented as millions of sperm per milliliter. The percentage of viable (membrane intact) sperm can then be calculated using the formula at the beginning of the chapter.

Additional Comments

There are many techniques available to estimate sperm concentration. The main clinical advantage of the NucleoCounter® is the ability to determine sperm concentration in stallion semen samples diluted in opaque extenders such as milk-based extenders used for cooled-transported semen and all freezing extenders. The alternative technique, manual hemocytometer counting of sperm, is less expensive to perform but is time consuming and may be inaccurate unless very detailed procedures are followed. The NucleoCounter® can subsequently be used to determine sperm concentration on a shipment of cooled semen or after thawing a dose of frozen semen. The sperm concentration value, along with volume and total/progressive motility, can then be used to determine the total number of motile sperm inseminated into a mare.

"Sperm viability" is an ambiguous but commonly used term. Most measures of sperm viability refer to the integrity of the sperm plasma membrane. Techniques used to measure sperm viability rely on penetration of special stains

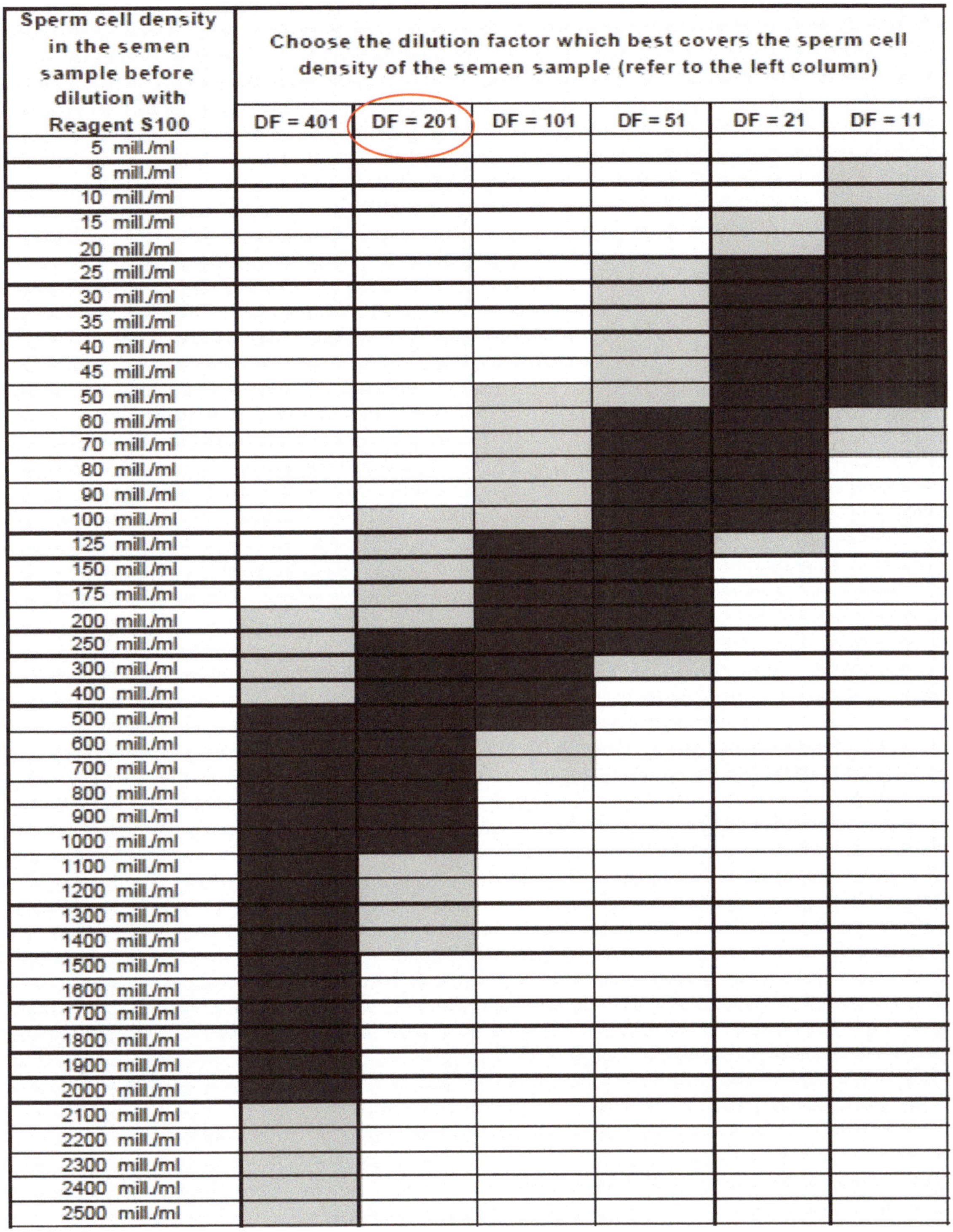

Figure 129.1 Semen dilution chart for the NucleoCounter®. The most commonly used dilution is dilution factor (DF) = 201 (red circle).

How to obtain a Dilution Factor of 401:

Sample	50 µl	25 µl	10 µl
Reagent S100	20.0 ml	10.0 ml	4.0 ml

To minimize pipetting errors, sample volumes smaller than 50 µl are not recommended

How to obtain a Dilution Factor of 201:

Sample	100 µl	50 µl	25 µl	10 µl
Reagent S100	20.0 ml	10.0 ml	5.0 ml	2.0 ml

How to obtain a Dilution Factor of 101:

Sample	200 µl	100 µl	50 µl	25 µl	10 µl
Reagent S100	20.0 ml	10.0 ml	5.0 ml	2.5 ml	1.0 ml

How to obtain a Dilution Factor of 51:

Sample	400 µl	200 µl	100 µl	50 µl	25 µl	20 µl
Reagent S100	20.0 ml	10.0 ml	5.0 ml	2.50 ml	1.25 ml	1.00 ml

How to obtain a Dilution Factor of 21:

Sample	1000 µl	500 µl	200 µl	100 µl	50 µl	25 µl
Reagent S100	20.0 ml	10.0 ml	4.0 ml	2.0 ml	1.0 ml	0.5 ml

How to obtain a Dilution Factor of 11:

Sample	1000 µl	500 µl	200 µl	100 µl	50 µl	25 µl
Reagent S100	10.0 ml	5.0 ml	2.0 ml	1.0 ml	0.5 ml	0.25 ml

Figure 129.2 How to dilute stallion semen according to dilution factor (DF) selected.

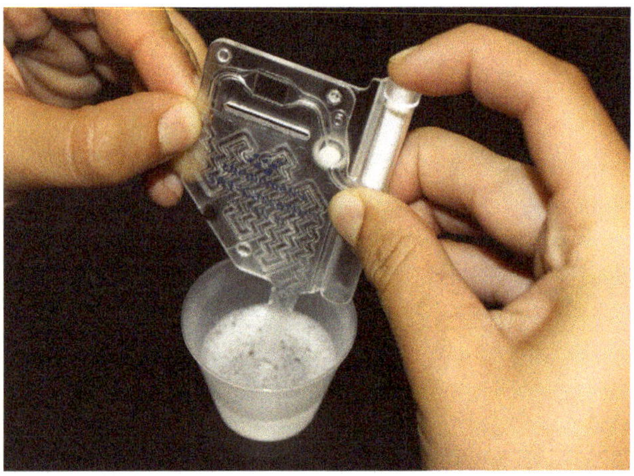

Figure 129.3 Loading the SP1 cassette with sperm diluted in the lysis/dilution buffer.

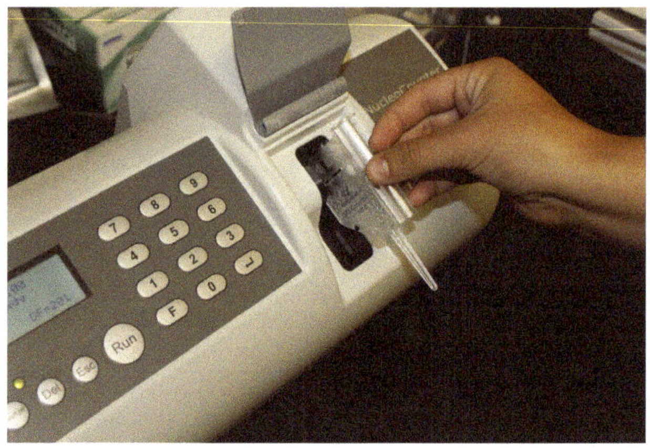

Figure 129.4 Placing the loaded SP1 cassette into the NucleoCounter®.

such as eosin or propidium iodide. Differences in sperm viability values determined by EN staining versus PI staining may reflect differences in penetration rates or a subjective interpretation of degree of staining in EN staining.

Sperm viability measurements are usually correlated with estimates of sperm motility. However, there appear to be populations of sperm that are non-motile yet contain an intact plasma membrane (i.e., "viable").

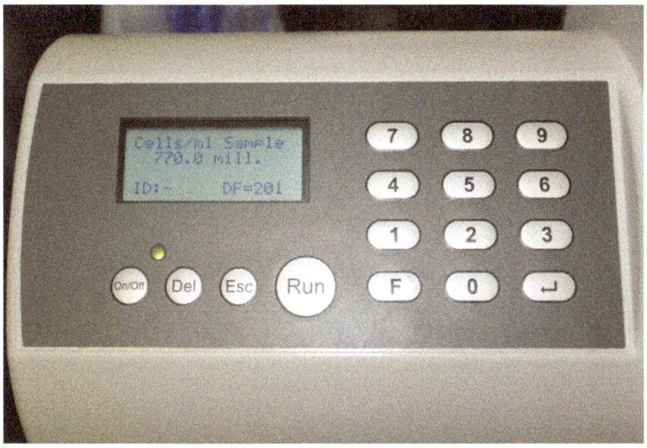

Figure 129.5 Display of sperm concentration on the NucleoCounter®.

Further Reading

Johansson CS, Matsson FC, Lehn-Jensen H, Nielsen JM, Petersen MM. 2008. Equine spermatozoa viability comparing the NucleoCounter SP-100 and eosin-nigrosin stain. *Anim Reprod Sci* 107: 325–6.

Love CC. 2013. Measurement of concentration and viability in stallion sperm. *J Eq Vet Sci* 32: 4464–6.

130

Visual Evaluation of Sperm Motility

Patrick M. McCue

Equine Reproduction Laboratory, Colorado State University, USA

Introduction

Fresh gel-free semen should be extended as soon as possible to preserve the viability of the spermatozoa and to permit observation of individual sperm motility characteristics. In addition, spermatozoa in a "raw" or undiluted semen sample are often highly concentrated and tend to clump or agglutinate, making an accurate estimate of motility in raw semen difficult or impossible.

Motility evaluation of extended cooled semen should be performed after allowing a small aliquot of semen to warm to approximately 37°C (98.6°F) for approximately 10 minutes. If the extended semen is not warmed properly, the motility values may be underestimated.

It is important that all materials that come in contact with the semen are clean, dry, and warmed to approximately 37°C (98.6°F). Ideally, estimates of sperm motility should be made as soon as possible after semen collection.

Table 130.1 Volume of semen extender to add to a standard volume of raw semen (180 μl) to provide a final concentration of approximately 25 million sperm/ml, when the original sperm concentration in the ejaculate is known.

Sperm Concentration (millions per ml)	Raw Semen Volume (μl)	Extender Volume (ml)
100	180	0.5
150	180	1.0
200	180	1.5
250	180	2.0
300	180	2.0
350	180	2.5
400	180	3.0
450	180	3.5
500	180	3.5
550	180	4.0
600	180	4.5
650	180	4.5
700	180	5.0
750	180	5.5
800	180	6.0
850	180	6.0
900	180	6.5
950	180	7.0
1,000	180	7.5

Equipment and Supplies

Semen extender, pipette, microscope with stage warmer, microscope slides, coverslip, 2–15 ml plastic disposable tubes, disposable pipettes, incubator, slide warmer.

Technique

- Semen is obtained from the stallion and the volume and concentration are determined.
- A small volume of semen is diluted into warmed semen extender. Ideally, semen should be evaluated at a consistent concentration of 25 million sperm per milliliter. A convenient method to dilute semen to this concentration is to add 180 μl of raw semen to an appropriate volume of warm extender (Table 130.1) to yield a final concentration of 25 million sperm/ml.
- Alternatively a 1:20 (semen : extender) dilution can be prepared by adding 0.25 ml of semen to 4.75 ml of warmed extender.

Equine Reproductive Procedures, Second Edition. Edited by John Dascanio and Patrick McCue.

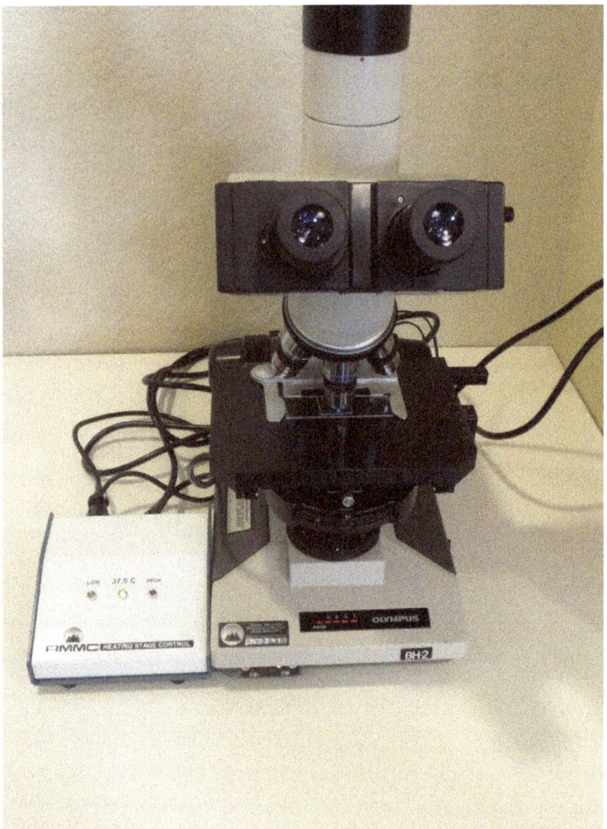

Figure 130.1 Light microscope with slide warmer.

- A small drop (6–10 μl) of extended semen is placed on a clean glass slide and covered with a clean coverslip. The quality of the examination is enhanced if the glass slides and coverslips are maintained at approximately 37°C using a slide warmer. Care should be taken to avoid trapping air bubbles in the semen when applying the coverslip.
- The slide is placed on the stage of a good quality light microscope, preferably a phase-contrast microscope equipped with a stage warmer (Figure 130.1). It is essential that the specimen be kept warm or the percentage of progressive sperm motility will be underestimated.
- Immediately after the slide is prepared, it is examined microscopically at a magnification of 200× to 400×. Five microscope fields should be examined and the results averaged.
- Generally, two motility estimates are determined when examining a semen sample:
  - *Total motility* refers to the percentage of sperm that exhibit any type of movement, and includes sperm moving in a straight line, circling, and/or twitching.
  - *Progressive motility* refers to sperm that exhibit forward motility across the microscopic field or are moving in a large circular path.
- Estimates of total and progressive motility should be evaluated from multiple visual fields and a representative average recorded.

Additional Comments

- Sperm motility estimates should be made quickly and efficiently after semen collection, especially if the microscope stage is not heated.
- The edge of the coverslip should be avoided where drying of the specimen and an artificial reduction in sperm motility may occur.
- Visual assessment of sperm motility is subjective, prone to bias, and may vary between examiners. Computer-assisted sperm analysis (CASA) systems have been developed to provide a more objective assessment of total and progressive motility (see Chapter 131)
- In general, most fertile stallions should have a progressive sperm motility of at least 60%.
- Spermatozoa may normally swim in a large circular path due to an abaxial attachment of the midpiece to the sperm head.

Further Reading

Hodder ADJ, Liu I. 2011. Spermatozoal motility. In: McKinnon AO, Squires EL, Vaala WE, Varner DD (eds). Equine Reproduction, 2nd edn. Ames, IA: Wiley Blackwell, pp. 1292–6.

131

Computer-Assisted Sperm Analysis

John J. Dascanio[1] and Lynda M. J. Miller[2]

[1]*School of Veterinary Medicine, Texas Tech University, USA*
[2]*College of Veterinary Medicine, Lincoln Memorial University, USA*

Introduction

Computer-assisted (or automated) sperm analysis or CASA is an objective way to evaluate spermatozoal motility. Modern CASA systems also advertise the ability to assess spermatozoal morphology, concentration, and viability. However, CASA units are not as accurate as traditional methods of morphology and concentration assessments. CASA employs the use of a microscope, a video camera, and computer software for the analysis. The system records multiple images of sperm movement (60 frames per second with 40 frames analyzed) to provide data that the computer system then uses to "connect the dots" resulting in a linear path of individual sperm movement (Figures 131.1 and 131.2). The dots marked on the computer screen are referred to as centroids and mark the location of the sperm head. In order for the computer to distinguish between debris and actual spermatozoa, certain gates or parameters must be pre-set in the software so that only cells of a certain size are evaluated and so that motility estimation may be performed based on velocity measurements. The gates are usually pre-set by the manufacturer for a particular species, but can be adjusted by the end user.

A special microscope slide is recommended for use in the CASA system that has a predefined volume (10 or 20 μm depth chamber). The fixed volume is sufficient to allow free movement of spermatozoa, but limits the depth so that the optics can focus on a group of spermatozoa. Regular microscope slides and coverslips may be used, but this may result in uneven slide depth and more variation between samples as the depth of field varies. Depth of the chamber will influence results, so a notation should be made as to the size of chamber that was used in the analysis.

Some systems accommodate fluorescent labeling of spermatozoa to avoid interference from debris in the sample, such as particulate matter in semen extenders. This makes analysis of frozen-thawed semen samples possible in samples with unclarified egg yolk extenders. Most equine skim milk-type semen extenders used for cooled semen transport do not interfere with motility readings and may be used to dilute semen for CASA analysis.

Equipment and Supplies

CASA machine (microscope, video camera, monitor, computer, software), mechanical pipettes and tips, CASA microscope slides, printer.

Technique

- Obtain a semen sample and filter to remove any gross debris and the gel fraction.
- Determine the spermatozoal concentration in the raw sample.
- Dilute the semen with commercial semen extender to obtain a final concentration of 25–50 million spermatozoa/ml. The extender should be free of debris that could interfere with the sample measurement. Dilution is important in order to avoid contact between spermatozoa and cross-over artifacts in which one spermatozoon moves across the path of another spermatozoon, which could potentially confuse the software as to the true path of an individual spermatozoon.
- Mix the sample thoroughly just prior to sampling.
- Using a mechanical pipette and attached tip, load the chamber on the CASA microscope slide with the appropriate volume.
- Place the slide on a heated microscope stage (37°C, 99°F) on the CASA machine. Variations in temperature will have a significant effect on motility estimates so a heated microscope stage is a requirement for analysis.

Equine Reproductive Procedures, Second Edition. Edited by John Dascanio and Patrick McCue.

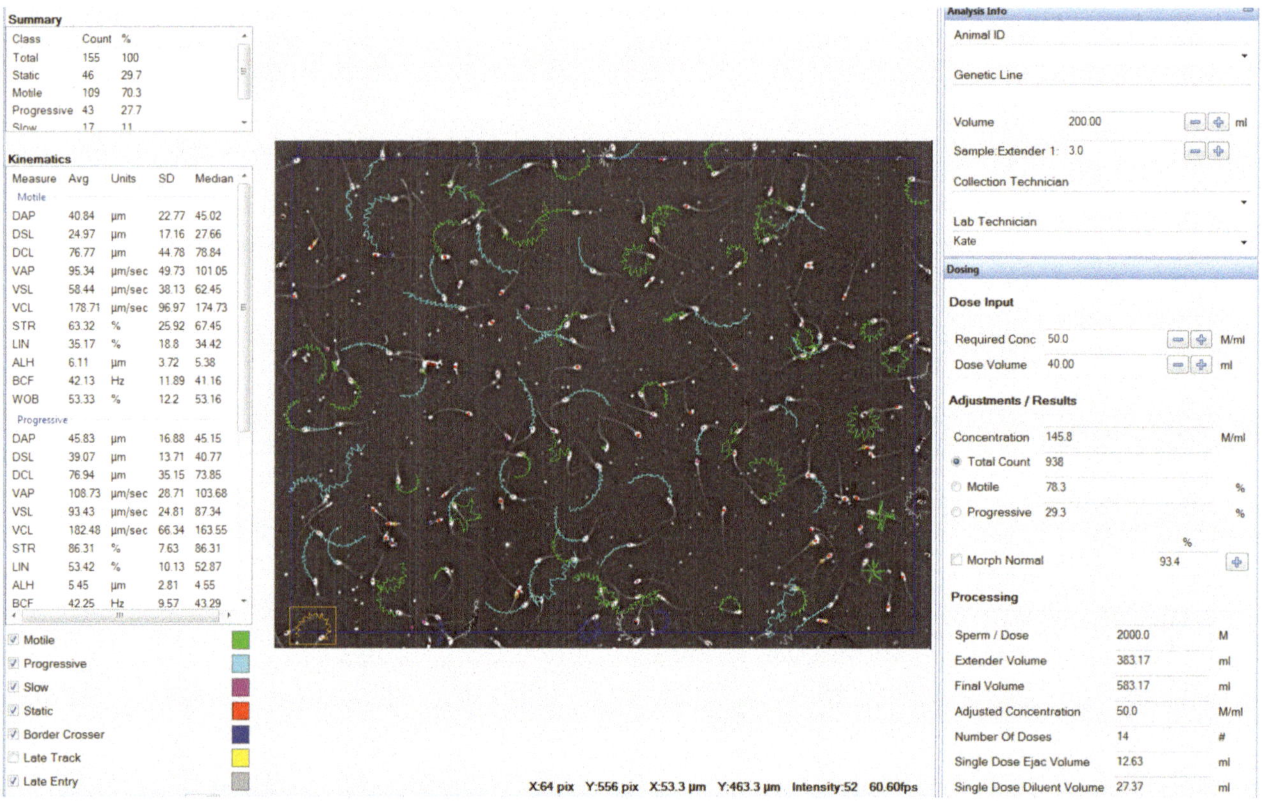

Figure 131.1 Screen image from the monitor of a Hamilton-Thorne® CASA machine demonstrating the curvilinear paths of spermatozoa over 40 frames. Refer to the text for an explanation of abbreviations.

- Orientate the slide on the stage so that the objective is located in the central region of the coverslip chamber. It is important to avoid the edges of the chamber where spermatozoa may not be as motile due to drying of the sample or interaction with the wall of the chamber.
- Ensure that there is no flowing movement to the liquid on the slide by observing the spermatozoal movement on the monitor. If all spermatozoa are moving the same direction independent of tail movement, the slide may have been overfilled. Either wait a few seconds to see if the sample stabilizes or make a new slide.
- Initiate the software to evaluate spermatozoal motility. Typically five or more separate fields are read to provide an average assessment of motility. Avoid regions of the slide with large amounts of debris. Also, avoid bias in the selection of fields in which sperm appear more or less motile.
- Each slide chamber is to be used only once and then discarded. However, the slide has two to eight chambers that may be used to independently assess multiple different semen samples. Only one chamber should be used per stallion. A permanent marker can be used to "X" out a used chamber to avoid accidental refilling.

Interpretation

A minimum of 400 motile or 1,000 total spermatozoa should be counted. A number of measurements of spermatozoal motility are provided by the software. Total and progressive motility are the two parameters most commonly reported. Other parameters are described below and shown in Figure 131.3.

- DAP – distance of the average path (µm).
- DCL – curvilinear distance (µm).
- DSL – straight line distance (µm).
- VAP – average path velocity. This is the velocity of the spermatozoa along a smoothed path calculated using various algorithms from the curvilinear path (µm/s).
- VCL – curvilinear path velocity. This is the velocity of the spermatozoa along the actual path of the sperm from the dots connected from the various images obtained (µm/s).
- VSL – straight line path velocity. This is the velocity along the path drawn in a straight line from the first to the last sperm head location (µm/s).
- LIN – linearity. This is calculated from VSL/VCL.
- STR – straightness. This is calculated from VSL/VAP.
- WOB – wobble. This is calculated from VAP/VCL.

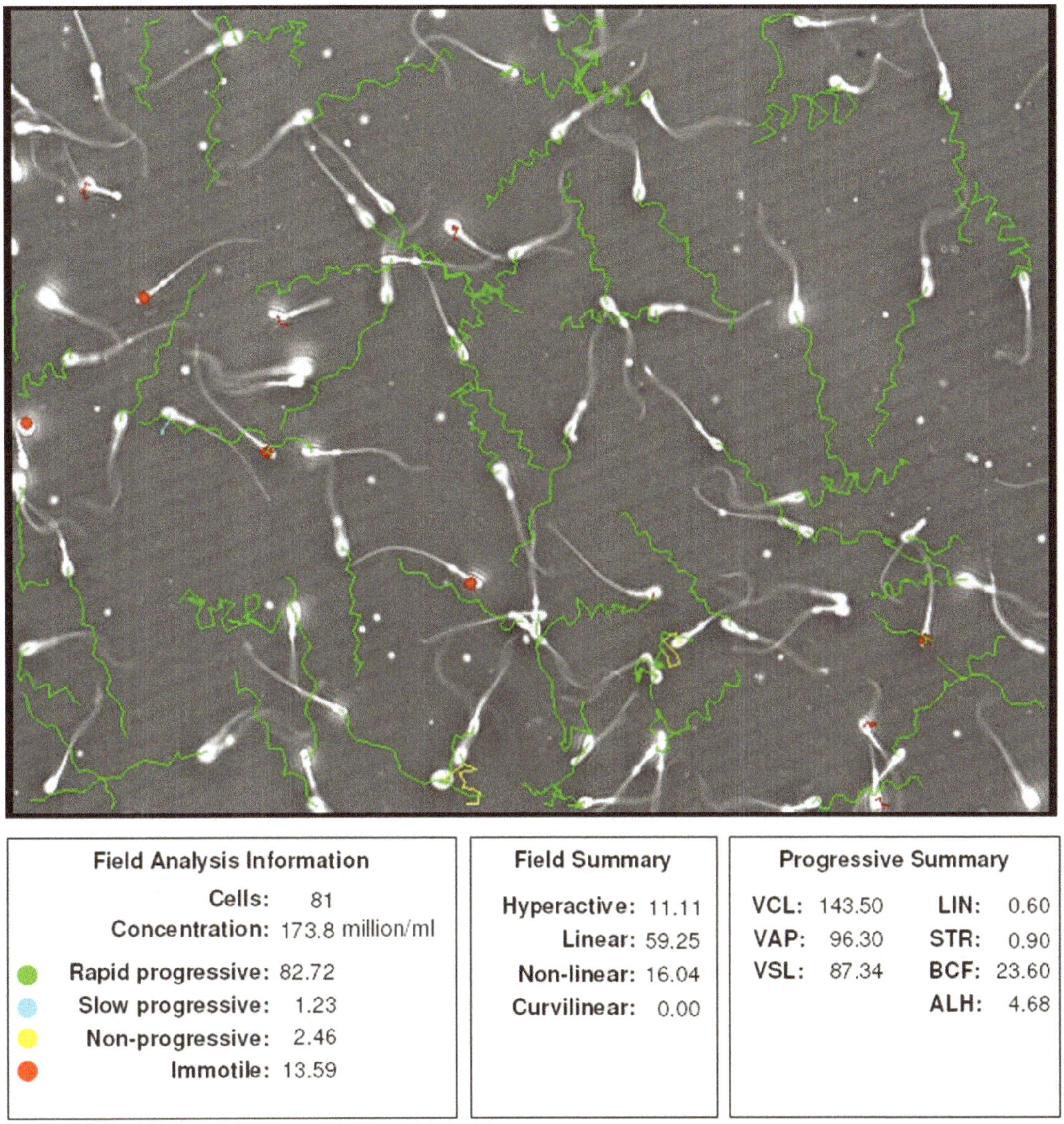

Figure 131.2 Screen image from the monitor of a MiniTube SpermVision® CASA machine demonstrating the curvilinear paths of spermatozoa over 30 frames (60 frames/s). Refer to the text for an explanation of abbreviations.

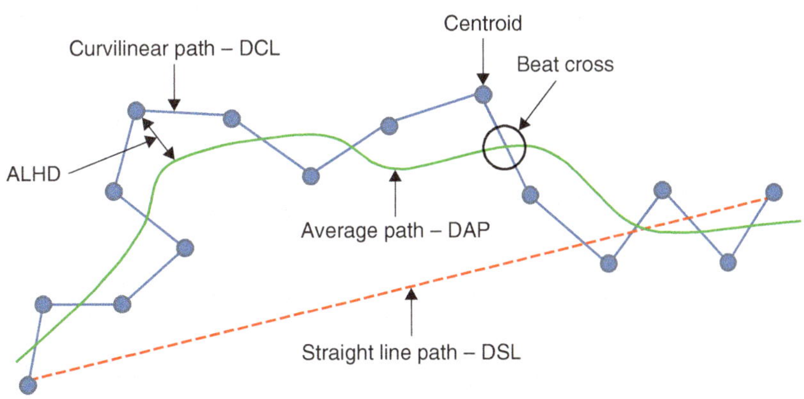

Figure 131.3 Spermatozoal motility measurements as assessed by CASA. Centroid refers to the center location of the sperm head to the amplitude of lateral head displacement (ALHD). Refer to the text for an explanation of abbreviations.

- ALH/ALHD – amplitude of lateral head displacement. This is the mean deviation of the sperm head from its average path (μm).
- BCF – beat cross frequency. Frequency that the actual path crosses the average path expressed as intersections per second (Hz).

Algorithims used to calculate these indices may vary between CASA software resulting in potentially different results for the same semen sample when using different systems. In addition, variations in the settings for spermatozoal head size and others may also yield differing results. Thus, it is important to report all settings when publishing results.

Motility estimation is performed slightly differently with different CASA machines based on the age of the software/hardware and the manufacturer. Settings for analysis should be documented. Some methods to estimate motility are presented here.

Motility Estimation Method 1

- Equine spermatozoa should have an average path velocity of >50 μm/s with a straightness of >75% to be considered progressively motile. Spermatozoa with an average path velocity <20 μm/s are considered non-motile. Sperm with an average path velocity between 50 and 20 μm/s are considered slow moving.

Motility Estimation Method 2 (SpermVision®)

- Sperm head size is identified by cells that range from 14 to 80 μm^2. This variation allows sperm to change orientation without the software losing the cell.
- Motility is divided into immotile, local motile, or progressively motile. Immotile cells have an average orientation change of less than 9.5 μm. Locally motile cells have a DSL <6 μm. All others are considered progressively motile.
- Progressively motile cells are evaluated for classification as hyperactive, linear, or non-linear. Progressively motile cells that exhibit a VCL >80 and LIN <0.65 and ALHD >6.5 are categorized as hyperactive. Hyperactive cells display enhanced motility moving somewhat erratically. In some species this is considered a sign of capacitated spermatozoa. Progressively motile cells that exhibit a STR >0.9 and LIN >0.5 are categorized as linear. Progressively motile cells that exhibit a STR <0.9 and LIN <0.5 are categorized as non-linear.

Additional Comments

The reader is directed to the references for more detail on the validation of systems. Accu-Beads® (Hamilton-Thorne, Beverly, MA, USA) are small latex beads (4 μm diameter) that may be used to check the performance of the optical system and computer image processing. Different concentrations are used during the analysis to check the machine's capability for determining concentration. This method does not analyze motility capability.

Further Reading

Amann RP, Waberski D. 2014. Computer-assisted sperm analysis (CASA): capabilities and potential developments. *Theriogenology* 81: 5–17.

Hoogewijs MK, De Vliegher SP, Govaere JL, De Schauwer C, De Kruif A, Van Soom A. 2012. Influence of counting chamber type on CASA outcomes of equine semen analysis. *Eq Vet J* 44: 542–9.

Loomis PR, Graham JK. 2008. Commercial semen freezing: individual male variation in cryosurvival and the response of stallion sperm to customized freezing protocols. *Anim Reprod Sci* 105: 119–28.

132

Eosin-Nigrosin Staining in the Evaluation of Sperm

Julie T. Cecere

Virginia-Maryland College of Veterinary Medicine, USA

Introduction

Morphologic evaluation of stallion semen is essential to any breeding soundness examination. The percentage of morphologically normal sperm is positively correlated with pregnancy rates in all species. Many methods have been developed to determine the quality of spermatozoa including sperm chromatin integrity, acrosomal reaction and capacitation, and special stains. A stain used routinely for semen evaluation across species is eosin-nigrosin, otherwise known as Hancock's stain. The eosin component will penetrate through the plasma membrane of dead sperm cell and is excluded from live cells. Nigrosin provides background contrast to evaluate morphology and differentiate between live and dead sperm. Cells that are dead will stain red, whereas live cells are white ("red is dead"). The ease with which this stain is utilized for determining the morphologic characteristics of spermatozoa makes it a widely used stain in reproductive practice. Phase-contrast microscopy, electron microscopy, and differential interference contrast microscopy are other methods for evaluation of spermatozoal morphology.

Equipment and Supplies

Pipettes, glass slides, warming plate (37°C, 99°F), eosin-nigrosin stain, Kimwipes®, microscope, immersion oil, cell counter.

Semen Staining Technique

- Warm a glass slide on a warming plate set at 37°C (98.6°F). This is to prevent cold shocking of the spermatozoa.

Technique 1

- With the slide still on the warmer and placed flat, place one drop of the stain, approximately 20–30 µl, on the end of the slide, leaving enough room for a drop of semen to be placed adjacent to the stain without touching.
- Place one drop of the semen, the same or slightly less than the volume of stain, on the slide (Figure 132.1). Do not touch the stain drop with the dropper of the semen.
- With the edge of a clean slide gently rock the edge between the drops of semen and stain to mix them together on the lower slide. Do not use a circular motion as you can cause damage to the spermatozoa (Figure 132.2).
- Once the drops are mixed and you have a uniform layer on the upper slide, pick up your slide from the sample.

Technique 2

- This technique is used with semen samples that are more concentrated as it results in dilution of the spermatozoa to allow for optimal evaluation (less overlying spermatozoa).

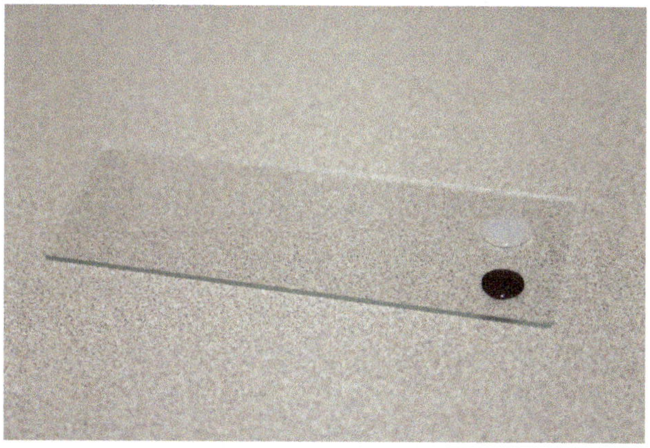

Figure 132.1 A drop of eosin-nigrosin stain is placed on a slide with a drop of semen.

Equine Reproductive Procedures, Second Edition. Edited by John Dascanio and Patrick McCue.

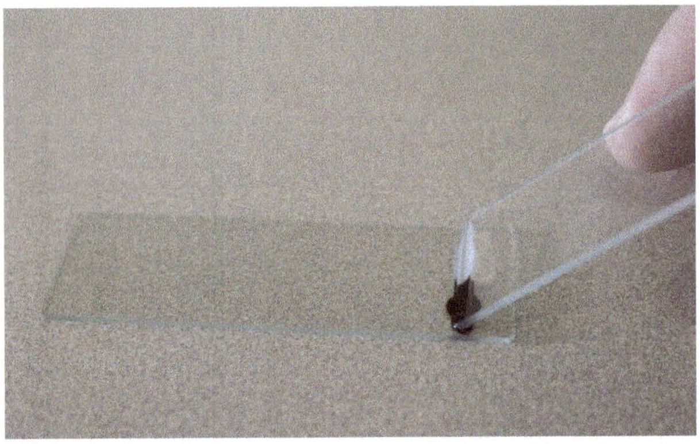

Figure 132.2 The end of an additional slide is dipped into the two drops. The upward slide may be gently rocked to mix the two drops together.

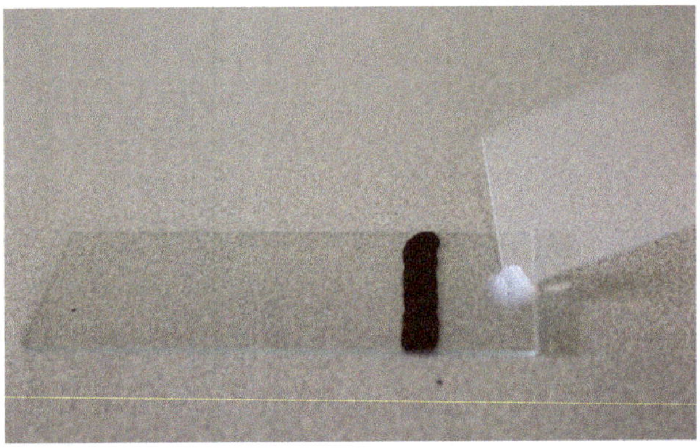

Figure 132.3 The upward slide may be dipped into a semen drop placed behind a line of eosin-nigrosin stain.

- With the slide still on the warmer, place a thin line of eosin-nigrosin stain perpendicularly across the glass slide at one end of the slide.
- Place a small drop of semen on the slide between the end of the slide and the line of stain.
- Take just the corner of a clean slide and touch it into the semen drop (Figure 132.3). This will pick up a smaller volume of semen than technique 1. Place this end of the slide into the line of stain so that the entire end of the clean slide with the semen sample is in contact with the entire line of stain (Figure 132.4).
- The slide may be gently rocked to mix the sperm with the stain. Once this is accomplished, lift the upper slide from the lower slide.

Semen Smearing Technique

- Place the upper slide back down on a clean part of the lower slide, about 0.5 cm (0.25 inch) away from the mixed sample, at a 45-degree angle.
- Now push (or pull) the 45-degree slide out to the end of the lower first slide. Make sure to keep even pressure on the slides at all times (Figure 132.5). This is the same technique as used for making a blood smear, although a feathered edge is not necessary.

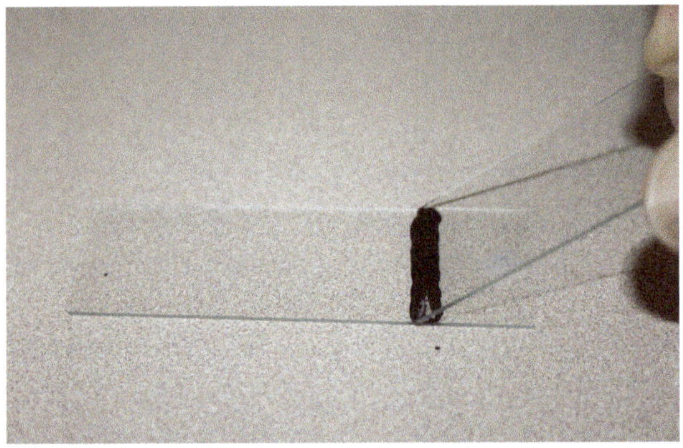

Figure 132.4 The upward slide is then laid into the line of stain and pushed forward to create a smear.

- While pushing the slide to make the smear, you may alter the speed (faster and slower) so that lighter and darker regions are created to allow the examiner options when looking at the slide.
- If you have a uniform sample, wipe off the excess sample from the initial drops from the end of the slide and allow it to dry on the warming block.
- If you want to make multiple slides you can take a fresh slide, gently mix the excess sample from the original slide, and smear on a new warm slide as before.
- If the sample is very concentrated (i.e., your first slide does not allow you to see individual sperm cells) you can dilute the sample with semen extender or mix a smaller drop of semen with a larger drop of stain or use technique 2.
- Once the slide has dried you can place it on the microscope and view with the 10× objective to focus. Once spermatozoa are found, refocus using the 20×.

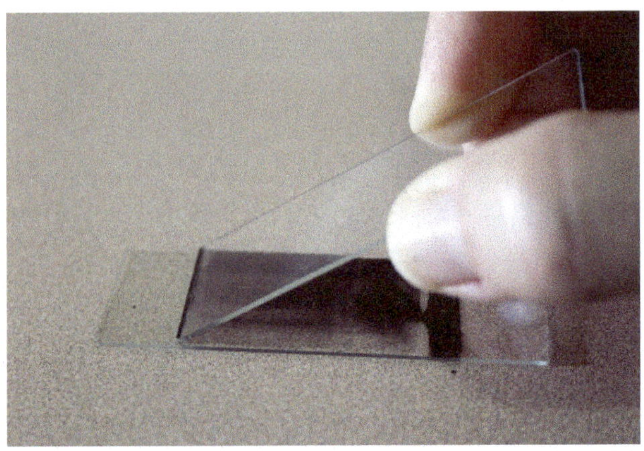

Figure 132.5 The upward slide may be lifted and placed ahead of the mixed stain/semen and pushed forward to create a smear.

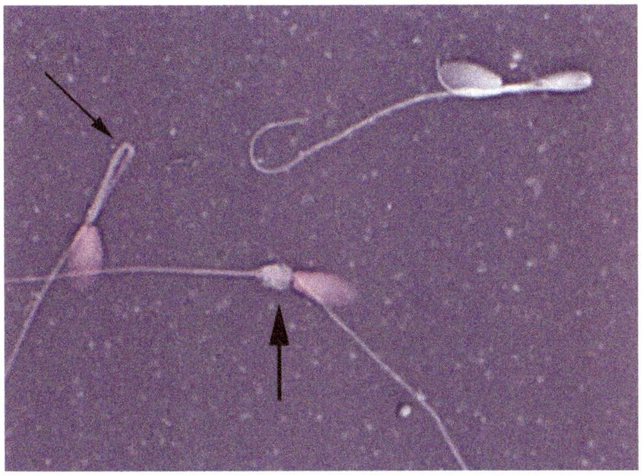

Figure 132.6 Stallion spermatozoa with a bent midpiece (thin arrow) and proximal droplet (large arrow) stained with eosin--nigrosin at 1,000×.

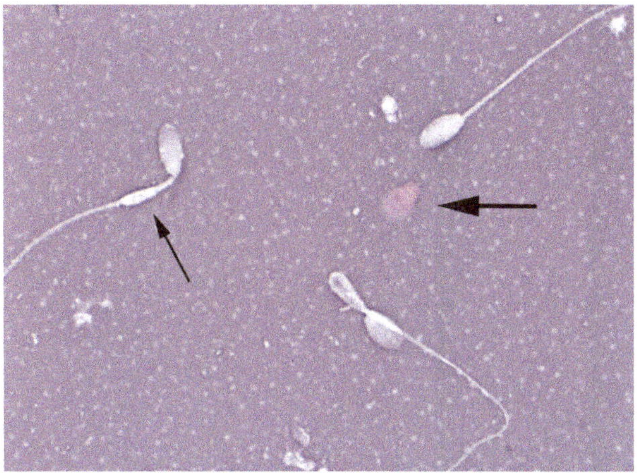

Figure 132.7 Stallion spermatozoa. Note the detached head (large arrow) and thickened midpiece (thin arrow) stained with eosin-nigrosin at 1,000×.

- Once you are ready to move onto 100×, place one drop of immersion oil on the slide and move the 100× oil objective into place. Take care not to drag other objectives through the oil.
- Live sperm will be gray to white in color (no stain uptake) and dead cells will be pink to purple (with stain uptake).
- At least 100 live cells should be counted for an evaluation. The number and percentages of various sperm abnormalities should be recorded with a cell counter (Figures 132.6 and 132.7). The more spermatozoa that are counted, the more accurate the result.
- Sperm may be classified by different methods such as primary or secondary abnormalities depending on where in the testes or outflow tract the defect is thought to originate; major or minor defects affecting fertility; or just by the type of morphologic abnormality (proximal droplet, detached head, etc.).
- Document each specific abnormality present in each cell (see Chapter 133). This is to ensure complete recording of the stallion's abnormalities for potential future comparisons. Some types of abnormalities may be linked to certain conditions or may change over time, such as detached heads related to processing issues or to ampullary blockage.

Interpretation

- Once 100 or more cells have been counted the number is reported as a percentage. This number should be included in the calculation of the total number of progressively motile, morphologically normal spermatozoa in the ejaculate.
- Some defects may require alternative processing such as phase contrast, differential interference contrast, or transmission electron microscopy to be observed properly, such as vacuoles in the spermatozoal head or acrosomal defects.
- It is important to always put the stain on the slide first and semen second so that the stain does not become contaminated.
- If the sample is too concentrated, spermatozoa will overly each other, making evaluation of morphology difficult. The sample should be appropriate diluted to allow examination of individual spermatozoa.

Further Reading

Brito LFC. 2007. Evaluation of stallion sperm morphology. *Clin Tech Eq Pract* 6: 249–64.

Brito LFC, Greene LM, Kelleman A, Knobbe M, Turner R. 2011. Effect of method and clinician on stallion sperm morphology evaluation. *Theriogenology* 76: 745–50.

Morrell JM, Johannisson A, Dalin AM, Hammar L, Sandebert T, Rodriguez-Martinez H. 2008. Sperm morphology and chromatin integrity in Swedish warmblood stallions and their relationship to pregnancy rates. *Acta Vet Scand* 50: 2.

Swanson EW, Bearden HJ. 1951. An eosin-nigrosin stain for differentiating live and dead bovine spermatozoa. *J Anim Sci* 10: 981–7.

Varner DD. 2008. Developments in stallion semen evaluation. *Theriogenology* 70: 448–62.

133

Evaluation of Sperm Morphology

Leonardo Brito

Stgenetics, USA

Introduction

Sperm morphology evaluation is an essential component of semen analysis and provides the clinician with valuable information for assessing the breeding soundness of a stallion and the potential fertility of individual semen samples. The most widespread (and dangerous) misconception regarding the evaluation of stallion sperm morphology is the assumption that morphology is not important or that it is less important than sperm motility. Sperm morphology greatly impacts fertility in all species studied, and it would not be expected to be any different in horses.

Proper evaluation of sperm morphology is a considerable technical challenge as the process is subjective and results are largely dependent on the proficiency and experience of the evaluator. As a consequence, significant differences in results can be observed among different clinicians. Formal training by a skilled clinician and proficiency testing are especially important for those performing evaluations. In addition, evaluators should be familiar with the distinctive appearance of sperm prepared using different methods as this might affect the ability to identify abnormalities.

Equipment and Supplies

Conventional light microscope with 10×, 40×, and 100× (oil immersion) objectives for evaluating eosin-nigrosin (EN) stained slides or a microscope equipped with a phase-contrast or differential interference contrast (DIC) optical system if evaluating unstained wet mount semen samples; differential cell counter. Access to reference publications containing descriptions and images of sperm abnormalities while conducting the exam is advisable.

Technique

- Filter the semen to remove debris and the gel fraction from the ejaculate. Gel interferes with the ability to visualize the sperm. Properly prepared specimens are absolutely essential; poor quality slides will generate poor results.
- Prepare either a wet mount slide (phase-contrast or DIC microscopy) (see Chapter 136) or an eosin-nigrosin (EN) stained slide (conventional light microscopy) (see Chapter 132) for morphologic assessment.
- Although the pattern per se is not important, the evaluator should follow a predefined pattern scanning the slide to avoid examining the same sperm twice. Detached sperm heads should be evaluated, but loose tails are not counted.
- It is especially helpful to move the fine focus control in order to better observe all sperm detail during the evaluation.
- A minimum of 100 sperm should be examined and the results tallied using a differential cell counter.
- Sperm morphology is preferably examined at 1,000× magnification under oil immersion. Lower magnification (600×) may be satisfactory when using DIC objectives. Examining sperm at lower magnifications is not advisable as some defects will be missed.

Classification of Sperm Abnormalities

Several classification systems have been reported in stallions and the nomenclature used for specific defects varies widely. The present Society for Theriogenology forms for

Equine Reproductive Procedures, Second Edition. Edited by John Dascanio and Patrick McCue.

stallion breeding soundness evaluation (BSE) have the following categories listed in the differential spermiogram: normal sperm, abnormal acrosome, abnormal head, detached head, proximal droplets, distal droplets, abnormal midpieces, and bent/coiled tails (see Appendix 1). The presence of other cells (round germ cells, white blood cells, red blood cells, etc.) should also be indicated. Ideally, the specific defects of these different sperm regions should also be enumerated.

- Acrosome defects include knobbed, roughed, and detached acrosomes.
- Head defects include microcephalic (small, underdeveloped, or dwarf), macrocephalic (large or giant), pyriform (narrow at the base), tapered (narrow), nuclear vacuoles (pouches or craters), and multiple heads.
- Midpiece defects include distal midpiece reflex (simple bent or folded midpiece), segmental aplasia of the mitochondrial sheath (or roughed), fractured (hairpin), swollen (thick), swollen/roughed/broken (Dag-like), disrupted sheet (filamentous), duplicated, pseudodroplet, and stump tail.
- Bent or coiled tails refer to those sperm in which both the midpiece and the principal piece are bent or coiled, or the distal part of the principal piece is coiled.
- The percentage of normal and abnormal detached heads (tailless or separated heads) could be recorded separately and teratoids ideally should be classified as a complete separate category.

Some authors have used a sperm morphology evaluation system in which defects are prioritized (usually the most proximal defect) so that only one is recorded per spermatozoon. This system is based on the assumption that certain defects are more important or more deleterious to fertility than others, which is an assumption not necessarily based on scientific evidence. Furthermore, it is not possible to record the distribution of sperm defects in the ejaculate and to track changes in specific defects, so that the use of this system is discouraged.

It is preferable to enumerate all the defects on a single spermatozoon to track the changes in the patterns and associations of specific sperm defects. This provides the clinician with a better overall picture of the condition and enhances the ability to determine breeding soundness. To enumerate multiple defects simultaneously, the evaluator presses the keys for the defects simultaneously on a cell counter so that this only advances the total cell count one number. Using this system, the percentages of sperm defects when added to the percentage of normal sperm will not total 100%.

Abnormal Sperm Morphology

Stallion sperm consists of a head, neck, and tail. The tail is the longest part of the sperm and consists of the midpiece, principal piece, and end piece (Figure 133.1a). The length of the sperm is approximately 60 μm. The sperm head is oval and elongated with the anterior third being the widest part. The head is relatively flat and a longitudinal section has an approximately elliptical shape with a slightly thicker posterior end. Head length, maximum width, and width at the base are approximately 6, 3, and 1.45 μm, respectively. The variation in the shape and size of normal stallion sperm heads is considerable, ranging from somewhat thinner and elongated to shorter and broader forms (Figure 133.1b–d).

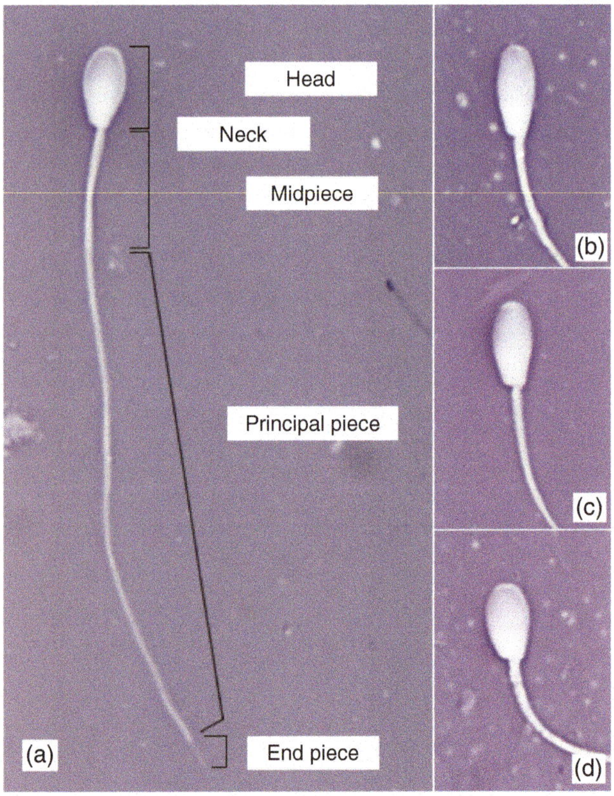

Figure 133.1 (a) Stallion sperm consists of a head, neck, and tail. The tail is the longest part of the spermatozoon and consists of a midpiece, principal piece, and end piece. (b–d) There is considerable variation in the shape of normal stallion sperm heads, from somewhat thinner and elongated to shorter and broader forms. Eosin-nigrosin stain.

Head Defects

The incidence of sperm head defects is relatively high and these are usually the most prevalent defects in the ejaculate. Sperm head defects involve acrosome defects, abnormal shape and/or size, and nuclear vacuoles.

The most common defect of the acrosome is the knobbed acrosome; its appearance on light microscopy varies from bead-like thickening on the sperm head apex (sometimes protruding from the head ridge) to indentation and flattening of the apex (Figure 133.2a–d).

Distinct abnormalities of sperm head shape include tapered and pyriform heads. The distinction between these defects is that while with the former the entire sperm head is tapered (narrow), tapering is observed only in the post-acrosomal region with the latter (Figure 133.2e, f). The head can also be considered to be abnormally small (microcephalic sperm) or large (macrocephalic sperm). Although these are "clear cut" classifications, the reality is that shape/size defects can include a wide array of variations (Figure 133.2g, h). In addition, because there is considerable variation in sperm head shape and size among stallions, comparison among several spermatozoa to establish what the "normal" is for an individual stallion is necessary for correct classification of sperm without obvious, extreme head shape/size abnormalities.

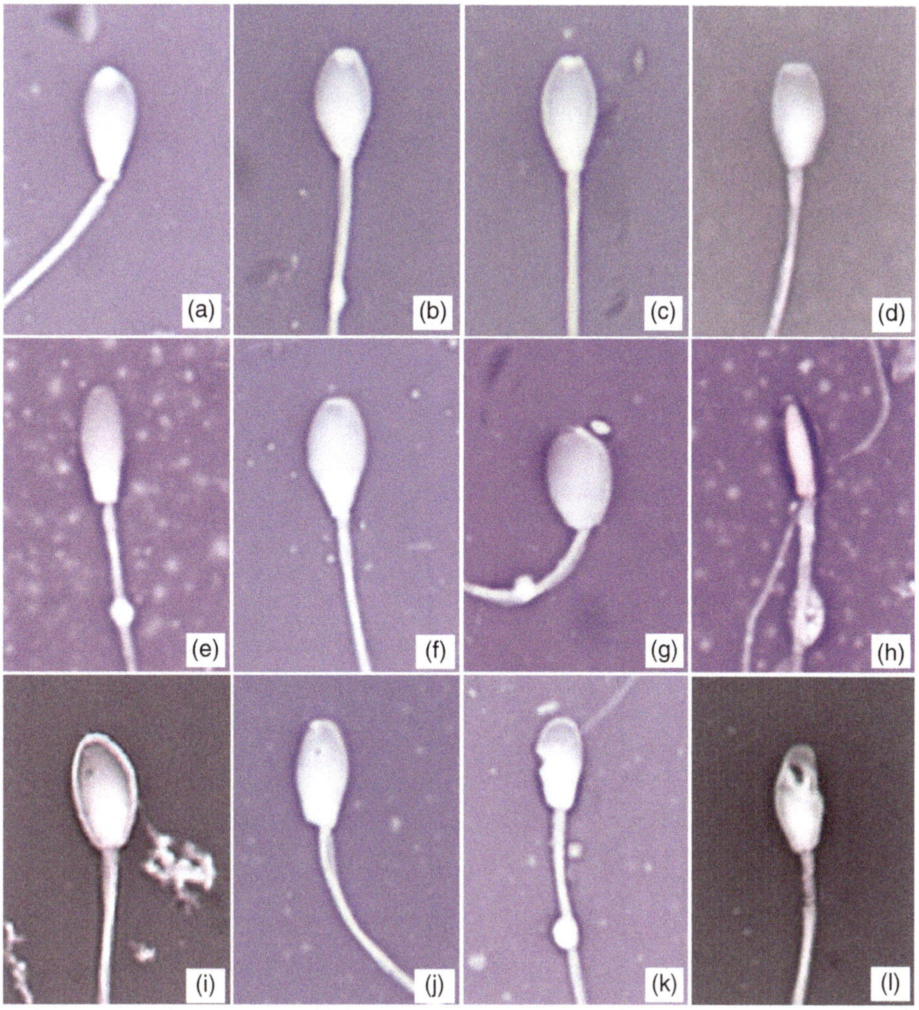

Figure 133.2 (a–d) The appearance of the knobbed acrosome defect varies from bead-like thickening on the sperm head apex, sometimes protruding from the head ridge, to indentation and flattening of the apex. (e, f) Tapered heads are narrow along the entire long axis, whereas pyriform heads show tapering only in the post-acrosomal region. (g, h) A wide variety of sperm head shape/size defects can be observed in the ejaculate. (i, j) Nuclear vacuoles appear as dark dots in eosin-nigrosin-stained samples and can be observed anywhere on the sperm head. (k, l) Larger vacuoles might result in abnormal head contour and/or shape. Eosin-nigrosin stain.

Single or multiple nuclear vacuoles can be observed anywhere on the sperm head. The appearance of nuclear vacuoles range from dark dots in EN-stained smears (Figure 133.2i, j), to clear dots in wet mounts examined under phase contrast, to what appears as depressions (craters) in wet mounts examined with DIC. In the author's experience, this is the most difficult defect to observe, and carefully adjusting the micrometer focus up and down during the examination facilitates the detection of this abnormality. Larger vacuoles might result in abnormal sperm head contour and/or shape (Figure 133.2k, l).

Midpiece Defects

A common midpiece defect is the distal midpiece reflex (DMR), which on light microscopy appears as a bend in the distal region of the midpiece in the shape of the letter "J" (Figure 133.3a). A distal cytoplasmic droplet is nearly always entrapped in the bend. Double bends of the midpiece usually accompany coiling of the principal piece with retention of cytoplasmic material (Figure 133.3b, c). The difference between the DMR or bent/coiled tails and the Dag-like defect is that with the former, the midpiece is smooth and complete, whereas with the latter, the bending and coiling involving the midpiece or the entire tail is associated with a rough, incomplete mitochondrial sheet usually accompanied by fractures and shattering of the axonemal fibers (Figure 133.3d).

Segmental aplasia of the mitochondrial sheet might be observed in a low percentage of sperm in varying degrees; some sperm lack a small part of the sheet, whereas others seem to miss the mitochondrial sheet completely (Figure 133.3e, f).

Cytoplasmic droplets appear as small, spherical masses attached to the neck region (proximal droplet) or to the distal portion of the midpiece adjacent to the annulus (distal droplet) (Figure 133.3g, h). The location, size, and contour differentiate cytoplasmic droplets from other midpiece defects.

Swollen and roughed midpieces might involve abnormalities of the mitochondrial sheet or accumulation of microtubular masses (Figure 133.3i, j).

Principal Piece Defects

Simple bend or coiling with retained cytoplasm (Figure 133.3k, l), and less commonly aplasia or abnormal development, are some of the defects involving only the principal piece.

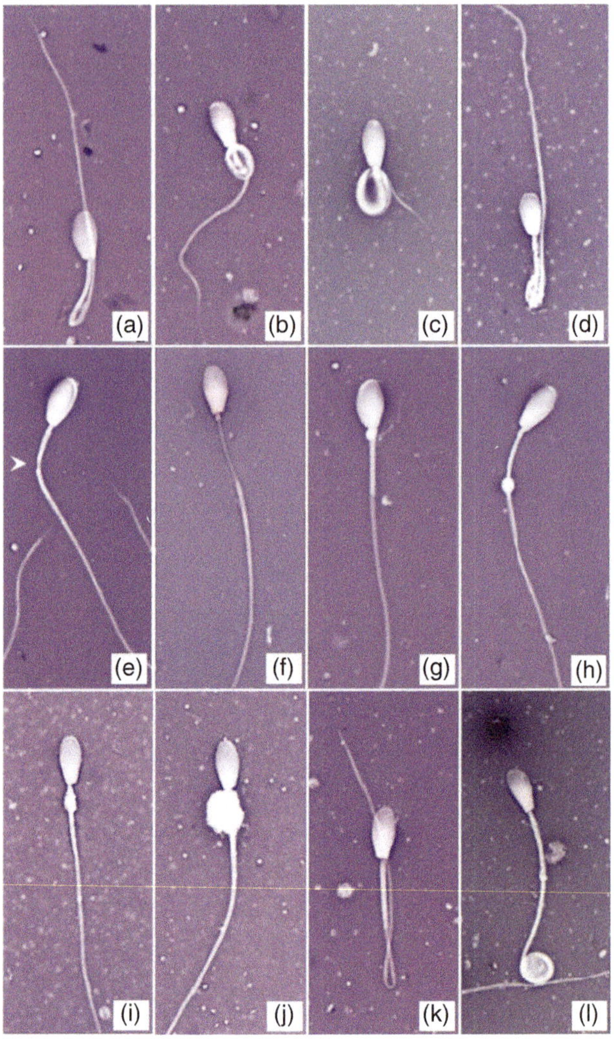

Figure 133.3 (a) The distal midpiece reflex is a common defect that appears as a bend in the distal region of the midpiece in the shape of the letter "J." (b, c) Double bends or coiling of the midpiece usually accompanies coiling of the principal piece with retention of cytoplasmic material. (d) The Dag-like defect also involves bending and/or coiling of the midpiece or the entire tail, but is associated with a rough, incomplete mitochondrial sheet and fractures. (e, f) Segmental aplasia of the mitochondrial sheet might be observed in varying degrees from small segments in some sperm (arrowhead in (e)) to the apparent complete lack of mitochondria in others. (g, h) Cytoplasmic droplets appear as small spherical masses attached to the neck region (proximal droplet) or to the distal portion of the midpiece adjacent to the annulus (distal droplet). (i, j) The location, size, and contour differentiate cytoplasmic droplets from other midpiece defects that might involve abnormalities of the mitochondrial sheet or accumulation of microtubular masses. (k, l) Simple bend or coiling with retained cytoplasm are some of the defects involving only the principal piece. Eosin-nigrosin stain.

Tail Defects

Duplication of the tail is an uncommon defect that is associated with duplication of the implantation fossa and replication of the distal centriole. Sperm with multiple heads and tails might have normal head structures with normal DNA content, but abnormalities of nuclear shape in one or more heads might also be observed. The heads are usually completely separated, and in the tail independent axial filament complexes are kept together by a common mitochondrial or fibrous sheet. Detached sperm heads are commonly observed in low percentages (<5%) in the ejaculate, but might be present in very high numbers in cases of sperm accumulation in the excurrent tract. Abnormal detached heads indicate more severe disturbance of spermatogenesis than normal detached heads. The tail stump defect might occasionally be observed in a low percentage of sperm in stallions. On light microscopy, the initial impression may be of a detached head, but close examination reveals that the tail is replaced by a small stump. The term teratoid has been used to describe sperm that are so severely deformed that the cell is barely recognized as sperm. In most cases, the head has an abnormal shape and the tail is tightly coiled around or over the head; these invariably take up eosin, indicating disruption of the plasmalemma. Attention should be paid to not confuse those with debris or other cells.

Other Cells

Other cells that might be found in the ejaculate include blood cells, round germ cells, and Sertoli cell mantles. Proper classification of these cells requires the use of different staining techniques that could include Giemsa or Diff-Quick®.

Interpretation

There is a wide variation in sperm morphology among breeding stallions, but in general the average stallion has approximately 50% morphologically normal sperm. Sperm morphology can vary considerably during the breeding season and routine evaluations (every 2–4 weeks) should be performed to determine sperm morphology characteristics of a particular stallion. More than 30% sperm head defects, >25% proximal cytoplasmic droplets, or <40% normal sperm are reasons for concern.

In North America, the BSE guidelines from the Society for Theriogenology were developed with the intent to select stallions that could render at least 75% of 40 or more mares pregnant when bred naturally or 120 mares when bred artificially. According to these guidelines, a satisfactory prospective breeder should produce a minimum of 1 billion morphologically normal, progressively motile sperm in each of two ejaculates collected 1 hour apart.

Effects on fertility may vary with each defect. Defects involving the ability of the spermatozoa to swim will have an obvious negative effect on fertility (coiled tails, bent midpiece or tail, etc.). Not all defects have been studied extensively in stallions, thus the information below is a compilation from the stallion and other species.

- *Micro and macro head defects.* These may have abnormal chromatin content, thus there may be effects on embryonic development.
- *Knobbed acrosomes or acrosomal defects.* These may predispose to premature sperm capacitation and spontaneous acrosome reaction. Sperm are not able to bind and penetrate the zona pellucida.
- *Nuclear vacuoles.* Sperm may have a reduced ability to bind and penetrate the zona pellucida. Abnormal chromatin may lead to decreased fertilization.
- *Tapered or pyriform head.* Sperm may have a reduced ability to bind to the zona pellucida.
- *Midpiece defects.* Mitochondrial defects can affect sperm motility and thus fertility.
- *Proximal cytoplasmic droplets.* Sperm may not be able to bind and penetrate the zona pellucida or they may result in abnormal embryonic development.
- *Distal cytoplasmic droplets.* These have little to no effect on fertility.
- *Detached heads.* Moderate numbers will reduce fertility.

Additional Comments

Although the Society for Theriogenology has no guidelines regarding the absolute percentage of abnormal sperm or the percentage of specific defects in the ejaculate, the correct classification and quantification of specific sperm defects can provide valuable information regarding potential fertility of a stallion or ejaculate and help to formulate a diagnosis and prognosis for reproductive problems.

In addition, the guidelines have not taken into account the concept of uncompensable sperm traits. Sperm with uncompensable traits compete with "competent" sperm for fertilization, but are unable to sustain normal embryonic development. Therefore, pregnancy rates cannot be increased by increasing sperm numbers in the breeding dose. Very different pregnancy rates would be expected with ejaculates/breeding doses with very different percentages of abnormal sperm even if both contained the same number of morphologically normal, progressive motile sperm. Clinicians should be cautious not to rely on total sperm numbers alone, but to also pay close attention to the existence and prevalence of specific sperm abnormalities.

Further Reading

Bielanski W, Kaczmarski F. 1979. Morphology of spermatozoa in semen from stallions of normal fertility. *J Reprod Fertil Suppl* 27: 39–45.

Brito LFC. 2007. Evaluation of stallion sperm morphology. *Clin Tech Eq Pract* 6: 249–64.

Card C. 2005. Cellular associations and the differential spermiogram: making sense of stallion spermatozoal morphology. *Theriogenology* 64: 558–67.

Dott HM. 1975. Morphology of stallion spermatozoa. *J Reprod Fertil Suppl* 23: 41–6.

Kenney RM (ed.). 1983. Manual for Clinical Fertility Evaluation of the Stallion. Hastings: Society for Theriogenology.

134

Determination of Daily Sperm Output

Patrick M. McCue

Equine Reproduction Laboratory, Colorado State University, USA

Introduction

Determination of daily sperm output (DSO) may be beneficial in the reproductive evaluation of an individual stallion. Evaluation of semen collected twice on one day approximately 1 hour apart can be used to estimate DSO. Actual DSO requires the collection of semen daily for a minimum of 5–7 days to deplete the extragonadal sperm reserves in the epididymides, ductus deferens, and ampulla. Thereafter, the total number of sperm *collected* each day will be relatively constant and represents the number of sperm *produced* each day. It is expected that a normal fertile stallion will produce approximately 4–6 billion or more spermatozoa each day. Determination of DSO can be used to estimate the number of mares that may be bred per day and therefore the number of mares that may be booked to a stallion for a season.

Equipment and Supplies

Artificial vagina and associated supplies, graduated cylinders to measure volume, spectrophotometer to estimate concentration, microscope, microscope slides, coverslips, and disposable pipettes to determine motility.

Technique

- Semen is collected from the stallion once each day for 5–7 days or more. It may be beneficial to collect the stallion more than once per day for the initial 2–3 days to help deplete the extragonadal sperm reserves.
- Standard semen analyses are performed, including measurement of volume, sperm concentration, spermatozoal motility (total and progressive), and sperm morphology.
- The total number of sperm in each ejaculate is calculated by multiplying the volume (ml) by the concentration (millions of sperm/ml).
- Semen collections continue until the total numbers of sperm in the ejaculate reach a relatively stable number each day (Figure 134.1).

Additional Comments

Sperm production potential is based on testicular size, with larger testes expected to produce a greater number of spermatozoa. Ultrasound measurements of testicular size can be used to calculate total testicular volume, which in turn can be used to estimate potential sperm production (see Chapter 135).

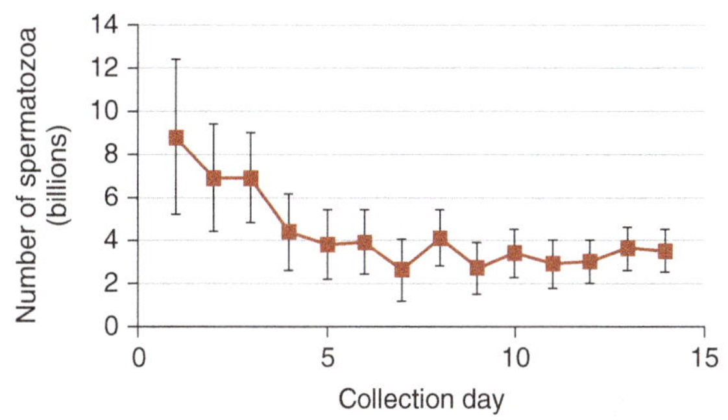

Figure 134.1 Total number of sperm (mean ± 95% confidence intervals) in the ejaculate of 11 stallions during 14 days of semen collection. Daily sperm output was reached after 4–5 days of collection. Source: From Gebauer MR, Pickett BW, Voss JL, Swierstra EE. 1974. Reproductive physiology of the stallion: daily sperm output and testicular measurements. *J Am Vet Med Assoc* 165: 711–13. Reproduced with the permission of American Veterinary Medical Association.

Equine Reproductive Procedures, Second Edition. Edited by John Dascanio and Patrick McCue.

The extragonadal sperm reserves should be depleted of sperm and the number of sperm in subsequent ejaculates should stabilize by day 7 to 10 and reflect the number of sperm produced each day.

An estimation of DSO can be made by collecting semen twice in one day, approximately 1 hour apart. The number of sperm in the second ejaculate will approximate the daily sperm output. In general, it is expected that the volume of semen in the two ejaculates will be similar, but the number of sperm in the second ejaculate will be approximately 50% of the number of sperm in the first ejaculate. Motility scores on the second ejaculate are often higher than that of the first ejaculate.

Reference

Gebauer MR, Pickett BW, Voss JL, Swierstra EE. 1974. Reproductive physiology of the stallion: daily sperm output and testicular measurements. *J Am Vet Med Assoc* 165: 711–13.

Further Reading

Pickett BW, Amann RP, McKinnon AO, Squires EL, Voss JL. 1989. *Management of the Stallion for Maximum Reproductive Efficiency. II.* Animal Reproduction Laboratory Bulletin No. 05. Fort Collins, CO: Colorado State University.

Squires ER, Pickett BW. 2011. Factors affecting sperm production and output. In: McKinnon AO, Squires EL, Vaala WE, Varner DD (eds). *Equine Reproduction,* 2nd edn. Ames, IA: Wiley Blackwell, pp. 1344–61.

135

Measurement of Testicular Size and Estimation of Daily Sperm Output

Patrick M. McCue

Colorado State University, USA and Equine Reproduction Laboratory

Introduction

Testes of mature stallions are normally capable of producing approximately 18–20 million sperm per gram of testicular tissue per day. Larger testes are expected to produce a greater number of spermatozoa than smaller testes. Since testicular weight cannot be obtained in a live, intact stallion, daily sperm production potential is estimated from total testicular volume. Measurement of testicular size is performed to estimate potential daily sperm production.

Historically, total scrotal width (TSW) was measured as an index of testicular size and the minimal accepted TSW expected for a mature light horse breeding stallion was 8.0 cm. Total testicular volume (TTV) has more recently been used to estimate daily sperm production potential. Testicular volume is considered to be a more accurate predictor of sperm production potential than measurement of total scrotal width.

Equipment and Supplies

Examination gloves, scrotal calipers, ultrasound machine, lubricant, alcohol swabs.

Technique

- The stallion should be restrained and attention paid to the safety of the examiner.
- Disposable gloves should be worn and discarded after the examination to prevent the transfer of any contagious/infectious diseases between stallions. Equipment should also be wiped with alcohol after use.
- The scrotal contents should initially be investigated by manual palpation to examine for any abnormalities. One example would be an older stallion with small testicular size from testicular degeneration that would present with a wrinkled tunica albuginea.
- Ultrasound examination of the testes and other scrotal contents may also be performed in stallions to identify lesions within the epididymis/testes or characterize fluid within the scrotum (see Chapter 165).
- Each testis should be examined for size, shape, and consistency.
- The morphology and location of each epididymal tail should be determined to note a non-pathologic partial testicular torsion or epididymitis.
- The spermatic cord should be palpated for size and morphology.
- TSW can be measured with scrotal calipers (Figure 135.1). The procedure should be repeated three times and the

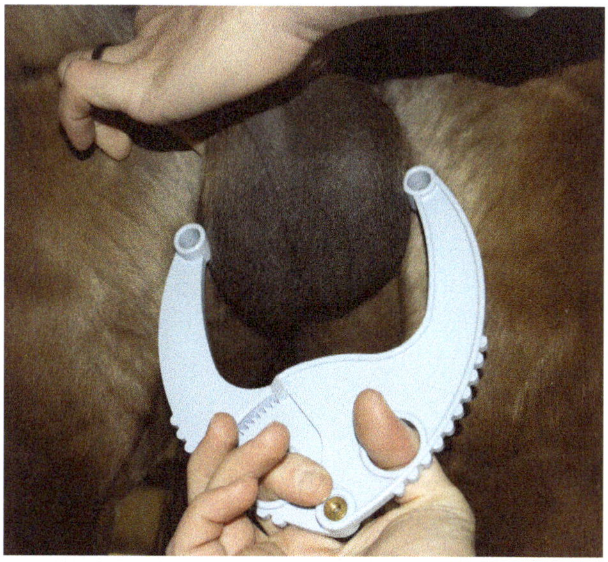

Figure 135.1 Measurement of total scrotal width using calipers.

Equine Reproductive Procedures, Second Edition. Edited by John Dascanio and Patrick McCue.

results averaged. The testes are gently and evenly held in the ventral scrotum and the calipers are used to determine the widest measurement across both testes. Care should be taken to not artificially widen the scrotal contents. TSW is correlated with both testes' weight and daily sperm production. The minimum acceptable TSW for light horse stallions is 8.0 cm. Actual minimal TSW is age dependent (8.1 cm for 2–3 year olds, 8.5 cm for 4–6 year olds, and 9.5 cm for light horse stallions >7 years old).

- The length, width, and height of each individual testis are measured by ultrasound (preferably) (Figures 135.2 and 135.3) or calipers and the data recorded in centimeters. Ultrasound measurement calipers should be placed on either side of the testicle on the hyperechoic tunica albuginea. It is important to not exert pressure on the testicle with the probe, thus altering the true diameter. The screen should be frozen for measurements at the point where the ultrasound image is just about to be lost due to loss of probe contact. Often this is a point where the left and right sides of the screen have lost the testicular image, but the central screen still has clearly delineated upper and lower testicle edges.
- TTV is subsequently calculated and used to estimate daily sperm production potential.

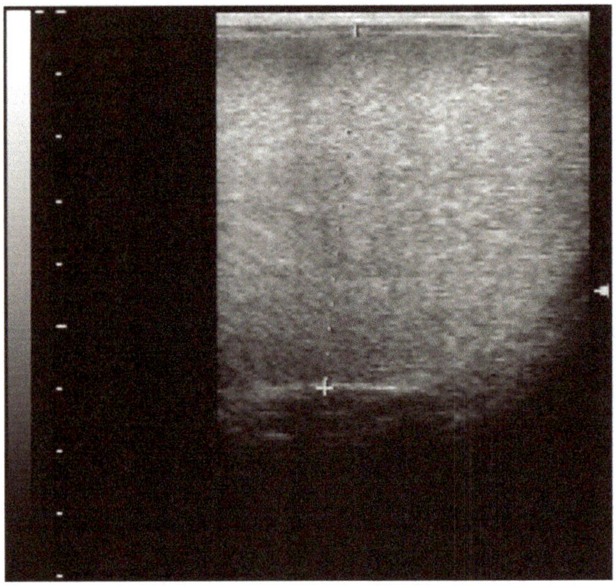

Figure 135.3 Ultrasound image of a testis showing measurement of testicular height.

Interpretation

Testicular measurements are used to calculate testicular volume and to subsequently estimate potential daily sperm production. Testicular volume (in cubic centimeters) of each testis can be determined using the following formula:

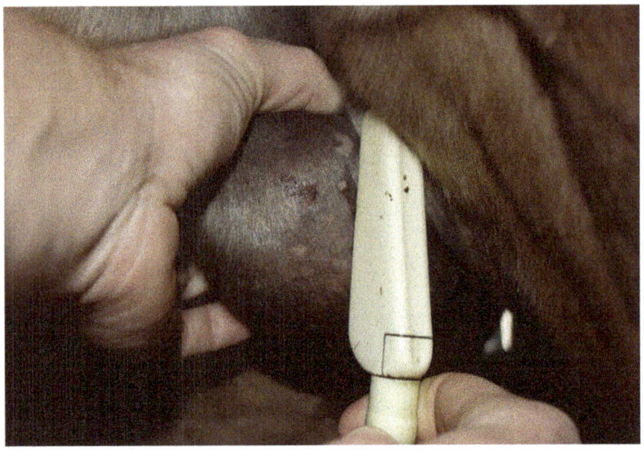

Figure 135.2 Measurement of testicular width using ultrasonography.

$$\text{Testicular volume (cm}^3) = 0.5233 \times \text{Length (cm)} \times \text{Width (cm)} \times \text{Height (cm)}$$

The calculated volume of each testis is added together to obtain the TTV (cm^3). Expected daily sperm production (in billions of sperm per day) can subsequently be estimated using the following formula:

$$\text{Expected daily sperm output} = (0.024 \times \text{Total testicular volume in cm}^3) - (1.26)$$

Spermatogenic efficiency can then be determined by comparing the actual number of sperm produced each day (daily sperm output) with the calculated daily sperm production rate based on testicular volume (Box 135.1). Stallions with an actual daily sperm output that is less than the predicted daily sperm production based on testicular volume should be evaluated for disease or dysfunction of the testes, epididymides, ductus deferens, or accessory sex glands. The relationship between testicular volume and predicted daily sperm output is presented in Figure 135.4.

Box 135.1 Example of a Daily Sperm Output Calculation

The length, width, and height of the left and right testes of a stallion are measured by ultrasound.

Measurement	Left testis	Right testis
Length	9.8 cm	10.2 cm
Width	6.0 cm	5.5 cm
Height	8.2 cm	7.5 cm

The ultrasound measurements of testicular size are used to calculate the total testicular volume (TTV), which is subsequently used to estimate daily sperm output.

Calculation	Formula
Total testicular volume in cm^3	Testicular volume (TV) = $0.5233 \times L \times W \times H$ (for each testis) Add volume of each testes together for TTV Left TV = $0.5233 \times 9.8 \times 6.0 \times 8.2$ Left TV = 252.3 cm^3 Right TV = $0.5233 \times 10.2 \times 5.5 \times 7.5$ Right TV = 220.2 cm^3 TTV = 252.3 + 220.2 TTV = 472.5 cm^3
Expected daily sperm output (DSP) in billions of sperm	DSP = $0.024 \times$ TTV – 1.26 DSP = 0.024×472.5 – 1.26 DSP = 10.1 billion spermatozoa

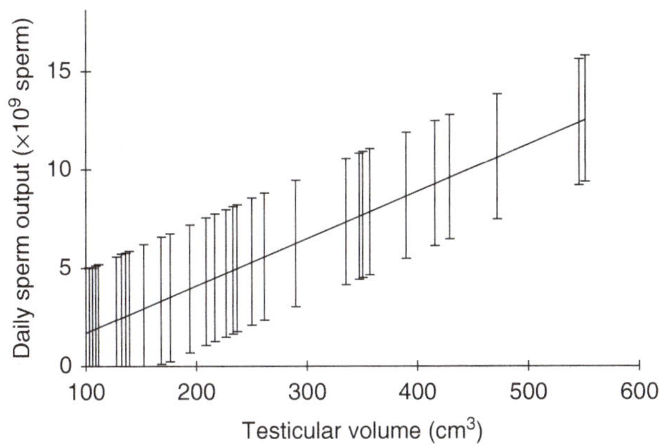

Figure 135.4 Relationship between testicular volume and daily sperm output in stallions. Source: From Love CC, Garcia MC, Riera FR, Kenney RM. 1991. Evaluation of measures taken by ultrasonography and caliper to estimate testicular volume and predict daily sperm output in the stallion. *J Reprod Fertil Suppl* 44: 99–105. Reproduced with the permission of Journal of Reproduction and Infertility.

Reference

Love CC, Garcia MC, Riera FR, Kenney RM. 1991. Evaluation of measures taken by ultrasonography and caliper to estimate testicular volume and predict daily sperm output in the stallion. *J Reprod Fertil Suppl* 44: 99–105.

Further Reading

Love CC, Garcia MC, Riera FR, Kenney RM. 1990. Use of testicular volume to predict daily sperm output in the stallion. *Proc Annu Conv Am Assoc Eq Pract* 36: 15–21.

Sertich PL. 2011. Examination of external genitalia. In: McKinnon AO, Squires EL, Vaala WE, Varner DD (eds). Equine Reproduction, 2nd edn. Ames, IA: Wiley Blackwell, pp. 1458–61.

136

Wet Mount Evaluation of Sperm

John J. Dascanio

School of Veterinary Medicine, Texas Tech University, USA

Introduction

The use of phase contrast and differential interference contrast (DIC) microscopy enhances the observation of structural detail within a cell. These methods impart contrast to cellular features in an otherwise transparent cell; such transparent cells would not be visible with standard bright field microscopy. This may make certain spermatozoal features, such as defects in the acrosome, more visible. Phase-contrast microscopy is more widely available to veterinarians than DIC microscopy due to the higher cost of the DIC equipment.

Assessment of spermatozoal morphology is most commonly performed in practice with a background stain such as an eosin-nigrosin stain. The semen sample is smeared out over a slide and air-dried for preparation, potentially causing some defects during processing such as detached heads or broken tails. Wet mount preparation, as used in phase-contrast and DIC microscopy, causes less physical damage to spermatozoa.

Phase-contrast and DIC techniques make use of phase and amplitude modulations or differential modulation of the light, respectively, to obtain contrast. Phase contrast produces a flatter image with darker cellular features ranging from black to white (Figure 136.1), whereas DIC produces an image with more uniform grays (Figures 136.2 and 136.3). DIC produces a higher resolution image of fine structures than phase contrast. DIC also causes the cell to have some topographic enhancement, creating an illusion of a slightly three-dimensional cell. With phase contrast a "halo effect" around cells may be present that may obscure some detail.

Equipment and Supplies

Formal buffered saline, microscope slides, coverslips, pipettes, microcentrifuge tubes, phase-contrast or DIC microscope.

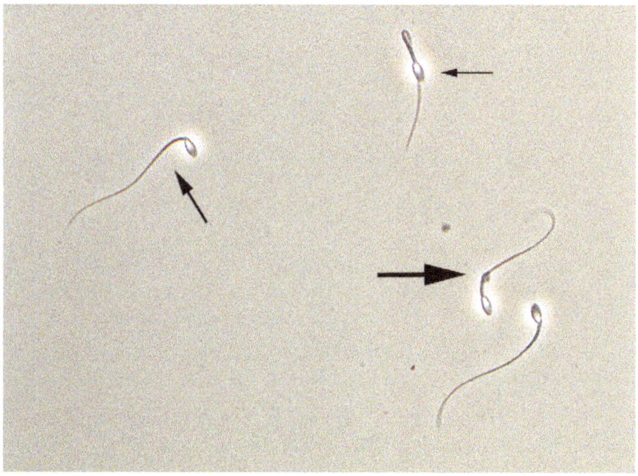

Figure 136.1 Stallion spermatozoa with a normal spermatozoon (medium arrow), distal cytoplasmic droplet (large arrow), and bent tail (small arrow) (phase contrast; 400×).

Preparation of a Wet Mount

- Fix the spermatozoa in 10% formal buffered saline. This is an isotonic solution that will not damage the spermatozoal cell.
- The recipe for formal buffered saline is: 100 ml of 40% formalin mixed with 900 ml of distilled water to which 4.5 g sodium phosphate monobasic dihydrate ($NaH_2PO_4 \cdot 2H_2O$) and 6.5 g of monosodium phosphate (NaH_2PO_4) is added. This should result in a 10% formal saline with a pH of 7.0.
- Place 100 µl of semen into 900 µl of formal buffered saline in a 2 ml microcentrifuge tube and mix thoroughly with gentle inversion of the tube. A similar 1:9 dilution may be made with other total volumes if desired. The resultant mixture should allow for visualization of

Equine Reproductive Procedures, Second Edition. Edited by John Dascanio and Patrick McCue.

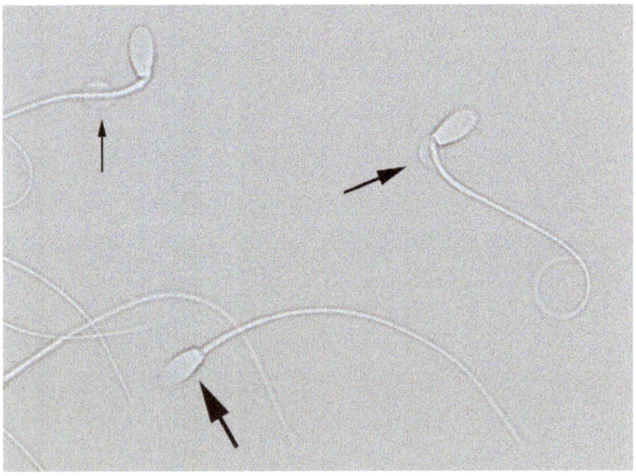

Figure 136.2 Stallion spermatozoa with a normal spermatozoon (large arrow), proximal cytoplasmic droplet (medium arrow), and distal cytoplasmic droplet (small arrow) (DIC; oil immersion, 1,000×).

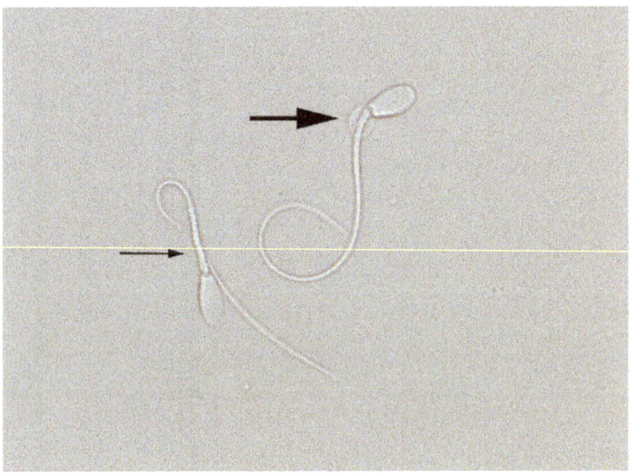

Figure 136.3 Stallion spermatozoa with proximal cytoplasmic droplet (large arrow) and roughened midpiece (small arrow) (DIC; oil immersion, 1,000×).

individual spermatozoa. If the sample is too concentrated or dilute, adjust the dilution ratio accordingly.

- Place approximately 30 μl of the semen solution on a glass microscope slide and cover with a coverslip.

Differential Interference Contrast Microscopy

- A DIC microscope has a polarizer between the light source and condenser, a DIC beam-splitting prism in the condenser turret, a DIC beam-combining prism just past the objective, and an analyzer in the space before the tube lens. The light beam is split, passes through the sample, and is then recombined.
- If the split beams pass through the sample without interfering with each other, a gray image appears. If the two beams pass through an edge of a structure, one beam will not be equal to the other. When they recombine they will be constructively recombined producing a bright spot or destructively recombined producing a dark spot. This provides the contrast to make a transparent cell's structure visible.

Phase-Contrast Microscopy

- A phase-contrast objective contains a phase plate or ring and a condenser annulus instead of a diaphragm. The different objectives require different-sized annulus rings. Phase contrast makes use of the differences in the refractive index of tissues to make them visible.
- When a new phase objective is put into place, the corresponding sized condenser annulus must be properly matched.
- The objective phase ring and condenser annulus must be aligned to produce an image.

Interpretation

- Sperm morphology should be evaluated under 400× magnification or higher.
- If the sample is too concentrated, spermatozoa will overlie each other, making evaluation of morphology difficult. The sample should be appropriately diluted to allow examination of individual spermatozoa.

Further Reading

Centonze Frohlich V. 2008. Phase contrast and differential interference contrast (DIC) microscopy. *J Vis Exp* 18:e844.

Cross NL, Meizel S. 1989. Methods for evaluating the acrosomal status of mammalian sperm. *Bio Reprod* 41: 635–41.

Varner DD. 2008. Developments in stallion semen evaluation. *Theriogenology* 70: 448–62.

137

Diff-Quik® Evaluation of Round Cells and Sperm

John J. Dascanio[1] *and Lynda M. J. Miller*[2]

[1] School of Veterinary Medicine, Texas Tech University, USA
[2] College of Veterinary Medicine, Lincoln Memorial University, USA

Introduction

Spermatozoa are visually assessed for morphologic defects using either a wet mount with phase-contrast microscopy or using a dry mount with an eosin-nigrosin stain. Differential interference contrast microscopy provides greater detailed assessment, but is not widely available in veterinary practices due to cost. Typically, 100–200 spermatozoa are counted to identify abnormalities. In addition to spermatozoa, round cells or bacteria may be noted. Diff-Quik® is a proprietary brand of a Romanowski-type stain that consists of a light blue fixative (triarylmethane dye), a red stain (eosin, xanthene-type dye), and a blue stain (thiazine dye). Diff-Quik® stain has been used primarily to assess round cells in a semen sample, but may also be used, with some modification in staining technique, to assess spermatozoal morphology. Diff-Quik® or similar generic stains are used commonly in equine reproduction to assess uterine cytologic samples.

Cellular material on slides should be fixed as soon as practical to retain cellular architecture. Cells may appear degenerative if not fixed in a timely manner. Nuclei from degenerating cells may lose spherical shape, becoming irregular and staining pink due to a decreased affinity for basic dyes.

Staining with Diff-Quik® stain offers an alternative to the more common eosin-nigrosin stain for the evaluation of sperm morphology. However, the staining procedure outlined for Diff-Quik® takes more time than eosin-nigrosin and sperm morphology may be adversely affected by the staining technique.

Since eosin-nigrosin is a negative stain, the round cells can be noted, but they cannot be differentiated. Staining with Diff-Quik® stain may be done following evaluation of the sample in eosin-nigrosin stain, if round cells are noted, to determine what type(s) of round cell(s) are present.

Equipment and Supplies

Diff-Quik® stain, paper towels, sink and water faucet, microscope, microscope slides, blot paper, disposable pipettes, immersion oil, manual cell counter.

Technique

Assessment of Round Cells

- A drop of semen should be placed at one end of a glass microscope slide.
- A second slide is held at a 45-degree angle to the first slide and the slide edge is dipped into the existing semen drop. The upper slide is then slid across the lower slide, creating a smear.
- This slide is then allowed to air-dry for about 10 minutes or until dried.
- The dried slide is dipped into and out of the light blue fixative (triarylmethane dye) 7–10 times. While holding the slide vertically, the end of the slide is then touched to a paper towel to remove excessive fixative.
- The slide is then immediately immersed into the red stain (eosin, xanthene-type dye), again dipping it 7–10 times. The slide is once again touched to a paper towel as before.
- The slide is then immediately immersed into the blue stain (thiazine dye), again dipping it 7–10 times. The slide is once again touched to a paper towel as before.

Assessment of Spermatozoal Morphology

- A smear is created as above and allowed to air-dry.
- For staining of spermatozoa, a much longer staining time in each stain type is required. The best results seem to be achieved with staining the air-dried slide once for

Equine Reproductive Procedures, Second Edition. Edited by John Dascanio and Patrick McCue.

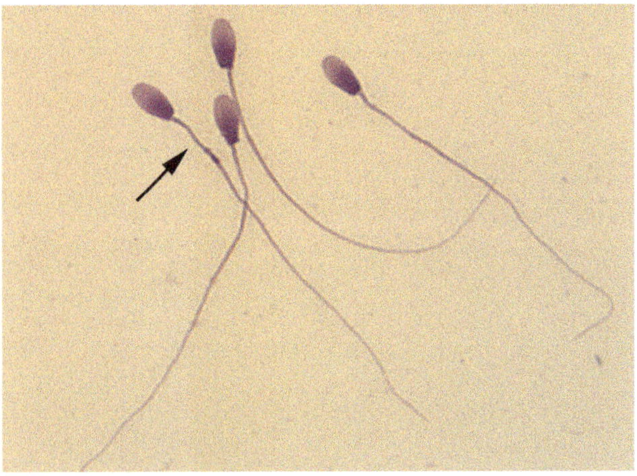

Figure 137.1 Stallion spermatozoa stained with Diff-Quik® stain. Note the abnormal or roughened midpiece (arrow).

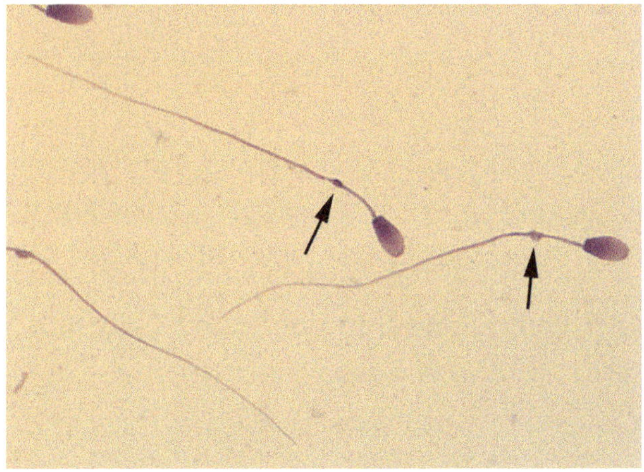

Figure 137.2 Stallion spermatozoa stained with Diff-Quik® stain with distal cytoplasmic droplets (arrows).

2 minutes in the fixative and then a consistent 30 minutes in the red solution followed by 30 minutes in the blue solution.

Rinsing of the Slides

- The slide is then rinsed with tap water or distilled water using a very gentle stream. The slide is once again touched to a paper towel as before to remove excess water.
- The slide is allowed to air-dry before being assessed. Alternatively, the slide may be blotted dry with blot paper taking care to not wipe the slide clear of material.

Interpretation

- Assessment of cells should be performed under high power (400× dry and 1,000× oil immersion).
- Round cells may be premature germ cells or inflammatory cells. Round cells should not be present or only occur in extremely few numbers in a normal ejaculate.
- A minimum of 100 spermatozoa should be observed and evaluated for morphologic characteristics. The percentage of spermatozoa with normal morphology and percentages of sperm with various morphologic defects are recorded.
- The prolonged exposure to the Diff-Quik® stains may result in slight dehydration of the spermatozoa and may adversely affect the appearance of defects such as cytoplasmic droplets (Figures 137.1 and 137.2).

Further Reading

Pozer MA, Zambrano GL, Runcan E, Macpherson ML. 2012. Usefulness of dip quick stain in evaluating sperm morphology in stallions. *Proc Annu Conv Am Assoc Eq Pract* 58: 506–10.

Varner DD. 2008. Developments in stallion semen evaluation. *Theriogenology* 70: 448–62.

138

Electron Microscopy of Constituents of Seminal Ejaculates

D. N. Rao Veeramachaneni

Animal Reproduction and Biotechnology Laboratory, Colorado State University, USA

Introduction

Standard techniques to evaluate equine semen include measurement of ejaculate volume, sperm concentration, total and progressive sperm motility, and light microscopic evaluation of sperm morphology. Routine light microscopic techniques include use of bright field optics for stained smears (i.e., eosin-nigrosin or toluidine blue) or phase-contrast optics or differential interference contrast (DIC) optics for wet smears (see Chapters 132, 133, and 136). It is not always possible to detect subtle, yet significant, morphologic sperm defects with these conventional techniques.

Transmission electron microscopy (TEM) has been used to critically evaluate ultrastructural features of sperm organelles that are pivotal in fertilization, in addition to other cellular debris not uncommon in seminal ejaculates of subfertile or infertile stallions. TEM can also be used to identify molecular events that underlie damage to sperm constituents, i.e., structural integrity of nuclear chromatin, mitochondrial cristae, and axonemal components. Semen has thus been used as 'biopsy material' for evaluation of the health status of the stallion reproductive tract.

Equipment and Supplies

Centrifuge, plasticizing ovens, microtome, refrigerator and incubator, light and transmission electron microscopes; fixative: 6% glutaraldehyde (in 0.1 M sodium cacodylate buffer, pH 7.4, with 0.15 M sucrose); wash buffer: sodium cacodylate buffer (0.1 mol/l); post-fixation: osmium tetroxide (1%) in cacodylate buffer (0.1 M); dehydration: graded series of ethanol propylene oxide; embedding material: Poly/Bed® 812 (Polysciences, Warrington, PA, USA); glass slides for thick sections, nickel grids (300 mesh) for thin sections, toluidine blue stain for thick sections, uranyl acetate (8 g/100 ml of 75% ethanol) and lead citrate stains for thin sections, immunogold staining of thin sections for targeted antigens: primary antibody of interest, biotinylated secondary antibody, and streptavidin-immunogold conjugate.

Technique

- A semen ejaculate is collected using traditional techniques.
- A 5 ml of gel-free semen sample is fixed in 10 ml of fixative for 36–48 hours.
- The fixed sample is centrifuged for 5 minutes at 300× g.
- The supernatant is removed and the pellet is re-suspended in 10 ml sodium cacodylate wash buffer.
- 100 µl of the suspension is added to 1 ml of distilled water in a glass vial and kept refrigerated (5°C (40°F)) for light microscopic evaluation of wet or stained dry smears.
- The remaining suspension is centrifuged again and the pellet is fixed in a solution of 1% osmium tetroxide in cacodylate buffer (0.1 M) for 90 minutes, centrifuged, and the pellet washed three times in cacodylate buffer.
- The sample is then dehydrated through a graded series of ethanol solutions (50%, 70%, and three times in 95% and 100%).
- Dehydrated pellets are rinsed in propylene oxide (three times for 15 minutes each time) and then embedded in Poly/Bed® 812.
- Using a microtome, 1 µm thick sections are cut and mounted on glass slides for light microscopy to ensure optimal cut surface and also to facilitate initial evaluation of cell pellets.
- 80 nm thin sections are cut and mounted on nickel grids and stained with uranyl acetate and lead citrate for characterization of ultrastructural defects.
- Grids with 80 nm thin sections are incubated overnight at 4°C (39°F) in primary antibody, followed by biotinylated secondary antibody at room temperature (30 minutes), and then with streptavidin-immunogold conjugate (60 minutes) for localization of the binding sites (structures of interest).

Equine Reproductive Procedures, Second Edition. Edited by John Dascanio and Patrick McCue.

Additional Comments

Traditional light microscopy of a stallion semen sample does not always detect subtle defects in spermatozoa or defects at the organelle level. TEM allows for critical qualitative evaluation of spermatozoal morphology at an ultrastructural level along with identification of any other somatic cellular constituents of a seminal ejaculate. The most common sperm abnormalities identified in cases of idiopathic infertility include lesions of the plasma membrane, acrosomal defects, premature acrosome reaction, nuclear chromatin abnormalities, and mitochondrial defects (Figure 138.1).

In addition to identifying ultrastructural abnormalities, TEM also facilitates identifying potential molecular events such as sperm DNA fragmentation and oxidative stress on various sperm components by means of antigen-immunogold labeled antibody staining techniques (Figure 138.2). Furthermore, cellular remnants from the lining of the genital tract following inflammatory conditions and even pathogens (that might otherwise simply be dismissed as stain deposits or debris at light microscopic level) can be discerned (Figure 138.3).

In each of these instances a precise identification of the problem can be accomplished to arrive at strategies for therapeutic intervention.

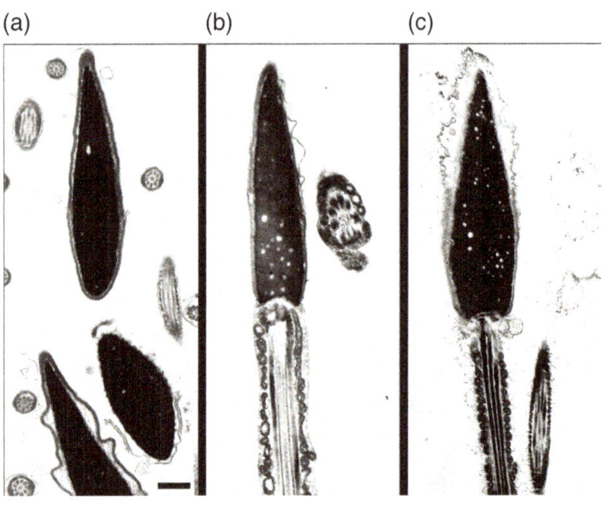

Figure 138.1 Transmission electron micrographs of equine spermatozoa showing: (a) plasma membrane and acrosomal defects (lower two profiles; compare with normal sperm head on top); (b) incomplete chromatin condensation and mitochondrial swelling; and (c) premature acrosome reaction. Scale bar: 1 μm.

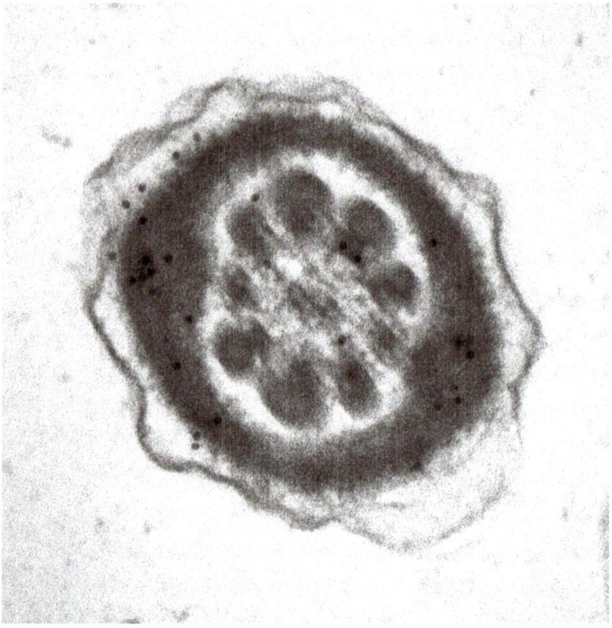

Figure 138.2 Transmission electron micrograph of a cross-section of the principal piece of sperm tail stained with streptavidin-conjugated 10 nm colloidal gold particles in an antigen–primary antibody–biotin-labeled secondary antibody reaction. The targeted antigens in this instance are glycotoxins that are associated with oxidative stress. Visualization of colloidal gold markers (black dots) reflect the localization of advanced glycation end products on the fibrous sheath (outermost ring underneath the plasma membrane), outer dense fibers, as well as the axonemal microtubule proteins (innermost ring), suggesting an inflammatory condition.

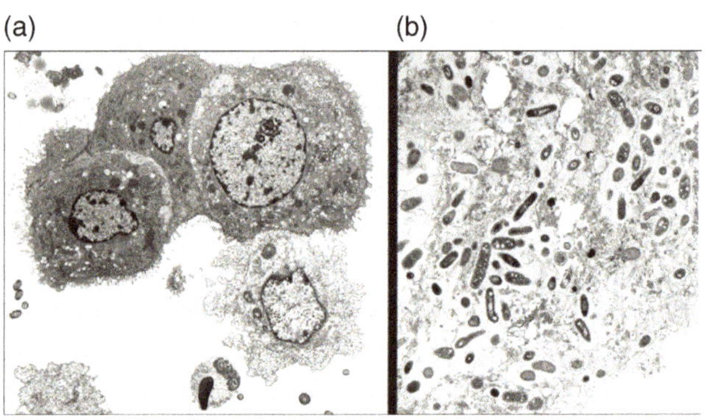

Figure 138.3 Transmission electron micrographs of exfoliated degenerative epithelial cells from accessory sex organs (a) and bacteria embedded in cellular detritus (b). Identification of such constituents in a seminal ejaculate facilitates localization of the underlying cause of infertility.

In summary, TEM can be used as an adjunctive diagnostic technique in the evaluation of stallion semen in cases of undiagnosed infertility.

References

Pesch S, Bostedt H, Failing K, Mergmann M. 2006. Advanced fertility diagnosis in stallion semen using transmission electron microscopy. *Anim Reprod Sci* 91: 285–98.

Veeramachaneni DNR. 2011. Spermatozoal morphology. In: McKinnon AO, Squire EL, Vaala WE, Varner DD (eds). Equine Reproduction, 2nd edn. Ames, IA: Wiley Blackwell, pp.1297–307.

Veeramachaneni DNR. 2017. Utility of testing sperm DNA fragmentation: an all-in-one diagnostic tool to address a multi-pronged clinical problem. *Transl Androl Urol* (Suppl 4): S462–4.

Veeramachaneni DNR, Moeller CL, Pickett BW, Shiner KA, Sawyer HR. 1993. On processing and evaluation of equine seminal samples for cytopathology and fertility assessment: the utility of electron microscopy. *J Equine Vet Sci* 13: 207–15.

Veeramachaneni DNR, Moeller CL, Sawyer HR. 2006. Sperm morphology in stallions: ultrastructure as a functional and diagnostic tool. *Vet Clin North Am Eq Pract* 22: 683–92.

Veeramachaneni DNR, Sawyer HR. 1996. Use of semen as biopsy material for assessment of health status of the stallion reproductive tract. *Vet Clin North Am Eq Pract* 12: 101–10.

139

Bacterial Culture

John J. Dascanio

School of Veterinary Medicine, Texas Tech University, USA

Introduction

Cultures of the stallion's external genitalia and semen may be performed as part of a routine breeding soundness examination, as a requirement for import or export purposes, as a routine procedure prior to the start of the breeding season, or performed as part of an infertility assessment. Bacterial and/or fungal cultures of a stallion may include culturing semen, the urethra pre-and post-ejaculation, the penile shaft, the prepuce, the urethral fossa, and the urethral sinus. If cost is an issue then the urethral fossa and the shaft of the penis should be preferentially cultured as they tend to be the areas most represented in stallions with infectious infertilities.

A sterile cotton-tipped culture swab is used to acquire samples. A prepackaged swab with culture media may be purchased for convenience for shipment of samples to a laboratory or swabs may be directly plated onto culture media (blood agar plate, MacConkey's agar plate) for aerobic culture (see Chapter 14).

Equipment and Supplies

Sterile culture swabs, transport media, examination gloves.

Technique

Culturing a Stallion's External Genitalia

- The stallion should be adequately restrained to prevent movement and to ensure a safe working environment. The stallion's right side may be placed against a solid wall while having the handler and the veterinarian on the stallion's left side.
- Only enough stimulation should be provided for the stallion to extend his penis from the prepuce and to obtain an erection. Overexcitation may make acquiring samples more difficult as the stallion may not want to stand quietly.
- Disposable examination gloves should be worn. Approaching the stallion from the left shoulder, the back of the hand may touch his shoulder and with the back of the hand remaining in contact with the stallion's thorax and then abdomen, the penis is gently grasped. Minimal pressure should be placed on the shaft and glans to prevent thrusting activity.
- A culture swab is used to obtain a culture of the preputial tissue folds and separately for the penile shaft prior to any rinsing of the penis (Figure 139.1).

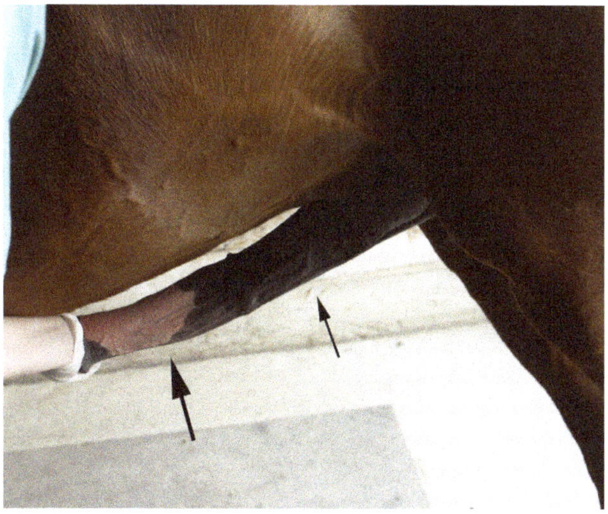

Figure 139.1 Sites for the collection of culture samples from the penis (large arrow) and prepuce (smaller arrow). Note the preputial ring of raised tissue separating the two areas.

Equine Reproductive Procedures, Second Edition. Edited by John Dascanio and Patrick McCue.

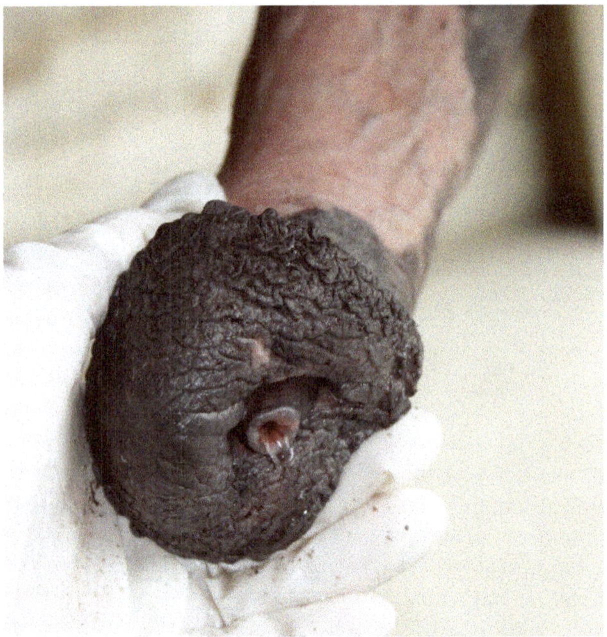

Figure 139.2 Glans penis of a stallion after teasing, demonstrating pre-ejaculatory fluid from the distal urethra.

- The stallion's penis should not be washed with a soap solution before cultures are obtained as this will adversely affect culture results. The penis may be rinsed with clean water and dried with a paper towel if a large amount of debris is present, but this should be avoided if possible.
- If the stallion has been adequately teased prior to culturing, clear pre-ejaculatory fluid may be evident from the urethra (Figure 139.2). If this is not present, gentle pressure with a cupped hand over the glans penis will often stimulate the flow of pre-ejaculatory fluid. This culture is a partial reflection of the bacteria present in the urethra and accessory sex glands. A clean culture swab is placed into the distal urethra to obtain a culture of this fluid.
- An additional swab is obtained from the urethral fossa.
- Semen is then collected from the stallion using an artificial vagina. Disposable artificial vagina liners and sterile/disposable equipment should be used for semen collection
- The distal end of the urethra is cultured again after semen collection.
- A culture is then obtained from the semen in the collection vesicle.

Culturing Fresh Cooled Semen

- Semen that has been processed for cooled storage should be cultured at 24 hours post-processing to determine if the antibiotics present in the semen extender have controlled bacterial growth.

Culturing Frozen Semen

- Semen that has been processed for frozen semen should be cultured just prior to loading the semen into straws for freezing. Freezing and thawing of semen will not kill bacteria.

Interpretation

- There is a normal flora of bacteria present on the stallion's external genitalia. These organisms must be differentiated from potentially pathogenic bacteria based on type, colonization numbers, and associated fertility issues. Typically, finding bacteria in pure culture with a high number of colony-forming units makes their isolation more significant in the causation of pathology. Isolation of the same bacteria from a mare bred to the stallion cultured offers more evidence of potential pathogenicity, especially if clinical signs of infection are present.
- Isolation of *Taylorella equigenitalis* (contagious equine metritis) or *Trypanosoma equiperdum* (dourine) is considered pathologic and must be reported to veterinary health officials.
- Bacteria that are commonly associated with pathology include *Klebsiella* species and *Pseudomonas* species. There are both pathologic and non-pathologic strains of *Klebsiella* that are identified by their capsule type. There are more than 70 capsule types identified. Types K1, K2, and K5 are most frequently associated with pathology.
- Bacteria that have been associated with pathologic issues include *Streptococcus equi* subspecies *zooepidemicus* and *Escherichia coli*; however, these organisms may be isolated from normal stallions as well. *Streptococcus* species, *Staphylococcus* species, and *E. coli* have been isolated from normal stallions, especially in mixed growth cultures.
- Occasionally, fungi may be isolated from normal stallions. Up to about 9% of normal stallions have been reported to culture positive for fungi without associated infertility.

Further Reading

Bowen JM, Tobin N, Simpson RB, Ley WB, Ansari MM. 1982. Effects of washing on the bacterial flora of the stallion's penis. *J Reprod Fertil* 32: 41–5.

Conboy HS. 2007. Significance of bacteria affecting the stallion's reproductive system. In: Samper JC, Pycock JF, McKinnon AO (eds). Current Therapy in Equine Reproduction. St Louis, MI: Saunders Elsevier, pp. 231–6.

Rota A, Calicchio E, Nardoni S, *et al.* 2011. Presence and distribution of fungi and bacteria in the reproductive tract of healthy stallions. *Theriogenology* 76: 464–70.

140

Evaluation of pH and Osmolarity of Semen

Patrick M. McCue

Equine Reproduction Laboratory, Colorado State University, USA

Introduction

pH is a measure of the acidity or alkalinity of a solution and measurement of the pH of semen is part of a complete breeding soundness evaluation of a stallion. Ideally, a calibrated pH meter should be used to obtain an accurate measurement of pH. Measurement with pH paper will be less precise.

The pH of raw semen should be determined as soon as possible after collection. Incubation of a semen sample for a prolonged period of time may lead to a lower pH due to the accumulation of metabolic by-products, such as lactic acid.

Osmolality is the concentration of a solution in terms of osmoles of solute particles per kilogram of solvent. An osmole refers to the number of moles of ions that contribute to a solution's osmotic pressure (i.e., 1 mol/l of NaCl corresponds to an osmolarity of 2 osmol/l as the NaCl dissociates into individual Na^+ and Cl^- ions in solution). Osmolality can be measured in either raw semen or seminal plasma.

Equipment and Supplies

pH meter, pH kit (standards, etc.), sample tube or vial, osmometer, osmolarity kit (standards, etc.), pipetter and tips, distilled or deionized water in a rinse bottle.

Technique

pH Measurement

- A sample of raw semen is collected for evaluation.
- The pH meter should be standardized prior to use to obtain an accurate reading using the instructions that come with the meter.
- The electrode is rinsed with distilled or deionized water prior to evaluation of the test sample.
- The electrode is placed down into the sample until the pH is determined by the meter (Figure 140.1).

Osmolarity Measurement

- A 20 µl sample of raw semen or seminal plasma is obtained and transferred into the bottom of a sample tube. The tube may be tapped lightly to eliminate air bubbles and to unite the fluid sample in the bottom of the tube.
- The loaded sample tube is placed into the sample well of the osmometer.
- The measuring head is lowered into the sample tube (Figure 140.2).
- The osmolarity test is initiated.

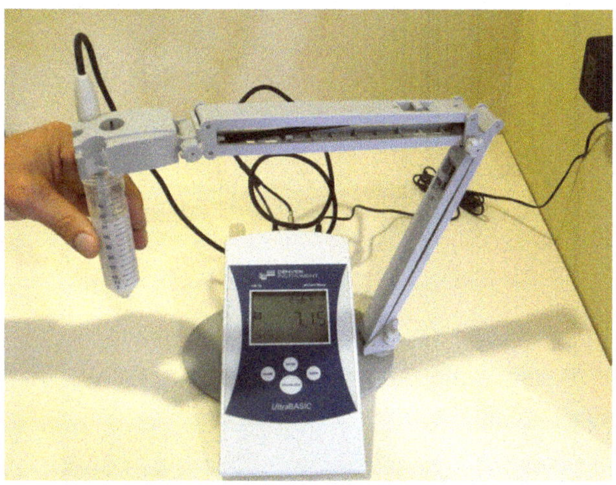

Figure 140.1 Measurement of pH of a sample of stallion raw semen.

Equine Reproductive Procedures, Second Edition. Edited by John Dascanio and Patrick McCue.

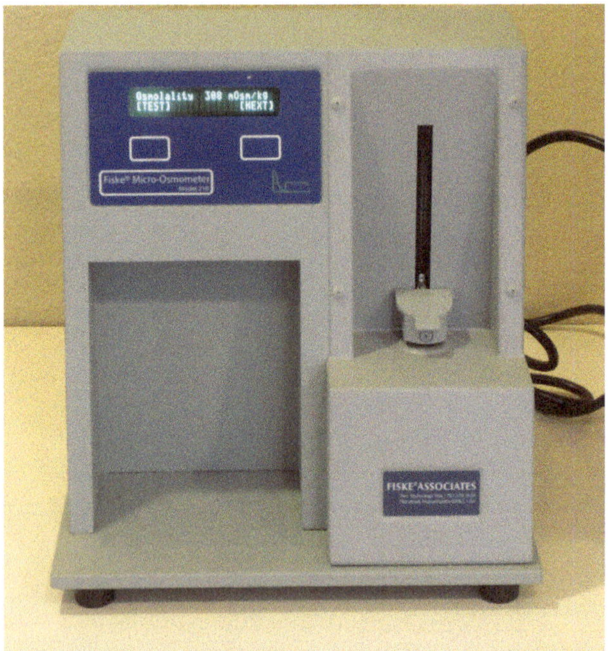

Figure 140.2 Measurement of osmolality of a sample of stallion semen.

- The probe should be wiped clean after each test and rinsed with distilled water or alcohol.

Additional Comments

The normal pH of raw (unextended) equine semen ranges from 7.2 to 7.7. The pH of normal stallion semen can be affected by season, frequency of ejaculation, and sperm concentration. A slight increase in pH (approximately 0.10) has been noted between the first and second ejaculates from stallions. It has been suggested that if the pH of the first ejaculate is equal to or higher than the second, the first ejaculate may have been incomplete or abnormal. The pH of accessory gland fluid devoid of epididymal contributions is approximately 8.0 (range 7.8–8.2). Semen samples with low sperm concentration may have a higher pH than a complete ejaculate. An elevation in semen pH may indicate urine contamination, inflammation within the reproductive tract, or contamination of the ejaculate with soap.

The osmolality of equine seminal plasma varies considerably by stallion. There is no significant difference in osmolality between the first and second ejaculates or difference due to season. The osmolality of stallion semen has been reported to be 331–336 mOsm. An elevation in osmolality may be indicative of sample contamination with urine or water-soluble lubricants.

Significant alterations in pH and/or osmolality may be associated with a reduction in sperm motility and potentially a reduction in fertility.

Further Reading

Griggers S, Paccamonti DL, Thompson RA, Eilts BE. 2001. The effects of pH, osmolarity and urine contamination on equine spermatozoal motility. *Theriogenology* 56: 613–22.

Pickett BW, Faulkner LC, Seidel GE, Jr, Berndtson WE, Voss JL. 1976. Reproductive physiology of the stallion. VI. Seminal and behavioral characteristics. *J Anim Sci* 43: 617–25.

141

Alkaline Phosphatase: A Marker for Ejaculation

Patrick M. McCue

Equine Reproduction Laboratory, Colorado State University, USA

Introduction

Alkaline phosphatase (AP) is a dephosphorylating enzyme active in multiple tissues in the body. Seminal plasma of many species has been reported to have AP activity. The site of origin of AP activity within the reproductive tract varies amongst domestic animal species. In the stallion, AP activity originates in the testes and epididymis and is concentrated to very high levels in the epididymal tail. Spermatozoa in the ejaculate do not contribute to AP activity. The measurement of seminal AP activity may be used as a sperm-independent marker for ejaculation in stallions.

Equipment and Supplies

Artificial vagina and accessories, storage tube or vial, centrifuge, disposable pipettes, serum chemistry analyzer, diluent (7% bovine serum albumen in reagent grade water).

Technique

- Semen is collected from the test stallion using an artificial vagina. An aliquot of the ejaculate is analyzed for AP activity.
- Centrifugation of the semen at 16,000× *g* for 20 minutes will result in sperm pellet formation.
- An aliquot of the seminal plasma supernatant can be collected for analysis of AP activity.
- Levels of AP activity above the dynamic range of the analyzer (i.e., >1,500 IU/l) are indicative of ejaculation.
- If specific values are desired, the semen sample should be diluted with a 7% bovine serum albumen solution and reanalyzed. The results are subsequently multiplied by the dilution factor to obtain the AP activity of the original sample. For example, if a 100 µl sample of semen is diluted with 900 µl of diluent (creating a 1:9 dilution or a 10-fold dilution), the assayed value would be multiplied by 10 to obtain the true activity in the original sample.
- It is recommended that semen not immediately analyzed for AP activity be stored at 4°C (39°F) for less than 24 hours.
- If a longer interval is anticipated, it is suggested that the samples be centrifuged and the supernatant frozen at −20°C (−4°F) until assayed.

Interpretation

The measurement of seminal AP activity is primarily used to determine if ejaculation occurred in instances where no sperm are present in the fluid recovered.

- High levels of AP in the presence of spermatozoa indicate that ejaculation occurred.
- A high level of AP activity in seminal fluid in the absence of spermatozoa is indicative of azospermia.
- In contrast, low levels of AP and the absence of spermatozoa suggest either failure of ejaculation or bilateral blockage of the ampullae.
- Levels of AP activity in pre-seminal fluid and semen from normal stallions are noted in Table 141.1.
- The guidelines given in Table 141.2 are recommended in interpreting AP levels in stallion semen.

Equine Reproductive Procedures, Second Edition. Edited by John Dascanio and Patrick McCue.

Table 141.1 Alkaline phosphatase (AP) activity in pre-seminal fluid and semen of normal stallions.

	AP Activity (IU/l)	
Sample	**Average ± SD**	**Range**
Pre-seminal fluid	30.4 ± 22.2	14–90
Semen	23,498 ± 11,889	6,390–48,700

From Turner (1996).

Table 141.2 Recommended guidelines to interpret alkaline phosphatase (AP) levels in stallion semen.

AP Level (IU/l)	Interpretation
>1,000	True ejaculation
100–1,000	Partial ejaculate or partial blockage
<100	Ejaculatory failure or blockage

Reference

Turner RM. 1996. Alkaline phosphatase in stallion semen: characterization and clinical applications. In: *Proceedings of the Society for Theriogenology*, pp. 284–93.

Further Reading

Turner RM, Sertich PL. 2001. Use of alkaline phosphatase activity as a diagnostic tool in stallions with azoospermia and oligospermia. In: *Proceedings of the 3rd International Symposium on Stallion Reproduction*, p. 35.

142

Diagnosis and Management of Urospermia

John J. Dascanio

School of Veterinary Medicine, Texas Tech University, USA

Introduction

Urine contamination of semen can lead to decreased conception rates due to the toxic effects of the urine on spermatozoa and possible inflammation induced in the uterus from components in the urine. Total and progressive spermatozoal motility will decrease with urine contamination in a dose-dependent manner. Causes of urospermia are not well defined. Neurologic abnormalities such as cauda equina neuritis, equine protozoal myeloencephalitis, equine herpesvirus 1, and sorghum toxicosis, as well as medical conditions such as hyperkalemic periodic paralysis, cystitis, and urolithiasis, can all cause urospermia. In addition, some cases do not appear to be associated with a specific pathologic or medical condition and are often considered to be behavioral in origin.

Methods for the prevention of urospermia include selective collection of the sperm-rich fraction of the ejaculate fluids with an open-ended artificial vagina, medications to augment bladder sphincter control, management to induce urination prior to breeding or collection, and centrifugation of semen after urine contamination.

Simple dilution of semen with a skim milk-based semen extender will decrease the adverse effects of urine on spermatozoal function and this should be done immediately after recognizing that contamination has occurred. Centrifugation and re-extension of semen, however, may still be advocated since it will aid in the removal of urine crystals/solids, thus decreasing possible inflammation induced in the mare's uterus. Both standard centrifugation and cushioned centrifugation have been demonstrated to be beneficial to decrease the adverse effects of urine contamination.

Assessment of semen for the presence of urine using Azostix® should be done before addition of the extender, as smaller amounts of urine contamination may be undetectable in extended samples. An Azostix® can also be used in extended semen samples, providing significant urine contamination is present. If the semen has been already diluted with semen extender, detection of urine may require laboratory analysis for urea nitrogen and creatinine.

Equipment and Supplies

Sterile urine cup, Azostix®, centrifuge, 50 ml centrifuge tubes, disposable plastic pipettes, semen extender.

Testing for Urospermia

- The first indication of urospermia is often a yellow discoloration to the ejaculate (Figure 142.1). There may also be a noticeable smell of urine (ammonia) in the ejaculate.
- The ejaculate may be tested for the presence of urea nitrogen by use of a diagnostic indicator strip (Azostix®) (Figure 142.2). Upon exposure to contaminated semen, the Azostix® turns from yellow to green within 10 seconds. The Azostix® may be immersed in the semen sample for 60 seconds, after which it should be rinsed with distilled water and evaluated. This is a semiquantitative test and can provide evidence of urine contamination of semen.
- The semen may be submitted for laboratory assessment of urea nitrogen and creatinine levels. A urea nitrogen >30 mg/dl or a creatinine value >2.0 mg/dl are indicative of urine contamination.
- In addition, pH and osmolality of the semen may both be significantly elevated in an ejaculate containing urine (Table 142.1).

Equine Reproductive Procedures, Second Edition. Edited by John Dascanio and Patrick McCue.

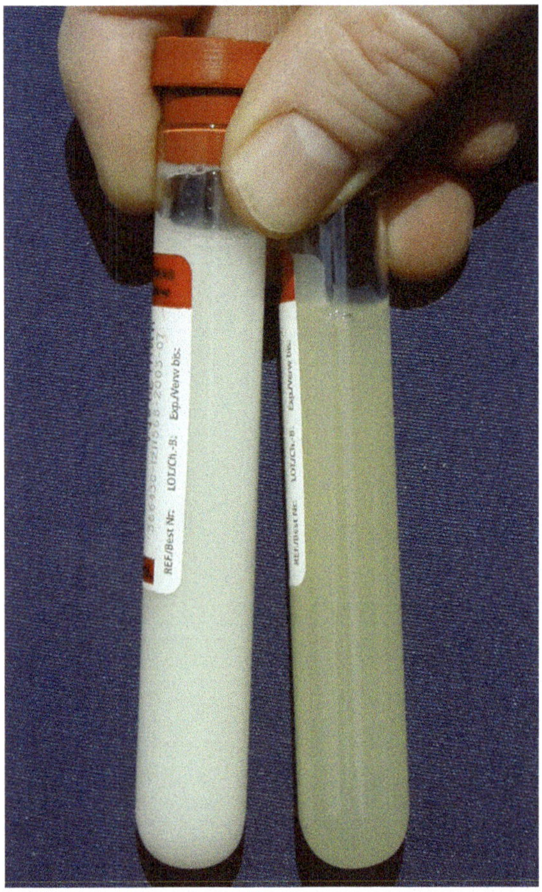

Figure 142.1 The tube on the left is from a stallion with a normal ejaculate for comparison. The tube on the right is from a stallion with urospermia; note the yellow discoloration.

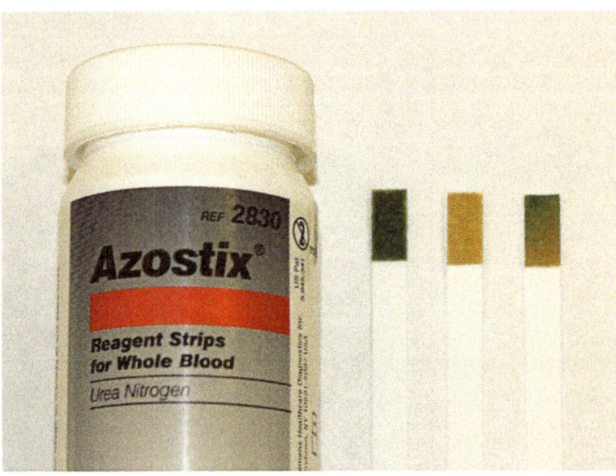

Figure 142.2 Evaluation of urea nitrogen in semen samples from a stallion using an Azostix® test strip (left, urospermia; center, unused test strip; right, normal ejaculate).

Table 142.1 Semen characteristics of a stallion's ejaculate with urospermia and a subsequent normal collection in which the stallion was induced to urinate prior to the collection attempt.

Semen Parameter	Ejaculate with Urospermia	Normal Ejaculate
Total motility (%)	40	89
Progressive motility (%)	30	83
pH	7.94	7.25
Osmolality (mOsm)	773	321

Technique for the Management of Urospermia

- A thorough physical examination should be performed to determine if there are neurologic or medical issues that may be contributing to the urospermia.
- The best management practice for a stallion with apparent behavior-associated urospermia is to have the stallion urinate prior to collection. This may be achieved by placing him in the stall of another stallion. In most instances, a stallion will urinate onto the fecal pile of the other stallion within a few minutes.
- Another technique to stimulate urination prior to collection is to remove the stallion from his stall, place new bedding in his stall, and then return him to his original stall. Most stallions will urinate to mark their territory within a few minutes. This technique works well if the stallion is turned out into an exercise paddock for 30–45 minutes and then returned to his cleaned stall just prior to semen collection.
- Minor urine contamination (i.e., a slight discoloration) may be managed by diluting the affected semen with a commercial semen extender to a concentration of 25–50 million spermatozoa/ml.
- If contamination is significant, the semen should be mixed with an equal volume of semen extender and centrifuged (see Chapter 149). A majority of the supernatant is removed (poured off or aspirated off), leaving approximately 5–10% of the seminal plasma, and additional semen extender is added to re-suspend the semen pellet. If there is evidence of urine crystals/debris below the semen pellet, care should be used to only re-suspend the semen pellet and not the lower urine debris (Figure 142.3).

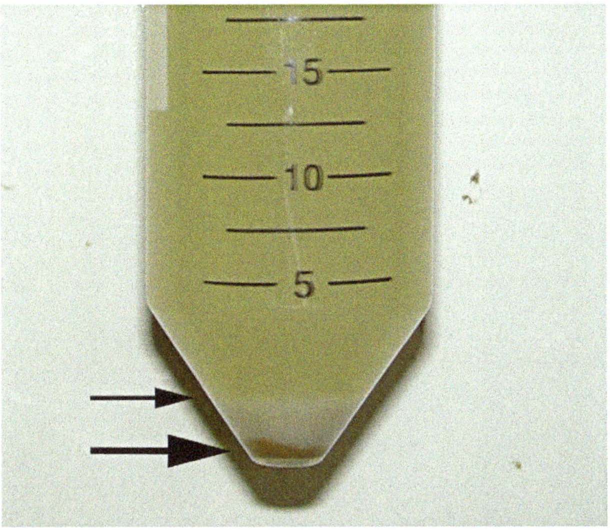

Figure 142.3 A urospermic stallion's ejaculate after centrifugation. The sperm pellet starts at the interface between the yellow seminal plasma and the white semen pellet (small arrow). There are significant urine crystals/debris at the bottom of the tube (large arrow).

- Alpha-adrenergic agonists may be administered in an attempt to augment bladder sphincter control. These include imipramine hydrochloride (0.8 mg/kg PO, 2–4 hours prior to semen collection) and phenylpropanolamine (0.35 mg/kg PO, b.i.d.).
- Diuretics, such as furosemide, have been used to dilute the urine and to potentially cause urination. While this may not eliminate urospermia, it may somewhat decrease toxic effects.

Interpretation

- Urine contamination of semen can lead to decreased conception rates due to the toxic effects of the urine on spermatozoa and possible inflammation induced in the uterus from components in the urine. In addition, the pH and osmolarity of the semen may be negatively affected by urine contamination.
- With proper preparation, urine contaminated semen may be used for fresh, cooled, or frozen semen breeding. Highly contaminated semen, however, may not be suitable for freezing due to a decrease in motility.
- The lower limit of sensitivity of Azostix® has been reported to be 39 mg/dl; thus samples below this limit may have slight urine contamination, but a negative Azostix® test result.
- Some stallions that urinate into their ejaculate will continue to do so constantly or intermittently during their entire breeding career. A complete neurologic examination should be performed on stallions with urospermia to rule out a treatable condition.

Further Reading

Dascanio JJ, Witonsky SG. 2005. Theriogenology question of the month: urospermia. *J Am Vet Med Assoc* 227: 225–7.

Ellerbrock R, Canisso I, Feijo L, Lima F, Shipley C, Kline K. 2016. Diagnosis and effects of urine contamination in cooled-extended stallion semen. *Theriogenology* 85: 1219–24.

Ellerbrock RE, Honorato J, Curcio BR, *et al.* 2018. Effect of urine contamination on stallion semen freezing ability. *Theriogenology* 117: 1–6.

Griggers S, Paccamonti DL, Thompson RA, *et al.* 2001. The effects of pH, osmolarity and urine contamination on equine spermatozoal motility. *Theriogenology* 56: 613–22.

Oristaglio Turner RM, Love CC, McDonnell SM, *et al.* 1995. Use of imipramine hydrochloride for treatment of urospermia in a stallion with a dysfunctional bladder. *J Am Vet Med Assoc* 207: 1602–6.

143

Hemospermia

Patrick M. McCue

Equine Reproduction Laboratory, Colorado State University, USA

Introduction

Hemospermia refers to the presence of blood in the semen. Fertility may be normal with mild cases of hemospermia, but significant hemorrhage will result in reduced fertility. Stallions may bleed during semen collection or during a live cover mating. Causes of hemospermia in stallions include:

- Lesion on the glans penis:
  - Trauma.
  - Laceration.
  - Squamous cell carcinoma.
  - Cutaneous habronemiasis.
- Lesion on the external urethral process (same causes as for glans penis lesion)
- Seminal vesiculitis.
- Rent in the proximal urethra.
- Other potential causes include epididymitis, urethritis, and trauma to the shaft of the penis.

A small laceration on the end of the glans penis or distal urethral process may be sustained during mating by friction against tail hairs of the mare or on breeding equipment such as a phantom. Active bleeding from these sites may not be evident unless a full erection is present. Bleeding in these regions may also be associated with the presence of cutaneous habronemiasis lesions ("summer sores") or squamous cell carcinoma lesions.

Another site of bleeding during mating or semen collection is from a rent or tear in the proximal urethra. A further potential site of blood loss from the penis of a stallion during mating is the seminal vesicles. Inflammation of the seminal vesicles (seminal vesiculitis) due to bacterial infection may result in the presence of blood within the gel fraction of the ejaculate.

Equipment and Supplies

Artificial vagina, sterile obstetrical lubricant, graduated cylinder, videoendoscope, examination gloves, microscope, glass slides, Diff-Quick® stain.

Technique

- Initial discovery of the presence of blood in the semen is usually made as a stallion dismounts from the mare after a live cover or is based on the color of the ejaculate obtained during semen collection (Figure 143.1). The differential diagnosis for blood on the end of the penis following a live cover includes issues associated with the mare (disrupted hymen, trauma to the vagina or cervix, bleeding from a vaginal varicose vein, etc.) or with the stallion.
- Identification of the site of bleeding from a stallion includes close examination of the glans penis, urethral process, urethral diverticulum, and shaft of the penis. Additional diagnostic tests may include collection of semen in an open-ended artificial vagina, transrectal palpation and ultrasonography of the seminal vesicles, and endoscopic examination of the proximal urethra.
- Visual examination of the distal end of the penis should be performed as soon as possible after live cover or semen collection. Lesions of the glans penis or urethral process resulting in blood loss are most visible immediately after ejaculation. Examination at a later time may not yield a correct diagnosis. External lesions may be located on the tip of the urethral process, along the rim of the glans penis, anywhere on the distal glans penis, or (rarely) along the shaft of the penis (Figures 143.2 and 143.3).
- A videoendoscopic examination of the urethra should be considered if there are no obvious lesions present on the glans penis or urethral process (see Chapter 163).

Equine Reproductive Procedures, Second Edition. Edited by John Dascanio and Patrick McCue.

(a) (b)

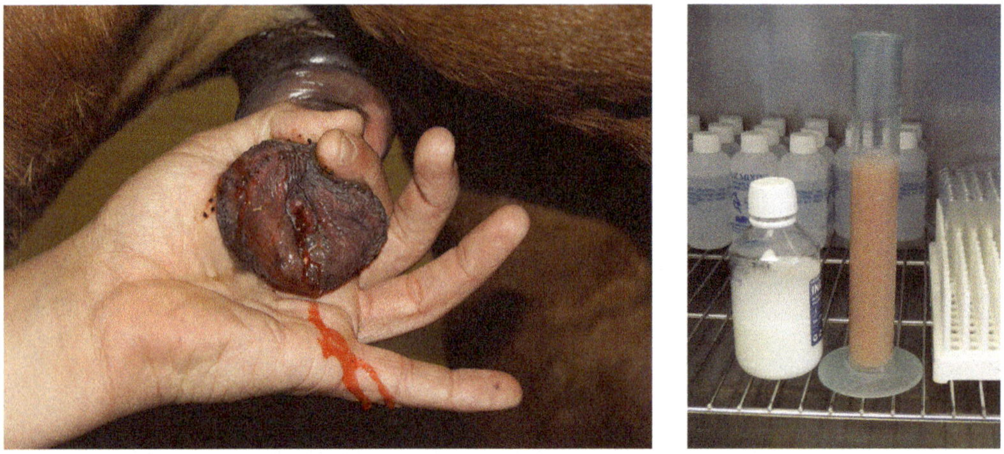

Figure 143.1 (a) Blood exiting the urethra of a stallion with hemospermia and (b) blood contamination of semen after collection.

(a) (b)

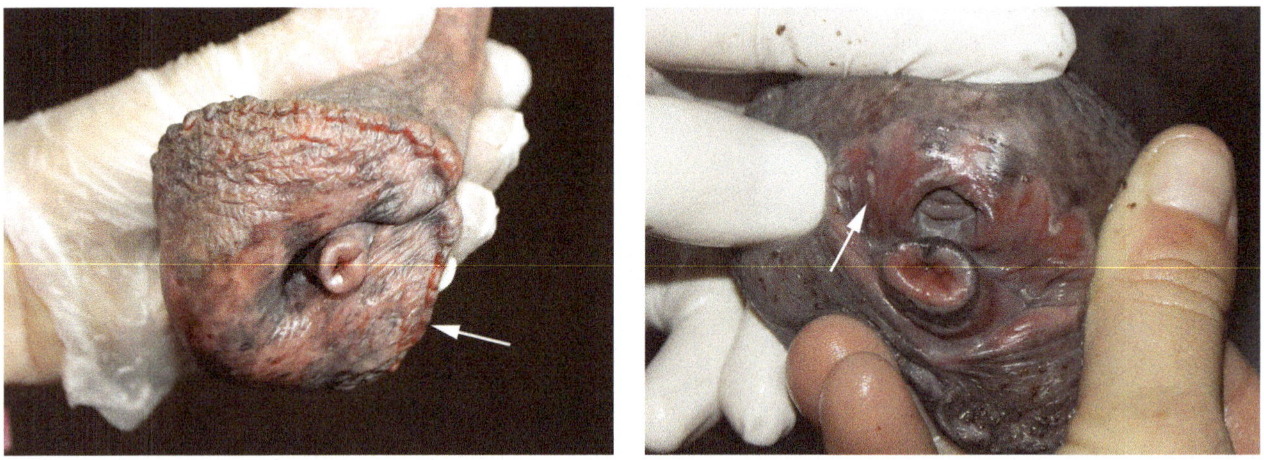

Figure 143.2 (a, b) Small lesions (arrows) on the glans penis resulting in hemospermia.

(a) (b)

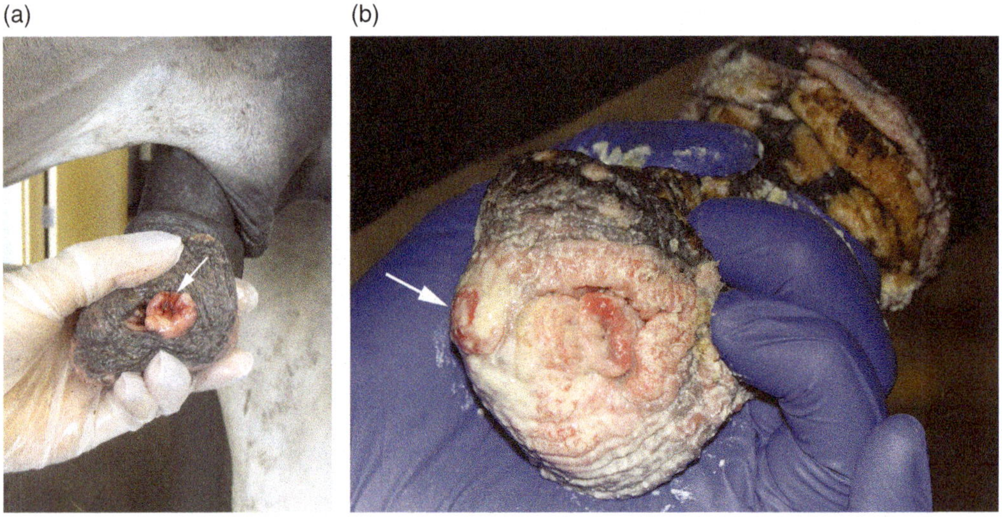

Figure 143.3 (a) Lesion on the distal urethral process (arrow) and (b) squamous cell carcinoma lesion on the glans penis (arrow).

- The stallion should be sedated and properly restrained (preferably in examination stocks). One common sedation protocol consists of a combination of detomidine (~0.015 mg/kg) plus butorphanol tartrate (~0.01 mg/kg), administered intravenously.
- When the stallion is sedated, his penis will usually extend out of the sheath and can be washed thoroughly with a non-residual soap, rinsed with clean water, and dried with disposable paper towels (see Chapter 123).
- A small amount of sterile obstetrical lubricant is applied to the outside of the near-distal end of the videoendoscope, taking care to not apply lubricant onto the camera or light. The endoscope is slowly passed proximately up the urethra, taking note of any lesions that are visible. If the hemospermia is due to a urethral rent, the lesion is almost always located 6–10 cm distal to the seminal colliculus on the caudo-dorsal convex surface of the urethra at the level of the ischial arch (Figure 143.4).
- Seminal vesiculitis can be diagnosed as the cause of hermospermia by a combination of techniques:
- The first is collection of semen using an open-ended artificial vagina and confirming that first 2–4 jets of semen are free of blood and that the blood is confined to the gel-fraction at the end of ejaculation.
- A second technique is transrectal palpation and ultrasonography to determine if one or both seminal vesicles are enlarged (see Chapter 166).
- A third technique is direct cannulation of the seminal vesicles using a videoendoscope and collection of samples for culture and cytologic evaluation (see Chapter 164).
- A final technique that is suggestive of seminal vesiculitis is the presence of white blood cells in the semen. The latter technique should be interpreted with caution as inflammation or infection of other parts of the reproductive tract (orchitis, epididymitis, ampullitis, etc.) could also lead to the presence of white blood cells in the semen.

Interpretation

An accurate diagnosis of the source of blood is important as the location and cause of the bleeding will determine the optimal course of management or therapy as well as the prognosis for recovery. Small lacerations on the urethral process or glans often heal with a short period of sexual rest (i.e., 5–10 days) with or without topical application of an antiseptic or antibiotic ointment.

Habronema lesions are rare in stallions under good health management protocols that include routine anthelmintic administration. Larvae of *Draschia megastoma*, *Habronema muscae*, or *Habronema microstoma* are deposited onto the glans penis or urethral process by flies. Active

(a) (b)

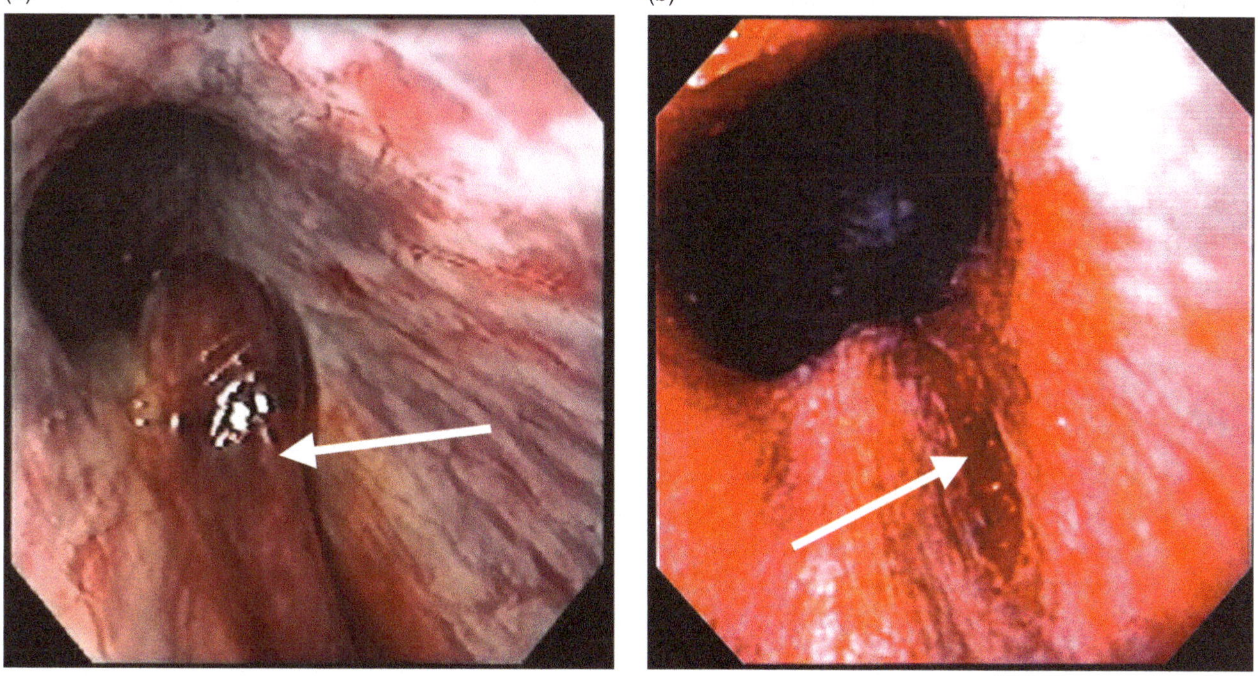

Figure 143.4 (a, b) Rents in the proximal urethra of two stallions with hemospermia (arrows). A hematoma is present over the rent in (a).

lesions are recognized as raised granulomatous, ulcerated, or caseous masses comprised of eosinophils, necrotic debris, and parasitic larvae. Therapy for clinical cases includes killing the parasites by systemic administration or topical application of ivermectin in conjunction with reducing inflammation by topical and/or systemic administration of corticosteroids. Prevention includes fly control at the premises, insect repellant application, and regular administration of ivermectin.

Squamous cell carcinoma of the glans, urethral process, or shaft of the penis is often locally invasive and multicentric. Treatment options include surgical debulking or debridement along with adjunctive procedures such as cryotherapy, radiofrequency hyperthermia, radiation therapy, photodynamic therapy, topical or intratumoral chemotherapy, immunomodulators, and other treatments. Local or intralesional therapy may be beneficial in reducing systemic side effects of treatments.

Management of hemospermia due to a urethral rent includes a prolonged period of sexual rest (i.e., 6–12 months) and potentially a temporary perineal urethrotomy or similar surgical procedure. A perineal urethrotomy consists of an incision into the urethra below the perineal region, which would allow urine to exit at that location and bypass the distal aspect of the penis, theoretically resulting in reduced pressure on the proximal urethral lesion. Other surgical procedures include a perineal approach without incising into the urethra, a buccal mucosal urethroplasty, and laser ablation of the rent. All surgical procedures include a prolonged period of sexual rest. A recently described technique for treatment of urethral rents in stallions is infusion of 100 ml of 4% policresulen solution, a topical hemostatic and antiseptic agent, into the proximal urethra via a catheter once per day for 4–7 days to "chemically cauterize" the lesion in conjunction with prolonged sexual rest.

Treatment of seminal vesiculitis may include irrigation of the affected seminal vesicle(s) using a cannula passed through a videoendoscope followed by infusion of antibiotics directly into the affected vesicle, plus systemic administration of antibiotics. The choice of antibiotics should be based on culture results and antimicrobial sensitivity tests. Additional reproductive management may include incubation of semen from an affected stallion in a semen extender containing an appropriate antibiotic.

Further Reading

Hackett ES, Bruemmer J, Hendrickson DA, McCue PM. 2009. Buccal mucosal urethroplasty for treatment of recurrent hemospermia in a stallion. *J Am Vet Med Assoc* 235: 1212–15.

Madron M, Schleining J, Caston S, Reinertson E, Evans L. 2013. Laser treatment of urethral defects in geldings and stallions used as the primary treatment or in combination with a temporary subischial incision: eight cases (2003–2011). *Eq Vet Educ* 25: 368–73.

Pearson LK, Campbell AJ, Tibary A. 2013. How to diagnose and treat hemospermia: a review and case series. *Proc Am Assoc Eq Pract* 59: 40–50.

Sancler-Silva YF, Silva-Junior ER, Fedorka CE, *et al.* 2018. New treatment for urethral rent in stallions. *J Eq Vet Sci* 64: 89–95.

Schumacher J, Varner DD, Schmitz DG, Blanchard TL. 1995. Urethral defects in geldings with hematuria and stallions with hemospermia. *Vet Surg* 24: 250–4.

144

Semen Extenders and Sperm Media

Patrick M. McCue

Equine Reproduction Laboratory, Colorado State University, USA

Semen Extenders

Raw semen should be diluted with an appropriate semen extender as soon as possible after collection and initial evaluation of gel-free volume and sperm concentration. The goal of an extender is to protect the spermatozoa from cold shock, to provide metabolizable substrate(s), to inhibit microbial growth, and to provide optimized spermatozoal survival during the period between collection and insemination. The integrity of the spermatozoa and survival during short-term storage are affected by the type of extender as well as the cooling rate, storage temperature, concentration of seminal plasma, and oxygen exposure.

Equine semen extenders should have the following characteristics:

- Osmolarity of 300–350 mOsm/l.
- pH of 6.8–7.0.
- Components that stabilize pH (buffers).
- Energy source(s) for spermatozoa.
- Components that control microbial growth.
- Components that protect the membranes and metabolic function of sperm.
- Components that neutralize metabolic byproducts.

Extender Components

One of the first media designed for use with stallion spermatozoa was a skim milk glucose extender. Variations of the "Kenney extender" formulation have been developed that differ in the percentage of ingredients, contain an additional sugar such as sucrose, or utilize different type(s) of antibiotics. Other extenders contain only native phosphocaseinate, a fractionated component of milk, or egg yolk. Milk components and egg yolk help protect sperm plasma membranes, provide buffering capacity, and provide antioxidative properties to the extender. Buffers that are added to some semen extenders include sodium bicarbonate, sodium citrate, and HEPES. Table 144.1 lists some commonly used extenders. E-Z Mixin® CST, a traditional Kenney-type extender, and INRA 96, which contains native phosphocaseinate, are depicted in Figure 144.1.

Antimicrobial agents

Antimicrobial agents that are commonly incorporated into an equine semen extender include amikacin (1 mg/ml) alone, a combination of amikacin and potassium penicillin G (1,000 U/ml), or ticarcillin sodium plus clavulanic acid (1 mg/ml). Longevity of spermatozoa from an individual stallion during cooled storage may vary with the type of antimicrobial agent used. Consequently, a cooling trial is recommended to determine which antimicrobial agent may be optimal for a given stallion (see Chapter 147).

Table 144.1 Commercial stallion semen extenders for cooled storage of stallion semen. Some of these extenders have variable combinations of antibiotics and other ingredients for specific conditions.

Product Name	Company
BotuSemen	Botupharma USA, Phoenix, AZ, USA
EquiPlus, EquiPro, Gent	Minitube, Verona, WI, USA
E-Z Mixin®	Animal Reproduction Systems, Ontario, CA USA
INRA 96	IMV Technologies USA, Maple Grove, MN, USA
Next Generation®	Exodus Breeders Corporation, York, PA, USA
VMD-Z™ Extender	Breeder's Choice, Rochester Hills, MI, USA

Equine Reproductive Procedures, Second Edition. Edited by John Dascanio and Patrick McCue.

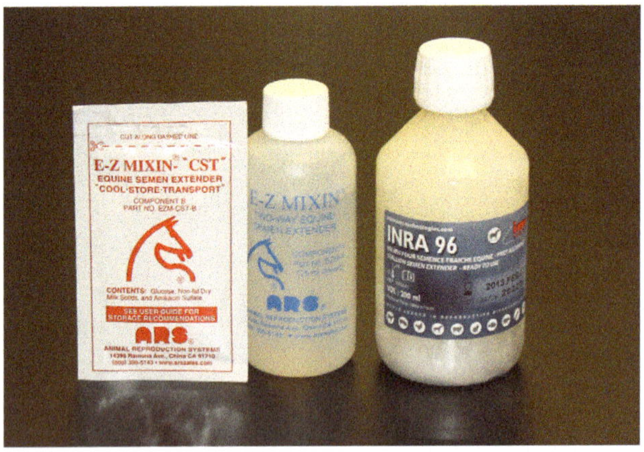

Figure 144.1 Two types of extenders commonly used to dilute equine semen.

Seminal plasma

High concentrations of seminal plasma are detrimental to sperm motility during cooled storage. Consequently, the addition of a semen extender to raw semen will dilute the concentration of seminal plasma. Ideally, the final concentration of spermatozoa after addition of semen extender will be 25–50 million spermatozoa per milliliter. Centrifugation of semen and subsequent removal of a majority of the seminal plasma will enhance the longevity of the spermatozoa during cooled storage of "poor cooler" stallions (see Chapter 149). After centrifugation and removal of seminal plasma, the concentration of spermatozoa after the addition of semen extender may exceed 50 million/ml without detriment to longevity.

Skim Milk Glucose Extender

Ingredients

All the ingredients for skim milk glucose extender (Table 144.2) can be obtained from Sigma-Aldrich Chemical Co., St Louis, MO, USA. Instant non-fat (skim) milk (e.g., Sanalac®) can be obtained in most grocery stores.

Table 144.2 Ingredients for skim milk glucose semen extender.

Ingredient	Amount
Instant non-fat dry milk	2.4 g
Glucose	4.9 g
Sodium bicarbonate stock solution (7.5 g/100 ml)	2 ml
Optional antibiotic: gentamycin sulfate stock solution 50 mg/ml	2 ml
Distilled water	92 ml

Preparation

- Mix all the ingredients in a sterile container and stir until completely mixed.
- Adjust the pH as needed to 7.0 by adding either an acid (i.e., HCl) or a base (i.e., NaOH).

Sperm Media

In some instances, it may be advantageous to dilute stallion spermatozoa in media that does not contain milk products or egg yolk. Examples of two such media are presented here.

Sperm TALP (Parrish *et al.* 1988)

Ingredients

All the ingredients can be obtained from Sigma-Aldrich Chemical Co., St Louis, MO, USA. The molecular weight (MW) is included so the correct chemical with the associated water molecules or type of chemical preparation can be purchased. Note that lactate is sold as a 60% syrup and you measure the amount with a pipette; alternatively you can weigh out the amount as 0.368 ml = 0.486 g and 3.68 ml = 4.86 g based on a specific gravity of 1.321. The buffer HEPES is purchased as a free acid powder; ensure the MW is correct. Pyruvate is sold as a sodium salt, but that is taken into account with the MW, so the amounts are correct. The bovine serum albumin is fraction V. Gentamicin is supplied as a powder preparation, but could be made from a purchased solution using appropriate conversions. Large amounts of preservative are not added to the sperm TALP (Tyrode's albumin–lactate–pyruvate medium) as this can kill sperm.

Preparation

- Place either 90 or 900 ml of water in a container (for 100 ml or 1 liter final volume) and add the components in the order listed in Table 144.3 with mixing. If you alter the order – specifically $CaCl_2 \cdot 2H_2O$, and $NaHCO_3$ – precipitates will form that will not dissolve.
- Adjust the pH to 7.4 with 1 N NaOH.
- Add sufficient water to adjust final volume to 100 ml or 1 liter.
- Solution can be used as is or it can be sterile filtered with a 0.22 μm filter into a sterile bottle.
- The solution of sperm TALP can be stored at 5°C (40°F; refrigerator temperature) for up to a week in the non-sterile form or for several months in the sterile version. Note that the pH of the solution will change over time if exposed to air due to the high level of $NaHCO_3$.
- The antibiotic can be changed or omitted if desired.

Table 144.3 Ingredients for sperm TALP.

Ingredient	Amount per 100 ml
$CaCl_2 \cdot 2H_2O$	0.029 g
KCl	0.023 g
$MgCl_2 \cdot 6H_2O$	0.008 g
$NaH_2PO_4 \cdot H_2O$	0.004g
NaCl	0.584 g
Lactate (sodium salt)	368 µl
Pyruvate	0.011 g
HEPES	0.238 g
$NaHCO_3$	0.210 g
Bovine serum albumin	0.600 g
Gentamycin	0.005 g

Table 144.4 Ingredients for SMED.

Ingredient	Amount per 100 ml
NaCI	0.216 g
KCl	0.075 g
KH_2PO_4	0.016 g
$NaHCO_3$	0.300 g
$MgSO_4$ anhyd.	0.029 g
HEPES	0.24 g
$CaCl_2 \cdot 2H_2O$	0.025 g
Fructose	1.52 g
Glucose	0.1 g
Sodium pyruvate	0.002 g
Sodium lactate	0.37 ml
Bovine serum albumin	0.3 g

Sperm Medium (SMED) (Wilhelm *et al.* 1996)

Ingredients

All the ingredients can be obtained from Sigma-Aldrich Chemical Co., St Louis, MO, USA.

Preparation

- Place 100 ml of sterile water in a container and add the components in the order listed in Table 144.4 with mixing.
- The pH should be approximately 7.0 and the osmolarity approximately 300 mOsm.
- Solution can be used as is or it can be sterile filtered with a 0.22 µm filter into a sterile bottle.
- The solution of SMED can be stored at 5°C (refrigerator temperature) for up to a week in the non-sterile form or for several months in the sterile version. Note that the pH of the solution will change over time if exposed to air due to the high level of $NaHCO_3$.
- The antibiotic can be changed or omitted if desired.

References

Parrish JJ, Susko-Parrish J, Winer MA, First NL. 1988. Capacitation of bovine sperm by heparin. *Biol Reprod* 38: 1171–80.

Wilhelm KM, Graham JK, Squires EL. 1996. Effects of phosphatidylserine and cholesterol liposomes on the viability, motility, and acrosomal integrity of stallion spermatozoa prior to and after cryopreservation. *Cryobiology* 33: 320–9.

Further Reading

Kenney RM, Bergman RV, Cooper WL, Morse GW. 1975. Minimal contamination techniques for breeding mares. Technique and preliminary findings. *Proc Annu Conv Am Assoc Eq Pract* 21: 327–36.

145

Preparation of Semen for Cooled Transport

Etta A. Bradecamp

Rood and Riddle Equine Hospital, USA

Introduction

Stallion semen may be cooled for transport to a distant location or to hold semen on the breeding farm until the next day. The use of cooled shipped semen for breeding is widespread in the equine industry and the proper preparation of the semen is imperative to maximize pregnancy rates. General guidelines have been established for processing equine semen for cooled transport. These guidelines include:

- A breeding dose of 1 billion progressively motile sperm (PMS).
- A ratio of extender to semen of at least 3:1 so as to dilute seminal plasma effects.
- The final volume (semen plus extender) should be less than 60 ml.
- The use of a semen extender containing an appropriate antibiotic.
- A final concentration of 25–50 million motile sperm per milliliter to maximize sperm viability.

It is recommended that a test cool be performed on semen from a stallion for which no cooled semen data are available. A test cool compares semen extenders and evaluates sperm motility/longevity following cooled storage of semen at a standardized sperm dilution (25–50 million spermatozoa/ml) in the same type of storage/shipping container to be used during the breeding season. The goal is to determine if semen from the stallion cools well and to identify the semen extender that best maintains motility after cooled storage. Semen extenders vary according to the type of protein source, type of sugar source, and antibiotic (see Chapters 144 and 147).

Stallions that are found to be "poor coolers" may benefit from the removal of a majority of the seminal plasma in the ejaculate by centrifugation. It is recommended that 5–20% of the seminal plasma should remain with the sperm pellet after centrifugation unless this is found to have a negative effect on motility.

Equipment and Supplies

Extender, 50 ml conical centrifuge tubes, calculator, densimeter, hemocytometer or NucleoCounter®, microscope, microscope slides, coverslips, pipettes, microcentrifuge tubes, warming plate.

Technique

- After collection, the gel portion of the ejaculate should be immediately removed from the sperm-rich fraction. This can be done by incorporating an in-line filter into the collection apparatus or by immediately passing the ejaculate through a filter after collection.
- Remove 0.5–1 ml of semen and place in a microcentrifuge tube for analysis of concentration, motility, and morphology.
- Place a single drop of raw semen on a warmed slide and cover with a coverslip to evaluate initial motility with a microscope.
- Measure the concentration using a densimeter (see Chapter 127), hemocytometer (see Chapter 128), or NucleoCounter® (see Chapter 129).
- A few drops of semen extender may be mixed with a drop of semen to assess progressive motility (see Chapter 130). A drop of this admixture is placed on a warm microscope slide with a coverslip and evaluated for progressive motility.
- A drop of raw semen can be mixed on a slide with a live-dead semen stain such as an eosin-nigrosin stain and smeared to create a slide for morphology analysis (see

Equine Reproductive Procedures, Second Edition. Edited by John Dascanio and Patrick McCue.

Chapters 132 and 133). Morphologic analysis is often not performed on routine semen shipments.
- If the concentration of the sample is less than 100 million/ml, the ejaculate should be extended and centrifuged (see Chapter 149). Centrifugation of raw semen with an initial concentration <100 million/ml is necessary as a minimum dilution of 3:1 would result in less than 25 million/ml spermatozoa in extended semen.

There are two main methods for determining how much extender to add to semen for cooled semen shipment. The first one calculates the dosage based on the total number of spermatozoa while the second method is based on the number of progressively motile spermatozoa. The following two examples are made using an ejaculate with 245 million sperm/ml and a progressive motility of 65%.

Total Spermatozoa Calculation

- This method assumes that the final product will be between 25 and 50 million spermatozoa/ml.
- The dilution ratio is calculated by dividing the current concentration by the desired concentration.
- Thus for a target of 33 million spermatozoa/ml (between 25 and 50 million/ml) the calculation is as follows.
- Dilution ratio factor = (Current concentration) ÷ (Desired concentration); i.e., dilution ratio factor = 245 ÷ 33 = 7.4.
- The dilution factor is rounded off to the nearest whole number = 7.4 = approximately 7.
- This results in a 1:6 dilution ratio: 1 part semen with 6 parts extender (subtract 1 from the dilution factor).
- The number of PMS per milliliter is: 245 × 0.65 (% prog motile) = 159.25 million PMS/ml.
- To provide 1 billion PMS: 1,000 (1 billion) ÷ 159.25 = 6.28 ml of semen is required.
- The final amounts to mix are calculated using the 1:6 dilution ratio from above: 6.28 ml of semen with 37.68 ml of extender.
- The resultant total volume is approximately 44 ml. The final volume should be kept to less than 60 ml.
- If the total volume is too high, divide the current concentration by a desired concentration closer to 50 million/ml final concentration, rather than 33 million/ml used in this example. If the volume is considered too low, then divide by a number closer to 25 million/ml.

Progressively Motile Spermatozoa Calculation

- The volume of raw semen needed to provide one breeding dose can be calculated using the following formula.
- Volume of raw semen needed = (Desired number of PMS) ÷ (Sperm concentration × Progressive motility).
- Volume of raw semen needed = 1,000 ÷ (245 × 0.65).
- Volume of raw semen needed = 6.28 ml.
- The volume of extender needed can be determined by the following formula.
- Volume of extender needed = (Final insemination volume) – (Volume of raw semen needed).
- Volume of extender needed = 40 – 6.28 = 33.72 ml.
- The resultant total volume is 40 ml.

Final Product

The two methods above use the same amount of semen, but the amount of extender differs slightly and probably has negligible effect. Both methods are appropriate and are used in clinical practice.

- The final product can be obtained by adding the extender to the raw semen or vice versa (Figure 145.1). This assumes that a commercial extender is used that is at the same temperature as the semen and is pH and osmotically balanced. If in doubt, add the extender slowly to the semen while mixing so as to not shock the spermatozoa. When pouring, run the liquid down the side of the container so as to not cause bubbling of the semen.

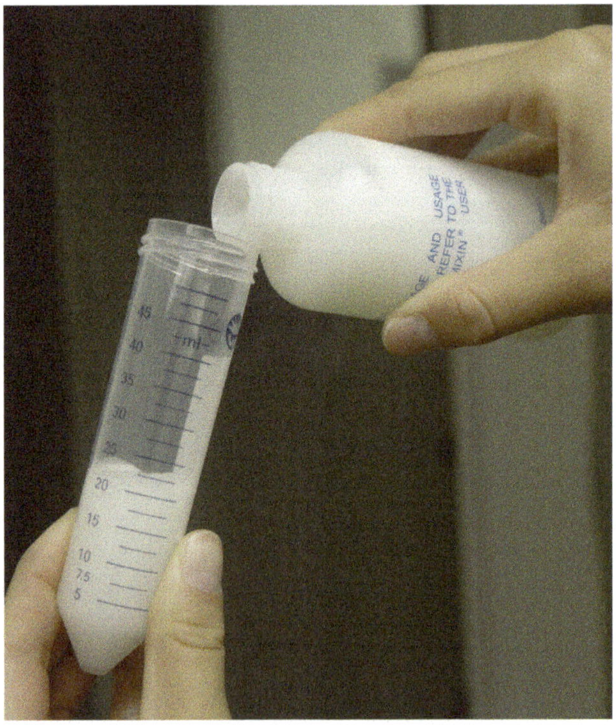

Figure 145.1 Addition of extender to semen.

- Cover the top of the graduated cylinder with a small amount of Parafilm® or place the top on the centrifuge tube and gently mix the contents. The insemination dose is now complete and can be packaged and placed into a passive cooling system.

Interpretation

- From the time of collection until the semen is packaged for shipment, it must be protected from light, sudden changes in temperature, and toxic substances.
- The ejaculate should not contain blood or urine as this will have a negative effect on motility/fertility.
- The semen extender should be warmed to approximately 37°C (99°F) prior to adding to raw semen.
- Motility should be evaluated before and after extending the semen to ensure that the addition of extender has not had an immediate detrimental effect on the semen.
- Equine spermatozoal web calculators are available to easily determine the amount of extender to add to semen.

Semen Extension Worksheet

This worksheet was created to aide in quick calculations for extension of semen (Box 145.1).

Box 145.1 Semen Extension Calculations

Rules

1) Ship 1 billion progressively motile sperm (PMS)
2) Minimum semen: extender ratio of 1:3 (1:4 is preferable)
3) Final extended concentration of 25–50 million sperm/ml
4) Final volume ⩽60 ml

Quick calculations

- Part A: satisfies rule no. 1
  - Concentration (million/ml) × % progressive motility = PMS/ml
  - 1,000/(PMS/ml) = volume semen (ml) needed to equal 1 billion PMS
- Part B: satisfies rules no. 2 and no. 3
  - If concentration is ⩾250 million/ml:
  - Concentration/50 million/ml = no. of parts (1 part semen to *x* parts extender)

  OR
  - If concentration is <250 million/ml:
  - Concentration/5 parts = final concentration (million/ml)

Note: if final concentration is less than 25 million/ml, centrifugation is required.

- Part C: preparation

  Using the results from above:
  - Volume of semen (ml) × (no. of parts – 1) = volume of extender
  - Volume of semen + volume of extender = dose of semen to be shipped

If the initial concentration is 245 million/ml and the progressive motility is 65% the calculations would look like this:

Quick calculations

- Part A: satisfies rule no. 1
  - Concentration (245 million/ml) × 65% progressive motility = 159.25 PMS/ml
  - 1,000/(159.25 PMS/ml) = 6.3 (ml) needed to equal 1 billion PMS
- Part B: satisfies rules no. 2 and no. 3
  - If concentration is ⩾250 million/ml:
  - Concentration/50 million/ml = no. of parts (1 part semen to *x* parts extender)

  OR
  - If concentration is <250 million/ml:
  - 245 million/ml/5 parts = final concentration of 49 million/ml

Note: if final concentration is less than 25 million/ml, centrifugation is required.

- Part C: preparation

  Using the results from above:
  - 6.3 ml × (5 – 1 = 4) = 25.2 ml (volume of extender)
  - 6.3 ml + 25.2 ml = 31.5 ml (dose of semen to be shipped)
  - If the dose is ~30 ml, semen may be shipped in all-plastic syringes or two doses can be shipped in a single 60 ml conical tube to eliminate any air in the tube.

Further Reading

Samper JC. 2011. Breeding with cooled transported semen. In: McKinnon AO, Squires EL, Vaala WE, Varner DD (eds). Equine Reproduction, 2nd edn. Ames, IA: Wiley Blackwell, pp. 1316–22.

Vanderwall DK. 2008. How to process dilute ejaculate of semen for cooled-transported insemination. *Proc Annu Conv Am Assoc Eq Pract* 54: 369–73.

146

Packing Semen for Cooled Transport

Etta A. Bradecamp

Rood and Riddle Equine Hospital, USA

Introduction

Proper packaging techniques should be followed to ensure that the highest quality product is received after the semen is cooled and shipped. After proper extension, semen may be packaged in plastic bags (Whirl-Pak®; eNasco, Fort Atkinson, WI, USA), heat-sealed plastic pouches (or baby bottle liners), all-plastic syringes (without rubber plungers), or plastic containers, such as conical centrifuge tubes. Semen should be packaged anaerobically when shipped at 5°C (40°F). Air should be eliminated from the shipping containers, thus if 60 ml conical centrifuge tubes are used, the dose should be adjusted to 60 ml by either shipping two doses in the same tube or a single larger dose in the tube.

There are several commercially available containers designed for the shipment of cooled semen. Reusable containers include the Equitainer® and Equitainer II® (Hamilton Research, South Hamilton, MA, USA) and the EST, EST XL, or EST H (Plastilite Corp., Omaha, NE, USA). Disposable containers designed for single use include the Bio-Flite (Animal Reproduction Systems, Chino, CA, USA), the Clipper (Hamilton Research), the Equine Express II (Exodus Breeders Supply, Ltd, York, PA, USA), and the ControliQ EquiSaver Omaha, EST, or EST XL (Plastilite Corp.). While the disposable containers are designed to cool the semen to approximately 5°C, research has shown that in extreme weather conditions some of the disposable containers may not maintain a stable temperature.

Documentation should be included in the shipping container, including the stallion's name and breed registration number, the date and time collected, initial semen motility, amount of progressively motile sperm (PMS) per dose, number of doses shipped, and the name of the mare to be inseminated and her breed registration number. Contact information for the person and facility that collected and processed the semen should also be included. A copy of this information should be kept in the stallion's records at the collection facility in case a shipment problem should occur. A second note is often included indicating if a disposable container should be returned to the original stallion station.

> **Equipment and Supplies**
>
> Extended semen, Whirl-Pak® bags, plastic tube roll, sterile baby bottle liners, syringes without rubber plungers or 50 ml conical centrifuge tubes, rubber bands, plastic syringe tips or a heat sealer, reusable or disposable shipping container with all of the required components, freezer cans or ice packs, semen evaluation form, zip ties, security tape.

Technique

- Prepare one or two doses of semen for cooled transport; each dose should initially contain 1 billion PMS and be diluted to a concentration of 25–50 million spermatozoa/ml (see Chapter 145). A minimum of 500 million PMS should be available for insemination upon delivery of the shipped semen when factoring in spermatozoal loss during cooled storage and shipment.
- Place the extended semen into Whirl-Pak® bags, sterile baby bottle liner, plastic syringes without rubber plunger, or 50 ml conical tubes. If a Whirl-Pak® or baby bottle liner is used, the bags should be double bagged so that if leakage occurs it will remain contained (Figure 146.1). Plastic bags can be closed with small rubber bands or sealed with a heat sealer (Figure 146.2). Rolled plastic tubing may also be used and heat sealed on both ends. The semen within a heat-sealed bag should not contact the heat sealer. In order to remove air from the bag prior to sealing, the bag may be draped over a sharp edge, such

Equine Reproductive Procedures, Second Edition. Edited by John Dascanio and Patrick McCue.

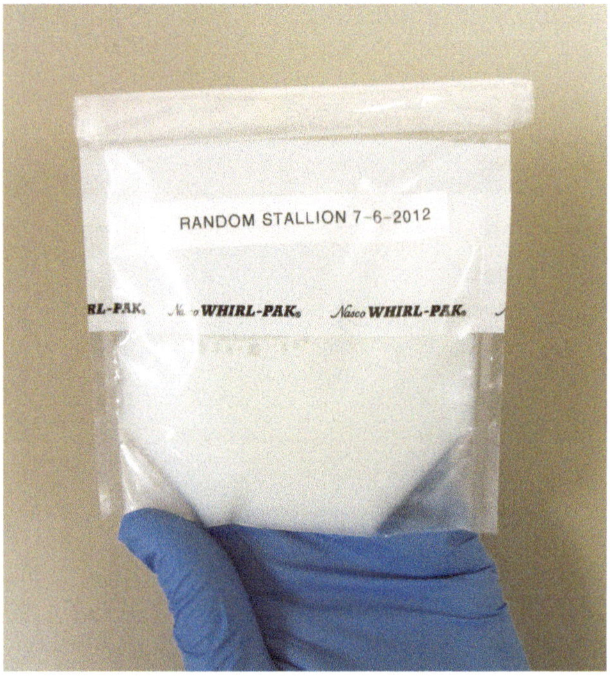

Figure 146.1 A Whirl-Pak® labeled with the stallion's name and date of collection. This pack should then be placed in a second Whirl-Pak® to prevent accidental leakage.

as a table edge, and lowered to remove air from the bag (Figure 146.3). It is important to keep the sides of the bag against each other to keep air from re-entering prior to sealing.

- Packages containing the extended semen should be labeled with the stallion's name and collection date.
- The package of extended semen is then placed into a shipping container.
- If an Equitainer® is used, coolant can(s) are first placed in the Equitainer® in the correct orientation (Figure 146.4). The coolant can(s) must have been previously stored in a freezer until completely frozen (for a minimum of 24 hours). These can(s) are stored with one end up in the freezer and placed in the Equitainer® with the other end orientated upward (Figure 146.5). The larger Equitainer I® requires two coolant cans and the smaller Equitainer II® requires one coolant can (Figure 146.6). The Equitainer I® with two cans can maintain cool temperatures for up to 70 hours, while the Equitainer II® with one can will maintain stable temperature for up to 48 hours.
- If the semen is packaged in plastic bags, the bags are placed in the plastic cup provided with the shipping container. A pre-warmed (37°C, 99°F) ballast bag may also be added to the cup if the packaged semen does not fill a majority of the cup (Figure 146.7). Each ballast bag contains 60 ml of diluent and the total volume of semen and

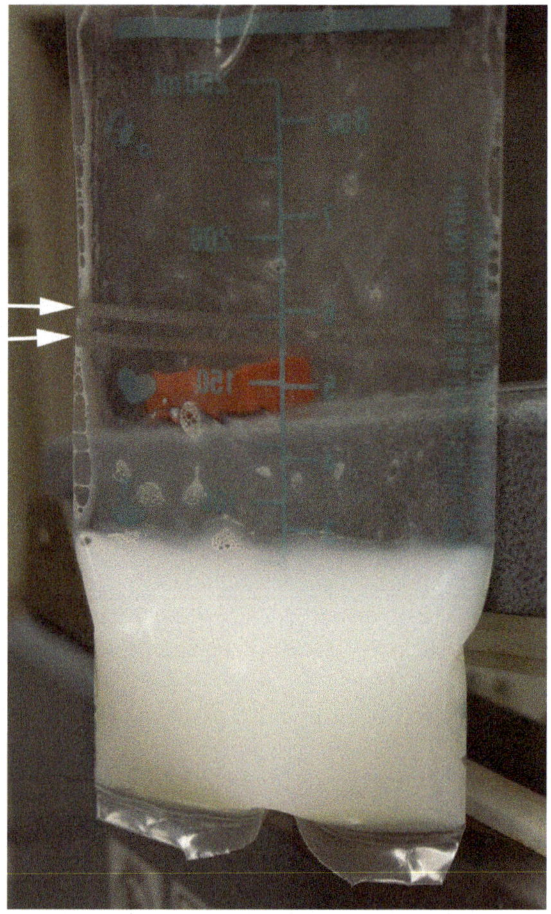

Figure 146.2 Heat-sealed bag. Notice that the bag was sealed twice (arrows) away from the semen and that minimal air is included.

ballast contained within the cup should be between 120 and 170 ml. If excess air space remains in the cup after placement of the semen, the air acts as an insulator and therefore prevents uniform cooling of the semen. Thus a ballast bag may be used to eliminate the dead space and minimize the amount of air in the cup. A lid is then placed on the plastic cup and the cup is placed inside a larger insulated cup (isothermalizer).

- The isothermalizer is then placed on top of the coolant cans and covered with a lid (Figure 146.8).
- If an isothermalizer that accommodates 50 ml centrifuge tubes is used, the volume of semen within the centrifuge tubes should be maximized so that there is minimal air space in the tube (Figure 146.9). This requires calculations for dilution ratio to factor in a total volume of 57.5 ml.
- The semen evaluation form should be placed inside a sealable plastic bag and placed inside the container before the Equitainer® is closed and sealed (Figure 146.10). The plastic bag will keep the paperwork from becoming wet from possible condensation.

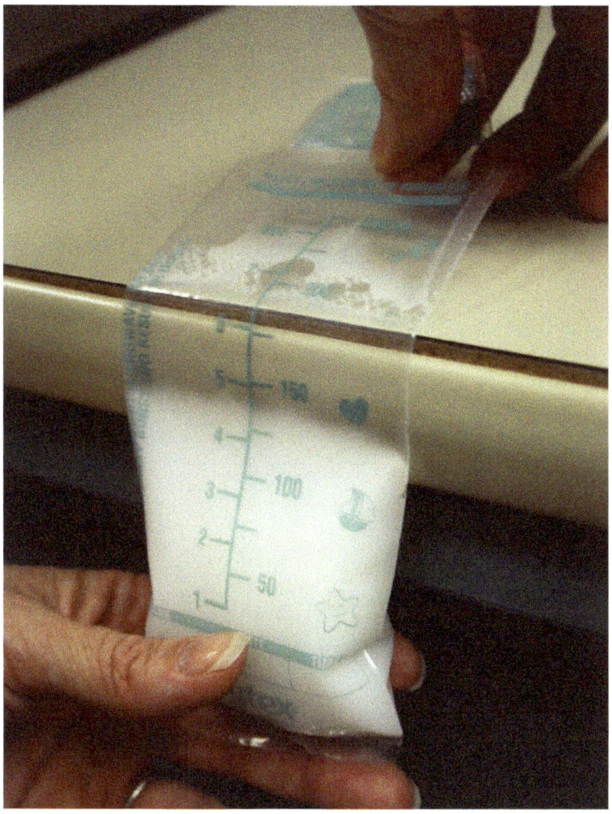

Figure 146.3 Technique for removal of air from bag. The bag is draped over a sharp edge and lowered to remove any air.

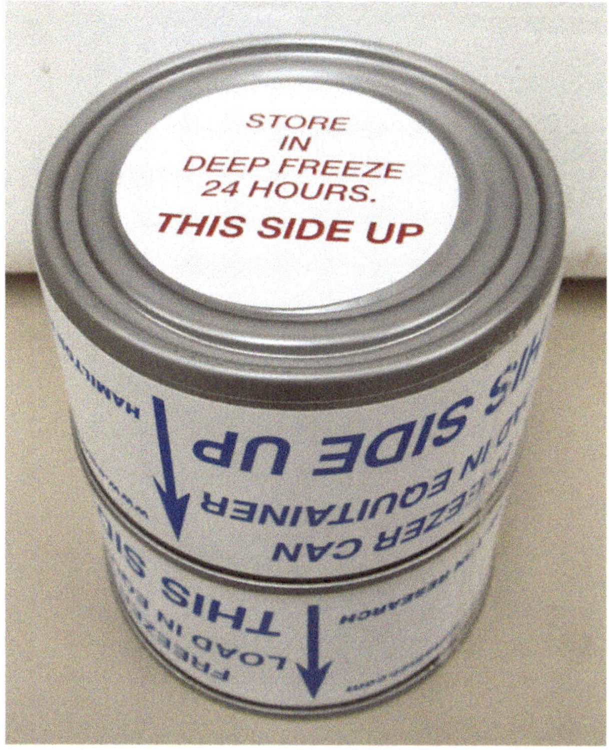

Figure 146.5 Equitainer® freezer cans should be stored in the freezer as directed and placed in the Equitainer® in the opposite orientation.

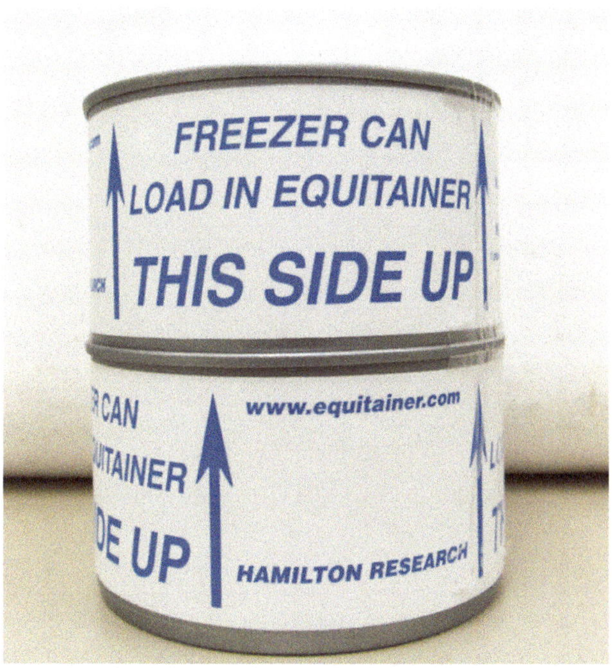

Figure 146.4 Two Equitainer® freezer cans ready to be loaded into an Equitainer®.

- To insure that the Equitainer® is not opened during shipment and the semen compromised, the latch should be secured with a zip tie and the lid taped shut (Figure 146.11). A signature may be written across the sealing tape over the closing latch work to provide proof of security.
- If semen is shipped in syringes, only syringes devoid of barrel lubricant or devoid of rubber plungers should be used (all-plastic syringes) so as to avoid negative effects on spermatozoal viability. Syringes should have a sealing cap placed on the needle port of the syringe to avoid leakage (Figure 146.12).
- If a disposable Styrofoam™ shipper is utilized, the semen is placed in the bottom of the container and covered with a plank of Styrofoam™ to separate the semen from the ice pack. A frozen ice pack, designed to fit the box, is then placed in the box and covered with the lid (Figures 146.13–146.15). The semen evaluation form and any other paperwork can be placed on top of the lid before the cardboard box lid is closed and secured with a zip tie and/or tape.

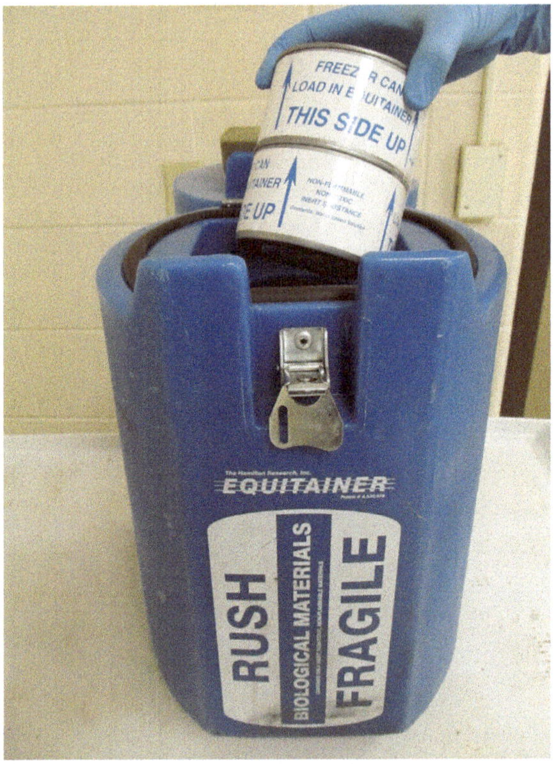

Figure 146.6 Loading the freezer cans into the Equitainer®.

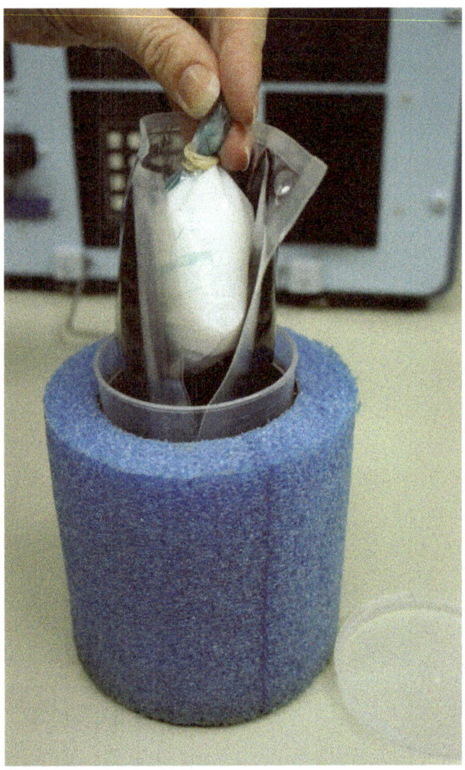

Figure 146.7 This insulated isothermalizer cup is designed to hold semen packed in small plastic bags. The purple ballast bag is used if the package of semen does not fill the cup.

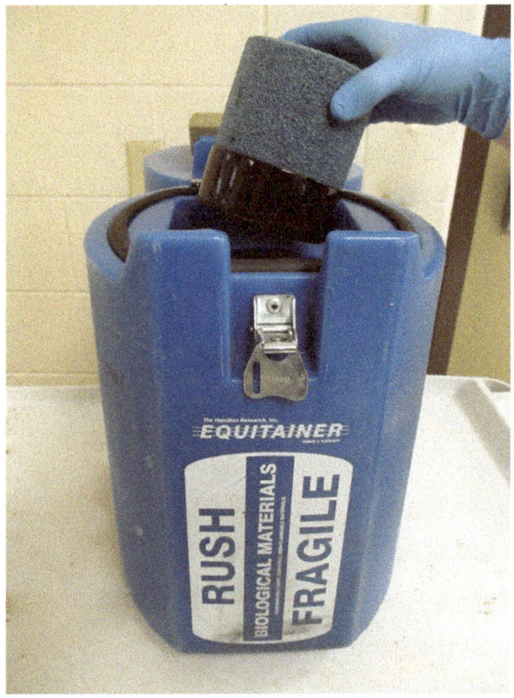

Figure 146.8 Insulated isothermalizer cup being loaded on top of coolant cans.

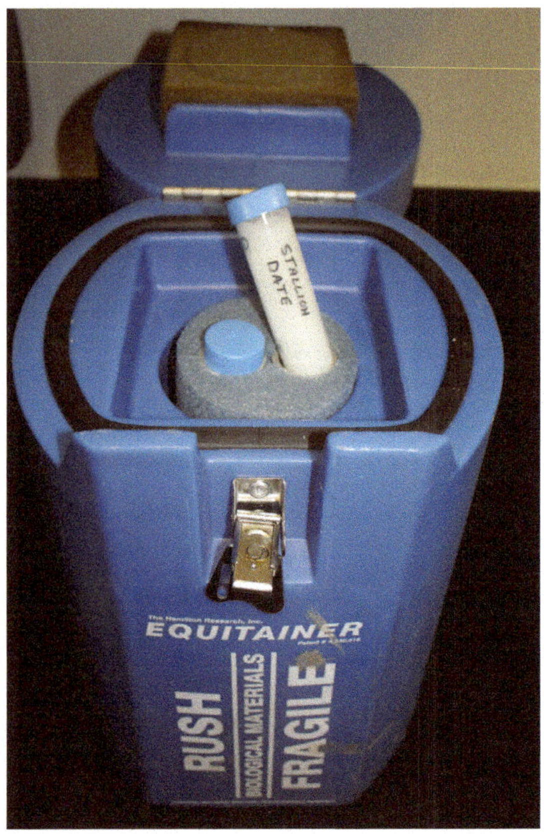

Figure 146.9 This isothermalizer cup is designed to hold two 50 ml conical tubes.

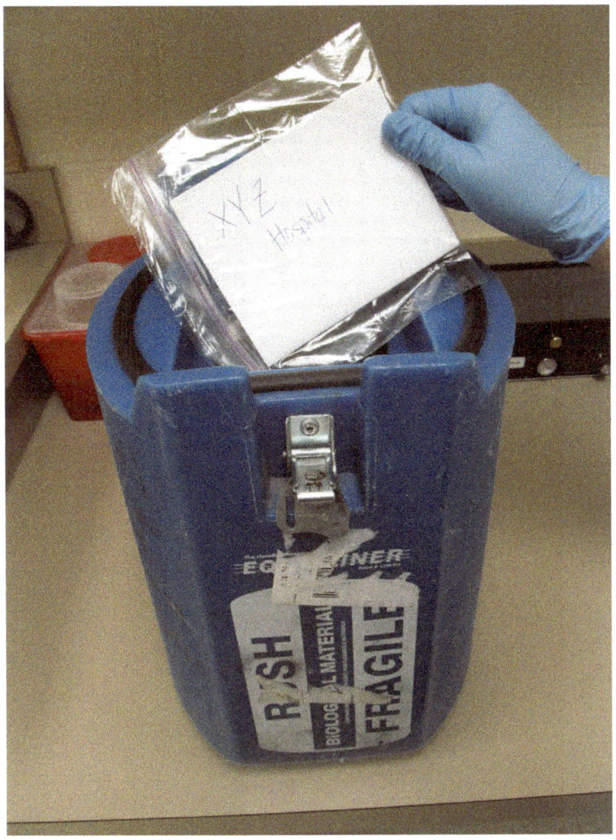

Figure 146.10 Include documentation that identifies the semen donor and the results of a semen evaluation.

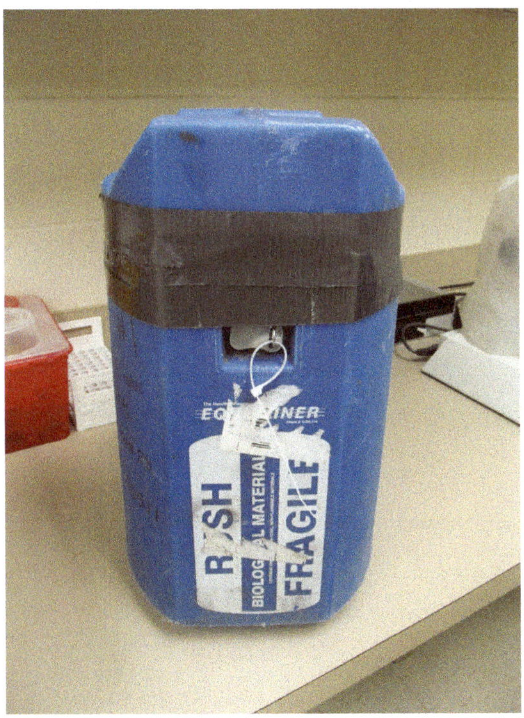

Figure 146.11 An Equitainer® sealed and ready for shipment.

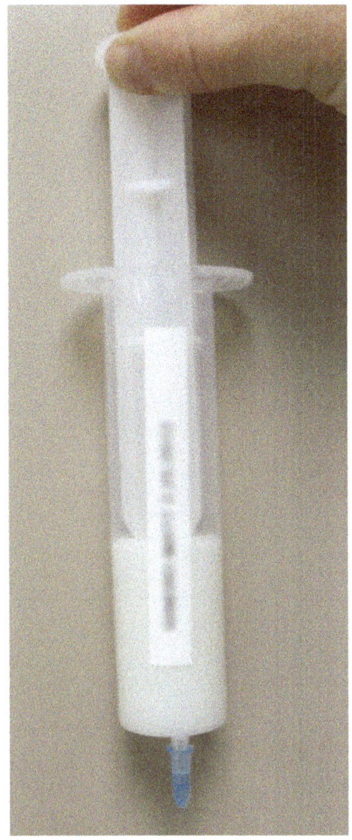

Figure 146.12 One dose of semen loaded into a labeled, air-tight syringe.

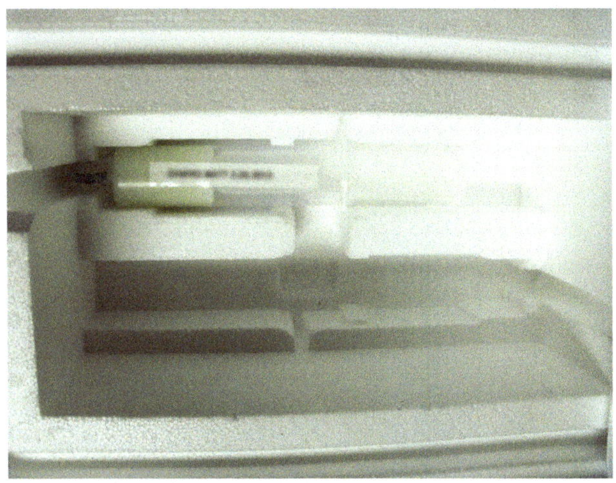

Figure 146.13 One dose of semen packaged into an air-tight syringe and loaded into a Styrofoam™ disposable shipper. If a second dose is not being shipped, a syringe filled with warm water and so labeled should be included to ensure the proper rate of cooling is maintained.

Interpretation

- Only containers specifically designed for cooled transport of equine semen should be used.

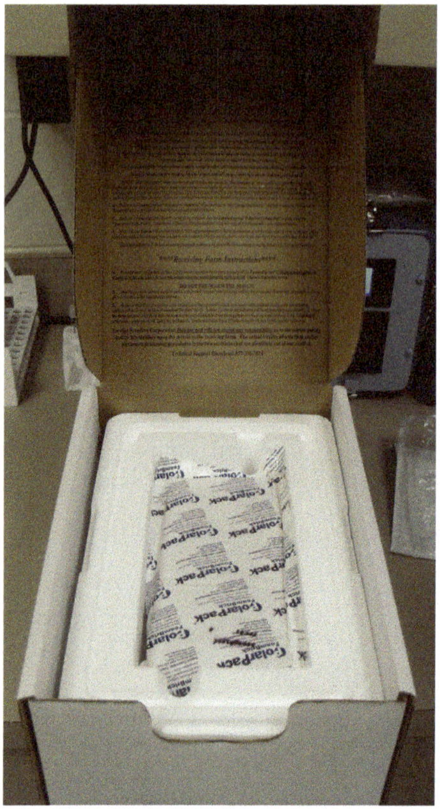

Figure 146.14 Disposable shipper loaded with the ice pack in place.

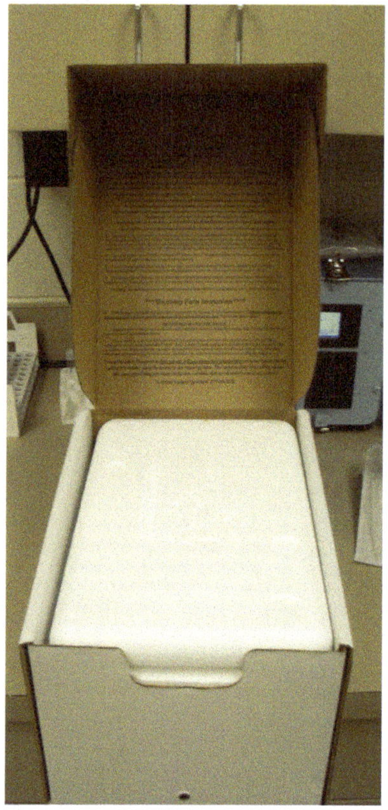

Figure 146.15 Disposable shipper with the lid in place.

- Extended semen should be packaged without any excess air left in the bag, syringe, conical tube, or plastic vial.
- Containers should be packaged as they were designed to be used to ensure that proper cooling of the semen occurs.
- Labels with the stallion's name and date should be placed on the packages of semen to eliminate any confusion at the receiver's end as to the identification of the semen.
- If the frozen cans/bricks/gel packs are not completely frozen at the time of packaging, the semen may prematurely warm, decreasing viability.
- A semen evaluation form should accompany the shipment so that the person receiving the shipment can compare the cooled sample with the parameters of the initial ejaculate.
- If unknown temperature extremes may be encountered during shipment, a semen shipment container rated for those conditions should be used.
- Variations may occur in packaging with different types of semen transport systems. Manufacturer's recommendations should be followed for packaging.
- Reused containers should be examined regularly for any disruption in the sealing mechanism that could result in premature warming of cooled shipped semen.

Further Reading

Blanchard TL, Varner DD, Schumacher J, Love CC, Brinsko SP, Rigby SL. 2003. Semen preservation. In: Blanchard TL, Varner DD, Schumacher J, Love CC, Brinsko SP, Rigby SL (eds). Manual of Equine Reproduction, 2nd edn. St Louis, MI: Mosby, pp. 165–72.

Samper JC. 2011. Breeding with cooled transported semen. In: McKinnon AO, Squires EL, Vaala WE, Varner DD (eds). Equine Reproduction, 2nd edn. Ames, IA: Wiley Blackwell, pp. 1316–22.

147

Longevity Testing of Sperm

John J. Dascanio

School of Veterinary Medicine, Texas Tech University, USA

Introduction

Prior to the beginning of each breeding season, the longevity of spermatozoa should be determined for breeding stallions. Storage may be at room temperature or at cooled semen shipment temperature and may be with or without a semen extender. For practical considerations, the longevity testing should be done under the same conditions as those under which the semen would be normally used. Thus for natural cover situations semen should be tested at room temperature without an extender, and for cooled semen transport the semen should be tested with an extender at 5°C (40°F) in a typical shipping container.

Equipment and Supplies

Microscope, microscope slides, coverslips, warming plate or heated microscope stage, pipettes, semen extender, equine semen shipping container, centrifuge tubes, aluminum foil.

Technique

- Semen should be collected in an artificial vagina and filtered to remove gel and debris.
- The semen should be assessed for volume, concentration, total motility, and progressive motility (see Chapters 127 and 130).

Raw Semen Longevity

- Place semen in a 15 ml centrifuge tube in a rack at room temperature (20°C, 68°F). The tube should be covered with aluminum foil to prevent the admittance of light.

Interpretation

- Good sperm longevity: >10% progressive motility at 6 hours post-collection when held at room temperature.
- Poor sperm longevity: <10% progressive motility at 3 hours post-collection when held at room temperature.

Cooled Extended Semen Longevity

- The semen should be diluted to between 25 and 50 million spermatozoa/ml with a commercial semen extender. If the stallion's semen has been shipped in previous breeding seasons with success, the same extender should be used for the longevity test. If this is the first longevity test for the stallion or if he had decreased longevity in the previous season, a series of longevity tests should be conducted with different extenders and antibiotic combinations.
- For an initial longevity test, different extenders, based on composition, should be tested:
  - A typical Kenney's extender with non-fat skim milk, glucose, and an antibiotic.
  - An extender with non-fat skim milk, glucose and sucrose, and an antibiotic.
  - An extender with native phosphocaseinates, glucose (or range of sugars), and antibiotics.
  - Proprietary commercial extenders known to maintain longevity.
- Different antibiotics may be added to semen extenders to prevent bacterial growth, which may have different effects on motility and longevity. Typically, a combination of amikacin and penicillin will maintain motility the best, but there are cases where other antibiotics, such as polymixin B, will work better. Potentially, a longevity test may be performed without an antibiotic, but this will result in significant bacterial overgrowth.

Equine Reproductive Procedures, Second Edition. Edited by John Dascanio and Patrick McCue.

- The diluted semen should be placed in a commercial equine shipping container with proper coolant and examined at 24, 48, and 72 hours post-collection (see Chapter 146). The container is held at room temperature.
- For evaluation, the semen sample from the shipping container should be gently mixed and a drop placed on a cool microscope slide to which a coverslip is added. Thus, cooled semen is placed on a cooled or room temperature slide to avoid temperature shock.
- The microscope slide should then be warmed to 37°C (98.6°F) for 2–3 minutes prior to evaluation for progressive motility.
- Alternatively, a small aliquot of cooled semen can be placed into a room temperature glass tube and stored in an incubator at 37°C (98.6°F) for 10 minutes prior to evaluation. In this case, warm semen would be placed on a warm slide for evaluation.

Interpretation

- Cooled extended semen with poor longevity has <10% progressive motility at 24 hours.
- Cooled extended semen with excellent longevity has >30% progressive motility after 72 hours.
- If longevity is less than desired, removal of most of the seminal plasma may increase sperm longevity. This is accomplished by centrifugation and re-suspension of the semen pellet in extender (see Chapter 149).

Additional Comments

- The lubricant used with an artificial vagina should be isosmotic and have a neutral pH without any preservatives. A specifically designed lubricant for use with spermatozoa should be used that has been tested against other lubricants for maintenance of longevity. It has been demonstrated that not all non-spermicidal lubricants will maintain semen longevity equally.
- Semen storage containers that are not disposable generally provide more stable environments and may enhance longevity for some stallions.

Further Reading

Pagl R, Aurich JE, Muller-Schlosser F, Kankofer M, Aurich C. 2006. Comparison of an extender containing defined milk protein fractions with a skim milk-based extender for storage of equine semen at 5°C. *Theriogenology* 66: 1115–22.

Samper JC, Garcia A, Burnett K. 2007. The effect of different lubricants on longevity of motility and velocity of stallion spermatozoa. *Theriogenology* 68: 496.

Varner DD, Scanlan CM, Thompson JA, Brumbaugh GW, Blanchard TL, Carlton CM, Johnson L. 1998. Bacteriology of preserved stallion semen and antibiotics in semen extenders. *Theriogenology* 50: 559–73.

148

Calculation of *g* Force for Centrifuging Semen

John J. Dascanio

School of Veterinary Medicine, Texas Tech University, USA

Introduction

A centrifuge that can be accurately programmed at a specific g force should be used to centrifuge equine semen. Some centrifuges may only vary the revolutions per minute (rpm) or do not provide any information on the actual rotational speed. Newer centrifuges may provide a button to change from rpm to relative centrifugal force (i.e., gravitational force: g force or × g). The formula to convert from rpm to g force is provided in this chapter; however, there are many on-line web calculators that will help perform this calculation. The centrifuge should be able to accommodate 15 or 50 ml conical centrifuge tubes.

Equipment and Supplies

Centrifuge, ruler in centimeters, calculator, optional nomograph.

Technique

Centrifuge with no Rotation Speed Gauge

- If there is no dial to provide rotational speed, then a test should be performed to estimate the speed needed to centrifuge semen.
- Semen should be placed in a conical centrifuge tube and spun at the best estimated speed, noting the position of the lever used to alter speed on the centrifuge.
- The semen pellet should not be extremely firm (too fast a rotor speed) or too soft (too slow a rotor speed).
- The semen pellet should be capable of being re-suspended into solution by admixing semen extender, yet only 20% or less of spermatozoa will remain in the supernatant. A test of the supernatant sperm concentration with a hemocytometer will confirm percent loss.
- Once the relative speed is determined, the lever used to alter speed should be marked as to its position so that it may be set for future centrifugation procedures.

Centrifuge with Revolutions per Minute Gauge but no *g* Force Designation

- The rotor arm radius should be measured in centimeters. The radius of the centrifuge is the distance from the center of the centrifuge rotor to the end of the centrifuge bucket (when extended horizontally) (Figure 148.1).
- The formula for the calculation of g force is: (0.00001118) × (Radius in centimeters) (rpm^2).

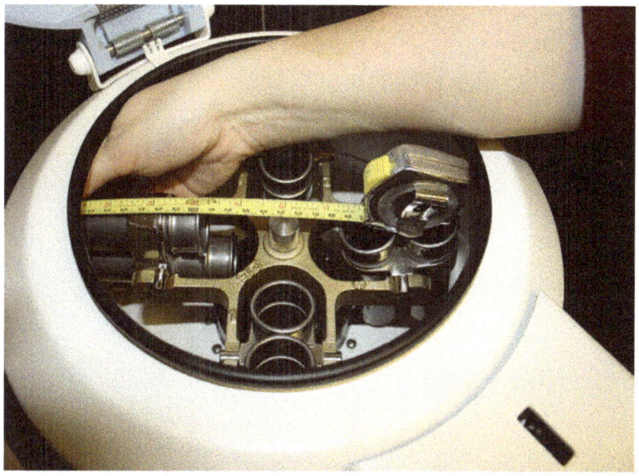

Figure 148.1 Measuring the rotating radius of a centrifuge from the center of the centrifuge to the end of the bucket when held horizontally.

Equine Reproductive Procedures, Second Edition. Edited by John Dascanio and Patrick McCue.

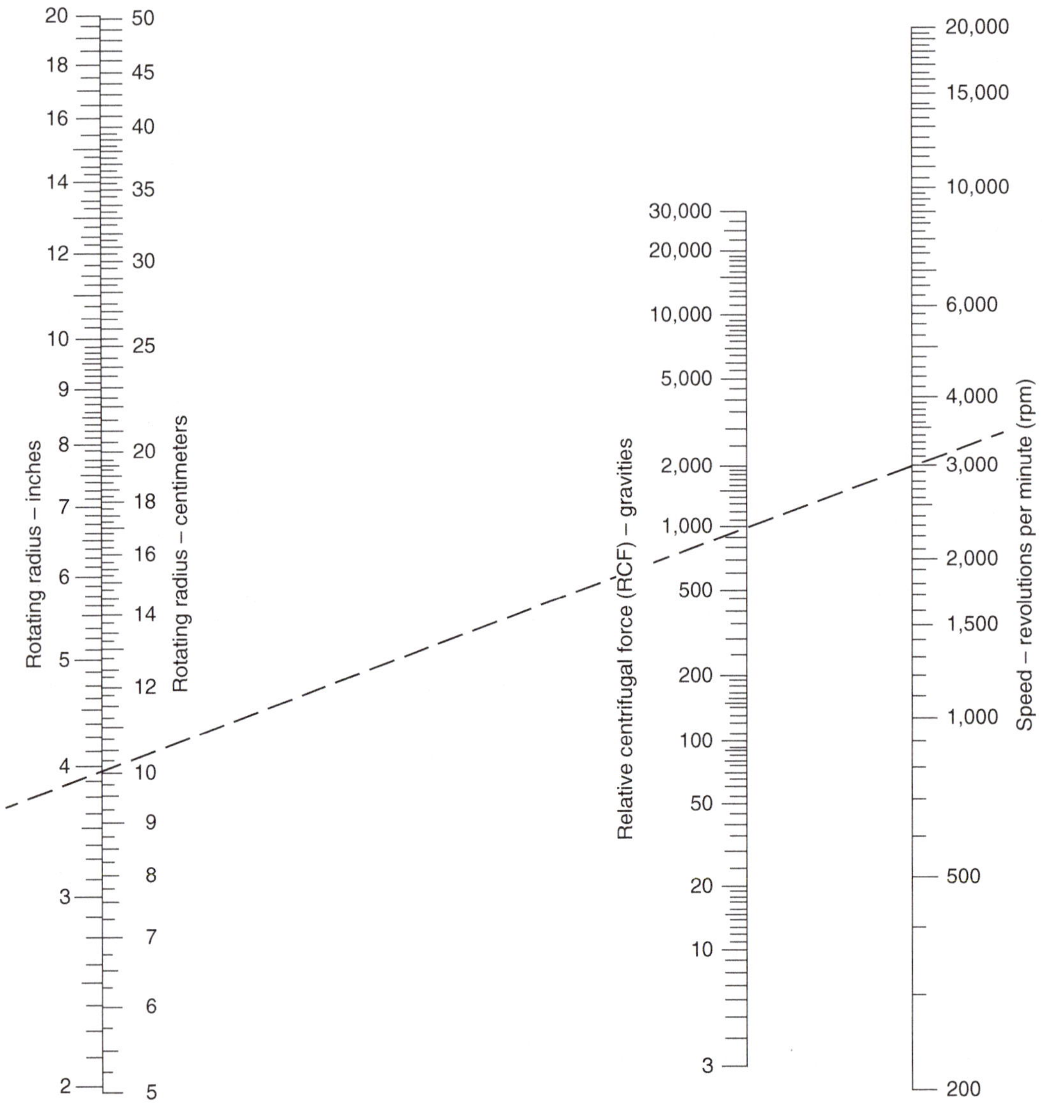

Figure 148.2 Nomograph for calculating the *g* force from known revolutions per minute and centrifuge rotating radius. In this example a 10 cm rotating radius and desired 1,000× *g* force would require 3,000 rpm setting on the centrifuge. From Vanderwall (2008).

- Usually, however, the g force to spin the semen is already known (typically 400–600× g) and the equation must be solved to provide the desired rpm to set the centrifuge. Thus, the formula to set the centrifuge for rpm speed for a desired g force would be:

$$= \sqrt{\frac{(\text{Desired } g \text{ force})}{0.00001118 * (\text{Radius in centimetres})}}$$

Thus for a desired g force of 500× g, with a radius of 10 cm, the centrifuge should be set to about 2,100 rpm (2,114.8 rpm).

- A nomograph may also be used that uses the rotating radius of the centrifuge and revolutions per minute to calculate g force. A ruler is place over the nomograph to line up the radius length with revolutions per minute, thus also lining up the resulting g force (Figure 148.2).

Reference

Vanderwall DK. 2008. How to process a dilute ejaculate of semen for cooled-transported insemination. *Proc Annu Conv Am Assoc Eq Pract* 54: 369–73.

149

Centrifugation of Semen: Standard Technique

Etta A. Bradecamp

Rood and Riddle Equine Hospital, USA

Introduction

Centrifugation is a processing technique that can be utilized if an ejaculate has a low initial concentration (less than 100 million sperm/ml) or if the stallion's seminal plasma has a detrimental effect on spermatozoal viability. Centrifugation is also utilized when processing semen for freezing or to remove seminal plasma that has been contaminated with urine during semen collection. Centrifugation will concentrate spermatozoa into a pellet. Subsequently, a majority or all of the seminal plasma can be removed and the sperm pellet re-suspended in an appropriate extender to the desired concentration.

Equipment and Supplies

Semen, 50 ml conical tubes, centrifuge equipped to hold 50 ml conical tubes with swinging buckets, semen extender, disposable pipettes, densimeter or hemocytometer or NucleoCounter®, microscope, microscope slides, coverslips, balance scale.

Technique

- Determine the volume, concentration, and motility of the sample prior to centrifugation (see Chapters 127 and 130).
- Dilute the ejaculate 1:1 with a commercial semen extender and divide the volume equally amongst the 50 ml conical centrifuge tubes. The semen extender helps to maintain spermatozoal viability during centrifugation.
- Determine the motility again after addition of the extender, but prior to centrifugation as a quality control step.
- Using a scale, each pair of tubes (along with the centrifuge buckets) must be weighed and balanced to ensure that the centrifuge is balanced once loaded (Figure 149.1). If there are an odd number of tubes containing extended semen, a conical tube filled with water can be used as a counter balance.
- The conical tubes are then loaded into the centrifuge opposite one another (Figure 149.2).
- The tubes are centrifuged at a specific combination of *g* force and time. Typical options include:
  - 400× *g* for 13–15 minutes.
  - 600× *g* for 10–12 minutes.
  - 900× *g* for 9 minutes.
- A sperm pellet should be readily visible in the bottom of the conical tube (Figure 149.3). It is estimated that approximately 20–25% of the original spermatozoa will

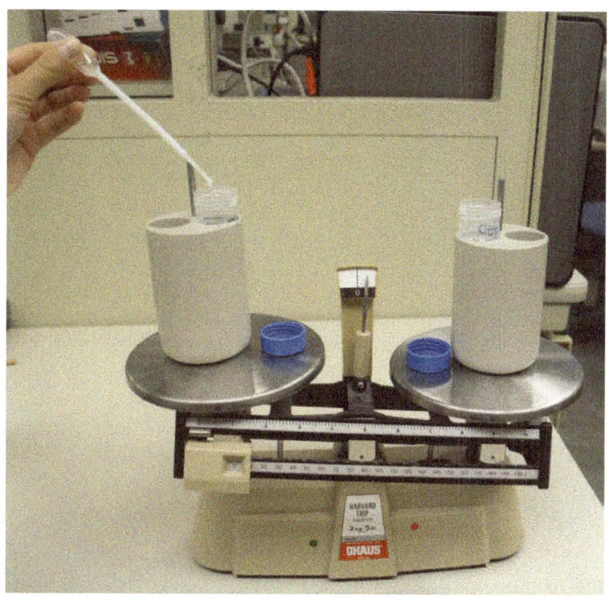

Figure 149.1 Balancing centrifuge tubes on a scale.

Equine Reproductive Procedures, Second Edition. Edited by John Dascanio and Patrick McCue.

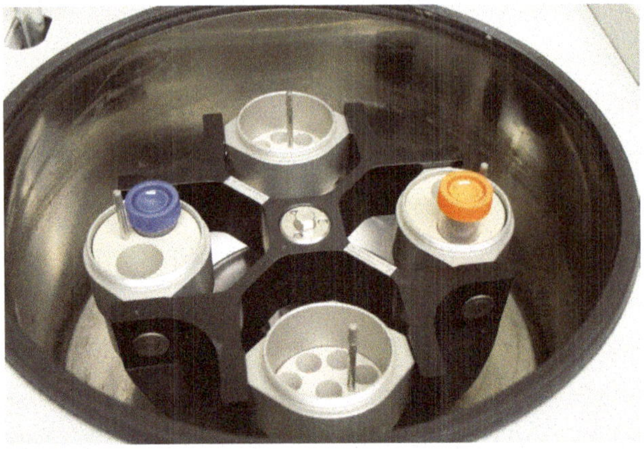

Figure 149.2 Location of centrifuge tubes opposite each other to balance the centrifuge.

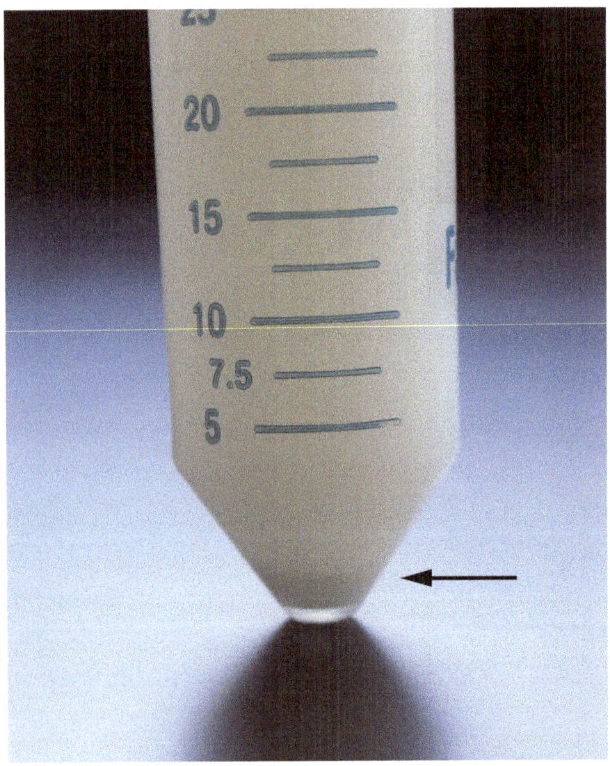

Figure 149.3 Sperm pellet after centrifugation of 1.0 billion spermatozoa diluted in a skim milk glucose extender. The arrow shows the demarcation between supernatant and pellet.

remain in the supernatant and will not be in the sperm pellet following traditional centrifugation. Use cushion media centrifugation to increase the spermatozoal recovery rate (see Chapter 150).

- The supernatant is removed using a pipette (Figure 149.4) or sink aspiration unit (Figure 149.5). It is advantageous to leave approximately 5–10% of the seminal plasma with the pellet to help modulate the uterine inflammatory

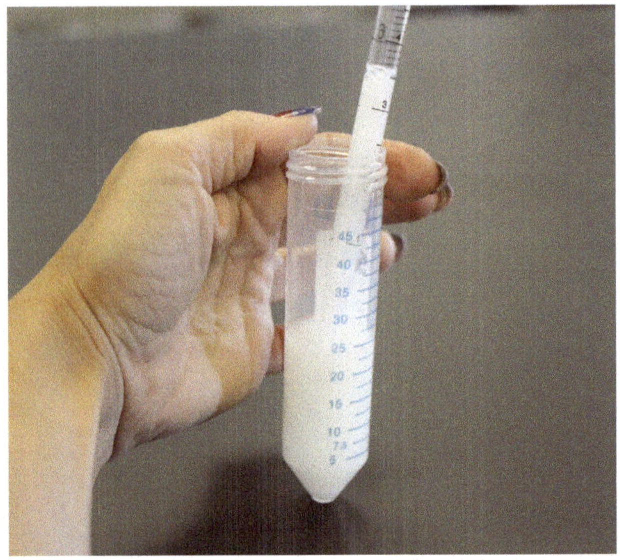

Figure 149.4 Aspiration of the supernatant after centrifugation using a pipette.

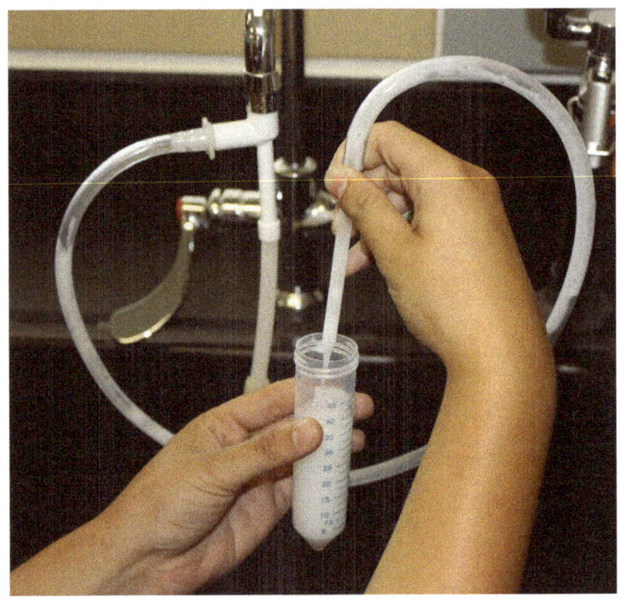

Figure 149.5 Use of a sink aspiration unit to remove the supernatant after centrifugation.

response to spermatozoa. However, in some instances, where seminal plasma is deemed to be toxic or for processing of frozen semen, it may be best to remove as much seminal plasma as possible.

Option 1: Removal of Most of the Supernatant

- The supernatant can be removed from each conical tube using a clean, disposable pipette or a sink aspiration unit, leaving a volume of approximately 5 ml in the bottom of the tube including the sperm pellet.

- Gently re-suspend the sperm pellet in the remaining supernatant. Aspirate some remaining liquid in a disposable pipette and gently "puff" that liquid against the pellet to re-suspend the pellet. Use the pipette to gently aspirate and expel the mixture to complete the re-suspension. Make sure to not bubble air through the liquid.
- Combine the contents of all the conical tubes, if more than one tube was used.
- Measure the volume of the combined re-suspended semen.
- Determine the sperm concentration by either a manual count with a hemocytometer (see Chapter 128) or with a NucleoCounter® (see Chapter 129).
- Calculate the volume of re-suspended semen needed to provide a minimum breeding dose of 500 million progressively motile sperm (PMS) for fresh insemination or 1 billion PMS for cooled storage and transport (Box 149.1).
- Combine the calculated volume of re-suspended semen needed with the optimal volume of additional semen extender to yield the final breeding dose (20 ml volume for a fresh insemination or 40 ml volume for a cooled insemination dose).
- A final motility estimate should be made after any additional semen extender is added as a final quality control.

Option 2: Removal of the Entire Supernatant (Seminal Plasma Plus Extender)

- If the seminal plasma has been found to be detrimental to spermatozoal survival, it is recommended that all of the supernatant be removed before re-suspending the pellet with semen extender.
- Remove the supernatant to the level of the sperm pellet using a clean, disposable pipette or a sink aspiration unit.
- Re-suspend the sperm pellet in each conical tube to a volume of 5 ml with warmed semen extender.
- Combine the contents of all conical tubes if more than one was used.
- Measure the final volume, sperm concentration, and sperm motility as noted for Option 1.
- Calculate and prepare breeding doses as noted for Option 1.

Alternative Technique

- If the concentration and progressive motility of spermatozoa in the original ejaculate are known, an estimate of 75% recovery can be used to predetermine the number of spermatozoa to be centrifuged in order to achieve the required breeding dose(s).
- The actual amount recovered may be more or less than 75% depending on the original sperm concentration, centrifugation speed, time, and possibly on other factors as well.
- The following number of PMS need to be centrifuged to achieve a final fresh or cooled breeding dose assuming a 75% recovery rate:
- Begin with 667 million PMS to yield 500 million PMS after centrifugation (fresh dose).
- Begin with 1.33 billion PMS to yield 1 billion PMS after centrifugation (cooled dose).
- If the entire ejaculate is centrifuged, the following formulas may be used to calculate a breeding dose. The volume of re-suspended semen required can be mixed with additional semen extender to prepare the final breeding dose(s).

Original volume × Concentration × Progressive motility
= Total PMS in the initial ejaculate

Total PMS in the initial ejaculate × 0.75
= Estimated total PMS recovered after centrifugation without a cushion

Estimated total PMS recovered after centrifugation ÷ Volume (ml) remaining after centrifugation and aspiration of supernatant
= Concentration of PMS per ml after centrifugation and resuspension

Desired PMS per breeding dose ÷ Concentration of PMS per ml after centrifugation and resuspension
= Volume of centrifuged semen needed

Final volume of insemination – Volume of centrifuged semen needed
= Amount of additional extender to provide final insemination dose

Interpretation

- Centrifugation is a necessary process for preparing cooled-shipped semen when a dilute ejaculate is obtained or when urine is present in the ejaculate (Figure 149.6).
- In cases where the longevity of the semen is poor, centrifugation to remove the seminal plasma can improve the quality/longevity of the semen for cooled storage.
- If the seminal plasma has been determined to be detrimental to spermatozoal survivability, it may be necessary

Box 149.1 Worksheet: Centrifugation Without a Cushion

Example

Original semen parameters *Volume = 85 ml*
Concentration = 78 million sperm per ml
Progressive motility = 65%

85 *ml ×* ***78*** *million sperm/ml ×* ***0.65*** *(% progressive motility) =* ***4,309.5*** *million progressively motile spermatozoa (PMS)*

4,309.5 *× 0.75 =* ***3,232.1*** *million PMS (estimated 75% recovery after centrifugation in 5 ml)*

3,232.1 *million PMS ÷ 20 =* ***161.6*** *million PMS/ml after centrifugation and re-suspension (4 tubes of 5 ml each = 20 ml)*

To prepare a fresh insemination dose of 500 million PMS in a final volume of 20 ml:

500 ÷ ***161.6 = 3.1*** *ml of re-suspended semen*

20 ml – ***3.1 = 16.9*** *ml extender to provide a 20 ml volume containing 500 million PMS at a concentration of 25 million PMS/ml*

To prepare a cooled insemination dose of 1.0 billion PMS in a final volume of 40 ml:

1,000 ÷ ***161.6 = 6.2*** *ml of re-suspended semen*

40 ml – ***6.2 = 33.8*** *ml extender to provide a 40 ml volume containing 1,000 million (1.0 billion) PMS, a concentration of 25 million PMS/ml*

Stallion: ________ **Collection date: ________**

Original semen parameters Volume = ____ ml
Concentration = ____ million sperm/ml
Progressive motility = ____ %

____ ml × ____ million sperm/ml × ____ (% progressive motility) = ____ million PMS

____ × 0.75 = ____ million PMS (estimated 75% recovery after centrifugation)

____ million PMS ÷ 20 = ____ million PMS/ml after centrifugation and re-suspension (4 tubes of 5 ml each)

To prepare a fresh insemination dose of 500 million PMS:

500 ÷ ____ = ____ ml of resuspended semen

20 ml – ____ = ____ ml extender to provide a 20 ml volume containing 500 million PMS at a concentration of 25 million PMS/ml

To prepare a cooled insemination dose of 1.0 billion PMS:

1,000 ÷ ____ = ____ ml of resuspended semen

40 ml – ____ = ____ ml extender to provide a 40 ml volume containing 1,000 million (1.0 billion) PMS, a concentration of 25 million PMS/ml

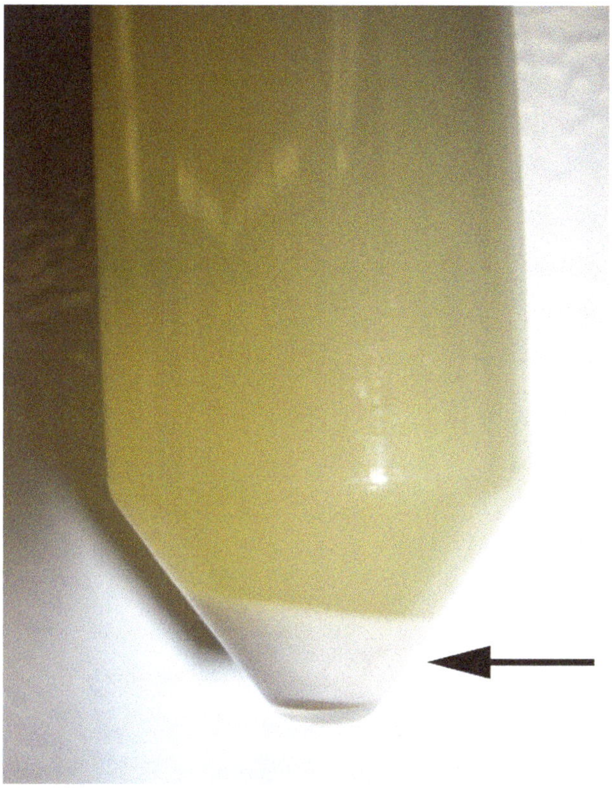

Figure 149.6 Pellet (arrow) from a stallion with urospermia after centrifugation. Note yellow supernatant.

to remove all of the supernatant before re-extending the pellet with seminal plasma from a fertile stallion or with semen extender.

- The supernatant should be removed as soon as the centrifuge stops. Spermatozoa will start to swim up out of the formed pellet once centrifugation stops, and are thereby lost when the supernatant is removed.
- If a higher g force is applied during centrifugation, the percentage of spermatozoa recovered will be increased. However, irreversible damage may be done to the spermatozoa and the pellet may be packed too tightly to be easily re-suspended.
- If the centrifugation g force is too low, an appropriate sperm pellet will not form. Adjustments in time and g force can be made for an individual stallion after an initial centrifugation procedure to optimize sperm recovery.
- Calculations to convert revolutions per minute (rpm) to a desired g force may be necessary if the centrifuge is only calibrated in rpm (see Chapter 148).
- An ideal sperm pellet should minimize spermatozoa in the supernatant; however, a very high centrifugation rate may result in a sperm pellet that is overly compacted and not easy to re-suspend, leading to possible spermatozoal damage.

Further Reading

Rigby SL, Brinsko SP, Cochran M, Blanchard TL, Love CC, Varner DD. 2001. Advances in cooled semen technologies; seminal plasma and semen extender. *Anim Reprod Sci* 68: 171–80.

Vanderwall DK. 2008. How to process dilute ejaculate of semen for cooled-transported insemination. *Proc Annu Conv Am Assoc Eq Pract* 54: 369–73.

Varner DD, Love CC, Blanchard TL, *et al.* 2010. Breeding-management strategies and semen-handling techniques for stallions. *Proc Annu Conv Am Assoc Eq Pract* 56: 215–26.

150

Centrifugation of Semen: Cushion Technique

Etta A. Bradecamp

Rood and Riddle Equine Hospital, USA

Introduction

Semen freshly collected from stallions is usually evaluated, extended, and either inseminated, cooled for short-term storage, or frozen. It is recommended that stallion semen be centrifuged if the ejaculate contains a low concentration of spermatozoa (i.e., less than 100 million sperm/ml) or if sperm motility is adversely affected by prolonged exposure to seminal plasma. Centrifugation of semen can be performed with or without the aid of a cushion medium. The purpose of the cushion is to allow the semen to be centrifuged at a higher *g* force to maximize the percentage of sperm harvested post-centrifugation without having a detrimental effect on the viability of the sperm.

Several non-ionic iodixanol-based cushions for the centrifugation of equine semen are commercially available (Table 150.1). The advantage of a cushion is that a higher g force can be used with less sperm damage and greater recovery rates (95–100% recovery). This is especially helpful when there are low numbers of spermatozoa in the ejaculate. The cushion is placed underneath the extended semen in a conical tube, the tube is centrifuged, and then the supernatant and cushion are both removed leaving a concentrated semen pellet in the tube.

Table 150.1 Iodixanol-based cushions for the centrifugation of equine semen.

Cushion	Source
Cushion Fluid™	Minitube International, Tiefenbach, Germany
Eqcellsire®	IMV Technologies USA, Maple Grove, MN, USA
E-Z Cushion™	Animal Reproduction Systems, Chino, CA, USA
OptiPrep™	Greiner Bio-One, Axis-Shield, Oslo, Norway

Equipment and Supplies

Cushion Fluid™, Eqcellsire®, E-Z Cushion™, or OptiPrep™; semen; 50 ml conical tubes; centrifuge equipped to hold 50 ml conical tubes with swinging buckets; semen extender; disposable pipettes; densimeter, hemocytometer, or NucleoCounter®; microscope; microscope slides; coverslips; balance scale.

Technique

- Collect semen and determine the gel-free volume, concentration, and motility of the sample prior to centrifugation (see Chapters 127 and 130).
- Extend the semen 1:1 with extender.
- Transfer the extended semen into one or more 50 ml conical centrifuge tubes.
- Add a cushion to the bottom of each conical tube below the extended semen:
- Draw up the appropriate volume (i.e., 0.5–3.0 ml) of cushion into a sterile pipette.
- Pass the pipette through the extended semen to the bottom of the conical tube.
- Gently deposit the layer of cushion material on the bottom of the tube, beneath the extended semen. Do not mix the two layers together.
- Using a scale, each pair of tubes (along with the centrifuge buckets) must be weighed and balanced to ensure that the centrifuge is balanced once loaded. If there are an odd number of tubes containing extended semen, a conical tube filled with water can be used as a counter balance.
- The conical tubes are then loaded into the centrifuge opposite one another.
- Centrifuge at 1,000× g for 20–25 minutes. At the end of centrifugation, the sperm will be compacted into a pellet on top of the cushion and below a supernatant of seminal plasma/extender (Figure 150.1).

Equine Reproductive Procedures, Second Edition. Edited by John Dascanio and Patrick McCue.

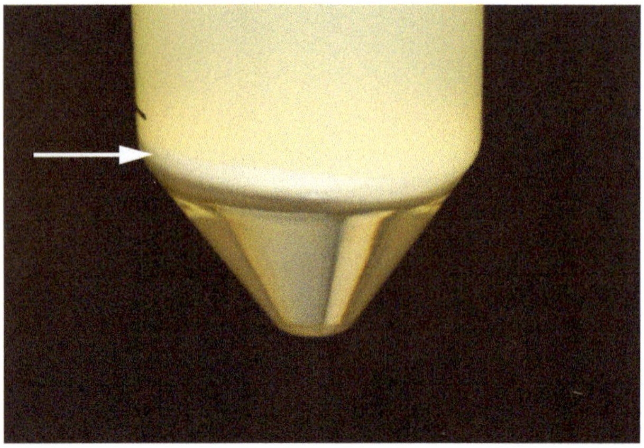

Figure 150.1 Sperm pellet (arrow) between the supernatant of seminal plasma/semen extender (above) and the centrifugation cushion (below).

- Aspirate off and discard most of the supernatant, leaving a total volume of approximately 7.5 ml. Removal of the supernatant can be accomplished using a pipette or a sink aspiration system.
- Gently aspirate a majority of the cushion from beneath the sperm pellet after removal of the supernatant. This may be accomplished manually using a glass pipette, a syringe attached to a 0.25 or 0.5 ml semen straw, an open-ended tomcat catheter, or a long spinal needle (Figure 150.2). The instrument must gently pass through the sperm pellet layer. Be careful to not disturb the sperm pellet layer during removal of the cushion.
- Re-suspend the sperm pellet in the small volume of seminal plasma/extender that remained in the conical tube. The total volume after removal of the cushion is approximately 5 ml.
- Combine the re-suspended semen from all the centrifuge tubes.
- Measure the volume of the combined re-suspended semen.
- Determine the sperm concentration by either a manual count with a hemocytometer (see Chapter 128) or with a NucleoCounter® (see Chapter 129).
- Calculate the volume of re-suspended semen needed to provide a minimum breeding dose of 500 million progressively motile sperm (PMS) for fresh insemination or 1 billion PMS for cooled storage and transport (Box 150.1).

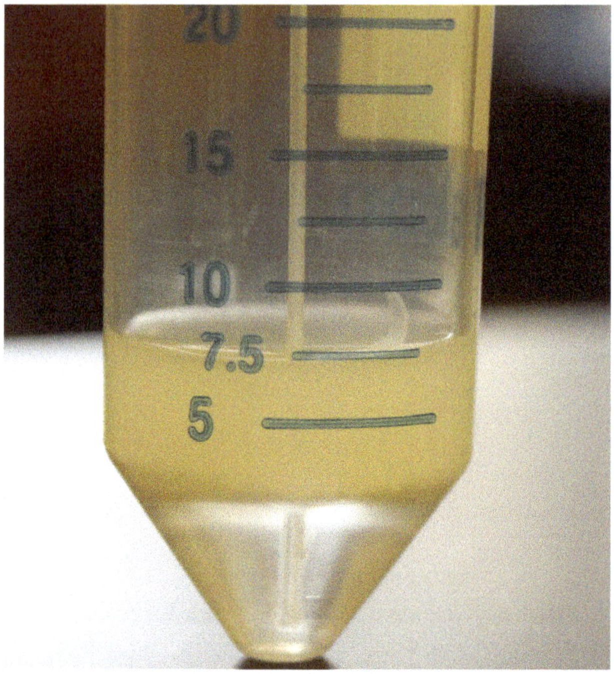

Figure 150.2 Aspiration of the cushion below the sperm pellet using a tomcat catheter.

- Combine the calculated volume of re-suspended semen needed with the appropriate volume of additional semen extender to yield the final breeding dose (20 ml volume for a fresh insemination or 40 ml volume for a cooled insemination dose).
- A final motility estimate should be made after any additional semen extender is added as a final quality control.

Additional Comments

Cushioned centrifugation allows a higher centrifugation force for a longer time than traditional centrifugation of semen without the risk of mechanical damage and with a higher sperm recovery rate.

The requirement to remove the cushion after centrifugation and removal of the supernatant is in debate. The presence of cushion material in the final re-extended semen sample does not appear to have a detrimental effect on spermatozoal function, the uterus of an inseminated mare, or fertility.

Box 150.1 Predictors and time frames in propensity modeling

Example

Original semen parameters — *Volume* = *85 ml*
Concentration = *78 million sperm per ml*
Progressive motility = *65%*

85 *ml × **78** million sperm/ml × **0.65** (% progressive motility) = **4,309.5** million progressively motile spermatozoa (PMS)*

4,309.5 *PMS ÷ 20 ml = **215.5** million PMS/ml after centrifugation and re-suspension* (4 tubes of 5 ml each =20 ml). *Assumes 100% sperm recovery and approximately 5 ml of sperm pellet and supernatant in each tube. This may be adjusted if a greater volume is present in each tube*

To prepare a fresh insemination dose of 500 million PMS:

*500 ÷ **215.5** = **2.3** ml of re-suspended semen is needed to provide 500 million PMS*

*20 ml – **2.3** = **17.7** ml extender to provide a 20 ml volume containing 500 million PMS at a concentration of approximately 25 million PMS/ml*

To prepare a cooled insemination dose of 1.0 billion PMS:

*1,000 ÷ **215.5** = **4.7** ml of re-suspended semen*

*40 ml – **4.7** = **35.3** ml extender to provide a 40 ml volume containing 1,000 million (1.0 billion) PMS at a concentration of c. 25 million PMS/ml*

Stallion: ________ **Collection date:** ________

Original semen parameters — Volume = ____ ml
Concentration = ____ million sperm/ml
Progressive motility = ____ %

____ ml × ____ million sperm/ml × ____ (% progressive motility) = ____ million PMS

____ million PMS ÷ ____ ml* = ____ million PMS/ml after centrifugation and re-suspension (4 tubes of 5 ml each).
*Refers to the total volume of re-suspended semen after all tubes are combined

To prepare a fresh insemination dose of 500 million PMS:

500 ÷ ____ = ____ ml of re-suspended semen

20 ml – ____ = ____ ml extender to provide a 20 ml volume containing 500 million PMS at a concentration of 25 million PMS/ml

To prepare a cooled insemination dose of 1.0 billion PMS:

1,000 ÷ ____ = ____ ml of re-suspended semen

40 ml – ____ = ____ ml extender to provide a 40 ml volume containing 1,000 million (1.0 billion) PMS at a concentration of 25 million PMS/ml

Further Reading

Hoogewijs M, Rijsselaere T, De Vliegher S, *et al*. 2010. Influence of different centrifugation protocols on equine semen preservation. *Theriogenology* 74: 118–26.

Waite JA, Love CC, Brinsko SP, Teague SR, Salazar JL, Jr, Mancill SS, Varner DD. 2008. Factors impacting equine sperm recovery rate and quality following cushioned centrifugation. *Theriogenology* 70: 704–14.

151

Centrifugation of Semen: Selection of Motile Sperm Using a Single Layer Colloid Technique

Etta A. Bradecamp

Rood and Riddle Equine Hospital, USA

Introduction

Single layer centrifugation is a process by which semen is passed through a colloidal, silanized, silica particle solution during centrifugation to select sperm with good motility, morphology, and chromatin quality. This procedure is utilized to improve fertility and pregnancy rates from stallions with decreased fertility due to a high proportion of morphologically abnormal sperm in the ejaculate. Due to the differences in the isopycnic values (density) of the normal and abnormal sperm, the abnormal sperm are trapped within the silica particle solution during centrifugation, while the normal sperm are able to pass through and collect in a pellet at the bottom of the centrifugation tube. Removal of the supernatant and colloid solution will leave a pellet containing a high concentration of morphologically normal sperm in the bottom of the tube. This technique can be used to improve the quality of sperm recovered from fresh semen, cooled semen, or frozen-thawed semen, but is often associated with a low percentage of sperm recovered.

There are several colloid solutions commercially available for the centrifugation of equine semen including EquiPure™ (Nidacon, Mölndal, Sweden) and AndroColl™ (Minitube, Verona, WI, USA) (Figure 151.1). The following protocol describes the use of EquiPure™.

Equipment and Supplies

Extender, colloid centrifugation media (EquiPure™), 50 or 15 ml conical centrifuge tubes, centrifuge equipped to hold 50 and 15 ml conical tubes with swinging buckets, dispensing pipette and disposable tips, Pasteur pipettes, densimeter or hemocytometer or NucleoCounter®, microscope, microscope slides, coverslips, disposable pipettes.

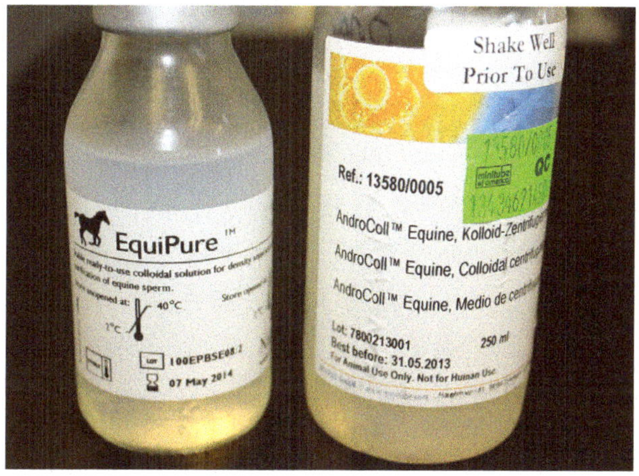

Figure 151.1 EquiPure™ and AndroColl™ equine products for single layer centrifugation.

Technique

- Measure the sperm concentration with a densimeter (see Chapter 127), hemocytometer (see Chapter 128), or a NucleoCounter® (see Chapter 129).
- Extend the ejaculate 1:1 (v:v) with a commercial semen extender. Pre-warm the semen extender to 37°C (99°F).
- Pre-warm the EquiPure™ solution to 37°C.
- The following procedure details were provided by the manufacturer, Nidacom.
- Add 10–20 ml EquiPure™ at ambient temperature to a 50 ml centrifuge tube.
- Add an equal volume of extended semen to the tube above the EquiPure™ layer using a Pasteur pipette or disposable syringe. Add the diluted semen slowly making sure not to mix the EquiPure™ solution and semen (Figure 151.2). Important: the maximum total number of sperm must not exceed 3 billion.

Equine Reproductive Procedures, Second Edition. Edited by John Dascanio and Patrick McCue.

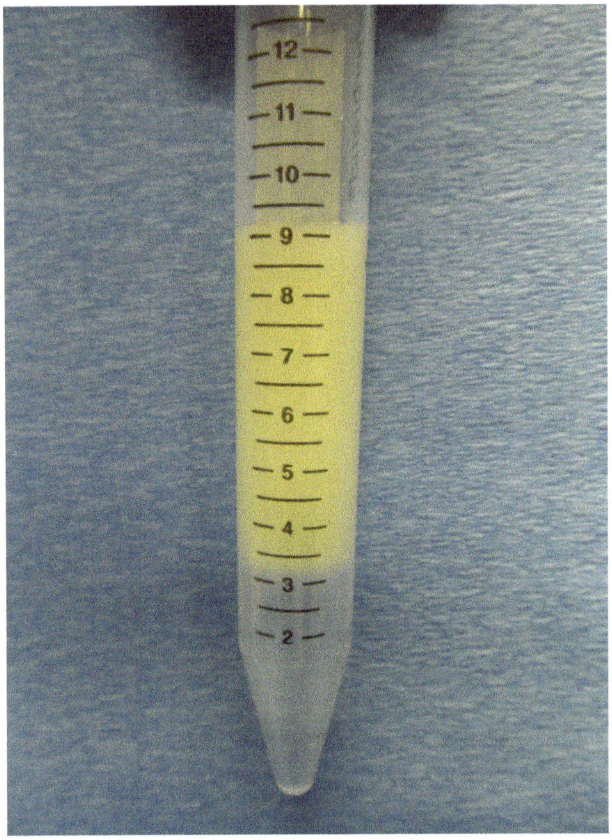

Figure 151.2 Layering of extended semen (yellow layer) over a density gradient medium (bottom clear fluid).

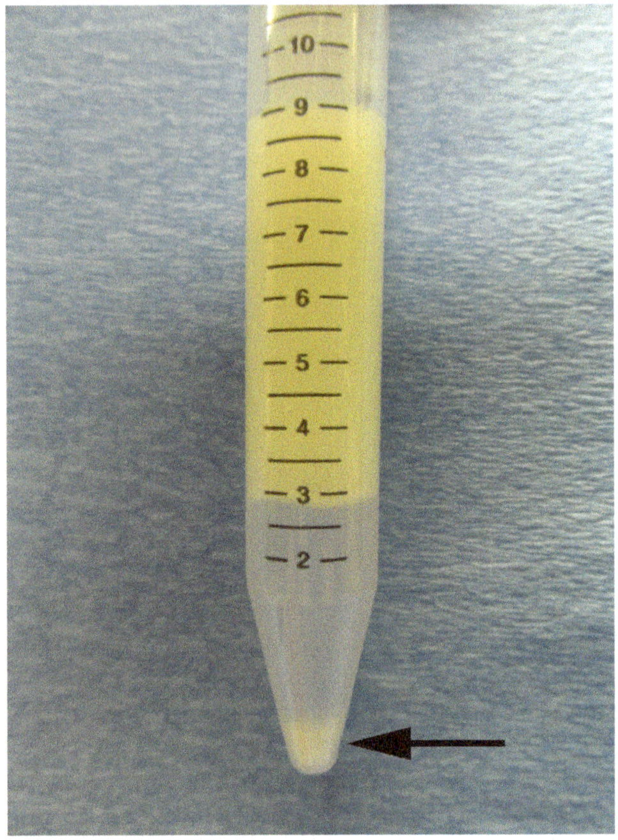

Figure 151.3 Pellet (arrow) formed after centrifugation through a density gradient medium.

- Using a scale, each pair of tubes (along with the centrifuge buckets) must be weighed and balanced to ensure that the centrifuge is balanced once loaded. If there are an odd number of tubes containing extended semen, a conical tube filled with water can be used as a counter balance.
- The conical tubes are then loaded into the centrifuge opposite one another.
- Centrifuge at 400× g for 20 minutes; do not use the brake.
- After centrifugation, remove the ejaculate and most of the EquiPure™ using a Pasteur pipette.
- Using a new pipette retrieve the pellet (Figure 151.3) and transfer to a new tube.
- Re-suspend to a concentration of 50×10^6 sperm/ml. Sperm recovery after selection with EquiPure™ largely depends on the initial sperm quality, but on average ranges around 40%.

Interpretation

- Centrifugation through a colloidal yields a sample of sperm with good motility, morphology, and chromatin quality.
- Due to the potential for loss of a large percentage of spermatozoa during processing, the final sample is typically utilized for low dose, deep-horn insemination or other assisted reproduction procedures.
- Do not pre-centrifuge the ejaculate prior to processing with single layer centrifugation due to the possible agglutination of sperm cells.
- Do not place more than 45 ml of extended semen in a conical centrifuge tube when processing.
- Use 15 ml conical tubes for extended semen volumes of less than 10 ml.

Further Reading

Morrell JM, Rodriguez-Martinez H, Johannisson A. 2010. Single layer centrifugation of stallion spermatozoa consistently selects the most robust spermatozoa from the rest of the ejaculate in a large sample size. *Eq Vet J* 42: 579–85.

Varner DD, Love CC, Blanchard TL, *et al.* 2010. Breeding-management strategies and semen-handling techniques for stallions. *Proc Annu Conv Am Assoc Eq Pract* 56: 215–26.

152

Use of a SpermFilter

Marco A. Alvarenga and Lorenzo G. T. M. Segabinazzi

School of Veterinary Medicine, São Paulo State University, Brazil

Introduction

Sperm concentration is an important step for cryopreservation of stallion semen and a useful tool to improve sperm quality of cooled semen or of semen from subfertile stallions. The most common technique to concentrate sperm is centrifugation. However, beyond the need of a centrifuge machine, which is not always available in ambulatory practice, this procedure can also be harmful to spermatozoa. In contrast, a SpermFilter is an effective alternative for sperm concentration. This technique reduces the negative effects of centrifugation, is inexpensive, and is a practical approach. In addition, concentrating sperm using a SpermFilter also decreases bacterial contamination in the semen, since the sperm is retained in the filter, but the majority of bacteria flow through the filter with the supernatant.

The SpermFilter consists in a synthetic hydrophilic membrane with 2 μl pores, which allows the flow of seminal plasma and extender through the membrane but retains the sperm (Figure 152.1). Surface tension allows the flow of the supernatant through the filter membrane, while the sperm concentrate stays above the filter.

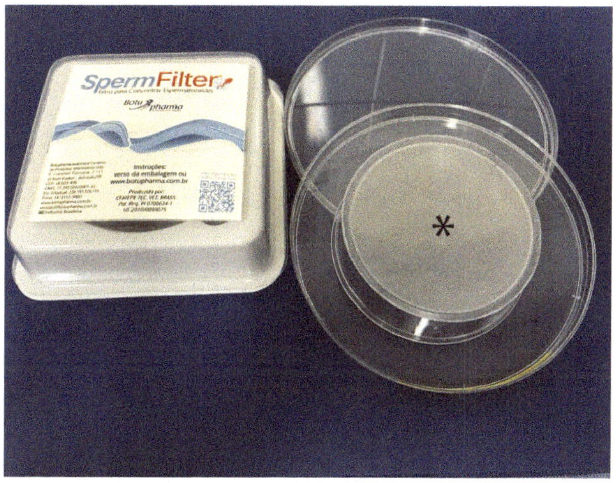

Figure 152.1 Equipment for semen filtration (SpermFilter®)

Equipment and Supplies

SpermFilter (Botupharma USA, Phoenix, AZ, USA), 15 cm (6 inch) Petri dish, semen extender, all-plastic syringes (3–20 ml), Pasteur pipette, 100 ml beaker (optional), 15 or 50 ml tube (optional).

Technique

- The SpermFilter should be placed in a 15 cm Petri dish and loaded with a small amount of extender to wet the membrane.
- To filter a raw semen sample, the semen should be extended 2:1 (v:v, semen:extender) in a skim milk or casein-based extender. If cooled semen is being filtered, the semen sample can be immediately placed in the SpermFilter.
- The SpermFilter should be gently tapped against the Petri dish to release fluid through the pores (Figure 152.2). It may also be placed on a 30-degree inclination surface to increase the outflow of the supernatant and to concentrate sperm (Figure 152.3). Gently swirl the diluted semen around the filter and repeatedly touch the bottom of the Petri dish until a viscous liquid (concentrated sperm) is evident on the membrane (Figure 152.2).
- A predetermined volume of the chosen extender should be used to re-suspend the sperm cells.
- The extender should be placed in the SpermFilter, and using a Pasteur pipette or circular movements, the filter

Equine Reproductive Procedures, Second Edition. Edited by John Dascanio and Patrick McCue.

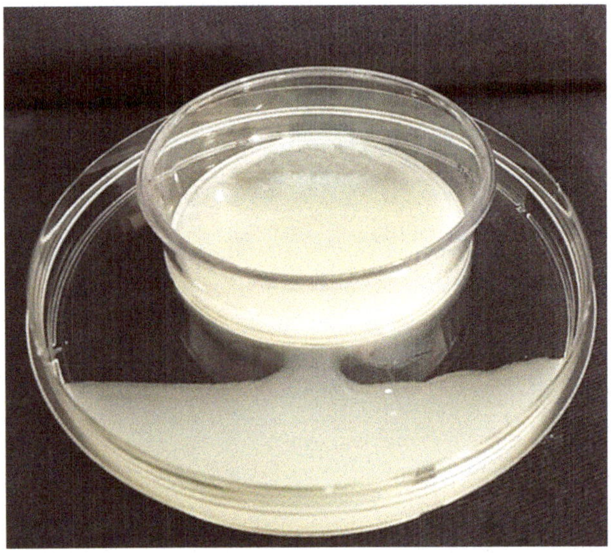

Figure 152.2 Sperm is placed on a surface with a 30-degree inclination.

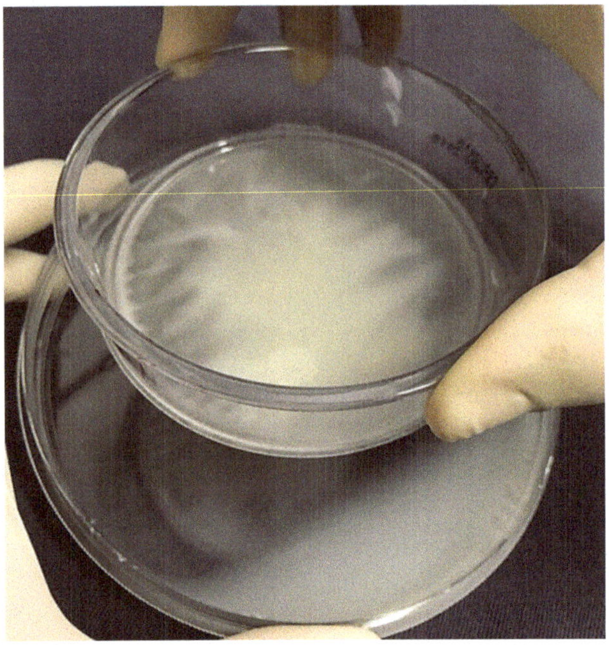

Figure 152.3 Sperm concentrated on the filter.

membrane must be washed to recover the sperm cells (Figure 152.4) into a clean Petri dish.

- After washing the filter, the extended semen should be collected into a beaker or 50 ml conical tube and used for cooled storage, freezing, or immediate insemination.

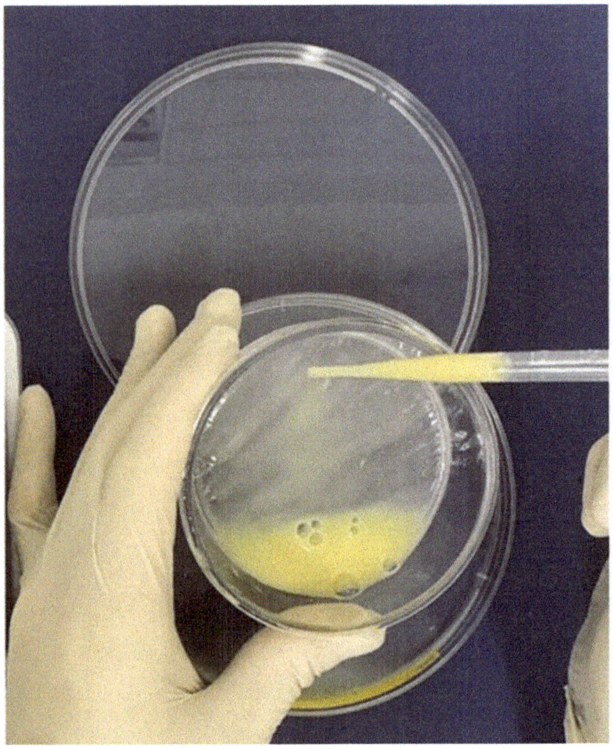

Figure 152.4 Washing the filter membrane for sperm recovery using a semen extender and a Pasteur pipette.

Additional Comments

- The entire filtration takes 5–10 minutes, depending on the amount of semen being processed.
- After semen manipulation, the SpermFilter can be carefully washed using clean water, with 70% isopropyl alcohol added on the filter. The filter can be placed, upside down to avoid filter membrane damage, in an incubator at 37°C (99°F) to dry and then at 50°C (122°F) to sterilize. The membrane should not be touched with needles or other objects, it can only touch the Petri dish or the inside of its own commercial box.
- The same filter can be reused several times to process semen from the same stallion without detrimental effects on sperm quality and recovery.
- The expected sperm recovery using the SpermFilter is 90% of the initial sperm concentration. A study comparing the sperm filters and cushion centrifugation (see Chapter 150) showed that the cell recovery rate was close to 100% using a cushion, whereas the SpermFilter achieved 93%.

Further Reading

Alvarenga MA, Papa FO, Ramires Neto C. 2016. Advances in stallion semen cryopreservation. *Vet Clin North Am Eq Pract* 32(3): 521–30.

Ramires Neto C, Monteiro GA, Soares RF, Pedrazzi C, Dell'Aqua JA, Jr, Papa FO, Alvarenga MA. 2013. Effect of removing seminal plasma using a sperm filter on the viability of refrigerated stallion semen. *J Eq Vet Sci* 33: 40–3.

Ramires Neto C, Monteiro GA, Soares RF, *et al.* 2013. New seminal plasma removal method for freezing stallion semen. *Theriogenology* 79: 1120–3.

Roach J, Schnobrich M, Ellerbrock R, *et al.* 2016. Comparison of cushioned centrifugation and SpermFilter filtration on longevity and morphology of cooled-stored equine semen. *Vet Rec* 10: 241.

153

Semen Freezing

Patrick M. McCue

Equine Reproduction Laboratory, Colorado State University, USA

Introduction

The main advantages of frozen semen are long-term preservation of genetic material, insurance against unanticipated loss of a stallion, access to frozen semen if fresh or cooled semen is not available, and ability to ship semen worldwide. Unfortunately, the spermatozoa from some stallions do not freeze well. In addition, pregnancy rates for mares bred with frozen semen are often slightly less than those of fresh or cooled semen.

Stallion semen is usually diluted to either 200 or 400 million sperm per milliliter in freezing extender and packaged in 0.5 ml straws containing a total of either 100 or 200 million sperm per straw. A typical breeding dose would consist of either eight or four straws containing a total of 800 million spermatozoa. It is also generally accepted that the post-thaw motility should be *at least* 30%.

Equine semen can be processed for cryopreservation either with or without use of a cushion in the centrifugation step. Standard centrifugation techniques result in the recovery of approximately 75% of spermatozoa in the initial sample. The advantage of incorporating a cushion centrifugation technique is that the cushion allows for increased centrifugation speed and duration, which ultimately results in enhanced sperm recovery (i.e., >95%) without a detrimental effect on sperm motility or morphology (see Chapter 150).

Equipment and Supplies

Semen extender (for initial centrifugation), cushion for centrifugation, graduated cylinder (50 ml), conical centrifuge tubes and caps, balance scale, hemacytometer kit or NucleoCounter®, centrifuge, sink aspirator, glass pipettes, all-plastic syringes (no rubber plunger), bubbler comb, 0.5 ml semen straws, sealing powder/sealing balls, clay, freezing extender, disposable glass pipette (5 ml), rack, Styrofoam™ box with freezing rack or computerized cell freezer, liquid nitrogen, thermo-protective gloves, safety glasses.

Technique for Loading Straws with Extended Semen

- Collect and evaluate the semen.
- Extend the raw semen 1:1 with centrifugation medium or extender. Fill conical centrifuge tubes with 40 ml of extended semen.
- Slowly deposit 0.5–3 ml of cushion medium to the bottom of each conical tube beneath the extended semen by passing a pipette through the extended semen.
- Balance the centrifuge tubes by weight using a balance scale.
- Centrifuge at 1,000× g for 20–25 minutes at room temperature. The sperm pellet will be suspended between the supernatant on top and the cushion below (Figure 153.1).
- Aspirate the supernatant. This may be accomplished easily using a sink aspiration kit (Figure 153.2), or

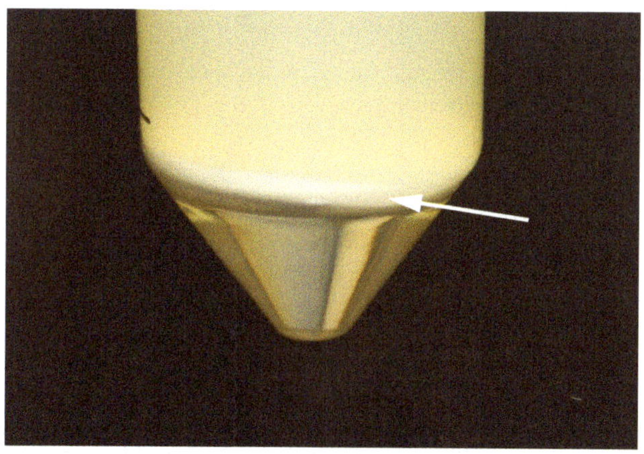

Figure 153.1 Sperm pellet (arrow) between the cushion (the clear layer at the bottom of the tube) and supernatant (above). Note the volume of cushion in this photo is 3.0 ml; a smaller volume of cushion (i.e., 0.5 ml may also be used).

Equine Reproductive Procedures, Second Edition. Edited by John Dascanio and Patrick McCue.

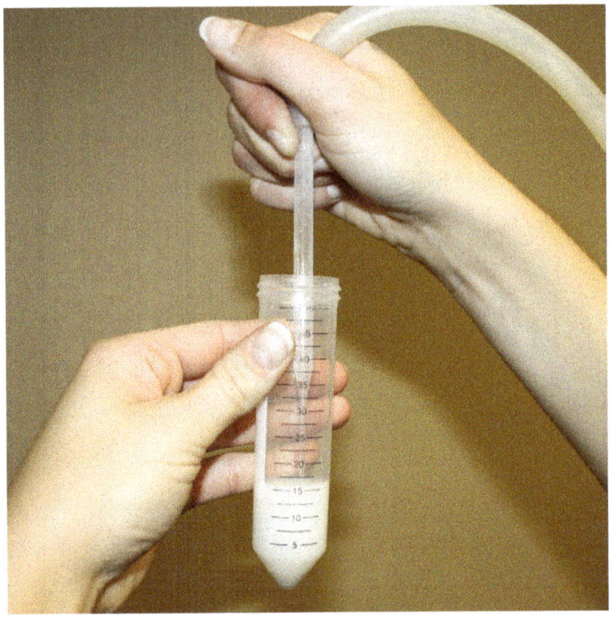

Figure 153.2 Aspirate the supernatant above the sperm pellet after centrifugation.

Box 153.1 Calculations

Total number of sperm recovered = New concentration × New volume
Total volume required = Total number of sperm recovered ÷ 400 (or 200)
Volume of extender to add = Total volume required − New volume

alternatively an open-ended tomcat catheter or similar device may be used.
  - The sperm pellet (approximately 3 ml) will remain on top of the cushion.
- Remove a majority of the cushion by passing a pipette through the pellet and aspirating the cushion.
- Re-suspend the pellet in each tube with 1.0 ml of freezing extender.
- Pool the re-extended semen from all the tubes into one tube. Measure the new volume. This may be done by aspirating the contents into an all-plastic syringe or pipette.
- Perform a sperm count using either a hemocytometer or NucleoCounter® to determine the new concentration (see Chapters 128 and 129).
- Add additional freezing extender to achieve a concentration of 200 or 400 × 10^6/ml (Box 153.1).
- Label the 0.5 ml straws (with the stallion's name, extender, concentration, date, and facility) (Figure 153.3). The number of straws required will equal twice the volume of the extended semen in milliliters (i.e., 6 ml will require 12 straws). Laser-printed straws may be commercially ordered with advance notice.

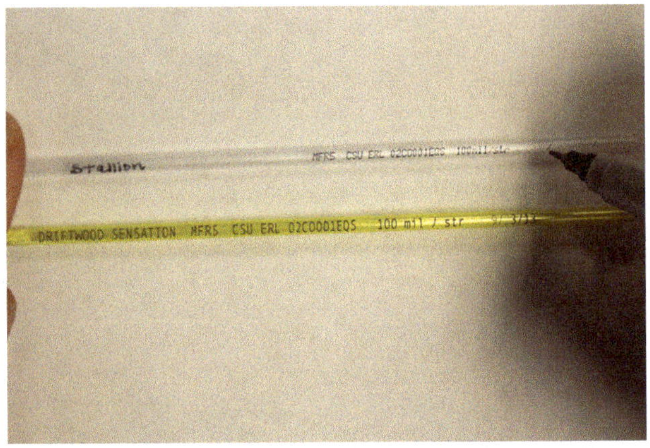

Figure 153.3 Label the straws with the stallion's name, date, extender, facility, and concentration (top straw). Pre-labeled straws can also be ordered or produced ahead of time with all pertinent information (bottom straw).

- Load the extended semen into the straws. One option is to use a manual straw-filling device that attaches to a thumbwheel pump to load five straws at a time (Figure 153.4). A second option is to use a disposable, white plastic, cow teat cannula attached to a syringe to load individual straws. The teat cannula is placed into the end of the straw with the cotton pledgets/polyvinyl chloride powder. The straw is then lowered into the extended semen and the syringe plunger pulled to pull semen into the straw. The semen should be pulled into the straw so that the polyvinyl chloride powder in between the two cotton pledgets is completely wetted to seal that end of the straw. A third option is to use an automated straw-filling machine (Figure 153.5).
- Create a bubble within the straws using a disposable bubbler comb (Figure 153.6) or pull the straw out of the semen while aspirating once the semen contacts the first cotton pledget so that an air bubble will remain in the straw. The air bubble is compressible during the liquid expansion of the freezing protocol, preventing the straw from rupturing or the sealed ends from becoming dislodged.
- Seal the open end of the straws with sealing powder (Figure 153.7) or use sealing balls (plastic or stainless steel). If no sealing powder or sealing balls are available, clay used to seal microhematocrit tubes may be used.
- Flick the straws to move the air bubble to the center of the straw. This allows equal expansion of the liquid within the straw during freezing.
- Freeze the semen (see next technique).

Technique for Freezing Straws of Extended Semen

Straws of extended semen may be frozen in a Styrofoam™ box or a programmable liquid nitrogen cell freezer. The

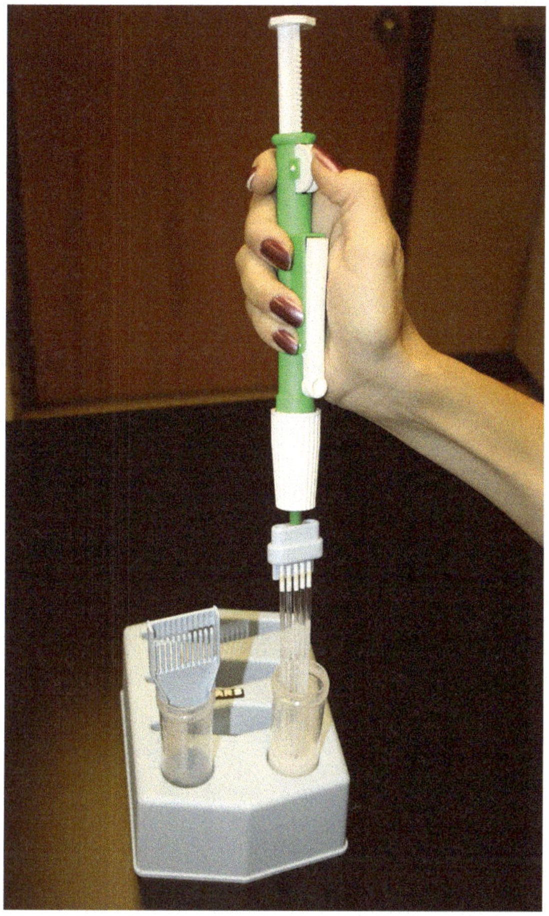

Figure 153.4 Loading five 0.5 ml straws using a manual straw-filling device.

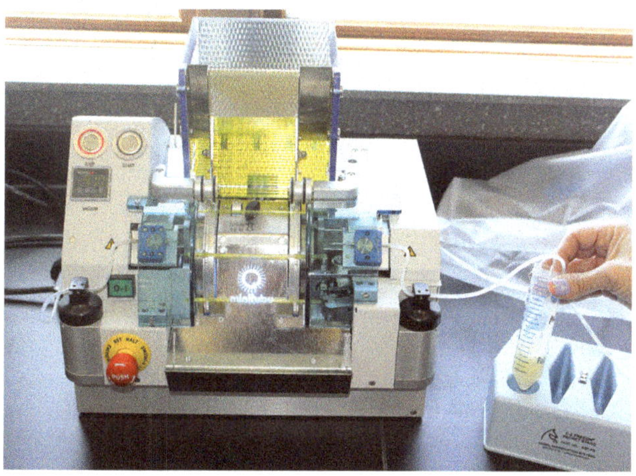

Figure 153.5 Automated straw-filling machine loading straws with extended semen.

techniques described here are for freezing stallion semen in a Styrofoam™ box. The liquid nitrogen should be poured into the Styrofoam™ box and the lid loosely placed to allow outgassing and to equilibrate the Styrofoam™ to the temperature prior to placement of the straws. The rack used to freeze the

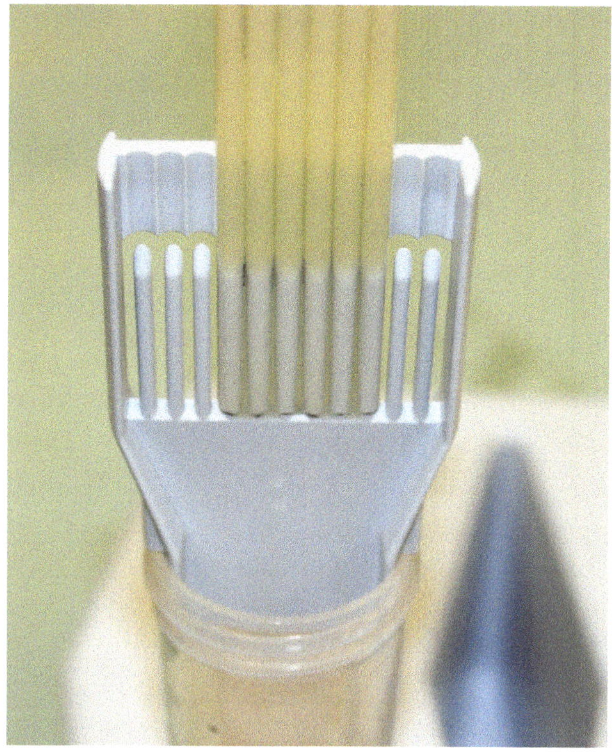

Figure 153.6 Removal of a small amount of extended semen from 0.5 ml straws using a bubbler comb to provide an air pocket.

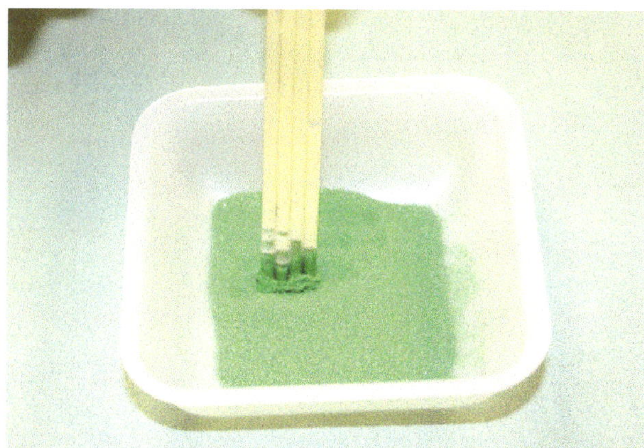

Figure 153.7 Sealing the open end of loaded semen straws with straw sealant.

straws should be at the same temperature as the straws that are placed on them and is then lowered into the cooled Styrofoam™ box. Canes and goblets should be lowered into the liquid nitrogen in the Styrofoam™ box to cool prior to loading them with frozen straws. Frozen straws should be loaded into the goblets within the liquid nitrogen.

Lactose-EDTA Extender

Semen diluted in lactose-EDTA-based (LE) extenders (i.e., the original LE extenders with a single cryoprotectant and modified LE extenders with dual cryoprotectants) do not need to be cooled prior to freezing. However, some opt to cool semen diluted in LE-type extenders for 30 minutes prior to freezing. The technique for freezing semen in extended in lactose-EDTA is as follows.

- Place the loaded straws on a room temperature stainless steel floating rack (Figure 153.8).
- (Optional) Place the loaded rack into a refrigerator for 30 minutes for pre-cooling prior to freezing (Figure 153.9).
- Gently transfer the loaded rack into a Styrofoam™ box containing liquid nitrogen; the straws should be 3 cm above the surface of the liquid nitrogen (Figure 153.10).
- Allow 10 minutes equilibration or until the temperature reaches −120°C (−185°F).
- Plunge the straws into the liquid nitrogen.
- Place the straws into goblets that are already fixed onto canes and store in a liquid nitrogen tank.

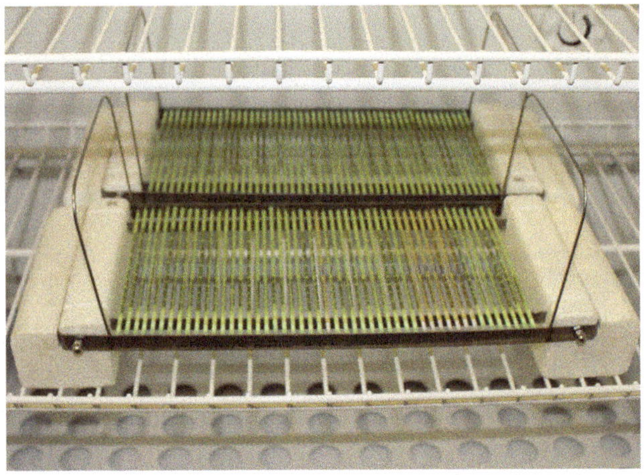

Figure 153.9 Racks of loaded straws in a refrigerator for pre-cooling prior to freezing (optional).

Skim Milk/Egg Yolk Extender

Semen diluted in skim milk/egg yolk freezing extenders (i.e., the original modified French formula 5 (MFR5) type extenders with a single cryoprotectant and the modified MFR5-type extenders with dual cryoprotectants) require a 1–2 hour pre-cooling step prior to freezing to optimize post-thaw motility characteristics. The technique for freezing semen extended in skim milk/egg yolk is as follows.

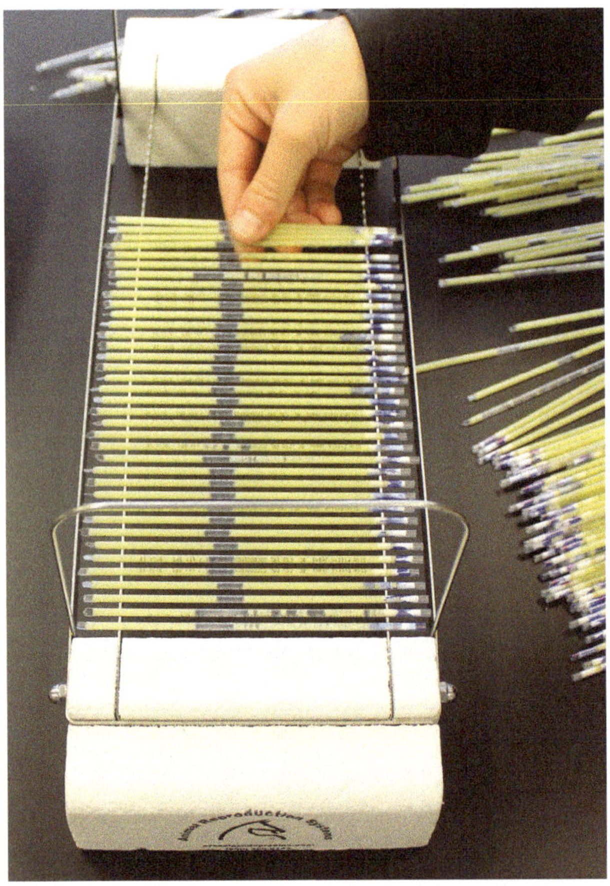

Figure 153.8 Loading straws of extended semen onto a floating rack prior to freezing.

Option 1: Cool the semen after loading into straws

- Place the loaded straws on a room temperature stainless steel floating rack (Figure 153.8)
- Place the loaded rack into a refrigerator for 60–120 minutes for pre-cooling prior to freezing (Figure 153.9)
- Transfer the loaded rack into a Styrofoam™ box containing liquid nitrogen (Figure 153.10); allow 10 minutes equilibration and then plunge straws into the liquid nitrogen.

Option 2: Cooling the entire aliquot of semen prior to loading into straws

- Place the centrifuge tubes (sealed with caps) filled with extended semen into a beaker of room temperature water filled to the level of the semen.
- Place the beaker in the refrigerator to cool for 1–2 hours or until the semen reaches 5°C (40°F).
- Label, load, bubble, and seal the straws as described earlier in a cold room at 5°C.
- Place the loaded straws on a pre-cooled rack (at 5°C) and then place the rack so that the straws are 3 cm above the liquid nitrogen.
- Allow 10 minutes equilibration or until the temperature reaches −120°C.
- Plunge the straws into liquid nitrogen.
- Place the straws into goblets that are already fixed onto canes, and store in a liquid nitrogen tank.

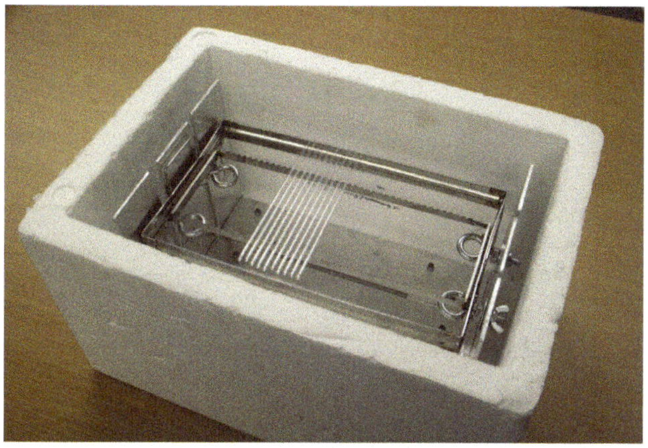

Figure 153.10 Straws on a rack placed in a freezing box above liquid nitrogen. The Styrofoam™ box lid is placed on top after the rack has been placed into the box.

Additional Comments

A test freeze should be performed the first time that semen from an individual stallion is frozen. The test freeze can compare post-thaw motility and viability characteristics between two or more freezing extenders, centrifugation techniques, cooling rates, sperm concentrations, and possibly different straw sizes and thawing rates. The goal is to identify a customized cryopreservation protocol to maximize sperm survival after freezing and thawing.

Pregnancy rates per cycle for mares inseminated with frozen-thawed semen are highly variable due to differences between stallions, freezing extenders, insemination dose, timing of insemination, number of inseminations, and reproductive status of the mare. Pregnancy rates can range from <10% per cycle for some stallions to >50% per cycle for other stallions. However, in general it is assumed that pregnancy rates with frozen semen will range between 30% and 45% per cycle. Based on the results of several studies, it has been estimated that approximately 25–35% of stallions are "good freezers," 40–50% are "satisfactory freezers," and 25–30% are "poor freezers" with regard to both post-thaw motility characteristics and fertility rates (i.e., pregnancy rates per cycle).

Further Reading

Sieme H. 2011. Freezing semen. In: McKinnon AO, Squires EL, Vaala WE, Varner DD (eds). Equine Reproduction, 2nd edn. Ames, IA: Wiley Blackwell, pp. 2972–82.

154

Refreezing Semen

Patrick M. McCue

Equine Reproduction Laboratory, Colorado State University, USA

Introduction

Stallion semen is commonly cryopreserved in 0.5 ml straws at a concentration of 200–400 million sperm per milliliter. Traditional artificial insemination with frozen semen may use one to eight straws per dose. Intracytoplasmic sperm injection (ICSI) has made it possible to produce embryos and subsequent pregnancies utilizing a single motile sperm.

Thawing a single straw containing 100 or 200 million total spermatozoa in order to obtain one motile spermatozoa is wasteful if the remainder of the spermatozoa are discarded. In addition, in many clinical situations, the stallion may either be deceased, no longer producing viable spermatozoa, or no longer commercially available – making every straw of frozen semen valuable and essentially irreplaceable.

Several strategies have been investigated as to how to optimize the use of frozen semen for ICSI. One strategy consists of cutting off a very small portion of a frozen straw while still under liquid nitrogen and only thawing the cut portion. A second strategy is to initially freeze semen from valuable stallions in "ICSI doses," each straw of which contains a low number of spermatozoa.

A third strategy is to thaw individual straws of semen, remove a very small aliquot for immediate use for ICSI and refreeze the remainder. An adjunct to this strategy is to dilute the thawed semen in additional cryopreservation extender, aliquot the diluted semen into multiple straws containing smaller total numbers of sperm per straw, and refreeze all the straws for future use.

Equipment and Supplies

Straws of frozen semen, freezing extender, 50 ml conical tubes, pipettes, semen straws, liquid nitrogen, semen freezing rack, Styrofoam™ box, thermo-protective gloves, safety glasses.

Technique

- Straws of frozen semen are initially maintained in tanks of liquid nitrogen. A single straw containing frozen semen from the appropriate stallion is removed from the liquid nitrogen tank (Figure 154.1) and thawed in a 37°C (99°F) water bath for 30 seconds. The straw is subsequently removed and the outside dried with a paper towel.
- The contents of the straw are then transferred into a sterile 50 ml conical tube containing, for example, 49.5 ml of fresh cryopreservation extender (i.e., CryoMax™ LE; Animal Reproduction Systems, Ontario, CA, USA), resulting in a 100-fold dilution of spermatozoa. The contents of the conical tube are gently, but thoroughly mixed.
- The diluted semen is loaded into 0.5 ml polyvinylchloride straws, sealed, and loaded onto floating straw racks

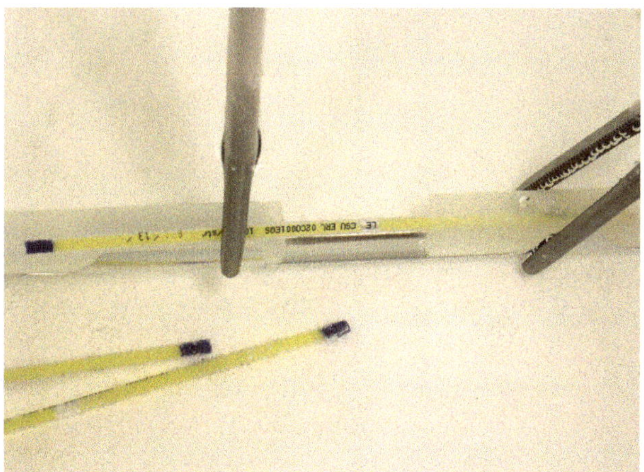

Figure 154.1 Selecting a straw to thaw while immersed in a bath of liquid nitrogen.

Equine Reproductive Procedures, Second Edition. Edited by John Dascanio and Patrick McCue.

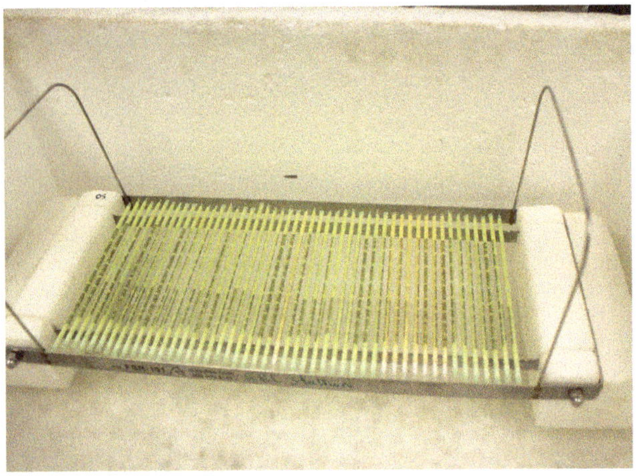

Figure 154.2 Loading straws onto a floating rack.

(Figure 154.2). The racks are placed in a refrigerator and cooled at 4°C (39°F) for 30 minutes.

- The racks are then placed into a Styrofoam™ box containing liquid nitrogen, with the straws maintained 3 cm above the liquid nitrogen for 10 minutes, after which the straws are plunged into liquid nitrogen for long-term storage.
- It is important to label the new straws with the stallion's name, the new sperm concentration, the fact that the straw contains refrozen semen, and other pertinent information.
- If the original straw was frozen at a concentration of 200 million total sperm/ml, or 100 million sperm per straw, the new straws will contain approximately 1 million sperm each.
- A straw of the refrozen stallion semen can subsequently be selected and a 2–4 mm piece cut with a scalpel blade under liquid nitrogen and the remainder of the cut straw returned to the tank.
- The cut piece can be transferred into a droplet of medium at 38.5°C (101°F) to thaw. After 10 minutes, a small aliquot of supernatant can be removed and a progressively motile, morphologically normal spermatozoon selected for ICSI.
- Incorporating a cut-straw approach to a straw of diluted refrozen semen will only "waste" a few thousand spermatozoa instead of several million. Ultimately, thawing a single straw of valuable stallion semen, diluting it in additional freezing extender, transferring the diluted semen into multiple new straws and refreezing can provide an almost unlimited supply of spermatozoa for assisted reproduction techniques such as ICSI.

Interpretation

- Thawing, diluting, and refreezing stallion semen results in significantly lower total and progressive motility, plasma membrane integrity, and acrosome integrity after the second freeze as compared with after the initial freeze. However, refreezing does not result in an increase in sperm chromatin structure damage.
- Stallion semen initially frozen in one cryopreservation extender can be thawed and diluted in a different extender and refrozen without significant detriment to the spermatozoa.
- Several studies have shown that diluting stallion semen, initially frozen in an extender containing glycerol alone, in an extender containing both glycerol and methylformamide results in better post-thaw motility after refreezing than diluting with extender-only containing glycerol.
- Refrozen stallion semen is currently used in commercial ICSI programs to generate embryos that are transferred into recipient mares resulting in the birth of live healthy foals.
- Refrozen semen has also been used in ICSI to produce embryos that are subsequently cryopreserved for transfer at a later date.
- Frozen stallion semen has even been thawed, sex-sorted by flow cytometry, refrozen, and subsequently used for ICSI to generate embryos and live sex-selected foals.
- Even the small number of motile spermatozoa obtained after thawing a small piece of a frozen straw (i.e., a cut-straw technique) can be diluted in freezing extender and refrozen.

Further Reading

Carnevale EM, Graham JK, Suh TK, Stokes JE, Squires EL. 2008. Foals produced after ICSI using frozen, sex-sorted, refrozen sperm. *Reprod Fertil Develop* 21: 228.

Choi YH, Love CC, Varner DD, Hinrichs K. 2006. Equine blastocyst development after intracytoplasmic injection of sperm subjected to two freeze-thaw cycles. *Theriogenology* 65: 808–19.

Gonzalez-Castro R, Amoroso-Sanches F, Rossi M, Graham JK, Carnevale EM. 2016. Effect of extenders on the refreezing of stallion semen for ICSI. *J Eq Vet Sci* 43: S70.

Leisinger CA, Pinto CR, Cramer E, Love CC, Paccamonti DL. 2017. Effects of repeated partial thaw and refreeze on post-thaw parameters of stallion semen cryopreserved in cryovials. *J Eq Vet Sci* 49: 19–24.

McCue PM, Moore AI, Bruemmer JE. 2003. Refreezing stallion spermatozoa for assisted reproduction. *Reprod Fertil Develop* 16: 176–7.

Sielhorst J, Hagen C, Behrendt D, Schuette B, Burger D, Martinsson G, Sieme H. 2016. Effect of multiple freezing of stallion semen on sperm quality and fertility. *J Eq Vet Sci* 40: 56–61.

155

Thawing Frozen Semen

John J. Dascanio

School of Veterinary Medicine, Texas Tech University, USA

Introduction

Frozen semen should be thawed immediately before use. Typically, thawing instructions are provided by the person or facility that initially froze the semen. Frozen semen in North America is most commonly packaged in 0.5 ml semen straws, but may also be packaged in 5 ml straws, 2.5 ml straws, glass vials, or ampules.

Equipment and Supplies

Semen storage tank, thermo-protective gloves, safety glasses, two pairs of long-handled forceps, water bath, straw cutter, paper towels, examination gloves.

Technique

- Move the water bath and the semen storage tank near each other.
- Prepare a water bath that is at the correct temperature for the type of semen to be thawed. The shipper of the semen should provide thawing directions. Typically 0.5 ml semen straws are thawed at 37°C (99°F) for 30 seconds, and 2.5 or 5 ml semen straws are usually thawed at 50°C (122°F) for 45 seconds. There may be variations to these two protocols depending on the facility that initially froze the semen. Read and follow the thawing instructions that accompany the frozen semen.
- The water bath should have a volume of water present that will not cool off with the expected number of straws to thaw. An electric temperature-controlled water bath is ideal, but any leak-proof vessel can be used. A thermometer should be placed in the water bath to confirm the temperature.
- The water bath should allow for the complete immersion of the straw. With 5 ml straws, confirm that the thawing vesicle is long enough to accommodate the length of the straw – usually a minimum of a 30 cm (12 inches) length.
- Determine the correct tank, canister, and cane where the frozen semen is located.
- Wear thermo-protective gloves and protective eye glasses when handling liquid nitrogen.
- Make sure that you are in an area that has good ventilation and air circulation. Nitrogen vapor displaces oxygen and can lead to asphyxiation in a closed room.
- Clothing and shoes should not be capable of absorbing liquid nitrogen as this could lead to freezing injury if a spill of liquid nitrogen were to occur.
- To remove a semen straw from the tank, first remove the Styrofoam™ cork/plug. Lift the canister upward, but make sure that the semen straws remain below the frost line in the tank neck (Figure 155.1). Canisters are usually numbered sequentially around the top of the tank neck.
- Remove the semen straws from the appropriate goblet/cane/canister location (Figure 155.2) and transfer into the water bath with as little delay as possible. The Styrofoam™ cork/plug in the top of the semen tank should be replaced as soon as the semen has been removed from the tank to avoid liquid nitrogen loss.
- Identify the appropriate cane from information written on the top of the cane.
- Using long-handled forceps, grasp the appropriate cane and elevate it from the canister so that a semen straw may be grasped with a second pair of forceps. Be careful to not bend the straw during extraction as it may fracture in the frozen state. Make sure to keep the remaining semen straws below the frost line in the tank neck. The top of the cane may be bent upward to facilitate removal of straws without bending them.

Equine Reproductive Procedures, Second Edition. Edited by John Dascanio and Patrick McCue.

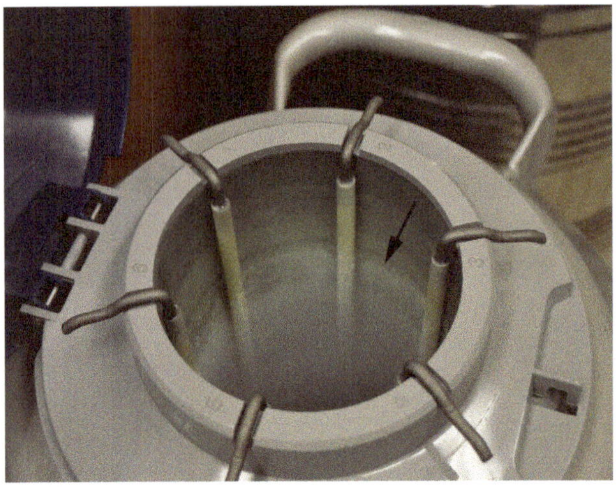

Figure 155.1 Frost line inside the neck of a semen tank (black arrow). Make sure to keep semen straws below this during manipulations.

- Being careful to not drop the straw, transfer it immediately to the prepared water bath. Caution should be exercised to ensure that liquid nitrogen does not come into contact with the water bath as it will immediately vaporize, possibly causing injury. With multiple straws, a goblet may be completely removed from the cane, the straws dumped onto a paper towel, and then the straws immediately placed into the water bath. The paper towel will absorb any liquid nitrogen preventing it from coming into contact with the water bath.
- Alternatively, the cane containing the straws of frozen semen may be transferred into a Styrofoam™ box filled with a 2–3 cm (0.75–1 inch) depth of liquid nitrogen. This will allow for an opportunity to select the individual straws to be thawed and to also verify the name of the stallion. The appropriate straws can then be moved into the water bath and the cane with the remaining straws transferred back into the original storage tank. Ideally, all long-handled forceps to be used for handling straws of frozen semen should be pre-cooled by immersing the working end in a bath of liquid nitrogen.
- Allow the straws to remain in the water bath for the appropriate amount of time. Then remove the straw(s) and dry them with a paper towel. Water must be removed from the outside of the straw as it may be harmful to the spermatozoa.
- Read the label carefully on each straw to double check that it is from the appropriate stallion.
- Shake the air bubble in the straw toward the end that will be cut. This is the end that has been sealed with polyvinyl chloride powder, heat-sealed, or plugged with a metal ball.
- Cut the correct end of the straw. The other end of the straw with the cotton plug or pledget usually remains intact so that a direct straw insemination method may be used. The straw can be cut with a sharp instrument such as a scalpel blade or a commercial semen straw cutter rather than scissors (Figure 155.3). Scissors may crimp or crush the straw end, resulting in an oblong opening that will not seal as well within the insemination pipette if a direct transfer is to be performed. If a commercial semen straw cutter is used, make sure it is taken apart and cleaned/disinfected regularly to remove potential semen deposits and bacterial/fungal overgrowth.

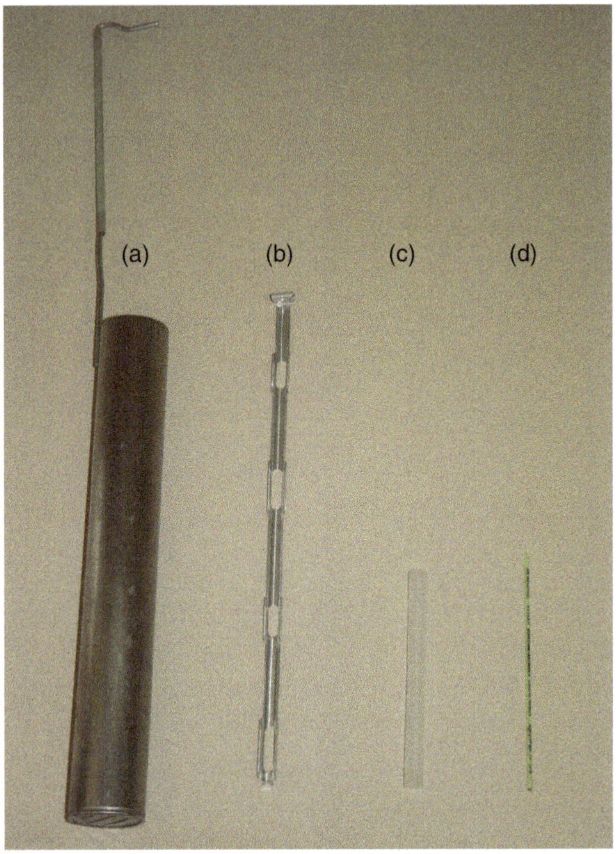

Figure 155.2 Organizational scheme for the storage of semen showing a canister (A), cane (B), goblet (C), and semen straw (D). The straw(s) is(are) placed into the goblet. Up to two goblets are snapped onto the cane and the cane is placed into the canister. Usually a few canisters, each with multiple canes, are present within a semen tank.

- Semen straws may be used directly for insemination or may be emptied into a small container (sterile glass test tube, red-top Vacutainer® tube) from which semen can be aspirated into a pipette for insemination.

Interpretation

- Semen straws should be placed into a water bath within 6–8 seconds after their removal from a storage tank. This

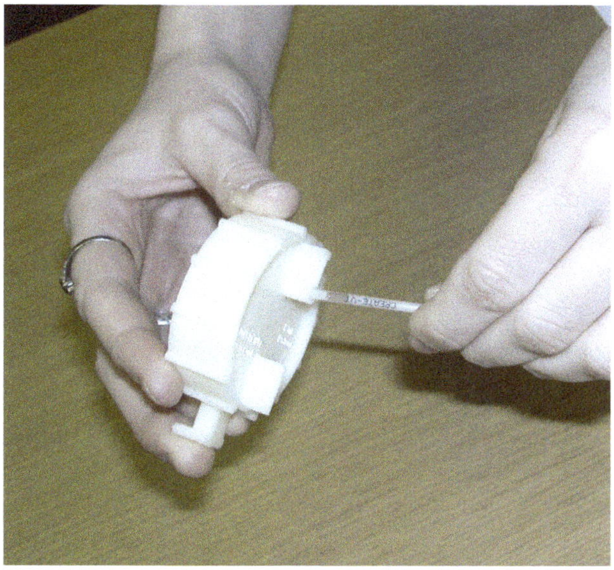

Figure 155.3 Commercial straw cutter. Make sure to clean the internal aspect of the cutter regularly to prevent mold/bacterial growth contaminants.

is approximately the time that a straw will remain frozen at room temperature.

- If the plug in the end of the semen straw becomes completely displaced during thawing, carefully plug the end of the straw with a gloved finger to prevent water in the water bath from entering the semen straw.
- The cut end of the semen straw should not be squished or crimped whilst removing the plug/ball bearing from the straw end. A crimped straw will not seat properly within an insemination gun during direct insemination, possibly causing leakage of semen within the apparatus. Crimping most often occurs when scissors are used to cut the straw.
- Occasionally, a single, small, cotton plug will eject out of a semen straw end during the transfer of semen between tanks or from a tank into a water bath. Usually this is not a concern, as the polyvinyl chloride powder in that end of the straw is most likely intact. The reason the cotton plug was dislodged was due to the fact it was not wet during the initial freezing process and has subsequently absorbed liquid nitrogen that expanded when warmed, causing the effective blowout of the plug.
- If it is known that frozen semen from a particular stallion (i.e., from one freeze date) has a tendency to have the straws crack or the ends blowout during freezing, the straws can be placed into a sealed plastic bag (e.g., Ziploc® bag) that is subsequently immersed in the water bath for thawing.

Further Reading

Dascanio JJ, Kasimanickam R. 2008. Breeding the mare with frozen semen. *Eq Vet Educ* 20: 667–72.

156

Semen Processing for Intracytoplasmic Sperm Injection

Patrick M. McCue

Equine Reproduction Laboratory, Colorado State University, USA

Introduction

Stallion spermatozoa for intracytoplasmic sperm injection (ICSI) can be acquired from fresh, cooled-transported, frozen, refrozen, and even lyophilized semen. Appropriate processing of semen is critically important in order to optimize ICSI success. This chapter discusses laboratory techniques for processing semen for ICSI.

A majority of clinical ICSI procedures are performed using frozen-thawed semen from a stallion selected by the owner of the oocyte donor mare. Frozen semen may be available as a traditionally cryopreserved dose (i.e., either 100 or 200 million total sperm per 0.5 ml straw), or initially cryopreserved as "ICSI doses" (variable; often ~1 million total sperm per straw), or a traditionally cryopreserved straw may be thawed, further diluted with additional cryoprotectant, and refrozen as "ICSI doses" with a variable number of spermatozoa per straw (see Chapter 154).

Equipment and Supplies

Liquid nitrogen tank, canes with goblets, water bath with thermometer, timer, long-handled tongs, sperm TALP, pipetters and tips, centrifuge, 15 ml centrifuge tubes, scissors, glycidoxypropyltrimethoxysilane-coated silica colloid, synthetic oviductal fluid–*in vitro* fertilization (SOF-IVF) medium, polyvinylpyrrolidone, phosphate buffered saline, thermo-protective gloves, safety glasses.

Sperm Processing Techniques

Although it is possible to thaw an entire straw of frozen semen to obtain a few motile spermatozoa for one ICSI session, it is common in commercial ICSI programs to cut off a small portion of a straw while under liquid nitrogen. Only the small cut portion is thawed in order to optimize the use of the entire frozen semen straw. In many cases only a limited quantity of frozen semen is available. The remainder of the straw is placed back into a labeled goblet, attached to a labeled cane, and replaced into a storage tank of liquid nitrogen. It is common practice at some ICSI facilities to place a second "inverted" goblet over the open end of the goblet containing the cut straw so that the straw does not float out of the goblet during subsequent storage once placed into a liquid nitrogen tank.

The most common techniques for processing frozen stallion semen for ICSI are swim-up, washing, single layer centrifugation, density gradient centrifugation, microfluidic sorting, or a combination of the procedures. Each clinical ICSI laboratory will have their own variations on semen processing related to equipment used, sperm media preferred, centrifugation speeds and time, and the number of swim-up or centrifugation steps. In addition, some ICSI laboratories tailor sperm processing procedures for individual stallions.

Swim-Up

Whole straw

- If an entire straw of frozen is to be used, the semen is placed into a water bath at 37–38.2°C (99–101°F) for 30 seconds. The thawed semen is subsequently layered beneath 1.0 ml of sperm media (Tyrode's albumin–lactate–pyruvate medium, also known as sperm TALP, or similar medium) and allowed to incubate for approximately 20 minutes (see Chapter 144).
- The top ~0.5 ml of medium containing live motile spermatozoa that have moved up out of the thawed semen is subsequently collected and washed by one to two rounds of centrifugation at 300–350 × g for 3–5 minutes and resuspended in sperm media.

Equine Reproductive Procedures, Second Edition. Edited by John Dascanio and Patrick McCue.

- After the last centrifugation, the pellet containing spermatozoa is resuspended a final time in sperm media.
- A small volume of this sperm suspension is collected, out of which one or more spermatozoa are identified for subsequent ICSI.

Cut straw

- If a cut-straw approach is used, the small (<5 mm) section of straw removed, while under liquid nitrogen, is transferred into a sterile 5 ml plastic tube containing 1.0 ml of sperm media and the tube is subsequently placed into a CO_2 incubator at 38.2°C (100.8°F). After a 15-minute incubation period, a 0.5 ml volume of the supernatant is removed and transferred into a 15 ml conical tube.
- The conical tube is subsequently centrifuged at 300–350 × *g* for 3–5 minutes to pellet the spermatozoa in the bottom of the tube. An incubation period of 5–20 minutes is used to allow motile spermatozoa to swim up out of the pellet into the supernatant.
- A small volume of supernatant is subsequently collected and spermatozoa identified for ICSI.

Washing

In a washing technique, thawed semen is diluted directly into sperm media followed by centrifugation at 300–350 × *g* for 3–5 minutes.

- The supernatant is removed and the sperm pellet resuspended in fresh sperm media.
- This process is repeated two additional times; after the third round of centrifugation, the supernatant is removed and the sperm pellet again resuspended in sperm media for eventual use in ICSI.

Density Centrifugation

Single layer procedure

- A single layer centrifugation procedure can be used to clean up the frozen semen and yield a pellet containing a high concentration of motile, morphologically normal, and DNA intact spermatozoa.
- A 3–4 ml volume of glycidoxypropyltrimethoxysilane-coated silica colloid (e.g., AndroColl-E™, Swedish University of Agricultural Sciences, Uppsala, Sweden; EquiPure™, Nidacon International AB, Mölndal, Sweden) is dispensed into a 15 ml conical tube.
- A single 0.5 ml straw of semen is thawed and the entire volume is layered onto the top of the colloid. The tube is centrifuged at approximately 300 × *g* for 20 minutes or 200 × *g* for 30 minutes.
- The sperm pellet is recovered from the bottom of the tube and washed twice as described previously in sperm media prior to use in ICSI.

Density gradient procedure

- Alternatively, a density gradient centrifugation procedure can be used by preparation of 45% and 90% colloid fractions.
- The 90% colloid is dispensed into the bottom of a centrifuge tube and the 45% colloid is gently applied above the 90% layer.
- The thawed semen is gently added to the top.
- The tube is subsequently centrifuged at 700 × *g* for 40 minutes, after which the sperm pellet is resuspended in TALP and washed as previously described.

Density Centrifugation Plus Swim-Up

- A volume of thawed semen is applied to the top of a 3.0 ml column of colloid within a 15 ml conical tube and centrifuged for 30 minutes at 200 × *g*.
- The sperm pellet is resuspended in 50 µl of sperm media, which is subsequently applied to the bottom of a 1.0 ml volume of fresh sperm media.
- Motile sperm are allowed to swim-up into the supernatant for 20 minutes. A small volume of the supernatant is subsequently collected and motile sperm identified for ICSI.

Final Sperm Preparation

After the final wash, sperm pellets are resuspended in synthetic oviductal fluid-*in vitro* fertilization (SOF-IVF) medium and subsequently diluted in polyvinylpyrrolidone 12% (Sigma-Aldrich, Milan, Italy) in phosphate buffered saline before ICSI.

Additional Comments

The specific technique(s) used for sperm processing in an ICSI program will depend on the number of straws of frozen semen available, number of sperm per straw, requirement for use of the cut-thaw approach, post-thaw motility, previous fertility history with the frozen semen, individual laboratory preferences, and other factors.

References

Choi YH, Chung YG, Walker SC, Westhusin ME, Hinrichs K. 2003. In vitro development of equine nuclear transfer embryos: effects of oocyte maturation media and amino acid composition during embryo culture. *Zygote* 11: 77–86.

Colleoni S, Lagutina I, Lazzari G, Rodriguez-Martinez H, Galli C, Morrell JM. 2011. New methods for selecting stallion spermatozoa for assisted reproduction. *J Eq Vet Sci* 31: 536–41.

Morris LH, Maclellan LJ. 2019. Update on advanced semen-processing technologies and their application for in vitro embryo production in horses. *Reprod Fertil Dev* 31: 1771–7.

157

Preparing a Vapor Shipper

Julie T. Cecere[1] *and Paul Loomis*[2]

[1] *Virginia-Maryland College of Veterinary Medicine, USA*
[2] *Select Breeders Services, USA*

Introduction

Vapor shippers, or dry shippers, are used on a daily basis to ship cryogenically preserved specimens between facilities. These containers can maintain an internal temperature of −180°C (−300°F) for 1–3 weeks, while eliminating the hazards associated with shipping liquid nitrogen. Most vapor shippers used today contain a hydrophobic absorbent that can resist moisture and humidity, but absorb liquid nitrogen. These absorbents are crucial to the shipper's functionality and if damaged result in the contamination or loss of samples and possibly the container itself.

Proper disinfection, filling, and packing of these shippers is essential. International shipment of samples may require a higher level of disinfection than domestic shipment. It is important to understand all shipment and importation requirements prior to the date of shipment. The vapor shipper should be filled and packaged in accordance with the manufacturer's specifications. Advanced notice should be provided to the semen storage facility for shipment of frozen semen in order to ensure adequate time to clean and charge the vapor shipper.

Equipment and Supplies

30% bleach solution, examination gloves, sterile gauze, sterile water, liquid nitrogen, digital weight scale, metal funnel, thermo-protective gloves, safety glasses, vapor (dry) shipper, vapor shipping mailing container.

Disinfection Technique

- Choose which shipper you are going to use and determine the disinfection level, filling capacity, and weight when fully charged of that shipper. This information should be provided by the manufacturer.
- Remove the tank from its shipping container.
- If a lower level of disinfection is desired, or the shipper has been used recently, wiping the inside and outside of the canister down with a 30% bleach solution is sufficient.
- If shipping internationally, if a known contamination has occurred, or if a higher level of disinfection is required one of the following must be done:
  - Fill the vapor shipper to top of the neck with a bleach solution and allow it to sit for 30 minutes. Pour out the bleach and wash the shipper by filling it with sterile water and emptying three times. Allow the container to drain upside down until completely dry.
  - Gas sterilization of the entire tank with ethylene oxide at a local hospital or other facility is also acceptable.
- Disinfectants that cannot be used with a hydrophobic absorbent membrane are Viralex™ (Alda Pharmaceuticals Corp., Vancouver, Canada) and 70% ethanol. These will irreversibly damage the membrane and render your shipper unusable.

Filling Technique

- Wear thermo-protective gloves (Figure 157.1) and protective eye glasses when handling liquid nitrogen.
- Make sure that you are in an area that has good ventilation and air circulation. Nitrogen vapor can lead to asphyxiation in a closed room as it can rapidly displace oxygen.
- Porous clothing, such as canvas shoes, should be avoided when working with liquid nitrogen to avoid absorption/penetration of coolant.

Equine Reproductive Procedures, Second Edition. Edited by John Dascanio and Patrick McCue.

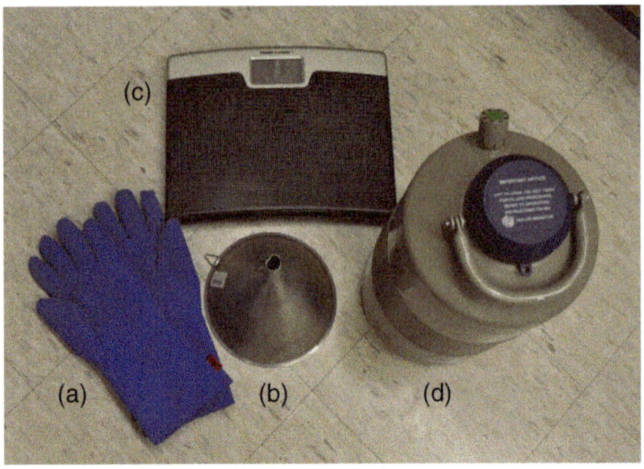

Figure 157.1 Filling supplies, showing thermo-protective gloves (A), a funnel for pouring liquid nitrogen into the vapor shipper (B), a digital scale to weigh the vapor shipper after filling (C), and a vapor shipper (D).

- Remove the vapor shipper out of the protective shipping container. A round top protective container or a square top container of hard plastic usually protects the actual vapor shipper (Figures 157.2 and 157.3).
- Remove the top of the shipper and insert a stainless steel funnel. If you are using a pressurized tank with a cryogenic phase separator nozzle to fill the vapor shipper, the funnel is not necessary as the nozzle fits nicely into the canister opening.
- When filling the vapor shipper, do not position yourself over the neck of the container as nitrogen vapor will forcefully exit a warm container and there is potential for splashing of liquid nitrogen out of the tank.
- Fill the canister to the top with liquid nitrogen without the liquid nitrogen overflowing the container and contacting the seal at the top of the container. This can crack the material and render it useless.
- With the Styrofoam™ plug in place, allow the liquid nitrogen to absorb into the shipper's wall (Figure 157.4). A completely warm tank may need to be refilled several times before it reaches the manufacturer's specified weight and liquid remains visible in the canister.
- Once the liquid nitrogen level remains static and no more liquid nitrogen will absorb into the wall of the shipper, all of the liquid nitrogen should be poured off.
- It is critical that no liquid remains in the vapor shipper. Since it is being shipped without a hazardous materials classification there cannot be any liquid nitrogen in the container. If there is residual liquid nitrogen in the container then the shipper is liable for shipping dangerous goods without proper documentation and if detected the fines can be considerable.

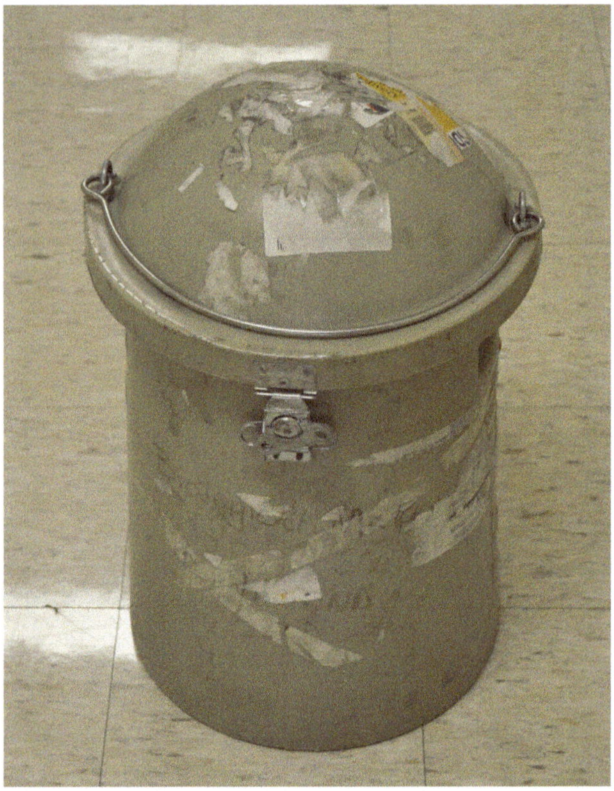

Figure 157.2 Mushroom top protective shipping container (with the vapor shipper inside). The round top inhibits someone from turning the tank upside down, allowing the tank to be stored in an upright position only, and protecting the tank from damage or premature warming. Even though it is a vapor shipper and contains no liquid nitrogen, the nitrogen gas is heavier than air and if tipped on its side the gas in the container will "pour" out, minimizing the holding time of the shipper.

- When replacing the Styrofoam™ cork back into the neck of the container take care to make sure there is no moisture from condensation in the grooves of the cork that the canister handle passes through. If there is moisture present, it can freeze when placed in the neck of the container trapping the canister handle in ice and making it difficult to open without damaging the cork.
- Place the Styrofoam™ plug in the vapor shipper and place it back into its shipping container.

Interpretation

- Examine the Styrofoam™ plug insert for wear. It should fit without gaps, as gaps will result in premature warming of the shipper.
- Check the vapor shipper weight at 12 hours. Add liquid nitrogen if it has not maintained its proper weight. The

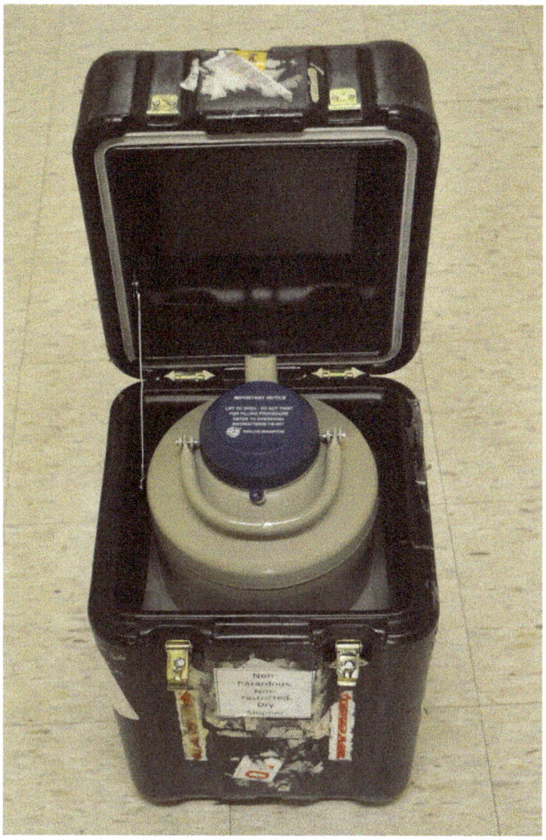

Figure 157.3 Square protective container with a vapor shipper in place.

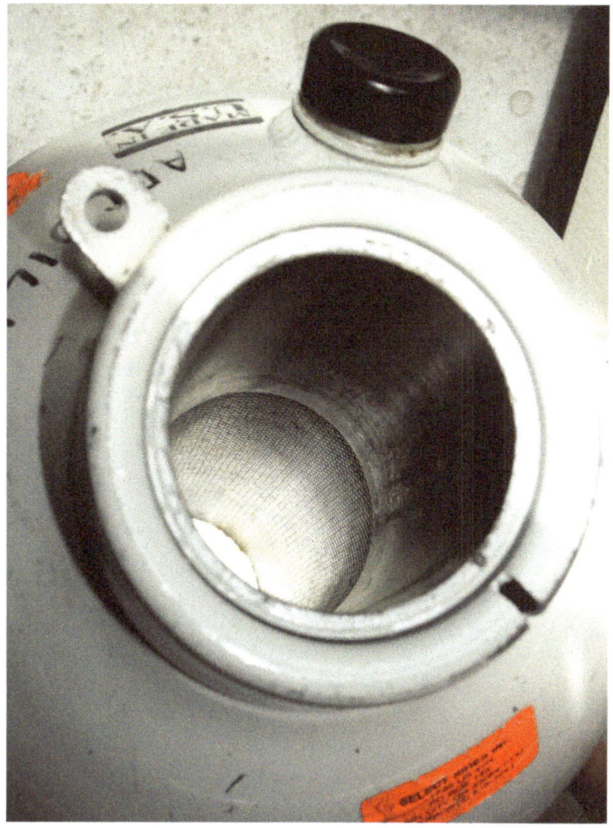

Figure 157.4 View inside a vapor shipper demonstrating the mesh in the lower part of the tank that liquid nitrogen passes through to be absorbed into the wall.

manufacturer should provide a filled or charged weight and a dry weight for the vapor shipper.

- Check the vapor shipper weight again at 24 hours to make sure it is maintaining its weight and is not prematurely warming. A "puff" of vapor may be seen exiting a charged tank (Figure 157.5).
- In general, most vapor shippers are good for at least 7 days, with a quoted static holding time from 8 to 21 days under controlled conditions. Time frames vary drastically depending on the type of tank, shipping conditions, and outer packaging. Be sure to check on the type of tank you are using for guidelines on the time frame to hold a charge to prevent loss of semen due to premature thawing.
- The semen should be transferred into a permanent semen storage tank upon arrival or used within 24–72 hours.
- The shipping container must be maintained in an upright orientation or the vapor shipper will lose the liquid nitrogen charge and prematurely warm.
- All vapor shippers must be evaluated prior to the breeding season. This involves filling the shipper followed by daily evaluation of weight and temperature. This ensures that the vapor shipper is maintaining its specified static holding time. Refer to the shipper's manual for instructions.

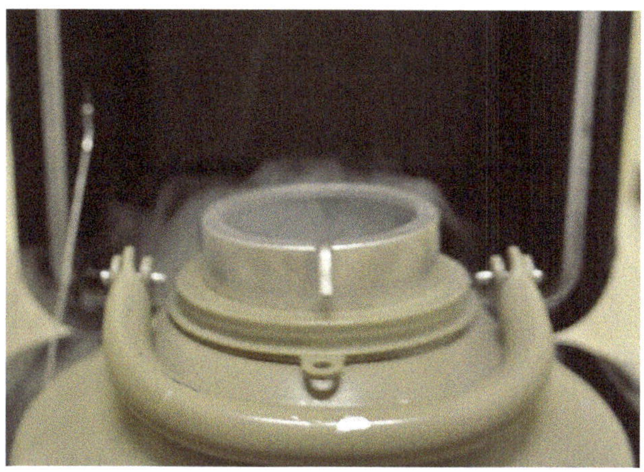

Figure 157.5 Liquid nitrogen vapor "puff" in a charged dewar.

Further Reading

Bielanski A. 2005. Experimental microbial contamination and disinfection of dry (vapour) shipper dewars designed for short-term storage and transportation of cryopreserved germplasm and other biological specimens. *Theriogenology* 63: 1946–57.

158

Loading a Vapor Shipper

Julie T. Cecere[1] *and Paul Loomis*[2]

[1] *Virginia-Maryland College of Veterinary Medicine, USA*
[2] *Select Breeders Services, USA*

Introduction

Once you have charged your vapor shipper properly, loading the shipper with the frozen semen should be fast and simple. On average you have less than 10 seconds of exposing the frozen semen to room temperature before the sample starts to thaw. A general rule of 5–8 seconds maximum at room temperature will prevent premature thawing. Repeated chilling and thawing is detrimental to any cryopreserved sample. Prepare containers side by side prior to transferring frozen semen to minimize the chances of inadvertently thawing the semen.

Paperwork included in a shipment of frozen semen should include:

- Thawing instructions.
- Facility that froze the semen.
- Name of the stallion and registration number.
- Collection/freeze date.
- Lot number or straw ID code.
- Post-thaw motility.
- Number of breeding doses.
- Number of straws per dose.
- Total number of sperm per dose.
- Equine viral arteritis (EVA) status of stallion and/or semen.
- Name of the mare and registration number.
- Instructions for return of container.
- Policy regarding unused semen.
- Breed registry certificates (if needed).

Equipment and Supplies

Liquid nitrogen, long-handled hemostats (at least two), shallow Styrofoam™ container large enough to fit one standard cane, thermo-protective gloves, safety glasses, cotton plug, vapor shipper.

Technique

- Place the vapor shipper next to the long-term liquid nitrogen storage dewar.
- Determine the number of samples (straws, vials, etc.) you are sending. If the entire cane is not to be shipped, you must prepare another cane and goblet prior to sample transfer.
- If you are transferring an entire cane, open the tops of each container and transfer the cane directly into the vapor shipper from the long-term storage dewar using forceps.

Preparing a Goblet or Cane for Loading When Only Sending a Partial Goblet

- Don protective apparel.
- Pour liquid nitrogen into the bottom of a shallow Styrofoam™ container to a depth of 2.5–5 cm (1–2 inches).
- Label the top of an empty cane with the appropriate identifying information.
- Plunge the empty cane and a goblet into the liquid nitrogen to allow the materials to equilibrate to liquid nitrogen temperature. The liquid nitrogen will stop boiling when the temperatures of the objects equilibrate.
- Remove the lid from the permanent storage tank and locate the straws to be transferred. Make sure to keep the canister below the frost level in the tank.
- Once the sample is located, grasp the cane with a long-handled hemostat and slowly lower the canister so it can recess into the tank. Keep the canister centered in the tank in case the cane is accidently dropped. Keep the cane below the frost line (Figure 158.1).
- Straws are fragile at this temperature. Make sure not to bend the straw too sharply during the transfer. The tab

Equine Reproductive Procedures, Second Edition. Edited by John Dascanio and Patrick McCue.

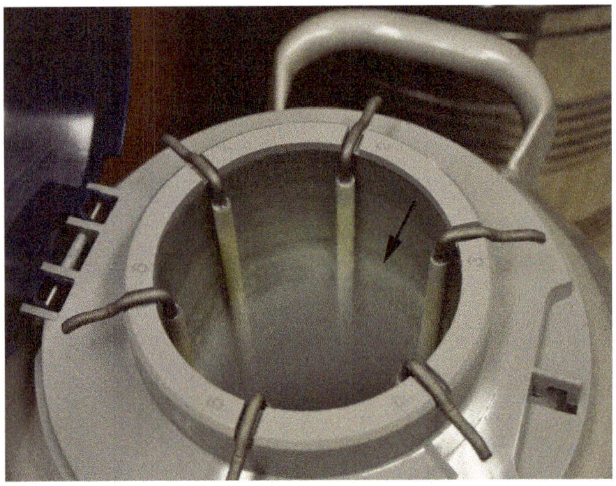

Figure 158.1 Frost line in a long-term storage tank.

on the top of the cane may be bent outward to slightly straighten it so that it is easier to remove straws from a goblet.

- With another pre-cooled hemostat, one at a time, pull out the straw(s) needed and plunge them into the liquid nitrogen in the Styrofoam™ container. Make sure they are submerged in liquid nitrogen.
- Place the originating cane and canister back in its place and put the lid back on the permanent storage tank.
- While working in the liquid nitrogen in the Styrofoam™ box, use hemostats to place the straws that are going to be shipped into the appropriate goblet/cane pair. Make sure all straws stay within the liquid nitrogen. Use this time to inspect the individual straws to verify the stallion name and lot number or freeze date on the straws and ensure that there are no cracks or extruded sealing balls or cotton plugs.
- Remove the Styrofoam™ plug from the vapor shipper. Grasp the cane to be transferred with a hemostat and place it into the canister of the vapor shipper.
- Loose cotton can be placed inside the canister, on and around the cane, to prevent the straws from dislodging during shipment or the cane from moving around inside the cannister.
- Once all your samples are within the vapor shipper, replace the Styrofoam™ plug and secure the lid to the tank with a zip tie.

Interpretation

Vapor shippers should be evaluated on a regular schedule. International shipment from the United States requires that semen be collected, processed, and frozen at a US Department of Agriculture approved collection center. Individual countries (e.g., Australia) or geopolitical units (e.g., European Union) have their own regulations regarding the importation of frozen semen. Therefore, it is critical that these regulations be fully understood prior to freezing. Specialized blood tests, cultures, and a quarantine period are often required. The complete regulations and requirements can be accessed at http://www.aphis.usda.gov/regulations/vs/iregs/animals/ (last accessed Oct 2020).

Further Reading

Loomis PR. 2011. Storage management and distribution of frozen semen. In: McKinnon AO, Squires EL, Vaala WE, Varner DD (eds). Equine Reproduction, 2nd edn. Ames, IA: Wiley Blackwell, pp. 3005–14.

Loomis PR, Squires EL. 2005. Frozen semen management in equine breeding programs. *Theriogenology* 64: 480–91.

Metcalf ES. 2011. Import and export of frozen semen. In: McKinnon AO, Squires EL, Vaala WE, Varner DD (eds). Equine Reproduction, 2nd edn. Ames, IA: Wiley Blackwell, pp. 3029–35.

159

Maintaining a Long-Term Frozen Semen Storage Tank

John J. Dascanio

School of Veterinary Medicine, Texas Tech University, USA

Introduction

Long-term storage of semen should be managed by a facility that has the capability to continuously monitor liquid nitrogen levels in the semen tanks. Tanks should be monitored a minimum of once per week for liquid nitrogen level and should be examined daily for any signs of failure. A monitoring and refilling log should be kept next to the tank, recording tank number/name, level of liquid nitrogen in centimeters, date/time, and person performing the measurement.

The tank should be locked to prevent unintended access to the contents. A detailed semen log should be kept identifying the location of each semen dose, laboratory that prepared the semen, date of freezing, stallion's registration information, along with thawing instructions, and post-thaw evaluation. The canisters containing the canes, goblets, and semen straws should be all easily read and properly labeled.

Semen tanks are designed for different storage capacities and holding times with both small and large capacity tanks. The larger neck diameter tanks are easier to get samples out of, but will also result in increased liquid nitrogen usage through evaporation. The number of times semen is accessed in a tank will also influence liquid nitrogen loss.

Equipment and Supplies

Long-term storage tanks, locks, recording paperwork or software, plastic measuring stick, stainless steel funnel, source of liquid nitrogen from a dewar or commercial service.

Technique

- Semen tanks should be stored in a room that has good ventilation and air circulation. Nitrogen vapor can displace air and lead to asphyxiation in a closed room. The tank should not be stored in direct sunlight to avoid inadvertent tank heating and should not be in direct contact with a concrete floor to prevent corrosion.
- Wear thermo-protective gloves and protective eye glasses when handling liquid nitrogen.
- Porous clothing, such as canvas shoes, should be avoided when working with liquid nitrogen to avoid absorption/penetration of coolant.
- Unlock the semen tank to be examined.
- Insert a plastic measuring stick into the tank so that it contacts the bottom of the tank. Be careful that the stick is not on top of any metal guides for canisters and is actually on the bottom of the tank. Hold the stick in place until it has cooled to the internal temperature. This is determined by the cessation of nitrogen "bubbling" that occurs with the insertion of a warm object into liquid nitrogen. Be careful not to look directly down the neck of the tank while performing the measurement in case liquid nitrogen bubbles upward.
- Pull the stick out of the tank and swing the stick in the air a few times to cause frosting of the stick. Immediately read the length of the frost on the stick (Figure 159.1). This corresponds to the height of liquid nitrogen within the storage tank. Record the depth on a log sheet.
- Refill the tank as needed to keep the liquid level more than half full at all times. Do not overfill the tank as this may result in premature failure of the seal in the neck of the tank from liquid nitrogen exposure.

Equine Reproductive Procedures, Second Edition. Edited by John Dascanio and Patrick McCue.

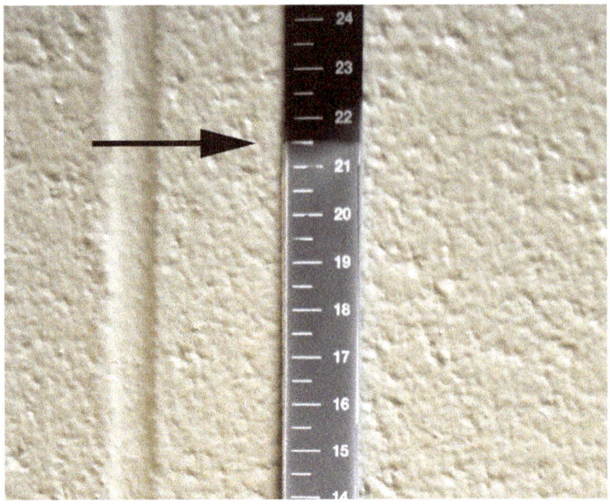

Figure 159.1 Frost line on a measuring stick. The level of liquid nitrogen in the tank measured would be approximately 21.5 cm (arrow).

Additional Comments

- Plan to have an alternative location to store semen in case of a tank failure. A failing tank is one that is losing or has lost the vacuum within the wall of the tank and thus has lost its insulating capability.
- The tank may be failing if the time between refilling is becoming shorter. This is demonstrated by the liquid nitrogen level inside the tank falling faster than normal during monitoring examinations. If condensation is noted on the outside of the tank, the contents should be immediately transferred to another tank as this tank is failing.
- Examine the monitoring/refilling log for trends in increased liquid nitrogen usage.
- Examine the Styrofoam™ plug insert for wear. It should fit without gaps, as gapping will result in premature warming of the tank contents. Frosting outside the plug on the neck of the tank may also indicate a failing tank or ill-fitting plug.
- Tanks more than 10 years of age should be considered for replacement prior to their failing.
- The tank should not be in direct contact with the ground as this may increase rusting and deterioration of the tank. Ideally, the tank should be on rollers to allow movement for filling and distribution of semen straws and to allow for air flow around the tank (Figure 159.2).

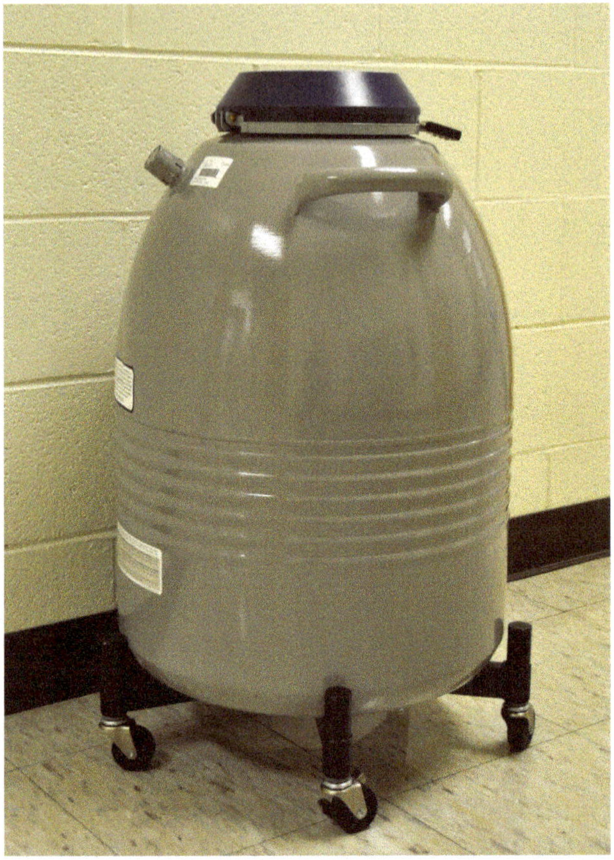

Figure 159.2 Semen tank on rollers.

- The numbers on the outside of the semen tank are often linked to the quantity of liquid nitrogen that the tank holds and how many weeks the tank will hold liquid nitrogen between refilling. Thus, a 34/18 tank will hold 34 liters of liquid nitrogen for 18 weeks between fills. This holding time frame assumes a closed tank that is not regularly accessed. If an additional number is present on the tank, it refers to the number of canisters present within the tank.
- A "V" on the tank will indicate that it is a vapor shipper and not intended for long-term storage of semen.
- Alarm systems are commercially available to either continuously monitor the temperature with liquid nitrogen tanks or to send an alert in the event of an excessive loss of liquid nitrogen.

Further Reading

Loomis PR. 2001. Storage, handling and distribution of frozen equine semen. *Proc Annu Conv Am Assoc Eq Pract* 47: 296–301.

160

International Transport of Frozen Semen

Paul Loomis

Select Breeders Services, USA

Introduction

A major advantage of frozen semen is that it allows breeders access to superior genetics from stallions located in other countries. However, with the increased use of frozen semen in the equine industry, veterinary and agricultural agencies are concerned about possible disease transmission through global distribution of frozen semen. Successful cryopreservation of spermatozoa requires suspension of sperm in special diluents followed by controlled cooling and freezing in liquid nitrogen. The same process will also preserve vectors of potential venereal disease such as bacteria and viruses. In order to minimize this risk, most countries have established regulations that must be met for semen to be imported into the country. Prior to undertaking a semen freezing program for international distribution, one should understand the regulations that must be adhered to for semen to qualify for importation into the country of choice.

Unfortunately, there is no single set of regulations that applies to all countries, and authorities may change regulations or completely close borders for the import of stallion semen at any time and for any reason. This chapter focuses primarily on the regulations for collection and freezing of semen for export from the United States to member states of the European Union (EU). Although many other countries employ similar regulations, they are not exactly the same and may require different health testing protocols, collection center specifications, or donor stallion residency requirements. Ultimately, the best way to ensure compliance is for the importer to apply for an import permit with that country's Ministry of Agriculture (or equivalent body). If granted, the permit should specify what conditions must be met for the semen to be qualified.

For current regulations published by the US Department of Agriculture (USDA), health certificate templates, and lists of approved facilities, consult the USDA Animal and Plant Health Inspection Service (APHIS) IRegs and select the country of interest under the "IRegs for LIVE Animals" tab at the bottom of the page (https://www.aphis.usda.gov/aphis/ourfocus/animalhealth/export/iregs-for-animal-exports/ct_iregs_animal_exports_home; last accessed December 2020). Regulations for semen are also located here.

Equipment and Supplies

USDA endorsed health certificates, import permit, commercial invoice, vapor shipper, protective shipping carton, USDA seals, transaction reports.

Qualification as an Approved Semen Collection Center

Regulations for most countries state that the semen must be collected and processed by a center that is "approved" and under the supervision of an official center veterinarian. For some countries there is little further specific definition about what is required to be approved and who is responsible for such approval. However, the EU, Australia, and New Zealand all have very specific requirements which must be met for a facility to be approved. These countries and others have negotiated with USDA to inspect and recommend for approval facilities in the United States that meet the requirements set forth by those countries.

For the EU, specific requirements and inspection checklists for approval as a semen collection center, storage center, as well as health certificate templates can be found at https://www.aphis.usda.gov/aphis/ourfocus/animalhealth/export/international-standard-setting-activities-oie/regionalization/sa_by_country/sa_e/ct_animal_european_union (last accessed November 2020).

Equine Reproductive Procedures, Second Edition. Edited by John Dascanio and Patrick McCue.

To view the complete EU legislation on the matter, visit the website of EU law at https://eur-lex.europa.eu/homepage.html (last accessed November 2020). There you can search for the specific directives that address semen collection centers.

General Guidelines for Approval as an EU Equine Semen Collection Center

Note: this is just a general summary of main points of the regulations and is not meant to be a comprehensive or complete list. It is strongly recommended that you contact your regional USDA federal veterinary medical officer (VMO) prior to starting a freezing program, to discuss the details of the inspection and qualification process as it applies to your specific facility. A list of contacts can be found at the APHIS website (https://www.aphis.usda.gov/aphis/banner/contactus/sa_animal_health/; last accessed November 2020).

1) Only semen from approved semen collection centers (SCCs) may be exported to the EU.
2) SCCs shall be inspected by an official veterinarian at least once every calendar year.
    a) In the USA, APHIS notifies the European Commission (EC) of an inspected and approved facility, then the EC adds the name of the facility to the list of approved centers on the EU website. Semen can be collected and frozen as soon as APHIS approves the center, but semen cannot be exported until the center appears on the EU website. SCCs cannot stay on the list without annual inspection. SCCs cannot stay on the list and skip inspections even if they are not actively collecting for export.
3) The center must be under the direct supervision of a licensed veterinarian who is authorized by the competent authority. This means an accredited veterinarian who is ultimately responsible for all operations of the collection center not just animal health.
4) The center must have stabling that is lockable and be separated from collection facilities and semen processing and storage rooms.
5) The collection facilities must have slip-proof footing that can be readily cleaned and disinfected.
6) The center must have a separate room for cleaning and disinfection of equipment. The room must be separate from laboratory/processing areas. This cannot just be a sink in the laboratory.
7) The semen processing room must be separate from collection, storage, cleaning, or administration areas.
8) The semen storage area must be a separate, lockable room or cabinet. EU qualified semen must be stored separate from non-EU qualified semen, not just in separate tanks but also in a separate room.
9) The center must be constructed to prevent contact with outside livestock or horses that have not been tested to demonstrate "like health status".
10) The entire center (excluding the office and exercise areas) should be constructed of materials that can be readily cleaned and disinfected.
11) The entry of unauthorized persons into the center must be controlled (sign in/out log, restricted areas, signage, etc.).
12) Staff must be trained in disinfection and hygiene techniques and this training must be documented.
13) The center should have written standard operating procedures for all activities (cleaning and disinfection, semen processing, etc.). Inspectors will want to review these.
14) The center must keep detailed records of all horses entering the center to include species, breed, date of birth, ID number, health history, diagnostic test results, treatments, vaccination history, etc. These records must be readily accessible and well organized.
15) The center must keep written logs or a computerized database of all semen collection records, straw identification, storage records, and distribution records. It must be able to produce all records associated with any given dose of EU qualified semen. This would include all stallion entry records, health testing, collection record, storage location, and/or shipment record.

Health Testing Requirements for Horses at the Collection Center

1) Donor stallions and any tease mares at the center must not have been used for natural breeding during the period of 30 days prior to the first semen collection or during the entire collection period.
2) Donor stallions can not have shown any signs of infectious disease at the time of admission or at any time during the collection period. This must be documented by the center veterinarian.
3) The center must obtain written attestation from the attending veterinarian at a prior location that the donor stallion was not resident at a location or had contact with horses at a location that was under restriction for several reportable diseases (see Directive 2009/156/EC of the European Commission Code for details). The center should obtain attestation from the attending veterinarian where the horse resided for 6 months prior to entry to the SCC.
4) The center also needs written attestation from the attending veterinarian that the donor stallion has not been kept for 30 days prior to entry to the SCC in any holding where any equine has shown any clinical signs

of equine viral arteritis (EVA) or contagious equine metritis (CEM) during that period.

5) Depending on the donor residency status (resident, temporarily absent, or walk-on), stallions must undergo testing according to one of three different protocols for equine infectious anemia (EIA), EVA, CEM (and in some cases vesicular stomatitis) (see sections 4.7.1, 4.7.2, and 4.7.3 of EC Directive 2009/156/EC for the details of these testing protocols).
6) Frozen semen must be stored in approved conditions for a minimum 30-day period after collection and prior to dispatch to the EU.

Semen Processing Requirements

1) All instruments or equipment that come into contact with the semen or the donor animal during collection and processing must be new and disposable, or properly disinfected or sterilized prior to use.
2) Any products of animal origin that are used in diluents or extenders must "present no animal health risk or be treated prior to use that such risk is prevented." For example, specific pathogen-free or pasteurized egg yolks, pasteurized milk, and bovine serum albumin that is safety tested.
3) Antibiotics in semen diluents are required for equine semen and must have a bactericidal activity equivalent to EU standards.
4) Straws must be clearly and properly labeled to include the date of collection (or collection code), species, breed, ID number and SCC approval number. Printed straws are recommended as some countries will not accept any handwritten information on straws.
5) Upon approval, the SCC will be assigned an EU approval number. This number cannot be placed on straws that contain semen that does not fully comply with EU regulations.
6) Liquid nitrogen must not have been used previously for other products of animal origin.
7) Storage and transport containers must be properly disinfected or sterilized before use for storage or shipment of EU qualified semen. The centerust keep a standard operating procedure and log book of protocol and dates.

Export Documentation

Once the SCC has produced the export qualified semen and is prepared to ship internationally, there are several steps that must be followed to ensure that the shipment will be accepted upon inspection by veterinary authorities and customs at the port of entry. It is suggested the SCC contacts their regional USDA VMO or USDA office to inform them that an export shipment is being prepared as the health certificate must be endorsed by the USDA and the tank must be sealed with an official USDA embossed metal seal. In some cases, the tank will have to be brought to the USDA office to be sealed, while in other cases the center veterinarian may be permitted to apply the seal.

1) Determine if an import permit is required by the destination country. If so, a copy may need to accompany the shipment.
2) The center veterinarian must prepare and sign the appropriate model health certificate. The EU has four different models depending on when the semen was frozen and where it is dispatched from. Templates can be found at https://www.aphis.usda.gov/aphis/ourfocus/animalhealth/export/international-standard-setting-activities-oie/regionalization/sa_by_country/sa_e/ct_animal_european_union (last accessed November 2020).
   - Model 1: semen collected after September 30, 2014.
   - Model 2: semen collected after August 31, 2010 and before October 1, 2014.
   - Model 3: collected before September 1, 2010 and dispatched after August 31, 2010.
   - Model 4: semen dispatched from a storage center.
3) Health certificates must be endorsed by a USDA federal veterinarian based on attestation by the official center veterinarian and examination of health testing results for the donor stallions.
4) Depending on the importing country and requirements of certain breed registries, it may be necessary to include a commercial invoice with the shipment as well as various certificates. All required documents should be completed before loading and sealing the container. As a precaution against rejection of the shipment, it is advisable to forward a copy of all documents to the importer or broker to verify that all conditions have been met and the required paperwork is in order. Entire consignments may be rejected for failing to provide the exact documents required. In this case veterinary authorities may refuse to admit the container and send it immediately back, hold it until the issue is resolved, or even destroy the semen all together.
5) Once an endorsed health certificate is obtained and all documents are in order, the container should be loaded in a fully charged vapor shipper (as described Chapter 158), the USDA seal applied, and arrangements made for the container to be shipped. Commercial express delivery services such as FedEx, UPS, and DHL can act as freight forwarder/brokers or a broker that is experienced in shipment of frozen animal semen can be

used. When transporting semen internationally we recommend using a vapor shipping container with as long a holding time as possible. It is not uncommon for there to be significant delays in clearing customs and veterinary inspection at the port of importation and such delays can be potentially damaging to the semen if the container temperature is not maintained properly.

EU Approved Semen Collection Centers vs Semen Storage Centers

As an approved SCC, donor semen can be collected, processed, stored, and distributed to member states of the EU. However, an approved SCC can only export semen that was collected and frozen at that center. Semen cannot be transferred from one approved SCC to another approved SCC prior to export unless the receiving facility is an EU approved semen storage center (SSC). Requirements for approval as an SSC are different than for an SCC and involve semi-annual inspections rather than annual inspections by USDA. Only an approved SSC can receive EU qualified semen for storage, consolidation, or future export. An approved SSC does not also need to be an approved SCC although in many cases the facility is approved for both.

Moving qualified semen from an SCC to a SSC must be done correctly or the semen may lose its qualification status. The following are presented as guidelines only – the appropriate regional/federal VMO should be contacted before initiating a transfer to ensure compliance.

1) The EU semen must never come into contact with non-EU semen, there must be a complete paper trail, and the center veterinarian for the SSC must document EU eligibility of the consignment so that it can be stored with EU qualified semen.
2) The center veterinarian for the original SCC must issue the appropriate initial (model 1, 2, or 3) health certificate to accompany the shipment to the SSC. This health certificate does not require endorsement by USDA/APHIS. However, a USDA official seal must be applied to the container by the SCC accredited veterinarian.
3) Upon receipt at the SSC, the center veterinarian breaks the seal and records the date, seal number, container identification, and initial model 1, 2, or 3 health certificate.
4) The semen can then be consolidated with other EU qualified semen for shipment or placed into storage at the SSC for future dispatch.
5) At the time of dispatch from the SSC, the original SCC veterinarian issues a final model 1, 2, or 3 health certificate that reflects only the doses in the actual export consignment, which may not be the entire amount sent to the SSC. This model 1, 2, or 3 health certificate must be endorsed by USDA/APHIS.
6) The SSC veterinarian then issues a model 4 heath certificate and attaches the final (endorsed) model 1, 2, or 3 health certificate issued by the SCC veterinarian.
7) The SSC veterinarian seals the container and the semen is shipped.

Additional Comments

This chapter provides the reader with some guidelines regarding the process for freezing, storage, and distribution of frozen equine semen. The example of distribution of semen from the USA to the EU was used to illustrate the complexity of the process.

Frozen semen has been successfully exported from the USA to numerous other countries since the mid-1980s, however it is still not a simple process and must be done carefully and with adequate planning and foresight. Each country has different regulations and those regulations may change without notice, therefore it is critical to establish a good working relationship with the regional USDA VMO, stay abreast of current regulations, and work with breeders or agents in the importing countries to make sure that you are aware of the most current regulations for import of frozen equine semen.

161

Harvesting and Shipping Testes

John J. Dascanio

School of Veterinary Medicine, Texas Tech University, USA

Introduction

The unexpected death of a stallion may result in the loss of genetic material if the owners do not have previously frozen semen. It is possible to harvest the testes and to isolate spermatozoa from the tail of the epididymis and vas deferens for assisted reproductive techniques or for artificial insemination from a stallion prior to euthanasia or immediately at death. When harvesting the testes, as much of the associated vas deferens (ductus deferens) should remain attached. The quicker the testes arrive at a processing facility, the greater the number of viable spermatozoa that can be recovered. It is recommended that testes be processed within 12 hours after removal for best results and no more than 24 hours for adequate recovery of viable sperm. If this is a terminal procedure for a stallion, then euthanasia should be performed after testicle harvest. It is unknown the degree to which euthanasia solution administration affects epididymal spermatozoa, but viable spermatozoa have been isolated after euthanasia.

Equipment and Supplies

Fresh cooled equine semen shipping container, 2-0 suture, sterile obstetrical sleeve, lactated Ringer's solution, syringes, surgical pack for castration.

Technique

- The stallion should be placed under general anesthesia.
- The anesthetized stallion should be castrated using routine procedures.
- As much of the vas deferens as possible should be salvaged along with the epididymides and testes. Care should be exercised to keep the epididymis and vas deferens intact without any breaks in their tubular structure that would allow spermatozoa to leak out.
- The excised vas deferens should be ligated with 2-0 suture material so that spermatozoa do not leak from the cut end during shipment (Figure 161.1).
- The testes, epididymis, and vas deferens should be rinsed with warm (37°C, 99°F), sterile lactated Ringer's solution to remove any tissue debris and blood.
- The tissues should be placed into a sterile plastic bag such as a sterile obstetrical sleeve. The testes should remain slightly wet during transport so that the tissues do not dry out; 5 ml of lactated Ringer's solution may be included in the transport bag. All air should be removed and the bags tied or sealed. The packaged tissues may then be placed into a second bag in case the first bag leaks.

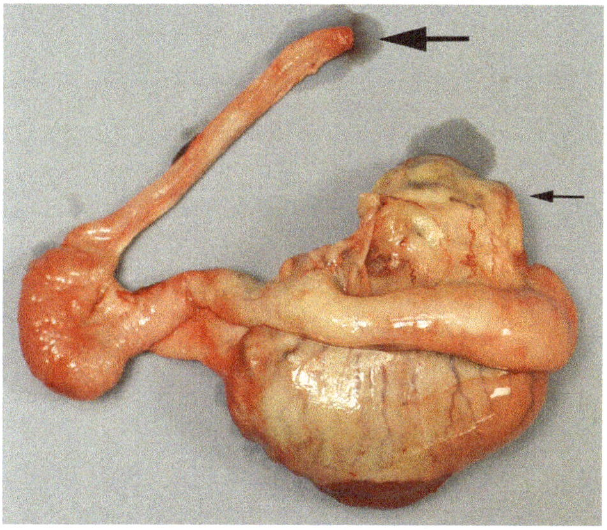

Figure 161.1 The vas deferens should be ligated as proximally as possible (large arrow), while the vascular structures may be excised close to the testes (small arrow).

Equine Reproductive Procedures, Second Edition. Edited by John Dascanio and Patrick McCue.

- The packaged testicles should be placed into a shipping container that is typically used for shipping fresh cooled equine semen. Properly frozen gel packs or canisters should be included in the container, but should not come into direct contact with the testes. Packing material or a small towel should separate the tissues from the ice packs so that testicular tissue/spermatozoa do not freeze.
- If the testes are to be processed locally, but there is a delay in processing, the packaged testes may be placed into a beaker of room temperature water which may be placed into a refrigerator until processing. This will slowly cool the water in the beaker and thus slowly cool the testes.
- The container is then sent to a processing laboratory by the quickest possible route. That may be counter-to-counter airline shipment (same day delivery) or by overnight courier service.
- Include the appropriate information with the shipment, including the registered name of the stallion, breed registration number, date and time of castration, and any previous history of semen cryopreservation such as types of extender(s) used. Also include any pertinent recent medical history for the stallion.
- Owner information should also be included with the shipment, such as name, address, phone numbers, email address, and other pertinent contact information.

Interpretation

- The motility/velocity of epididymal spermatozoa is typically lower than for ejaculated spermatozoa due to the absence of accessory sex gland fluid (seminal plasma). Mixing of seminal plasma that is devoid of spermatozoa from a stallion with excellent fertility may enhance the motility and fertilization capability of the epididymal spermatozoa.
- The best results will be obtained with processing of the epididymal spermatozoa within 12–24 hours after removal of the testes.
- Recovery of viable sperm may be poor in stallions with a chronic medical condition or a potential exposure to endotoxins or certain medications.

Further Reading

Braun J, Sakai M, Hochi S, Oguri N. 1994. Preservation of ejaculated and epididymal stallion spermatozoa by cooling and freezing. *Theriogenology* 41: 809–18.

Eichelberger AC, Troedsson MH, Pozor MA, Macpherson ML. 2007. How to collect, handle and process post-mortem epididymal sperm for breeding or assisted reproductive techniques. *Proc Annu Conv Am Assoc Eq Pract* 53: 583–6.

Johnson AEM, Coutinho da Silva MA. 2008. Effects of recovery technique, freezing extender and antioxidants on motility parameters of cryopreserved stallion epididymal sperm. *Theriogenology* 70: 579–80.

162

Epididymal Sperm Recovery

John J. Dascanio[1] *and Lynda M. J. Miller*[2]

[1]*School of Veterinary Medicine, Texas Tech University, USA*
[2]*College of Veterinary Medicine, Lincoln Memorial University, USA*

Introduction

Spermatozoa can be recovered from a stallion that sustained a catastrophic injury, or experiences severe colic or other life-threatening medical condition. The epididymis contains billions of spermatozoa that can be harvested and cryopreserved for future use. In most instances, spermatozoa will survive and maintain capacity for fertilization for 12–24 hours after the stallion's death. However, it is recommended that sperm be harvested and cryopreserved as soon as possible following death, euthanasia, or elective castration of a stallion.

Approximately 10–15 billion sperm can be harvested from the paired epididymides of most stallions for cryopreservation. A total of 12–20 breeding doses (eight straws per dose, with each straw containing 100 million sperm) are usually obtained. Mares may be inseminated with one or two doses of frozen semen per estrous cycle.

Equipment and Supplies

Surgical instruments, scalpel blades, Petri dishes, warmed semen extender, bovine teat infusion cannulas or tomcat catheters, syringes, sterile surgical gloves, gauze sponges, suture, centrifuge, 5 ml macrotubes, 5 and 1.2 μm in-line syringe filters.

Technique

- The testes, epididymides, and vas deferens should be harvested, packaged, and shipped according to recommended guidelines (see Chapter 161).
- All further processing occurs at room temperature in a clean environment. Sterile instruments, sterile drapes, and sterile equipment should be used.
- Working in a large disposable Petri dish, dissect the tail of the epididymis, with the attached vas deferens, from the body of the epididymis (Figure 162.1). A hemostat should be placed at either end of the dissected tissue to prevent the loss of semen, one at the ligated end of the vas deferens and one at the junction between the tail and body of the epididymis. The testes and the remaining portions of the epididymis (head and body) may be discarded.
- Any remaining fascia may now be removed while straightening the major sections of the coiled tail of the epididymis. The majority of the epididymis will not be uncoiled. Care should be taken to not break the tubular structure.
- Any blood remaining on the surface should be rinsed off with warmed lactated Ringer's solution and the testicle blotted with gauze to remove excess liquid.
- The vas deferens and tail of epididymis are transferred to a new Petri dish.

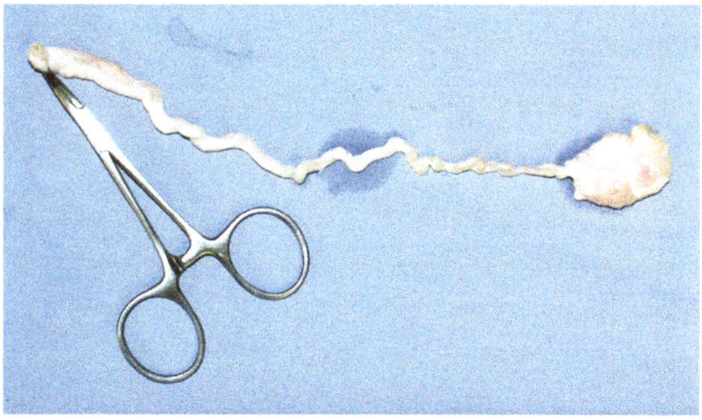

Figure 162.1 Isolated vas deferens (with hemostat attached) and tail of the epididymis.

Equine Reproductive Procedures, Second Edition. Edited by John Dascanio and Patrick McCue.

Harvesting Epididymal Sperm: Option 1

- A 20 ml syringe is filled with 5 ml of warmed seminal plasma, previously collected from a stallion of known fertility, and air.
- The syringe is then attached to a bovine teat cannula, tomcat catheter, or modified pipette tip.
- The cannula or catheter is inserted into the open end of the vas deferens and gentle but firm pressure is applied to flush the intact vas deferens and epididymal tail with the seminal plasma and air volume into a clean glass beaker or other container (Figure 162.2).
- Subsequently, the tract is flushed with 10–20 ml of air as needed to evacuate the tract of spermatozoa.
- The tract could also be flushed with 5–10 ml of warmed semen extender. This would necessitate a subsequent centrifugation step when processing the semen.

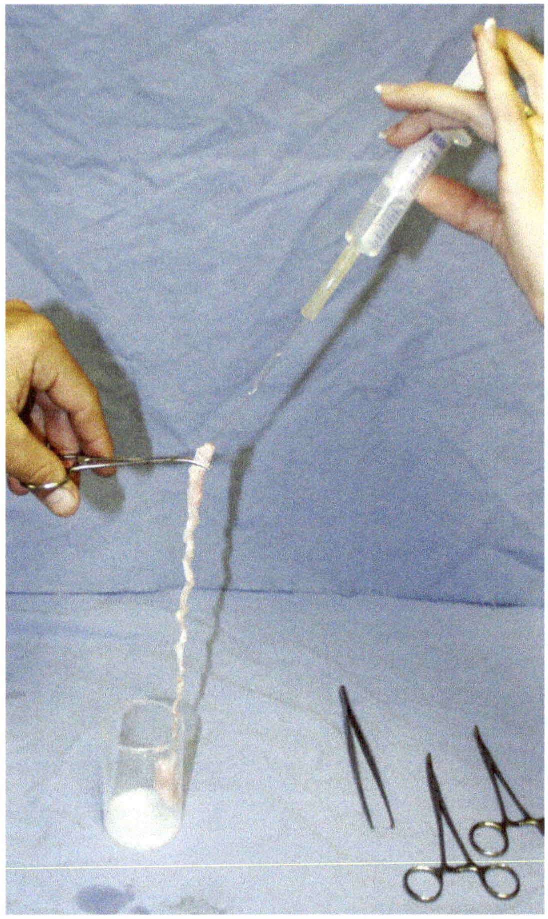

Figure 162.2 Flushing of the vas deferens and tail of the epididymis.

Harvesting Epididymal Sperm: Option 2

- The vas deferens is cleanly cut from the tail of the epididymis as close to the epididymis as possible, so that you have a long length of tubular tissue intact.
- The end of the vas deferens with the hemostat is cleanly cut, keeping the cut end of the vas deferens within a 50 ml conical centrifuge tube.
- A 20 ml syringe is filled with warmed semen extender and a bovine teat cannula is attached to the syringe.
- The teat cannula is threaded into the proximal portion of the vas deferens and may be secured with 2-0 suture. If the bovine teat cannula will not fit within the lumen of the vas deferens, an open-ended tomcat urinary catheter may be used or even an appropriate gauge injection needle. Care should be taken if using a needle to not puncture the wall of the vas deferens.
- With gentle pressure on the syringe plunger, semen extender is pushed through the vas deferens, catching the effluent in a 50 ml pre-warmed centrifuge tube or similar container. This effluent is sperm-rich and should be saved for further processing.
- The tail of the epididymis is placed into a clean Petri dish with about 5–10 ml of warmed semen extender. The tail of the epididymis is minced into small pieces within the semen extender using two scalpel blades, each working in opposite directions. White clumps of spermatozoa will be seen floating amongst the minced tissue.
- Leave the minced epididymis in the semen extender for 10–15 minutes to allow further egress of spermatozoa from the minced tissue (swim-up procedure).
- Place an expanded piece of a sterile gauze sponge over the previously filled 50 ml centrifuge tube. Push the center of the gauze down into the centrifuge tube so that it forms a funnel shape. Pour the minced tissue and semen extender from the Petri dish through the gauze and into the 50 ml centrifuge tube. Rinse the Petri dish and gauze sponge with warmed semen extender into the centrifuge tube to remove any retained spermatozoa. Alternatively, a commercial mesh filter such as that used for semen collection may be used as a filter.
- The isolated spermatozoa are subsequently processed for semen freezing using standard techniques (see Chapter 153).
- An additional step may be taken prior to freezing whereby isolated spermatozoa are centrifuged for 400–600× g for 12 minutes to reduce the amount of semen extender. The supernatant is removed and the semen pellet is re-suspended in 5 ml of seminal plasma (see next section) and then processed for semen freezing using standard techniques.

Alternative Seminal Plasma Processing

- Seminal plasma may be flushed through the vas deferens (option 1) or may be added to the isolated spermatozoal pellet (option 2) to enhance spermatozoal motility and to provide substrates that may enhance fertility.
- Seminal plasma is obtained in advance and frozen from a stallion of known good fertility whose semen has been determined to freeze well. The stallion should test negative for equine arteritis virus, equine infectious anemia, and contagious equine metritis, and have negative bacterial cultures on isolated seminal plasma.
- Seminal plasma is isolated by performing routine semen collection and then centrifuging the semen at 1,000× *g* for 20 minutes in 50 ml conical centrifuge tubes.
- The seminal plasma supernatant is removed from the pellet and used for further processing. The pellet is discarded.
- Seminal plasma is then passed sequentially through 5 and 1.2 μm in-line syringe filters to remove any residual sperm. The seminal plasma is placed within 5 ml macrotubes and snap frozen in liquid nitrogen. When needed, the seminal plasma is thawed at 50°C (122°F) for 40 seconds and added to epididymal spermatozoa.

Interpretation

- Frozen-thawed epididymal spermatozoa may have a lower total and progressive motility if no seminal plasma has been added.
- Frozen-thawed epididymal spermatozoa typically have lower fertility rates than fresh cooled or frozen semen when used for artificial insemination. Pregnancy rates can be increased by optimizing mare management and timing insemination relative to ovulation. Factors such as the health status of the stallion prior to castration or euthanasia, the interval from castration to harvest of epididymal spermatozoa, post-thaw motility, and the reproductive status of mares that are bred all influence fertility with epididymal semen.
- Frozen-thawed epididymal spermatozoa may also be used with assisted reproductive techniques such as intracytoplasmic sperm injection (ICSI) to conserve spermatozoa, as the procedure requires the injection of only one spermatozoon into an oocyte. Frozen epididymal semen yields an equivalent pregnancy rate to frozen ejaculated semen when using ICSI.

Further Reading

Braun J, Sakai M, Hochi S, Oguri N. 1994. Preservation of ejaculated and epididymal stallion spermatozoa by cooling and freezing. *Theriogenology* 41: 809–18.

Eichelberger AC, Troedsson MH, Pozor MA, Macpherson ML. 2007. How to collect, handle and process post-mortem epididymal sperm for breeding or assisted reproductive techniques. *Proc Annu Conv Am Assoc Eq Pract* 53: 583–6.

Johnson AEM, Coutinho da Silva MA. 2008. Effects of recovery technique, freezing extender and antioxidants on motility parameters of cryopreserved stallion epididymal sperm. *Theriogenology* 70: 579–80.

Morris LHA, Tiplady CA, Allen WR. 2002. The in vivo fertility of caudal epididymal spermatozoa in the horse. *Theriogenology* 58: 643–6.

163

Endoscopic Examination of the Urethra

Patrick M. McCue

Equine Reproduction Laboratory, Colorado State University, USA

Introduction

Visualization of the lumen of the urethra, seminal colliculus, seminal vesicles, and urinary bladder may be indicated in cases of hemospermia, hematuria, obstruction, infection, and discomfort during urination and/or ejaculation. Endoscopic examination of the urogenital system of horses has become relatively common, in part due to the availability of quality videoendoscopes in private practices, referral centers, and universities. Endoscopic examination of the urethra and associated structures may also facilitate the collection of samples for microbacteriological culture and tissue samples for histology as well as providing a means for local treatment.

Equipment and Supplies

Sedation (xylazine hydrochloride 0.22–0.66 mg/kg, butorphanol tartrate 0.01–0.02 mg/kg, detomidine hydrochloride 0.01–0.02 mg/kg), disinfectant soap, roll cotton, bucket, clean water, 2.4% glutaraldehyde disinfectant, sterile saline, sterile lubricant, videoendoscope (100 cm long, 6 mm or less OD), sterile saline, glutaraldehyde solution.

Technique

- The stallion is sedated with a combination of xylazine and butorphanol, or detomidine and butorphanol, administered intravenously and is restrained in a set of stocks. Phenothiazine tranquilizers (i.e., acepromazine) are to be avoided because of the possibility of paraphimosis.
- The sheath and distal penis are cleaned with mild soap and then rinsed with water (see Chapter 123).
- One person should wear disposable examination gloves and hold the distal penis.
- The endoscope is sterilized in an activated solution of 2.4% glutaraldehyde (Cidex®) and then rinsed thoroughly with 0.9% sterile saline.
- Sterile lubricant is applied along the side of the endoscope, with care not to apply lubricant to the end where the camera is located so as to not obscure the camera.
- The endoscope is passed into the urethra and advanced proximally. It may be beneficial to insufflate the urethra slightly as the scope is passed.
- The distal penis should be grasped firmly around the endoscope, forming a seal that allows distension of the urethra with air. Care should be exercised to not overinflate the lumen of the various structures. On rare occasions, stallions have become neurologic and collapsed in stocks during this procedure, possibly owing to an air embolus or thrombus formation. The use of CO_2, instead of room air, may provide a safer means of insufflation.
- The endoscope is passed proximally up the urethra until the seminal colliculus is visualized. The endoscope may be passed into the seminal colliculus using a probe passed through the biopsy channel of the endoscope as a guide. The probe is passed into the seminal colliculus and the endoscope is advanced along the probe to help guide the endoscope into the lumen in a similar manner to that used to examine a guttural pouch.
- The endoscope is subsequently advanced proximally up the urethra to visualize the entrance to the bladder.
- In most cases, the endoscope is passed into the bladder to allow for a thorough examination.

Equine Reproductive Procedures, Second Edition. Edited by John Dascanio and Patrick McCue.

Interpretation

The normal mucosal surface of the distal urethra is pale pink in color with slight longitudinal folds. The submucosal vasculature is more prominent in the proximal urethra. Visual aspects of the urethral mucosa should be noted during the initial pass of the endoscope, which may cause transient irritation and hyperemia. The urethra curves dorsally and then cranially as it passes around the ischial arch.

Two rows of bulbo-urethral gland ducts are located along the dorsal aspect of the pelvic urethra (Figure 163.1). The seminal colliculus (Figure 163.2) is located on the dorsal aspect of the pelvic urethra approximately 3 cm proximal to the bulbo-urethral gland duct openings. The slit-like common openings of the ductus deferens and seminal vesicles are located on the caudal surface of the colliculus seminalis, which is more prominent in stallions than in geldings. Excretory ducts of the prostate gland are located lateral to the seminal colliculus. The internal urethral orifice is located proximal to the seminal colliculus (Figure 163.3).

Urethral rents or tears usually occur in the proximal urethra on the dorso-caudal (convex) aspect of the proximal urethra just before it begins to curve around the ischial arch (Figure 163.4). Urethral lesions, such as rents, tears, or hematomas, are typically 1–2 cm in length, longitudinal in orientation, and easy to visualize with the endoscope. Treatment consists of a prolonged period of sexual rest and, possibly, a perineal urethrotomy or related surgical procedure.

Additional Comments

Hematuria and hemospermia may be caused by defects or tears in the dorso-caudal aspect of the proximal urethra at or just above the ischial arch. Other causes of blood in the

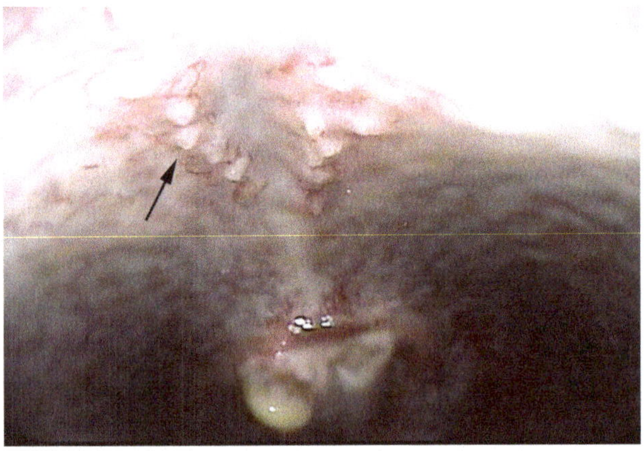

Figure 163.1 Bulbo-urethral gland ducts (arrow) viewed through a videoendoscope.

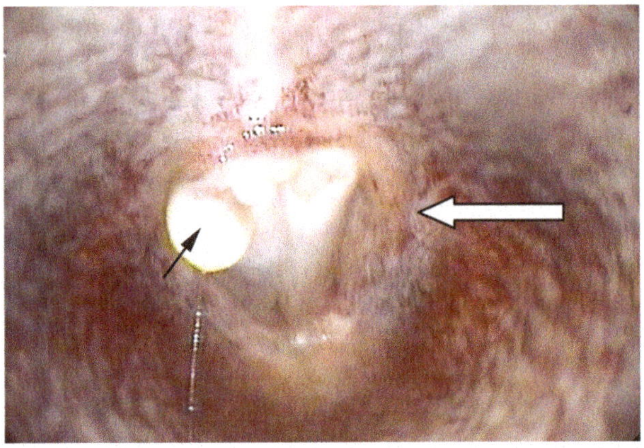

Figure 163.2 Seminal colliculus viewed through a videoendoscope; discharge is evident from the left orifice (small arrow). The location of the excretory ducts of the prostate is indicated by the open arrow.

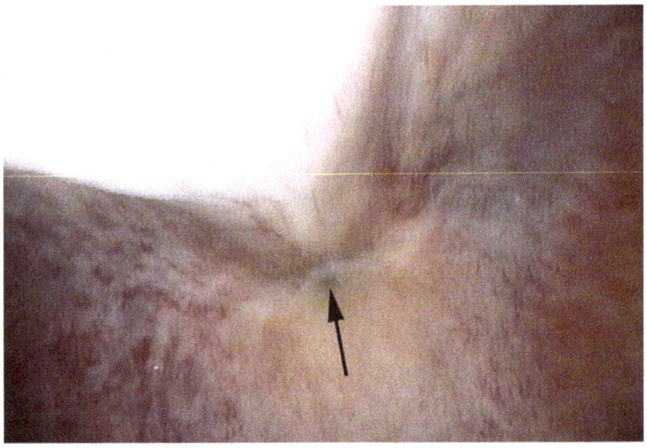

Figure 163.3 Internal urethral orifice (arrow) viewed through a videoendoscope.

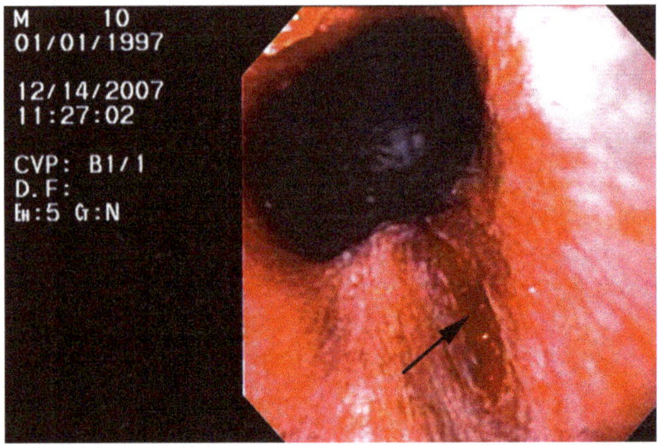

Figure 163.4 Urethral tear (arrow) in a stallion viewed through a videoendoscope.

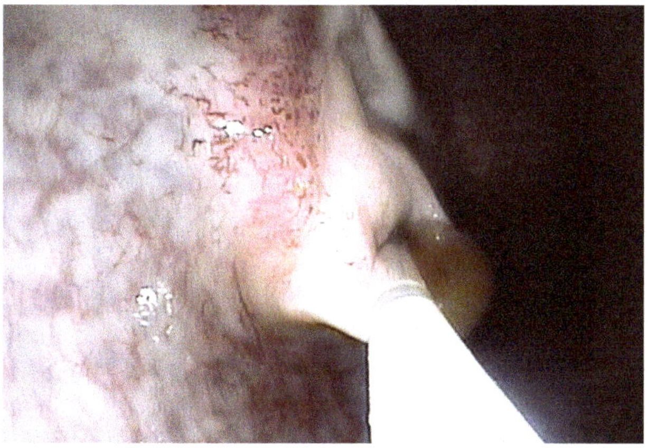

Figure 163.5 Cannulation of the seminal colliculus. The endoscope can be passed into the seminal vesicle using the cannula as a stylet.

ejaculate include lesions on the glans penis or distal urethra and seminal vesiculitis. The detection of a urethral defect by endoscopy and the exclusion of other causes is critical in formulating treatment options, which may include prolonged sexual rest and a temporary subischial urethrotomy. Urethral lesions may be caused by rupture of the corpus spongiosum penis into the urethra due to increased pressure during ejaculation and urination. Urethrotomy or incisions into the corpus spongiosum penis without entering the urethra via a perineal urethrotomy approach have been successful in resolving these lesions.

Seminal vesiculitis is an uncommon clinical disease in stallions that may be associated with the culture of bacteria from semen samples. Confirmation of seminal vesiculitis may be made by a combination of transrectal ultrasonography and the passage of an endoscope through the colliculus seminalis into the gland lumen using a long cannula as a stylet (Figure 163.5). Samples for bacterial culture may be collected using guarded culture instruments designed for use with an endoscope. Treatment may involve extensive lavage of the gland(s) via the endoscope and infusion of appropriate antibiotics.

Further Reading

Lloyd KCK, Wheat JD, Ryan AM, Matthews M. 1989. Ulceration in the proximal portion of the urethra as a cause of hematuria in horses: four cases (1978–1985). *J Am Vet Med Assoc* 194: 1324–6.

Schott HC, Varner DD. 1997. Urinary tract. In: Traub-Dargatz JL, Brown CM (eds). Equine Endoscopy, 2nd edn. St Louis, MI: Mosby, pp. 187–203.

Schumacher J, Varner DD, Schmitz DG, Blanchard TL. 1995. Urethral defects in geldings with hamaturia and stallions with hemospermia. *Vet Surg* 24: 250–4.

164

Endoscopic-Guided Cannulation of the Seminal Vesicles

Patrick M. McCue

Equine Reproduction Laboratory, Colorado State University, USA

Introduction

Infection of the seminal vesicles of stallions is uncommon, but when present can be challenging to treat. Clinical signs associated with seminal vesiculitis include reduced fertility and endometritis in mares bred, as well as the presence of white blood cells, inflammatory debris, and blood in the ejaculate of affected stallions. A majority of cases are associated with *Pseudomonas aeruginosa* or *Klebsiella pneumoniae* infections, but other bacterial organisms such as *Streptococcus* species, *Staphylococcus* species, *Proteus vulgaris*, *Actinobacter calcoaceticus*, and *Brucella abortus* have also been reported.

Systemic antibiotic therapy is not often successful as most antibiotics do not diffuse across the internal mucosal border of the seminal vesicles. Another option for treatment is irrigation of the affected seminal vesicle(s) using a cannula passed through a videoendoscope, followed by infusion of antibiotics directly into the affected vesicle. The choice of antibiotics should be based on culture results and antimicrobial sensitivity tests, but may include ticarcillin-clavulanic acid, ampicillin, procaine penicillin, or imipenem-cilastatin if needed.

Equipment and Supplies

Videoendoscope (100 cm length, 6 mm OD, or 120 cm length, 10 mm OD), 2.4% glutaraldehyde disinfectant, sterile saline, sterile cannula (180 cm length, 1.8 mm OD, or 240 cm length, 2.3 mm OD), sterile obstetrical lubricant, examination gloves, sedation.

Technique

- The stallion should be restrained in examination stocks and sedated with a combination of detomidine (~0.015 mg/kg) plus butorphanol tartrate (~0.01 mg/kg) administered intravenously.
- Once extended, the penis is firmly grasped while wearing exam gloves and the thoroughly washed with a non-residual soap, rinsed with clean water and dried with disposable paper towels (see Chapter 123).
- The endoscope is sterilized in an activated solution of 2.4% glutaraldehyde (Cidex®). The endoscope is then rinsed thoroughly with 0.9% sterile saline or sterile water.
- A small amount of sterile obstetrical lubricant is applied to the outside of the distal end of the videoendoscope, taking care to not apply lubricant onto the camera or light.
- The endoscope is slowly passed proximately up the urethra to the level of the seminal colliculus (Figure 164.1). If a 6 mm diameter endoscope is used, a 180 cm washing catheter 1.8 mm in diameter can be passed through the biopsy channel of the videoendoscope. If a 10 mm endoscope is used, a slightly larger 2.3 mm diameter cannula can be passed through the scope.
- The distal penis should be grasped firmly around the endoscope, forming a seal that allows distension of the urethra with air. Care should be exercised to not overinflate the lumen of the various structures. On rare occasions, stallions have become neurologic and collapsed in stocks during this procedure, possibly owing to an air embolus or thrombus formation. The use of CO_2, instead of room air, may provide a safer means of insufflation.
- The cannula is advanced until it is visualized protruding through the end of the scope. The endoscope is then positioned so that the cannula can be passed into the seminal colliculus on the affected side (Figure 164.2).
- The interior of the seminal vesicle can be lavaged to remove inflammatory debris by slowly infusing sterile saline or lactated Ringer's solution through the cannula. After the lavage, antibiotics can be infused into the

Equine Reproductive Procedures, Second Edition. Edited by John Dascanio and Patrick McCue.

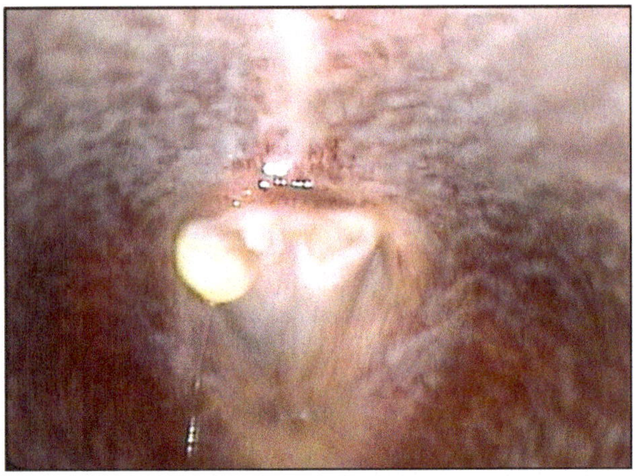

Figure 164.1 Videoendoscopic view of the seminal colliculus of a stallion with infection of the left seminal vesicle.

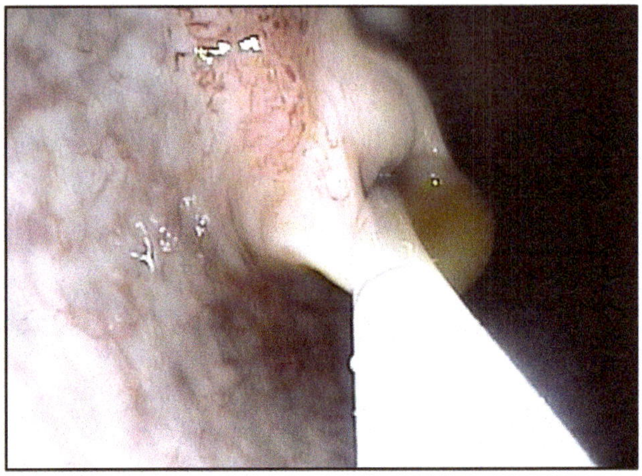

Figure 164.2 Cannulation of the affected seminal vesicle.

affected vesicle through the cannula. The procedure can be repeated on subsequent days as needed.

- In some cases, the endoscope can be passed directly into the lumen of the seminal vesicle for direct visualization of the interior, aspiration of contents for culture, and medical treatments including lavage and antibiotic infusion.

Interpretation

Cannulation of infected seminal vesicles using a videoendoscope passed proximately up the urethra, followed by therapeutic lavage and infusion of appropriate antibiotics, appears to be the most effective way to treat clinical cases of seminal vesiculitis in stallions. The choice of antibiotics is critical, as the organisms associated with seminal vesiculitis may be resistant to antibiotics commonly used in the treatment of infectious endometritis in mares. Consequently, an antimicrobial susceptibility test should be performed to determine the most appropriate antibiotic.

An additional management procedure for stallions with seminal vesiculitis is collection of semen and subsequent dilution with an extender containing an appropriate antibiotic based on an antimicrobial susceptibility test. In affected stallions managed in a live-cover breeding program, semen extender containing an appropriate antibiotic can be infused into the uterus immediately before or after natural service.

Further Reading

Ball BA. 2008. Diagnostic methods for evaluation of stallion subfertility: a review. *J Eq Vet Sci* 28: 650–65.

Blanchard TL, Varner DD, Hurtgen JP, *et al.* 1988. Bilateral seminal vesiculitis and ampullitis in a stallion. *J Am Vet Med Assoc* 192: 525–6.

Pinto MR, Neild DM, Benegas D, Vieyra DH, Miragaya MH. 2014. Successful treatment of seminal vesiculitis with imipenem-cilastatin in a stallion. *J Eq Vet Sci* 34: 544–8.

Varner DD, Blanchard TL, Brinsko SP, Love CC, Taylor TS, Johnson L. 2000. Techniques for evaluating selected reproductive disorders of stallions. *Anim Reprod Sci* 60: 493–509.

165

Palpation and Ultrasonography of the Testis, Epididymis, and Spermatic Cord

Sofie Sitters

Amsterdam, The Netherlands

Introduction

Thorough clinical inspection and palpation of external genitalia of a stallion provides information about breeding potential and permits the detection of reproductive abnormalities. In addition, ultrasonography of the external genitalia is now used routinely as an adjunct to the routine breeding soundness examination of a stallion and is an excellent diagnostic tool in the evaluation of suspected reproductive pathology.

Safety and Restraint

- Safe and effective examination of the scrotal contents of the stallion by palpation and ultrasonography requires adequate restraint and handling techniques. A good time to perform the examination is after ejaculation as most stallions will be more tolerant of the procedure at this time.
- The stallion may be restrained in an open area with just a halter and lead shank with a chain or placed into examination stocks.
- A twitch may be applied or chemical restraint administered as necessary. Use of phenothiazine tranquilizers such as acepromazine should be avoided because of the potential for development of priapism or paraphimosis.

Equipment and Supplies

Ultrasound machine: a linear array or microconvex 5.0 MHz transducer is acceptable, but 7.5–10 MHz transducers are more useful for imaging details of more superficial structures like the epididymis and to detect more subtle pathology; ultrasound coupling gel; methanol or alcohol; mineral oil or water-soluble gel; halter and chain; twitch and/or sedation.

- All personnel handling and examining the stallion should wear a protective helmet, appropriate footwear, and disposable examination gloves. A protective safety vest should also be considered.

Technique

- Perform the examination from the left (near) side of the horse. It is important that the stallion handler and the examiner both stand on the same side.
- The person performing the exam should stand in contact with the stallion's left shoulder. The right hand should be used to gently stroke the ventral abdomen to help relax the animal prior to actual palpation of the scrotal contents.
- Slowly move the right hand caudally over the ventral abdomen towards the stallion's inguinal region whilst staying in contact with the stallion's left shoulder. Do not to pull on the skinfold of the stallion's flank during the examination as this is generally a sensitive area and may cause an unwanted reaction.
- Systematically examine the scrotal skin and both testes, epididimydes, and spermatic cords both visually and manually to detect abnormalities prior to the ultrasound examination (Figure 165.1 and 165.2).
- For the ultrasound examination, the ultrasound unit should be placed in a safe location out of reach of the stallion or be hand held by an assistant. One hand of the examiner should be used to grasp and stabilize a testis and the other used to hold the transducer.
- Lubricant or an ultrasound gel should be applied to the probe and scrotal skin to ensure good contact between the transducer and scrotal skin.
- Place the transducer vertically on the lateral surface of a testis and obtain cross-sectional images of the testicular

Equine Reproductive Procedures, Second Edition. Edited by John Dascanio and Patrick McCue.

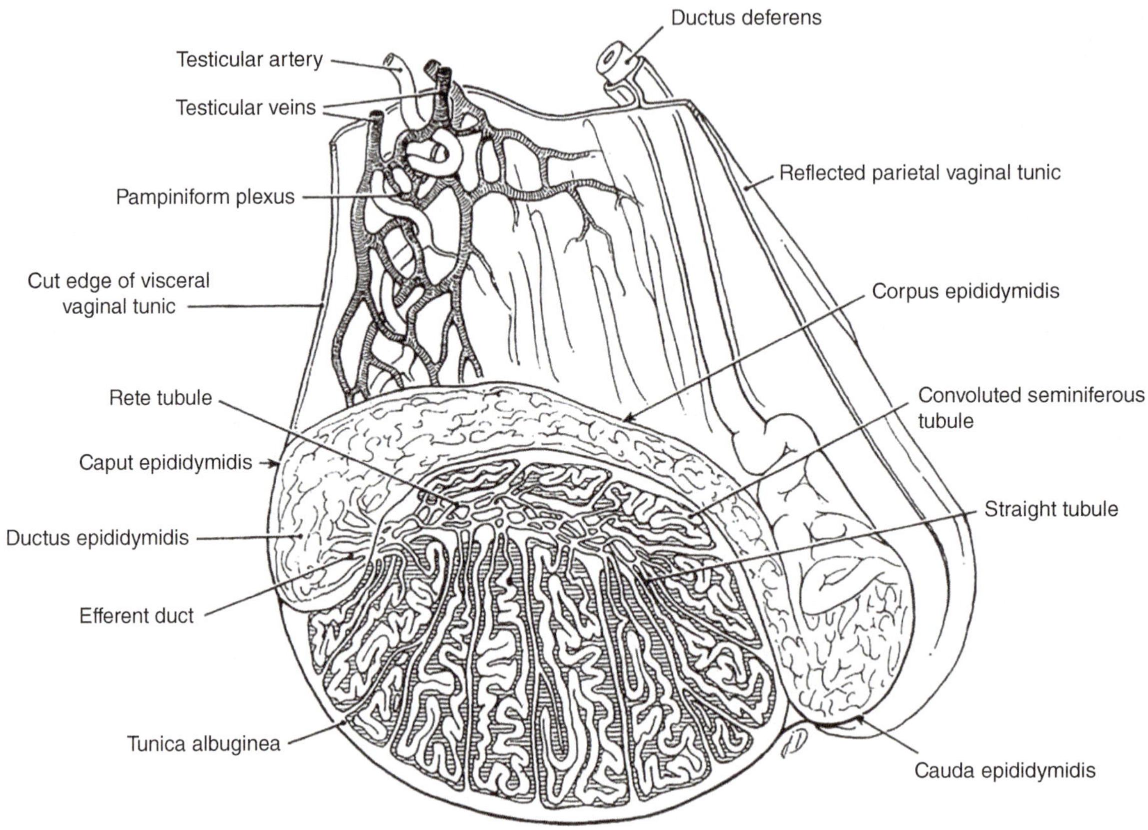

Figure 165.1 Anatomy of the testis, epididymis, and spermatic cord. Source: From Pickett BW, Voss JL, Squires EL, Amann RP. 1989. *Management of the Stallion for Maximum Reproductive Efficiency II*. Animal Reproduction Laboratory Bulletin No. 05. Colorado State University 1989. Reproduced with the permission of Colorado State University.

parenchyma by slowly moving the transducer over the entire surface of the testicle.

- The width, height, and length of each testis should subsequently be measured by ultrasonography. First, hold the transducer on the lateral surface of the testis and measure the widest part of the testis. Next, place the transducer on the ventral surface of the testis and direct the beam dorsally at a 90-degree angle to the long axis of the testis and measure the greatest height. Finally, place the transducer on the most cranial part of the testis and direct the beam caudally to measure the length. The epididymis should not be included in the length measurement.
- The head, body, and tail of the epididymis may be imaged by placing the transducer initially on the dorso-lateral surface of the testis and imaging caudally along the length of the epididymis. The epididymal tail by itself can be imaged by placing the transducer just cranial to the tail on the testis and directing the beam caudally or by placing the transducer on the caudal aspect of the scrotum and directing the beam cranially.
- The spermatic cord can be imaged by gently, but firmly, pulling a testis ventrally and positioning the transducer dorsally on the proximal aspect of the cord. Cross-sectional images of the spermatic cord are obtained by holding the transducer parallel to the ground and moving it up and down the cord as far as possible.

Interpretation

Palpation

- The scrotum is an outpouching of skin composed of the two scrotal sacs separated by the scrotal septum. A stallion's scrotum and its contents are located high in the inguinal region and are normally pendulous, but may be drawn toward the body wall during palpation because of voluntary contractions of the cremaster muscles. The scrotum should be thin and elastic, with a distinct neck. The scrotal skin should be smooth, free from evidence of trauma, inflammation, or other lesions and should slide loosely and freely over the underlying testicles. The median raphe can be found externally ventral to the scrotal septum.
- The testes should be ellipsoid, approximately equal in size and shape, and positioned horizontally within the

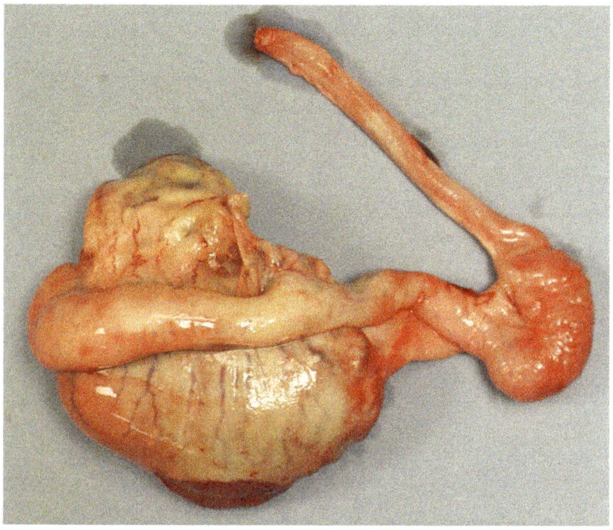

Figure 165.2 Testis, epididiymis, and ductus deferens (vas deferens).

scrotum with a spermatic cord attachment cranially. The testes should have a firm to turgid, resilient consistency on palpation. A testis that is obviously smaller, softer, or firmer may have a degenerative, neoplastic, or traumatic condition. Each testis should be evaluated independently as one testis may be affected while the other testis may be normal. Stallions with testicular degeneration and a decrease in testicular parenchyma present with a wrinkling of the tunica albuginea on palpation.

- A bulge on the lateral surface of the testes in adult stallions, more than 5 years old, can be associated with the presence of a lateral branch of the testicular artery. This anatomic vascular variation has been shown to be present in approximately 20% of stallions. The affected testis will have a pear-like shape, detectable visually or by palpation.
- The epididymis is a highly convolute duct and consists of a head, body, and tail. Spermatozoa undergo maturation in the head and body of the epididymis and the tail is the main storage site for matured sperm. In the stallion, the epididymis lies on the dorso-lateral aspect of the testis with the flattened head firmly attached to the cranial pole of the testis. The corpus (body) is more loosely attached and positioned laterally across the dorsal surface of the testis. The prominent tail is firmly attached to the caudal pole of the testis by the proper ligament. A second ligament, the ligament of the tail of the epididymis, attaches the tail to the scrotum. The epididymal head is soft and not easily identifiable manually. The body of the epididymis is firmer and easier to palpate. The tail is readily palpable and care should be taken to palpate the ligament of the tail of the epididymis (a remnant of the gubernaculum) with its distinctive firm ($\pm$1 cm flat) character. This ligament is an obvious landmark that can be used to determine the position of the testicle within the scrotum.
- Examination may reveal a 180-degree rotation of the testicle in the scrotum. Mild rotations may occur intermittently or permanently and are not necessarily associated with clinical problems or alterations in seminal parameters. Some stud books will not accept stallions that exhibit spontaneous rotation. The presence of this condition should be noted on any report when encountered. In the case of a spermatic cord torsion, the twist in the cord could be great enough to interfere with blood flow to and/or from the testicle. The stallion will have a painful, swollen testis and may demonstrate acute signs of pain (colic or lameness) and be at risk for testicular compromise.
- The spermatic cord contains the deferent duct, testicular artery, testicular veins (pampiniform plexus), lymphatic vessels, nerves, and cremaster muscle.

Ultrasonography

- The appearance of the testicular parenchyma should be homogeneous, gray, and slightly granular throughout (Figure 165.3). Diffuse increased echodensity may indicate testicular fibrosis, whereas diffuse decreased echodensity may indicate edema. Differences in echogenicity between the testes may indicate pathology. Focal variations should also be noted because they may be associated with possible pathologies such as tumors (Figures 165.4 and 165.5), hematomas, or abcessation. Testicular cysts are sometimes identified in fertile stallions and do not seem to negatively affect fertility.
- The central vein of the testis can be imaged as an anechoic line traversing the center of the testicular parenchyma. The vein is widest where it joins the spermatic cord cranio-dorsally and narrowest caudo-ventrally. Normal width measurements of the vein vary from 1 to 4 mm.
- The testicular artery is embedded in the tunica albuginea and runs dorsally around the caudal pole before it runs back cranially along the ventral border on a tortuous course. Small branches of this artery (<5 mm in diameter), the arcuate arteries, can be imaged near the surface of the testis with a 7.5 MHz or higher frequency transducer. These vessels are largest and most prominent at the caudal aspect of the testis.
- The parietal vaginal tunic is imaged as a thin echoic layer lining the vaginal cavity. Normally, a small volume of non-echoic fluid will be visible in the vaginal cavity, particularly along the dorsal surface of the testis. A thickening of the vaginal tunic or an increased volume of fluid

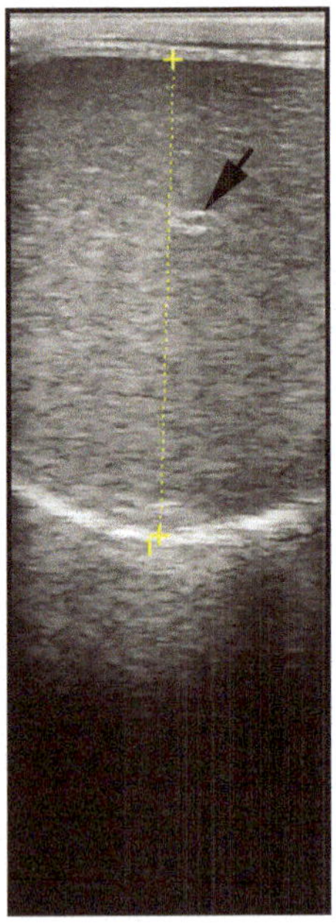

Figure 165.3 Normal echodenisty of an equine testicle. Testicular height can be measured by ultrasound. The arrow marks the central testicular vein.

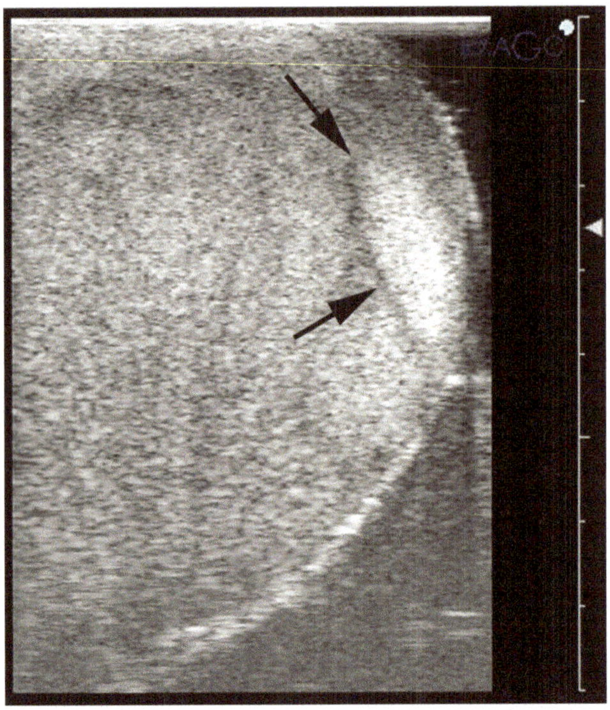

Figure 165.4 Testicular tumor from a 21-year-old stallion with unilaterally enlarged testes. The main parenchyma of the testicle was involved in a Sertoli cell tumor giving it a somewhat mottled increased echogenicity. There was also a more hyperechoic demarcated area present (arrows) that was a seminoma.

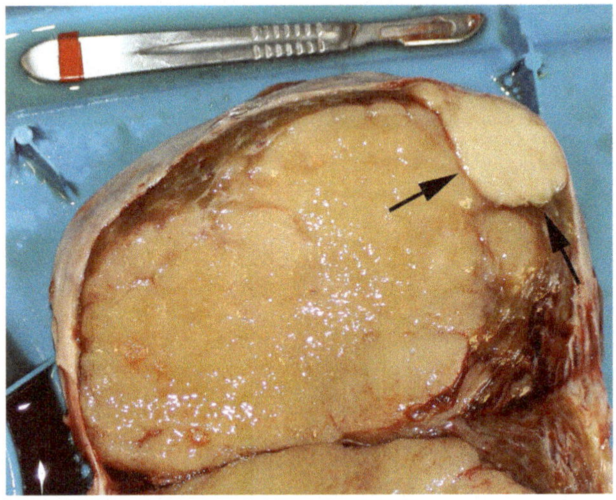

Figure 165.5 Testicle from the stallion in Figure 165.4 demonstrating diffuse infiltration of a Sertoli cell tumor throughout the testicle and an isolate seminoma focus (arrow).

in the vaginal cavity (hydrocele, hematocele, pyocele) is abnormal and may be associated with a decreased semen quality (Figures 165.6 and 165.7).

- Testicular size in post-pubertal stallions ranges considerably and depends on breed, season, age, and reproductive status. Average testes measure 80–140 mm in length and 50–80 mm in width. Daily sperm production and output (DSO) is highly correlated with testis parenchymal weight. Testis parenchymal weight is correlated with testicular volume and total scrotal width. A satisfactory prospective breeder should have a total scrotal width of at least 8 cm. Sperm output is more accurately predicted by calculating testicular volume using the dimensions of width, height, and length acquired using either calipers or ultrasonography.

$$\text{Volume} = 4/3\pi \times W/2 \times H/2 \times L/2 = 0.523\left(W \times H \times L\right)$$

$$\text{Predicted DSO}\left(\times 10^{9}\right) = \left(\text{Total testicular volume} \times 0.024\right) - \left(0.76 \text{ to } 1.26\right)$$

- The appearance of the epididymis is a "swiss cheese" pattern owing to the fact that the epididymis is composed of a single, highly convoluted, fluid-filled duct. The lumen is narrowest in the head and widest in the tail, making the epididymal tail the easiest to visualize and differentiate from the testicular parenchyma. Prominent dilation of the epididymal duct can be due to chronic accumulation of sperm or may indicate a disease process such as epididymitis or testicular torsion. Cystic structures may be found in the tail and head; the latter may be associated with ejaculatory dysfunction.

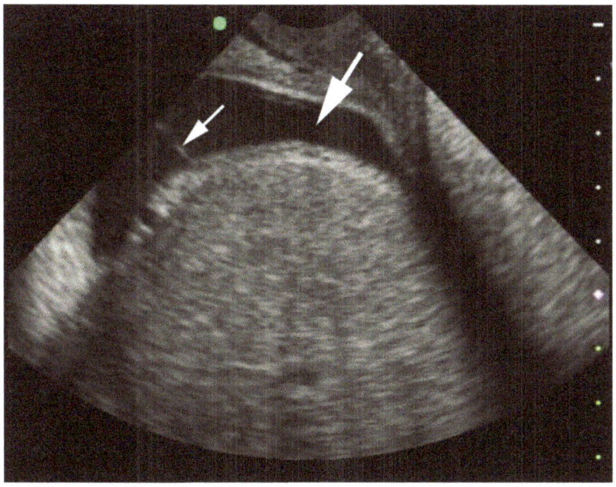

Figure 165.6 Hydrocele (large arrow) with fibrin tags (small arrow) in a stallion with a swollen scrotum. The affected testicle is below the large arrow, with the second testicle just to the right of the image.

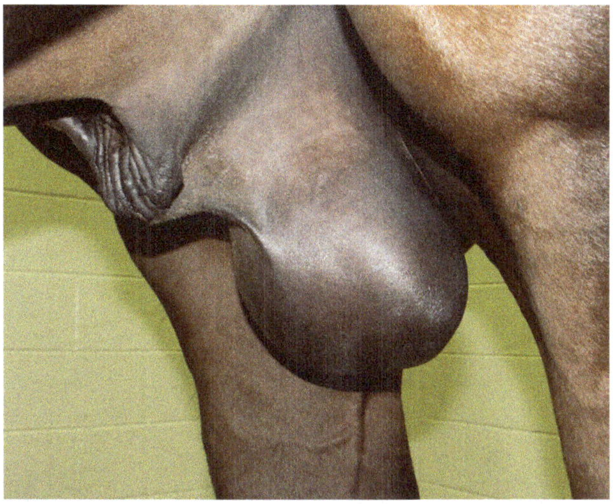

Figure 165.7 Stallion with a swollen scrotum, orchitis, and hydrocele (same stallion as seen in Figure 165.6).

- The spermatic cord should have a heterogenous appearance with anechoic circular areas surrounded by more hyperechoic regions in cross-section. Enlargement of the venous vessels within the pampiniform plexus (varicocele) or within the lymphatic vessels (lympangiectasis) may be found. The presence of a varicocele may be associated with the distension of the central vein and have a negative effect on semen characteristics. If torsion of the spermatic cord is suspected, ultrasonography can be used to help confirm the diagnosis, especially using Doppler functions.

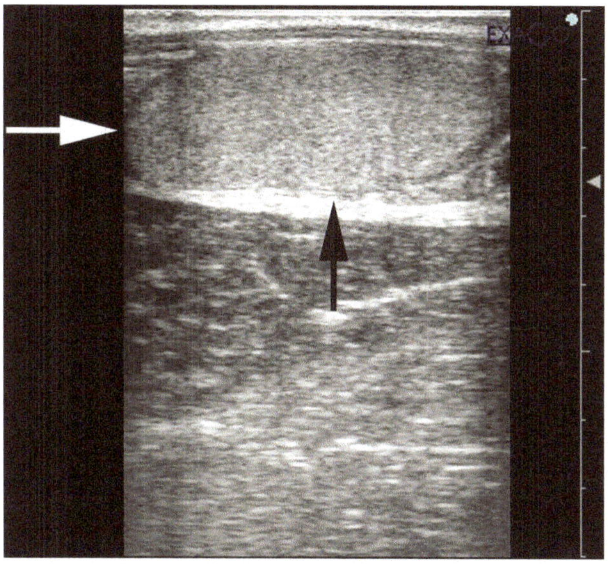

Figure 165.8 Ultrasound image of a small cryptorchid testis (arrows).

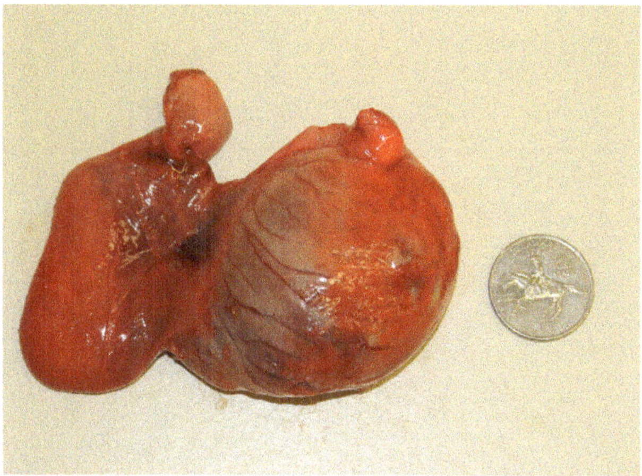

Figure 165.9 Cryptorchid testis after surgical removal. The coin in the figure is a US Quarter for size reference.

- Ultrasound may also be used to help locate cryptorchid testes, owing to the distinctive oval homogeneous echogenity of the testes (Figures 165.8 and 165.9).

Additional Comments

Doppler and color Doppler ultrasonography have been used to evaluate testicular vasculature in stallions and reference values are available for normal stallions (see Chapter 76). Furthermore, a variety of testicular pathologies have also been evaluated knowing that vascular disorders play an important role in male infertility. These studies suggest that this technique provides an important clinical reference and preferably should be included in the stallion breeding soundness exam and certainly in the diagnostic workup of scrotal diseases.

Also, three-dimensional ultrasonography and image analysis have been performed successfully on the equine testes and have, for instance, been shown to lead to more accurate volume predictions then when using measurements from conventional two-dimensional ultrasound or calipers, increasing precision when predicting the breeding potential (DSO) of a stallion.

Reference

Pickett BW, Voss JL, Squires EL, Amann RP. 1989. Management of the Stallion for Maximum Reproductive Efficiency II. Animal Reproduction Laboratory Bulletin No. 05. Fort Collins, CO: Colorado State University.

Further Reading

Love CC, Garcia MC, Riera FR, Kenney RM. 1991. Evaluation of measures taken by ultrasonography and caliper to estimate testicular volume and predict daily sperm output in the stallion. *J Reprod Fertil Suppl* 44: 99–105.

Love CC, Varner DD. 1998. Ultrasonography of the scrotal contents and penis of the stallion. In: Rantanan NW, McKinnon AO (eds). Equine Diagnotic Ultrasonography. Baltimore: Williams and Williams, pp. 253–69.

Pozor MA. 2005. Diagnostic applications of ultrasonography to stallion's reproductive tract. *Theriogenology* 64: 505–9.

Pozor MA, Harnik S. 2016. Lateral branched of the testicular artery affect testicular shape in adult stallions. *J Eq Vet Sci* 36: 90–6.

Pricking S, Bollwein H, Spilker K, *et al*. 2017. Testicular volumetry and prediction of daily sperm output in stallions by orchidometry and two- and three-dimensional sonography. *Theriogenology* 104: 149–55.

Sertich PL. 2011. Examination of external genitalia. In: McKinnon AO, Squires EL, Vaala WE, Varner DD (eds). Equine Reproduction, 2nd edn. Ames, IA: Wiley Blackwell, pp. 1458–61.

Turner RM. 2011. Ultrasonography of the genital tract. In: McKinnon AO, Squires EL, Vaala WE, Varner DD (eds). Equine Reproduction, 2nd edn. Ames, IA: Wiley Blackwell, pp. 1469–87.

166

Palpation and Ultrasonography of the Accessory Sex Glands

Sofie Sitters

Amsterdam, The Netherlands

Introduction

The stallion accessory sex glands include the paired ampullae of the ductus deferens, the paired vesicular glands (previously termed seminal vesicles), the prostate gland, and the paired bulbourethral glands (Figure 166.1). Secretions of these accessory sex glands are collectively referred to as seminal plasma and make up approximately 95% of the ejaculate volume.

Examination of the stallion's accessory sex glands should be part of a routine breeding soundness evaluation and may provide valuable information in a stallion with fertility issues. The examination is performed by a combination of palpation and ultrasonography per rectum. A majority of stallions tolerate the procedures well with minimal restraint (i.e., palpation stocks) and light sedation.

Although pathology of the accessory sex glands is uncommon, it is advisable to become accustomed with the ultrasonographic technique and normal appearance of the accessory glands so that pathology can be identified more easily should it occur.

Anatomy

- The *ampullae* are prominent circumferential enlargements in the terminal (distal) segment of the deferent ducts. Their diameter measures 1–2 cm (0.4–0.75 inches) and they are 10–25 cm (4 to 10 inches) long. The ampullae converge caudally over the neck of the bladder, taper sharply, and form two excretory ducts that merge with the two ducts of the vesicular glands forming two short common ejaculatory ducts.
- The *vesicular glands* lie laterally to the ampullae and are elongated, slightly pyriform, thin-walled sacs that produce the gel fraction of the stallion ejaculate. During sexual stimulation, secretory products are emitted into the glands' lumen causing them to expand. When fully extended they can reach 5 cm (2 inches) in diameter and 15–20 cm (6 to 7.8 inches) in length. However, when empty, the glands conform closely to the surrounding structures (ampullae, bladder, digestive tract). The duct of each vesicular gland merges with the ipsilateral deferent duct to form the common ejaculatory duct. The seminal colliculus is the anatomic site where the ejaculatory ducts of the ampullae and vesicular glands enter into the lumen of the pelvic urethra.
- The *prostate gland* is composed of a left and right pyramidal lobe and a connecting isthmus located at the cranial level of the urethralis muscle, and has a nodular spongy character. Each lobe measures 5–8 cm (2–3 inches) in length, 2–4 cm (0.75–1.5 inches) in width, and can be 1–2 cm (0.4–0.75 inches) thick. The isthmus borders the dorsal edge of the pelvic urethra as a thin, traverse band. Multiple excretory ductules emerge from the prostatic lobes, each individually opening into the lumen of the pelvic urethra on the lateral sides of the colliculus. The prostatic contribution to the ejaculate appears mainly in the sperm-rich fraction of the ejaculate.
- The *bulbourethral* are ovoid in shape and lie caudal to the prostate gland on the dorso-lateral surface of the pelvic urethra at the ischial arch. Each gland measures 3–4 cm (1–1.5 inches) in length and 2–3 cm (0.75–1 inches) in width and has several excretory ducts that enter the urethral lumen near the ventral midline distal to the seminal colliculus. These glands produce the majority of the pre-ejaculatory fluid.

Equipment and Supplies

Ultrasound machine: a linear array 7.5 MHz transducer is preferred, although a 5 MHz transducer can be used but some detail will be lost; non-sterile obstetrical lubricant, non-sterile obstetrical sleeves, halter and chain, twitch, sedation, and *N*-butylscopolammonium bromide (Buscopan®).

Equine Reproductive Procedures, Second Edition. Edited by John Dascanio and Patrick McCue.

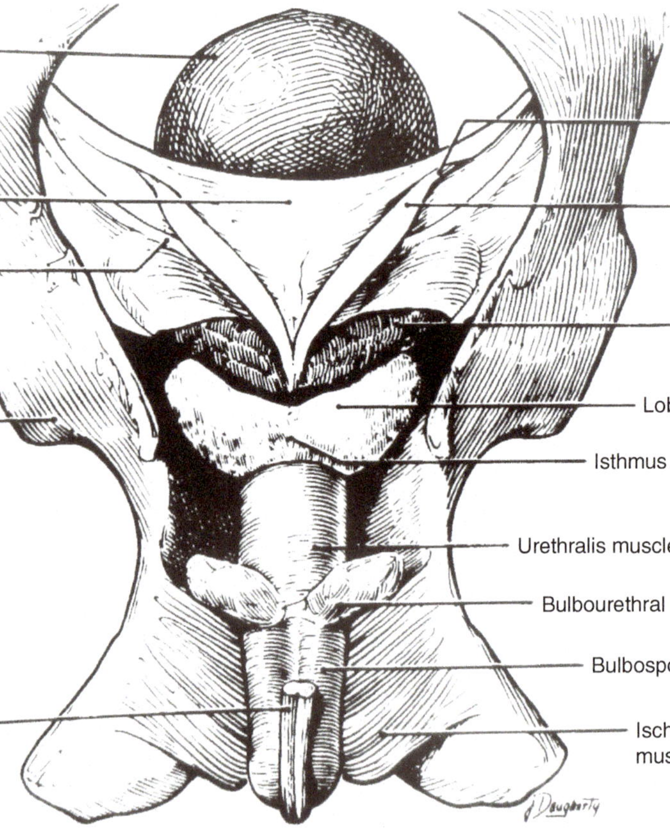

Figure 166.1 Anatomy of the accessory sex glands of the stallion. Source: From Pickett BW, Voss JL, Squires EL, Amann RP. 1989. *Management of the Stallion for Maximum Reproductive Efficiency II.* Animal Reproduction Laboratory Bulletin No. 05. Colorado State University 1989. Reproduced with the permission of Colorado State University.

Safety and Restraint

Preferably place the stallion in stocks as most stallions will not be accustomed to being palpated per rectum. Restrain the animal appropriately with the use of an experienced handler and/or with the use of a twitch and sedation. If sedation is required, phenothiazine tranquilizers such as acepromazine should not be used as stallions may develop priapism or paraphimosis as a result. Sexual excitement should be avoided while under the influence of a tranquilizer. Administration of *N*-butylscopolammonium bromide may be indicated to facilitate a safe transrectal examination.

Technique

- Using copious lubricant, slowly introduce your hand into the rectum and evacuate all fecal material.
- Manually locate each of the accessory glands starting cranially:
  - Identify the *ampullae* that are located dorso-lateral to the bladder and medial to the vesicular glands.
  - Moving slightly laterally and caudally locate the *vesicular glands*. Whether or not they are easily palpable will depend on the amount of fluid in their lumen.
  - After localizing the vesicular glands move further caudal to the *prostate gland,* located on the ventral midline of the pelvis with lobes just caudal to the corresponding vesicular glands.
  - Moving further caudal locate the *bulbourethral glands*. They can be found just inside the anus, to the right and left of the ventral midline. Withdraw your wrist and the palm of your hand from the rectum, palpating mainly with your fingers. Sometimes the glands can be isolated between the thumb and fingers, with the thumb held outside the anus, at the 5 and 7 o'clock positions.
- After manually locating an accessory sex gland examine it thoroughly for shape, size, consistency, symmetry, possible abnormalities, and pain. Take note of any abnormalities encountered in order to further examine these in more detail by ultrasonography. Remove your hand from the rectum and re-enter with an ultrasound transducer.

- Proceed by positioning the transducer on each of the previously located accessory glands and systematically examine them ultrasonographically:
  - Start by obtaining images of the individual *ampullae* in a sagittal plane by placing the transducer directly over each gland. Next try to obtain a transverse image by turning the transducer at a 90-degree angle to the long axis of each gland. However, this might be hard to accomplish in smaller stallions or with larger transducers. If you are successful at imaging the glands in cross-section, follow them caudally where they approach the midline and enter the urethra. While doing so the urethra will be visible ventral and medial to the ampullae.
  - Next move the transducer slightly laterally and caudally to the ampullae in order to obtain both sagittal and transverse images of the *vesicular glands* in the same way as described for the ampullae. Keep in mind that the vesicular glands are usually readily identifiable when fluid-filled, but when empty they can be difficult to distinguish.
  - Proceed to the isthmus of the *prostate gland* by moving the transducer caudally from the vesicular glands over the ventral midline of the pelvis. From that point on, both lobes can be viewed in cross-section by moving the transducer laterally to the left and right.
  - Finally, image the *bulbourethral glands* by moving the transducer caudally to the prostatic lobes. As described earlier, leave only your fingers holding the transducer just within the anal sphincter to properly place the transducer.

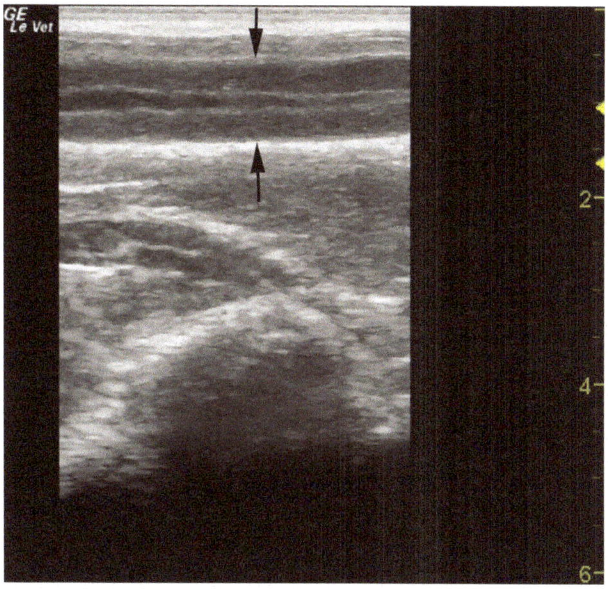

Figure 166.2 Sagittal (longitudinal) view of the normal ampulla denoted by the arrows. Note the more hypoechoic central lumen.

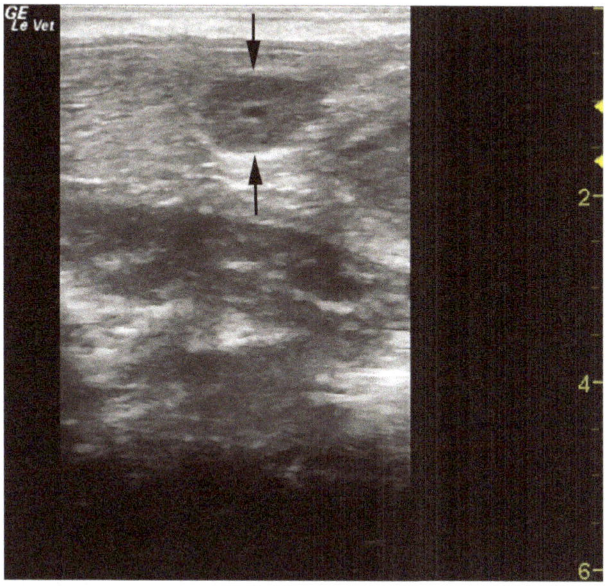

Figure 166.3 Transverse view (cross-section) of the normal ampulla denoted by the arrows. Note the more hypoechoic central lumen.

Interpretation

- The ampullae will be viewed as soft tissue bands in a sagittal plane with their centrally located lumen visible as a hypoechoic line when they contain fluid (Figure 166.2), or as a hyperechoic line when devoid of fluid. When visualized in cross-section the lumen that contains the fluid will appear as a hypoechoic circle (Figure 166.3), and the empty lumen as a broken hyperechoic line. The ampullar parenchyma has a mottled appearance in most stallions and echogenicity varies widely. Normally the diameter of the lumen, and therefore of the ampulla, will increase after sexual stimulation and decrease following ejaculation.
- The vesicular glands have smooth, slightly hyperechoic walls when viewed in a sagittal plane (Figure 166.4). The glands will be empty at sexual rest and will appear as flattened soft tissue structures with a somewhat irregular outline. When devoid of intraluminal fluid they can be quite hard to visualize. The amount of anechoic fluid in the lumen can vary depending on the amount of sexual stimulation. The glands can become quite large and extend into bladder-like shapes with a thin wall.
- The size and appearance of the prostate gland depends on the amount of sexual stimulation. In the sexually rested animal, the parenchyma will appear heterogenous gray-white and contains multiple small anechoic fluid-filled

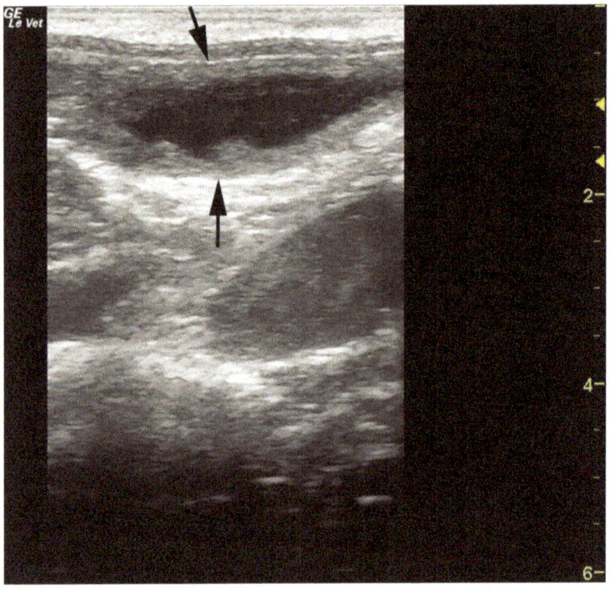

Figure 166.4 Sagittal (longitudinal) view of the normal vesicular gland outlined by the two arrows with hypoechoic fluid in the lumen.

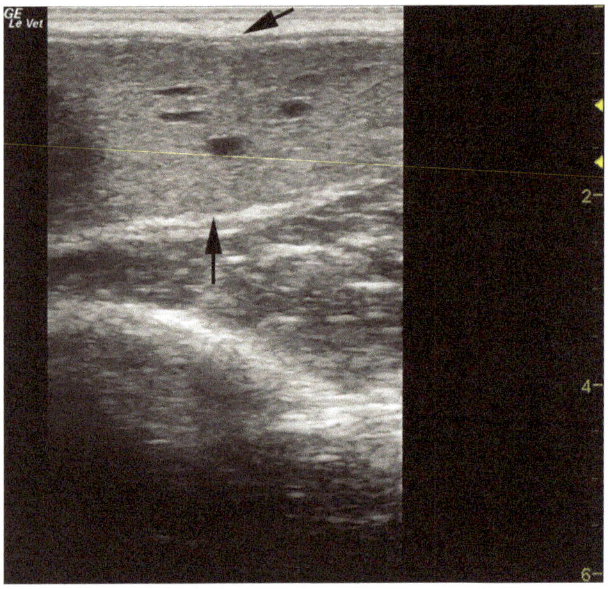

Figure 166.5 Sagittal (longitudinal) view of the normal prostate outlined by the two arrows.

pockets or bands radiating laterally (Figure 166.5). After teasing, the gland will increase in overall size and fluid content and this change can be quite dramatic.

- The bulbourethral glands, when imaged in a sagittal plane, have a mottled, isoechoic glandular parenchyma outlined by the bulboglandularis muscle appearing as a thin hypoechoic border. These glands will also increase in size and fluid content when the stallion is sexually stimulated and hypoechoic areas will appear throughout the parenchyma.

Pathology of the Accessory Sex Glands

Pathology of the accessory sex glands of the stallion are uncommon and primarily consist of blocked or plugged ampullae or infection of the vesicular glands.

Plugged ampullae may be associated with complete or incomplete occlusion of the ampullar lumen. A stallion with complete bilateral blockage will be azoospermic. Diagnosis is based on a combination of an absence of sperm in the ejaculate, low alkaline phosphatase levels in fluid recovered during the collection attempt, and palpation and ultrasonography of the ampullae per rectum. Enlarged and rigid ampullae may be detected on palpation. Ultrasonography may reveal a distended lumen with either hypo- or hyperechoic contents, or the ampullae may have a normal appearance.

Treatment consists of frequent collection attempts to remove the accumulated spermatozoa, manual massage of the ampullae per rectum, and administration of oxytocin to stimulate ampullar smooth muscle contractions. Eventual release of the plugged ampullae yields an initial ejaculate with very high sperm numbers, casts of densely packed spermatozoa (Figures 166.6 and 166.7), poor sperm motility, and many sperm with detached heads. Seminal parameters will generally improve upon subsequent collections.

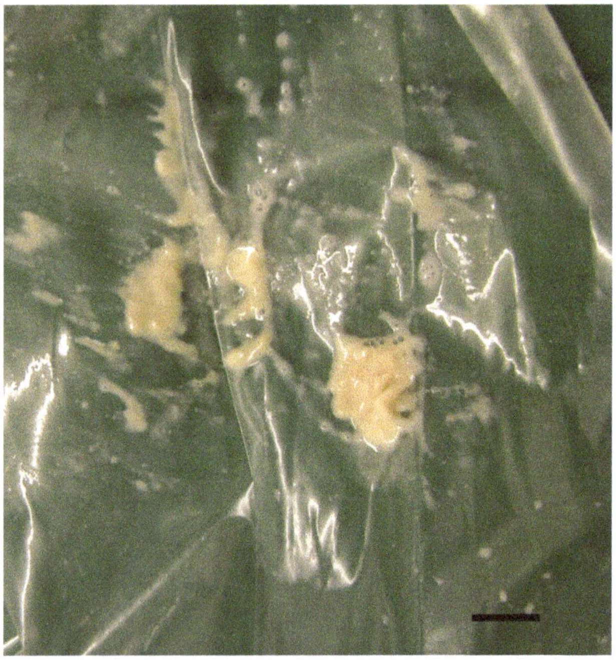

Figure 166.6 Inspissated semen within an artificial vagina liner after the clearance of an ampullar blockage (bar = approximately 1 cm).

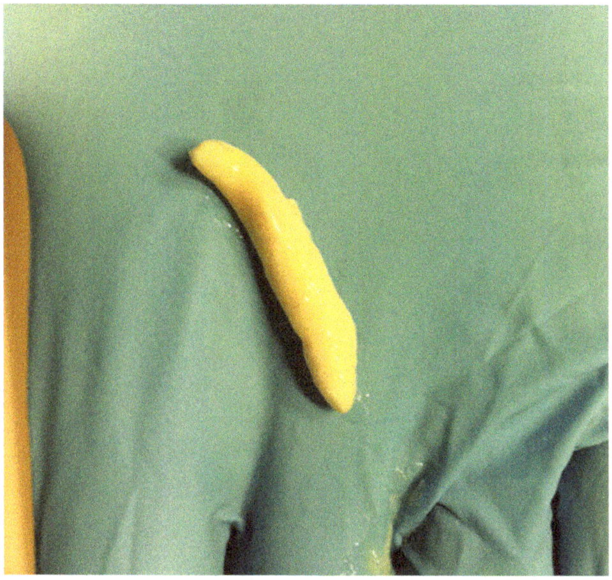

Figure 166.7 Inspissated semen plug after the clearance of an ampullar blockage, lying in a gloved hand.

Seminal vesiculitis is a less common, but quite persistent, abnormality reported in stallions. Bacterial organisms play an important role in the etiology, but the pathogenesis is unclear. Signs of seminal vesiculitis include poor semen quality, subfertility, and the presence of neutrophils and bacteria in the ejaculate. Grossly, the semen samples may be discolored due to blood contamination. Pus and debris will be associated with the gel fraction of the ejaculate. Examination of the affected vesicular glands by palpation per rectum may reveal enlarged, painful, lobulated and firm structures or the glands may feel normal. Ultrasonographic examination can be very helpful and may reveal anechoic to hyperechoic fluid containing debris or fibrin tags within an irregular lumen with hyperechoic edges. Chronically affected glands are often devoid of fluid. Cytologic evaluation and bacterial culture of vesicular gland secretions aid in the diagnosis of this abnormality. The contents of the glands may be sampled directly through catheterization guided rectally or with the help of a flexible endoscope (urethroscopy) (see Chapter 163). The glands may be lavaged prior to the deposition of antibiotics using a flexible endoscope and catheter passed through the biopsy channel. Surgical removal of infected vesicular glands has been described, but is not an easy procedure.

Additional Comments

If visualization of the accessory sex glands during ejaculation is desired, it has been shown that stallions can be trained to tolerate transrectal ultrasonography during ejaculation, resulting in acceptable visualization of their accessory sex glands and excurrent ducts (Weber & Woods 1991).

References

Pickett BW, Voss JL, Squires EL, Amann RP. 1989. Management of the Stallion for Maximum Reproductive Efficiency II. Animal Reproduction Laboratory Bulletin No. 05. Fort Collins, CO: Colorado State University.

Weber JA, Woods GL. 1992. Transrectal ultrasonography for the evaluation of stallion accessory sex glands. *Stallion management. Vet Clin North Am Eq Pract* 8: 183–90.

Further Reading

Little TV, Woods GL. 1987. Ultrasonography of the accessory sex glands in the stallion. *J Reprod Fertil Suppl* 35: 87–94.

Love CC, Riera FR, Oristaglio Turner RM, Kenney RM. 1992. Sperm occluded (plugged) ampullae in the stallion. In: *Proceedings of the Annual Meeting of the Society for Theriogenology, pp.* 117–25.

Pozor MA, McDonnell SM. 2002. Ultrasonographic measurements of accessory sex glands, ampullae and urethra of normal stallions of various size types. *Theriogenology* 58: 1425–33.

Turner RM. 2011. Ultrasonography of the genital tract. In: McKinnon AO, Squires EL, Vaala WE, Varner DD (eds). Equine Reproduction, 2nd edn. Ames, IA: Wiley Blackwell, pp. 1469–87.

Varner DD, Schumacher J. 2011. Abnormalities of the accessory sex glands. In: McKinnon AO, Squires EL, Vaala WE, Varner DD (eds). Equine Reproduction, 2nd edn. Ames, IA: Wiley Blackwell, pp. 1113–18.

167

Radiographic Examination of the Penis

Patrick M. McCue

Equine Reproduction Laboratory, Colorado State University, USA

Introduction

The stallion or gelding penis may be evaluated by contrast radiography in order to detect or confirm the presence of specific disorders. Contrast radiography may allow urethral abnormalities such as strictures, space-occupying masses (i.e., calculi), ulcerations, fistulas, and other conditions to be visualized. In addition, contrast radiography may allow for the detection of shunts within the corpus cavernosum and rupture or laceration of the tunica albuginea.

Equipment and Supplies

Contrast media (i.e., barium sulfate or iohexol), radiography unit, sedation, non-residual soap, povidone-iodine scrub, sterile saline, paper towels, examination gloves, syringes, needles, urethral catheter.

Technique

Urethral Evaluation

- The stallion should be sedated with a combination of xylazine or detomidine plus butorphanol.
- The penis is extended and washed thoroughly with a non-residual soap and rinsed with water (see Chapter 123).
- Approximately 180 ml of a suspension of barium sulfate is slowly infused into the urethra using a urethral catheter and syringe.
- Lateral and (if possible) dorso-ventral views of the penis are radiographed.
- The barium is allowed to drain from the urethra and air is infused. Another series of radiographs are taken to provide a double-contrast effect.
- The testes should be shielded from the X-ray beam with lead shielding.

Corpus Cavernosum Evaluation (Caverosography)

- The dorsal aspect of the penis should be thoroughly cleaned with povidone-iodine scrub and rinsed with 0.9% sterile saline.
- Approximately 100–200 ml of iohexol, a 24% water-soluble, organic, iodine radiographic contrast medium, is injected into the corpus cavernosum penis (CCP).
- A series of radiographs are taken for evaluation.
- If vascular shunts are present, contrast medium will appear in the nutrient vessels of the penis and prepuce.
- Damage to trabeculae of the CCP is identified by incomplete filling of the sinusoidal spaces with contrast medium.
- Rupture of the tunica albuginea is recognized by leakage of contrast medium out of the CCP.

Additional Comments

Contrast radiography may only be beneficial in a select few clinical cases. It is likely that a lesions or abnormalities of the urethra could be diagnosed more efficiently with a videoendoscope.

Equine Reproductive Procedures, Second Edition. Edited by John Dascanio and Patrick McCue.

Further Reading

Schumacher J. 2006. Penis and prepuce. In: Auer JA, Stick JA (eds). Equine Surgery, 3rd edn. St Louis, MI: WB Saunders, pp. 811–35.

Voss JL, McKinnon AO. 1993. Hemospermia and urospermia. In: McKinnon AO, Voss JL (eds). Equine Reproduction. Baltimore: Williams and Wilkins, pp. 864–70.

Weaver AD. 1968. Midline laparotomy in a gelding for removal of large vesical calculus. *Br J Urol* 40: 459–63.

168

Testicular Biopsy and Aspiration

John J. Dascanio

School of Veterinary Medicine, Texas Tech University, USA

Introduction

Testicular biopsy may be performed to assess areas of suspected pathology and to evaluate testicular function by monitoring morphologic aspects of spermatogenesis. There are three methods to obtain testicular tissue for diagnostic purposes: incisional (wedge) biopsy, split needle biopsy, and fine needle aspiration. An automated split needle biopsy is usually the technique of choice due to ease of use and minimal trauma caused to the testicle. Manual palpation and ultrasound examination are used to identify specific areas for biopsy collection. General anesthesia is recommended to safely perform the technique.

Equipment and Supplies

Sterile surgical gloves, surgical scrub, 2% lidocaine, sterile gauze, scalpel blades, needles, syringes, sedatives, Tru-Cut® biopsy instrument, Bard® biopsy system, formalin, sterile container, sedation, general anesthesia, antibiotics, non-steroidal anti-inflammatory drugs, Diff-Quik® stain, microscope slides, microscope.

Technique for an Incisional (Wedge) Biopsy

- Incisional or wedge biopsies provide the largest tissue sample for diagnostic analysis. However, they also may lead to the most complications. The tunica albuginea must be incised for sample collection and sutures used to close the incision. Adhesion formation and bleeding from the surgical site may occur after the procedure.
- The stallion is placed under general anesthesia. The scrotum is aseptically prepared for surgery and draped. A skin incision is made and a 0.5 cm incision is made in the tunica albuginea at an avascular site. The testicular tissue will protrude or bulge through the incision and a scalpel blade can be used to excise tissue to just below the level of the tunica albuginea. The tunica albuginea, parietal vaginal tunic, and scrotal skin are closed separately using 4-0 absorbable sutures.
- The testicular sample is placed in formalin and submitted for histologic analysis.
- The stallion may be administered a non-steroidal anti-inflammatory drug and antibiotics after the procedure to minimize inflammation and to prevent potential infection at the biopsy site.

Technique for a Split Needle Biopsy

- There are two techniques employed for split needle biopsy: an automated technique using a 14 gauge Bard® biopsy system (Monopty® Split Needle Biopsy Instrument; Bard Biopsy Systems, C.R. Bard, Inc., Tempe, AZ, USA), which is a spring-loaded instrument, and a manual technique using a 14 gauge 7.5 cm (3 inch) Tru-Cut® biopsy instrument.
- The procedure may be performed with the standing stallion restrained and under sedation, typically with xylazine, romifidine, or detomidine plus butorphanol tartrate.
- The scrotum is aseptically prepared.
- Wearing sterile surgical gloves, the testicle is held ventrally within the scrotum by placing the hand above the testes, around the spermatic cord. The scrotal skin should be tight across the testicle.
- The cranio-lateral aspect of the testes should be sampled to avoid vasculature. Ultrasound may also be used to identify and avoid vascular structures prior to biopsy if an alternative site is chosen.
- The site of puncture should be infiltrated subcutaneously with 2–3 ml of 2% lidocaine.

Equine Reproductive Procedures, Second Edition. Edited by John Dascanio and Patrick McCue.

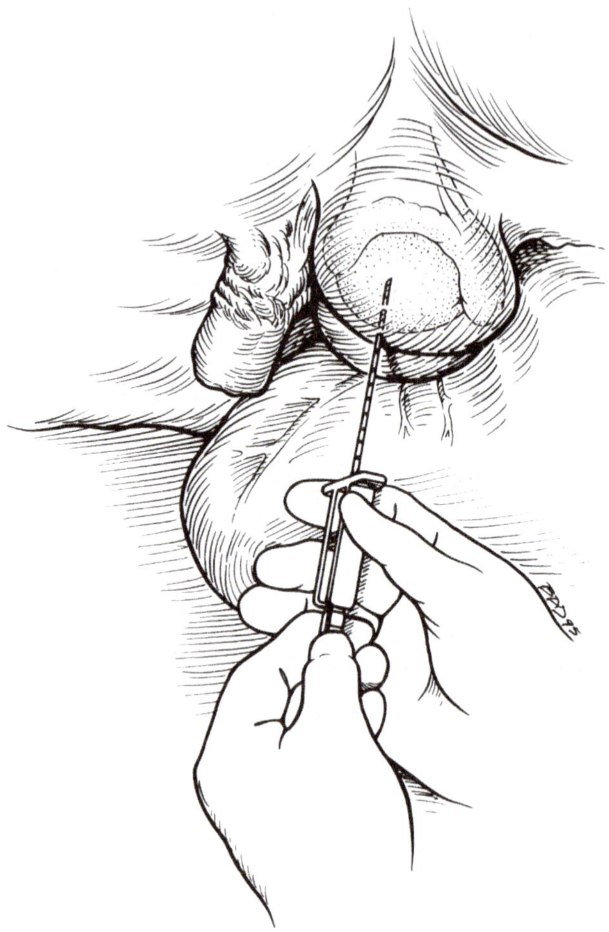

Figure 168.1 Biopsy of a stallion testes using a Tru-Cut® biopsy instrument. Source: From Dascanio JJ. 1999. Examination of the scrotum, testes, prepuce and penis. In: Wolfe DF, Moll HD (eds). *Large Animal Urogenital Surgery Text.* Baltimore: Williams and Wilkins, pp. 17–21. Reproduced with the permission of Lippincott Williams and Wilkins.

- A no. 15 scalpel blade is used to make a 2–3 mm incision in the scrotal skin. It is possible to take the biopsy without the skin incision, but the incision makes placement of the needle easier.
- The tip of the biopsy instrument is inserted through the skin incision perpendicular to the testicle.
- With the Bard® biopsy instrument in contact with the testicle, a button is depressed on the instrument to fire the split needle to acquire a sample. Alternatively, the Bard® instrument may be advanced through the tunica albuginea and then fired.
- With the Tru-Cut® system, the tip of the needle is advanced into the testicular parenchyma just past the tunica albuginea (Figure 168.1). The inner needle is advanced, keeping the outer shaft stationary. The outer shaft is then advanced over the stationary inner needle to obtain the tissue sample. The Tru-Cut® needle is then removed from the testes keeping the inner needle and outer shaft together. The inner needle may be advanced to reveal the tissue sample within the 20 mm sample notch. An assistant will need to stabilize the testicle for this procedure.
- After the biopsy is collected, manual pressure may be applied to the puncture site with sterile gauze to prevent excessive hemorrhage at the site.
- The testicular biopsy sample is placed in formalin and submitted for histologic analysis. The entire needle may be put into the formalin solution and gently moved about to dislodge the tissue sample to preserve its architecture.
- The scrotal skin incision may be left open to heal or a 4-0 suture may be placed to oppose the skin.
- The stallion may be given a non-steroidal anti-inflammatory drug and antibiotics after the procedure to minimize inflammation and the potential for infection at the biopsy site.

Technique for Fine Needle Aspiration

- Fine needle aspiration is performed with the stallion standing and sedated with xylazine, romifidine, or detomidine plus butorphanol tartrate.
- The scrotum is aseptically prepared.
- An ultrasound examination may be performed to identify a relative non-vascular testicular site for needle puncture.
- Wearing sterile surgical gloves, the testicle is held ventrally within the scrotum by placing the hand above the testes, around the spermatic cord.
- A 22 gauge needle on a 5 ml syringe is slowly advanced into the testicular parenchyma perpendicular to the testes. The central testicular vein, epididymis, and lateral testicular artery should be avoided. The needle is usually inserted into the cranio-lateral quarter of the testes.
- The syringe plunger is pulled outward to generate a vacuum, pulling tissue into the needle. With continuing vacuum, the needle may be moved forward and backward slightly a few times to aid in obtaining a diagnostic sample.
- The syringe plunger is released to discontinue the vacuum.
- The syringe is removed from the needle prior to removal of the needle from the testes. This may help to avoid getting blood within the needle upon removal. The needle is then removed from the testes and pressure applied to the needle puncture site with sterile gauze to prevent excessive hemorrhage at the site.
- The syringe is filled with air and reattached to the needle. The plunger is gently pushed with the needle over a

glass microscope slide to discharge the contents, forming a drop on the slide. A second slide is used to create a smear by laying the second slide parallel to the first and drawing it outward to create a smear.
- The two smeared slides are allowed to air-dry. One slide may be stained with Diff-Quik® stain (modified Wright Giemsa stain) and the other held for alternative staining, pending initial review.
- Slides are examined under high dry (400×) and oil immersion (1,000×) objectives.

Interpretation

- A fine needle aspiration will provide a sample for cytologic analysis, but in a less organized fashion than a histologic sample.
- If the sample obtained by the various needle techniques is not of diagnostic quality, additional samples may be collected without causing significant testicular trauma.
- Scrotal edema may occur secondary to the various biopsy procedures, but usually resolves within a few days.
- Hemorrhage, infection, or adhesions are potential complications with more invasive procedures and should be discussed with the stallion owner prior to performing the procedure.
- With incisional (wedge) biopsies, spermatogenesis and potentially fertility may be adversely affected for a period of weeks until the surgical site heals. Once inflammation is resolved, approximately 2 months is required to produce non-affected spermatozoa.

Reference

Dascanio JJ. 1999. Examination of the scrotum, testes, prepuce and penis. In: Wolfe DF, Moll HD (eds). Large Animal Urogenital Surgery Text. Baltimore: Williams and Wilkins, pp. 17–21.

Further Reading

Faber NF, Roser JF. 2000. Testicular biopsy in stallions: potential diagnostic and effects on prospective fertility. *J Reprod Fertil Suppl* 56: 31–42.

Hillman RB, Casey PJ, Kennedy PC, *et al.* 1994. Testicular biopsy in stallions. In: *Proceedings of the 6th International Symposium on Equine* Reproduction, pp. 145–6.

Leme DP, Papa FO. 2010. How to perform and interpret testicular fine needle aspiration in stallions. *J Eq Vet Sci* 30: 590–6.

Pearson LK, Rodriguez JS, Tibary A. 2011. How to obtain a stallion testicular biopsy using a spring-loaded split-needle biopsy instrument. *Proc Annu Conv Am Assoc Eq Pract* 57: 219–25.

169

Assessment of Sperm Plasma Membrane Integrity and Viability: Propidium Iodide/SYBR-14

Amanda I. Glazar[1] *and Patrick M. McCue*[2]

[1] *Kynectiv, Inc., USA*
[2] *Equine Reproduction Laboratory, Colorado State University, USA*

Introduction

Spermatozoa are considered as viable when they have an intact plasma membrane. SYBR-14 is a fluorescent stain that can penetrate all cells, membrane damaged or intact, and bind to DNA. SYBR-14 is used in the evaluation of semen to identify spermatozoa from other non-cellular debris in the sample. Propidium iodide (PI) is a fluorescent stain that cannot penetrate an intact plasma membrane and therefore can only enter spermatozoa and bind to DNA of spermatozoa with a damaged plasma membrane (i.e., a non-viable sperm).

A dual stain of PI and SYBR-14 is commonly used to evaluate the viability of stallion spermatozoa. The two stains are added to an aliquot of spermatozoa and when excited by a laser, non-viable cells will fluoresce red from the PI and live, membrane-intact cells will fluoresce green with SYBR-14 (Table 169.1). Fluorescent stains allow for greater contrast and interpretation between viable and non-viable cells as compared with dried smears with an eosin-nigrosin (Hancock) stain.

Equipment and Supplies

Live-dead sperm viability kit (Molecular Probes, Eugene, OR, USA), fluorescent microscope or flow cytometer, sperm TALP media, dimethyl sulfoxide (DMSO) (99%), glass test tubes (12 × 75 mm), glass slides, coverslips, microcentrifuge tubes, pipetters and tips (200 and 1,000 μl).

Stock Solutions

Stock solutions of SYBR-14 can be prepared and stored in small aliquots until used. To prepare the stock solution add 900 μl of dimethyl sulfoxide (DMSO) to the 100 μl of SYBR-14 that comes in the viability kit. An aliquot of 30 μl can then be placed into microcentrifuge tubes and stored at −20°C (−4°F) until use. To make a working solution to stain cells, add 270 μl DMSO to the thawed 30 μl aliquot of SYBR-14 stock solution. This results in a final concentration of 10 μM SYBR-14 and will remain stable at 5°C (40°F) for 3–4 weeks.

Stock solutions of PI do not have to be made if using the Molecular Probes sperm viability kit; however, the solution can be divided into smaller aliquots and stored at −20°C (−4°F) until use. Once thawed, the stain is stable at 5°C (40°F) for 4–8 weeks.

Technique

- Semen must first be diluted to a concentration of 25–50 × 10^6 sperm/ml in either a commercial skim milk/glucose semen extender or TALP diluent (see Chapter 144).
- In a glass test tube add 20 μl SYBR-14 (working solution), 10 μl PI, 200 μl TALP, and 100 μl diluted sperm. The samples should be incubated in a container protected from light exposure for 10–15 minutes at 20°C (68°F) before being read on a fluorescent microscope.

Equine Reproductive Procedures, Second Edition. Edited by John Dascanio and Patrick McCue.

Table 169.1 Fluorescent dyes to detect spermatozoal viability. The dyes are excited by a laser and emissions fluorescence is observed.

Fluorescent Dye	Excitation	Emission	Properties
Propidium iodide (PI)	488 nm	617 nm (red)	Cell impermeant
SYBR-14	488 nm	516 nm (green)	Cell permeant

- Two separate slides should be analyzed with a minimum of 200 cells counted per slide. Cells that fluoresce red are considered non-viable, while cells that fluoresce green are considered viable (Figure 169.1). These cells can also be analyzed via flow cytometry. Flow cytometry allows a large number of cells (>50,000) to be automatically analyzed.

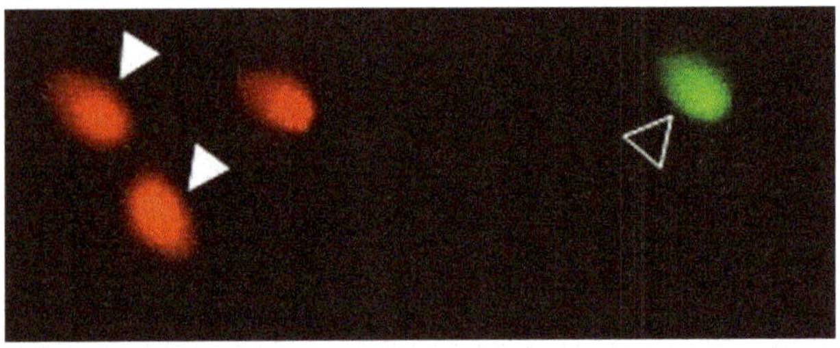

Figure 169.1 Stallion spermatozoa stained with SYBR-14 and propidium iodide (PI). Viable cells (open arrowhead) are stained with SYBR-14 and non-viable cells (white arrowheads) are stained with PI.

Interpretation

Assessment of stallion semen using SYBR-14 and PI fluorescent stains and flow cytometry allows for the rapid analysis of sperm viability (membrane integrity). Viability is usually highly correlated with spermatozoal motility. However, in some cases a significant percentage of sperm may be viable (membrane intact), but not motile. Unfortunately, sperm motility and/or viability alone do not necessarily correlate with fertility in a stallion.

Further Reading

Garner DL, Johnson LA. 1995. Viability assessment of mammalian sperm using SYBR-14 and propidium iodide. *Biol Reprod* 53: 276–87.

Graham JK. 1996. Analysis of stallion semen and its relation to fertility. *Vet Clin North Am Eq Pract* 12(1): 119–29.

Graham JK. 2001. Assessment of sperm quality: a flow cytometric approach. *Anim Reprod Sci* 68: 239–47.

Kirk ES. 2001. Flow cytometric evaluation of stallion sperm. MS thesis. Fort Collins, CO: Colorado State University.

Wilhelm KM, Graham JK, Squires EL. 1996. Comparison of the fertility of cryopreserved stallion spermatozoa with sperm motion analysis, flow cytometric evaluation, and zona-free hamster oocyte penetration. *Theriogenology* 46: 559–78.

170

Sperm Chromatin Structure Assay

Charles Love

College of Veterinary Medicine and Biomedical Sciences, Texas A&M University, USA

Introduction

The sperm chromatin structure assay (SCSA) was originally introduced and performed using flow cytometry in human sperm. The assay relies on the stain acridine orange, termed a metachromatic stain because it fluoresces different colors (orange or green) depending on whether it attaches to double-stranded (green) or single-stranded (orange) DNA/RNA. While sperm have some RNA, the levels are very low and considered insignificant when performing this assay.

The intent of the assay is to discriminate the proportion of double-stranded (native) from single-stranded (denatured) DNA by measuring the amount of green and orange fluorescence emitted by individual sperm. Unlike fluorescent assays that measure viability in which sperm fluoresce predominantly one color due to their plasma membrane status, sperm stained with acridine orange may stain both green and orange, denoting the presence of both double- and single-stranded DNA.

It is recommended that the SCSA be performed using a flow cytometer and not a fluorescent microscopy for the following reasons:

- Acridine orange is subject to bleaching and fading after a very short time period, therefore observing sperm under a microscope for an extended period of time will result in a loss of fluorescence.
- Additionally, when acridine orange bleaches, the DNA stained orange will convert to green, resulting in a higher percentage of sperm with "normal" DNA.
- The flow cytometer can detect gradations of green and orange fluorescence in individual sperm that the eye cannot discern, making the assay much more sensitive when a flow cytometer is used.

Equipment and Supplies

Mechanical pipettes, microcentrifuge tubes, acridine orange stain (Sigma-Aldrich, St Louis, MO, USA), flow cytometer (FACScan™; Bectin-Dickinson, Franklin Lakes, NJ, USA), buffer solution (0.186 g disodium EDTA, 0.790 g Tris-HCl, 4.380 g NaCl in 500 ml deionized water, pH 7.4), acid/detergent solution (2.19 g NaCl, 1.0 ml of 2 N HCl solution, 0.25 ml Triton-X, qs. 250 m deionized water), acridine orange solution (3.8869 g citric acid monohydrate, 8.9429 g Na_2HPO_4, 4.3850 g NaCl, 0.1700 g disodium EDTA, 4 µg/ml acridine orange stock solution (1 mg/ml), qs. 500 ml deionized water, pH 6.0).

Technique

- The SCSA can be performed on either fresh (raw or extended), flash frozen, or frozen-thawed sperm. Sperm should be frozen immediately after collection since holding at room temperature or especially in the incubator may induce DNA denaturation. Preferred freezing methods include liquid nitrogen, dry ice, or a –80°C (–112°F) frost-free freezer.
- The SCSA requires only 3–5 µl of a 100 million/ml semen sample. A larger sample (0.5–1.0 ml) should be frozen to ensure that there is only minimal sample exposure to air.
- It is recommended that Eppendorf tubes, cryovials, or straws be used for conventional freezing.
- Samples can be shipped to a laboratory performing the assay on dry ice or in a liquid nitrogen vapor container (dry shipper). Samples should be shipped by overnight delivery.
- The SCSA procedure is as follows:
  - A small aliquot (2–7 µl) of semen is diluted to 200 µl in buffer solution.

Equine Reproductive Procedures, Second Edition. Edited by John Dascanio and Patrick McCue.

- This is mixed with 400 μl of acid/detergent solution.
- 30 seconds later, 1.2 ml of acridine orange solution is added.
- The sample is covered in aluminum foil and placed in the flow cytometer.
- Fluid is allowed to pass through the tubing for 2 minutes before evaluating the cells.

Interpretation

The SCSA is used to complement other sperm quality assays so the clinician can offer an opinion about a stallion's fertility status. In general, stallions with high quality sperm are, or should be, fertile. While there are exceptions to this rule the clinician should strongly pursue other reasons for reduced fertility, such as mare and management considerations, when a stallion is presented with a fertility problem in the face of high sperm quality.

Causes of poor DNA quality include intrinsic production of poor quality sperm DNA in the testes and acquired causes. While stallions that produce poor quality DNA tend to have other sperm quality values that are also reduced, this is not always the case. There are individuals that appear to produce sperm quality (motility, morphology) sufficient to render a higher pregnancy rate than they are achieving and their lower level can only be explained when the SCSA is performed.

Acquired causes of reduced sperm DNA quality are due mostly to semen handling and storage conditions. The primary cause of an inadequate storage condition is excessive seminal plasma in samples that are cooled and stored. Some seminal plasma appears to have a more deleterious effect on DNA quality than others. This problem can be diagnosed by comparing a sperm sample at the time of collection with the same sample that has been extended and stored. In addition, the problem can usually be easily corrected by reducing seminal plasma concentration by centrifugation of the semen prior to storage (see Chapter 149).

Fertility generally decreases as the mean$_{\alpha t}$ and %COMP$_{\alpha t}$ in a stallion sperm sample increases. The SCSA has been able to detect differences in fertility (seasonal pregnancy rate, first cycle pregnancy rate, overall pregnancy rate per cycle) in a group of stallions with no history of reduced fertility. In these stallions, fertility decreased as the mean$_{\alpha t}$, SD$_{\alpha t}$, and %COMP$_{\alpha t}$ increased (Figures 170.1 and 170.2; Table 170.1).

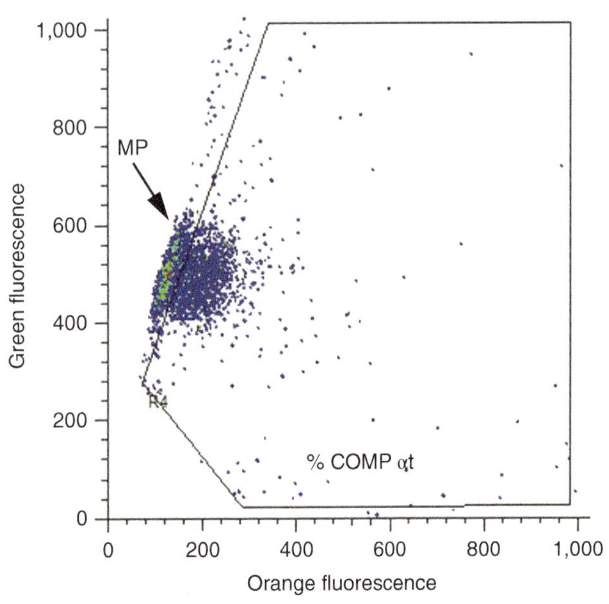

Figure 170.1 Scattergram showing the distribution of sperm following evaluation on the flow cytometer. The main population (MP) identifies those sperm with normal DNA (i.e., high green and low orange fluorescence). The five-sided region is the %COMP$_{\alpha t}$ (cells outside the main population), also termed the DNA fragmentation index (DFI). This region identifies those sperm that exhibit a higher orange fluorescence (single-stranded DNA) compared with the main population.

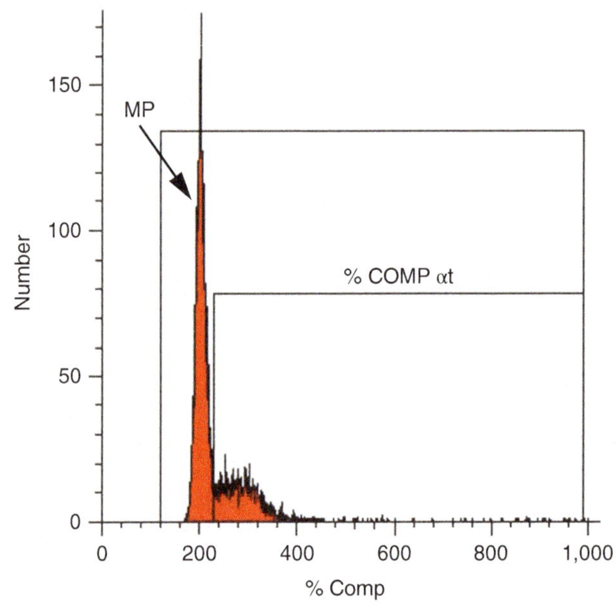

Figure 170.2 Histogram that represents the αt values from each sperm in Figure 170.1. The αt value represents the amount of orange fluorescence divided by the total fluorescence (orange + green) emitted from each sperm. The %COMP$_{\alpha t}$ (cells outside the main population) can be calculated from either the scattergram or the histogram, but the mean$_{\alpha t}$ and standard deviation of αt (SD$_{\alpha t}$) can only be calculated from the histogram. This often requires a software program such as WinList (Verity Software House, Inc., verity@vsh.com).

Table 170.1 The levels of $\%COMP_{\alpha t}$ associated with different levels of fertility.

		Fertility Parameter	
Fertility Group	Seasonal Pregnancy Rate (%)	First Cycle Pregnancy Rate (%)	$\%COMP_{\alpha t}$
1	90 ± 6	89 ± 9	13 ± 6 [a]
2	58 ± 21	58 ± 7	17 ± 7 [a]
3	NA	25 ± 18	27 ± 14 [b]

A higher level of abnormal DNA ($\%COMP_{\alpha t}$) does not necessarily reduce a stallion's fertility by itself, but it does signal that a stallion with a higher level requires a greater degree of veterinary involvement to overcome the depressing effects of the lesser DNA quality. In addition, reduced DNA quality may be cumulative, with reductions in other measures of sperm quality (motility, morphology, viability, sperm numbers). As an example, a stallion with average sperm motility and morphology and normal DNA would have higher fertility than a stallion with the same level of motility and morphology with more sperm with abnormal DNA (e.g., a 20–25% $COMP_{\alpha t}$).

Further Reading

Evenson DP, Darzynkiewicz Z, Melamed MR. 1980. Relation of mammalian sperm chromatin heterogeneity to fertility. *Science* 240: 1131–3.

Kenney RM, Evenson DP, Garcia MC, Love CC. 1995. Relationships between sperm chromatin structure, motility, and morphology of ejaculated sperm, and seasonal pregnancy rates. *Biol Reprod Mono* 1: 647–53.

Love CC, Kenney RM. 1998. The relationship of increased susceptibility of sperm DNA to denaturation and fertility in the stallion. *Theriogenology* 50: 955–72.

171

Hypo-Osmotic Swelling Test

Patrick M. McCue

Equine Reproduction Laboratory, Colorado State University, USA

Introduction

The goal of the hypo-osmotic swelling (HOS) test is to evaluate the functional integrity of the plasma membrane of spermatozoa. The test is simple to perform, accurate, and consistent, with good reliability and repeatability. It has been validated for spermatozoa of stallions and several other species.

The basis of the test is the exposure of spermatozoa to a hypo-osmotic solution, such as a 50–100 mOsm lactose or sucrose solution. Fluid from the hypo-osmotic solution will be transported across the plasma membrane. Spermatozoa with intact plasma membranes will exhibit characteristic swelling and/or coiling of the tail as water enters the intact sperm cell. Sperm with plasma membrane damage do not swell or exhibit coiling of the tail since fluid is not confined within the sperm cell.

The HOS test can be used to evaluate sperm plasma membrane integrity in lieu of more expensive diagnostic tests, such as supravital stains (SYBR-14 and propidium iodide) which require fluorescent microscopy or a flow cytometer (see Chapter 169).

Equipment and Supplies

Semen sample (raw), hypo-osmotic solution: 100 mOsm sucrose (1.712 g sucrose dissolved in 50 ml of sterile deionized water); mechanical pipettes (50–200 µl and 200–1,000 µl) and tips (200 and 1,000 µl non-filter), 1.5 ml microcentrifuge tube, glass microscope slides, coverslips, microscope (compound) with 10× eye piece and 100× (oil immersion) objective and either bright field, differential interference contrast, or phase-contrast optics.

Technique

- A 100 µl volume of raw semen is added to 1.0 ml of pre-warmed hypo-osmotic solution in a glass test tube or microcentrifuge tube.
- The contents are gently mixed.
- The sample is incubated at 37°C (99°F) for 30–60 minutes.
- A small drop of sample (approximately 30 µl) is placed onto a glass slide and a coverslip applied.
- Sperm morphology is evaluated in the wet mount sample at 400× or 1,000× using either bright field, differential interference contrast (DIC), or phase-contrast optics (Figure 171.1).
- The percentage of sperm with swollen or coiled tails (HOS+) is determined (Figure 171.2) to acquire the percentage of plasma membrane-intact spermatozoa.

Additional Comments

There is a high correlation between the HOS test and progressive motility. However, the relationship between the HOS test and fertility is not well established in the horse. One study reported that stallions with a "low swelling score" (<40%) had doubtful fertility. It has been suggested that the HOS test may be especially valuable in the evaluation of membrane integrity of frozen-thawed equine spermatozoa.

Equine Reproductive Procedures, Second Edition. Edited by John Dascanio and Patrick McCue.

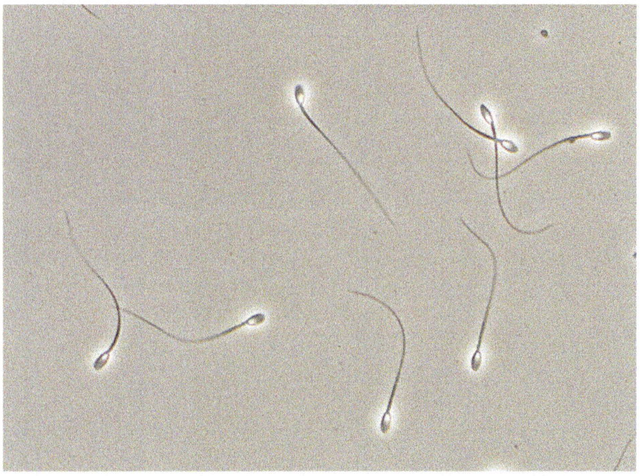

Figure 171.1 Normal stallion spermatozoa before the hypo-osmotic swelling test. Phase-contrast image (400×).

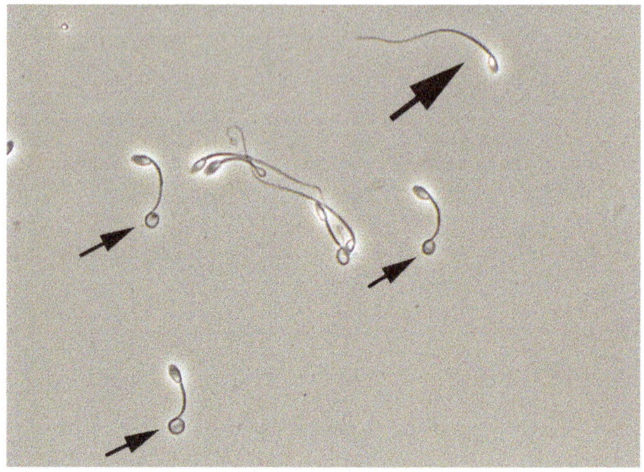

Figure 171.2 Normal stallion spermatozoa in a hypo-osmotic solution of sucrose exhibiting swollen or coiled tails (small arrows) and a spermatozoa with a non-intact plasma membrane (large arrow). Phase-contrast image (400×).

Further Reading

Neild DM, Chaves MG, Flores M, Miragaya MH, Gonzalez E, Agüero A. 2000. The HOS test and its relationship to fertility in the stallion. *Andrologia* 32: 351–5.

Neild DM, Chaves MG, Flores M, Mora N, Beconi M, Agüero A. 1999. Hypoosmotic test in equine spermatozoa. *Theriogenology* 51: 721–7.

Nie GJ, Wenzel JGW. 2001. Adaptation of the hypoosmotic swelling test to assess functional integrity of stallion spermatozoal plasma membranes. *Theriogenology* 55: 1005–18.

172

Assessment of Sperm Acrosomal Status: PE-PNA

Amanda I. Glazar[1] *and Patrick M. McCue*[2]

[1] *Kynectiv, Inc., USA*
[2] *Equine Reproduction Laboratory, Colorado State University, USA*

Introduction

Equine sperm that have been freshly ejaculated are unable to fertilize an oocyte without undergoing a series of cellular modifications known as capacitation. Changes occurring in the spermatozoa during capacitation include loss of cholesterol from the plasma membrane, hyperactivated motility, and increases in intracellular calcium, pH, and cyclic adenosine monophosphate. The phenomenon of capacitation opens receptor sites on the spermatozoon, which allows binding to the zona pellucida of the oocyte and the acrosome reaction to occur. The normal acrosome reaction will only occur in fully capacitated sperm, and will be triggered by the sperm binding to the zona pellucida.

The acrosome is an enzymatic cap that is located on the rostral end of the sperm's head. The acrosomal enzymes are released during the acrosome reaction, which digest a hole through the zona pellucida, allowing the sperm to pass through the zona pellucida, bind to the oocyte plasma membrane, and ultimately fertilize the oocyte. The acrosome reaction is an exocytotic event in which the plasma membrane fuses with the outer acrosomal membrane leading to small, separate, membrane-bound vesicles, thereby releasing the enzymatic contents of the acrosome. Once acrosome-reacted, the lifespan of the sperm is very short and if fertilization does not occur the sperm will die.

The process of cooling and freezing equine semen can damage either the plasma or acrosomal membrane and can render a sperm infertile by causing a loss of intracellular molecules or premature release of the acrosomal contents, respectively. Conventional dried smear staining techniques cannot be used to detect the acrosomal status of stallion sperm, because of its small size relative to the sperm's head and the lack of an acrosomal ridge that is present on the sperm of many other species. However, fluorescent microscopy can be used to accurately detect the integrity of the acrosome. Certain lectins, plant proteins, bind only to the enzymatic contents of the acrosome. These proteins are large and cannot pass through an intact membrane. These lectins can be tagged with fluorescent probes and if membrane damage has occurred, they will contact and bind to any acrosomal enzymes adhering to the sperm head, causing the acrosomal area to fluoresce. Sperm that have intact acrosomes, however, will not allow any lectin binding and will not fluoresce.

Two lectins are commonly used for these analyses; the common pea plant (*Pisum sativum*) agglutinin (PSA) and the peanut (*Arachis hypogea*) agglutinin (PNA). These lectins each bind to different sugar groups that are attached to proteins, and while both bind to proteins of the acrosome, PNA binds to fewer non-acrosomal proteins scattered over the entire sperm surface, making damaged acrosomes stand out much brighter than the rest of the sperm.

Lectins must be conjugated to fluorescent molecules in order to view them under a fluorescent microscope. Many different probes can be used, but fluorescein isothiocyanate (FITC), a molecule that excites at 488 nm and provides a green fluorescent emission at 518 nm, is most commonly used, as it fluoresces brighter than other probes. However, lectins conjugated to phycoerythrin (PE), which also excites at 488 nm but provides a yellow-orange fluorescence at 578 nm, can be used too. A triple staining procedure is used for the detection of acrosomal damage by fluorescent microscopy. Cells are stained with a combination of propidium iodide (PI), SYBR-14, and PE-PNA. The PI/SBYR-14 combination is necessary to differentiate between live and dead cells, while PE-PNA is used to determine if acrosomal damage has occurred.

Equine Reproductive Procedures, Second Edition. Edited by John Dascanio and Patrick McCue.

Equipment and Supplies

Live-dead sperm viability kit (Molecular Probes, Eugene, OR, USA), peanut agglutinin conjugated with phycoerythrin (Phycoprobe R-PE-PNA, P44; Biomeda Corp., Foster City, CA, USA), fluorescent microscope (set up: 488 nm argon laser with 520 nm long pass filter), sperm TALP media, dimethyl sulfoxide (DMSO) (99%), glass test tubes (12 × 75 mm), glass slides, coverslips, microcentrifuge tubes, mechanical pipettes and tips (200 and 1,000 μl).

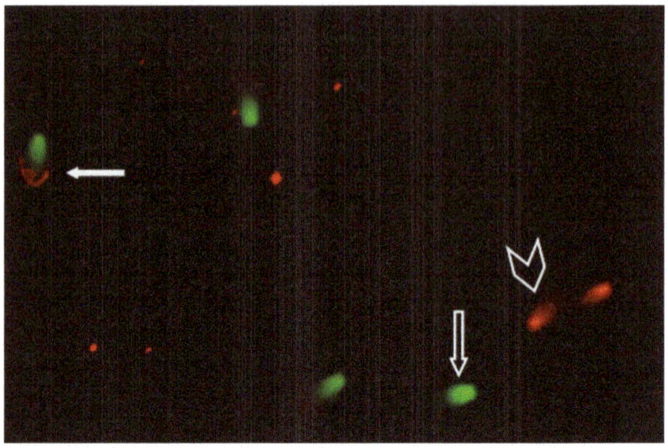

Figure 172.1 Stallion sperm stained with propidium iodide (PI), SYBR-14, and PE-PNA showing a viable acrosome-intact sperm (open arrow) stained green with SYBR-14 only, a viable acrosome-damaged sperm (solid white arrow) stained green with SYRB-14 and orange with PE-PNA, and a non-viable sperm (open arrowhead) stained red with PI.

Stock Solutions

- Stock solutions of SYBR-14 and PI should be prepared as described in the Chapter 169.
- Stock solutions of PE-PNA do not have to be made. Store the PE-PNA solution at 5°C (40°F), and do not freeze.
- Prepare a stock solution of sperm TALP media (see Chapter 144).

Technique

- Semen must be diluted to a concentration of 25–50 × 10^6 sperm/ml in the TALP diluent.
- In a glass test tube add 20 μl SYBR-14 (working solution), 10 μl PI, 5 μl PE-PNA, 200 μl TALP, and 100 μl diluted sperm. The samples should be incubated for 10–15 minutes at 20°C (68°F) before being read on a fluorescent microscope.
- Two separate slides should be analyzed with a minimum of 200 cells counted per slide. There will be three separate populations of sperm analyzed (Figure 172.1): viable, acrosome-intact sperm (fluoresces green), viable, acrosomal-damaged sperm (fluoresces green with orange acrosome cap), and non-viable sperm (fluoresces red). The acrosomal status of the non-viable sperm is hard to discern because of the similar fluorescence of PI and PE-PNA.

Interpretation

Equine sperm must possess an intact acrosome when it reaches the oocyte in order for fertilization to occur. If the acrosome is lost or damaged during processing, cryopreservation, or in transit through the female reproductive tract, the sperm cannot bind to the zona pellucida and fertilization will not occur. Therefore it is necessary to have intact acrosomal membranes at the time of insemination.

Measuring acrosomal integrity as a single attribute has been poorly correlated with a stallion's potential fertility. However, it can be expected that samples containing a high percentage of acrosome-damaged sperm (>10% of the population) will most likely exhibit reduced fertility. One potential way to increase the fertility of these frozen samples would be to inseminate an increased number of sperm into the mare compared with the normal insemination dose. This increase in sperm numbers will increase the number of viable, acrosome-intact sperm present in the oviduct during the time of fertilization. Changes in the processing and cryopreservation of sperm from a stallion that experience an increase in acrosomal damage after thawing may also improve the integrity of the acrosome and fertility. Sperm from individual stallions respond differently to cryopreservation and changes in the freezing extender, cryoprotectant, centrifugal force, and freeze rate may be necessary to preserve the acrosome.

Further Reading

Amann RP, Graham JK. 1993. Spermatozoal function. In: McKinnon AO, Voss JL (eds). Equine Reproduction. Philadelphia: Lea and Febiger, pp. 712–48.

Graham JK. 1996. Analysis of stallion semen and its relation to fertility. *Vet Clin North Am Eq Pract* 12: 119–29.

Kirk ES. 2001. Flow cytometric evaluation of stallion sperm. MS thesis. Fort Collins, CO: Colorado State University.

Nagy S, Jansen J, Topper EK, Gadella BM. 2003. A triple-stain flow cytometric method to assess plasma-and acrosome-membrane integrity of cryopreserved bovine sperm immediately after thawing in presence of egg-yolk particles. *Biol Reprod* 68: 1828–35.

173

Assessment of Sperm Mitochondrial Function: JC-1 and Rhodamine 123

Amanda I. Glazar[1] and Patrick M. McCue[2]

[1]*Kynectiv, Inc., USA*
[2]*Equine Reproduction Laboratory, Colorado State University, USA*

Introduction

Visual or computer-assisted sperm analysis (CASA) assessment of spermatozoal motility is not always correlated with the estimated fertility of a stallion. The energy source for motility is produced in the mitochondria of the middle piece of a spermatozoon. Changes in mitochondrial membrane potential may result in changes in sperm motility and be more indicative of spermatozoal function. Rhodamine 123 (R123) is the most widely used mitochondrial probe. R123 excites with visible light (488 nm) and emits a green fluorescence at 515–575 nm. This probe has been validated for stallion sperm; however, this stain cannot differentiate between high and low mitochondrial membrane potential, only the presence of mitochondria. The lipophilic probe JC-1 (5,5′,6,6′-tetrachloro-1,1′,3,3′-tetraethylbenzimidazolyl carbocyanine iodide) has been reported as distinguishing sperm cells with high or low mitochondrial membrane potential. JC-1 is excited by visible light (488 nm) and accumulates in the mitochondria of the sperm. With an increase in transmembrane electrical potential, JC-1 forms aggregates that will cause the mitochondria to fluoresce orange (590 nm). However, if the sperm has low membrane potential, JC-1 will form monomers in the mitochondria which will fluoresce green (530 nm). It is hypothesized that sperm with high mitochondrial membrane potential are more functionally correct and are able to produce the necessary adenosine triphosphate (ATP) energy to provide sperm motility.

Equipment and Supplies

JC-1 fluorescent probe (T-3168; Molecular Probes, Eugene, OR, USA), dimethyl sulfoxide (DMSO) (99% solution), fluorescent microscope (set up: 488 nm argon laser with 520 nm long pass filter), sperm TALP media, glass test tubes (12 × 75 mm), glass slides, coverslips, microcentrifuge tubes, mechanical pipette and tips (200 and 1,000 µl).

Stock Solutions

- Stock solutions of JC-1 are made by dissolving 5 mg of JC-1 powder into 1.094 ml of DMSO.
- To make a working solution, place 11 µl of the stock solution into a microcentrifuge tube and add 189 µl of DMSO. This working solution can be frozen at −20°C (−4°F) until use.
- Sperm TALP (Tyrode's albumin-lactate-pyruvate) medium consists of 37 mM NaCl, 10 mM KCl, 1 mM KH_2PO_4, 36 mM $NaHCO_3$, 2.4 mM $MgSO_4$, 10 mM HEPES, 2 mM $CaCl_2$, 84 mM fructose, 6 mM glucose, 182 µM Na-pyruvate, 0.37 ml/l Na-lactate, and 3 g/l bovine serum albumen (BSA), with the pH adjusted to 7.2.

Technique

- Semen must first be diluted to a concentration of 25–50 × 10^6 sperm/ml in a commercial skim milk/glucose diluent or TALP diluent.
- In a glass test tube add 20 µl JC-1 (working solution) and 500 µl of diluted sperm. Incubate sperm in a 37°C (99°F) water bath or incubator for 20 minutes.
- After incubation add 250 µl of JC-1-stained sperm to 250 µl TALP in a separate glass test tube and mix gently.
- The sperm can now be read using a fluorescent microscope. Two separate slides should be analyzed with a minimum of 200 cells counted per slide.

Equine Reproductive Procedures, Second Edition. Edited by John Dascanio and Patrick McCue.

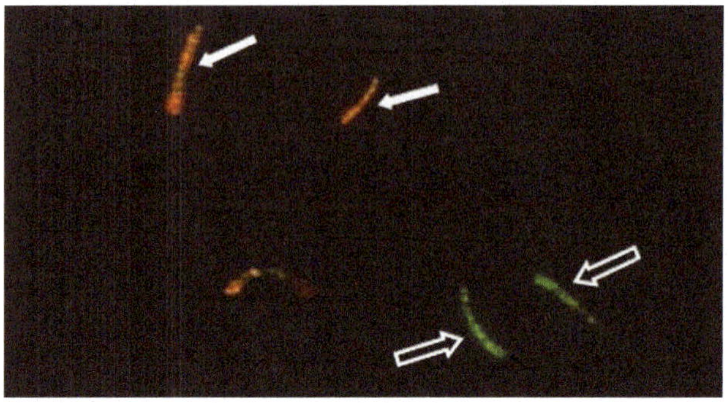

Figure 173.1 Stallion sperm stained with JC-1. Sperm with high mitochondrial potential (white arrows) stain orange, and sperm with low mitochondrial potential (open arrows) stain green.

- Two populations of sperm can be visualized (Figure 173.1): cells with the mitochondrial midpiece fluorescing orange (high mitochondrial potential) and cells with the mitochondrial midpiece fluorescing green (low mitochondrial potential).

Interpretation

The evaluation of sperm motility has been an important standard method of assessing sperm quality. The mitochondria of sperm provide the energy source for motility and any changes in mitochondrial function may be reflective of changes in sperm motility. With the use of JC-1, two distinct sperm populations can be observed. The percentage of cells fluorescing orange indicates the amount of sperm in the sample that contains functioning mitochondria. A higher percentage of functioning mitochondria in the sample provides information that the sperm are able to produce the energy needed for motility. An increase in the percentage of cells staining green may indicate a functional loss in motility and fertility may be compromised. Changes in the procedures used to cryopreserve these sperm cells may help to increase the amount of cells with high mitochondrial membrane potential after thawing.

Further Reading

Graham JK. 1996. Analysis of stallion semen and its relation to fertility. *Vet Clin North Am Eq Pract* 12(1): 119–29.

Gravance CG, Garner GL, Baumber J, Ball BA. 2000. Assessment of equine sperm mitochondrial function using JC-1. *Theriogenology* 53: 1691–703.

174

Equine Viral Arteritis Testing

G. Reed Holyoak[1] and Udeni B. R. Balasuriya[2]

[1] Oklahoma State University, USA
[2] School of Veterinary Medicine, Louisiana State University, USA

Introduction

Equine viral arteritis is a highly contagious disease whose etiology was defined in the early 1950s. The virus was named equine arteritis virus (EAV), and the disease equine viral arteritis (EVA), because of the distinctive vascular lesions found on histopathologic examination of acutely infected cases (Doll *et al.* 1957a, 1957b). During the 1984 Kentucky EVA outbreak, it was discovered that persistently infected stallions served as the natural reservoir within the equine population. Following natural infection, 10–70% of stallions can become persistently infected carriers of EAV and continuously shed virus in their semen (Timoney *et al.* 1987). While EVA is a disease almost exclusively of the horse, antibodies against EAV have been identified in donkeys in South Africa and other countries, and the virus was associated with a case of abortion in an alpaca (demonstrated by reverse transcription polymerase chain reaction, RT-PCR) (Balasuriya *et al.* 2013). All horses appear to be susceptible to EAV infection; however, there are considerable differences in seroprevalence between different breeds. While breed-specific differences might reflect inherent genetically conferred resistance or susceptibility to infection, they are more likely reflective of different cultural and management factors.

Clinical signs of EVA vary considerably among individual horses and among outbreaks (Timoney *et al.* 1987). A substantial percentage of all infections are subclinical, especially those that occur in mares bred to persistently infected stallions. Typically, clinical cases of EVA have an incubation period of 2–14 days (6–8 days following venereal exposure), with the most consistent clinical features of EAV being pyrexia and leukopenia. Typical cases of the disease can present with all or any combination of the following signs: fever up to 41°C (105.8°F) (2–9-day duration), anorexia, serous nasal discharge, conjunctivitis, urticaria, leukopenia, edema of the lower limbs, scrotum, prepuce, eyelids, ventral body wall, and udder, abortion in the mare, fatal interstitial pneumonia, or pneumoenteritis in young foals. However, a vast majority of naturally infected animals are asymptomatic.

Following natural EAV infection, the majority of stallions will become persistently infected and continuously shed virus in their semen for either a short period (ranging from several weeks to <1 year, defined as short-term shedders (STS) or short-term carriers) or a long period of time (>1 year to lifelong, defined as long-term persistently infected (LTPI) shedders or carriers without adverse effects on semen quality or reproductive capacity) (McCollum *et al.* 1971). The virus persists exclusively in the male reproductive tract despite the presence of high levels of neutralizing and mucosal antibodies. Moreover, maintenance of EAV LTPI status is testosterone dependent and, therefore, does not cause persistent infection in mares, foals, and sexually immature colts.

Recently, it has been demonstrated that establishment of EAV LTPI status correlates with the *in vitro* susceptibility of a subpopulation of $CD3^+$ T lymphocytes to EAV infection, and, consequently, stallions with the $CD3^+$ T-lymphocyte susceptibility phenotype are at higher risk of becoming LTPI carriers compared with those that lack this phenotype. A genome-wide association study demonstrated that these phenotypes are associated with the *CXCL16* gene located in equine chromosome 11 (ECA11). Subsequently, studies have identified two allelic variants of *CXCL16* (*CXCL16S* and *CXCL16R*) that differ by four non-synonymous nucleotide substitutions in exon 1, and show a very strong association with the two $CD3^+$ T-lymphocyte phenotypes (susceptible and resistant) and with either the establishment of LTPI status (*CXCL16S*) or the early viral clearance (STS) in stallions (*CXCL16R*).

Equine Reproductive Procedures, Second Edition. Edited by John Dascanio and Patrick McCue.

Risk factors associated with EAV transmission are summarized in Figure 174.1, with EVA transmitted among horses in five ways:

- Respiratory: primary route of transmission in acute cases of infection, and common at racetracks, shows, and sales.
- Venereal: the virus is shed in the semen of a carrier stallion (cooled or frozen semen can be infectious, and potentially from embryos of subclinically infected mares).
- Other bodily secretions: fetal fluids, urine, feces, etc.
- *In utero:* the virus passes across the placenta from an acutely infected mare to her unborn foal.
- Indirect contamination: tack and/or equipment shared among horses.

There is a very real risk of EAV being transferred indirectly via personnel and fomites. Special care should be taken when handling semen and equipment in laboratories prior to insemination or preparation for shipping of semen (frozen and cold).

The differential diagnosis of EVA includes other viral respiratory tract infections such as:

- Equine herpesviruses 1 and 4.
- Equine influenza virus.
- Equine rhinitis A and B viruses.
- Equine adenovirus.
- Getah virus.
- It may also include equine infectious anemia, African horse sickness, purpura hemorrhagica, and urticaria and toxicosis due to hoary alyssum (*Berteroa incana*).

Technique

- Suitable clinical samples to attempt virus isolation or detection of viral nucleic acid include nasopharyngeal swabs or nasal washings, conjunctival swabs, and whole blood (in EDTA or citrate).
- In seropositive stallions with no known vaccination history, a semen sample may be submitted for virus isolation and viral nucleic acid detection.
- Tissue samples from foals and aborted fetuses could also be submitted for histopathologic and immunohistochemical evaluation in 10% neutral buffered formalin.
- The laboratory diagnosis of EVA is currently based on following laboratory tests:

- Virus isolation.
- Viral nucleic acid detection (molecular techniques):
  - standard RT-PCR, real-time RT-PCR) or reverse transcription insulated isothermal PCR (RT-iiPCR)
  - *in situ* hybridization (conventional or RNAscope®).

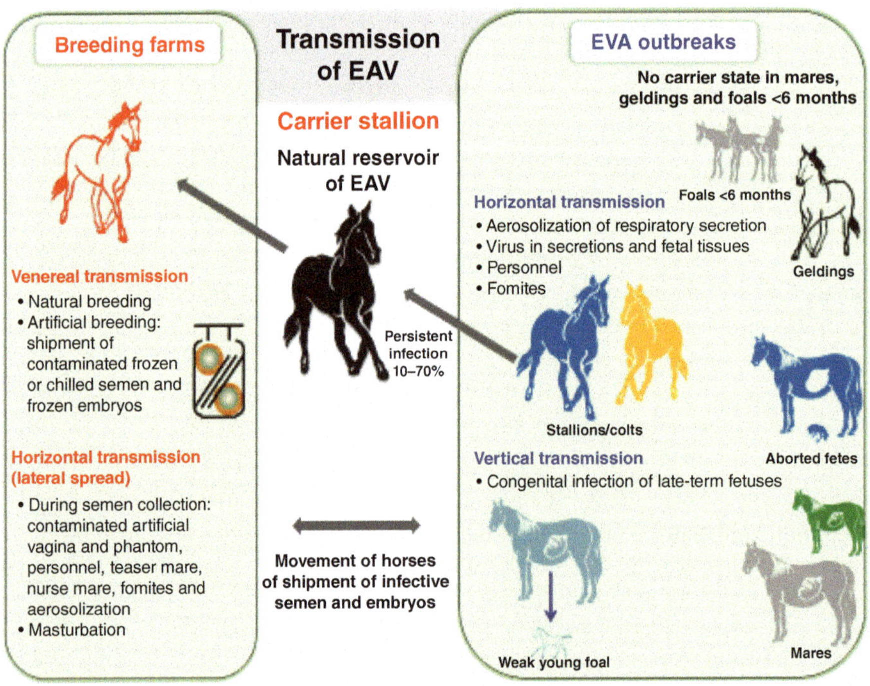

Figure 174.1 Transmission of equine viral arteritis (EAV) between horses. The persistently infected stallions play a central role in the maintenance, perpetuation, and evolution of the virus in the horse population. Source: From Balasuriya. 2017. *Fenner's Veterinary Virology*, 5th edn. Reproduced with the permission of Elsevier.vbhgg

- Virus isolation is the gold standard for detection of EAV in samples, including semen, and the OIE (World Organization for Animal Health or Office International des Epizooties) prescribed test for international trade. However, the performance of RT-qPCR and RT-iiPCR described in the literature showed equal or higher sensitivity compared with virus isolation in semen samples. Therefore, molecular assays could be used as an alternative method for EAV diagnosis.
- Viral antigen detection (immunohistochemistry).
- Serology. For serologic diagnosis of acute EAV infection, paired acute and convalescent sera should be collected 3–4 weeks apart, and tested for either seroconversion or a four-fold or greater increase in serum antibody titer. The virus neutralization assay remains the gold standard for the detection of serum antibodies to EAV. However, a competitive enzyme-linked immunosorbent assay (cELISA) was recently developed and validated for the detection of EAV-specific antibodies and could be considered as an alternative assay for the serologic diagnosis of EVA.

Treatment

- The main goal for treatment of EVA is for the recovery from infection and avoidance of virus spread.
- Treatment of EVA is general supportive care until the acute phase passes. Adequate rest should be provided, particularly to breeding stallions and to horses in training.
- Use of systemic antibiotics is unrewarding and usually contraindicated, except in pneumonitic foals at risk of secondary bacterial infection.
- Repeated vaccination has no impact on affecting the clearance of virus in persistently infected stallions.
- Antagonists of gonadotrophin-releasing hormone (GnRH) and GnRH vaccinations have been used to eliminate persistent infection and viral shedding with varying levels of success. However, no conclusive therapies have been developed.

Outcome and Prognosis

- Abortion is a frequent outcome in naïve pregnant mares, and generally occurs 10–30 days after exposure to EAV and at any time between 3 and 10 months of gestation.
- 10–70% of exposed stallions become persistently infected with EAV and shed virus in their semen, sometimes for life.
- Older foals acutely infected with EAV may develop a secondary bacterial infection. Prophylactic administration of antibiotics may be indicated.
- With the major exception of the persistently infected stallion, there are no long-term difficulties after the resolution of EAV infection. Immunity is long-lasting and protective over multiple years.
- In cases of persistent infection in stallions, they are asymptomatic and may shed large numbers of virus in their semen. The virus can survive semen processing for cooled shipment and cryopreservation, remaining infectious and readily transmitted to naïve mares at the time of insemination.

Prevention

For all venereal diseases in the horse, biosecurity is paramount (Balasuriya *et al.* 2019). Horses and/or semen arriving without appropriate health certification paperwork should not be unloaded or examined. Before semen is collected and shipped, appropriate health parameters must be evaluated and paperwork certifying the health status of the stallion and semen must accompany the shipment.

- Effective strategies for control and prevention include:
  - Biosecurity – a major factor in determining the success of any control program is minimizing or eliminating direct or indirect contact of susceptible horses with the secretions/excretions of EAV-infected animals:
    - determine the serologic and virologic status of all stallions, especially those contributing sperm to both cooled shipped and cryopreserved semen AI programs before they are vaccinated with modified live virus (MLV) or inactivated EAV vaccines. Testing should be done at least 60 days prior to use in breeding
    - non-vaccinated seropositive stallions (with no vaccination history) for EAV (virus neutralization test titer ≥1:4) should be tested for the presence of EAV by virus isolation or molecular testing of two separate semen samples derived from two separate collections or by test breeding. If semen samples are negative for EAV by virus isolation or molecular testing, identify stallions as EAV non-carriers
    - if seronegative (titer <1:4), stallions should be vaccinated with the MLV vaccine after collecting a serum sample as proof. The vaccination needs to be officially recorded
    - pre-pubertal colts could be genetically tested for the presence of the CXCL16 genotype (*CXCL16SS* or *CXCL16SR*) using an allelic discrimination real-time PCR. Colts that carry the susceptible genotype (*CXCL16S*) should be vaccinated after 6 months of age. If no genetic testing is to be performed, all colts should be vaccinated between 6 and 12 months of age
    - establish AI industry standards.

- Prevent the establishment of the carrier state in stallions and post-pubertal colts:
  - vaccinate colts after 6 months and before 10 months of age (before puberty)
  - prevention of the carrier state will eliminate the disease.
- There are effective and safe vaccines available against EAV:
  - Arvac® (Zoetis, Kalamazoo, MI, USA), a MLV vaccine available in the United States.
  - Artervac® (Zoetis), a killed virus vaccine available in the European Union.
- The MLV vaccine is both safe and effective for use in breeding mares and stallions, in early gestational pregnant mares, geldings, fillies, and colts.
- Late-term pregnant mares should not be vaccinated unless the risk of natural exposure is sufficient to offset the risk of potential complications of a MLV vaccine.
- All seronegative mares being bred to a persistently infected stallion should be vaccinated 21 days prior to natural breeding or AI. Those previously vaccinated should be given a booster immunization.
- There is no evidence that a vaccinated stallion will develop the carrier state with vaccine virus.
- Horses that travel for competitions or are co-mingled with outside horses should be vaccinated.
- For EVA and other reportable diseases, more widespread screening of stallion populations and tighter quality controls over laboratories providing diagnostics would increase the detection rate of carrier stallions.

Client Education

Critical to the prevention and control of EVA is the observance of sound practices that will reduce the risk of viral spread. Horse owners should understand that the reservoir is the carrier stallion and prevention and detection of persistent infection are critical. There are a number of specific measures aimed at minimizing the spread of the virus:

- Isolate new entries and test all stallions.
- Screening for EAV seropositive stallions without a vaccination history.
- Certify/test imported semen.
- Institute an appropriate vaccination protocol.
- Especially vaccinate all colts prior to puberty.
- Genetic test potential breeding stallions

The vaccination of stallions may preclude their importation into some countries. Any potential international movement of animals should be determined prior to vaccination.

References

Balasuriya UBR. 2017. Fenner's Veterinary Virology, 5th edn. Amsterdam: Elsevier.

Balasuriya UBR, Carossino M, Mekuria Z, Holyoak GR. 2019. Genetic predisposition for developing equine arteritis virus carrier state: adopting proper biosecurity measures when breeding mares to a persistently infected stallion. *Clin Theriogenol* 11(3): 369–78.

Balasuriya UBR, Go YY, MacLachlan NJ. 2013. Equine arteritis virus. *Vet Microbiol* 167: 93–122.

Doll ER, Bryans JT, McCollum WH, *et al.* 1957a. Isolation of a filterable agent causing arteritis of horses and abortion by mares; its differentiation from the equine abortion (influenza) virus. *Cornell Vet* 47: 3–41.

Doll ER, Knappenberger RE, Bryans JT. 1957b. An outbreak of abortion caused by the equine arteritis virus. *Cornell Vet* 47: 69–75.

McCollum WH, Prickett ME, Bryans JT. 1971. Temporal distribution of equine arteritis virus in respiratory mucosa, tissues and body fluids of horses infected by inhalation. *Res Vet Sci* 12: 459–64.

Timoney PJ, McCollum WH, Murphy TW, *et al.* 1987. The carrier state in equine arteritis virus infection in the stallion with specific emphasis on the venereal mode of virus transmission. *J Reprod Fertil Suppl.* 35: 95–102.

Further Reading

Balasuriya UBR, MacLachlan NJ. 2007. Equine viral arteritis. In: Sellon DC, Long MT (eds). Equine Infectious Diseases, 2nd edn. St Louis, MI; Saunders Elsevier, pp.153–64.

Broaddus CC, Balasuriya UBR, White JLR, Timoney PJ, Funk RA, Holyoak GR. 2011. Safety considerations of vaccinating mares against equine viral arteritis in mid and late pregnancy and in the immediate postpartum period. *J Am Vet Med Assoc* 238: 741–50.

Burger D, Janett F, Imboden I, Zientara S, Timoney P, Thun R. 2004. Treatment of an equine arteritis virus-shedding stallion by immunization against GnRH. In: 15th International Congress on Animal Reproduction, Vol. 1, Porto Seguro, Brazil, p. 281 (abstract).

Burger D, Janett F, Vidament F, Stump R, Fortier G, Imboden I, Thun R. 2006. Immunization against GnRH in adult stallions: effects on semen characteristics, behaviour and shedding of equine arteritis virus. *Anim Reprod Sci* 94: 107–11.

Fortier G, Vidament M, DeCraene F, Ferry B, Daels PF. 2002. The effect of GnRH antagonist on testosterone secretion, spermatogenesis and viral excretion in EVA-virus excreting stallions. *Theriogenology* 58: 425–7.

Holyoak GR, Balasuriya UBR, Broaddus CC, Timoney PJ. 2008. Equine viral arteritis: current status and prevention. *Theriogenology* 70: 403–14.

175

Diagnostic Endocrinology: Baseline Hormone Levels

Patrick M. McCue

Equine Reproduction Laboratory, Colorado State University, USA

Introduction

Endocrine evaluation of the hypothalamic–pituitary–testicular axis should begin by monitoring the blood levels of pituitary and testicular hormones in unstimulated stallions over time. Unfortunately, concentrations of endogenous gonadotropin-releasing hormone (GnRH) cannot be measured in peripheral blood. It is theoretically possible to measure blood GnRH levels if a cannula is placed into the cavernous sinus via the facial vein. However, this technique is not practical for routine clinical evaluations. As a consequence, hypothalamic function is monitored by observing patterns of luteinizing hormone (LH) and follicle-stimulationg hormone (FSH) secretion from the anterior pituitary.

Testicular endocrine function is evaluated by measuring endogenous levels of testosterone, estradiol 17β, and/or estrogen conjugates and inhibin. In general, it is best to collect multiple samples at set intervals during a day and evaluate patterns of change than to rely on hormone levels in a single sample. Anti-Müllerian hormone (AMH) can also be used to evaluate testicular function. Concentrations of AMH are low in geldings and elevated in cryptorchid stallions and intact stallions.

Equipment and Supplies

Vacutainer® tubes (10 ml, without anticoagulant), Vacutainer® needles, Vacutainer® needle guide, centrifuge, disposable pipette, sterile vial for serum, appropriate shipping container.

Technique

- The daily rhythm of hormone secretion can be monitored by serial collection of jugular venous blood for 6–8 hours.
- One protocol entails the collection of blood every 30 minutes beginning at 8:00 am and continuing for 8 hours.
- A second protocol calls for blood collection once per hour from 10:00 am until 3:00 pm.
- With either protocol, the occurrence of a midday rise in LH would be detected.
- In addition, the absolute amount of testosterone appearing in circulation after the LH rise may be used to determine whether the production of testosterone for testicular function is adequate.
- Blood samples should be allowed to clot and then centrifuged at 1200× g for 10 minutes at room temperature.
- The serum should be stored at −20°C (−4°F) until assayed for LH, FSH, testosterone, estradiol 17β, and inhibin.
- It may be beneficial for interpretation to submit blood samples collected in an identical manner from one or two normal stallions along with samples from the test stallion.

Additional Comments

Gonadotropin-releasing hormone is secreted in a pulsatile manner from the hypothalamus. Pulses of GnRH cause pulsatile release of LH and FSH from the anterior pituitary. LH stimulates the production and release of testosterone and estrogens from the Leydig cells of adult stallions. FSH binds with Sertoli cells to stimulate the release of inhibin, activin, androgen-binding protein, and other factors needed for spermatogenesis. Secretion of GnRH, LH, and FSH are modulated by feedback from the testicular hormones. Pituitary LH secretion is stimulated by estradiol 17β and suppressed by testosterone, while FSH secretion is suppressed by estradiol 17β, inhibin, and testosterone. In addition, the administration of exogenous progestagens

Equine Reproductive Procedures, Second Edition. Edited by John Dascanio and Patrick McCue.

such as altrenogest induces an immediate and dramatic decrease in LH and testosterone concentrations.

Concentrations of pituitary gonadotropins and testicular hormones vary with the time of day. Serum levels are lowest in the morning and rise to peak concentrations around midday. Consequently, if a single blood sample is collected for evaluation, the time of day the blood was collected may dramatically influence the results and, potentially, the interpretation. There is also a marked seasonal variation in hormone levels in stallions. Concentrations of gonadotropins, testicular steroids, and inhibin are highest in the late spring and summer (March to September) and lowest in the fall and winter (October to February) in North America. Hormone levels should be interpreted using normal ranges provided by the diagnostic laboratory performing the assays.

The association between the midday rise of LH and the rise of testosterone indicates that LH is stimulating the testes to produce testosterone. A stallion with a testicular problem may exhibit a rise in LH without a concomitant rise in testosterone. Elevation in FSH concentrations may be noted in stallions with decreased testicular function due to a decrease in negative feedback from testicular steroids and inhibin. An increase in serum FSH may be a more consistent change in subfertile stallions than the decrease in LH, testosterone, estrogen, and inhibin which may be variably present in some individual horses with testicular dysfunction. Stallions with declining fertility usually exhibit alterations in hormone patterns in the following order:

- Increased levels of FSH.
- Decreased levels of estradiol and inhibin.
- Decreased levels of LH.
- Decreased levels of testosterone.

Further Reading

Burns PJ, Douglas RH. 1985. Reproductive hormone concentrations in stallions with breeding problems: case studies. *J Eq Vet Sci* 5: 40–2.

Claes AN, Ball BA, Almeida J, Conley AJ. 2011. Detection of serum anti-Müllerian hormone concentrations as a method for diagnosis of cryptorchidism in the horse. *Proc Annu Conv Am Assoc Eq Pract* 57: 56.

Nett TM. 1993. Reproductive endocrine function testing in stallions. In: McKinnon AO, Voss JL (eds). Equine Reproduction. Baltimore: Williams and Wilkins, pp. 821–4.

Roser JF. 2001. Subfertility in stallions: endocrine diagnostics. In: *Proceedings of the West Coast Equine Reproduction Symposium*, pp. 16–24.

Roser JF, McCue P, Hoye E. 1994. Inhibin activity in the mare and stallion. *Dom Anim Endocrinol* 11: 87–100.

176

Diagnostic Endocrinology: GnRH Stimulation Tests

Patrick M. McCue

Equine Reproduction Laboratory, Colorado State University, USA

Introduction

Gonadotropin-releasing hormone (GnRH) produced in the hypothalamus stimulates the secretion of luteinizing hormone (LH) and follicle-stimulating hormone (FSH) from the anterior pituitary. Pulses of GnRH induce pulsatile secretion of LH and FSH which, in turn, regulate testicular function. Native GnRH is a peptide comprised of 10 amino acids and its composition is identical between mammalian species.

Administration of GnRH to a stallion will stimulate the synthesis and secretion of LH and FSH and may be used as a test of pituitary function. Test strategies include the administration of a physiological dose of GnRH (i.e., 10–25 μg) to measure pituitary function and the administration of a pharmacological dose of GnRH (i.e., 1 mg) to measure pituitary content of LH and FSH. In either situation, it is recommended that a normal fertile stallion be tested along with a subfertile stallion to evaluate and compare pituitary responses.

Equipment and Supplies

Vacutainer® tubes (10 ml, without anticoagulant), Vacutainer® needles, Vacutainer® needle guide, GnRH (i.e., luteinizing hormone-releasing hormone (LHRH); www.sigmaaldrich.com) or Cystorelin® (Merial LLC, Diluth, GA, USA), 1 ml syringe, 20 gauge needle.

Technique

- If the GnRH (LHRH) obtained is lyophilized, it must be reconstituted to a "working dilution." For example, if 5 mg of GnRH powder is available, it may be reconstituted with 10 ml of sterile saline in a sterile empty vial to achieve a stock concentration of 500 μg/ml. The addition of 1 ml of stock to an additional 19 ml of sterile saline in a new, sterile, empty vial will achieve a working dilution of 25 μg/ml. Cystorelin® is commercially available at a concentration of 50 μg/ml.
- The *low dose, single pulse GnRH stimulation test* is used to assess pituitary and potentially testicular responsiveness.
  - Blood samples are collected 30 minutes prior and immediately prior to intravenous administration of 25 μg of GnRH. Additional blood samples are collected at 30-minute intervals up to 120 minutes.
  - It is recommended that the GnRH be administered at or before 9:00 am when levels of LH are low prior to the normal midday rise.
  - Blood samples are allowed to clot and the samples are subsequently centrifuged at 1200× g for 10 minutes. The serum is stored at −20°C (−4°F) until assayed for LH and testosterone.
- The *high dose, single pulse GnRH stimulation test* is used to evaluate the pituitary–gonadal axis in stallions previously determined to have an endogenous testosterone value below the normal range. A maximum stimulatory dose of GnRH (2 μg/kg body weight) is administered intravenously.
  - Blood samples should be collected prior to and at 30-minute intervals after the GnRH challenge for 8 hours. An increase in circulating levels of testosterone into the normal range after the GnRH challenge indicates that both the pituitary gland and testes are capable of responding to stimulation by their respective trophic hormones.
- The *three pulse GnRH challenge test* evaluates the ability of the pituitary to be "primed" by a series of GnRH pulses.
  - Blood samples are collected every 10 minutes for 30 minutes prior to the first administration of GnRH at 9:00 am.

Equine Reproductive Procedures, Second Edition. Edited by John Dascanio and Patrick McCue.

- Three small doses of GnRH (5 µg each) are given intravenously at 1-hour intervals. Additional blood samples are collected every 10 minutes for 1 hour after each GnRH challenge.
- The entire process takes 210 minutes. Blood samples are handled as described previously and assayed for LH concentration.

Additional Comments

The GnRH stimulation test is a sensitive test used to evaluate pituitary function. The low dose, single pulse test is more physiological than the high dose test and is meant to mimic the normal response of the pituitary to an endogenous GnRH pulse. The high dose test evaluates pituitary gonadotropin content and reflects pituitary response to maximal stimulation. In the three pulse test, a priming effect is noted when the GnRH-induced LH release is higher after each challenge. The test is most sensitive when administered in the non-breeding season when the hypothalamic–pituitary–testicular axis activity is at its lowest. Subfertile stallions have a significantly lower response to the second and third challenges of GnRH in the non-breeding season than fertile stallions.

Stallions with a normal GnRH-induced LH response, but a low testosterone response, may have a primary testicular disorder. Stallions with low circulating LH levels, but a good pituitary response to exogenous GnRH, may have decreased hypothalamic function (i.e., hypogonadotropic hypogonadism).

Further Reading

Nett TM. 1993. Reproductive endocrine function testing in stallions. In: McKinnon AO, Voss JL (eds). Equine Reproduction. Baltimore: Williams and Wilkins, pp. 821–4.

Roser JF. 1997. Endocrine basis for testicular function in the stallion. *Theriogenology* 48: 883–92.

Roser JF. 2001. Subfertility in stallions: endocrine diagnostics. In: *Proceedings of the West Coast Equine Reproduction Symposium*, pp. 16–24.

177

Diagnostic Endocrinology: hCG Stimulation Test

Patrick M. McCue

Equine Reproduction Laboratory, Colorado State University, USA

Introduction

Human chorionic gonadotropin (hCG) is a large glycoprotein hormone produced by syncytiotrophoblast cells of the developing human embryo. hCG has luteinizing hormone (LH) biological activity in most species and the administration of hCG to stallions stimulates an increase in the synthesis and secretion of testosterone from the Leydig cells of the testes. The hCG stimulation test is primarily used to determine if testicular tissue is present (or absent) in cryptorchid horses and geldings exhibiting stallion-like behavior. The hCG stimulation test is also occasionally used to evaluate testicular function in intact stallions. Typically, one or more blood samples are collected prior to the administration of hCG and then one or more samples are collected after hCG is given to evaluate testicular response. Testosterone concentration is measured using either serum or plasma.

Equipment and Supplies

Vacutainer® tubes (10 ml, without anticoagulant; i.e., serum tubes), Vacutainer® needles, Vacutainer® needle guide, centrifuge, disposable pipette, sterile vial for serum, appropriate shipping container, hCG (10,000 IU).

Technique

- A *paired sample hCG stimulation test* is most commonly performed to determine the presence or absence of testicular tissue in suspected cryptorchid stallions.
- A single pre-treatment blood sample is collected for baseline analysis of testosterone concentration.
- A total of 10,000 IU of hCG is administered intravenously.
- One or two blood samples are subsequently collected 1–2 hours after hCG administration. Additional blood samples may be collected 24 and 48 hours after hCG administration.
- Diagnosis of the presence of testicular tissue is dependent on a rise in plasma testosterone following hCG administration (Table 177.1).
- The degree to which testosterone increases in the second sample in a cryptorchid stallion is quite variable and may range between a 50% increase to a four-fold increase (Table 177.2; Figures 177.1 and 177.2). Consequently, clinical interpretation of the laboratory results should be made with caution.
- The hCG stimulation test is most diagnostic when administered in the morning, prior to the midday rise in LH and testosterone.
- A *multiple sample hCG stimulation test* may be performed to evaluate testicular endocrine function in subfertile stallions.

Table 177.1 Plasma testosterone concentrations in 10 normal stallions prior to and 1 hour after administration of 10,000 IU of human chorionic gonadotropin (hCG) (mean ± SEM).

Sample	Testosterone (ng/ml)
Pre-hCG	0.51 ± 0.07
1 hour post-hCG	3.89 ± 0.54

Table 177.2 Testosterone concentration prior to and 1 hour after administration of 10,000 IU of human chorionic gonadotropin (hCG) to a cryptorchid stallion.

Sample	Testosterone (ng/ml)
Pre-hCG	0.177
1 hour post-hCG	0.250

Equine Reproductive Procedures, Second Edition. Edited by John Dascanio and Patrick McCue.

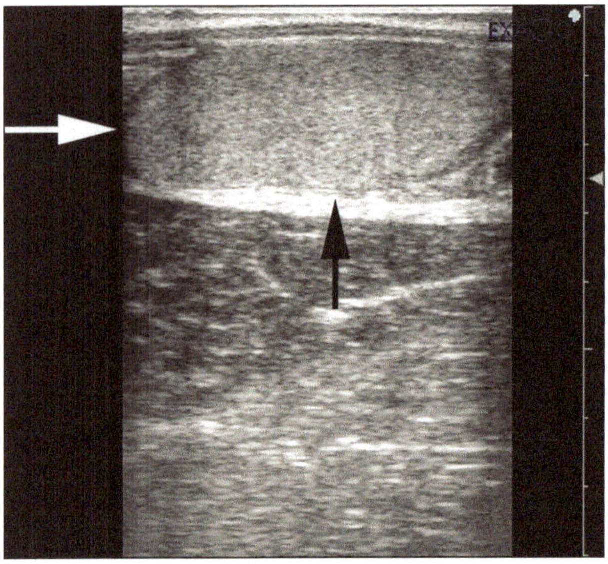

Figure 177.1 Ultrasound of the retained testis in a cryptorchid stallion subjected to the hCG stimulation test in Table 177.2. The arrows are pointing to the retained testes.

- Blood samples are collected 30 minutes prior to and immediately prior to the administration of 10,000 IU of hCG at 9:00 am.
- Additional blood samples are collected at 30-minute intervals for up to 3 hours after treatment.
- The blood is centrifuged and the serum or plasma stored at −20°C (−4°F) until assayed for testosterone.
- Normal stallions should have a marked increase in testosterone in response to hCG. Stallions with decreased Leydig cell function may have lower baseline testosterone levels and a reduced response to hCG.

Interpretation

Cryptorchidism does not inhibit steroid hormone production in the stallion to the degree that it inhibits spermatogenesis. Consequently, a majority of cryptorchid stallions can be identified from a single resting testosterone value. If a single sample test is to be performed, blood should be collected in the early afternoon, when circulating concentrations of testosterone are highest. Testosterone levels in normal stallions are usually greater than 0.5–1.0 ng/ml (500–1,000 pg/ml). Baseline levels of testosterone are influenced by season, with values lower in the winter than in the summer.

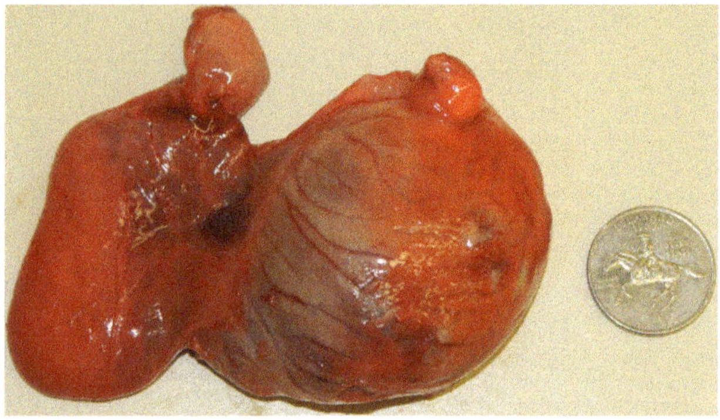

Figure 177.2 Post-surgery retained testis in the cryptorchid stallion from Figure 177.1 (US Quarter depicted for size).

In geldings, testosterone levels are usually less than 0.05–0.10 ng/ml (50–100 pg/ml). Cryptorchid stallions typically have testosterone levels in between those of geldings and normal stallions (i.e., 200–500 pg/ml). Cryptorchid stallions occasionally have testosterone levels between 50 and 200 pg/ml. The hCG stimulation test is most beneficial in identifying cryptorchid stallions where the resting testosterone level is not diagnostic.

The administration of hCG is used to bypass the influence of the pituitary and directly stimulate Leydig cells of the testes by virtue of the inherent LH activity. In contrast, a GnRH stimulation test depends on a functional anterior pituitary to synthesize and secrete gonadotropins that would subsequently affect testosterone production. A GnRH stimulation test, using agonists such as deslorelin or histrelin, is not as effective as an hCG stimulation test in eliciting a testosterone response in cryptorchid horses.

If a single blood sample is to be collected for evaluation of the presence of testicular tissue in a suspected cryptorchid horse, it is recommended that concentration of both testosterone and anti-Müllerian hormone be determined (see Chapter 179).

The term "proud cut" is often used to describe horses where the tail of the epididymis is inadvertently left in the horse during a castration procedure. Horse owners may claim that proud cut geldings retain stallion-like behavior. However, testosterone is not produced by the epididymis and therefore any residual stallion-like behavior that remains after castration is not due to the retained epididymis.

Further Reading

Arighi M, Bosu WTK. 1989. Comparison of hormonal methods for diagnosis of cryptorchidism in horses. *J Eq Vet Sci* 9: 20–6.

Nett TM. 1993. Reproductive endocrine function testing in stallions. In: McKinnon AO, Voss JL (eds). Equine Reproduction. Baltimore: Williams and Wilkins, pp. 821–4.

Roser JF. 2001. Subfertility in stallions: endocrine diagnostics. In: *Proceedings of the West Coast Equine Reproduction Symposium*, pp. 16–24.

178

Diagnostic Endocrinology: Estrogen Conjugate Assay

Patrick M. McCue

Equine Reproduction Laboratory, Colorado State University, USA

Introduction

Stallion testes produce large quantities of estrogens compared with males of most other species. Estrogens are secreted by both Leydig cells and Sertoli cells in the stallion testis. A majority of the estrogens produced are sulfo-conjugated and the primary testicular estrogen is estrone sulfate. In the stallion, circulating levels of estrogen conjugates (ECs) are approximately 200-fold higher than testosterone levels. Low levels of ECs have been correlated with low sperm production in subfertile stallions. Serum concentrations of EC have also been used to identify cryptorchid horses. Estrogens are excreted, in part, in the feces and consequently ECs can be measured in feces as well as in blood.

Technique

- Collection of one blood (or fecal) sample is generally sufficient. However, because of potential variability in hormone levels in individual animals, submission of paired samples collected at different times of the day or on subsequent days may be beneficial.
- Blood collected in a Vacutainer® tube without anticoagulant should be allowed to clot for 20 minutes. The tube should be centrifuged at 1200× g for 10 minutes and the serum aspirated with a disposable pipette and placed into a separate sterile tube for storage or shipment to an endocrine laboratory.
- Blood collected in a Vacutainer® tube containing an anticoagulant may be centrifuged immediately and the plasma subsequently transferred into a separate sterile tube using a disposable pipette.

Equipment and Supplies

Vacutainer® tubes (10 ml, without anticoagulant), Vacutainer® needles. Vacutainer® needle guide, centrifuge, disposable pipette, sterile vial for serum, appropriate shipping container, fecal cup, diagnostic laboratory.

Additional Comments

Reporting of absolute values for ECs and comparison of levels between laboratories is difficult due to the fact that different standards and antibodies are often used. Consequently, interpretation of EC values must be done using controls, and normal ranges established for the endocrine laboratory performing the assays.

Measurement of serum ECs has been reported to be approximately 95% accurate in differentiating cryptorchid stallions from true castrates if the horses are older than 3 years of age. Levels of serum CEs in donkeys of all ages and horses less than 3 years of age are much less than levels in horses >3 years of age. Consequently, the measurement of ECs is not recommended as a diagnostic test for young horses or donkeys of any age.

The administration of human chorionic gonadotrophin (hCG) does not consistently affect levels of ECs in blood. Measurement of fecal estrogens is also effective in differentiating geldings from cryptorchid stallions. The advantages in measuring fecal estrogens include non-invasive sample collection and the lack of need for a stimulation test. Estrogens are stable in feces for at least 1 week. A disadvantage of fecal testing of estrogens is the need to perform chemical extraction of the estrogen from the feces prior to testing and that the concentration of estrogens may vary with water content and organic matter in the sample, especially if wet feces are used in the extraction process.

Equine Reproductive Procedures, Second Edition. Edited by John Dascanio and Patrick McCue.

Further Reading

Arighi M, Bosu WTK. 1989. Comparison of hormonal methods for diagnosis of cryptorchidism in horses. *J Eq Vet Sci* 9: 20–6.

Cox JE, Redhead PH, Dawson FE. 1986. Comparison of the measurement of plasma testosterone and plasma oestrogens for the diagnosis of cryptorchidism in the horse. *Eq Vet J* 18: 179–82.

Palme R, Holzmann A, Mitterer T. 1994. Measuring fecal estrogens for the diagnosis of cryptorchidism in horses. *Theriogenology* 42: 1381–7.

179

Diagnostic Tests for Cryptorchidism

Patrick M. McCue

Equine Reproduction Laboratory, Colorado State University, USA

Introduction

Cryptorchid is a term derived from the Greek words *kryptos* and *orchis*, meaning "hidden testis." A stallion is considered to be a cryptorchid if one or both testes are not fully descended into the scrotum. Cryptorchid testes may be located anywhere from the caudal pole of the kidneys to adjacent to the inguinal rings. Cryptorchids may have one or both testes and associated epididymides located completely within the abdomen, partially within the inguinal canal, or located just outside of the inguinal canal ("high flankers"). Approximately 85% of affected horses are unilateral cryptorchids, while ~15% are bilateral. Left-retained testes are more likely to be located within the abdomen, while right-retained testes are more likely to be inguinal.

An accurate diagnosis of cryptorchidism is not difficult if the horse has had one owner and if adequate medical records have been maintained. However, it may be less obvious if a horse has had several owners or was purchased at auction as a gelding and began to show stallion-like behavior when exposed to mares at his new home. Suspect animals may be true geldings, bilateral cryptorchids, or unilaterally castrated cryptorchids.

Equipment and Supplies

Examination gloves, sedation, *N*-butylscopolammonium bromide (Buscopan®), obstetrical sleeve, obstetrical lubricant, ultrasound unit, syringes, needles, vacutainer tubes, human chorionic gonadotropin (optional).

Technique

Diagnostic evaluation of a male horse that may have one or two retained testes should begin with collection of a complete medical history, including age, breed, previous ownership, previous veterinary examinations, surgical procedures, and diagnostic tests. The second step should be an account of behavior(s) being exhibited by the horse in question and the context in which the behaviors are expressed (i.e., aggressive behavior around horses or people, herding behavior, gaining an erection around or mounting mares in estrus).

The third step would be a physical examination of the horse, beginning with a visual and manual examination of the inguinal region. It is often not possible to visualize an incision scar from a previous castration in normal geldings or suspect cryptorchids. Consequently, the next procedure is often deep manual palpation of the inguinal area in an attempt to detect either testicular or epididymal tissue located external to the inguinal ring or within the inguinal canal. In most cases, sedation is helpful to facilitate safe examination of the inguinal area. One effective sedation protocol is a combination of detomidine hydrochloride (~0.01–0.015 mg/kg) plus butorphanol tartrate (~0.01 mg/kg) administered intravenously. After manual examination, an external ultrasound examination of the inguinal region may be performed in an attempt to detect the presence of testicular tissue.

Often the next step is a transrectal palpation and ultrasound examination. Administration of *N*-butylscopolammonium bromide (Buscopan®; 0.1–0.2 mg/kg IV) in addition to adequate sedation and restraint may facilitate a safe transrectal examination. Abdominally cryptorchid testes may be located anywhere from just caudal to the kidneys to the inguinal canal. Palpation of the vas deferens entering the inguinal canal (vaginal ring) is indicative of either a normal descended (scrotal) testis or an inguinal location. Failure to detect the vas deferens entering the vaginal ring may be indicative of an abdominal cryptorchid testis.

A systematic and thorough ultrasonographic examination of the entire caudal abdomen from just in front of the

Equine Reproductive Procedures, Second Edition. Edited by John Dascanio and Patrick McCue.

pelvis to the kidneys, and from the ventral midline to the lateral flank, should be performed on both left and right sides. An alternative technique is to locate each ampulla, just lateral to the midline in the pelvic canal, and follow that structure cranially as it narrows into the vas deferens, which in turn should lead to a testis if one is present. A cryptorchid testis is usually significantly smaller than a normal scrotal testis, but has the same general ultrasonographic characteristics, including a prominent central vein or mediastinum (Figure 179.1), although some are slightly less echogenic.

An external transabdominal ultrasound examination of the flank region may also be useful to determine the presence and location of retained testes.

Endocrine testing may be indicated if testes cannot be located by palpation or ultrasound examination in a gelding exhibiting stallion-like behavior. As with any endocrine test, interpretation of endocrine values must be based on ranges of normal values established for the reference laboratory.

The most reliable endocrine assay for the presence of testicular tissue is measurement of anti-Müllerian hormone (AMH) levels in peripheral blood (Table 179.1). The advantages of AMH testing are:

- Only one blood sample is required.
- AMH levels are not as affected by age as testosterone levels.
- AMH levels are not as affected by season as testosterone levels.
- AMH levels are typically higher in bilateral cryptorchids than unilateral cryptorchids or normal intact stallions.

Table 179.1 Concentrations of anti-Müllerian hormone (AMH) in serum or plasma of geldings, cryptorchid stallions, and intact stallions. Values are from the Clinical Endocrinology Laboratory at the University of California, Davis.

Horse	AMH (ng/ml)
Gelding	Undetectable
Cryptorchid	>0.15 ng/ml
Intact stallion	>0.15 ng/ml

- AMH levels in most cryptorchids are markedly elevated over levels in true geldings.
- Sertoli cells of the testis are the only source of AMH.

Historically, an analysis of testosterone levels in a single blood sample was used to detect the presence or absence of testicular tissue in suspect cryptorchids. Geldings have very low blood testosterone levels, whereas cryptorchid stallions typically have moderately elevated levels, and intact stallions usually have very high testosterone levels. Unfortunately, evaluation of testosterone in a single blood sample is not always diagnostic.

Dynamic testing of testosterone levels before and after the administration of human chorionic gonadotropin (hCG) improves the diagnostic accuracy in the detection of testicular tissue. A blood sample is collected prior to and 1–2 hours after intravenous administration of 2,500–10,000 IU of hCG intravenously or intramuscularly. However, in some cases the elevation in testosterone did not occur until 24–72 hours after hCG administration. The

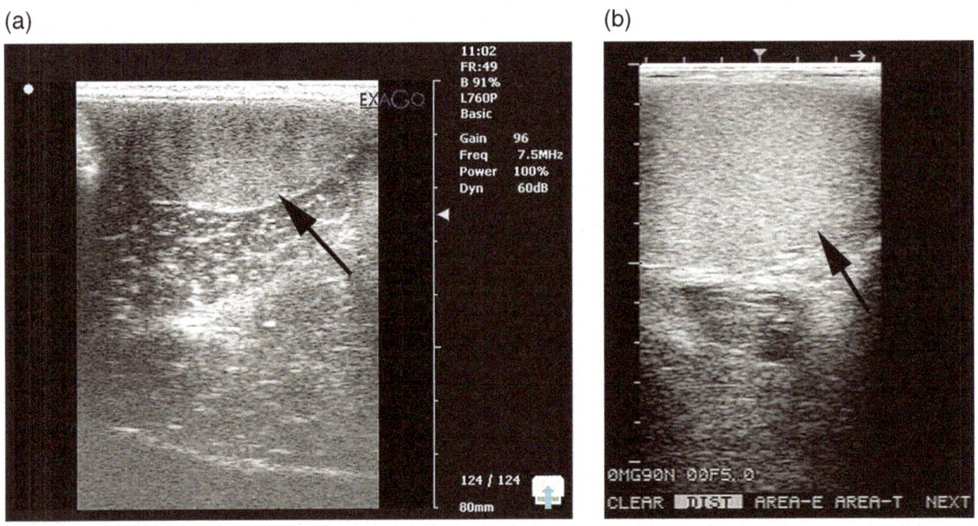

Figure 179.1 Ultrasound photo of a retained testis (arrow) within the abdomen of a cryptorchid stallion (a) and a normal descended testis (b; arrow).

Table 179.2 Testosterone levels in intact stallions, cryptorchid stallions, and geldings prior to and after administration of human chorionic gonadotropin (hCG). Values are from the Clinical Endocrinology Laboratory at the University of California, Davis.

	Testosterone (pg/ml)	
Horse	**Pre-hCG**	**Post-hCG**
Gelding	<50	No change
Cryptorchid	100–500	Increased
Intact stallion	800–2,000	Increased

physiological basis for the hCG stimulation test is that the luteinizing hormone-like biological activity of hCG will stimulate an increase in testosterone production from testicular Leydig cells. Consequently, testosterone levels in the second blood sample will be "significantly increased" over levels in the first sample if testicular tissue is present (Table 179.2).

Estrone sulfate and/or total estrogen levels have also been evaluated as a diagnostic test to differentiate between cryptorchid stallions and geldings (Table 179.3). Estrogen testing for cryptorchidism is not considered to be of diagnostic value in horses less than 3 years of age.

Table 179.3 Concentrations of estrone sulfate in serum or plasma of geldings, cryptorchid stallions, and intact stallions. Values are from the Clinical Endocrinology Laboratory at the University of California, Davis.

Horse	Estrone Sulfate (ng/ml)
Gelding	<0.1
Cryptorchid	35–60
Intact stallion	140–200

Interpretation

The absence of a history of castration in a male horse with either one or no scrotal testes is immediately indicative of unilateral or bilateral cryptorchidism, respectively. However, a vague history of a possible surgery or an incomplete or inaccurate history is not helpful. Behavioral traits exhibited by a suspect cryptorchid may be suggestive of retained testes, but some geldings exhibit aggressive behavior or may mount and even breed mares in heat. A thorough transrectal and/or transabdominal ultrasound examination can be successful in detection of retained testes in a majority of clinical cases. Endocrine assays are helpful when ultrasound evaluation is inconclusive or not available. Finally, laparoscopic examination may be the last diagnostic resort to differentiate monorchids (rare), cryptorchids, and true geldings.

Further Reading

Claes A, Ball BA, Almeida J, Corbin CJ, Conley AJ. 2013. Serum anti-Müllerian hormone concentrations in stallions: developmental changes, seasonal variation, and differences between intact stallions, cryptorchid stallions, and geldings. *Theriogenology* 79(9): 1229–35.

Lu KG. 2005. Clinical diagnosis of the cryptorchid stallion. *Clin Tech Eq Pract* 4(3): 250–6.

Pozor M. 2016. Application of various techniques in localizing retained testes in horses before cryptorchidectomy. *J Eq Vet Sci* 43: S45–8.

180

Probang Apparatus

Julie T. Cecere

Virginia-Maryland College of Veterinary Medicine, USA

Introduction

Paraphimosis is a serious condition of stallions and geldings and is an emergency that must be attended to quickly if the functionality of the penis is to be preserved. The longer the penis remains out of the prepuce, the more likely it is that the resulting edema will lead to impaired venous and lymphatic drainage. This increases the likelihood that the horse will be unable to withdraw his penis due to gross enlargement of the appendage. The increased weight of the penis proper will lead to muscular fatigue and may also affect pudendal nerve function, potentially causing penile paralysis. Further trauma can result from extended environmental exposure. As blood clots within the penile structures, manual removal of the clot will be necessary and additional trauma to the penis will ensue.

A thorough history must be obtained to determine the most likely cause, as well as an extensive physical examination of the stallion. Trauma, phenothiazine drugs, nutritional debilitation, and systemic diseases such as equine herpesvirus 1 or purpura hemorrhagica are potential causes. Ultrasound with Doppler assessment may be beneficial to identify the cause of any swelling and assess penile blood flow. The primary goal in treatment should be to remove edema and to replace the penis within the prepuce to limit further edema and trauma.

Equipment and Supplies

5 cm (2 inch) OD PVC piping 40–65 cm (15.5–25.5 inches) in length, an endotracheal tube or other flexible tubing that will fit into the PVC pipe (optional), roll cotton, clean examination gloves, nitrofurazone or other ointment of choice, 10 cm (4 inch) elastic adhesive tape, duct tape, 5 cm (2 inch) white adhesive tape.

The probang device is designed to be a round, blunt object that will physically keep the penis within the prepuce. The plastic tubing/pipe acts as a handle to push the larger knobbed end into the prepuce and also is an object around which to wrap adhesive tape in order to maintain its position. The stallion will urinate around the device, not through the lumen.

Technique

- The polyvinyl chloride (PVC) pipe and endotracheal tube are cut to an appropriate length, between 38 and 50 cm (15 and 20 inches), or long enough to be secured to the abdomen (Figures 180.1 and 180.2).
- Roll cotton is placed on one end of the PVC pipe, opposite that of the endotracheal tube if used, and held in place with adhesive tape. The endotracheal tube will allow for

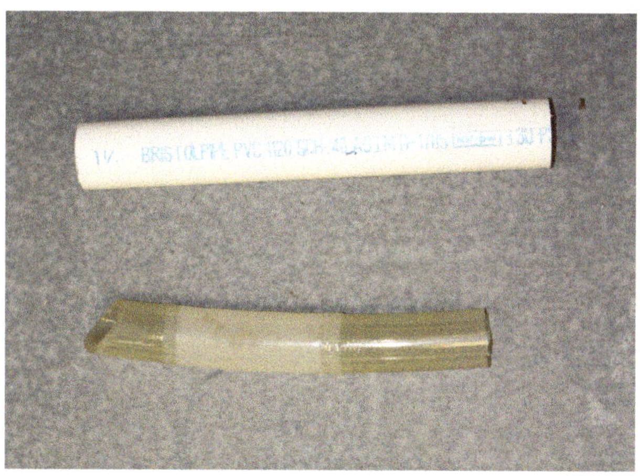

Figure 180.1 Cut lengths of PVC pipe and an endotracheal tube.

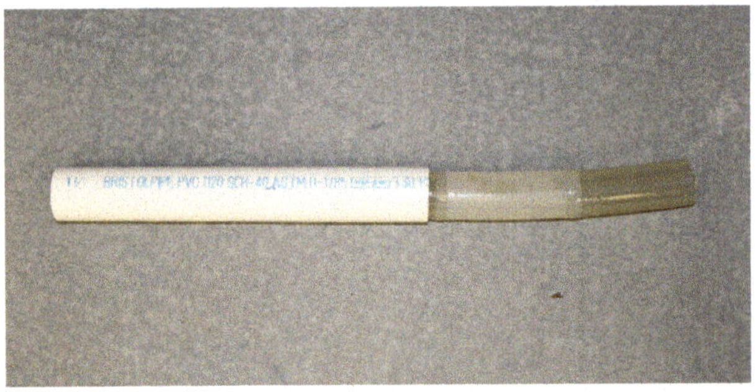

Figure 180.2 Endotracheal tube inserted part way into the PVC pipe.

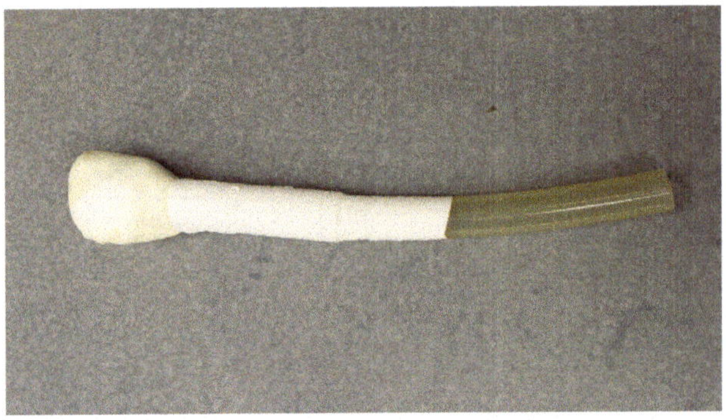

Figure 180.3 Assembled probang with cotton wrapped around the end of the PVC pipe, tape placed to hold the apparatus together, and a disposable glove over the end.

additional length of the device, and allow for a non-rigid structure to be taped to the abdomen.

- The amount of roll cotton used each time is going to depend on the size of the horse and the diameter of the preputial opening. The goal is to keep the mushroom top large enough to maintain the penis within the prepuce but to allow urine to flow around the probang.
- A glove is then placed over the cotton, so that the fingers remain inverted and are retained next to the cotton ball. This is to protect the cotton from urine as it flows around the device. Alternatively, a rectal sleeve could be used to protect the cotton.
- The glove is secured into place with adhesive tape (Figures 180.3 and 180.4).
- Nitrofurazone or another emollient is applied to the gloved end of the device.
- The prepuce and penis should be cleaned and inspected carefully, taking care not to further damage the tissues.
- Excessive edema should be removed from the penis, either with manual reduction, or the application of an elastic, non-adhesive bandage.
- Place the penis back within the prepuce and gently work the gloved end of the probang into the distal prepuce, until the cotton end is just within the orifice.

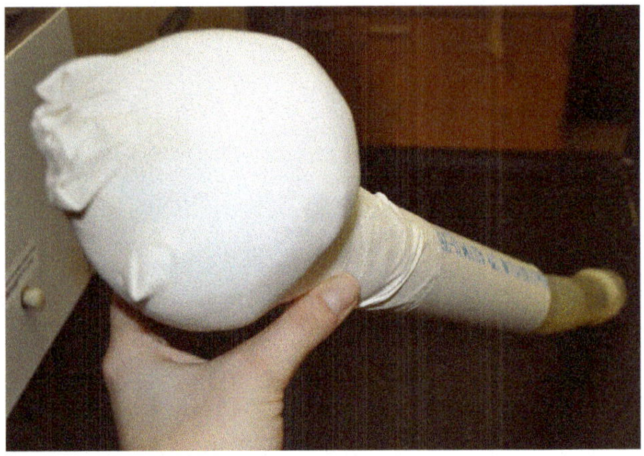

Figure 180.4 Assembled probang. Note that the fingers of the glove are not exposed on the surface of the mushroom.

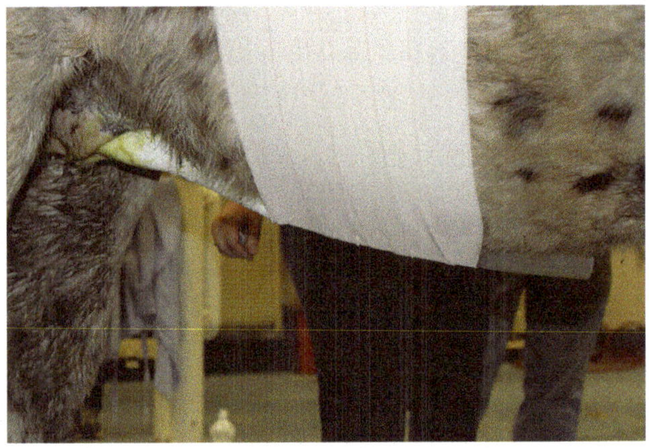

Figure 180.5 Probang device inserted into the prepuce and taped to the ventral abdomen.

- There should be enough room for urine to escape around the device but not to allow the penis to slip between the cotton and the prepuce.
- The PVC is then secured to the abdomen with elastic adhesive tape (Figure 180.5).

Interpretation

- The device should be checked at least twice daily and monitored closely for any slipping, failure to retain the penis, or ongoing trauma to the affected area.
- Reapplication of the device should be done once daily.
- Approximately 24 hours to 7 days may be required for the horse to regain its own ability to maintain the penis within the prepuce and retract his penis normally, if ever. This can be tested by removing the device and allowing the animal to prolapse his penis, and then

checking for retraction by gently flicking the shaft of the penis with your fingers, which should result in withdrawing of the penis.

- Ongoing paraphimosis, despite aggressive treatment, lasting over 1 week should be re-evaluated. Other methods of penile retention within the prepuce such as purse-string sutures around the preputial opening, a mesh sling, or a plastic bottle should also be considered (see Chapter 181). Surgical intervention may be required to salvage the use of the horse's penis in the face of prolonged paraphimosis.

Further Reading

Koch C, O'Brien T, Livesey M. 2009. How to construct and apply and penile repulsion device (probang) to manage paraphimosis. *Proc Annu Conv Am Assoc Eq Pract* 55: 338–41.

181

Support Apparatus for Paraphimosis

John J. Dascanio

School of Veterinary Medicine, Texas Tech University, USA

Introduction

Paraphimosis is a medical emergency in which a stallion is unable to retract his penis fully into the preputial cavity. If paraphimosis occurs, the penis must be supported to avoid dependent edema and further trauma. There are a number of devices designed to hold the flaccid penis upward near the ventral abdomen or within the prepuce, including the use of an open-ended bottle, a mesh support, purse-string sutures in the preputial opening, or a probang device (see Chapter 180).

The choice between procedures may be made considering previous experience, ability to replace the penis entirely into the prepuce, availability of supplies, or previous failure of one of the techniques. The mesh support works well when the penis will not easily return to the prepuce. The preputial purse-string suture is low maintenance and works if the penis can be completely reduced into the preputial cavity. The probang device is used when the penis can be returned to the prepuce and avoids a purse-string suture in the prepuce, allowing for easier examination/treatment of the penis/prepuce.

Equipment and Supplies

Tail wrap, non-irritant soap, roll cotton, stainless steel bucket, disposable liner for bucket, paper towels, exam gloves, 0.2% nitrofurazone ointment or a silver sulfadiazine ointment, non-steroidal anti-inflammatory drugs, gauze or silastic tubing, 500 ml plastic bottle, mesh material, umbilical tape or similar non-absorbable suture material, Buhner needle or large "S"-shaped cutting needle, lidocaine or carbocaine, needles, syringes.

Technique

- Prior to placing any support wraps or other devices, the affected penis should be cleaned and hydrotherapy performed as needed. The penis should then be dried and an ointment such as 0.2% nitrofurazone ointment or silver sulfadiazine applied over the entire penile surface. Additional management and therapeutic procedures would include daily exercise to reduce edema and the administration of a non-steroidal anti-inflammatory drug such as flunixin meglumine or phenybutazone.
- Make sure to examine the skin of the penis and prepuce thoroughly for any lacerations or abrasions that may need to be treated by removal of necrotic tissue, lavage, and administration of systemic antibiotics.
- If there is any question about the presence of blood clots, blood supply, abscesses, or soft tissue masses, ultrasound (with or without Doppler) may be used to delineate possible pathology.
- If there is significant edema (Figure 181.1) within the penile tissues, an elastic-type compression bandage may be placed from distal to proximal around the penis to reduce edema for about 15–20 minutes. It is removed prior to the placement of a support device.
- Large fluid accumulations may be drained with a 14 gauge needle prior to compression using an aseptic technique.
- A stallion should have complete sexual rest and separation from mares until resolution of the issue.

Bottle Technique

- Cut the closed end out of a 500 ml plastic round IV bottle. Remove the rubber plug from the open end of the bottle.
- Flame the cut plastic so that it becomes smooth.

Equine Reproductive Procedures, Second Edition. Edited by John Dascanio and Patrick McCue.

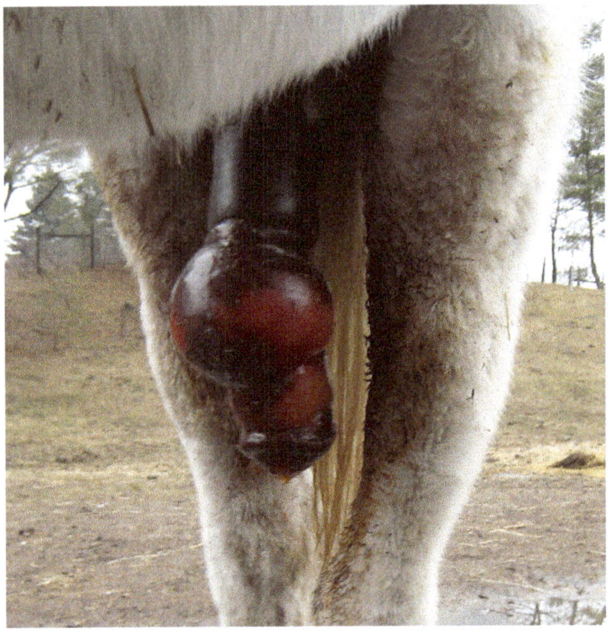

Figure 181.1 Paraphimosis in a debilitated gelding. The penis is extremely edematous below the preputial ring. A penile hematoma should be ruled out.

- Place a rim of cotton around the cut end of the bottle and overlie with 2.5 cm (1 inch) wide dressing tape (Figure 181.2).
- Tie the middle of two strands, with each end about 1.8 m (6 feet) in length (total of 3.6 m (12 feet) each), of gauze or silastic tubing around the neck of the bottle. These strands will be used to hold the bottle up against the preputial opening: one set of strands going over the back, one set of strands going backward between the hind legs. All four strands are tied together at the back.
- Place the cut open end of the bottle over the glans penis and secure the gauze or silastic tubing between the legs and over the back while pushing the bottle into the preputial opening, returning the penis to the prepuce. Only moderate pressure should be exerted to return the penis to the prepuce.
- 10 cm (4 inches) wide adhesive tape may be placed over the bottle near the smaller open end with the attached gauze or silastic tubing and wrapped around the abdomen. This will keep the bottle from everting and coming off the end of the penis (Figure 181.3).
- The stallion should be able to urinate out of the small open end of the plastic bottle when it is tied in place.

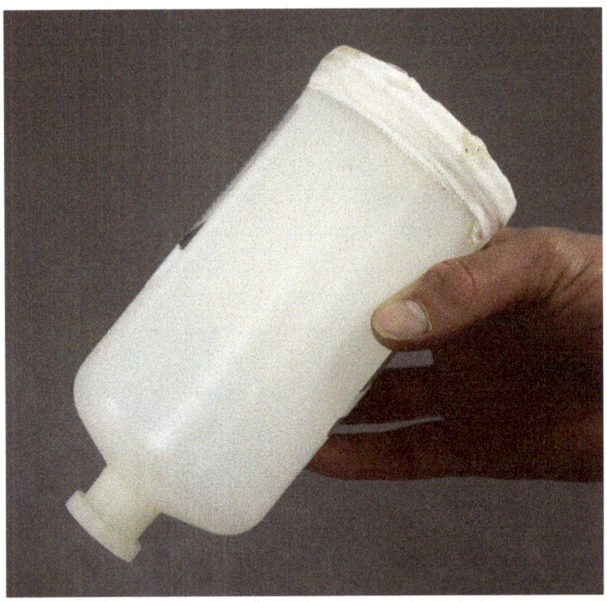

Figure 181.2 Bottle with the bottom cut off and wrapped with cotton and tape.

Mesh Technique

A 20 by 20 cm (8 × 8 inch) square or triangular piece of mesh material is cut out.

- Gauze or silastic tubing is tied to each end of the square or triangle and passed over the back and between the hind legs, securing the ends over the back (Figures 181.4 and 181.5).

Preputial Purse-String Suture

- The procedure may be performed standing or in a recumbent position.
- *Option 1* (standing). A local block with lidocaine or carbocaine is placed subcutaneously around the preputial opening.
- *Option 2* (general anesthesia). Placement of the horse under general anesthesia and then dorsal recumbency may help in replacement of the penis within the prepuce with the aid of gravity. It is also easier to work on the

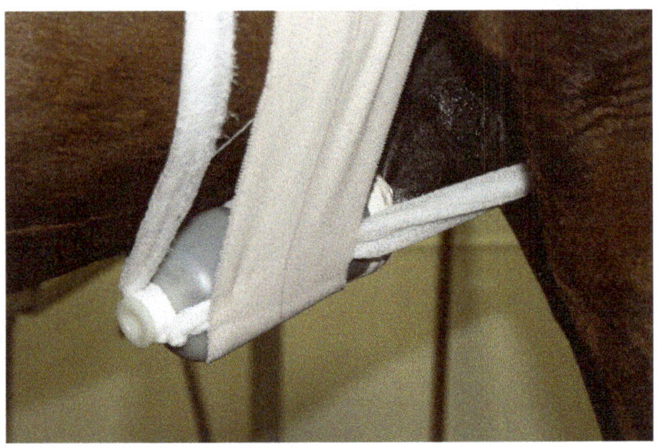

Figure 181.3 Bottle sling to support a penis with paraphimosis. The open end of the bottle allows urination.

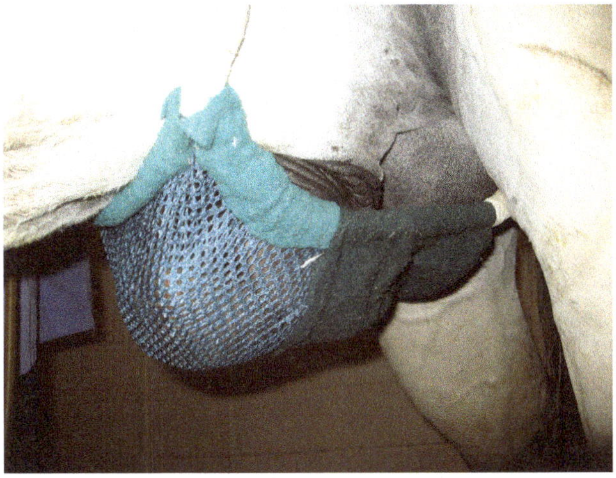

Figure 181.4 Mesh sling to support a penis with paraphimosis. Photo courtesy of Dr Rob Lofstedt.

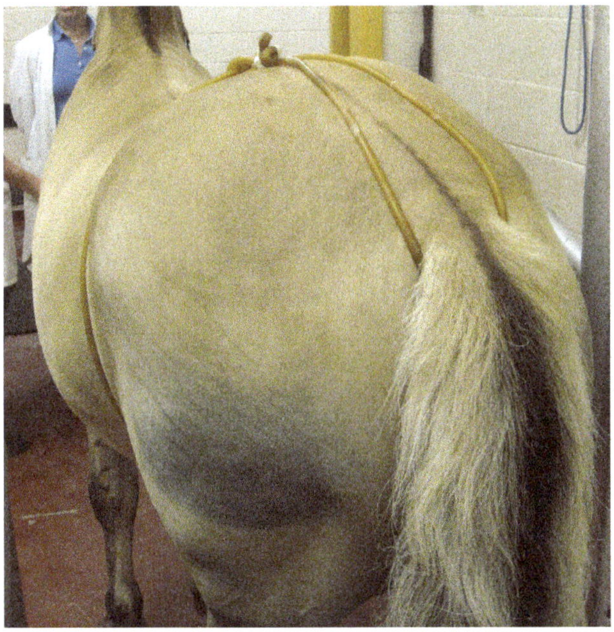

Figure 181.5 Silastic tubing tied over the back and passed between the hind legs and around the flank to hold the mesh supporting the penis. If tubing begins to migrate caudally, an additional strap may be placed going forward around the neck. Photo courtesy of Dr Rob Lofstedt.

horse in dorsal recumbency to place a compression bandage to reduce edema.
- Push the penis into the prepuce, being careful to not push with focused pressure over edematous tissue so as

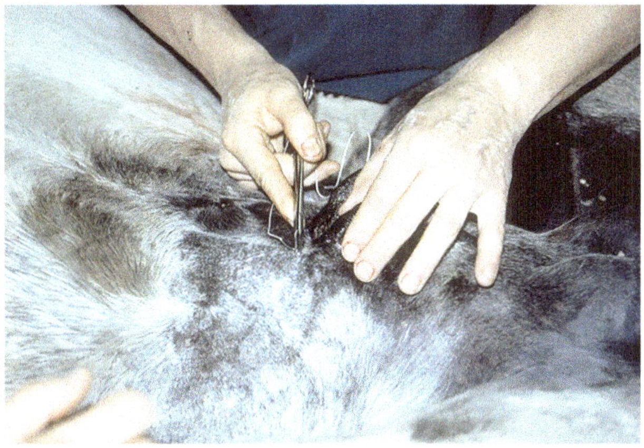

Figure 181.6 Placement of a purse-string suture around the preputial opening of a stallion in dorsal recumbency.

to avoid disrupting the tissue. Only broad-based pressure should be used.
- Soak umbilical tape in a 0.5% iodine solution. The length of the tape should allow for placement around the prepuce and a tie.
- Using a Buhner needle or large "S"-shaped cutting needle, place the umbilical tape or a similar non-absorbable suture material circumferentially around the preputial opening (Figure 181.6).
- The purse-string suture should be pulled tight enough to prevent prolapse of the penis, but not tight enough to prevent urination.
- The purse-string should be loosened in 14 days to determine if the penis and preputial tissue can be retained within the prepuce. The penis should be examined, cleaned, lubricated, and returned to the prepuce and the purse-string tightened if it is unable to be retained.

Interpretation

- With any support device, the penis and preputial tissues should be examined daily for abrasions or rub sores.
- Hydrotherapy with reapplication of an ointment should be performed daily.
- In the suture method, care should be taken that the penis does not extend through the tied purse-string, become swollen, and then have a constricting band where the purse-string is placed, leading to venous occlusion.
- Any abnormal discharge, swelling, or odor would be reason to re-examine the penis and prepuce.

Further Reading

Brinsko SP, Blanchard TL, Varner DD. 2007. How to treat paraphimosis. *Proc Annu Conv Am Assoc Eq Pract* 53: 580–2.

182

Equine Castration Techniques

Stacy Anderson

College of Veterinary Medicine, Lincoln Memorial University, USA

Introduction

Castration of a stallion is commonly performed for behavior modification and/or to treat lesions of the testicle and scrotum. It is important to inform clients that a small percentage of stallions may retain stallion-like behavior following castration. A newly gelded stallion should remain separated from mares for at least 1 week, as extragonadal spermatozoa are present within the remaining vas deferens and ampulla. In North America, equine castration is most commonly performed under general anesthesia, while in Europe the procedure is often performed under sedation in a standing patient. Castration may be performed as an open procedure, where the vaginal tunic is incised, or a closed procedure, in which the vaginal tunic is left intact. Generally, the scrotum is left open to heal by second intention, but it may be closed with or without ablation. Cryptorchidism is fairly common in horses and surgery should not be performed unless both testes are able to be successfully removed.

Equipment and Supplies

Safe environment with good footing, towel, ropes (3–3.6 m (10–12 feet), 4 cm (1.5 inch) diameter minimum), surgical scrub, stainless steel bucket with or without disposable plastic liner, rolled cotton or gauze squares, antiseptic solution and scrub (chlorhexidine or povidone-iodine), sterile surgical gloves, emasculators (White, Serra, Reimer, or Henderson castration tool), scalpel (no. 10 or no. 20 blade), sterile gauze squares, minor procedures surgical pack (in case of complications), USP 2-0 or 0 absorbable monofilament suture (optional), tetanus toxoid and/or antitoxin, anesthetic supplies: ketamine, α2-agonist (xylazine), butorphanol, lidocaine, benzodiazepine (optional; midazolam or diazepam), assortment of syringes and needles, non-steroidal anti-inflammatories (phenylbutazone or flunixin meglumine).

Technique

- Place a plastic disposable liner in a stainless steel bucket and fill with clean warm water. Add cotton from the cotton roll or gauze squares for scrubbing the surgical site. The antiseptic of choice will be placed on this material during surgical site preparation.
- Anesthetize the stallion or colt.
  - The common anesthetic protocol for castrating the horse is:
    - give pre-medication of 1.1 mg/kg xylazine IV (optional: add 0.02 mg/kg butorphanol)
    - induction with 2.2 mg/kg ketamine IV (optional: add 0.02 mg/kg benzodiazepine)
    - (optional) give intratesticular block with 5 ml of 2% lidocaine for small testicles (<8 cm (3 inches) diameter) or 10 ml for large testicles (>9 cm (3.5 inches) diameter) per testicle following an initial preparation of the scrotum
    - horses may be administered an additional dose of ketamine with or without xylazine, at one quarter to one half of the initial dose of each, during the procedure, if the plane of anesthesia proves to be inadequate.
  - Horses should be administered a non-steroidal anti-inflammatory drug (4–6 mg/kg phenylbutazone IV) and tetanus toxoid (and tetanus anti-toxin if vaccination status is unknown) peri-operatively. Non-steroidal anti-inflammatory durgs and tetanus toxoid/anti-toxin can be given before, during, or after the procedure. Antibiotics are generally considered unnecessary.
  - Dosages for donkeys and ponies may be increased 30–40% from those just listed.

Equine Reproductive Procedures, Second Edition. Edited by John Dascanio and Patrick McCue.

- Place a towel over the eyes of the horse to help maintain a quiet environment.
- Pull the down front leg forward to prevent radial nerve compression. Also ensure that the metal rings on the halter are not causing compression of the facial nerve.
- Using a 3–3.6 m (~10 feet), 4 cm (1.5 inches) cotton rope, tie the hind legs either with the horse remaining in lateral recumbency or so that the hind end is in dorsal recumbency to provide access to the surgical site (Figure 182.1 and 182.2).
- Wearing examination gloves, prepare the castration site.
  - The scrotum and caudo-ventral prepuce are prepared with an antiseptic scrub (povidone-iodine or chlorhexidine) using rolled cotton or gauze squares and rinsed with ethyl alcohol directly from the bottle or on gauze squares.
- Incise the scrotum.
  - Two 6–10 cm (2 to 4 inch) skin incisions are made along the ventral aspect of the scrotum over the right and left testicle. The incision length varies by the size of the horse's testicles. It should be at least the entire length of the testicle.
- Exteriorize the testicles.
  - For a closed technique, the parietal tunic is left intact. The subcutaneous tissues are incised until the parietal tunic is exposed. Then the fascia and scrotal ligament are stripped manually using sterile gauze squares to exteriorize the testicle and expose the spermatic cord.
  - For an open technique, the parietal tunic is incised, which removes the need to strip the fascia. However, the ligament of the tail of the epididymis must still be transected either sharply or bluntly to free the testicle from the parietal tunic and exteriorize the testicles and structures of the spermatic cord.
- Apply the emasculator.
  - Emasculators are applied at right angle to the spermatic cord. As the emasculator is being closed, release tension

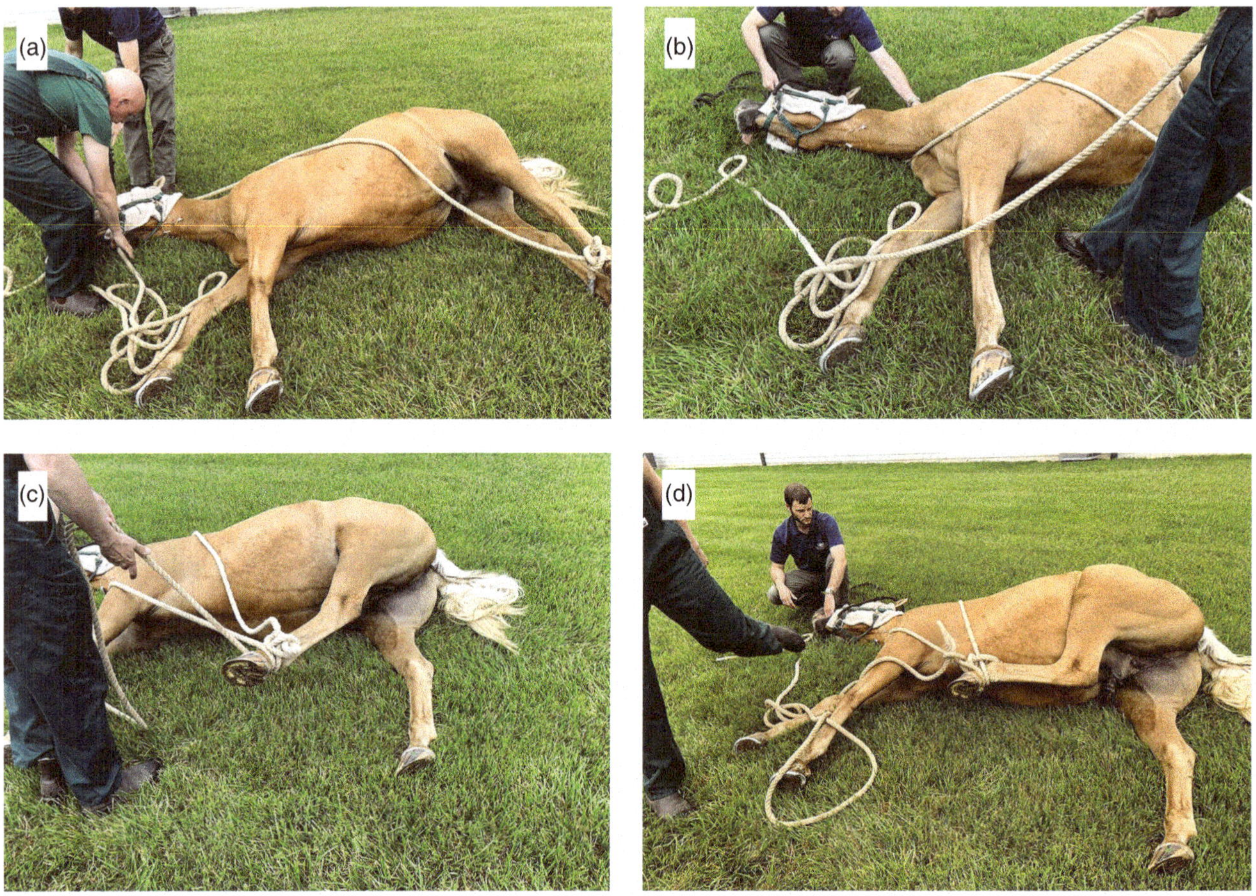

Figure 182.1 Securing the hind leg for positioning in lateral recumbency. (a) A quick release knot is tied around the pastern of the upper rear limb. (b) The rope is passed over then under the horse's head and neck. (c) The rope is passed under then over the upper rear limb pastern. (d) A quick release knot is tied to secure the upper leg in a cranial position. The end of the rope is passed toward the horse's head so that is may be pulled to release the upper hind limb if the horse suddenly attempts to stand.

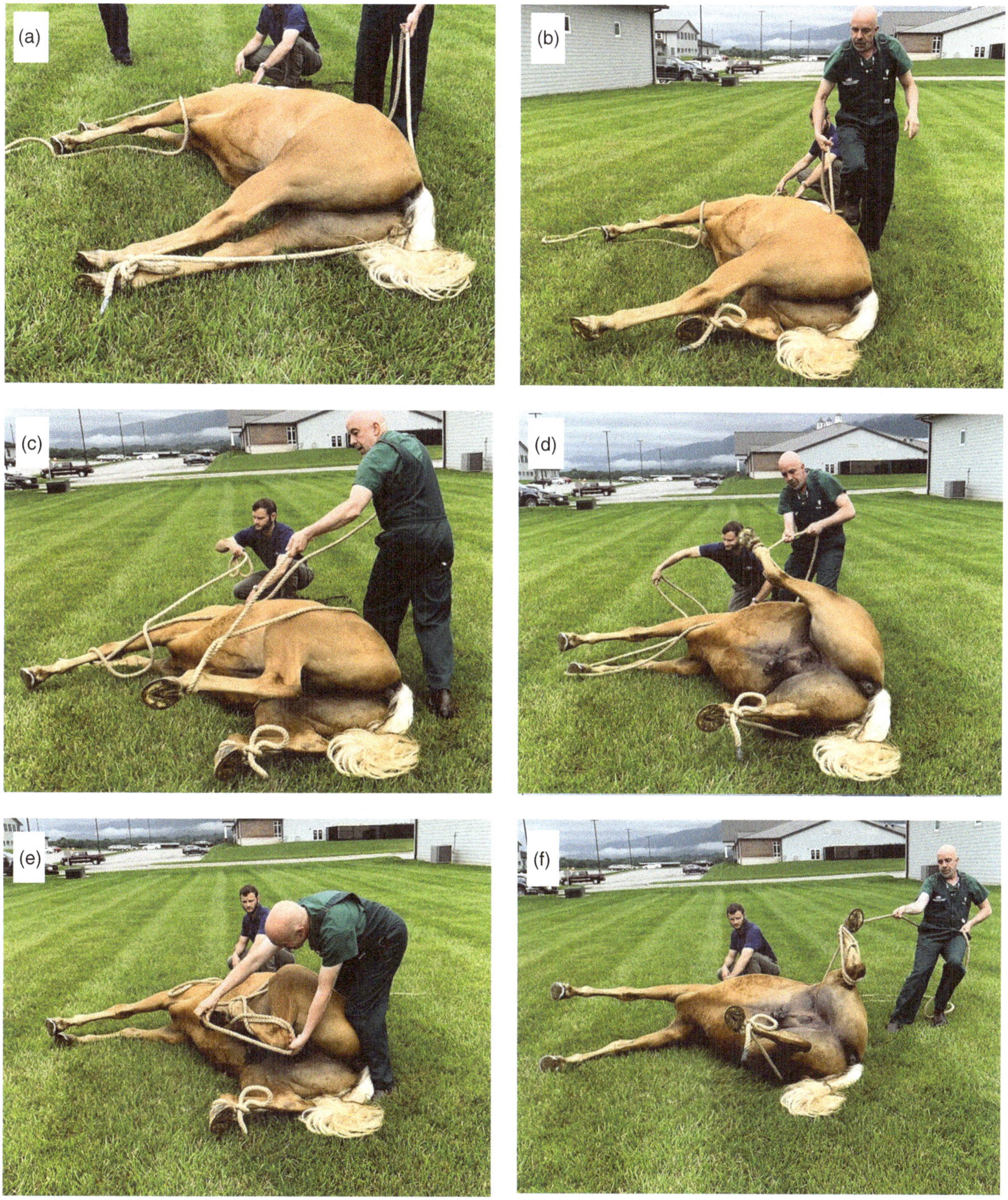

Figure 182.2 Securing the hind legs for positioning in dorsal recumbency. (a) A quick release knot is tied around the pastern of the lower rear limb. (b) The rope is passed under the haunches and the lower rear limb is flexed. (c) The rope is looped over the pastern of the upper rear limb. (d) The rope is pulled taut to flex the upper rear limb. (e) A figure of eight pattern is used to secure the upper rear limb in flexion. (f) An assistant pulls the end of the rope to keep the patient in dorsal recumbency. The rope under the horse should be in front of the pelvis and stifles to aid in retention if the horse moves.

on the cord to ensure the cord end remains within the emasculator. In emasculators that have a blade to cut, in addition to incising, the crushing part must be proximally orientated toward the horse. Commonly used emasculators, such as the Reimer and Serra, have a bolt and nut that hold the joint of the instrument together. The nut is on the side of the emasculator that has the cutting blade, so it should be orientated distally toward the testicle (i.e., "nut to nut").
 - The emasculators are applied and should be left in place a minimum of 2 minutes. In larger horses and donkeys, it is recommended to leave them on for at least 5 minutes.
 - When the emasculators are removed, the inguinal area should be should be observed for excessive hemorrhage. Optionally, a hemostat may be used to gently grasp the cord as it is being removed from the emasculator to aid in retrieval should ligation be required.
 - Optionally, a circumferential ligature may be placed proximal to the emasculators to aid in hemostasis using USP 2-0 or 0 absorbable monofilament suture.
- Trim excessive subcutaneous tissues.
 - For closed castration, there is often tissue left from stripping the testicle and spermatic cord that could hang down once the horse is standing. An emasculator may be used to incise the redundant tissue, or optionally a Rochester-Carmalt forceps or a large hemostat may be used to crush the tissue prior to excision with a scalpel blade.
- Leave the scrotal incision open or perform a primary closure.
 - The scrotal incisions are most commonly left open to heal by second intention. The author advises stretching the incisions manually by placing an index finger at each end of the incision and apply tension at the end of the procedure to make sure that the subcutaneous incision is the same length as the skin incision.
 - Scrotal incisions may be closed primarily or the scrotum may be ablated. These procedures should ideally be performed in a hospital setting with strict adherence to aseptic technique.
- Recovery from anesthesia.
 - The horse is left to recover from anesthesia on its own in either an enclosed or open space. If recovering in the open, a handler should be nearby to hold the horse after recovery. In either situation, a handler should be available to stabilize the horse once it stands if needed as it regains its balance.

Interpretation

- Horses should be administered tetanus toxoid at the time of surgery unless vaccinated within the past 30 days. Horses with no or an unknown vaccine history should receive an additional dose of tetanus anti-toxin.
- Castrated stallions should not be exposed to mares for at least 7 days following castration.
- Castration should ideally occur during the year when flies are less active, but if castration occurs during fly season, the incision site should be protected from flies.
- Horses should be stall-rested for 24 hours, then begin a program of forced exercise, such as lunging at the trot for 10–20 minutes, for 5–7 days postoperatively to reduce excessive swelling of the surgical site and promote drainage.
- Horses should be administered a non-steroidal anti-inflammatory drug (phenylbutazone or flunixin meglumine) perioperatively up to 3 days postoperatively as needed.
- Complications include excessive hemorrhage, excessive postoperative swelling, evisceration, funiculitis, hydrocele, penile damage, and continued masculine behavior.

Additional Comments

The decision to ligate the spermatic cord in the equine is generally based on the likelihood of evisceration and to reduce postoperative hemorrhage. Most commonly, it is performed in mature stallions (aged greater than 5 years) and donkeys. If excessive hemorrhage is noticed after removing the emasculators, the spermatic cord should be ligated to provide additional hemostasis.

Further Reading

Schumacher J. 2012. Testis. In: Auer JA, Stick JA (eds). Equine Surgery, 4th edn. St Louis, MO: Elsevier Saunders, pp. 804–40.

Searle D, Dart AJ, Hodgson DR. 1999. Equine castration: review on anatomy, approaches, techniques and complications in normal, cryptorchid and monorchid horses. *Aust Vet J* 77: 428–34.

183

Stallion Acupuncture

Rhonda A. Rathgeber

Hagyard Equine Medical Institute, USA

Introduction

Stallion reproductive disorders can be a costly and time-consuming issue in equine practice. Stallions with back pain would be good candidates for acupuncture treatment given the nature of their job. Any musculoskeletal pain can reduce a stallion's libido and ability to breed. It has been well documented that horses with back pain respond well to acupuncture. Pain during breeding can also affect the behavior of stallions. Behavior issues may or may not be addressed in an acupuncture treatment. Acupuncture may address hormonally based behavior by its effect on the hypophyseal–pituitary–gonadal axis. When acupoints are stimulated, sensory receptors stimulate impulses in the afferent nerves that carry information to the central nervous system. The central nervous system then activates the hypothalamic–pituitary axis. Gonadal function and sexual behavior are regulated by this axis. It is a complex pathway of hormonal cascades and feedback loops that originate in the hypothalamus. The hypothalamus processes many visual, auditory, olfactory, and tactile signals. Then it translates this information into secretion of gonadotropin-releasing hormone. This in turn causes the gonadal production of steroid hormones that affect spermatogenesis. An imbalance of this hormone cascade leads to reproductive dysfunction. For these reasons, a stallion with a history of poor breeding performance should have a thorough lameness and neurologic evaluation. Acupuncture may be a beneficial adjunct to conventional therapy, because it has been shown to relieve myofascial pain, relieve muscle spasms, and reduce inflammation.

There are increasing numbers of studies in men identifying the effects of acupuncture on fertility in humans. Since 2000, several research projects have examined the effect of acupuncture on male fertility with encouraging results. Many reproductive hormones can be altered by acupuncture. Endorphins in the brain, spinal cord, and blood increase after acupuncture. A series of acupuncture treatments given to men over 5 weeks was shown to increase the mean total motility and mean total vitality of sperm. Motility, density, and vitality of sperm are all encouraged by acupuncture treatments. Acupuncture can be effective without the side effects of many medications given for infertility. Acupuncture will increase the blood flow to the testicular artery; this leads to an increased blood flow to the testicles, with increased nutrients, better removal of waste products, and cooling of the scrotum.

In traditional Chinese medicine (TCM), symptoms of male infertility are a manifestation of an underlying qi imbalance. The imbalances usually involve the kidney and the liver. In TCM, the kidney stores the essence of qi which would be the reproductive cells, the sperm, and the semen in western medicine. The liver stores blood and regulates the flow of qi. Traditionally, male infertility patients are categorized into their pattern of qi disharmony or imbalance and treated accordingly with both acupuncture and with herbs. Formulations or collections of acupoints are used empirically that are associated with boosting fertility.

In conclusion, acupuncture helps infertility treatment by boosting blood flow to the reproductive organs, by balancing hormones through neurohormonal regulation, relieving stress, and relieving pain. Needling can increase sperm production, increase the percentage of healthy sperm, improve sperm motility, and improve the levels of hormones responsible for fertility.

Equipment and supplies

Sterile acupuncture needles (0.30 × 50 mm and 0.30 × 75 mm) (Figure 183.1), vitamin B_{12} (1,000 μg/ml) (Figure 183.2), sterile 25 gauge 4 cm (1.5 inch) hypodermic needles (Figure 183.3), electroacupuncture machine (Figure 183.4), moxa (Figure 183.5).

Equine Reproductive Procedures, Second Edition. Edited by John Dascanio and Patrick McCue.

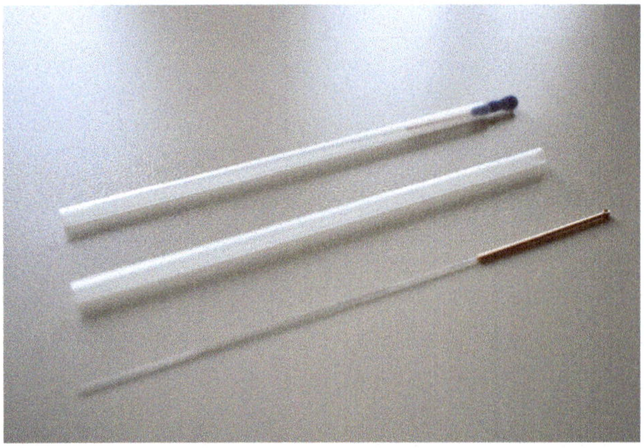

Figure 183.1 Sterile acupuncture needles.

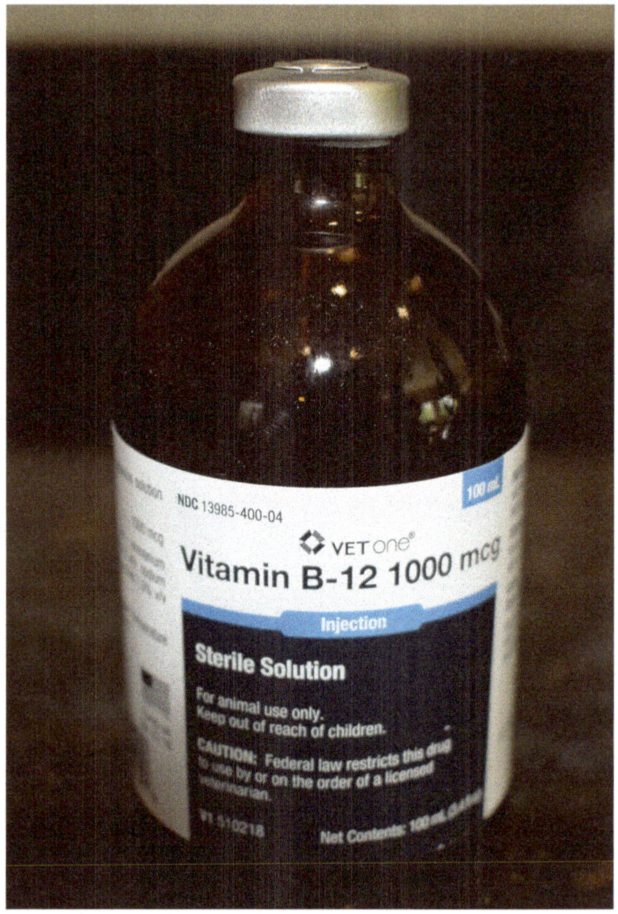

Figure 183.2 Vitamin B_{12}.

Technique

- Identify a certified veterinary acupuncturist in your area if you are not certified yourself. You can find a practitioner in your area at http://www.tcvm.com/ or https://www.ivas.org/ (last accessed November 2020) and enter your zip code.
- Perform a complete lameness and neurologic examination on the stallion. This will aid in acupuncture point selection as well as a western medicine treatment plan. Decreased libido in a breeding stallion may simply be musculoskeletal in origin and may respond very well to acupuncture directed to the musculoskeletal pain to make the horse more comfortable. TCM kidney qi deficiency may manifest as a weak and sore caudal back. Stallions with a history of infertility and that are reluctant to mount a mare may be suffering from back pain secondary to kidney qi deficiency. These cases respond very well to acupuncture.
- If indicated and practical, perform semen analysis on a sample from the stallion. Acupuncture can affect the gonadal paracrine and autocrine control of steroidogenesis and help with infertility. It may be helpful to monitor the progress with consecutive semen analysis.

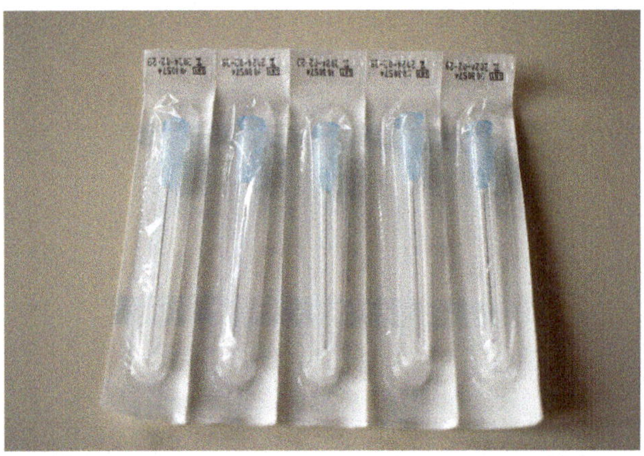

Figure 183.3 Sterile hypodermic needles.

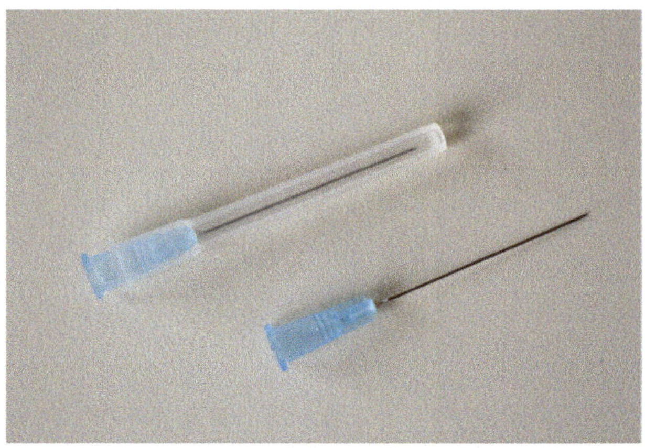

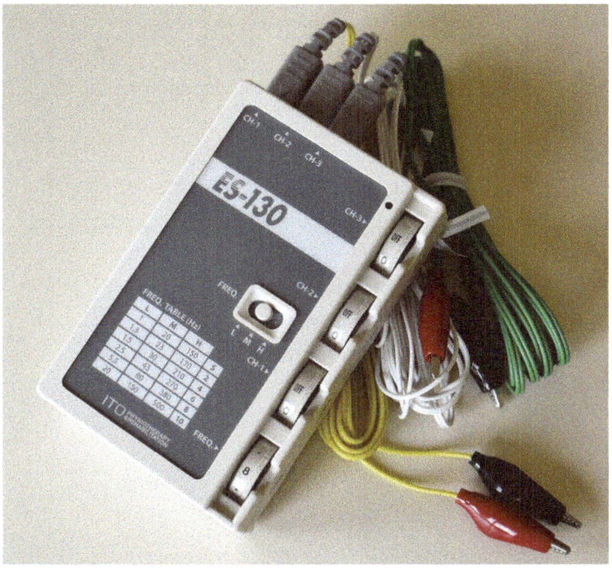

Figure 183.4 Electroacupuncture machine.

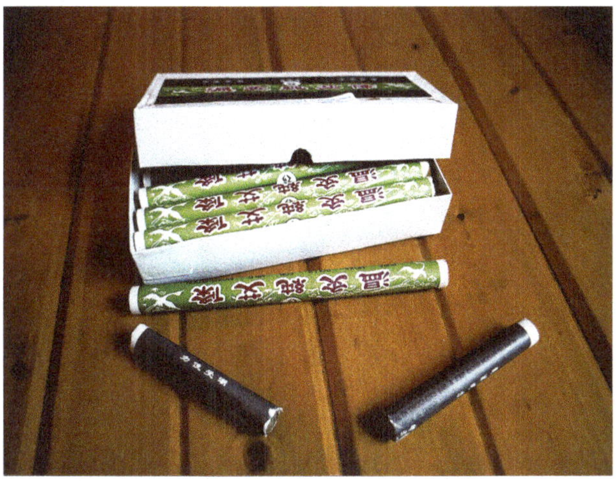

Figure 183.5 Moxa.

- Perform a TCM examination on the stallion to determine the pattern of imbalance; the most common patterns for stallion infertility are kidney yang/qi deficiency, kidney yin deficiency, and kidney jing deficiency. Musculoskeletal soreness may be causing decreased libido and unwillingness to breed and may present as a different pattern and require different point selection.
- Point selection:
  - Electroacupuncture can be used at the following pairs:
    - shen-shu, bilateral
    - shen-peng, bilateral
    - BL-24 to yan-chi, bilateral
    - BL-23, bilateral
  - KI-3, KI-7, KI-14, SP-6, SP-8, SP-9.
  - Qi and blood deficiency signs include worry, over-thinking, stress, chronic illness, impotence, low sperm count, short sperm life, and slow sperm mobility. Acupoints are ST-36, SP-6, BL-23, and HT-7.
  - Kidney deficiency acupoints include: KI-3, BL-23, KI-11, KI-6, BL-52.
  - Damp heat in genital system: SP9, liver 5, liver 11, ST-28, GB-41.
  - Orchitis: BL-20, ST-36, BL-23, BL-25, CV-1, KI-11, KI-12, bai hui, GV2.
  - Testicular disorders: BL-21, BL-22, BL-23, GV-4, GV-5, SP-6, ST-36.
  - Impotence/penile paralysis: bau hui, CV-1, GV-2, GV-1, GV-4, BL-29, BL-30, BL-31, BL-32, BL-33, BL-34, moxa.
  - Bai hui hundred meetings: location in the depression between the spinous process of L6 and S1; insertion is perpendicular 4–8 cm; can use moxibustion; used for back pain and urogenital problems.
  - Kai feng wind release: location in the depression between the spinous process of S3 and S4; insertion is perpendicular 2–3 cm; used for pelvic pain and urogenital problems.
  - Shen shu: location in the muscle groove 3–5 cm lateral to bau hui; insertion is perpendicular 2–4 cm; used for infertility and hind limb pain.
  - Shen men: location is in the depression between the spinous process of L3 and L4; insertion is perpendicular 2–3 cm; used for pain in back and hind quarters.
  - Ming men gate of life: location in the depression between the spinous process of L2 and L3; insertion is perpendicular 2–3 cm; indicated in urogenital disease.
  - Fei shu lung association point: location is about 6 cm lateral to the dorsal midline at the eighth intercostal space; insertion is perpendicular 2–3 cm; indicated for infertility, respiratory, or cardiac problems.
  - Hou hai caudal sea: location in depression between the anus and ventral base of the tail; insertion is 2–3 cm; used for prolapse or infertility.

Additional Comments

- Other patterns of male infertility in TCM are: liver qi stagnation, spleen oi deficiency, kidney yang deficiency, kidney yin deficiency, stomach qi deficiency, and blood stagnation.
- If you are not getting results with your first point selection after 3–4 weeks, repeat your TCM examination and try a different selection of points.
- If the client is interested, consult a veterinarian that specializes in Chinese herbs and add them to the regimen. They are very beneficial in infertility cases.

Further Reading

Gerhard I, Jung I, Postneek F. 1992. Effects of acupuncture on semen parameters/hormone profile in infertile men. *Mol Androl* 4: 9–25.

He Y, Chen CT, Qian LH, *et al.* 2015. [Acupuncture treatment of male infertility; a systematic review.] *Zhonghua Nan Ke Xue* 21(7): 637–45. (Abstract in English.)

Jerng UM, Jo JY, Lee S, Lee JM, Kwon O. 2014. The effectiveness and safety of acupuncture for poor semen quality in infertile males: a systematic review and meta-analysis. *Asian J Androl* 16(6): 884–91.

Pei J, Strehler E, Noss U, Abt M, Piomboni P, Baccetti B, Sterzik K. 2005. Quantitative evaluation of spermatozoa ultrastructure after acupuncture treatment for idiopathic male infertility. *Fertil Steril* 84(1): 141–7.

Siterman S, Eltes F, Wolfson V, *et al.* 1997. Effect of acupuncture on sperm parameters of males suffering from subfertility related to low sperm quality. *Arch Androl* 39: 155–61.

Siterman S, Eltes F, Wolfson V, *et al.* 2000. Does acupuncture treatment affect sperm density in males with very low sperm count? Pilot study. *Andrologia* 32(1): 31–9.

Part V

Newborn Foal

184

Birth Resuscitation

Patrick M. McCue

Equine Reproduction Laboratory, Colorado State University, USA

Introduction

Spontaneous respiration in most foals begins almost immediately after passage through the birth canal of the mare. However, some foals do not initiate spontaneous respiration after birth and emergency institution of resuscitation procedures may be indicated. Personnel involved in foaling and foal care should be trained in obstetrical intervention and birth resuscitation procedures. A foaling kit and emergency resuscitation equipment should be readily available. Emergency procedure codes and charts should be reviewed and posted in the foaling area.

Indications for resuscitation intervention in a newborn foal include: no respiratory movements evident at birth, no heart beat evident at birth, gasping for breath for longer than 30 seconds after birth, obvious respiratory distress, and a heart rate of less than 50 beats per minute (bpm).

Equipment and Supplies

Towel to dry and stimulate foal; birth resuscitation device: Ambu bag or similar device, Foal Resuscitator®, mask, or naso-tracheal tube; oxygen delivery system: E-tank, regulator, oxygen tube, nasal insufflation tube; stethoscope, epinephrine, doxapram, needles, syringes.

Birth Resuscitation Technique

- Establish an airway. Remove amnion from the nose if present. Suction mucus, meconium, etc. from the mouth/nose if needed. Intubate the foal if needed and inflate the cuff; typically 14–18 mm endotracheal tubes are used.
- Vigorously dry the foal with cloth towels for approximately 20 seconds. This will provide stimulation for the onset of breathing.
- Provide ventilation support (i.e., assisted breathing) if needed. The goal is to provide 10–20 breaths per minute (up to 40 breaths per minute). A resuscitation device may be attached to a naso-tracheal tube or mask. If a mask is available, place the mask firmly over the nose of the foal (Figure 184.1). Squeeze the Ambu bag with both hands to provide an adequate air volume (Figure 184.2). Observe for lifting or excursion of the chest with each compression of the Ambu bag. Mouth-to-nose ventilation can be provided if necessary. One nostril must be occluded when using this technique. If an extra person is available, occlude the esophagus with manual compression over the neck to prevent air from entering gastrointestinal tract. A brief pause should occur every 30 seconds to check if the foal is breathing on its own.

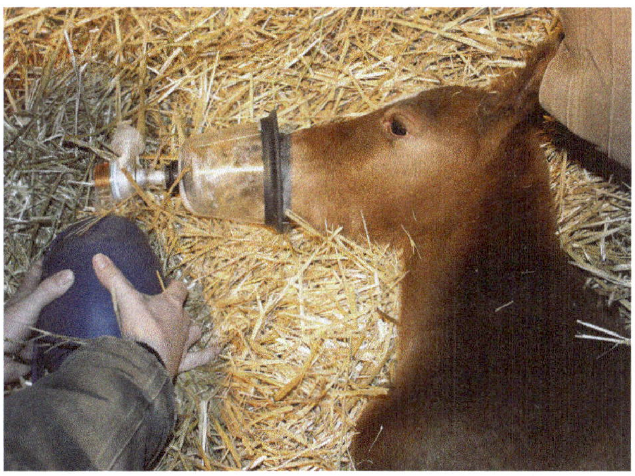

Figure 184.1 Placement of a mask over the nose of a foal.

Equine Reproductive Procedures, Second Edition. Edited by John Dascanio and Patrick McCue.

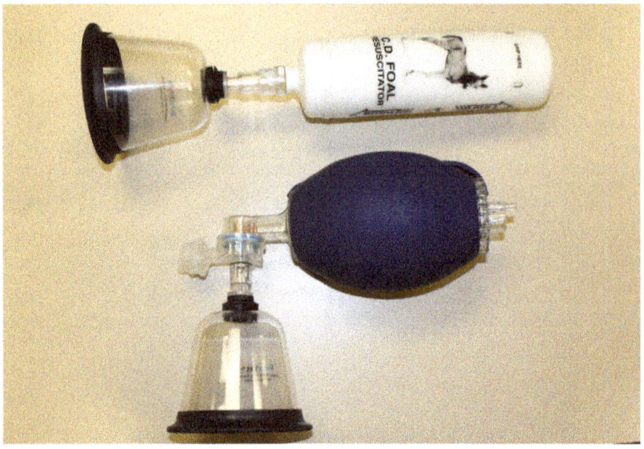

Figure 184.2 Foal Resuscitator® (top) and Ambu bag (bottom) each attached to a nose cone.

- Oxygen supplementation may be provided at a flow of 8–10 1/min (Figure 184.3); humidify the oxygen if the required equipment is available. The foal should be in right lateral recumbency, initially with its head on the floor to help brain perfusion when circulation is marginal. Adjust the foal to sternal recumbency when blood circulation is adequate; this will help ventilate both lungs.
- Provide circulatory support if needed. Assess the heart rate and rhythm with a stethoscope 30 seconds after starting assisted ventilation. Thoracic compressions should be initiated by the following conditions: absence of a heart beat or heart beat of less than 40 bpm. The goal is to apply approximately 80–120 compressions per minute. The recommended ratio is 2 breaths per 30 thoracic compressions. The foal should be in lateral recumbency during thoracic compression with its back against a wall. Care should be exercised to not fracture its ribs during compressions.

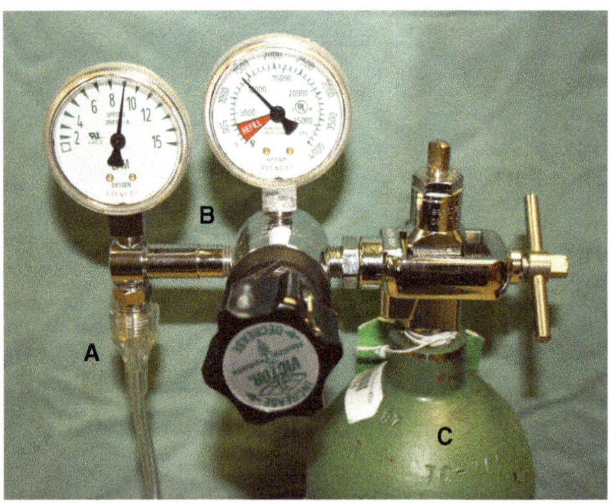

Figure 184.3 Oxygen tube (A) attached to a regulator (B) on an oxygen E-tank (C), set at a rate of 9 liters of oxygen per minute.

- Administration of selected medications may be indicated:
  - Epinephrine should be administered if the heart rate is <40 bpm and does not increase after 30 seconds of thoracic compressions and adequate ventilation. The intravenous dose is 0.01–0.02 mg/kg or 0.5–1.0 ml of a 1 mg/ml (1:1,000) solution for a 50 kg foal. Epinephrine should be administered every 3 minutes until adequate circulation is achieved.
  - Administration of doxapram is controversial in an apneic neonate. Ventilation is considered as effective in reversing primary apnea and is the only effective treatment of secondary apnea. If doxapram is to be administered in the emergency treatment of primary apnea in an equine neonate, the dosage range is 0.5–2.5 mg/kg IV.
- Fluid support via a jugular venous catheter may also be warranted. Place an 18 gauge 9 cm (3.5 inch) intravenous jugular catheter and initially administer 10–20 ml/kg lactated Ringer's solution as an initial bolus dose (i.e., 500–1,000 ml to a 50 kg foal). Glucose should be provided as needed; it is recommended to measure blood glucose levels first.
- Thermal support in the form of blankets or an external heat source may be warranted. Body temperature should be monitored. Care should be taken to avoid overheating.
- Birth resuscitation therapy should be discontinued when a heart rate of >60 bpm and spontaneous breathing is well established, or if no response is detected after approximately 10 minutes.
- Oxygen supplementation should be continued as needed.

Additional Comments

- Foals that survive after emergency birth resuscitation procedures are at risk of medical problems early in life. They often do not have a strong suckle instinct or response and are consequently prone to failure of passive transfer. It is common to provide these foals with supplemental colostrum and/or plasma. At-risk foals should be monitored closely, especially for the first 3–5 days of life, as medical complications are not uncommon. Prophylactic administration of anti-inflammatory drugs, free radical scavenger medications, and/or antioxidants may be considered for the prevention of hypoxic ischemic encephalopathy.
- Physical findings in a normal foal are listed in Box 184.1.

Box 184.1 Normal Foal Peri-parturient Physical Examination Findings

- Normal regular breathing should begin within 30 seconds of birth
- Heart rate should be regular and approximately 70–80 bpm
- Foals should have sensory awareness at birth
- Righting reflex should be evident within approximately 5 minutes of birth

Further Reading

Collins NM, Axon JE, Palmer JE. 2011. Resuscitation (foal and birth). In: McKinnon AO, Squires EL, Vaala WE, Varner DD (eds). Equine Reproduction, 2nd edn. Ames, IA: Wiley Blackwell, pp. 128–35.

Corley KTT, Axon JE. 2005. Resuscitation and emergency management for neonatal foals. *Vet Clin North Am Eq Pract* 21: 431–55.

185

Handling and Restraint

Undine Christmann

College of Veterinary Medicine, Lincoln Memorial University, USA

Introduction

Foals may need to be restrained for physical exams, treatments, diagnostic procedures, and sometimes for minor interventions. The veterinarian can use standing restraint while completing a physical exam or a handler can hold the foal while treatment is administered. Placing a foal in lateral recumbency is often used to perform abdominal ultrasound, to place a catheter, or to complete other procedures under sedation.

Contrary to adult horses, neonatal foals are not used to leading and have different reactions or defense mechanisms against restraint. Applying pressure or pulling results in the foal struggling to regain freedom and can lead to injury of the handler or the foal. Foals may also react by sinking or collapsing in the handler's arm and then suddenly kick out, leap, or rear. Restraining a foal requires patience, experience, and knowledge of common reactions to stimuli.

Veterinarians can also help owners learn proper restraint and care. In addition, they can guide owners in the use of imprinting techniques which can facilitate socialization of the foal with humans, learning to halter and lead, and getting used to several routine procedures including picking up feet, tolerating touch during a physical exam, and accepting use of clippers. Imprinting has been shown to result in learned behavior and to decrease self-defense responses from the foal.

Equipment and Supplies

Soft cotton lead rope, foal halter, foal harness, soft rope 1.5–2 cm (3/4 inch) in diameter and 5–5.5 m (~18 feet) in length.

Technique

Standing Restraint

The handler can use the following techniques for standing restraint:

- Technique 1. One arm is wrapped around the neck or the pectoral area and the other arm is placed around the hind end (Figure 185.1a).
- Technique 2. One arm is wrapped around the neck or pectoral area, elevating the tail or holding the tail head with the other hand (taking care not to pull on the tail or jacking it up) (Figure 185.1b).
- Technique 3. One arm is wrapped around the neck or pectoral area, keeping the foal's hind end against a wall or the corner of the stall (Figure 185.1c). This method is particularly useful if the veterinarian needs both hands to perform a task.

Leading the Foal

The handler can use the following techniques to lead the foal:

- Technique 1. Hold the foal with one arm wrapped around the neck or the pectoral area and the other arm placed around the hind end and walk with the foal following the mare (Figure 185.2a).
- Technique 2. Use a soft cotton lead rope around the foal's hind end to encourage forward movement while gently restraining the foal around the neck (Figure 185.2b).
- Technique 3. Place a harness or halter around the foal's chest to guide movements (Figure 185.2c). A halter should not be placed on the foal's head unless it has already been halter trained.

Equine Reproductive Procedures, Second Edition. Edited by John Dascanio and Patrick McCue.

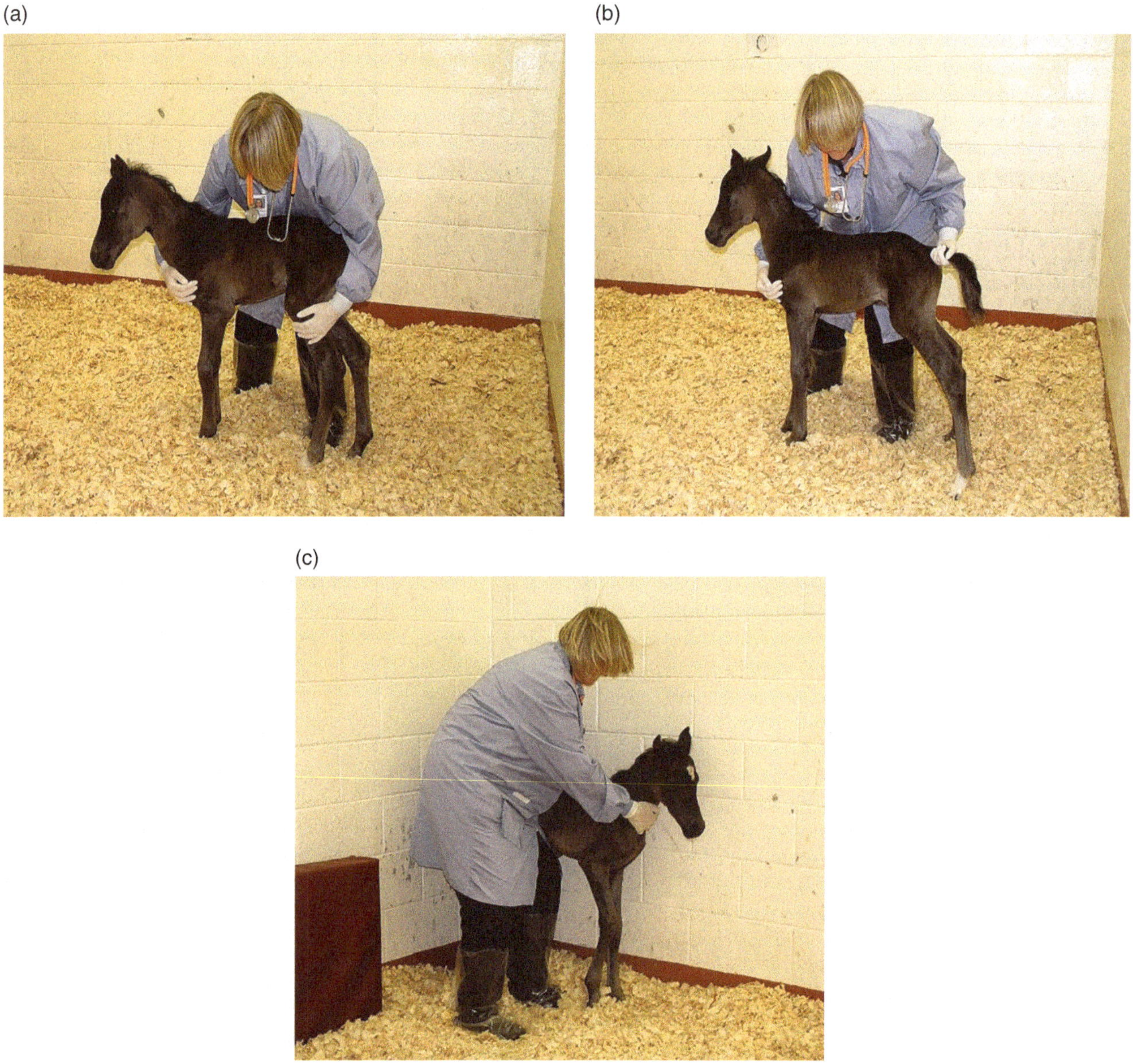

Figure 185.1 Standing restraint in the foal, with the handler holding (a) the foal's front and hind end; (b) the foal's front end and tail; and (c) the foal's front end while using a corner of the stall to retain the foal's hind end. Photos courtesy of Dr Virginia Buechner-Maxwell.

- Technique 4. Place a cotton or nylon rope around the chest and hind quarters of the foal in a "figure of eight" and grasp the rope where it crosses over the dorsal midline (Figure 185.2d).

Lateral Recumbency

The handler can use the following techniques to place the foal in lateral recumbency (folding):

- Stand on the lateral side of the foal (see technique 1 and 2 for standing restraint).
- Consider the following:
- The foal should always be laid down on a soft surface (i.e., thick layer of straw, blanket, pad).
- Sedation may be required in the healthy foal to avoid struggle.
- Care should be taken to cover the foal's eye on the down side to avoid corneal abrasions or ulcers. Covering the foal's eye also helps decrease visual stimuli.
- Technique 1. Pick the foal up around the chest and hind end and gently lay it down.

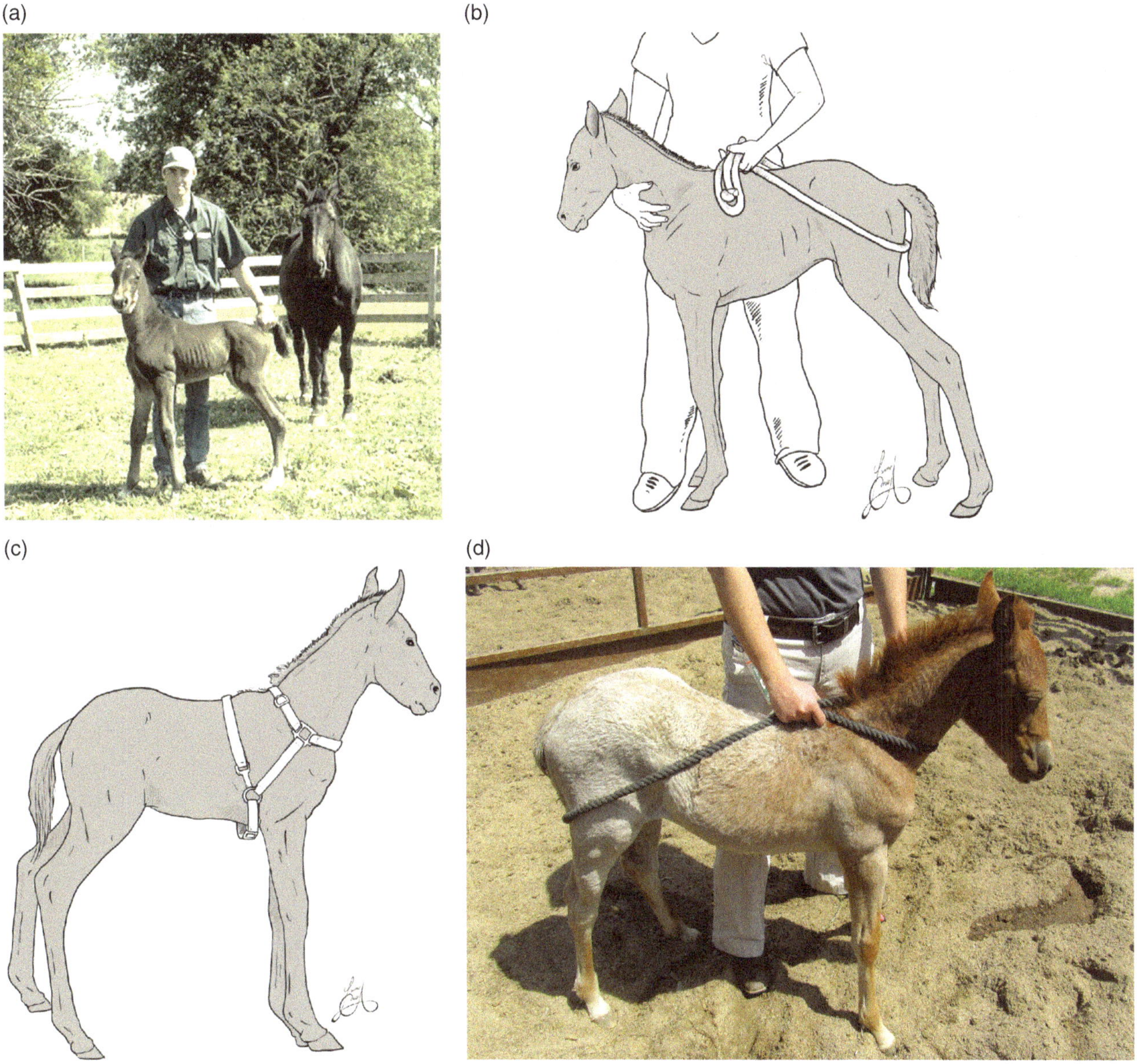

Figure 185.2 Leading the foal. (a) Leading the foal with the handler holding the foal's front end and tail. (b) Rope placement around the foal's hind end to encourage it to lead. (c) halter placement around the foal's chest to encourage it to lead. (d) Foal being restrained and lead using a cotton or nylon rope applied in a "figure of eight" pattern around the chest and hind quarters of the foal. (a) Photo courtesy of Dr Virginia Buechner-Maxwell. (b, c) Drawings courtesy of Dr Ismael Concha-Albornoz DVM, MVSc (www.anato.cl).

- Technique 2. Fold the head of the foal towards its chest and move the hind end towards the head and chest ("the foal is folded like a pretzel") while lifting the flank away from the handler (Figure 185.3a). Gently using the handler's knee to push the flank away from the handler can assist with this procedure. The foal is gently lowered down (Figure 185.3b).
- Restraint needs to continue while the foal is in lateral recumbency. The handler should always be behind the foal's back and away from its legs. Maintaining lateral recumbency may be achieved by preventing the foal from getting its nose on the ground by keeping its head in the air while maintaining pressure on the neck. The adage "where goes the head, so goes the body" is an important concept. The foal must use its head to counterbalance itself to stand. Holding the nose slightly upward with the neck bent prevents the foal from initiating the standing movement (Figure 185.3b). The other option is to hold a front and hind limb each.

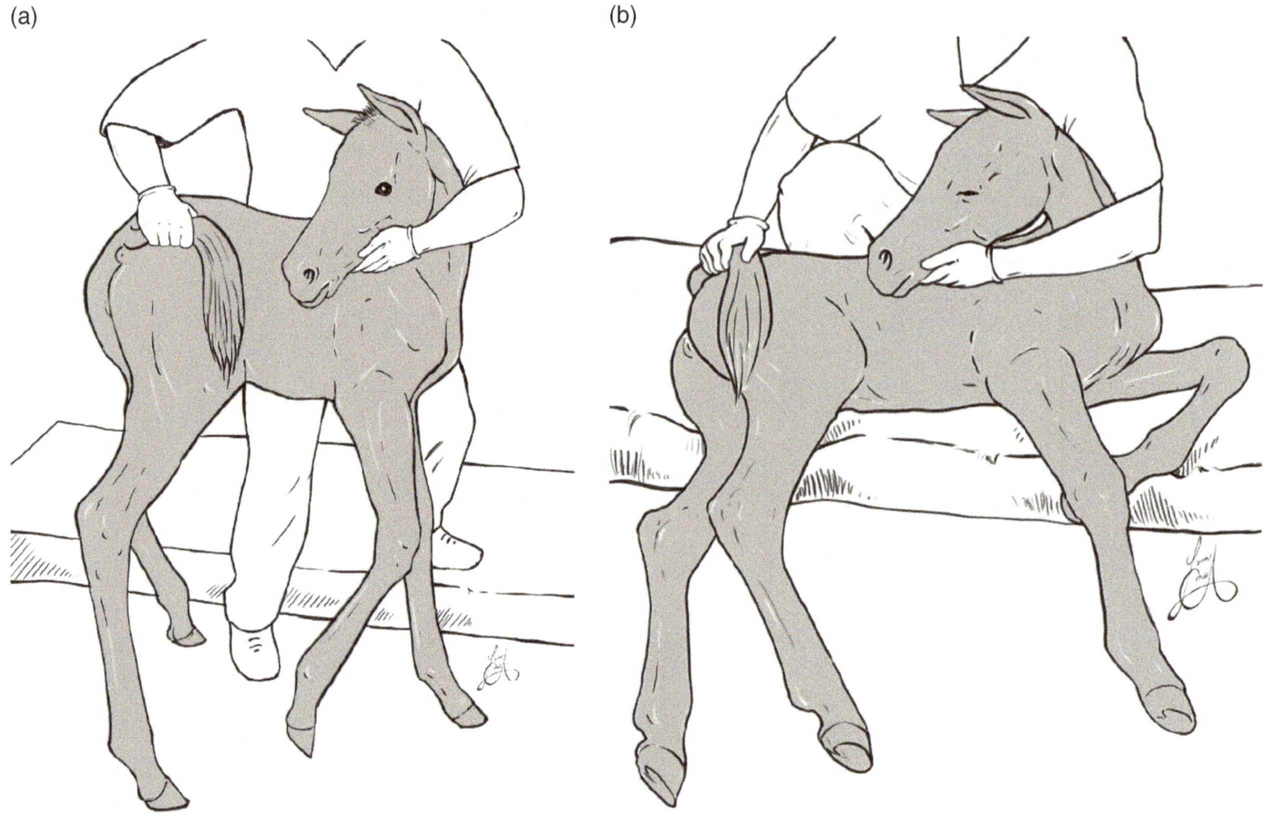

Figure 185.3 Lateral recumbency. (a) Handler positioning to lay a foal down (folding). (b) Handler positioning to restrain a foal in lateral recumbency. Drawings courtesy of Dr Ismael Concha-Albornoz DVM, MVSc (www.anato.cl).

- An additional foal position may be used once the foal is in lateral recumbency for such procedures as naso-gastric intubation for colostrum administration (see Chapter 188), whereby the handler positions themselves in a sitting position over the foal's back with either leg on each side of the foal. The foal is rolled into sternal recumbency and both front carpi are flexed. The handler then "mounts" the foal facing toward the foal's head. The handler's weight is on their knees and not on the foal's back. This allows the handler to use their hands for intubation and to hold the foal's head.

Madigan Squeeze Method

The Madigan squeeze method is an additional method that can be used to lay a foal down and keep it in lateral recumbency (see Chapter 186). It should only be performed by an experienced clinician and in relatively healthy foals less than 3 days of age. It requires a soft rope 1.5–2 cm (3/4 inch) in diameter and 5–5.5 m (~18 feet) in length. This is a method that was originally developed by Dr John Madigan to treat foals with neonatal maladjustment syndrome.

Imprint Training

Describing the details of the techniques used for imprint training is beyond the scope of this book chapter. In brief, imprint training involves getting foals desensitized to touch right after birth and repeating this training at regular intervals thereafter. Foals that have undergone imprint training get used to common procedures and may become easier to handle and less fractious compared to untrained foals.

Additional Comments

In cases where the foal becomes distraught and starts thrashing during restraint, it is sometimes best to just let go of the foal, providing that they are in a confined space, so that they do not flip over or otherwise injure themselves or the handlers. Care should be used to not injure the tail while using it as a point of restraint. Hold the tail closest to the body and use it to guide the foal. Do not lift the foal by the tail or excessively pull on the tail to avoid nerve, muscle, and skeletal damage. Sedation should be considered in foals that struggle excessively during restraint to facilitate the procedure and avoid injury.

Foals can start halter training very early on in their life. Halters should fit correctly and should not be left on a growing foal for longer than a week without adjustment. Using a halter on an unaccustomed foal may result in injury and a loose-fitting halter can result in the foal getting hung up on equipment or getting stuck in the halter with their hooves. Placing a well-fitted halter on the foal early on facilitates training to lead and to stand still.

If a foal needs to be trailered, it is best not to restrain the foal during transport. The foal should be led onto the trailer before the mare to encourage her to follow. In two-horse trailers the partition between the two sides should be removed. Trailers without a ramp should be unloaded in a grassy spot or an area with soft footing.

Further Reading

Cable CS. 2000. Foal handling and restraint. *The Horse* 3: 1–7.

Madigan J. 2018. Foal squeezing with "Madian squeeze." https://www.equineneonatalmanual.com/foalsqueezing (last accessed November 2020).

Miller RM. 1991. Imprint Training of the Newborn Foal. Colorado Springs, CO: Western Horseman Inc.

Nogradi N, Magdesian KG. Restraining the neonatal foal. In: Costa LRR, Paradis MR (eds). Manual of Clinical Procedures in the Horse, 1st edn. Hoboken, NJ: Wiley Blackwell, pp. 411–715.

186

Madigan Foal Squeeze Technique

John Madigan

School of Veterinary Medicine, University of California-Davis, USA

Introduction

The Madigan foal squeeze technique is a procedure in which thoracic pressure is applied to a young foal in order to induce recumbency and a slow-wave sleep. The procedure can be used as a method of restraint or as a treatment for foals exhibiting clinical signs of neonatal maladjustment syndrome.

The squeeze procedure is used routinely to provide drug-free restraint to neonatal foals less than 3 days of age for administration of plasma or in order to perform minor medical procedures and ultrasound exams. The advantage of the procedure is that the foal does not have to be heavily restrained or sedated or become fearful with the first encounters with a veterinarian.

Contraindications for use of the squeeze technique for restraint include rib fractures, respiratory distress, foals in septic shock, severe prematurity with floppy chests, severe neuromuscular disease compromising normal breathing, and congenital anomalies. In addition, the person(s) applying the squeeze should be experienced in handling neonatal foals and have an understanding of mare–foal behavioral interactions.

A majority of foals with maladjustment and septicemia have elevated levels of neurosteroids that affect behavior and other physiological states. Fetal physiology is controlled in part by these elevated neurosteroids. *In utero*, the fetus does not need to nurse, walk, bond to the mare, thermoregulate, have gut motility, breathe in response to low oxygen and elevated carbon dioxide, and have the brain chemistry for a flight animal. After birth, neonatal survival requires a quick switch in physiology. Persistence of elevated neurosteroids due to a failure to transition into consciousness at birth is a cause of many of the behavioral and physiological changes observed in the maladjusted foal and the septic foal. Therefore, use of the squeeze technique to simulate or repeat the birth canal influences for transition of consciousness can be attempted.

Equipment and Supplies

Soft rope 5–5.5 m (16–18 feet) long, 1.5–2 cm (3/4 inch) diameter, which slides easily, optional luggage scale pressure gauge.

Technique

- Tie a bowline knot and make a fixed loop so that the rope will slide through like a honda knot on a lariat. Instructions on how to tie the bowline knot are given at http://www.animatedknots.com/bowline/ (last accessed November 2020).
- Starting at the withers area, place the rope across the neck and between the front limbs, and bring the end of rope up to the withers area (Figure 186.1). Thread the

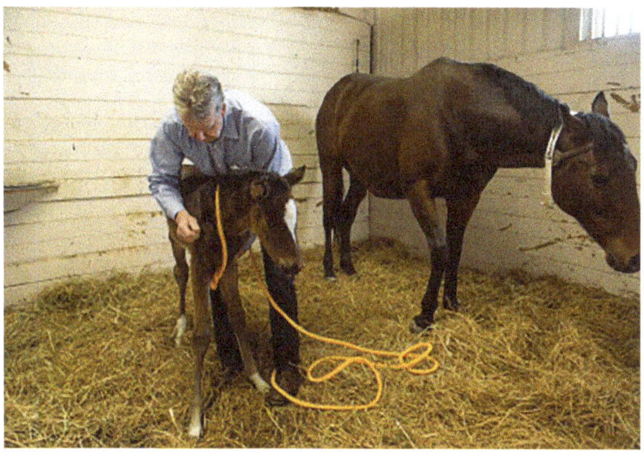

Figure 186.1 Step 1: put the rope over withers and between front limbs.

Equine Reproductive Procedures, Second Edition. Edited by John Dascanio and Patrick McCue.

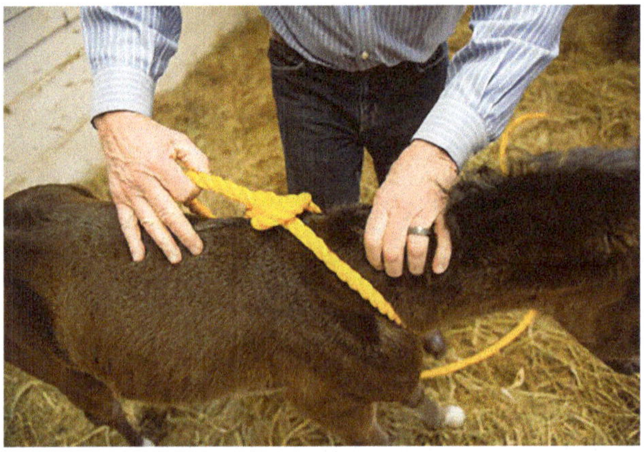

Figure 186.2 Step 2: run the rope through the loop at end of the rope and snug the rope.

end of the rope through the fixed loop and adjust to a snug fit so there is pressure on the chest, but no airway obstruction (Figure 186.2).

- Pass the rope over the foal and make a half hitch (Figure 186.3). Snug the rope just behind the elbow where a cinch would go on a saddle (Figure 186.4).
- Pass the rope over the foal's ribcage again, about 15 cm (6 inches) back from the first half hitch, forming a second half hitch, and snug it up (Figure 186.5).
- Have the assistant hold the foal, position yourself behind the foal, and put pressure on the rope until the foal begins to lie down (Figure 186.6).
- Allow the mare to stand close and within view of the foal so she does not whinny or arouse the foal.
- Protect yourself from the foal kicking or moving its head during the squeeze. Some foals seem to move once or twice during the 20 minutes of squeeze. The amount of pressure is just the amount needed to have the foal lie down.

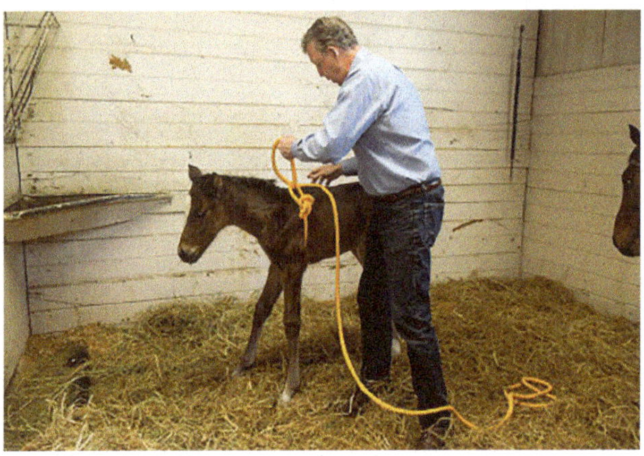

Figure 186.3 Step 3: begin by making the first half hitch around the chest, just behind the elbow.

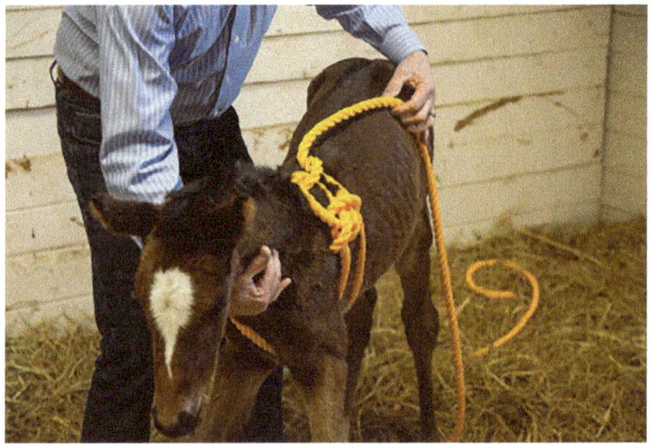

Figure 186.4 Step 4: keep the rope snug (first half hitch in place).

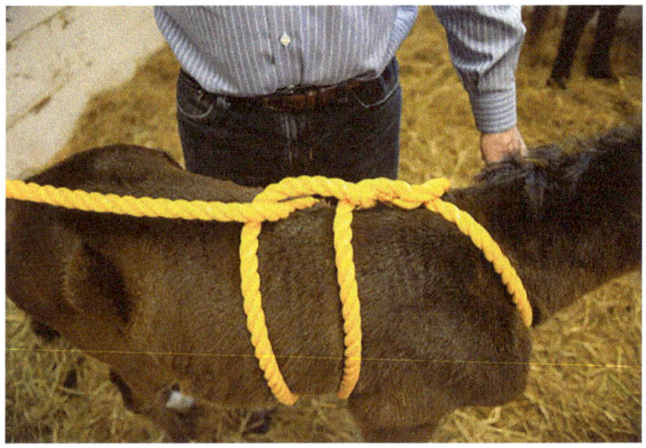

Figure 186.5 Step 5: two half hitches in place.

- Cover the foal's eyes with a soft towel.
- When you pull on the rope and the foal begins to lie down, keep that same pressure on for 20 minutes (Figure 186.7). Using a luggage scale, it should register at

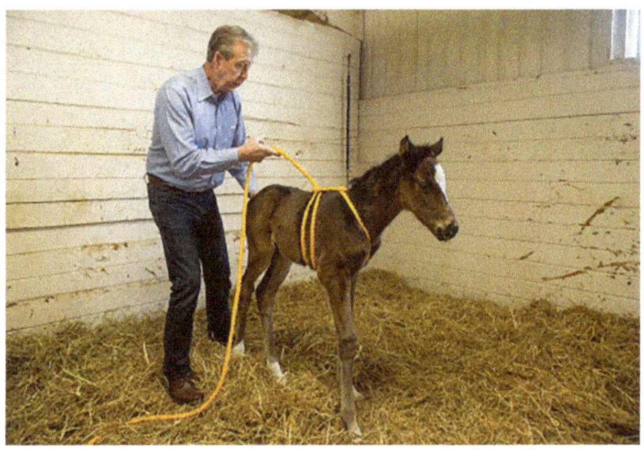

Figure 186.6 Step 6: stand behind the foal and begin to put tension on the rope. The foal will then lie down.

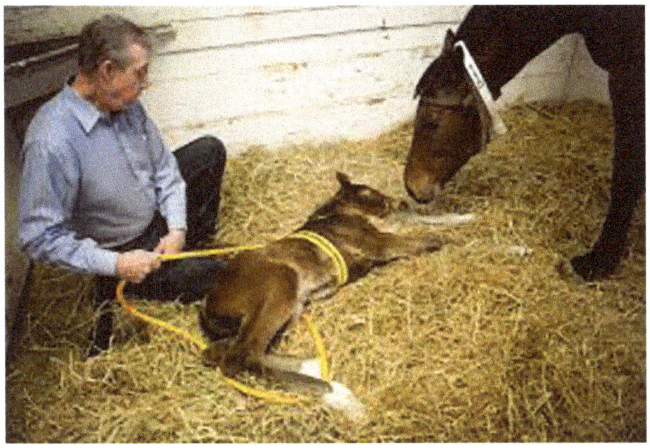

Figure 186.7 Step 7: when the foal is lying down, keep tension on the rope for the next 20 minutes and then release.

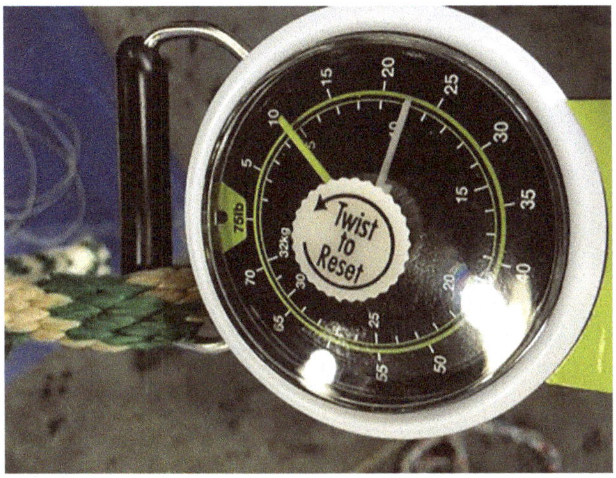

Figure 186.8 Luggage scale with rope attached showing the suggested pressure (green indicator).

about 4.5–9 kg (10–20 lbs) of pressure (Figure 186.8). If the foal moves, add a bit of pressure and allow the foal to resume sleeping.

- At the end of the 20-minute squeeze, release pressure on the rope and allow the foal to stay down or get up as it chooses.
- Slowly move the rope away from the foal. Do not force it to get up. Let the foal sleep more if it wants.
- One can eventually stimulate the foal by gently pinching the skin along the back to mimic a nip from the mare.
- When the foal gets up, allow it to do whatever it wants and observe. Do not attempt to assist nursing or push to the mare.
- Allow the foal to wander toward the mare's udder and observe for nursing. Most foals will latch on to the mare nipple with a coordinated tongue curl and suckle. Note the foal's ear position and alertness post-squeeze and observe over the next hour for any change. If the foal initially appears more alert, but does not quite get to the udder for a complete suckle of the mare, one can repeat the foal squeeze at 2–4-hour intervals until arousal is maintained. Some foals have been squeezed every 4 hours over a 24-hour period.
- Foals that require more than one squeeze procedure should have a veterinary evaluation and a more extensive workup.
- The squeeze is not contraindicated in a seizing foal and may lessen the seizure in some foals. Appropriate management of seizures should be carried out and the squeeze procedure used in refractive cases.
- Additional information can be found at: https://compneuro.vetmed.ucdavis.edu/sites/g/files/dgvnsk5376/files/inline-files/mfsm_instructions_0.pdf (last accessed November 2020).

Additional Comments

- The mare should be allowed to stand close to the foal. Mares seem to know the foal is asleep and will stand quietly. Some mares become aggressive after foaling and may need some degree of manual restraint or sedation for safety.
- The duration of the squeeze should be limited to 20–30 minutes.
- The foal's respiration, heart rate, and mucous membrane color should be monitored during the squeeze procedure.
- Remember, the foal is in slow-wave sleep and not anesthetized and may arouse during the squeeze procedure and could kick. Always position yourself behind the back of the foal and away from the limbs. The squeeze technique works best for foals from newborn to 3 days of age. After 3 days, the squeeze technique is inconsistent in producing recumbence and sleep.
- The squeeze procedure has been used for plasma administration for *Rhodococcus equi* prevention in over 200 Thoroughbred foals on one farm over a 4-year period without complication. The foals were treated within 24 hours of birth.
- In a study of use of the squeeze method in maladjusted foals over 30% of foals nursed within 1 hour. With conventional treatment only 4% of foals nursed within 1 hr.
- Some foals with maladjustment syndrome which were fully recumbent when the rope system was applied have responded by standing and nursing.
- The age of foals seems to be a factor in response to the squeeze. Foals less than 3 days of age are more consistent in their response. In slightly older, healthy foals

where the foal needs to be restrained, a low dose of xylazine (25–50 mg IV to an average size foal) may be administered prior to the squeeze procedure. Xylazine should never be used in septic neonatal foals or cardiovascularly compromised foals, and may induce hypovolemic shock.

Further Reading

Aleman M, Weich KM, Madigan JE. 2017. Survey of veterinarians using a novel physical compression squeeze procedure in the management of neonatal maladjustment syndrome in foals. *Animals (Basel)* 7(9): 69.

Toth B, Aleman M, Brosnan RJ, *et al.* 2012. Evaluation of squeeze-induced somnolence in neonatal foals. *J Vet Res* 73: 1881–9.

187

Evaluation of Passive Transfer

Patrick M. McCue

Equine Reproduction Laboratory, Colorado State University, USA

Introduction

Equine neonates are born immunologically näive since no significant transplacental transfer of antibodies occurs *in utero*. Consequently, a newborn foal is entirely dependent on maternal antibodies absorbed following the ingestion of colostrum from the dam in the first few hours of life for immune protection. Failure of passive transfer of maternal antibodies places the foal at significant risk of infectious diseases. The degree of risk depends on multiple factors, including exposure potential and management.

Failure of passive transfer has been subdivided into several levels dependent on serum immunoglobulin G (IgG) levels (Table 187.1). Complete failure of passive transfer (FPT) in foals has been defined as plasma IgG levels of <200 mg/dl. Partial failure of passive transfer (PFPT) has been described as plasma IgG levels of 200–400 mg/dl. Plasma IgG levels 400 mg/dl or greater may be adequate for healthy foals in a clean environment with minimal exposure to pathogens, but levels ≥800 mg/dl are considered optimal. A concentration of IgG between 400 and 800 mg/dl may be inadequate for compromised or systemically ill foals or for foals moved to new environments with different local pathogens.

Early testing for antibody levels in a neonatal foal can identify potential cases of FPT and allow for early intervention and medical management. It is recommended that a blood sample be collected from a newborn foal approximately 12 hours after birth to evaluate circulating IgG levels prior to "closure" of the gastrointestinal tract to antibody absorption. If IgG levels are <400 mg/dl at 12 hours, oral supplementation with frozen-thawed colostrum or a commercial colostrum substitute should be performed. If IgG levels are 400–800 mg/dl, the need for intervention and therapy is dependent on potential pathogen exposure and/or the medical condition of the foal.

Table 187.1 Antibody levels in foals with adequate passive transfer and failure of passive transfer of maternal immunity.

Foal Plasma IgG Concentration (mg/dl)	Interpretation
≥800	Optimal passive transfer
400–800	Adequate passive transfer
200–400	Partial failure of passive transfer
<200	Complete failure of passive transfer

Foals with *complete* FPT (<200 mg/dl) are in desperate need of antibodies in order to obtain immune protection from infectious diseases and require supplementation for survival. Foals with *partial* FPT (200–400 mg/dl) are at risk of developing infections and will benefit from IgG supplementation. In contrast, foals with *adequate* FPT (400–800 mg/dl) born into a clean environment with low pathogen exposure potential and good preventative management practices may not need supplemental IgG, but are often supplemented to provide additional antibody protection. Antibody levels of >800 mg/dl at 12 hours of age indicate that *optimal* passive transfer of immunoglobulins occurred and no additional testing or intervention is necessary under most management conditions.

Testing a foal at 24 hours of age or more will determine the final extent of passive antibody absorption. It is critical to understand that no significant amount of antibodies is absorbed if oral supplementation is provided after 24 hours of age. Foals more than 24 hours of age identified with FPT require intravenous administration of plasma to increase blood antibody levels. Although plasma transfusions are commonly performed in foals for disease prevention and medical therapy, oral administration of colostrum early in the first day of life is easier and possibly safer to perform.

Equipment and Supplies

Syringe and needle, Vacutainer® tube (with or without anticoagulant), IgG test (see options below).

Equine Reproductive Procedures, Second Edition. Edited by John Dascanio and Patrick McCue.

Technique

- Collect 1–3 ml of jugular venous blood from the foal using a syringe and needle.
- Transfer the blood to a Vacutainer® tube.
- If a red top tube (without anticoagulant) is used, allow the blood to clot and then harvest serum for testing.
- If a purple or green top tube is used (with EDTA or heparin, respectively), centrifuge and harvest plasma for testing; note that some tests use whole blood for IgG testing and do not require centrifugation.
- Perform an IgG test according to the manufacturer's directions.

Interpretation and Additional Comments

Diagnostic tests for the evaluation of plasma IgG levels in foals include single radial immunodiffusion (RID), glutaraldehyde coagulation (GC), zinc sulfate turbidity (ZST), latex agglutination test (LAT), enzyme immunoassay (EIA), and turbidimetric immunoassay (TIA) tests (Table 187.2).

Single Radial Immunodiffusion Test

The RID test is considered to be the most accurate test for quantitative measurement of serum or plasma antibody levels in foals and is used as the reference standard when other tests are evaluated. Unfortunately, results of the RID test are generally not available for 24 hours or more, making it impractical for routine use on a breeding farm or at a veterinary clinic when rapid results are required for therapeutic intervention.

Table 187.2 Screening tests for failure of passive transfer in foals.

Test Type	Name	Manufacturer
Radial immunodiffusion (RID) test	Immunocheck	VMRD, Inc., Pullman, WA, USA
Glutaraldehyde coagulation (GC) test	Gamma-Check® E	Veterinary Dynamics, Templeton, CA, USA
Zinc sulfate turbidity (ZST) test	Equi-Z	VMRD, Pullman, WA, USA
Latex agglutination test (LAT)	Foalcheck®	Centaur, Overland Park, KS, USA
Enzyme immunoassay (EIA)	SNAP test	Idexx Laboratories, Westbrook, ME, USA
Turbidimetric immunoassay (TIA)	ARS Foal-IgG test	Animal Reproduction Systems, Chino, CA, USA

Glutaraldehyde Coagulation Test

The GC test is based on the ability of glutaraldehyde to react with immunoglobulin and form a solid clot or gel. The test is performed by adding 0.5 ml of serum into each of two test tubes containing 50 μl of glutaraldehyde (10% and 20%, respectively) and mixing immediately. The time interval from the addition of serum to the formation of a solid coagulation gel is recorded for each tube (up to 60 minutes). A positive coagulation reaction using a 10% glutaraldehyde solution indicates a serum IgG concentration of ≥400 mg/dl. A negative reaction using the 10% solution, but a positive reaction (coagulation) using the 20% solution, suggests a PFPT (200–400 mg/dl). A negative reaction using both the 10% and 20% solutions indicates that complete FPT has occurred (<200 mg/dl).

In addition, the time required to form a positive reaction using a 10% solution may be used to estimate serum IgG levels. The time taken for a positive reaction to occur is inversely proportional to serum IgG levels. A positive reaction (clot formation) in less than 10 minutes is associated with a serum IgG level of >800 mg/dl and a positive reaction within 60 minutes suggests an IgG concentration of >400 mg/dl. The GC test has been used for many years to detect FPT in neonatal foals and is an inexpensive and practical semiquantitative test. Severe hemolysis has been reported to interfere with the GC test. Serum should be used for the test, as fibrinogen will also contribute to a positive reaction.

Zinc Sulfate Turbidity Test

The ZST test measures total antibody levels based on the formation of a precipitate when immunoglobulins combine with zinc ions. Quantitative assessment of IgG levels may be made with the ZST test by measuring the optical density (OD) of the zinc sulfate–serum mixture using a spectrophotometer. The OD value is compared against a standard curve produced by assessment of OD values of serum controls with known IgG levels measured by RID. If a spectrophotometer is not available, the detection of cloudiness or opacity in the tube is sufficient to indicate that the foal has absorbed colostral IgG. The ZST test is a simple and relatively rapid procedure, with test equilibration times reported from 15–60 seconds to 1 hour. The ZST test has been reported to overestimate IgG concentrations in serum with RID-determined values of ≤400 mg/dl and underestimate IgG levels in serum with antibody levels of 401–1,500 mg/dl. Hemolysis in serum samples may result in the overestimation of IgG content by increasing turbidity.

Latex Agglutination Test

The LAT estimates antibody concentration from the degree of agglutination between IgG in serum or whole blood and latex beads that are coated with anti-equine IgG antibodies. The presence or absence of agglutination in each of three test rings after 15–60 seconds of mixing is used to provide a semiquantitative estimate of IgG levels in the whole blood or serum. The LAT was reported to be accurate in the assessment of foal IgG levels in the ranges of ≤400 mg/dl and ≥1,501 mg/dl, and to underestimate IgG levels between 400 and 1,500 mg/dl. Consequently, a foal with barely adequate passive transfer could not be differentiated from a foal with high IgG using the LAT.

Enzyme Immunoassay

The SNAP test is a semiquantitative EIA that can use whole blood or plasma by a simple adjustment in technique. The test can be performed on a breeding farm or at a clinic and results are available in 7–10 minutes. A color change in a test spot is compared with the color of known calibrated IgG levels in two additional control spots. One control level is "set" at 400 mg/dl and the other control is "set" at 800 mg/dl. The colors in these control spots will turn light blue and medium blue, respectively. The color in the test spot (the foal IgG level) is compared with the color in the control spots (Figure 187.1).

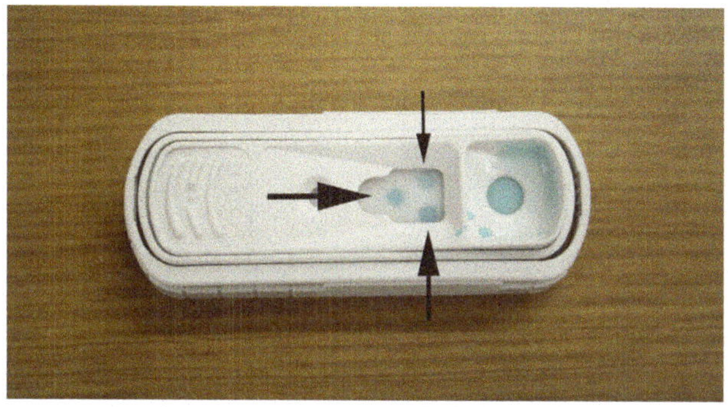

Figure 187.1 The SNAP test for evaluating foal IgG levels. The large horizontal arrow indicates the test sample, while the other two arrows show the 400 mg/dl (upper small arrow) and 800 mg/dl (lower medium arrow) internal standards.

Turbidimetric Immunoassay

TIAs are based on a specific antigen–antibody reaction in which a known quantity of goat anti-equine IgG is added to a specific dilution of foal plasma. The binding of goat antibody to foal IgG causes immune complexes to form in a quantity relative to the concentration of foal IgG in the original plasma sample. The assay is rapid, simple to perform, and uses a calibrated spectrophotometer already present on many breeding farms and veterinary clinics (Figure 187.2).

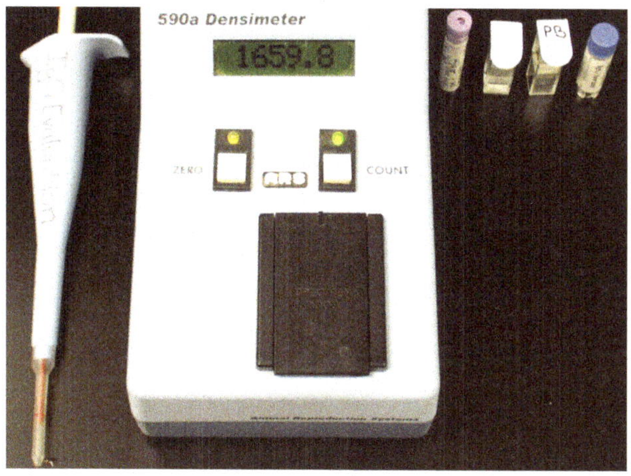

Figure 187.2 Turbidimetric immunoassay (ARS Foal-IgG test) for evaluating foal IgG levels.

Further Reading

Davis R, Giguere S. 2005. Evaluation of five commercially available assays and measurement of serum total protein concentration via refractometry for the diagnosis of failure of passive transfer of immunity in foals. *J Am Vet Med Assoc* 227: 1640–5.

McGuire TC, Crawford TB, Hallowell AL, Macomber LE. 1977. Failure of colostral immunoglobulin transfer as an explanation for most infections and deaths of neonatal foals. *J Am Vet Med Assoc* 170: 1302–4.

Vivrette SL. 2011. Assessment and modification of passive transfer. In: McKinnon AO, Squires EL, Vaala WE, Varner DD (eds). Equine Reproduction, 2nd edn. Ames, IA: Wiley Blackwell, pp. 346–52.

188

Colostral Administration via Naso-Gastric Intubation

John J. Dascanio

School of Veterinary Medicine, Texas Tech University, USA

Introduction

Foals are born without immune protection. Colostrum contains IgG-type antibodies critical for the survival of a newborn foal. Poor colostrum quality, limited quantity of colostrum, or inability of a newborn foal to suckle all may result in failure of passive transfer. Supplementation of colostrum to a foal by the passage of a naso-gastric tube may be indicated. The source of colostrum may be the foal's dam or thawed colostrum from a frozen colostrum bank.

Equipment and Supplies

Foal stomach tube or stallion catheter, sterile lubricant, gauze, 60 ml dose syringe or small funnel, colostrum.

Technique

- Banked colostrum should be thawed or, if the mare has adequate colostrum, she should be milked and the colostrum passed through a gauze filter to remove gross debris (see Chapters 105 and 106).
- A stomach tube may be passed with a foal standing or in sternal recumbency.
- Sternal recumbency may be achieved by standing on the left side of the foal and pulling its nose toward the right chest wall, while lifting outward on its right flank area, thus laying the foal in left lateral recumbency. The foal may then have its carpi flexed and is then rolled into sternal recumbency.
- The veterinarian assumes a sitting position over the foal's back. This keeps the foal from standing during the procedure and allows for control of the head. No significant weight is placed on the foal's back as the weight is born by the person's knees.
- Use a foal stomach tube or stallion urinary catheter of similar size (0.7 cm OD, or 22 Fr) and length of tubing (~137 cm (54 inches)). Lubricate the end of the tube with a small quantity of sterile lubricant.
- The tube may be marked with a black permanent marker at a level measured from the foal's nose to the medial canthus of the eye to estimate the distance to the pharynx. The tube may also be marked at a distance from the foal's nose to the last rib to approximate the tube length required to reach the stomach.
- Using the fingers, guide the tube medially and ventrally through the nasal passage.
- The tube has reached the pharynx once the appropriate length has been passed and a slight resistance is felt as the tube bumps against the larynx or dorsal pharyngeal recess.
- The tube should be rotated so that the curvature of the tube is upward toward the opening of the esophagus. The foal's head should be flexed downward to avoid passage of the tube into the trachea.
- By gently bumping the pharynx, the tube should be passed in coordination with the foal's swallowing to enter the esophagus. Many foals may not readily cough if the tube enters the trachea, so caution should be taken to check the proper placement of the tube prior to colostral administration.
- Confirmation of the tube's placement in the esophagus should be performed next. The two absolute ways to confirm that the tube is in the esophagus and not in the trachea are to either see the tube passing down the esophagus (typically on the left side of the neck) or manually feeling the tube pass down the esophagus. Other indicators of tube location, that are not absolute indicators, include elicitation of a cough (if in the trachea), resistance to passage (if in the esophagus), and ability to easily aspirate air when applying gently negative suction

Equine Reproductive Procedures, Second Edition. Edited by John Dascanio and Patrick McCue.

by mouth (if in the trachea). Once the tube is in the stomach, a small amount of air blown into the stomach by mouth may be heard within the stomach with a stethoscope placed on the abdomen or the smell of gastric contents may aid in confirmation.

- A 60 ml dosing syringe with the plunger removed may act as a funnel and is attached to the stomach tube or stallion catheter (Figure 188.1). If the colostrum has not been previously filtered through gauze, it may be done as it is poured into the open end of the dose syringe.
- For light breed horses, a minimum of 1–1.5 liters of good quality colostrum (>1.080 specific gravity and/or ≥20% Brix refractometer score) should be administered in 300–400 ml aliquots within the first 6–12 hours after foaling if no maternal source of colostrum is available (i.e., if the mare has no colostrum) to provide sufficient antibody protection.

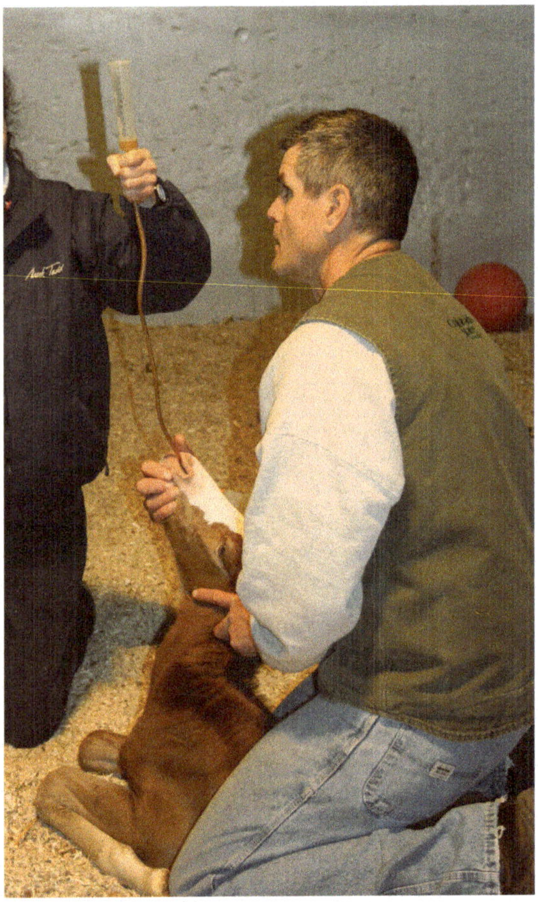

Figure 188.1 Foal in sternal recumbency and properly restrained. Colostrum is administered by gravity flow through a naso-gastric tube.

- If the foal is being supplemented and has ingested some colostrum from the dam, the administration of a single dose of 300–400 ml of good quality colostrum may be adequate to prevent failure of passive transfer.
- Remove the syringe from the tube and gently blow into the tube until any colostrum within the tube is pushed into the stomach and air flows easily into the stomach. Use enough air to clear the tube, but not insufflate the stomach. Immediately pinch or kink the tubing to prevent the back flow of colostrum into the tube and in a continuous movement gently remove the tube from the foal.

Interpretation

- The foal should be kept sternal or standing for 10–15 minutes post-intubation to prevent reflux of colostrum and possible inhalation. The foal should not be allowed to assume lateral recumbency.
- If colostrum starts to flow out the nostrils or mouth during gravity flow, the tube should be pinched or kinked to stop further flow and the position of the tube checked for proper placement. The tube may have pulled back into the esophagus and not be in the stomach, excessive colostrum may have been administered, the position of the foal's head and neck may be lower than the stomach, or the tube may not be within the esophagus.
- It is recommended that colostrum be provided by 6 hours after foaling.
- A blood sample should be collected from all foals, and certainly all foals at risk of failure of passive transfer, to evaluate IgG levels (see Chapter 187). Options include:
  - Collection of a blood sample 6–8 hours after the administration of colostrum.
  - Collection of a blood sample at 12 hours of age.
  - Collection of a blood sample at ≥24 hours of age.
- The collection and evaluation of a blood sample by 12 hours of age will still allow time to provide additional oral antibody supplementation. The evaluation of IgG level in a blood sample collected after 24 hours of age will provide the end result of passive transfer, but absorption of antibodies following oral supplementation will no longer occur.
- Adequate immunoglobulin transfer to the foal is indicated by a serum immunoglobulin concentration >800 mg/dl.

Further Reading

LeBlanc MM, McLaurin BI, Boswell R. 1986. Relationships among serum immunoglobulin concentration in foals, colostral specific gravity and colostral immunoglobulin concentration. *J Am Vet Med Assoc* 189: 57–60.

Raidal SL, McTaggart C, Penhale J. 2005. Effect of withholding macromolecules on the duration of intestinal permeability to colostral IgG in foals. *Aust Vet J* 83: 78–81.

189

Sedation

Undine Christmann

College of Veterinary Medicine, Lincoln Memorial University, USA

Introduction

Sedation in foals is used to facilitate diagnostic workup (e.g., radiographs, ultrasound) or to perform minor procedures (e.g., catheter placement, joint lavage). Factors that determine drug choice and dosage include age and temperament of the foal, the presence of disease and its severity, and the length and level of pain of the procedure to be carried out.

Foals are predisposed to hypothermia because they have less subcutaneous fat and a larger surface area compared with adults. Cardiac output is mainly determined by heart rate in foals and may decrease drastically with bradycardia. Arterial oxygen tension in foals is significantly influenced by body position (standing > sternal recumbency > lateral recumbency) and oxygen consumption in the neonatal foal is higher, leading to a higher metabolic rate. Foals also have lower energy stores and are susceptible to hypoglycemia. Newborn and premature foals are at risk of reverting to fetal circulation under conditions of hypoxia, hypotension, and bradycardia due to a reopening of the intracardiac (foramen ovale) and extracardiac (ductus arteriosus) shunts. These differences need to be taken into consideration when selecting drugs for sedation.

Benzodiazepines are the preferred sedative in foals younger than 2 weeks of age and premature or sick foals because of their minimal cardiovascular effects. Diazepam induces sedation, muscle relaxation, and recumbency and is well suited for minor procedures. Midazolam is less frequently used and has a shorter duration. Benzodiazepines do not provide analgesia and should always be associated with an opioid (e.g., butorphanol) if a painful procedure is to be performed. Alpha-2 agonists can be used safely in older healthy foals. However, they lead to more profound cardiovascular (i.e., bradycardia, hypotension), respiratory (i.e., altered respiratory rhythm, upper airway collapse), and temperature effects (e.g., hypothermia) in neonatal, premature, or sick foals. Butorphanol included with benzodiazepines or α2-agonists provides analgesia and leads to improved sedation.

Equipment and Supplies

Alcohol wipes, appropriate syringe size to measure injection volume, needles, sedative and/or analgesic of choice.

Restraint and Sedation

- A handler should restrain the foal.
- Administer appropriate restraint and sedation for the mare. The mare should be kept close to the foal to reduce separation anxiety, but should remain at a safe distance from the foal to avoid injury to personnel, foal, or equipment and to prevent contamination of materials and supplies.
- Common medications used to sedate foals are presented in Table 189.1.
- See Chapter 185 for more on the restrain of foals.

Additional Comments

Short term anesthesia may be needed to perform procedures such as joint lavage.

Antagonists are available for the majority of sedatives, but are rarely necessary.

Equine Reproductive Procedures, Second Edition. Edited by John Dascanio and Patrick McCue.

Table 189.1 Drug, route, dose, and indications for commonly used sedatives in foals.

Drug	Route	Dose (mg/kg BWT)	Dose for 50 kg foal (mg)	Indications
Benzodiazepines				
Diazepam	IV	0.1–0.2	5–10	Foals <2 weeks old Ill foals
Midazolam	IV	0.05–0.1	2.5–5	Foals <2 weeks old Ill foals
α2-agonists				
Xylazine	IV, IM	0.25–1	12–55	Healthy foals >2 weeks old
Detomidine	IV	0.01–0.02	0.5–1	Healthy foals >2 weeks old
Romifidine	IV	0.04–0.12	2–6	Healthy foals >2 weeks old
Opioids				
Butorphanol	IV	0.01–0.1	0.5–5	In combination with a diazepine or an α2-agonist
Phenothiazine tranquilizers				
Acepromazine				Not indicated in neonatal foals

BWT, body weight.

- Flumazenil is the antagonist for benzodiazepines and is given as a slow IV injection at a dose of 1 mg per 10 mg of diazepam administered.
- α2-antagonists for xylazine include yohimbine (given as slow IV injection at 0.1 mg/kg body weight) and tolazoline (2–4 mg/kg body weight).
- Naloxone (0.01–0.04 mg/kg body weight IV) may be used to antagonize butorphanol (1 ml or 0.4 mg diluted in 10 ml saline and given in 0.5–1 ml increments every 2–3 minutes IV to effect).

Further Reading

Fischer B. Clark-Price S. 2015. Anesthesia of the equine neonate in health and disease. *Vet Clin North Am Eq Pract* 31: 567–85.

Madigan JE. 2013. Sedation and anesthesia. In: Madigan JE (ed.). Manual of Equine Neonatal Medicine, 4th edn. Woodland, CA: Live Oak Publishing, pp. 261–6.

Robertson SA. 2005. Sedation and general anesthesia of the foal. *Eq Vet Educ* 7: 94–101.

190

Intravenous Catheter Placement

Undine Christmann

College of Veterinary Medicine, Lincoln Memorial University, USA

Introduction

Indications for intravenous catheter placement in foals include administration of fluids (i.e., fluids, plasma, blood, parenteral nutrition) or prolonged administration of intravenous drugs (i.e., antimicrobials). Neonatal foals, particularly compromised foals, are sensitive to development of sepsis and thrombophlebitis. Catheter placement should therefore be performed under sterile conditions.

The most frequent site for catheter placement is the jugular vein. Alternatively, the cephalic vein, saphenous vein, or lateral thoracic veins may be used.

Types of catheters used in foals differ based on material, method of placement, and number of lumens. Teflon catheters are the most thrombogenic and should only be used in relatively healthy foals needing one-time or short-term medication (e.g., a foal with failure of passive transfer needing a unit of plasma). Polyurethane or silicone catheters are less thrombogenic and are recommended in compromised foals requiring frequent treatments over an extended period. Teflon catheters should be removed in less than 72 hours, whereas polyurethane or silicone catheters can be used for 2–3 weeks if no complication develops. Over-the-needle Teflon catheters are the most commonly used in practice for a single treatment and are easy to place. Over-the-wire or peel away over-the-needle catheters are longer and softer and cause less irritation in the vein. These catheters are recommended in hospitalized foals needing prolonged treatment or that are at higher risk for thrombophlebitis. Their placement requires more skill and they are more costly. Catheters with more than one lumen are needed if the foal requires a dedicated line for parenteral nutrition.

Equipment and Supplies

Clippers, antiseptic scrub on 10 × 10 cm (4 × 4 inch) gauze sponges (povidone-iodine or chlorhexidine), 70% isopropyl alcohol on 10 × 10 cm gauze sponges, sterile gloves, 0.5–1 ml 2% lidocaine, catheter (16–20 gauge 5–12.5 cm (2–5 inch)), suture material, heparinized saline for flush (1 IU of heparin/ml saline), sedation for foal (optional), injection port. Optional: super glue, no. 15 scalpel blade, catheter introduction system (over-the-wire catheter or peel away), bandage material, extension system, surgical mask and cap.

Technique

Over-the-Needle Cathether

Preparation for catheter placement

- Sedate foal (optional): diazepam 0.1–0.2 mg/kg IV or xylazine 0.2–0.5 mg/kg IV in healthy foals >2 weeks old.
- Restrain the foal in lateral recumbency.
- Clip the hair in an area over the mid-neck jugular vein (Figure 190.1a).
- Perform a sterile site preparation alternating antiseptic and alcohol gauze sponges (Figure 190.1b).
- Administer 0.5–1 ml of 2% lidocaine under the skin where the catheter will be introduced using a 25 gauge needle (Figure 190.1c).
- Finalize the sterile site preparation.

Insertion of catheter

- Don sterile gloves.
- "Unlock" the catheter (briefly slide the catheter down on the stylet and back up) so that it will be easier to slide once in the vein.

Equine Reproductive Procedures, Second Edition. Edited by John Dascanio and Patrick McCue.

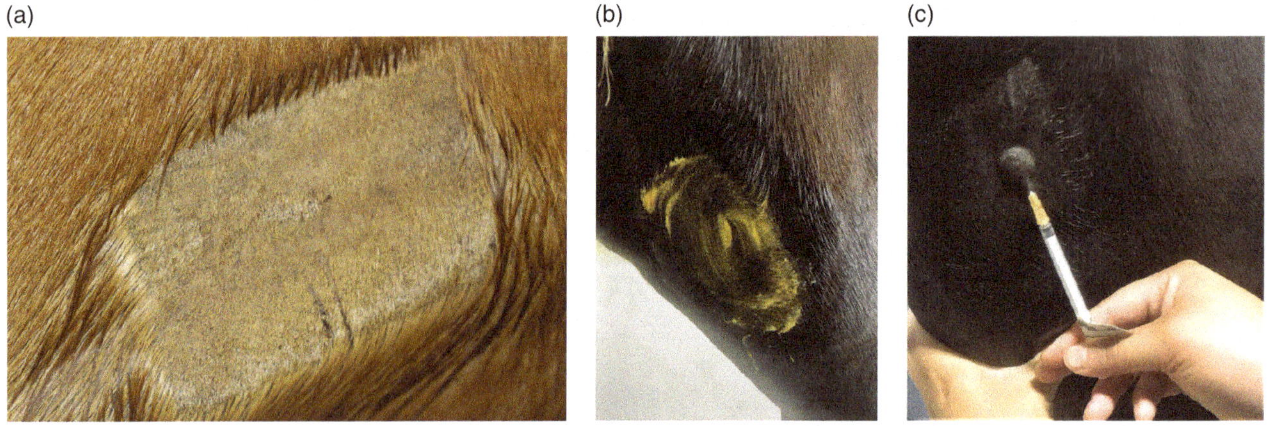

Figure 190.1 Preparation for placing an over-the-needle Teflon catheter. (a) Clipped area on the foal's upper neck. (b) Prepped area. (c) Placement of a lidocaine bleb.

- Flush the catheter with heparinized saline to prevent clotting within the catheter.
- Hold the vein off with the non-dominant hand.
- Grasp the catheter (hold the hub between the middle finger and thumb, and place the index finger on top of the stylet).
- Penetrate the skin and vein with the catheter at a 30-degree angle relative to the long axis of the vein. Note: foal veins have a tendency to roll and the catheter should be introduced in one swift motion (Figure 190.2a).
- Advance the catheter a few millimeters more once blood flashback is seen in the hub, while flattening the angle so that the catheter threads into the vein. Sometimes aspirating on the stylet with a syringe is needed to see blood to ensure that it is in the vein (Figure 190.2b).
- Hold the stylet in place while sliding the rest of the catheter into the vein up to the hub (Figure 190.2c).
- Remove the stylet (Figure 190.2d).
- Aspirate blood from the catheter to confirm placement and flush the catheter with 5–10 ml of heparinized saline.
- Attach an extension set and/or infusion plug.
- Suture the catheter in place by securing one suture into the suture groove on the catheter hub and a suture through the eyelet on each catheter wing. If an extension set is used it can be sutured in place using white tape as wings to attach it to the skin. The sutures should be placed so that the catheter hub is maintained snug against the skin and so that the catheter does not creep out of the vein at its insertion site when traction is applied (Figure 190.2e).
- Apply a drop of super glue where the catheter penetrates skin (optional) and/or apply antimicrobial ointment (optional).
- Use a sterile bandage over the catheter if the catheter needs to remain in place.

Over-the-Wire Catheter

- Wear a surgical face mask and cap.
- Put on set of sterile gloves (optional: use two sets of sterile gloves and remove the outer pair once the introducer is in the vein and before introducing the guidewire. This decreases the chances for contamination).
- Perform a stab incision through the skin with a no. 15 blade (optional).
- Flush the introducer needle or catheter with heparinized saline.
- Hold the vein off with the non-dominant hand.
- Insert the introducer (needle/catheter provided with kit or a large gauge needle (16 or 18 gauge) (Figure 190.3).
  - Penetrate the skin and vein at a 30–45-degree angle (Figure 190.4a).
  - Advance the introducer until a blood flashback is seen in the hub.
  - Remove the outer pair of gloves.
- Insert the guidewire (flexible J-tip) through the introducer needle or catheter. A guidewire straightener (supplied with the catheter kit) may be used to straighten the tip of the guidewire. The straightener is connected to the introducer needle and the wire is advanced into the vein (Figure 190.4b). Alternatively, some clinicians

(a) (b) (c) (d) (e)

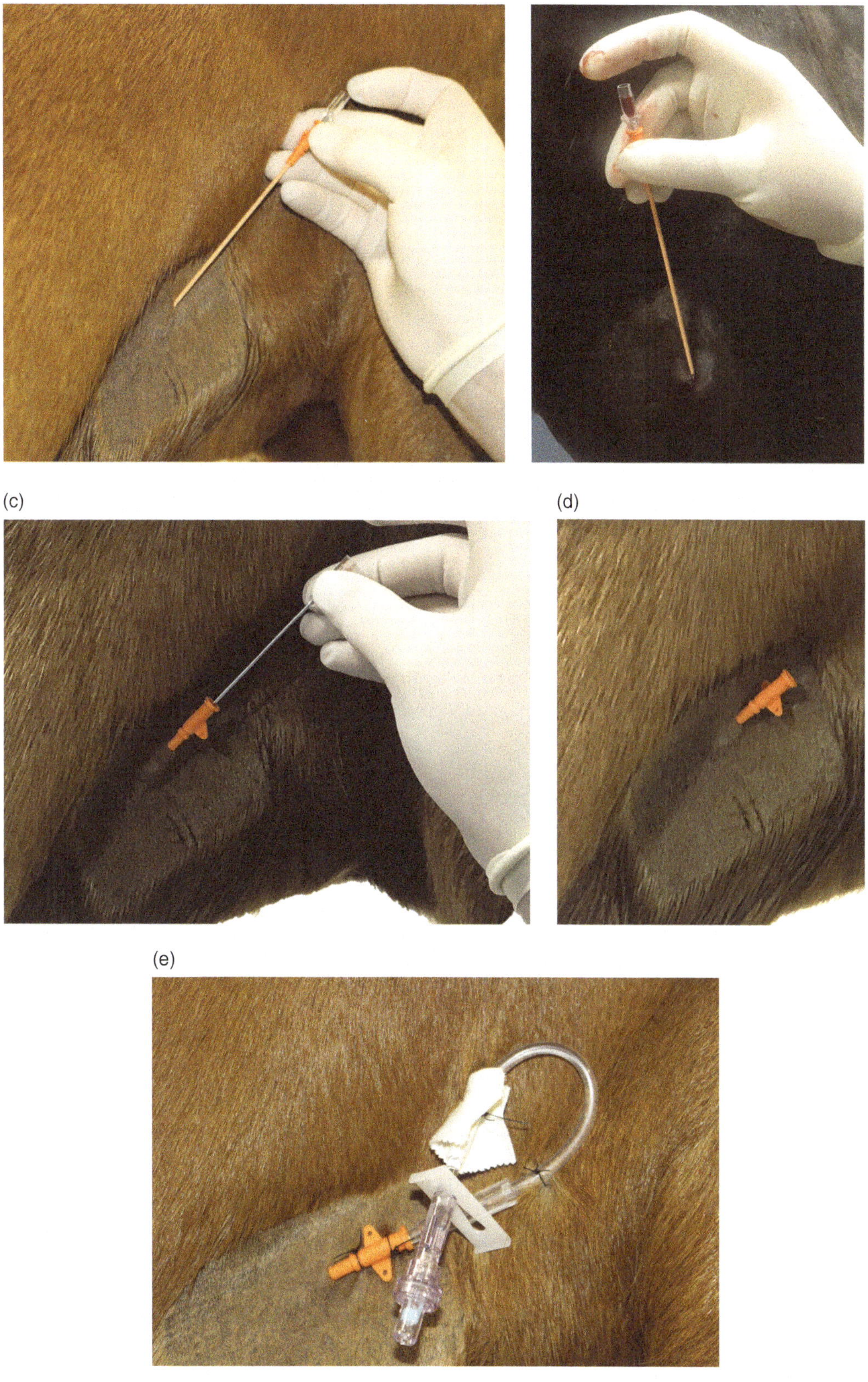

Figure 190.2 Insertion of an over-the-needle Teflon catheter. (a) Holding the catheter and stylet when penetrating the skin and vein. (b) Blood flashback in the catheter confirming penetration into the vein. (c) Sliding the catheter into the vein while maintaining the position of the stylet. (d) Catheter position in the vein. (e) Catheter with extension set sutured in place.

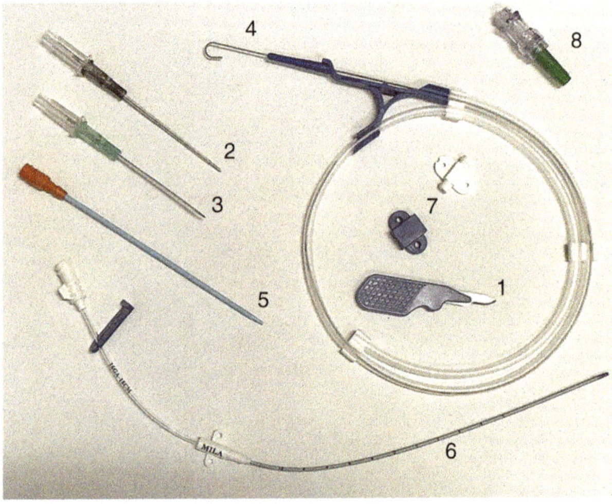

Figure 190.3 Components contained in an over-the-wire (long-term) venous catheter set. 1, Scalpel blade; 2 and 3, catheter over-the-needle introducers; 4, guidewire; 5, dilator; 6, antimicrobial polyurethane catheter; 7, catheter fasteners; 8, injection cap; and suture material (not represented in photo).

prefer to introduce the non-curved portion of the guidewire into the needle without using the straightener. In either case, the guidewire should be held, taking care not to let go of the wire or letting it touch non sterile areas. It should advance in the vein without resistance and should never be passed forcefully.

- Withdraw the introducer from the vein and guidewire (Figure 190.4c).
- Insert the dilator over the guidewire and advance a few centimeters into the vein using small rotating gestures (Figure 190.4d).
- Withdraw the dilator.
- Insert the intravenous catheter over the guidewire and advance all the way into the vein (Figure 190.4e).
- Withdraw the guidewire (Figure 190.4f).
- Aspirate blood from the catheter to confirm placement and flush the catheter with heparinized saline.
- Attach an extension set and/or infusion plug (Figure 190.4g).
- Suture the catheter in place, securing one suture into the suture groove on catheter hub and a suture through the eyelet on each catheter wing. If an extension set is used it can be sutured in place using white tape as wings to attach it to the skin (Figure 190.4h). The sutures should be placed so that the catheter hub is maintained snug against the skin and so that the catheter does not creep out of the vein at its insertion site when traction is applied.
- Apply a drop of super glue where the catheter penetrates the skin (optional) and/or apply antimicrobial ointment (optional).
- Use a sterile bandage if prolonged catheter use is needed.

Peel Away Catheter

- Put on sterile gloves.
- Flush the catheter with heparinized saline.
- Hold the vein off with the non-dominant hand.
- Grasp the introducer (hold between the middle finger and thumb and place an index finger on top of the stylet).
- Penetrate the skin and vein with the introducer at a 30–45-degree angle relative to the long axis of the vein. Advance the introducer until a blood flashback is seen in the hub.
- Withdraw the stylet.
- Maintain the introducer.
- Insert the catheter through the introducer.
- Peel away the introducer by grasping the tabs on either side (pull up and out).
- Advance the catheter in the vein if it has receded from the insertion site.
- Suture the catheter in place (see earlier sections).

Catheter Maintenance

- Injection cap:
  - Wipe with alcohol before any injection.
  - Replace every 24–48 hours.
- Flush the catheter four times per day with 5 ml of heparinized saline.
- Monitor the catheter site every day for swelling, heat, discharge, and migration outside the vein.
- Remove the catheter once intravenous treatments are discontinued or if infection, inflammation, or thrombosis is present.

Blood or Catheter Culture

- Blood for culture should be obtained immediately before placing a catheter or through the introducer during the process of catheter placement.
- The catheter tip may be cultured if infection is suspected.

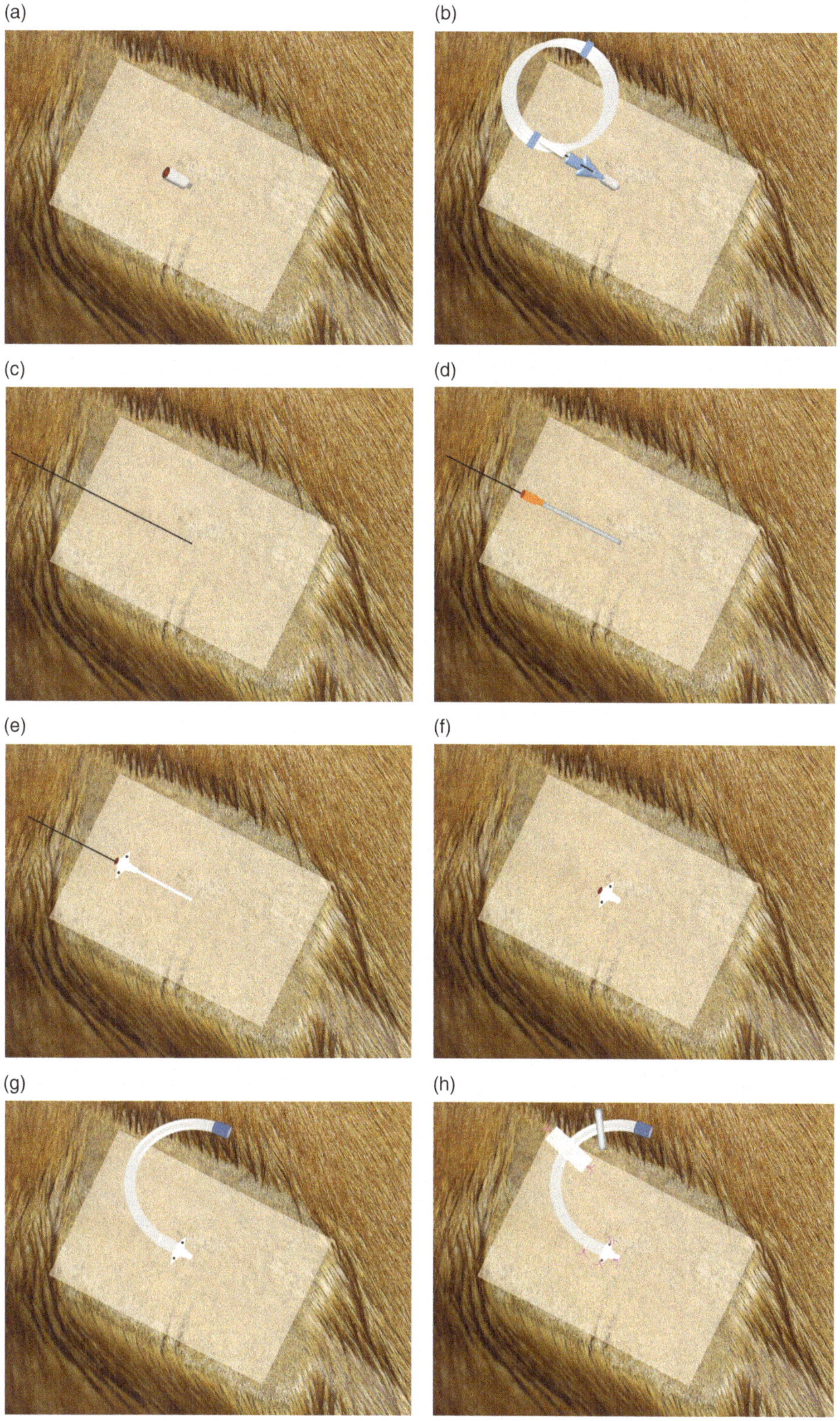

Figure 190.4 Schematic representation for over-the-wire catheter placement. (a) Introducer inserted in the vein. (b) Insertion of the guidewire with a wire straightener connected to the introducer. (c) Guidewire in the vein after the introducer and wire straightener are withdrawn. (d) Guidewire and the dilator partially introduced in the jugular vein. (e) Guidewire in place and the catheter sliding into the vein. (f) Catheter placed in the vein. (g) Catheter placed in the vein with the extension set and infusion plug. (h) Catheter and extension set sutured in place.

Additional Comments

Complications of intravenous catheter placement include thrombophlebitis (i.e., sepsis, contamination) extravascular or intra-arterial catheter placement, non-patent catheter (i.e., clot, kink), embolism (i.e., air, thrombus), and catheter embolism (i.e., sheared catheter tip, broken off catheter, lost guidewire).

Further Reading

Barakzai S, Chandler K. 2003. Use of indwelling intravenous catheters in the horse. *In Practice* 25(5): 264–71.

Madigan JE. 2013. Placement and management of intravascular catheter. In: Madigan JE (ed.). Manual of Equine Neonatal Medicine, 4th edn. Woodland, CA: Live Oak Publishing, pp. 261–6.

Nogradi N, Magdesian KG. Intravenous catheter placement in the neonatal foal. In: Costa LRR, Paradis MR (eds). Manual of Clinical Procedures in the Horse, 1st edn. Hoboken, NJ: Wiley Blackwell, pp. 46–71.

191

Plasma Therapy in the Foal

Undine Christmann

College of Veterinary Medicine, Lincoln Memorial University, USA

Introduction

Plasma therapy in foals is most frequently administered as a treatment for failure of passive transfer (FPT). In addition, plasma therapy is used to treat other neonatal diseases such as septicemia, to provide immunoprohylaxis against specific infectious diseases, and for the management for coagulopathies.

FPT is common in neonatal foals since the transfer of immunoglobulins must occur through ingestion of colostrum soon after birth. Any factor that interferes with the production of colostrum (i.e., absence, insufficient quantity, inadequate quality) and/or its ingestion by the foal (i.e., inability to get up, loss of suckle, hypoxic ischemic encephalopathy) may lead to FPT. Testing of foals for FPT has become standard practice since rapid stallside enzyme-linked immunoassay (ELISA) tests became available (e.g., SNAP foal IgG test; Idexx Laboratories, Westbrook, ME, USA) (see Chapter 187). These tests provide a semiquantitative measure of circulating immunoglobulin G (IgG) levels and whether a foal needs a plasma transfusion (Table 191.1). Intravenous plasma administration is strongly recommended in foals older than 12 hours with complete FPT. Plasma (or colostrum) administration by naso-gastric tube may be acceptable in foals younger than 12 hours, but does not guarantee adequate IgG absorption. Intravenous plasma administration is also recommended in foals with partial FPT, but this choice may depend on owner preference, financial means, and environmental conditions in which the foal and mare are kept. Guidelines for the administration of plasma in foals with FPT are shown in Table 191.1 and Figure 191.1.

Table 191.1 Example of interpretation using the SNAP test and treatment indication

SNAP Test Results	Passive Transfer	IV Plasma Administration
>800 mg/dl	Adequate	Not needed
400–800 mg/dl	Partial failure	Recommended
<400 mg/dl	Complete failure	Strongly recommended

The Animal and Plant Health Inspection Service/United States Department of Agriculture (APHIS/USDA) maintains updated information on licensed veterinary biological products: https://www.aphis.usda.gov/aphis/ourfocus/animalhealth/veterinary-biologics (last accessed October 2020). A list of companies with USDA licensed equine IgG products can be found following this link. Companies providing USDA licensed plasma for the treatment FPT are shown in Table 191.2. This plasma is sourced from healthy, vaccinated, tested, adult donor horses. Donor horses are blood typed and must lack the most common red blood cell antigens (A, Q, and C) to minimize the risk for neonatal isoerythrolysis in the foal. Donor horses must also test negative for known infectious diseases (equine infectious anemia, equine viral arteritis, piroplasmosis, brucellosis, dourine, glanders). USDA licensed plasma contains a minimum guaranteed amount of IgG and can be kept frozen for a period of up to 3 years. The American Association of Equine Practitioners (AAEP) published a white paper with detailed information on equine plasma and serum products for the equine practitioner (https://aaep.org/).

Fresh, "homemade", plasma can be used and collected from another horse on the farm. This plasma should be obtained from a suitable donor (negative for A, Q, and C red blood cell antigens) that is routinely vaccinated, and free of infectious disease. The main disadvantages of using "homemade" plasma are that the immunoglobulin content

Equine Reproductive Procedures, Second Edition. Edited by John Dascanio and Patrick McCue.

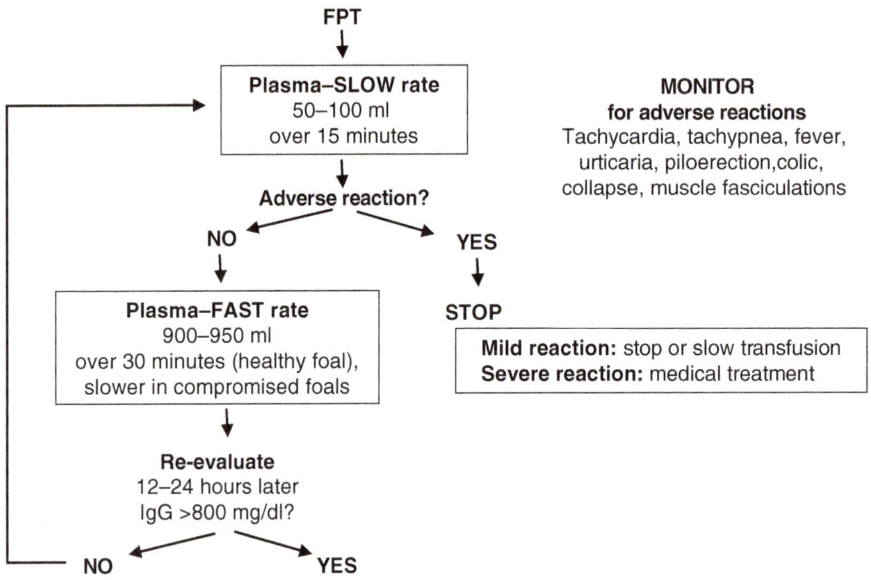

Figure 191.1 Decisional tree for plasma administration in foals with FPT.

is unknown, the immunogenicity is unpredictable, and it takes a significant amount of time to collect blood to acquire the plasma. The risk for anaphylaxis and infection is higher and the amount of plasma needed to achieve desired IgG levels in the foal is harder to predict. Foals with complete FPT require at least 1 liter of IV plasma. This need increases in foals that have other concurrent issues, such as septicemia (Figure 191.1).

Equipment and Supplies

Handler to restrain the foal, stethoscope and thermometer to record vital parameters, supplies for sterile site preparation and material for IV catheter placement, appropriate sedation (may or may not be needed), a blood administration set with in-line filter to avoid passage of clots, fibrins, or other debris (150–260 μm filter filter),desired amount of thawed plasma.

Technique

- Determine the amount of plasma required to correct the FPT. This amount depends on the foal's needs (weight, concurrent disease) and the plasma IgG concentration. Most foals with a simple FPT require 1 liter of plasma (sometimes 2 liters) to correct the FPT. Septic foals often require 2–3 times that amount of plasma transfusion.
- Thaw the plasma appropriately. Ideally, plasma is thawed immediately before administration (start thawing approximately 30 minutes before anticipated administration). This is achieved by placing the plasma bag inside another protective bag (to avoid contamination) and into a warm water bath or bucket (not to exceed 36.7–37.8ºC (98–100ºF)) and by running warm water into the bath or

Table 191.2 Commercial sources of plasma licensed for IV treatment of failure of passive transfer (FPT).

Company Information	USDA Licensed Product Name	Reported IgG Concentration According to Website
Lake Immunogenics, Inc., Ontario, NY, USA www.lakeimmunogenics.com (last accessed October 2020)	HiGamm USDA Licensed	≥2,800 mg/dl
Mg Biologics, Ames, IA, USA www.mgbiologics.com (last accessed October 2020)	High-Glo Equine IgG	Not reported on website
Plasvacc, Inc., Templeton, CA, USA www.plasvaccusa.com (last accessed October 2020)	EquiPlas® EquiPlasPlus®	≥1,500 mg/dl ≥2,700 mg/dl
Sera, Inc., Shawnee Mission, KS, USA www.seramune.com (last accessed October 2020)	Seramune IV™	>12,000 mg/dl

bucket until the plasma is thawed. Note: plasma should never be microwaved or thawed at high temperatures as this process denatures proteins including immunoglobulins.

- Check the plasma before administration. The plasma should be completely thawed and at body temperature. The plasma bag should be free of leaks and have an acceptable expiration date.
- Prime the plasma administration set. Connect the plasma bag to the blood administration set, prime the drip chamber half way, fill the administration line with plasma, check for air bubbles, and eliminate any air bubbles present.
- Place a catheter into the foal's jugular vein (see Chapter 190).
- Administer plasma at a slow rate (1 drop/s) for the first 15 minutes and then at a faster rate over the next 30 minutes.
- Monitor the foal closely for the first 15 minutes (take temperature, pulse, and respiration every 5 minutes) and then for the rest of the plasma administration (Figure 191.1).
- Treat adverse reaction as follows:
- Stop or slow administration for 5–10 minutes.
- If the transfusion reaction is mild, plasma administration can be started again slowly.
- If the transfusion reaction persists or is severe, administer treatment:
- Diphenhydramine 0.5–1 mg/kg IM or slow IV, once for mild reactions
- Corticosteroids (prednisolone sodium succinate 1–2.5 mg/kg IV once, or dexamethasone 0.05–0.1 mg/kg IV or IM once
- Epinephrine 0.01–0.02 mg/kg or 0.5–1 ml of 1:1,000 concentration slow IV, once for severe anaphylaxis and shock
- Note: administration of flunixin meglumine (1 mg/kg) may be sufficient to control mild discomfort in some foals.
- Recheck IgG concentration 12–24 hours later and repeat plasma administration as needed.

Additional Comments

Hyperimmune plasma may be used as part of the prevention or treatment against specific infectious diseases (*Rhodococcus equi*, *Escherichia coli*, *Salmonella* species. clostridial species such as botulinum, perfringens, and difficile, West Nile virus, *Streptococcus*, and others). Hyperimmune plasma is obtained from horses hyperimmunized against these specific agents. The benefits of hyperimmune plasma administration are still controversial and the amount of pathogen-specific IgG may be variable between lots of the same hyperimmune plasma product. Septic foals and critically ill foals are candidates for intravenous plasma administration as plasma provides antithrombin, coagulation factors, acute phase proteins, and complement in addition to IgG. Platelet-rich plasma is indicated in foals with thrombocytopenia.

Further Reading

Estell K, Magdesian KG. 2014. Use of fresh and frozen blood product in foals. In: Sprayberry KA, Robinson NE (eds). Robinson's Current Therapy in Equine Medicine, 7th edn. St Louis, MI: Elsevier, pp. 746–9.

Madigan JE. 2013. Plasma therapy. In: Madigan JE (ed.). Manual of Equine Neonatal Medicine, 4th edn. Woodland, CA: Live Oak Publishing, pp. 37–42.

Tennant-Brown B. 2011. Plasma therapy in foals and adult horses. *Compend Contin Educ Vet* 33(10): E1–4.

192

Acupuncture in the Neonate

Peter Morresey

Rood and Riddle Equine Hospital, USA

Introduction

The basis of the utility of acupuncture is the traditional Chinese medicine (TCM) theory that energy (Qi, pronounced "chee") travels through the body in channels associated with organ systems, known as *meridians,* along which exist acupuncture points. There are 12 defined fundamental meridians corresponding to the body's major functions, with these further divided between yin and yang. If this flow of Qi is obstructed (*stagnation of Qi*), due to local or systemic disease processes, loss of function and/or pain result.

The restoration of the free flow of Qi returns the body to a state of balance between yin and yang allowing normal physiological function to resume. This is achieved by physical manipulation near or along the obstructed meridians, considered releasing stagnation of Qi.

Housed within the kidney, *prenatal Jing* (literally essence) is present at birth and regulates the body's growth and development. It is inherited from the dam and sire. Throughout life Jing is depleted, working with Qi to protect the body from external pathogens. With Qi, Jing is considered to contribute to *shen*, or spirit. It can be considered therefore that any depletion of Jing will compromise the ability of the individual to grow, develop, protect itself, and maintain an appropriate level of vigor. Prenatal Jing can be replenished to some degree during life by Gu Qi (food-derived Qi), however the decrease in prenatal Jing cannot be completely eliminated and, when exhausted, death occurs. Signs of Jing deficiency in the neonate include poor growth, developmental orthopedic issues, and generalized loss of vitality.

The tenets of TCM are difficult to understand from a conventional perspective. However, physiological changes resulting from acupuncture have been demonstrated. Manipulation of acupuncture points leads to stimulation of sensory Aδ fibers causing segmental inhibition of pain impulses carried centrally in the slower unmyelinated C fibers. Opioid peptides and other neurotransmitters are measurably released. The hypothalamus and pituitary gland are also affected, thereby altering both central and peripheral neurotransmitter secretion. Immune functions may also be altered.

For successful treatment the practitioner needs an appreciation of TCM principles relating to diagnosis, Five Element Theory, and Zang-Fu physiology as well as a knowledge of acupuncture point location and correct needle insertion.

Equipment and Supplies

Stainless steel acupuncture needles of varying gauges (30–34) and lengths (1.3–2.5 cm (0.5–1 inches), electroacupuncture unit (if indicated), vitamin B_{12} injection (for use in aquapuncture, promotes chronic stimulation of selected acupuncture points) where indicated/applied, moxa (for moxibustion, burning the dried herb over acupuncture needles or acupuncture point), herbal therapies for ongoing treatment in conditions that tend to become chronic, or where needle placement meets with aversion behavior by patient.

Technique

- The selection of points is based upon the TCM pattern displayed by the patient. Assessment involves consideration of the constitution of the foal, appearance of the tongue and its coating, pulse character (depth, strength), and response to direct physical pressure stimulation of acupuncture points where the nature of the reaction indicates local Qi stagnation (indicating dysfunction of the associated organ system). Three categories of points are considered for stimulation during therapy.

Equine Reproductive Procedures, Second Edition. Edited by John Dascanio and Patrick McCue.

- *Constitutional*: seek to restore the overall physiology of the foal to an appropriate state, e.g., tonify Jing and Qi in a weakened neonate (seven back points, bladder-23, stomach-36, Qi-Hai-Shu).
- *Remote*: associated with an organ system or region of diagnosed dysfunction, however distant on the meridian of relevance, or associated with a related organ system, e.g., points associated with bone and musculoskeletal issues (small intestine-9, bladder-40, bladder-54, bladder-60).
- *Local*: directly affect the region or organ system displaying dysfunction, e.g., points on a weak limb directly associated with the area of diagnosed dysfunction.
- Indications in the neonate include obtundation from perinatal asphyxia syndrome (diminished appetite, suckle reflex, association with the mare), loss of function (ileus, musculoskeletal deficiencies resulting from parturient trauma such as fore limb weakness due to brachial plexus disruption), and generalized congenital weakness.
- The method of stimulation of acupuncture points depends on the desired result. In situations of neurologic or musculoskeletal dysfunction, electrical stimulation is appropriate. Pain also may benefit from both local supraspinal analgesia and central neurotransmitter release resulting from electrical stimulation. The character of response to electrical stimulation depends upon pulse amplitude and frequency. For generalized neonatal weakness, the addition of heat via moxibustion to the acupuncture point is directed towards the tonification of Jing.
- Insertion of the needle may induce "De Qi", literally the arrival of Qi. This is a prerequisite for a therapeutic effect. Dull pain indicates an appropriate response to placement of the needle, whereas sharp pain does not. It is likely the patient may react negatively to both, but particularly the latter, of these needle-associated responses.
- Location of acupuncture points is determined by regional topographic anatomy, distance from known landmarks (measured in Cun, pronounced "schwen"), and palpation of small surface depressions corresponding to acupuncture points.
- Some acupuncture points are well known due to established cross-species function, e.g. governing vessel-26 which is located on the upper gingiva, in the center of line between the lowest extent of the nares. Stimulation of this point is achieved by perpendicular insertion of a needle until resistance met. In the absence of an acupuncture needle, use a 1.3 cm (0.5 inches) 25 gauge hypodermic needle. Duration of residence is until spontaneous ventilation is maintained. The effect is enhanced by periodic repositioning and rotation of the needle. This point is useful in resuscitation situations to aid in stimulation of spontaneous breathing.

Additional Comments

- The goal of acupuncture is to return the patient to a state of normal function. No supraphysiological benefit will be gained from application to otherwise normal neonates.
- Response to acupuncture will be progressive. Serial treatments will be necessary.
- Acupuncture is best deployed as adjunctive therapy during acute episodes, and as long-term maintenance therapy with chronic conditions.
- Deleterious effects are unknown. Ensure the correct placement of needles near sensitive structures (e.g., joints, eyes).

Further Reading

Rathgeber R. 2001. Understanding Equine Acupuncture: Your Guide to Horse Health Care and Management. Eclipse Press.

Xie H, Preast V. 2013. Traditional Chinese Veterinary Medicine: Fundamental Principles. Reddick, FL: Chi Institute.

193

Routine Care

Patrick M. McCue

Equine Reproduction Laboratory, Colorado State University, USA

Introduction

The vast majority of foals are born without complications and unassisted. Intervention may be indicated in the absence of spontaneous breathing, if breathing is irregular or abnormal, in the absence of a heart beat, or if the newborn foal is flaccid and non-responsive. Foals born as a result of a dystocia, Cesarean section, induced labor, or born to mares with fescue toxicosis may be at increased need for resuscitation or immediate care.

An owner or foaling attendant should be trained, ready, and able to assist if necessary and should also understand when to call for professional assistance. A foaling kit, emergency contact list, telephone, emergency intervention protocol, and possibly even transportation should be readily available to the foaling attendant (see Appendix 4).

Equipment and Supplies

Stethoscope, disinfectant for umbilical stump, plastic container to dip umbilicus with, umbilical clamp (optional), umbilical tape and povidone-iodine (optional), sodium phosphate enema, acetylcysteine solution (optional).

"A-B-C Guidelines"

The "A-B-C guidelines" should be observed for newborn foals.

- *A – Airway*. The foal must be able to breathe on its own once it exits the protected environment of the uterus and is detached from the umbilical cord. Occasionally, a foal is born with the amnion still covering its nose, preventing normal respiration. An alert foaling attendant must quickly recognize this problem and immediately remove the amnion from the head and neck area. The amnion should not be covering the foal's nose once the foal's chest has been delivered through the mare's labia.

If there is visual evidence of yellow-brown meconium staining on the foal or the amnion, it is recommended that a veterinarian be consulted, as this may indicate that the foal may also have meconium in its airways and could have other issues related to pre- and/or intrapartum stress and hypoxia.

- *B – Breathing*. A newborn foal should take its first breath within a few moments after the chest has passed through the birth canal. If the foal has not initiated breathing immediately after it is born, the attendant should immediately call for assistance and begin resuscitation procedures (see Chapter 184). A normal foal should be trying to lift its head and should try to assume dorsal recumbency within minutes after birth.
- *C – Circulation*. A heart beat should be evident immediately after birth. The heart rate of a newborn foal is approximately 80–120 beats per minute (bpm). This will decrease over a few hours to 40–80 bpm. To check if the heart is beating in a newborn foal, place a stethoscope on the lower left side of the chest (behind the elbow) and listen for a heart beat or place a hand on the lower left side of the chest and manually feel for a heart beat. If a heart beat cannot be heard or felt in an obtunded foal, begin birth resuscitation procedures immediately.

The oral mucous membranes (i.e., gums) of a newborn foal should be pink, moist and, when blanched with firm digital pressure, should become pink again within 1–2 seconds (i.e., capillary refill time).

Equine Reproductive Procedures, Second Edition. Edited by John Dascanio and Patrick McCue.

Rupture of the Umbilical Cord and Umbilical Care

The umbilical cord normally breaks approximately 5 cm from the body wall of the foal when the mare stands or the foal struggles to rise (Figures 193.1 and 193.2). Manual disruption of the cord is not recommended, but may be necessary if the cord does not break on its own.

If it does become necessary to break the cord, manual rupture can be performed by firmly grasping the cord on either side of the normal breakpoint and tearing it. Do *not* attempt to break the cord away from the abdomen of the foal simply by pulling on it. Tearing is preferable to cutting since cutting does not allow the natural retraction and occlusion of the umbilical vessels, and has been associated with a higher incidence of excessive bleeding, patent urachus, and umbilical infections. Alternatively, an umbilical clamp (Figure 193.3) or umbilical tape, previously soaked in dilute povidone-iodine solution, can be applied to the cord approximately 5 cm from the body wall and a pair of scissors used to cut the cord distal to the clamp.

It is recommended that the umbilical stump be disinfected immediately after the cord has ruptured (Figure 193.4). This will decrease the likelihood of bacteria entering the open umbilical vessels and infecting the newborn foal. Choices for umbilical disinfectant treatment include 0.5% chlorhexidine, 1% povidone-iodine, and 2% tincture of iodine. It is currently recommended to use a diluted chlorhexidine solution to safely and effectively disinfect the umbilical stump of newborn foals as this type of disinfectant has been associated with less bacterial growth on umbilical cultures. Chlorhexidine umbilical dips will not, however, result in the cauterization of the umbilical stump as tends to occur with iodine solutions. Thus if you are familiar with iodine umbilical dips, when switching to chlorhexidine, the umbilicus may not shrink down quite as quickly. The umbilical stump should be completely immersed in a small container, such as a 12 ml syringe case or 50 ml centrifuge tube, of disinfectant for several seconds. Disinfectant treatment should be applied two or three times per day for 2–3 days.

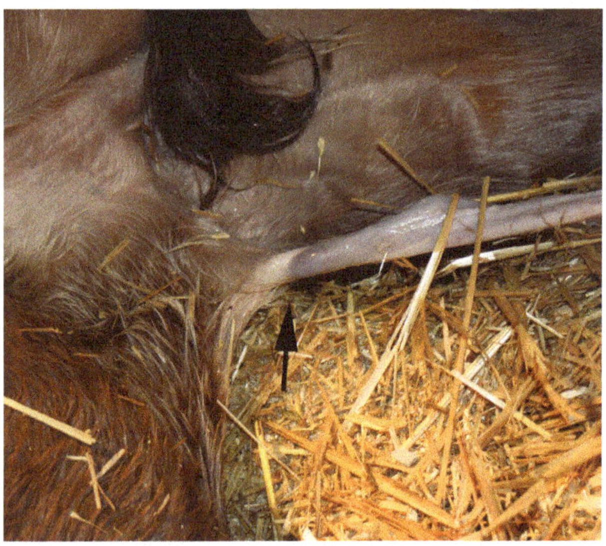

Figure 193.1 Umbilical cord still attached to a newborn foal. The area of normal disruption is indicated by the arrow.

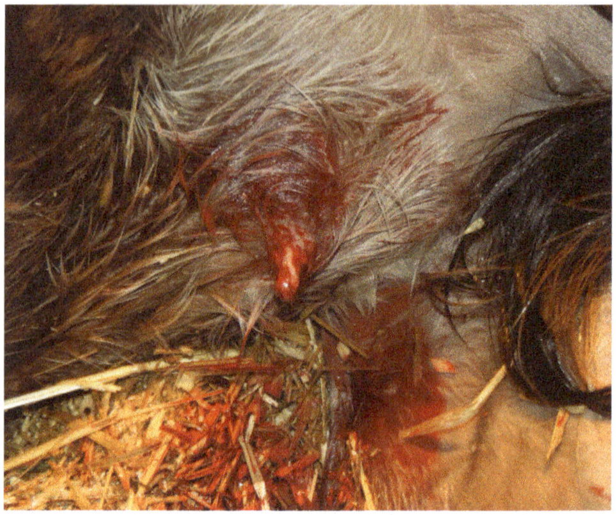

Figure 193.2 Umbilical stump after normal breakage of the cord.

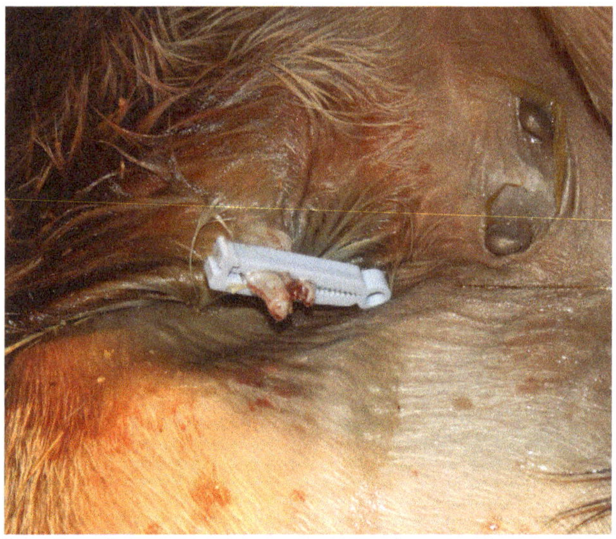

Figure 193.3 Umbilical clamp applied to the umbilical stump of a newborn foal.

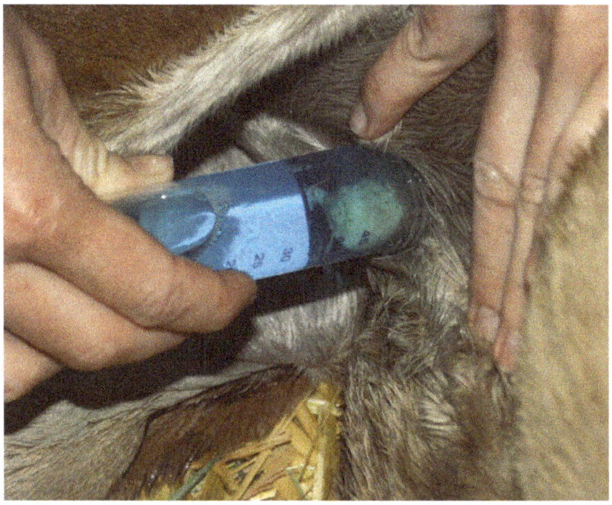

Figure 193.4 Dipping the navel of a foal with chlorhexidine solution.

Nursing and Ingestion of Colostrum

Nursing and ingestion of colostrum are critical to the well-being of a newborn foal. The foaling attendant and/or farm personnel should observe the foal to determine if it has stood and nursed on its own or if assistance is required. The vast majority of foals will stand and nurse unassisted within the first 1–2 hours after being born. A few foals will stand unassisted, but may need some guidance to find the udder. Observing dried milk on the face and nose of the foal and a full, tight udder on the mare suggests that the foal is not nursing effectively or maybe not at all. In some circumstances a young, inexperienced mare may not let her foal nurse and intervention may be needed, such as tranquilization of the mare, feeding the mare in a corner of a stall to decrease her movement, cross-tying the mare in the stall, or providing manual restraint.

Since mares have epitheliochorial placentation, newborn foals are entirely dependent on the passive transfer of maternal antibodies absorbed following ingestion of mare colostrum in the first few hours of life for protection against infectious diseases. Mares produce colostrum only during the last 1–2 weeks of gestation as antibodies are actively transported from their blood and concentrated in the mammary gland. After nursing colostrum, specialized cells that line the small intestine of the newborn foal absorb antibodies and transfer them into the foal's blood. Absorption of antibodies is greatest during the first 6–8 hours after birth, subsequently decreases, and stops completely by approximately 24 hours of age.

If the colostrum of a postpartum mare is tested and determined to be of marginal or poor quality (see Chapters 103 and 104), it would be beneficial to supplement the foal with frozen-thawed colostrum from another mare or to administer a colostrum substitute orally within the first few hours of life (see Chapter 188). Early intervention and oral supplementation (prior to approximately 12 hours after birth) can eliminate the need for intravenous plasma transfusion later.

Passage of Meconium and Meconium Impaction

Meconium is the first feces passed by a newborn foal and is comprised of digested amnionic fluid, gastrointestinal secretions, and cellular debris swallowed by the fetus while *in utero*. It is usually dark greenish brown or black in color, firm pellets to pasty in consistency, and is generally passed within the first 3–4 hours after birth. Failure to pass meconium results in significant abdominal pain in the neonate due to impaction.

A foal is considered to have retained meconium or a meconium impaction if frequent unsuccessful attempts to pass meconium occur within the first 12–36 hours of life. It has been estimated that 1.5% of all foals are affected by meconium impactions. Colt foals reportedly have a higher incidence of meconium impactions than filly foals.

Mild clinical signs are usually apparent within 6–24 hours after birth and include failure to completely pass meconium, a progressive increase in abdominal pain, and frequent posturing and straining to defecate (Figure 193.5). Affected foals may also be depressed and reluctant to nurse.

A common initial treatment for foals with a meconium impaction is the administration of an enema. A commercial sodium phosphate enema (Fleet® or a generic equivalent) is safe, easy to administer, and generally effective (Figure 193.6). Enemas should be warmed prior to use and

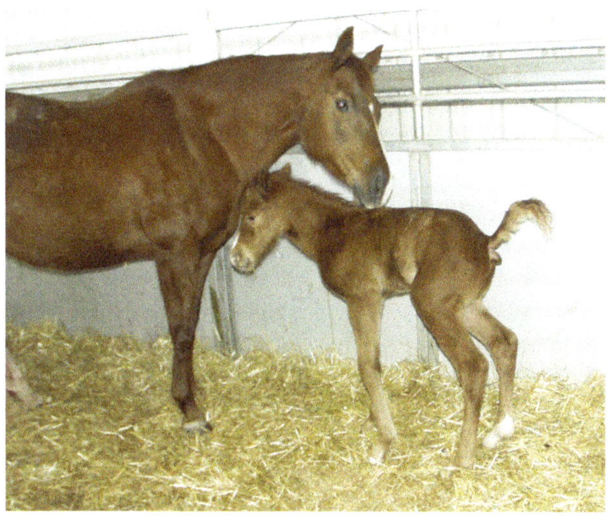

Figure 193.5 Newborn foal with meconium impaction straining to defecate.

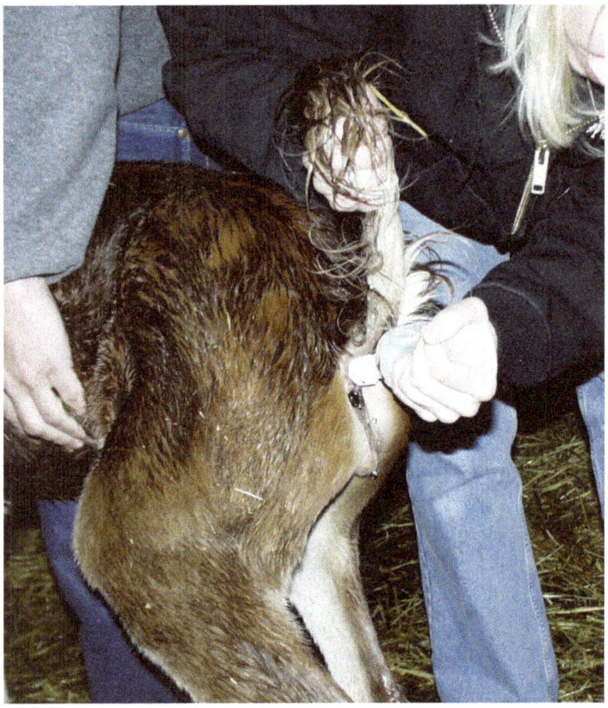

Figure 193.6 Administration of a sodium phosphate enema.

Box 193.1 Preparation of an Acetylcysteine Solution for a Foal Enema

- *Option 1.* Add 8 g acetylcysteine and 20 g baking soda ($NaHCO_3$) to 200 ml water.
- *Option 2.* Dilute a 20% commercial prepared solution of acetylcysteine to a 4% solution by adding 20 ml of the 20% solution to 80 ml of water for a total volume of 100 ml.

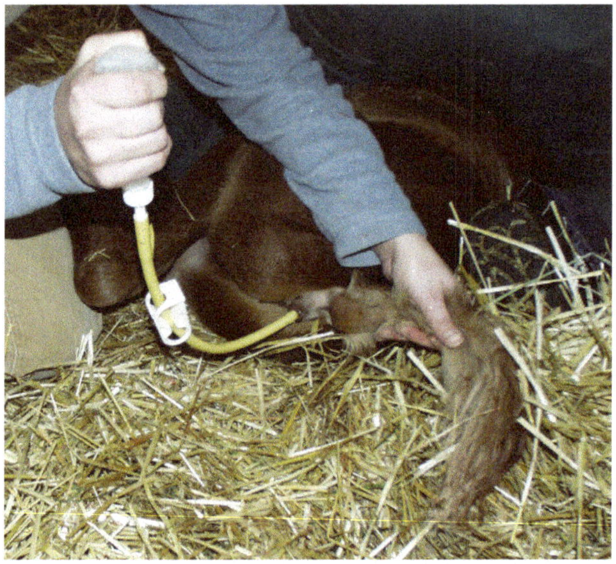

Figure 193.7 Acetylcysteine enema treatment.

may be kept in an incubator until needed or warmed to approximately 37°C (99°F) in a water bath. Proper restraint and careful passage of the applicator tip into the rectum are imperative to prevent trauma. Alternatively, 100–200 ml of warm water with a small amount of mild detergent soap may be used for an enema administered by a Foley catheter and gravity flow.

Breeding farms may choose to routinely give all newborn foals an enema within the first 1–2 hours after birth or may selectively administer enemas only to foals that do not pass meconium on their own. Foals that do not successfully pass meconium in the first few hours of life should be treated because of the potential for significant complications, including colic, failure to nurse adequately, and inflammation of the colon and rectum.

If the administration of one or two sodium phosphate enemas does not resolve a meconium impaction, the administration of an acetylcysteine retention enema may be successful in the medical resolution of meconium impactions (Box 193.1). An acetylcysteine solution is slowly infused into the rectum through a soft, flexible Foley-type catheter (Figure 193.7). The catheter is clamped shut and the solution allowed to remain in the rectum for 15–30 minutes before the clamp is opened and the catheter removed. The foal should be then be monitored for complete passage of the retained meconium and observations continued for the next 24–36 hours. The presence of yellow "milk stool" indicates that the meconium has passed completely and that digested colostrum is now being voided.

Additional therapy may be important in the management of a foal with meconium impaction. Colostrum intake should be monitored as it is a valuable source of antibodies required for passive transfer and has a strong laxative effect. Foals with colic associated with meconium impactions may not nurse as vigorously and may be at risk of failure of passive transfer. Additional veterinary treatments may include intravenous fluids, medications to provide pain relief, or other treatments. Rarely, but occasionally, a severe refractory case of meconium impaction may require surgical intervention.

"1-2-3 Rule"

As a general rule of thumb, critical events in the life of a newborn foal should occur by the following time periods: stand unassisted by 1 hour, nurse from the mare within

2 hours, and meconium passed within 3 hours. Often these events occur well before the 1–2–3 hour guidelines. In addition, the placenta should pass by 3 hours after foaling.

Antibiotics

Routine administration of one injection of an antibiotic to every foal immediately after birth is controversial. However, there are circumstances in which prophylactic or preventative administration of antibiotics to a newborn foal over a period of several days is warranted. These include: (i) if a foal is born to an unvaccinated mare, or if the vaccination history of the mare is unknown; (ii) if the mare leaked colostrum for several days prior to foaling; (iii) if the foaling was unattended or unexpected and it is unknown if the foal nursed an adequate amount of colostrum; and (iv) if the foal was born in an unsanitary environment and the risk of infection is high. In these situations, it may be warranted to administer antibiotics (as well as supplemental colostrum) to protect the newborn from infection.

In addition, newborn foals are occasionally administered antibiotics as a preventative measure on farms with a history of early foal disease or mortality due to specific infectious agents, such as *Rhodococcus equi* or *Clostridium perfringens.*

Plasma Therapy

Intravenous plasma transfusions may be administered to newborn foals as either prophylaxis to prevent the occurrence of a particular disease (e.g., *Rhodococcus equi* or *Clostridium botulinum*), as medical treatment of an ongoing infectious disease, or as medical management for failure of passive transfer (see Chapter 191).

Testing for Passive Transfer of Antibodies

Measurement of IgG levels in foals 12–24 hours of age can be very beneficial with regard to the evaluation of passive transfer and in the preventative management of neonatal infections. Early testing for antibody levels in a neonatal foal can identify potential cases of failure of passive transfer and allow for early intervention and medical management. Testing a foal at 24 hours of age or more will determine the final extent of passive antibody absorption. Methods for measurement of IgG levels are presented in Chapter 187.

Additional Comments

The newborn foal and dam should be observed carefully by farm personnel for the first 2–3 days after foaling to monitor activity level, health, social bonding, and nursing. Normal foals nurse frequently and generally keep the udder of the mare drained. Foaling attendants and farm personnel should be instructed to specifically observe the newborn foal for normal urination and defecation and to alert appropriate personnel if the foal appears to have problems voiding urine, is urinating through the umbilicus, or is straining to defecate. The strength and activity level of the foal should progressively increase over time. Foals with medical conditions may become weak, depressed, and stop nursing over a very short time period. Early recognition of changes in the behavior or attitude of the foal may be critical.

Foals that were born following a difficult birth (dystocia) or in a red bag delivery should be closely monitored for behavior over the first 48–72 hours as hypoxemic events that occurred during foaling may not be immediately apparent. Foals may sustain fractured ribs during a dystocia, assisted foaling, or even an apparently uneventful foaling. Affected foals may exhibit localized swelling, pain, difficulty in breathing, or other problems.

The body temperature of the foal should be measured if the foal appears to be depressed, not nursing, reluctant to move, or less active than normal. The normal body temperature of a newborn foal ranges from approximately 37.2 to 38.7°C (99.0–101.6°F). A body temperature below or above this range is considered abnormal and appropriate personnel should be notified. Note that it is common for a newborn foal to shiver for 3–4 hours after birth to generate heat. In some instances, a young foal may need extra bedding (i.e., deep straw), a blanket, or heat lamps to help it keep warm. A small human sweatshirt may be placed onto the foal, with the foal's front legs through the arms of the sweatshirt, to aid in maintaining body heat.

The mare should also be examined after the birth of the foal for a second fetus, any tears to the reproductive tract, passage of the placenta, and presence of milk/colostrum within the udder. The mare may also experience colic post-foaling due to uterine contractions, which are often alleviated by the administration of a non-steroidal anti-inflammatory drug such as flunixin meglumine (1.0 mg/kg IV or orally).

It is recommended that a routine newborn foal examination be performed by a veterinarian within 12 hours after birth to evaluate health status and determine if medical therapy is indicated.

Further Reading

Acworth NRJ. 2003. The healthy neonatal foal: routine examinations and preventative medicine. *Eq Vet Educ* 15: 45–9.

Knottenbelt DC. 2003. The newborn foal. In: Knottenbelt DC, LeBlanc M, Lopate C, Pascoe RR (eds). Equine Stud Farm Medicine and Surgery. Edinburgh: Saunders, pp. 353–90.

Shepherd C. 2010. Post-parturition examination of the newborn foal and mare. *In Practice* 32: 97–101.

194

Foal Rejection

Patrick M. McCue

Equine Reproduction Laboratory, Colorado State University, USA

Introduction

Rejection of a foal by its dam can take several forms. The mare may: (i) avoid the foal; (ii) prevent the foal from nursing; or (iii) become aggressive toward the foal. Mares in the latter category may assume a threatening posture, pin their ears back when the foal approaches, charge or chase the foal, squeal at the foal, or in more serious cases may kick at or bite the foal. Mares have, on rare occasions, seriously injured or killed their foals in the first few days after giving birth.

Foal rejection may occur in any horse breed, but has been reported to be most common in Arabians. Rejection is most likely to occur in primiparous mares giving birth to their first foal. Mares that have rejected a foal in the past have an increased chance of rejecting a subsequent foal. Mares that are separated from their foal for a prolonged time interval in the early postpartum period have an increased risk of foal rejection. In addition, foals with behavioral or medical issues or are otherwise debilitated may be at higher risk of being rejected by their dam.

Mares that ultimately reject their foals are not as likely to express normal maternal behaviors in the early postpartum period, such as licking their foals, nickering to their foals, and standing guard over or next to their foals (i.e., the "recumbency response"). Failure to allow nursing will result in an inability of the foal to acquire the maternal antibodies from colostrum necessary to protect itself against pathogenic disease organisms. In addition, affected foals will be deprived of important nutritional support in the neonatal period.

Equipment and Supplies

Halter and lead rope, twitch, sedation (acepromazine, xylazine, detomidine, butorphanol), bucket with grain, nursing chute, altrenogest, non-steroidal anti-inflammatory drugs, prostaglandins, oxytocin, supplies to wash the perineum of the mare (optional), sterile obstetrical sleeve (optional), sterile lubricant (optional).

Technique

- Mares exhibiting a tendency toward foal rejection should be monitored closely for the first 48 hours or more after foaling. The vast majority of rejection-type behavioral interactions occur within the first 12 hours after birth. Therefore, it is best to avoid interruption of the developing mare–foal bond that naturally occurs early in the postpartum period.
- Management of foal rejection may initially include restraint of the mare by hand, judicious use of a twitch, hobbles, or cross-ties, or by placing the mare behind a bar or within a nursing chute to allow the foal to have an unimpeded and safe opportunity to suckle (Figures 194.1 and 194.2).
- In mild cases, distraction of the mare with hay or grain may be sufficient to allow the foal time to nurse without the mare becoming nervous and moving away. If the foal

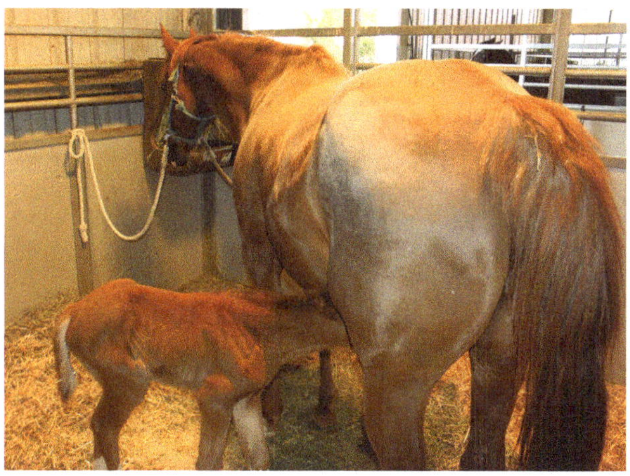

Figure 194.1 Foal nursing from a mare restrained in cross-ties.

Equine Reproductive Procedures, Second Edition. Edited by John Dascanio and Patrick McCue.

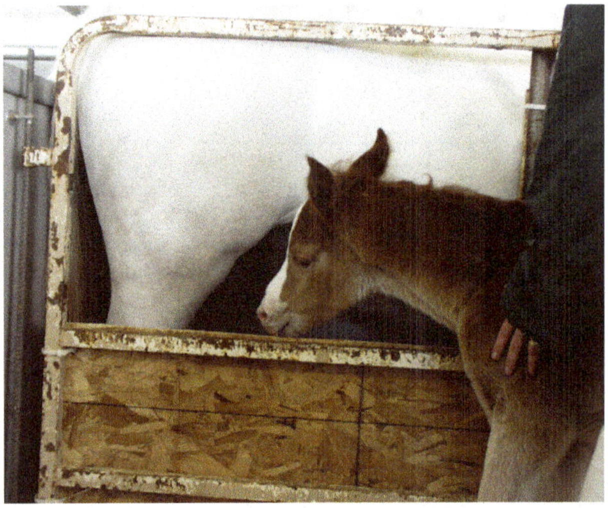

Figure 194.2 Foal approaching a mare restrained behind a nursing chute.

does not or cannot nurse, colostrum from the mare should be milked out and fed to the foal by bottle or by naso-gastric tube.

- In some instances, the mare may need to be muzzled to prevent biting of the foal.
- The mare may also need to be tranquilized periodically during the first few days postpartum with acepromazine (0.044–0.066 mg/kg IV) or sedated with a combination of detomidine (0.0088–0.011 mg/kg IV) and butorphanol (0.011–0.022 mg/kg IV) to decrease aggression.
- Administration of the oral progestin altrenogest (0.044–0.088 mg/kg PO, every 24 hours) has also been used in cases of foal rejection in an attempt to suppress or modulate aggressive behavior.
- Treatment of the mare with a non-steroidal anti-inflammatory drug, such as flunixin meglumine (1.1 mg/kg IV, every 12 hours), may be indicted if the mare appears to be rejecting nursing attempts by the foal due to post-foaling pain or mammary gland discomfort. With nursing, oxytocin release occurs causing uterine contractions that may be painful to some postpartum mares. Inflammation of the mammary gland, or mastitis, may contribute to the refusal of a mare to allow nursing.
- Administration of oxytocin (10–20 IU IM or IV) is sometimes advocated to stimulate milk let down.
- Administration of prostaglandins to "reprogram" the maternal behavior of the mare (i.e., concaveation method – see Chapter 195) is sometimes used.
- Manual vaginal/cervical stimulation of the mare with the foal present may also enhance acceptance. The mare's perineum should be washed and dried and a sterile obstetrical sleeve with sterile lubricant used for the procedure.
- If other techniques are not successful, some breeders advocate turning out a mare exhibiting mild foal rejection behavior and her foal into a paddock adjacent to another mare in the hope that natural maternal protective instincts will enhance acceptance of her foal.
- Prevention of foal rejection may be attempted by early acclimation of a primiparous mare to the foaling stall, desensitization of her udder to touch prior to foaling, and exposure of the at-risk mare to other mares with foals to observe normal maternal behavior.

Additional Comments

It may take several days of patient, diligent work to assist the mare to accept her foal. However, if the process is unsuccessful the foal may be fostered onto a nurse mare (see Chapter 195). If a nurse mare is not available, lactation can be hormonally stimulated in a non-pregnant mare to create nurse mares for orphan foals (Figure 194.3) (see Chapter 101). Hand-rearing the rejected foal as an orphan is a labor intensive and often ill-advised alternative if the mare does not eventually accept her foal or if a nurse mare is not available.

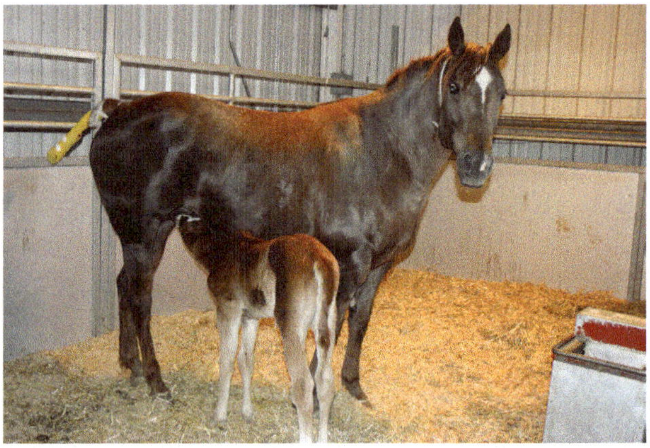

Figure 194.3 Fostering a foal onto a mare induced to lactate.

Further Reading

Daels PF, Bowers-Lepore J. 2007. How to induce lactation in a mare and make her adopt an orphan foal: what 5 years of experience have taught us. *Proc Annu Conv Am Assoc Eq Pract* 53: 349–53.

Daels PF, Duchamp G, Porter D. 2002. Induction of lactation and adoption of foals by non-parturient mares. *Proc Annu Conv Am Assoc Eq Pract* 48: 68–71.

Houpt KA, Olm D. 1984. Equine behavior: foal rejection: a review of 23 cases. *Eq Pract* 6: 38–40.

Juarbe-Diaz SV, Houpt KA, Kusunose R. 1998. Prevalence and characteristics of foal rejection in Arabian mares. *Eq Vet J* 5: 424–8.

Vaala WE. 2011. Foal rejection. In: McKinnon AO, Squires EL, Vaala WE, Varner DD (eds). Equine Reproduction, 2nd edn. Ames, IA: Wiley Blackwell, pp. 117–20.

195

Fostering a Foal onto a Nurse Mare

Peter F. Daels[1] *and Pouya Dini*[2]

[1] *Faculty of Veterinary Medicine, University of Gent, Belgium*
[2] *School of Veterinary Medicine, University of California-Davis, USA*

Introduction

Managing and feeding an orphan foal can be challenging. A mare that has recently lost her foal at an early age or from which the foal has recently been weaned can be an inexpensive and effective candidate to raise an orphan foal. However, a mare that has very recently lost her foal tends to have an instinctive aversion towards any other foal that is not hers, and fostering the orphan foal can be challenging, even dangerous to the foal and handlers, and occasionally impossible. The use of a mare with induced lactation that has neither foaled nor raised a foal in the current foaling season can be a convenient, safe, and effective alternative. The protocol for induction of lactation is a well-established, safe technique that takes about 1 week. The maternal behavior of a mare with induced lactation is identical to that of mares that raise their own foals. Most importantly, the fostering of a foal to a mare with an induced lactation is generally safe, quick, and simple.

A prospective nurse mare should not be pregnant, should be tractable, and preferably gentle with people and other horses. She must have foaled and successfully raised at least one foal in the past and preferably not be in seasonal anestrus. After successful fostering of the foal, she can be subsequently bred without a decrease in fertility or a negative effect on lactation. While bringing the foster mare to a sufficient level of lactation, which may take up to 1 week, the orphan foal can be fed a commercial equine milk replacer. If the orphan foal has never nursed from its natural mother (i.e., was separated at birth), then it is recommended to feed the foal with a bottle to maintain a good suckling reflex and, if needed, to be able to guide the foal with the help of the milk bottle under the abdomen of the foster mare. This can greatly facilitate training the naïve foal to look for the udder under the mare. Foals that have previously nursed from their natural mother may be fed from a bucket as their nursing instinct perseveres and they will quickly find their way to the udder.

Equipment and Supplies

Prostaglandin $F_{2\alpha}$, syringes, needles, sturdy halter and lead rope for the mare, feeding bottle for the foal, standard size foaling stall without direct contact with other horses.

Technique

- Some advocate placing the foster mare and foal in adjacent stalls so that they can see and smell one another during the days prior to the adoption procedure to facilitate bonding. However, the authors have not observed any advantage of doing so and routinely introduce the orphan foal for the first time to the foster mare at the time of the adoption procedure.
- About 15-20 minutes before the adoption, administer 3–4× the labeled luteolytic dose of prostaglandin $F_{2\alpha}$ ($PGF_{2\alpha}$) intramuscularly. The authors use 750–1,000 μg cloprostenol sodium (3–4 ml Estrumate®) intramuscularly as it produces strong side effects that are presumed to be important for the successful triggering of maternal behavior. Occasionally, other veterinarians have reported success using large doses of other $PGF_{2\alpha}$ preparations. The use of oxytocin in combination or instead of $PGF_{2\alpha}$ is ineffective and not recommended.

Equine Reproductive Procedures, Second Edition. Edited by John Dascanio and Patrick McCue.

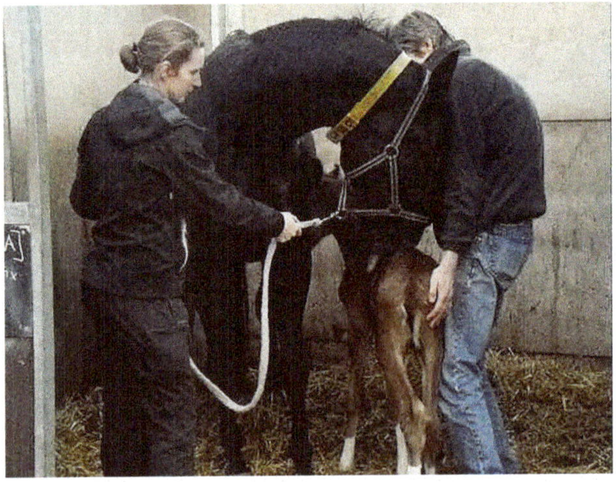

Figure 195.1 The foal has been introduced to the foal 15 minutes after prostagland $F_{2\alpha}$ administration. The mare actively licks the foal while the foal is gradually moved to the flank of the mare.

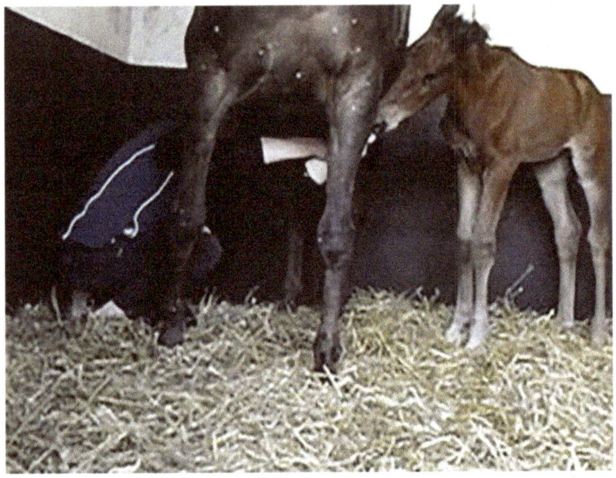

Figure 195.2 The foal has been adopted by the mare but the foal has not found the mammary gland yet. With the aid of a milk bottle, the foal is teased under the abdomen of the mare towards the udder.

- Wait until obvious side effects of PGF administration are apparent, such as sweating, unrest, and mild colic (about 15 minutes).
- While restraining the mare at a short distance with a lead rope, introduce the foal to the front of the mare and allow the mare to smell and lick the foal. Do not place a twitch on the mare or sedate the mare.
- Allow the mare to freely smell and lick the foal and look for signs of maternal behavior or signs of aggression. Typically, the mare will show impulsive licking and smelling of the foal, as well as the typical nickering that is often observed immediately after foaling.
- Gradually move the foal alongside the mare in the direction of the abdomen and mammary gland (Figure 195.1). Facilitate contact between the foal and the flanks of the mare to stimulate maternal behavior in the mare and suckling reflex in the foal.
- With foals that have never nursed a mare it is advised to use a milk bottle to guide the foal under the abdomen into the warm and dark area around the udder to trigger the nursing instinct in the foal (Figure 195.2).
- In general, the adoption of the foal, characterized by a total appropriation and actively protecting the foal, takes less than 15 minutes, at which time the mare and foal can be allowed to freely move together in the box stall.
- In less than 10% of attempts, the maternal behavior does not occur. A second attempt within 12–24 hours with the same mare and foal is often successful and is therefore clearly warranted.

Interpretation

- Within 0–1 minutes the mare should take a directed, active interest in the foal and start to smell and lick the foal.
- Within 5–10 minutes, the licking behavior intensifies and the mare should allow the foal to touch the flank and udder.
- Within 5–10 minutes, the foal is allowed to suckle from the mare without any restraint of the mare. The mare will often instinctively lick the foal's hindquarters in an attempt to stimulate nursing behavior.
- Within 15 minutes, the mare should show overt maternal behavior including following the foal, taking the typical posture to present the mammary gland to the foal during nursing, and showing protective, aggressive behavior towards other horses.
- When in doubt about the maternal bond with the foal, remove the foal gradually out of sight. If the maternal bond is established, the mare will display separation anxiety and attempt to follow the foal.

Further Reading

Daels PF. 2018. Fostering of foals. *In: Proceedings of the British Equine Veterinary Association BEVA Congress* 66.

Paradis MR. 20212. Feeding the orphan foal. *Proc Annu Conv Am Assoc Eq Pract* 58: 402–6.

Stoneham S, Morresey P, Ousey J. 2017. Nutritional management and practical feeding of the orphan foal. *Eq Vet Educ* 29: 165–73.

196

Entropion

John J. Dascanio

School of Veterinary Medicine, Texas Tech University, USA

Introduction

Entropion is a condition manifested in newborn foals in which one or both of the eyelid margins are rolled inward causing irritation of the cornea (Figure 196.1). Inversion of the lower eyelid is much more common than inversion of the upper eyelid and the condition may be unilateral or bilateral. In some cases entropion may be related to dehydration. The initial signs are blepharospasm and epiphora. Given time, the skin may tighten and the condition may resolve on its own; however, due to potential associated eye pathology, early intervention is warranted. The main complication is creation of a corneal ulcer from eyelashes or hair rubbing on the cornea with secondary ophthalmic complications. Intervention may consist of ophthalmic lubricant application and manual eversion of the affected eyelid(s), injection of a subcutaneous bleb of fluid to roll the skin outward, sutures to accordion excess skin, or surgery to remove excess skin.

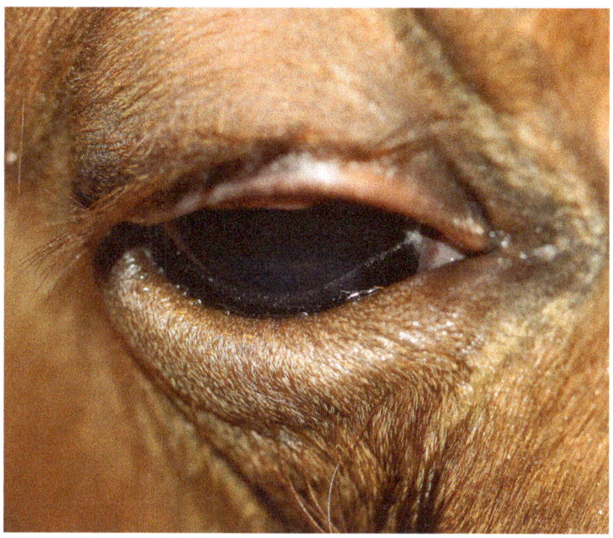

Figure 196.1 Entropion of the lower eyelid in a newborn foal.

Any newborn foal that is squinting should have a complete ophthalmologic examination to determine the cause and any related pathologies.

Equipment and Supplies

Needles, syringe, sedation, procaine penicillin G, small sterile suture pack, sedation, 4-0 suture, sterile scrub gauze, alcohol swabs, examination gloves, sterile surgical gloves, ophthalmoscope, fluorescein strip, sterile ophthalmic eye wash.

The foal should have a complete ophthalmic examination, including staining of the cornea with fluorescein dye to identify if a corneal ulcer present.

Penicillin Bleb Technique

- Sedate or adequately restrain the foal (see Chapter 189).
- Clean the skin area below the lower eyelid with alternating surgical scrub and alcohol swabs, being careful to not get any into the foal's eye.
- Using a 20 gauge needle, place 1–2 ml of procaine penicillin G in a line parallel to the lower lid margin about 1 cm from the lid margin in the primary area of the excessive skin folds (Figure 196.2). Place enough liquid to evert the rolled lid margin back to a normal margin.
- The foal must be adequately restrained to prevent accidental injury to the eye.

Suture Technique

- Sedate or adequately restrain the foal (see Chapter 189).
- Clean the skin area below the lower eyelid with alternating surgical scrub and alcohol swabs, being careful to not get any into the foal's eye.

Equine Reproductive Procedures, Second Edition. Edited by John Dascanio and Patrick McCue.

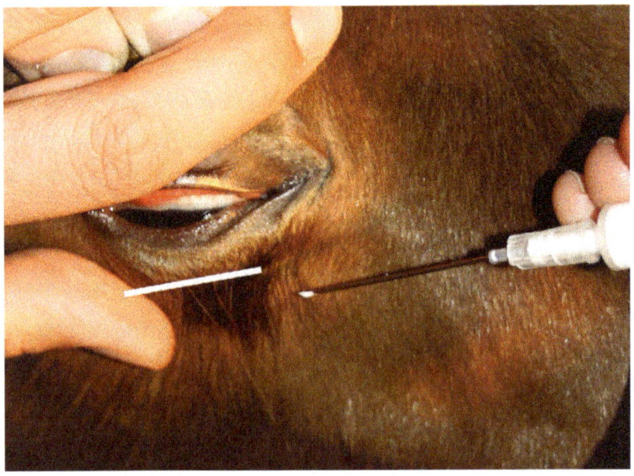

Figure 196.2 Direction for needle placement for subcutaneous injection of procaine penicillin to correct lower eyelid entropion. The white line indicates the area for penicillin placement.

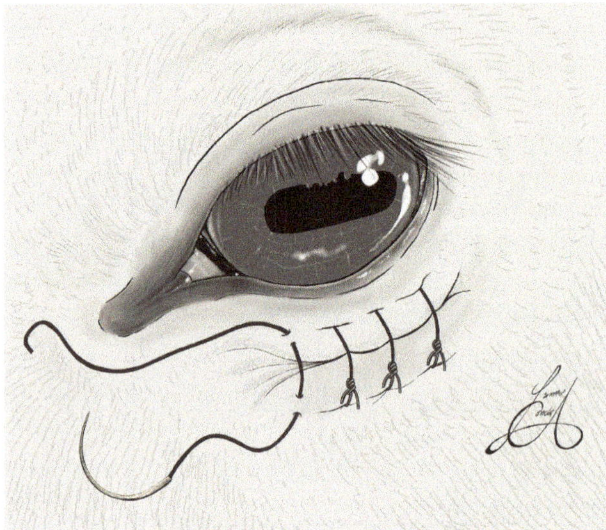

Figure 196.3 Location for placement of vertical mattress sutures. Drawing courtesy of Dr Ismael Concha-Albornoz DVM, MVSc (www.anato.cl).

- Using a 25 gauge needle, place a line of 2% lidocaine or similar solution in the area for suture placement. Determine the relative suture placement prior to the placement of lidocaine as it will roll the eyelid out from the fluid volume.
- Using 4-0 non-absorbable monofilament suture, place 2–3 vertical mattress sutures to evert the lower eyelid margin (Figure 196.3). A central suture should be first placed and then sutures on either side. The first bite should be 2–3 mm from the lid margin. The next bite will determine how much the lower eyelid margin is rolled back out. In addition, the tightness of the suture will also determine the amount of eyelid rolled outward. Pre-placement of all sutures prior to final knot completion can aid in assuring proper tension to roll the lower eyelid margin out. All sutures can then be tensioned before any final knot tying.
- Cut the suture end of the suture closest to the eye short to avoid corneal irritation.
- Removal of skin with subsequent placement of sutures should be avoided in the first few days post-foaling as overcorrection could occur as the foal grows. This procedure should be considered at a later date if the above techniques do not result in permanent correction.
- Usually a topical antibiotic or lubricating ointment is placed into the affected eye 4–6 times per day for a few days post-procedure.

Interpretation

- Correct any medical conditions that may result in dehydration.
- With procaine penicillin use, the lid margin may roll inward again in 24–48 hours. A repeat procedure may be considered.
- Monitor the site for suture dehiscence, excessive rubbing, or continued irritation to the eye(s).
- Ensure that, if sutures are used, the suture ends do not go toward the cornea, causing irritation. In addition, ensure that the foal can blink and close the eyelids and that the sutures are not preventing eyelid closure, in which case the sutures would need to be repositioned.
- Sutures should be removed in 10–14 days.

Further Reading

Leiva M, Pena T. 2017. Ophthalmic diseases of foals. In: Gilger BC (ed.). Equine Ophthalmology, 3rd edn. Ames, IA: Wiley Blackwell, pp. 112–50.

197

Umbilical Ultrasound

Undine Christmann

College of Veterinary Medicine, Lincoln Memorial University, USA

Introduction

Umbilical ultrasound is used to assess visible or palpable umbilical abnormalities and to explore suspected or covert infection of umbilical structures. Visible or palpable umbilical abnormalities include heat, swelling, pain, drainage, or patency. Umbilical ultrasound examination is also warranted in foals with failure of passive transfer, fever of unknown origin, and with laboratory abnormalities indicative of inflammation or infection (i.e., elevated white blood cell count, fibrinogen, or serum amyloid A).

An umbilical ultrasound examination allows the clinician to evaluate which structures are affected and to gauge the extent and severity of the issue. It is a valuable tool to monitor response to medical therapy, to decide if a foal should undergo surgery, and to establish a prognosis. Abnormalities visible on umbilical ultrasound include structural size changes (e.g., enlarged umbilical vessels), alterations in shape (e.g., urachal diverticulum), and modifications in appearance, such as thickening of walls, fluid accumulation, and presence of hypo- or hyperechogenic material.

The umbilical remnants that can be evaluated in the foal are listed in Table 197.1 with their respective fetal function, fate after birth, and location. An illustration of these structures and corresponding ultrasound views are shown in Figures 197.1 and 197.2.

Equipment and Supplies

Assistant to restrain the foal, ultrasound machine with linear array transducer (10–12 MHz) or transrectal linear array probe (5–7.5 MHz), alcohol or coupling gel, clippers (optional), sedation (optional).

Technique

- Prepare the ultrasound machine with a linear (10–12 MHz) or a transrectal (5–7.5 MHz) transducer.
- Restrain the standing foal or place the foal in lateral recumbency. Sedation may be needed in some foals (see Chapter 189).
- Clip the hair from the xyphoid process to the inguinal area, clean, and cover the skin with coupling gel. Alternatively, simply wet the area with alcohol.
- Perform a systematic scan of the umbilical structures including a minimum number of views (Figure 197.2), and transverse and longitudinal images of the structures evaluated.

Umbilical Vein

- Follow the umbilical vein cranially from the umbilical stump to the liver, along the midline, and close to the skin surface. Measure the horizontal and vertical diameter of the vein in transverse views.
- Document three views (Figure 197.1a, b):
  1) Cranial to the umbilical stump (view 2) (Figure 197.2a).
  2) Mid distance between the umbilical stump and the liver (view 3) (Figure 197.2b).
  3) Caudal to the liver (view 4) (Figure 197.2c).
- *Normal appearance*: the diameter of the umbilical vein should be under 1 cm; the wall of the umbilical vein appears thin; the vein may contain homogeneous, hypoechoic material which corresponds to a blood clot potentially visible during the first week of age. Age should be considered when evaluating umbilical structures as their size decreases significantly in the weeks following birth.

Equine Reproductive Procedures, Second Edition. Edited by John Dascanio and Patrick McCue.

Table 197.1 Umbilical structures or remnants visible on ultrasound examination in the foal with their respective function in the fetus, their fate after birth, and their location.

Structure(s)	Fetal Function	Fate	Location
Single umbilical vein	Transports blood from placenta to liver	Round ligament Liver	Cranially from umbilical stump to liver Along midline Close to skin surface
Paired umbilical arteries	Transports blood from foal to placenta	Round ligament Bladder	Caudally from umbilical stump to bladder Urachus located in between Depart to lateral aspect of bladder
Urachus	Transports urine from bladder to allantois	Median ligament Bladder	From umbilical stump to apex of the bladder

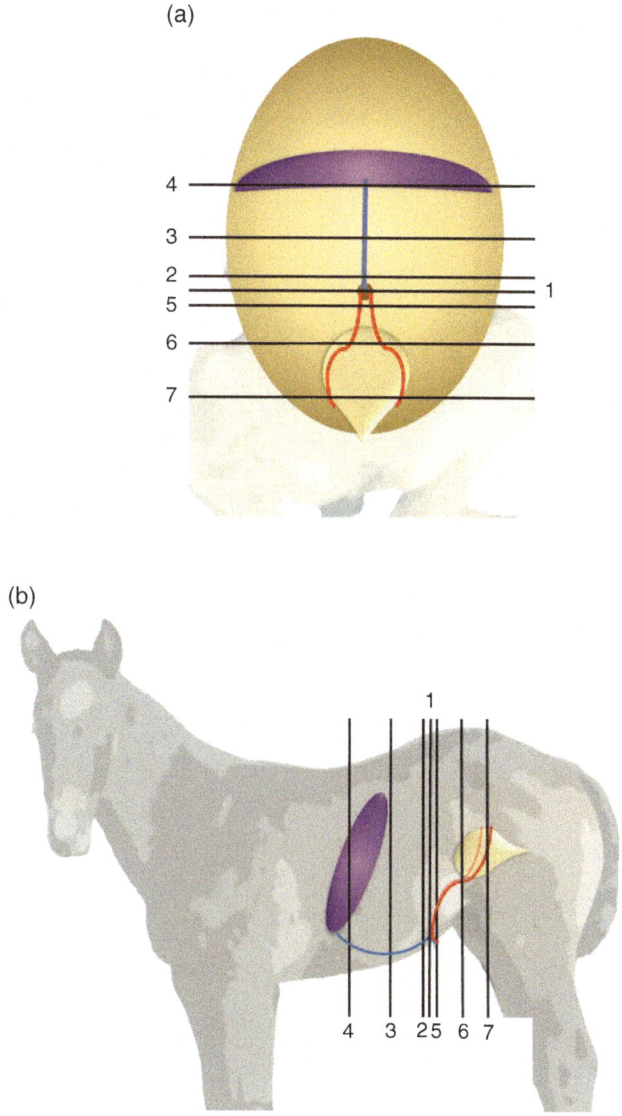

Figure 197.1 Schematic representation of ultrasound views obtained with (a) a foal in dorsal recumbency and (b) a standing foal or foal in lateral recumbency with depiction of the following structures: liver (purple), umbilical vein (blue), umbilical arteries (red), and bladder (yellow).

Umbilical Stump and Urachus

- Obtain an image just caudal to the umbilical stump and visualize the urachus between the two umbilical arteries. Measure the horizontal and vertical diameter of the arteries in transverse views.
- Document three views (Figure 197.1a and 197.1b):
  1) Cross-section of the umbilical stump (view 1).
  2) Cross-section of the urachus and the arteries just caudal to the umbilical stump (view 5) (Figure 197.3a).
  3) Longitudinal view of the urachus and the apex of bladder.
- *Normal appearance*: the diameter of the stump alone is less than 1.6 cm; the combined diameter of urachus with the two arteries is under 2.5 cm ("ET" view); all structures have thin walls; hypoechoic material may be visible within the arteries corresponding to a blood clot potentially visible in foals less than 1 week of age. A recent study identified significant variations in the appearance the urachus on longitudinal views.

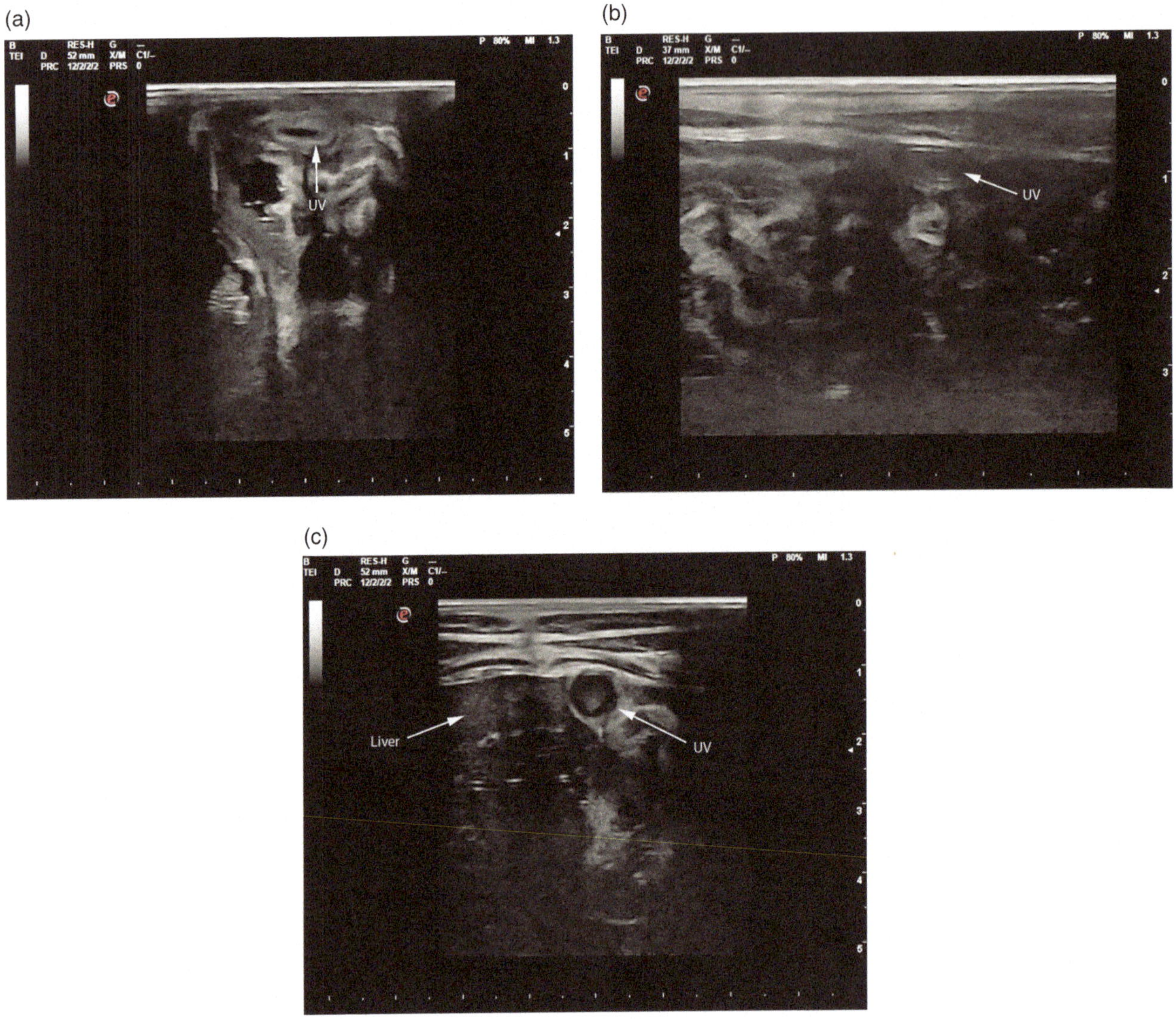

Figure 197.2 Transverse ultrasound images of the umbilical vein (UV) in a normal foal at <24 hours after birth. (a) Cranial to the umbilical stump (view 2). (b) At mid distance between the umbilical stump and the liver (view 3). (c) In proximity to the liver (view 4). Note the diameter of <1 cm, thin walls, ovoid shape, and homogenous appearance. Images courtesy of Dr Annette McCoy.

Umbilical Arteries

- Visualize the urachus between the umbilical arteries ("ET" view) and follow each artery to the lateral aspect of the bladder and towards the inguinal region.
- Document three views (Figure 197.1a and 197.1b):

  1) Cross-section of the urachus and the arteries just behind the umbilical stump (view 5) (Figure 197.3a).
  2) Arteries close to the apex of the bladder (view 6) (Figure 197.3b).
  3) Arteries close at the midpoint of the bladder (view 7) (Figure 197.3c, d).

- *Normal appearance*: diameter of arteries is less than 1.3 cm; walls of the arteries are thin (≤3 mm); hypoechoic material may be visible within the arteries corresponding to a blood clot potentially present in foals under 1 week of age. A size difference may be noted between the left and right umbilical arteries.

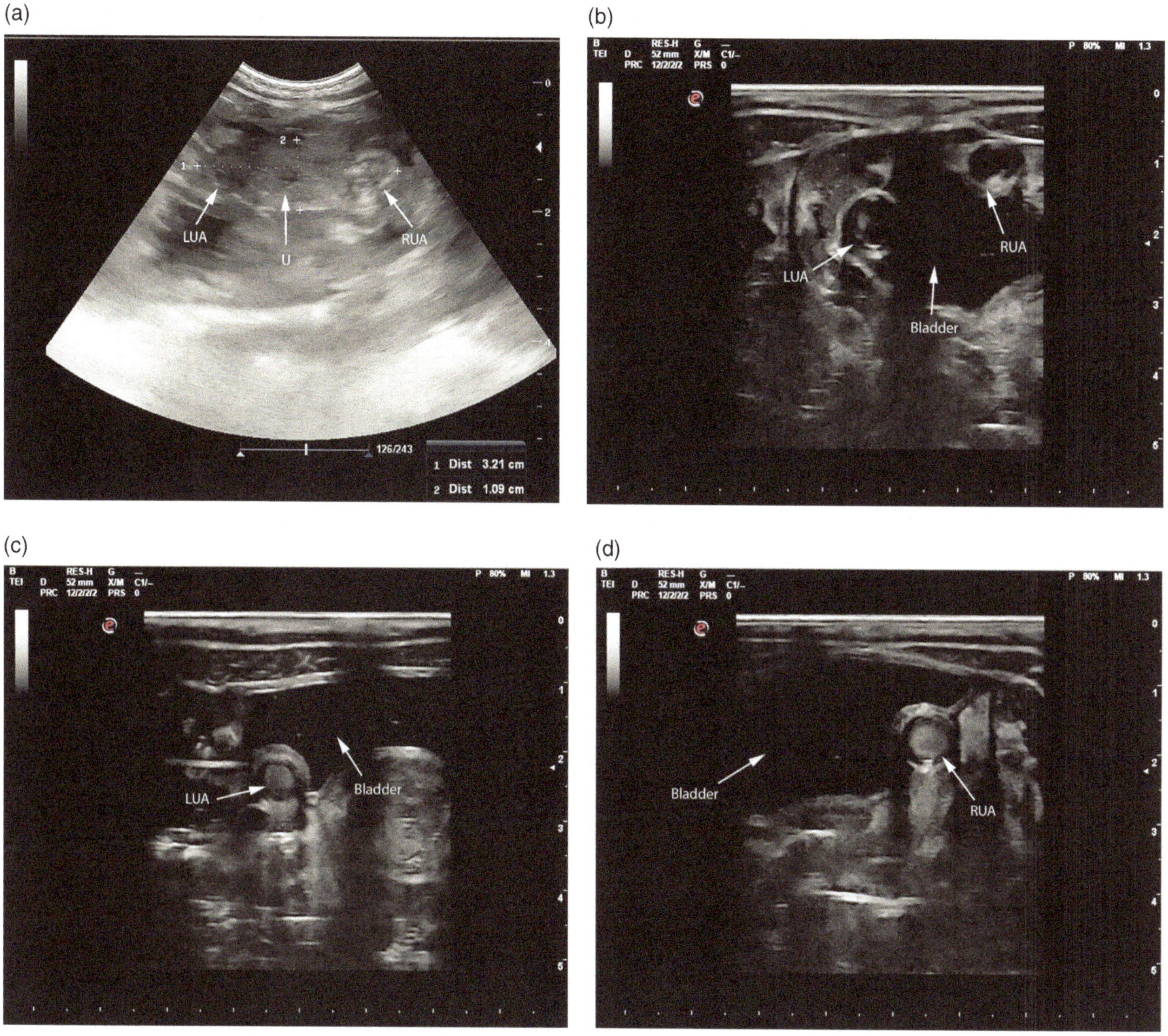

Figure 197.3 Transverse ultrasound images of the umbilical arteries in a normal foal at <24 hours after birth. (a) Caudal to the umbilical stump (view 5) with the urachus (U) and umbilical arteries on either side (LUA, left umbilical artery; RUA, right umbilical artery). (b) At the apex of the bladder (view 6). (c) LUA at the midpoint of the bladder (view 7). (d) RUA at the midpoint of the bladder (view 7). Images courtesy of Dr Tóth Balázs (a) and Dr Annette McCoy (b–d).

Interpretation

- Infection of the umbilical structures is a frequent issue in neonatal foals either as a primary infection (local spread) or secondary to bacteremia or septicemia (systemic spread). Infected structures appear enlarged in diameter, have a thickened wall, and accumulation of echogenic material. Infection may include any of the following structures: the umbilical vein (omphalophlebitis) (Figure 197.4a), the urachus (Figure 197.4b), or umbilical arteries (omphaloarteritis) (Figure 197.4c).
- A patent urachus is also common in neonatal foals and is encountered as a lack of atrophy or secondary to another pathology. If visible on ultrasound examination, the patent urachus appears as an anechoic lumen between the umbilical arteries that can be followed to the bladder (Figure 197.4b). Obtaining a longitudinal image is important in determining if an urachal diverticulum is present (tipped extension of bladder towards body wall).

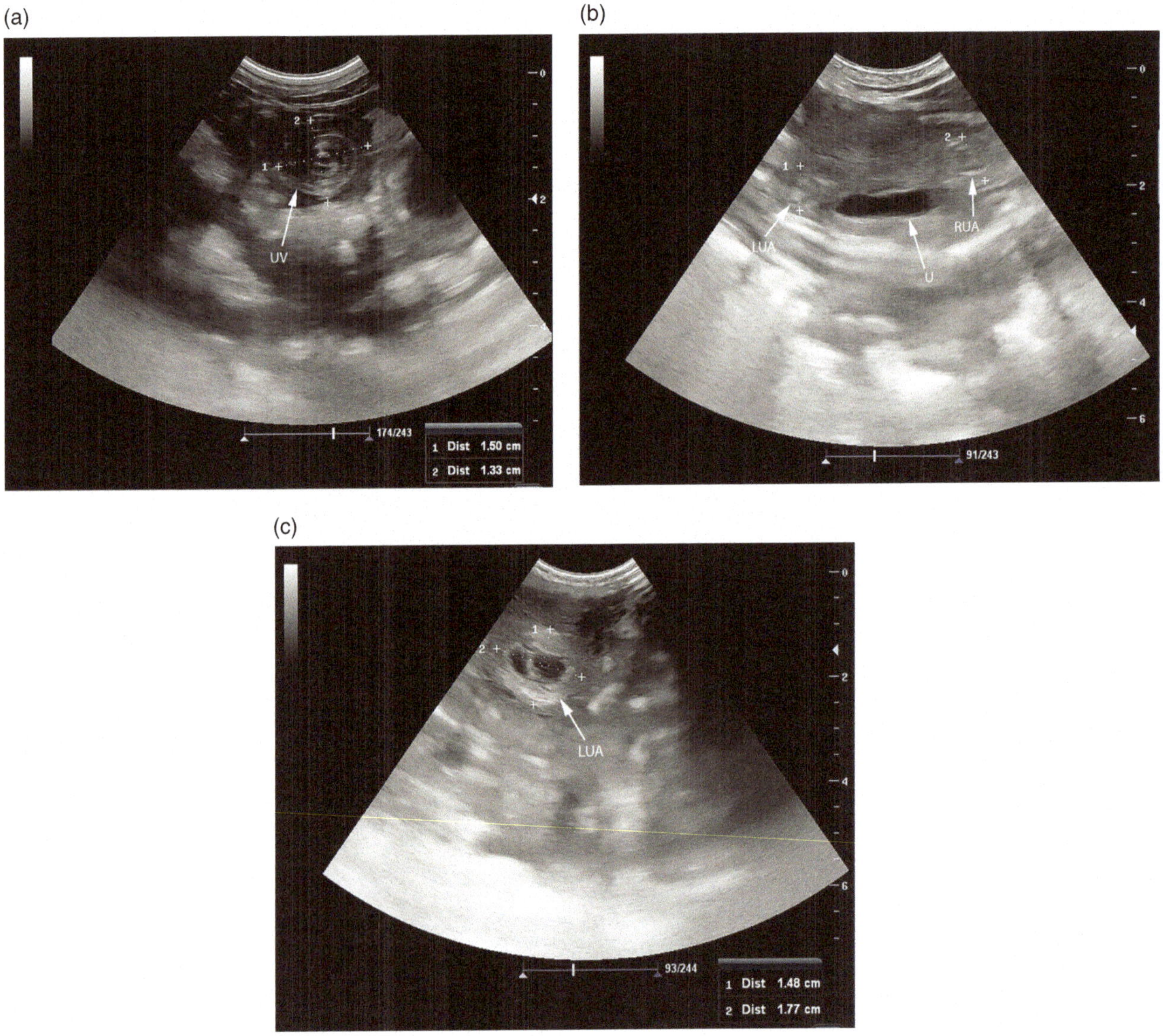

Figure 197.4 Transverse ultrasound images of abnormal umbilical structures. (a) Abnormal umbilical vein (UV) (omphalophlebitis) visualized mid distance between the umbilical stump and the liver (view 3). Note the enlarged diameter and thickened wall of the vein. (b) Patent urachus (U) imaged immediately caudal to the umbilical stump (view 5). Note the enlarged anechoic area between the two umbilical areas (LUA, left umbilical artery; RUA, right umbilical artery). (c) Abnormal umbilical artery (omphaloarteritis) visualized in proximity to the apex of the bladder (modified view 6). Note the enlarged diameter, thickened wall, and heterogenic content of the artery. Images courtesy of Dr Tóth Balázs.

Further Reading

Franklin RP, Ferrell, EA. 2002. How to perform umbilical sonograms in the neonate. *Proc Annu Conv Am Assoc Eq Pract* 48: 261–5.

Lavan RP, Craychee T. 1997. Practical method of umbilical ultrasonographic examination of one-week old foals: the procedure and the interpretation of age-correlated size ranges of umbilical structures. *J Eq Vet Sci* 17: 96–101.

McCoy AM, Lopp CT, Kooy S, Migliorisis A, Austin SM, Wilkins PA. 2020. Normal regression of internal umbilical remnant structures in Standardbred foal. *Eq Vet J* 00:1-8. https://doi.org/10.1111/evj.13267.

198

Management of Soft Tissue Laxity

Stacy Anderson

College of Veterinary Medicine, Lincoln Memorial University, USA

Introduction

Laxity of the flexor tendons and other soft tissues of the limb in foals is relatively common and can be quite severe. However, the overall prognosis is quite good with appropriate nursing care. The etiology of tendon laxity is unknown, but is often associated with dysmaturity and/or prematurity. The goal of caring for foals with tendon laxity is to prevent trauma to the delicate skin overlying important structures, such as joints. It is important not to over-support the foal's limb with splints as this usually exacerbates the laxity issue.

Equipment and Supplies

Bandage materials: combi-roll, sheet cotton, or rolled cotton; brown gauze, elastic cohesive bandage (Vetrap™), tongue depressors or glue-on shoes with extension, epoxyacrylic, area to confine foal (3.5 × 3.5 m (12 × 12 feet).

Technique

- The mare and foal should be confined to a stall or pen, no larger than 3.5 × 3.5 m (12 x 12 ft) until laxity improves.
- Controlled exercise in the form of short (10 minutes) walks may be used once or twice daily to strengthen soft tissues.
- Application of light-weight bandages are recommended to protect the limb, particularly if the fetlock hyperextends to the point that the proximal sesamoids bones are touching the ground. However, heavier support bandages are contraindicated as they do not allow for a normal increase in muscle–tendon tone.
- In cases of carpal laxity, restricted exercise is critical to prevent joint damage. No other treatment is generally necessary.
- Heel extensions may be used in cases of fetlock or coffin joint laxity, to increase the palmar/plantar-bearing surface of the foot in order to make the suspensory apparatus of the digit more effective (Figure 198.1). Heel extensions may be created from taped on tongue depressors, glue-on shoes, or epoxy acrylic (Figures 198.2 and 198.3).
- Glue-on heel extensions need to be removed after approximately 10 days and no more than 14 days after application and the foal re-evaluated.
- Note: some farriers advocate that glue-on shoes should not be applied to foals before they are at least 7–9 days of age as there is potential for damage from the heat generated by the epoxy methyl methacrylate acrylic glue.

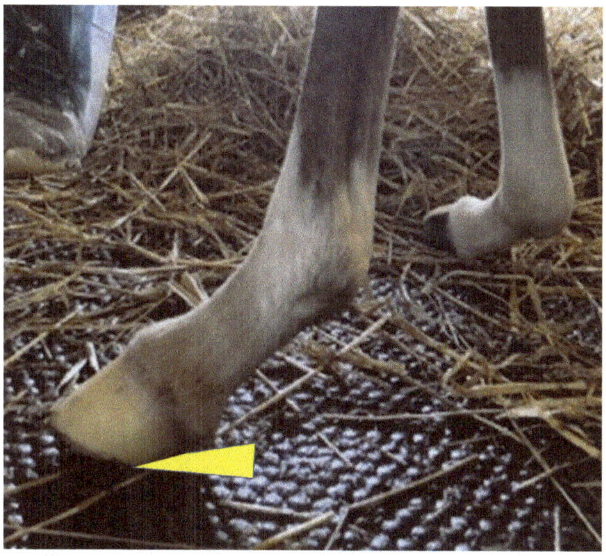

Figure 198.1 Foal with tendon laxity. A heel extension (represented by yellow wedge) would prevent the toe from lifting off the ground and allow the foal to bear weight on the bearing surface of the hoof.

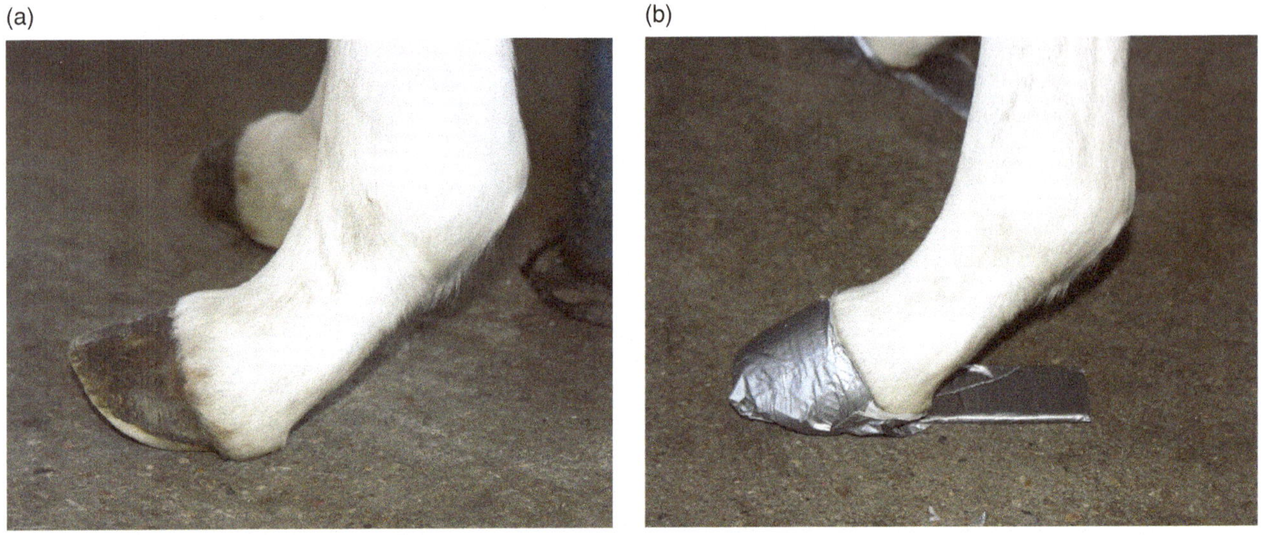

Figure 198.2 Foal with tendon laxity. Note the elevation of the toe (a). A temporary heel extension was applied using tongue depressors and duct tape (b). Unfortunately, taped-on heel extensions rarely remain in place longer than a few hours.

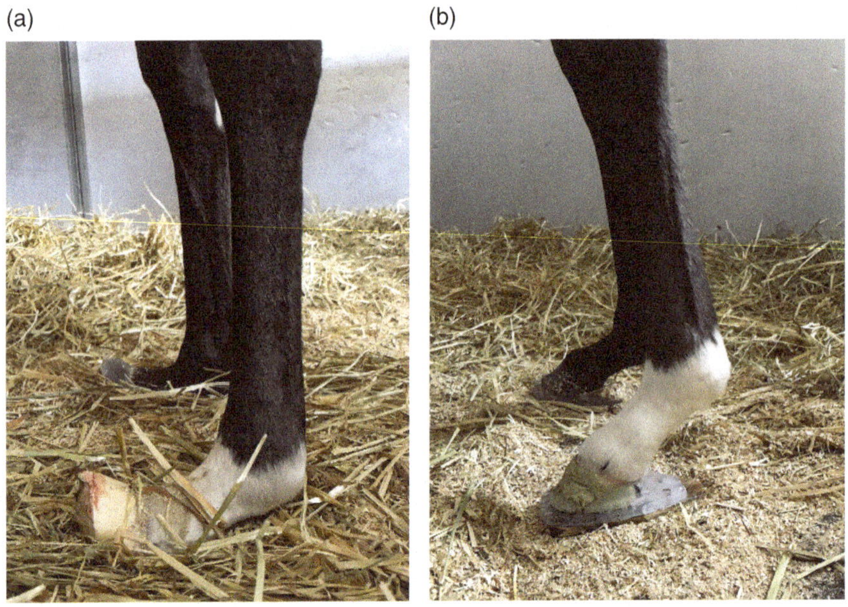

Figure 198.3 Foal with extreme tendon laxity at 20 hours of age. The foal is essentially standing on its heel bulb and pastern (a). A glue-on heel extension was subsequently applied (b).

- Joint laxity should improve within a few days of birth. It is critical to observe foals for the development of sores and to treat any open wounds appropriately with dressings using aseptic technique.

Additional Comments

- Foals with tendon laxity need to be monitored and managed closely over the first few days of life to prevent injury.
- Radiographs are usually not necessary; however, in some cases radiographs may be indicated to evaluate ossification of cuboidal carpal or tarsal bones or if a fracture of the sesamoid bones is suspected.
- Foals with tendon laxity so severe that they are unable to stand should be managed in a hospital setting.

Further Reading

Coleman MC, Whitfield-Cargile C. 2017. Orthopedic conditions of the premature and dysmature foal. *Vet Clin Eq* 33: 289–97.

199

Management of Angular Limb Deformities

Stacy Anderson

College of Veterinary Medicine, Lincoln Memorial University, USA

Introduction

Angular limb deformities (ALDs), deviation of the limb distal to a joint in the frontal plane, are very common in foals. Most common joints with ALD are the metacarpo(tarso)-phalangeal joint, carpus, and tarsus. Deviation of the limb laterally distal to the joint is termed valgus and deviation of the limb medially distal to the joint is termed varus (Figure 199.1).

Foals may be born with an ALD, or it may develop over time. Congenital ALDs are most commonly associated with perinatal complications, such as premature birth or dysmaturity, which leads to incomplete ossification of the cuboidal bones of the carpus or tarsus. When the foal bears weight on the partly cartilaginous bones, they may be crushed, resulting in a permanent deformity of the joint. It is important to differentiate incomplete ossification of the cuboidal bones from excessive joint laxity or limb deviation from lack of muscle using radiography. The etiology of acquired ALDs is unknown, but unbalanced nutrition, rapid growth, trauma, and pain may likely play a substantial role.

Regardless of the cause, if an ALD is not corrected within an appropriate time frame when growth is occurring at the physis, then the horse may have a permanently crooked leg and increased risk of unsoundness in the future. An ALD is best corrected when the physis proximal to the affected joint is going through rapid growth (Table 199.1); however, in cases with extreme deviation of the limb (>12 degrees) then intervention may be warranted earlier.

Equipment and Supplies

Radiography equipment, towel, sedation (benzodiazepine (midazolam or diazepam) 0.05 mg/kg IV, xylazine 0.3 mg/kg IV), farrier rasp, glue-on hoof cuffs with extensions, epoxy-acrylic, casting or splinting materials, area to confine foal.

Technique

- Determine which joint is affected through physical examination. The joint should be palpated for laxity. The foal should be observed standing still and plumb lines used to assess for deviations. It is also advised to watch the foal walk in order to observe for deviations in motion.
- Acquire a dorso-palmar (plantar) radiographic view of the affected joint to determine the point of deviation (Figure 199.2) and to ascertain that the bones are ossified. A lateral view, and potentially oblique views, should also be acquired to survey for bone abnormalities. On the dorso-palmar (plantar) view, two lines should be drawn

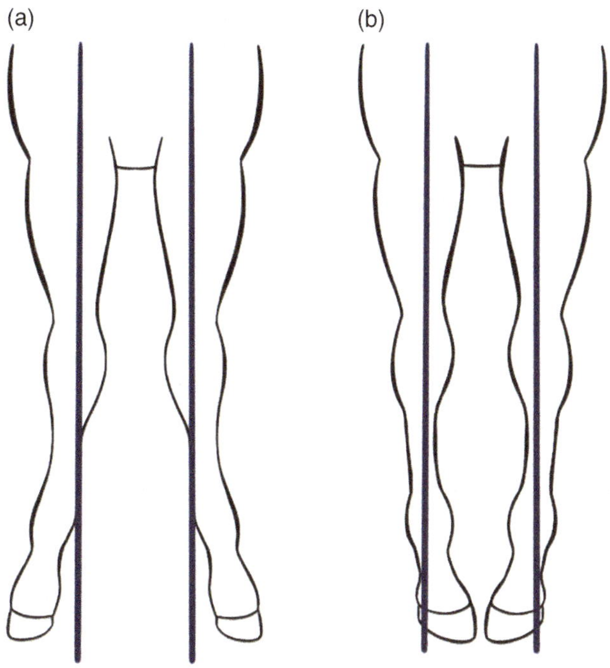

Figure 199.1 (a) A foal with carpal valgus. (b) A foal with fetlock varus.

Equine Reproductive Procedures, Second Edition. Edited by John Dascanio and Patrick McCue.

Table 199.1 Rapid growth period and physeal closure time for commonly affected physes.

Physis	Rapid Growth	Growth Complete
Distal radius	3–6, 8–10 months	15 months
Distal tibia	4–6 months	12 months
Distal metacarpus (tarsus)	2–3 months	5–7 months

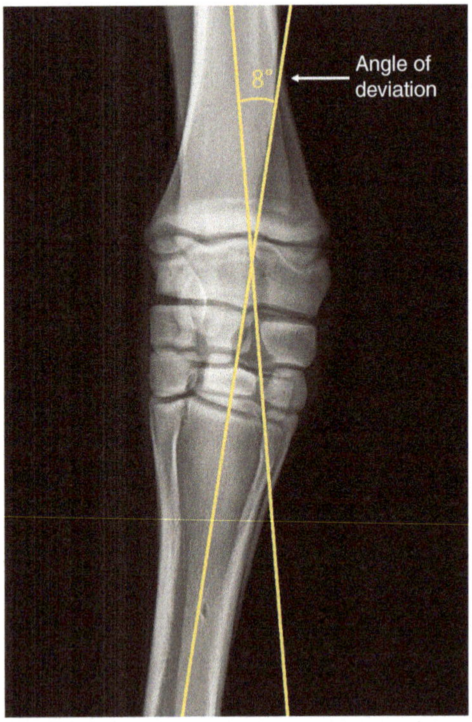

Figure 199.2 Dorso-palmar radiograph of the carpus demonstrating lines bisecting the radius and third metacarpal bone. In this image, the deviation of the limb occurs at the distal radial physis.

in the center of the long bone on either side of the affected joint. The point at which the lines bisect approximates the point of deviation. Deviation that occurs at a physis is amenable to intervention; whereas deviation that occurs within a complex joint is generally associated with malformation of that joint and carries a more guarded prognosis. The degree of deviation is used to guide treatment, with deviations greater than 12 degrees requiring more aggressive treatment, such as surgical intervention.

Management of Congenital ALDs

Management of foals with peri-articular ligament laxity or incomplete ossification of the cuboidal bones involves restricting exercise while the soft tissues gain strength or the bones continue to ossify, respectively. Sleeve casts or splints may be applied to reduce the development of angular limb deformities from crushed cuboidal bones with foals with incomplete ossification. Casts and splints are contraindicated for foal with peri-articular tendon laxity or to make a crooked leg straight as restricted movement will strengthen the peri-articular structures. Foals should improve within a few weeks.

To apply a sleeve cast:

- Sedate the foal (e.g., 0.05 mg/kg benzodiazepine IV).
- Place the foal in lateral recumbency, place a towel over the face to help quiet the foal, and protect the down eye from trauma.
- An assistant should hold the limbs in an anatomically correct position.
- A stockinette is applied in a double layer that should be smooth and fits snuggly. The cast will extend from the distal aspect of the elbow to proximal to the proximal sesamoid bones.
- Felt padding is wrapped circumferentially around the limb at the top and bottom aspects of the cast. The felt padding should be placed without tension and without gaps.
- Casting tape is wrapped evenly without tension, distal to proximal. At least three layers of cast material should be applied. The width of casting tape depends on the size of the foal, but should be 5–7.5 cm (2–3 inch) width on the first layer, with 7.5–10 cm (3–4 inch) width on subsequent layers.
- Following application, the foal must be monitored closely for development of cast sores by observing the foal for lameness and the cast for signs of discharge or strike-through. The cast should be replaced every 10–14 days until the cuboidal bones appear ossified on radiographs (this may take up to 4 weeks).
- When the cast is removed, soft tissue laxity will likely be present. The foal should be confined with restricted exercise until the soft tissue laxity improves.

Management of Acquired ALDs

Management of acquired ALDs in foals consists of altering the bearing surface of the hoof to change how the limb is loaded, which, in turn, alters growth at the physeal plate. The bearing surface may be altered through trimming or with hoof extensions. For trimming, the side of the hoof opposite to the direction of deviation is trimmed (Table 199.2). Similarly, hoof extensions are added on the side of the hoof opposite to the direction of deviation, or on the side of the leg that it should turn toward (Table 199.2 and Figure 199.3).

Table 199.2 Examples of locations for trimming and extensions in common cases of congenital angular limb deformities (ALDs).

ALD	Location of Extension	Side of Wall to Trim
Fetlock varus	Lateral	Medial
Carpal valgus	Medial	Lateral

To apply hoof cuffs shoes (Ibex Baby Cuffs; Anvil Brand, Lexington, IL, USA) with extensions:

- Clean and trim the hoof thoroughly. Rasp or dremel the periople from the hoof wall. For neonates, sand paper (180 grit) may also be used to remove the periople.
- Determine the type of extension and trim the plastic shoe accordingly with nippers or rasp. Fit the shoe to the foal's hoof.
- Apply epoxyacrylic product to the hoof and shoe. Follow the manufacturer's instructions. Generally, there are chemicals (acetone) that are applied to the hoof prior to the epoxyacrylic product to clean the hoof and to remove any oils.
- Alternatively, epoxyacrylic (Vettec Equi-Pak™; Vettec Animal Health, Orange, CA, USA) can be used to build the extension completely (Figure 199.3).
- The shoes or epoxyacrylic generally fall off on their own with wear, or should only be left on for 10–14 days as they will restrict hoof growth. Regardless, they should be removed once the limb straightens.

Surgical Management of ALDs

In foals with severe ALD (>12 degrees) or those nearing the end of the rapid growth phase at an affected physis (Table 199.1), surgical procedures are recommended. There are two different methods: growth acceleration or growth retardation.

- Growth acceleration is performed on the side of the limb that the distal deviation is toward (e.g., lateral side of a foal with a valgus deformity). Periosteal stripping is mostly commonly used to promote growth at the physis.
- Growth retardation is performed on the opposite side of the limb from the direction of the distal deviation (e.g., medial side of a foal with a valgus deformity). Growth retardation is most commonly achieved with a transphyseal bridge using metal implants, such as a single transphyseal screw or a transphyseal bridge (Figure 199.4). When implants are placed, it is critical that the foal is observed for correction of the deviation as the implants must be removed at that time to prevent over-correction.

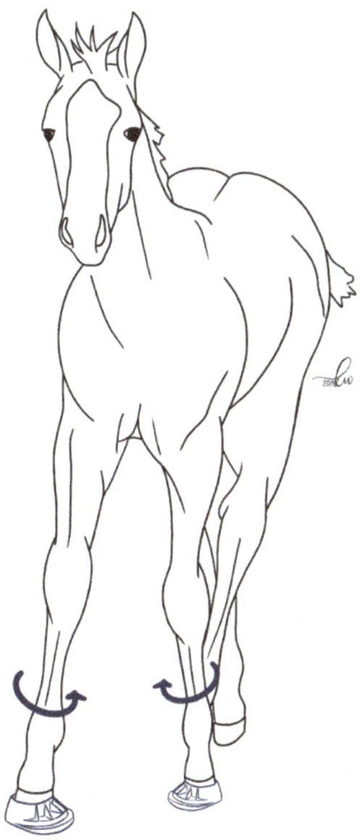

Figure 199.3 Foal with carpal valgus where medial extensions were applied to cause the limb to turn medial with each step. Drawing courtesy of Kaitlyn Wooton.

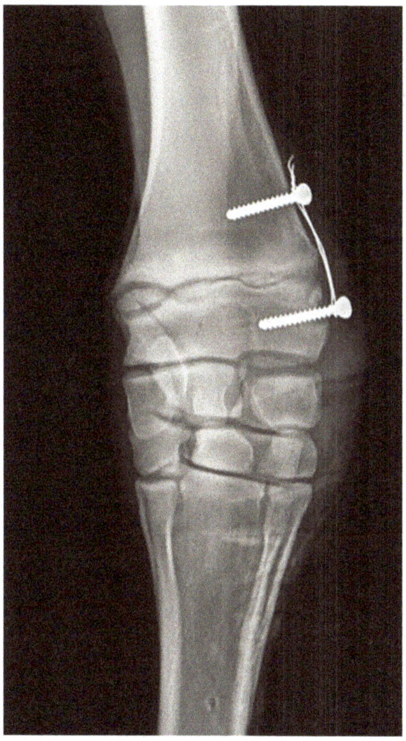

Figure 199.4 Radiographic image of a transphyseal bridge of screws and wires across the distal radial physis. Image courtesy of Dr Chris Bell.

Additional Comments

Owner compliance is critical to successfully managment of foals with ALDs. It is advised to frequently examine foals that are being treated for ALDs in order to have the best outcome. The frequency of examination depends on the severity of the ALD and the age of the foal. For severely affected foals, weekly examinations are advised.

There is also considerable difference of opinion on the management of ALDs among veterinarians, including the published literature.

Further Reading

Auer HA. 2012. Angular limb deformities. In: Auer JA, Stick JA (eds). Equine Surgery, 4th edn. St Louis, MO: Elsevier Saunders, pp. 1201–21.

García-López J. 2017. Angular limb deformities: growth augmentation. *Vet Clin Eq* 33: 343–51.

McCarrel TM. 2017. Angular limb deformities: growth retardation. *Vet Clin Eq* 33: 353–66.

200

Management of Congenital Flexural Limb Deformities

Stacy Anderson

College of Veterinary Medicine, Lincoln Memorial University, USA

Introduction

Flexural limb deformities may be congenital or acquired. The etiology for congenital flexural limb deformities is unknown, but could be due to uterine positioning, abnormal fetal development, or other perinatal factors. Acquired flexural limb deformities are associated with rapid growth and pain and will not be discussed further here. In the neonate, moderate to severe flexural deformities require aggressive treatment for maximum success. As a foal ages, the ability to correct deformities diminishes and once growth has ceased correction of flexural limb deformities is not possible. Flexural deformities that result in joint hyperextension are always congenital (see Chapter 198).

Flexural limb deformities are described by the joint affected. The most common joints affected are the coffin joint, fetlock joint, and carpus. The pastern joint may be affected, along with a fetlock deformity. The biomechanical properties of the affected joint or joints largely determines the techniques used to treat the problem. Carpal flexural deformities are often self-limiting (Figure 200.1) and may be associated with rupture of the common digital extensor tendon. Congenital fetlock flexural deformities are rare as a single problem and are often associated with carpal deformities. Coffin joint flexural deformities often require intervention due to impact on long-term soundness. Any cases of congenital flexural deformity that are not manually reducible are candidates for medical or, as a last resort, surgical intervention.

Neonatal foals (ideally within 3–5 days of birth) may be treated with oxytetracycline to correct congenital flexural deformities (Figure 200.2). It is thought that oxytetracycline chelates circulating calcium, which then reduces muscle contractility to relax the flexor muscles

Equipment and Supplies

Oxytetracycline (44 mg/kg), 1 liter sterile physiologic solution and intravenous administration set, intravenous catheter supplies, PVC pipe, oscillating saw, bandage materials (combi-roll, sheet cotton, or rolled cotton; brown gauze; VetRap™ or similar bandaging tape (optional)), duct tape, white medical tape or elastic adhesive bandage, epoxyacrylic or glue-on shoes with extensions, area to restrict foal (no larger than 3.5 × 3.5 m (12 × 12 feet), non-steroidal anti-inflammatory medication (ketoprofen, phenylbutazone, flunixin meglumine, firocoxib, or meloxicam), gastrointestinal protectants (omeprazole with or without) ranitidine, or sucralfate.

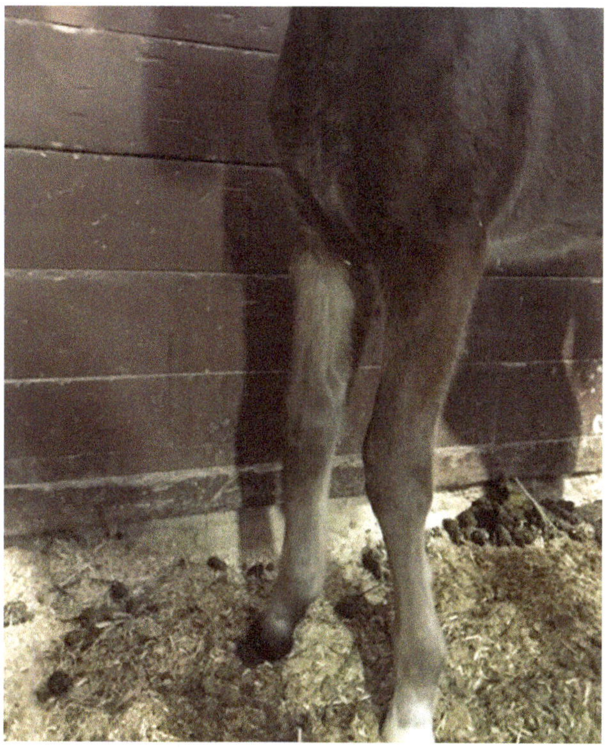

Figure 200.1 Foal with moderate carpal flexural limb deformity. Image courtesy of Dr Chris Bell.

Equine Reproductive Procedures, Second Edition. Edited by John Dascanio and Patrick McCue.

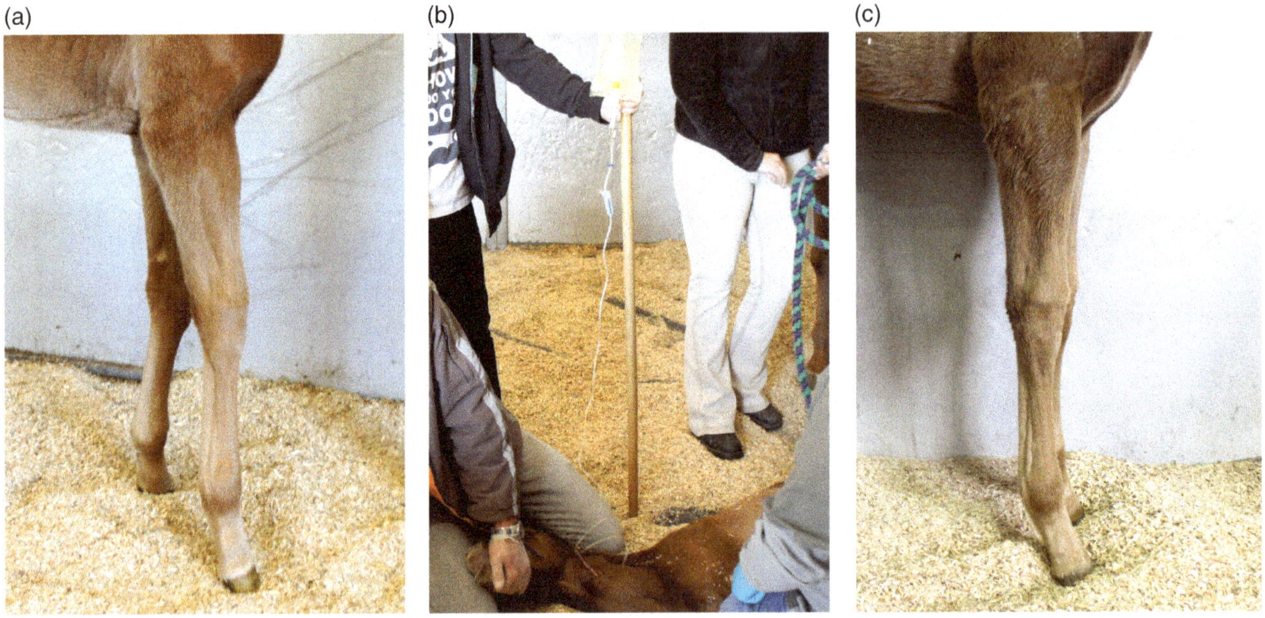

Figure 200.2 Foal with contracted tendons immediately before (a), during (b) and 48 hours after (c) oxytetracycline therapy.

Technique

- Examine the patient to determine the location of the flexural deformity. This may require physical manipulation of the limb with the foal recumbent if it cannot stand.
- Administer oxytetracycline:
  - Prior to administering oxytetracycline, a serum chemistry should be analyzed to determine that renal values (blood urea nitrogen and creatinine) are within normal limits.
  - Oxytetracycline is administered at 44 mg/kg IV in 1 liter of saline over 30–60 minutes. It may be repeated up to three times once daily within the first week of life.
- Pain management:
  - Full weight bearing is critical for the correction of flexural limb deformities, thus pain control is important.
  - Non-steroidal anti-inflammatory drugs (NSAIDs) should be used with caution in neonatal foals along with gastrointestinal protectants such as omeprazole (4 mg/kg orally once daily) in combination with ranitidine (6.6 mg/kg orally three times per day or 2 mg/kg IV twice daily) or sucralfate (4 g orally twice daily).
  - It is critical to acquire an accurate weight of the foal and use a single NSAID. Drugs and dosages for a neonatal foal are:
    - ketoprofen: 1.1–2.2 mg/kg IV once or twice daily
    - phenylbutazone: 1.1 mg/kg IV once or twice daily
    - flunixin meglumine: 1.1 mg/kg IV once or twice daily
    - firocoxib: 0.1 mg/kg (after 2.0 mg/kg loading dose) orally once or twice daily
    - meloxicam: 0.6 mg/kg orally twice daily.

Managing Flexural Deformities of the Carpus and Fetlock

- Bandaging and splinting are used for flexural deformities of the carpus and fetlock.
- Splints should be used when a flexural deformity is not manually reducible.
- Bandages should be thick enough to protect from pressure sores that can occur from splint application. Any materials may be used. It is best to use a secondary bandage layer of combi-roll, sheet cotton, or roll cotton, secured with a tertiary layer of brown roll gauze with or without a final layer of elastic cohesive bandage (VetRap™).
- Splints may be purchased commercially or made from material such as polyvinyl chloride (PVC) pipe. PVC pipe may be bought in different diameters that best conform to the foal's leg(s). An oscillating (i.e., cast) saw may be used to cut the pipe to fit the foal's bandaged leg. Casting tape may also be used to make a custom splint, although it has a tendency to break and bend more easily than PVC.
- Splints are placed on the flexor surface of the limb after a bandage is applied (Figure 200.3). For carpal deformities, a full limb splint is used. For fetlock deformities, a half

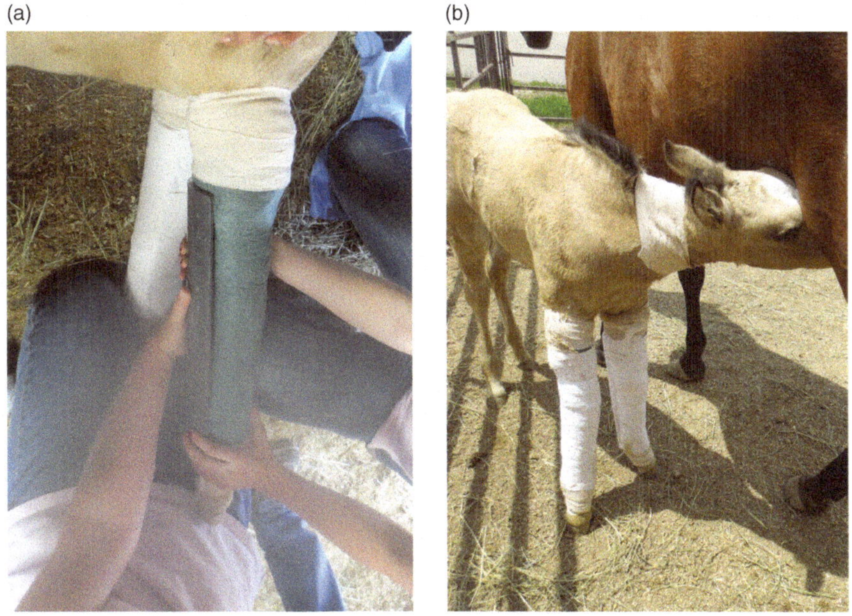

Figure 200.3 (a) Application of a splint on a foal with contracted tendons. (b) Same foal nursing from her mare while wearing splints.

limb splint is used. Splints may be held in place with duct tape, medical tape, or elastic adhesive bandage. If splints are held in place with duct tape, the entire limb should not be taped as the tape will cause the limb to sweat. The limb may need to be forced into the splint and held in place while an assistant tapes it in place.

- It is advisable to give the foal a break from the splints, depending on the severity of contracture. For example, the foal may be splinted for a 6–12 hours over a 24-hour period.

Managing Flexural Deformities of the Coffin Joint

- Toe extensions are used to address coffin joint flexural limb deformities.
- Toe extension may be made out of epoxy acrylic or glue-on shoes with toe extensions (Figure 200.4).
- To make an extension out of epoxy acrylic, a surface, such as cardboard, is place under the foot and extends beyond the toe farther out than the desired size of the toe extension. The foot is prepared by lightly rasping the periople and applying a drying agent, such as acetone. The epoxy acrylic is applied to the hoof and extended dorsally on the cardboard to the desired length of the toe extension.

Physical Therapy

- Exercise should be restricted for foals to prevent increased pain. If pain is not well controlled, exercise often causes the flexural deformity to become more severe. The mare and foal should be kept in a stall or small pen (3.5 × 3.5 m) while undergoing treatment.

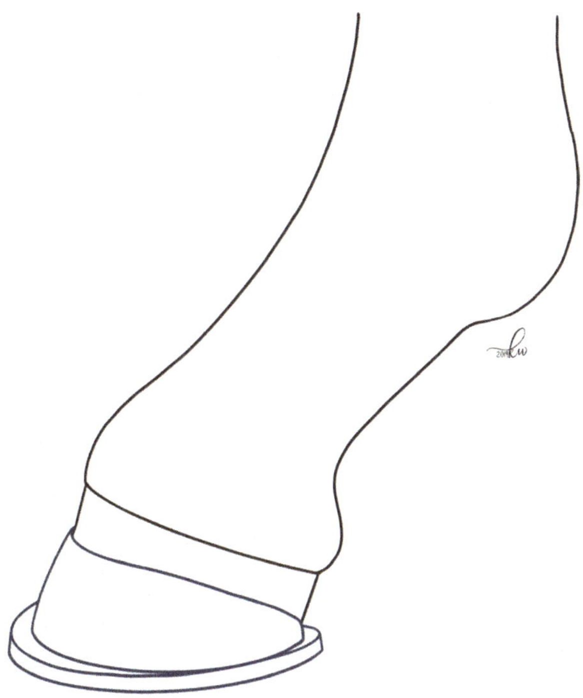

Figure 200.4 Coffin joint flexural deformity treated with a toe extension to encourage extension of the joint.

- Controlled exercise:
  - The foal may be allowed to follow its dam for exercise if pain is controlled and the flexural deformity is not severe.
- Massage:
  - The muscles of the caudal antebrachium can be massaged periodically (every 4–6 hours), particularly prior to stretching exercises.
- Stretches:
  - Standing the foal on the affected leg for 2–3 minutes at a time.
  - Manual extension of the flexed joints until the foal resents the stretch, for 15–30 seconds with repetition over 10–15 minutes a few times per day.

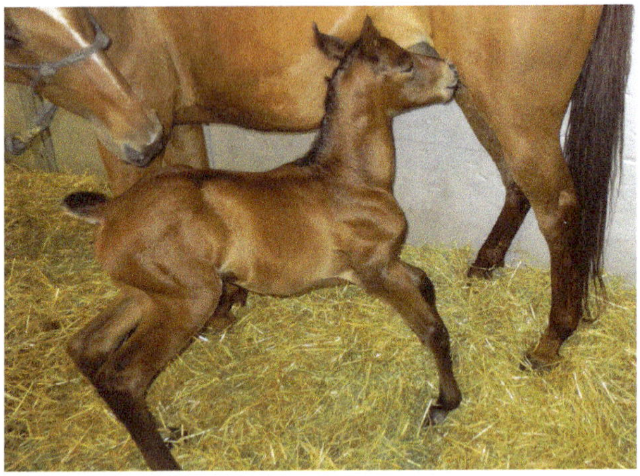

Figure 200.5 Foal with severely contracted tendons.

Additional Comments

Foals with severely contracted tendons (Figure 200.5) may not be able to nurse, which requires intensive management that is best done in a hospital. Surgical transection of the accessory ligament of the deep or superficial digital flexor tendon, or as a last resort the flexor tendons themselves, may be warranted in severe cases. The prognosis for athletic use in this cases is guarded.

Further Reading

Caldwell FJ. 2017. Flexural limb deformity of the distal interphalangeal joint. *Vet Clin Eq* 33: 315–30.

Gaughan EM. 2017. Flexural limb deformities of the carpus and fetlock in foals. *Vet Clin Eq* 33: 331–42.

Kidd JA. 2012. Flexural limb deformities. In: Auer JA, Stick JA (eds). Equine Surgery, 4th edn. St Louis, MO: Elsevier Saunders, pp. 1221–39.

Part VI

Appendices

Appendix A

Society for Theriogenology Stallion Reproductive Evaluation Form

Society for Theriogenology — Veterinarians Dedicated to Animal Reproduction

Society for Theriogenology

FOR USE BY MEMBERS ONLY

Stallion Reproductive Evaluation	
Owner Information	
Name:	Boarding Farm:
Address:	
Telephone:	Fax:
Stallion Information	
Name:	Age:
Breed:	Color/Tattoo:
Current Use:	Microchip:
Intended Use:	
Date of Evaluation:	
Location of Evaluation:	
Evaluator:	
History:	
General Physical Findings:	

Genital Physical Findings		
Method of Measurements:		
	Left Testicle	Right Testicle
Length (cm)		
Width (cm)		
Height (cm)		
vol = $\frac{4}{3}\pi$ x ½L x ½W x ½H Volume (cc)		
	Total Volume:	
	Total Scrotal Width:	

Equine Reproductive Procedures, Second Edition. Edited by John Dascanio and Patrick McCue.

Stallion: 2

Semen Evaluation			
Method of Semen Collections:			
Use of Jump Mare/Phantom:			
Computer Assisted Semen Analysis:	Yes	No	
Use of Semen Extender:	Yes	No	Type:

	Ejaculate 1	Ejaculate 2	Ejaculate 3
Time			
Libido			
Erection			
Number of Mounts			
Breeding Ability			
Volume (gel free)			
Volume Gel			
Gross Appearance			
Concentration Method			
Concentration (x10^6/ml)			
Total Sperm Number			
Total Motility (%)			
Total No. Motile Sperm			
Progressive Motility (%)			
Total # Progressively Motile Sperm			
Method of Evaluating Morphology:			
% Normal Sperm			
% Detached Heads			
% Abnormal Heads			
% Abnormal Acrosomes			
% Abnormal Midpieces			
% Bent Midpieces			
% Tail Bent			
% Tail Coiled			
% Proximal Droplets			
% Distal Droplets			
% Round Cells			
% Other			

Consistency of Testicles:
Comments:
Penis:
Internal Evaluation of Accessory Sex Glands:

Stallion: 3

Sperm Longevity			**Method**		
1st Ejaculate			2nd Ejaculate		
Date:	% Total Motility		Date:	% Total Motility	
	% Prog. Motility			% Prog. Motility	
Date:	% Total Motility		Date:	% Total Motility	
	% Prog. Motility			% Prog. Motility	
Date:	% Total Motility		Date:	% Total Motility	
	% Prog. Motility			% Prog. Motility	
Date:	% Total Motility		Date:	% Total Motility	
	% Prog. Motility			% Prog. Motility	

Semen Cytology:

Aerobic Bacterial Cultures

Penis:

Fossa Glandis:

Pre-ejaculatory Urethra:

Post-ejaculatory Urethra:

EVA	Positive	Negative	Unknown
EIA	Positive	Negative	Unknown

Ancillary Tests or Procedures:

Misc. Observations:

Interpretive Summary:

Date of Report: **Evaluator:**

Appendix B

Mare Breeding Soundness Evaluation Form

Examination Date: ____________________

Registered Name: ________________________ **Owner Name**: ________________________
Registration #: ______________ Breed__________ Address: ________________________
Year of Birth: __________ Color: ______________ ________________________
Description: ________________________ Phone #: ________________________
________________________ Fax #: ________________________
________________________ Email: ________________________

Reproductive History:

Reproductive History: ____

____

Last Foal: ____________ # Foals (lifetime): _____ Breeding Management: ________________

Physical Examination:

Comments: ____

Teasing Behavior:

Current Status: In Heat / Out / Indifferent

Comments: ________________________

Perineal Conformation:

Vulva Angle: __________ Tone: __________

Comments: ________________ Caslick: Yes / No

Palpation and Ultrasonography (*per rectum*):

Ovaries: Left: ____________________ Right: ____________________
Uterus: ____________________ Cervix: ____________________
Comments: ____

____

Vaginal Speculum Examination:

Comments: ____________________

____

Digital Examination of Cervix:

Comments: ____________________

____

Uterine Culture:

Method: Swab / Brush / Lavage / Biopsy
Results: No growth / Positive Culture
Organism # 1: ____________________
Organism # 2: ____________________
Organism # 3: ____________________
Laboratory Report Attached

Endometrial Cytology:

Method: Swab / Brush / Lavage / Biopsy
Stain: Diff-Quick / Other: ______________
Results: Normal / Abnormal
Comments: ________________________

____

Laboratory Report Attached

Equine Reproductive Procedures, Second Edition. Edited by John Dascanio and Patrick McCue.

Endometrial Biopsy:

Fixative: ______________ # Biopsy Samples / Location: ______________

Interpretation: ______________

____

Grade: I / IIa / IIb / III (circle one) Other: ______________ Laboratory Report Attached

Additional Diagnostic Tests: (Hormone Analysis, Hysteroscopy, Karyotype, Other)

Test # 1: ______________

Results: ______________ Laboratory Report Attached

Test # 2: ______________

Results: ______________ Laboratory Report Attached

Test # 3: ______________

Results: ______________ Laboratory Report Attached

Summary of Breeding Soundness Evaluation:

____

____

____

____

____

Management or Treatment Plan:

____

____

____

____

____

Clinician Signature: ______________ Date: ______________

Clinician Name: ______________ (print)

Clinic Name: ______________

Address: ______________

____

____

Phone (Office): ______________ Fax #: ______________

Phone (Cell): ______________ email: ______________

Appendix C

Formulary for Equine Reproduction

The authors make no warranties concerning the accuracy of the information within this formulary. Some drugs may be used in an extra-label manner. The use of information in this formulary is the sole responsibility of the practitioner with a valid client–patient–veterinary relationship.

Hormones

Medication	Dosage, route, frequency	Indications
Altrenogest (2.2 mg/ml)	0.044 mg/kg orally, every 24 hours	Suppression of behavioral estrus, synchronization of estrus, maintenance of pregnancy
Altrenogest (2.2 mg/ml)	0.088 mg/kg orally, every 24 hours or 0.044 mg/kg orally, every 12 hours (double dose)	Maintenance of pregnancy in high risk mares
Buserelin	10–50 μg IM, every 6–12 hours	Gonadotropin-releasing hormone (GnRH) agonist; stimulation of follicular development in anestrous, transitional, or acyclic mares
Carbetocin	0.14 mg IV or IM, every 12 hours	Stimulation of uterine contractions (evacuation of uterine fluid); longer duration of action than oxytocin; half-life of carbetocin is 17.2 minutes vs 6.8 minutes for oxytocin
Cloprostenol (250 μg/ml)	250 μg IM, once 50 μg IM, every 24 hours, repeated on consecutive days for 2–3 treatments	Termination of luteal activity, synchronization of estrus, termination of pregnancy, stimulation of uterine contractions (evacuation of uterine fluid); should not be administered in the early post-ovulation period due to adverse effects on development of the corpus luteum. Low dose protocol may be indicated for mares with reaction to prostaglandin F or with health issues such as laminitis
Cloprostenol (250 μg/ml)	750–1,000 μg IM, once	Stimulation of maternal behavior in a potential nurse mare approximately 15–20 minutes prior to introduction of orphan foal
Clostrostenol (250 μg/ml)	250 μg, every 12 hours on days 0, 1, and 2 post-ovulation and then every 24 hours on days 3 and 4 post-ovulation	Antiluteogenic dose
Cloprostenol (250 μg/ml)	750–1,000 μg IM	Stimulation of maternal behavior
Deslorelin acetate (2.1 mg implant)	2.1 mg SQ, once	Sustained release implant preparation of the GnRH agonist (Ovuplant™) used for induction of ovulation; implant may be removed after ovulation is confirmed
Deslorelin acetate (1.5 mg/ml)	0.5–1.5 mg IM, once	Sustained release preparation of the GnRH agonist used for induction of ovulation; anecdotal reports suggest the effective dose range is 0.5–1.8 mg
Deslorelin (low dose)	10–50 μg IM, every 6–12 hours	Aqueous preparation of the GnRH agonist used to stimulate follicular development in anestrous, transitional, or acyclic mares

Equine Reproductive Procedures, Second Edition. Edited by John Dascanio and Patrick McCue.

Medication	Dosage, route, frequency	Indications
Dinoprost tromethamine (5 mg/ml)	5–10 mg IM, once 2 mg IM, every 24 hours, repeated on consecutive days for 2–3 treatments	Termination of luteal activity, synchronization of estrus, termination of pregnancy, stimulation of uterine contractions (evacuation of uterine fluid); should not be administered in the early post-ovulation period due to adverse effects on development of the corpus luteum. Low dose protocol may be indicated for mares with reaction to prostaglandin F or with health issues such as laminitis
Dinoprost tromethamine (5 mg/ml)	10 mg, every 12 hours on days 0, 1, and 2 post-ovulation and then every 24 hours on days 3 and 4 post-ovulation	Antiluteogenic dose
Domperidone (110 mg/ml)	1.1 mg/kg PO, every 24 hours 1.1 mg/kg PO, every 12 hours or 2.2 mg/kg PO, every 24 hours for 2–3 days	Dopamine antagonist; stimulation of lactation (agalactia) in postpartum mares, induction of lactation in non-pregnant mares, treatment of fescue toxicosis, induction of follicular development in transitional mares. Typically start 10–15 days prior to expected foaling date for fescue treatment. Higher dosages may be indicated for agalactic mares with no udder development after foaling
Estradiol (E_2)	5–10 mg IM, every 24 hours	Stimulation of behavioral estrus in ovariectomized mares; used in conjunction with progesterone for estrus synchronization; used in combination with domperidone for stimulation of lactation in nurse mares
Estradiol cypionate (ECP)	10 mg IM, as needed	Stimulation of behavioral estrus in ovariectomized mares (long acting)
Histrelin (1.0 mg/ml)	0.5 to 1.0 mg, IM, once	GnRH agonist; used for induction of ovulation
Histrelin (low dose)	10-50 µg IM, every 6–12 hours	GnRH agonist used to stimulate follicular development in anestrous, transitional, or acyclic mares
Human chorionic gonadotropin (hCG) (10,000 units/vial)	1,500–3,000 units IV or IM, once	Induction of ovulation
Human chorionic gonadotropin (hCG) (10,000 units/vial)	10,000 units IV or IM, once	hCG stimulation test to evaluate male horse for presence of testicular tissue (testosterone response); also administered once per week for 4 weeks in an attempt to induce testicular descent in cryptorchid stallions (rarely successful)
Gonadotropin-releasing hormone (GnRH), native	25–100 µg IV or IM, every 6–12 hours	Stimulation of follicular development in transitional mares
Gonadotropin-releasing hormone (GnRH), native	500 µg IV or IM, once, 1–2 hours prior to breeding or collection	Increase libido in stallions with low libido
Oxytocin (20 IU/ml)	20 IU IV or IM, every 6–24 hours or as needed	Stimulation of uterine contractions (evacuation of uterine fluid), treatment of retained placenta, milk letdown, induction of labor
Oxytocin (20 IU/ml)	60 IU IM, every 12 hours on days 7–14 post-ovulation	Suppression of behavioral estrus; mechanism of action is development of a persistent corpus luteum. Prevents luteolysis by inhibiting increase in endometrial oxytocin receptors thus preventing prostaglandin F secretion
Oxytocin (low dose) (20 IU/ml)	5–10 IU IV or IM, as needed	Low dose protocol for induction of labor: administer 5 units followed by 10 units 15 minutes later; a majority of full-term mares will rupture their chorioallantoic within 5–15 minutes after the second dose of oxytocin
Progesterone-in-oil (P_4) (50 mg/ml)	150 mg IM, every 24 hours	Suppression of behavioral estrus; synchronization of estrus and ovulation
Progesterone-in-oil (P_4) (50 mg/ml)	200 mg IM, every 24 hours	Maintenance of pregnancy
Progesterone (long acting) (150 or 300 mg/ml)	1,500 mg IM, every 7 days	Suppression of behavioral estrus, synchronization of estrus, maintenance of pregnancy

Medication	Dosage, route, frequency	Indications
Progesterone/ estradiol (P&E) (50 mg P_4/3.3 mg E_2)	150 mg P_4/10 mg E_2 IM, every 24 hours	Synchronization of estrus, "programming" time of ovulation in transitional mares, suppression of estrus
Prostaglandin E_1 (misoprostol) (100 or 200 µg/tablet)	1,000–2,000 µg, topically onto cervix, as needed	Cervical relaxation. Crush or dissolve tablets and place into sterile lubricant; place onto/into cervix with syringe and/or pipette
Prostaglandin E_1 (misoprostol) (100 or 200 µg/tablet)	200 µg	Dissolve tablet(s) into 3 ml of sterile saline; administer by deep horn infusion; used to resolve presumptive oviductal blockage
Prostaglandin E_2 (dinoprostone cervical gel) (0.2 mg/ml)	1.0 ml gel applied to surface of each oviduct	Applied to surface of oviducts via laparoscope to "unblock" oviducts suspected of luminal blockage with gelatinous masses that contain fibroblast cells
Sulpiride 5% suspension (50 mg/ ml)	0.5–1.0 mg/kg IM, every 12–24 hours	Dopamine antagonist; stimulation of lactation in postpartum mares, induction of lactation in non-pregnant mares, stimulation of follicular development in transitional mares

Intrauterine Therapy

Medication	Dosage, route, frequency	Indications
Acetylcysteine solution (20%) (200 mg/ml)	30 ml (6 g) diluted into 150 ml sterile saline infused into uterus	Mucolytic; management of chronic uterine inflammation
Amikacin sulfate (250 mg/ml)	1–2 g; buffer with equal volume of sodium bicarbonate (8.4%) then take the volume up to 50–100 ml with sterile saline	Antibiotic (Gram-negative spectrum)
Amphoteracin B (50 mg/vial)	100–200 mg, reconstitute in 50–100 ml sterile saline	Antifungal agent
Ampicillin (1 g vial)	1–2 g, reconstitute in 50–100 ml sterile saline	Antibiotic (Gram-positive spectrum primarily)
Ceftiofur (1 g vial)	1 g, reconstitute in 20–60 ml sterile water	Antibiotic (broad spectrum)
Ciprofloxacin	400–500 mg; reconstituted to 50–100 ml in sterile saline	Antibiotic (broad spectrum)
Clotrimazole	500–700 mg in 50–100 ml sterile saline	Antifungal agent
Fluconazole (200 mg/tablet)	100–250 mg in 50–100 ml sterile water; to reconstitute, add 5 ml dimethyl sulfoxide (DMSO) to 1 g (5 tablets) of fluconazole to dissolve; divide into four aliquots of 250 mg each; take the volume up to 50–100 ml with sterile water	Antifungal agent
Gentamicin (100 mg/ml)	1–2 g; buffer equal volume of 8.4% sodium bicarbonate; take the volume up to 50–100 ml sterile saline	Antibiotic (Gram-negative spectrum)
Kerosene (K-1)	250–500 ml (do not dilute)	Chemical curettage of the uterus: infuse into uterus with disposable tubing; lavage uterus the next day and daily thereafter as needed
Lufenuron (270 mg/ packet)	540 mg in uterus suspended in 60 ml sterile saline; 270 mg applied to vaginal vault and clitoral area	Treatment of fungal endometritis (specifically for yeast organisms with chitin in cell wall); inhibits chitin formation; most effective on early stages of fungal growth
Miconazole (1,200 mg insert)	1,200 mg insert deposited into uterus	Antifungal agent

Medication	Dosage, route, frequency	Indications
Nystatin (100,000 USP units/vial)	5 g or 500,000 USP units in 50–100 ml sterile saline	Antifungal agent
Penicillin (potassium) (5 million units/vial)	5 million units, reconstitute in 50–100 ml sterile saline	Antibiotic (Gram-positive spectrum)
Penicillin (procaine) (300,000 units/ml)	15 ml, dilute to 50–100 ml in sterile saline	Antibiotic (Gram-positive spectrum)
Ticarcillin/clavulanic acid (3.1 g/vial)	3.1 g, reconstitute to 50–100 ml in sterile saline	Antibiotic combination; clavulanate blocks penicillinase; used for Gram-positive organisms and *Pseudomonas aeruginosa*

Uterine Lavage and Infusion

Medication	Dosage, route, frequency	Indications
Ceragyn™	60 ml; uterine infusion	Antimicrobial peptide mimic; treatment of infectious endometritis; reduction of biofilm
Dimethyl sulfoxide (DMSO) (99%)	50–200 ml DMSO per liter saline; may repeat as needed; follow with lavage with 1 liter saline or lactated Ringer's solution (LRS)	Anti-inflammatory; uterine lavage to decrease mucus production; may enhance antibiotic penetration into endometrium; avoid concentrations >30% which may cause severe endometrial irritation
Hydrogen peroxide (3%)	60–120 ml infused into uterus; follow the next day with lavage using sterile saline or LRS	Treatment of fungal endometritis; reduction of biofilm; use only during estrus as foaming action of hydrogen peroxide may cause uterine distension with closed cervix
Lactated Ringer's solution (LRS)	1–4+ liters; repeat lavage until effluent fluid is clear	Uterine lavage (note: neutral pH)
Povidone-iodine solution	5–10 ml of 10% iodine added to 1 liter sterile saline	Treatment of bacterial or fungal endometritis; may also add povidone-iodine to tap water for uterine lavage of postpartum mare, mare with retained placenta, or mare with a pyometra
Saline (0.9%)	1–4+ liters; repeat lavage until effluent fluid is clear	Uterine lavage (note: acidic pH c. 5.5) Note: non-sterile saline (0.95%) can be made by adding 35 g of table salt (NaCI) into 4 liters of tap water
Tris-EDTA	250–500 ml infused into uterus; then lavage uterus with LRS	Chelator of heavy metals; used as uterine infusion prior to antimicrobial therapy to reduce chelation and subsequent inactivation of antimicrobial agents; reduction of biofilm Can be purchased commercially or prepared by dissolving a 20 g packet of disodium EDTA and 2-amino-2-hydroxymetheyl-1,3-propanediol in 3.78 liters of sterile distilled water over heat with constant stirring. Adjust pH to 7.1 with 1 N HCI. Store aliquots of 500 ml in sterile containers in the dark at 15–30°C (60–85°F) Alternative formula for Tris-EDTA: • Add 1.211 g Tris to 10 ml deionized water to yield 1 M Tris. Adjust pH to 7.5–8.0 • Add 0.37 g EDTA to 2 ml deionized water to yield 0.5 M EDTA. Adjust pH to 8.0 • Add the 10 ml of 1 M Tris plus the 2 ml of 0.5 M EDTA to 988 ml of deionized water • Mix with stir bar until homogenous
Vinegar (distilled white) (2%)	20–100 ml added to 1 liter sterile saline	Treatment of fungal endometritis

Systemic Antibiotics

Medication	Dosage, route, frequency	Indications
Amikacin	10 mg/kg IV or IM, every 24 hours	Antibiotic (Gram-negative spectrum); used in equine reproduction for treatment of bacterial endometritis; chronic administration or administration to a dehydrated horse may result in acute renal failure
Ceftiofur crystalline free acid (200 mg/ml)	6.6 mg/kg IM, two doses 4 days apart	Long-acting antibiotic (broad spectrum); used in equine reproduction for treatment of bacterial endometritis; maximum of 20 ml per injection site
Ceftiofur sodium (50 mg/ml)	2.2–4.4 mg/kg IV or IM, every 12–24 hours	Antibiotic (broad spectrum); used in equine reproduction for treatment of bacterial endometritis; potential for diarrhea with intravenous administration
Doxycyline 100 mg/tablet	10 mg/kg PO, every 12 hours	Variable Gram-positive and Gram-negative spectrum. Less associated with fetal affects when given during pregnancy than oxytetracycline (i.e., discolored deciduous teeth and delayed skeletal development)
Enrofloxacin (50 or 100 mg/ml)	5 mg/kg IV, every 24 hours or 7.5 mg/kg PO, every 24 hours	Antibiotic (broad spectrum); used in equine reproduction for treatment of bacterial endometritis, specifically for resistant *Pseudomonas* species. Note that intrauterine therapy is associated with severe necrosis and is not recommended
Gentamicin (100 mg/ml)	6.6 mg/kg IV or IM, every 24 hours	Antibiotic (Gram-negative spectrum); used in equine reproduction for treatment of bacterial endometritis; chronic administration or administration to a dehydrated horse may result in acute renal failure
Penicillin (potassium)	22,000 IU/kg IV, every 6 hours	Antibiotic (Gram-positive spectrum); used in equine reproduction for treatment of bacterial endometritis; often combined with aminoglycoside for broader antibiotic coverage
Penicillin (procaine) (300,000 units/ml)	22,000 IU/kg IM, every 12 hours	Antibiotic (Gram-positive spectrum); used in equine reproduction for treatment of bacterial endometritis; severe procaine reactions may be observed after administration to susceptible horses
Trimethoprim-sulfadiazine (400 mg/ml suspension; 400 mg/g powder)	24 mg/kg suspension PO, every 12 hours for 10 days or as needed	Antibiotic (broad spectrum); used in equine reproduction for treatment of mares with chronic endometritis or pregnant mares with bacterial placentitis
	30 mg/kg powder PO, every 24 hours for 5–7 days or as needed	
Trimethoprim-sulfamethoxasole (960 mg tablet)	30 mg/kg PO, every 12 hours	Antibiotic (broad spectrum); used in equine reproduction for treatment of mares with chronic endometritis or pregnant mares with bacterial placentitis

Systemic Antifungal Agents

Medication	Dosage, route, frequency	Indications
Fluconazole (200 mg/tablet)	14 mg/kg PO, loading dose, followed by 5 mg/kg, every 24 hours	Antifungal agent
Itraconazole	5 mg/kg PO, every 24 hours for 2–3 weeks or longer	Antifungal agent

Miscellaneous Medications

Medication	Dosage, route, frequency	Indications
Acepromazine (10 mg/ml)	10–20 mg IV, once	Sedation; relaxation of cervix prior to embryo transfer
Aminocaproic acid (250 mg/ml)	Loading dose: 40 mg/kg Maintenance dose: 10–20 mg/kg, every 6 hours	Blocks plasminogen; antifibrinolytic (management of ruptured uterine artery)
Benztropine (1 mg/ml)	8 mg IV, once	Priapism in stallions or geldings (administer early in course of disease)
Cabergoline	2–3 mg PO, every 12–24 hours for 500 kg mare	Suppression of lactation
Calcium gluconate (23% solution)	Add 100–150 ml to 1 liter of LRS; administer IV over 45–60 minutes	Adjunct treatment for retained placenta in hypocalcemic mares
Clenbuterol (72.5 μg/ml)	2.0 μg/kg PO, every 12 hours	Tocolytic agent; used to block uterine contractions during impending abortion or dystocia. May cause cervical relaxation. Higher doses are associated with signs of anxiety, increased heart rate, and sweating. Lower the dose or discontinue if these signs occur
Dexamethasone (2 mg/ml)	30–50 mg IV or IM, once at time of mating or insemination	Anti-inflammatory; management of persistent mating-induced endometritis
Diazepam (5 mg/ml)	0.05 mg/kg, 5–7 minutes before breeding or collection	Reduces anxiety in stallions with ejaculation problems
Firocoxib (57 mg tablet)	Loading dose: 0.3 mg/kg PO, once Daily dose: 0.1 mg/kg PO, every 24 hours	Non-steroidal anti-inflammatory drug; selective COX-2 inhibitor; used in treatment of placentitis
Flunixin meglumine (50 mg/ml)	1.1 mg/kg IV (injectable) or PO (paste), every 12–24 hours	Anti-inflammatory, antiprostaglandin; administered prior to transfer of an embryo; treatment of placentitis
Formal buffered saline (FBS) or phosphate buffered formalin (10%, pH 6.8–7.0)	A minimum 10:1 ratio of FBS to tissue is recommended; tissue size should be 1–3 cm^3	Fixation of tissue for histopathology, such as uterine biopsies. Can be purchased commercially or prepared using the following recipe: Formalin (40% formaldehyde solution) – 100 ml Distilled water – 900 ml $NaH_2PO_42H_2O$ – 4.5 g $Na2HPO_4$ – 6.5 g
Imipramine (50 mg/tablet)	1.76–2.2 mg/kg PO, administered 1–2 hours prior to xylazine	Used in chemical ejaculation of stallions; lowers the ejaculation threshold
Meclofenamic acid	2.2 mg/kg PO, every 12 hours	Prostaglandin inhibitor potentially used as adjunct therapy in embryo transfer
Mycobacterium cell wall fraction immunostimulant (1.5 ml vial)	1.5 ml via intrauterine infusion or IV injection during early estrus (repeat as needed)	Immunostimulant; administered to mares with endometritis caused by *Streptococcus equi* subspecies *zooepidemicus*. Therapeutic goal is to enhance the innate humoral immune response in affected mares
N-butylscopolammonium bromide (20 mg/ml)	0.08–0.12 mg/kg IV (40–60 mg) administered 5–10 minutes prior to palpation	Relaxation of smooth muscle in the rectum; used to facilitate safe palpation or ultrasonography of the reproductive tract per rectum; may also relax uterine and cervical smooth muscle when administered systemically

Medication	Dosage, route, frequency	Indications
N-butylscopolammonium bromide cream	Topical cream	Cervical relaxation
Naloxone	0.03 mg/kg IV	Postpartum hemorrhage
Pentoxifylline	8.4 mg/kg PO, every 6–8 hours	Management of placentitis
Pergolide	0.002–0.004 mg/kg (1–2 mg total dose) PO, every 24 hours for 500 kg mare	Treatment of equine Cushing disease; suppression of lactation
Perphenazine	0.3–0.5 mg/kg PO, every 8 hours	Fescue toxicosis
Phenylephrine hydrochloride (0.25%)	Topical in vaginal vault	Vasoconstrictive agent; topical treatment for bleeding vaginal varicose veins
Propanetheline bromide	30 mg IV, once	Rectal relaxation; wait 5–10 minutes after administration prior to palpation
Reserpine	0.006 mg/kg, IM; once every 2 to 3 weeks or 2.5 mg (adult horses), PO, once daily; as needed	Management of agalactia, and behavioral modification
Sodium bicarbonate (8.4%)	10–20 ml added to aminoglycoside antibiotic prior to intrauterine infusion	Used to balance pH of aminoglycoside antibiotic (highly acidic)
Squalane (25%)	Local infusion	Cerumenolytic agent; used to clean out clitoral sinuses if bacterial or fungal organisms are present and a nidus for subsequent reinfection
Xylazine (100 mg/ml)	0.44–0.66 mg/kg IV, 1–2 hours after imipramine	Used in chemical ejaculation of stallions; most stallions will ejaculate 1–5 minutes after administration

Appendix D

Foaling Kit and Associated Equipment and Supplies

Mare owners are encouraged to keep basic critical supplies on hand during the foaling season. The items in the following list are considered to be essential supplies needed for the routine management of foaling and immediate care of the newborn foal. It is recommended that owners receive specific instructions or training from their veterinarian regarding the appropriate use of equipment, recognition of complications of the foaling process, and medical care of the newborn foal.

Item	Use
Thermometer (fast reading)	Evaluation of body temperature of mare and/or newborn foal
Stethoscope	Evaluation of heart rate and respiratory rate in mare and/or newborn foal
Scissors	Multiple uses, including opening placenta in a "red bag" birth, cutting umbilical tape, tail wrap material, or occasionally cutting the umbilical cord
Flashlight with batteries	Most mares foal out at night; a small flashlight may be very handy at that time
Milk calcium test kit	As an aid in the prediction of foaling date
pH strips	As an aid in the prediction of foaling date
Tail wrap	To get tail hairs out of the way prior to and during foaling
Obstetrical sleeves (sterile)	Used if needed to check the position of fetus during the foaling process
Obstetrical lubricant (sterile)	Applied to sleeve prior to checking position of fetus (if needed)
Exam gloves	General purpose, non-latex gloves used when washing mare prior to foaling, handling placenta, etc.
Liquid soap	Used to wash udder and perineum of mare prior to foaling
Umbilical tape	To tie off the umbilical cord immediately after foaling (if needed; used as an alternative to an umbilical clamp)
Umbilical clamps	To clamp off the umbilical cord immediately after foaling (if needed; used as an alternative to umbilical tape); usually removed or will fall off after 2–3 days
Umbilical cord disinfectant	Used to dip the stump of the umbilical cord (navel) immediately after foaling to help seal the vessels within the cord and disinfect the area to reduce the probability of a bacterial infection (navel ill). Typically a dilute tincture of iodine or chlorhexidine solution
Towel	To dry off and stimulate respiration in newborn foal
Enema (sodium phosphate-type)	Administered to newborn foal at 1–2 hours of life to prevent or treat a meconium impaction. May be repeated if necessary; not always performed routinely
Colostrum refractometer	Used to evaluate quality of mare's colostrum after foaling
Foal IgG test	Measurement of antibody levels in neonatal foals to evaluate passive transfer
Measuring cup (600 ml, 20 oz) plastic cup with handle	Convenient when collecting a larger volume of colostrum from a mare immediately after foaling for freezing
Plastic bottle (500 ml)	Used for storage of colostrum in freezer. Convenient size and prelabeled
Cotton gauze 10 × 10 cm (4 × 4 inches) or cheesecloth	Used to strain colostrum to remove dirt and debris

Equine Reproductive Procedures, Second Edition. Edited by John Dascanio and Patrick McCue.

Item	Use
Catheter-tip syringe (60 ml)	Dose syringe that may be used to administer oral medications to foal under supervision or instruction of a veterinarian
Foal resuscitation unit	Emergency resuscitation of a newborn foal (if needed)
Oxygen tank (E-tank)	Delivery of oxygen to newborn foal (if needed)
Oxygen regulator	Delivery of oxygen to newborn foal (if needed)
Oxygen line	Delivery of oxygen to newborn foal (if needed)
Nasal insufflation set	Delivery of oxygen to newborn foal (if needed)
Obstetrical chains and handles or obstetrical straps	Used to assist with a vaginal delivery (under veterinary supervision)

Index

Equine Reproductive Procedures, Second Edition. Edited by John Dascanio and Patrick McCue.

l

m

n

o